AF782512

Atlas of Cardiac Catheterization and Interventional Cardiology

EDITED BY

Mauro Moscucci, MD, MBA
Chairman, Department of Medicine, Sinai Hospital of Baltimore
Baltimore, Maryland
Adjunct Professor of Medicine, University of Michigan Health System
Physician Consultant, Joint Commission Resources
Baltimore, Maryland

ASSOCIATE EDITORS

Mauricio G. Cohen, MD, FACC, FSCAI
Professor of Medicine
Cardiovascular Division, Department of Medicine
University of Miami Miller School of Medicine
Director, Cardiac Catheterization Laboratory
University of Miami Hospital and Clinics
Miami, Florida

Stanley J. Chetcuti, MD
Professor of Medicine
Eric J. Topol Professor of CVM
Director Cardiac Catheterization Laboratory
Co-Director Structural Heart Service
Division of Cardiovascular Medicine
Department of Internal Medicine
University of Michigan
Ann Arbor, Michigan

Wolters Kluwer

Philadelphia • Baltimore • New York • London
Buenos Aires • Hong Kong • Sydney • Tokyo

Acquisitions Editor: Sharon Zinner
Product Development Editor: Ashley Fischer
Editorial Coordinator: Louise Bierig
Editorial Assistant: Nicole Dunn
Marketing Manager: Rachel Mante Leung
Production Project Manager: Marian Bellus
Design Coordinator: Holly McLaughlin
Manufacturing Coordinator: Beth Welsh
Prepress Vendor: TNQ Technologies

Copyright © 2019 Wolters Kluwer

All rights reserved. This book is protected by copyright. No part of this book may be reproduced or transmitted in any form or by any means, including as photocopies or scanned-in or other electronic copies, or utilized by any information storage and retrieval system without written permission from the copyright owner, except for brief quotations embodied in critical articles and reviews. Materials appearing in this book prepared by individuals as part of their official duties as U.S. government employees are not covered by the above-mentioned copyright. To request permission, please contact Wolters Kluwer at Two Commerce Square, 2001 Market Street, Philadelphia, PA 19103, via email at permissions@shop.lww.com, or via our website at shop.lww.com (products and services).

9 8 7 6 5 4 3 2 1

Printed in China

Library of Congress Cataloging-in-Publication Data

ISBN-13: 978-1-4511-9516-3

Cataloging-in-Publication data available on request from the Publisher.

This work is provided "as is," and the publisher disclaims any and all warranties, express or implied, including any warranties as to accuracy, comprehensiveness, or currency of the content of this work.

This work is no substitute for individual patient assessment based upon healthcare professionals' examination of each patient and consideration of, among other things, age, weight, gender, current or prior medical conditions, medication history, laboratory data and other factors unique to the patient. The publisher does not provide medical advice or guidance and this work is merely a reference tool. Healthcare professionals, and not the publisher, are solely responsible for the use of this work including all medical judgments and for any resulting diagnosis and treatments.

Given continuous, rapid advances in medical science and health information, independent professional verification of medical diagnoses, indications, appropriate pharmaceutical selections and dosages, and treatment options should be made and healthcare professionals should consult a variety of sources. When prescribing medication, healthcare professionals are advised to consult the product information sheet (the manufacturer's package insert) accompanying each drug to verify, among other things, conditions of use, warnings and side effects and identify any changes in dosage schedule or contraindications, particularly if the medication to be administered is new, infrequently used or has a narrow therapeutic range. To the maximum extent permitted under applicable law, no responsibility is assumed by the publisher for any injury and/or damage to persons or property, as a matter of products liability, negligence law or otherwise, or from any reference to or use by any person of this work.

shop.lww.com

CCS1118

Dedication

To my many mentors and colleagues, and particularly to Kenneth Borow, John Carroll, Donald Baim, and William Grossman, recognizing their charismatic vision and support that put me on this pathway.

And to my wife Adriana for her continuous understanding, love, and support. Her willingness to continue to adapt her life to the many months of night and weekend work that were required to create this Atlas will be unforgettable.

Preface

The evolution of photography and more recently of medical imaging has been one of the major advances of this past century. An image can tell a story, even without caption, and there is nothing more powerful than images when introducing new technology, new techniques, and new processes.

In 2010, I had the privilege to be asked by Wolters Kluwer to take over the eighth edition of "*Grossman and Baim's Cardiac Catheterization, Angiography, and Intervention*". That new edition, capitalizing on the outstanding work from prior editions, had an additional emphasis on cardiac imaging. Yet, it looked like there was still an opportunity for a book fully dedicated to images. Thus, following further discussion with the Wolters Kluwer team, the idea for this Atlas was developed.

The purpose of this Atlas is to provide a visual overview of cardiac catheterization and interventional cardiology. Given the emphasis on imaging, the opening chapter is on integrated imaging modalities in the cardiac catheterization laboratory. We hope that our readers will enjoy the unique cases illustrated in this chapter. The remaining chapters can be divided into 2 main groups. Chapters 2-15 are focused on basic elements of cardiac catheterization and interventional cardiology including complications, vascular access, pressure measurements, pitfalls in the evaluation of hemodynamic data, pericardial disease, pediatric cardiac catheterization, coronary, peripheral, and pulmonary angiography, coronary anomalies, evaluation of myocardial blood flow, and intravascular ultrasounds. Chapters 15-25 cover key areas of interventional cardiology, from percutaneous transluminal coronary angioplasty (PTCA) to advanced epicardial access.

Our readers will notice that the chapters have 2 basic formats: (1) a clinical, case-based structure with images and (2) a primarily image-based structure. Given the diversity of topics, we felt that this flexible approach could provide the most value to our readers. In addition, the chapters on PTCA and coronary stenting focus on basic concepts, equipment characteristics, basic techniques, and clinical trials, rather than on clinical cases. The decision of how to structure these chapters was based on the fact that general training in interventional cardiology not always incorporates formal training about the history, the development, and engineering of interventional devices.

This book and the stories told through images would have not been possible without the work of the many pioneers who contributed to the development of cardiac catheterization and interventional cardiology. Our gratitude to them will continue to be immeasurable.

Mauro Moscucci. MD, MBA
Baltimore, Maryland

Acknowledgments

First and foremost, I would like to thank the many mentors who I was fortunate to have through my career in cardiology and interventional cardiology, including Dr. Kenneth Borow, Dr. John Carroll, Dr. Donald Baim, and Dr. William Grossman for their charismatic mentorship and guidance during my initial training in cardiology at the University of Chicago, and my 2 years of training at the Beth Israel Hospital in Boston in the early 1990s. Their continued friendship and support over the following decades have been inspiring. I would also like to thank Julie Goolsby, who as acquisition editor for Wolters Kluwer supported my initial proposal, and Sharon Zinner, who in her role as senior acquisition editor continued to provide an incredible support while we were developing the Atlas. In addition, I would like to thank Ashley Fischer, for her outstanding assistance and patience as the product development editor, and Louise Bierig, for her support as development editor. The incredible support of the Wolters Kluwer team was what that made this Atlas becoming true. Finally, I am extremely grateful to my associate editors, Dr. Stanley Chetcuti and Dr. Mauricio Cohen, and to all the authors and many colleagues and friends who have contributed to this Atlas.

Contents

Contributors

Karim M. Al-Azizi, MD
Structural Heart Disease Fellow
Department of Interventional Cardiology
The Heart Hospital–Baylor Scott & White
Plano, Texas

Carlos Enrique Alfonso, MD
Assistant Professor of Medicine
Cardiovascular Division
University of Miami Miller School of Medicine
University of Miami Hospital & Clinics
Miami, Florida

Philip L Auyang, MD
Resident Physician
Houston Methodist DeBakey Heart and Vascular Center
Houston, Texas

Barry A. Borlaug, MD
Associate Professor
Department of Cardiovascular Diseases
Mayo Clinic
Rochester, Minnesota

Samuel L. Casella, MD, MPH
Clinical Fellow
Department of Pediatrics
Harvard Medical School
Massachusetts Hall
Cambridge, Massachusetts
Department of Cardiology
Boston Children's Hospital
Boston, Massachusetts

Stanley J. Chetcuti, MD
Professor of Medicine
Eric J. Topol Professor of CVM
Director Cardiac Catheterization Laboratory
Co-Director Structural Heart Service
Division of Cardiovascular Medicine
Department of Internal Medicine
University of Michigan
Ann Arbor, Michigan

Kyung J. Cho, MD
Emeritus Professor of Radiology
University of Michigan Health System
Department of Radiology
Division of Interventional Radiology
Ann Arbor, Michigan

Mauricio G. Cohen, MD, FACC, FSCAI
Professor of Medicine
Cardiovascular Division, Department of Medicine
University of Miami Miller School of Medicine
Director, Cardiac Catheterization Laboratory
University of Miami Hospital and Clinics
Miami, Florida

André D'Avila, MD
Director
Cardiac Arrhythmia Service Hospital
SOS Cardio
Florianopolis, SC, Brazil

Carlos D. Davila, MD
General Cardiology Fellow
The Cardiovascular Center
Tufts Medical Center
Boston, Massachusetts

Michael David Dyal, MD
Interventional Cardiology Fellow
Department of Medicine
University of Miami
Miami, Florida

Michele Esposito, MD
Cardiovascular Disease Fellow
The Cardiovascular Center
Tufts Medical Center
Boston, Massachusetts

Peter J. Fitzgerald, MD, PhD, FACC
Professor Emeritus, Medicine & Engineering
Director, Stanford Center for Cardiovascular Innovation
Division of Cardiovascular Medicine
Stanford University School of Medicine
Stanford, California

Yasuhiro Honda, MD, FAHA, FACC
Clinical Professor of Medicine
Director, Stanford Cardiovascular Core Analysis Laboratory
Division of Cardiovascular Medicine
Stanford University School of Medicine
Stanford, California

Masayasu Ikutomi, MD, PhD
Division of Cardiovascular Medicine
Stanford University School of Medicine
Stanford, California

Allen Jeremias, MD, MSc
Director of Interventional Cardiology Research
Department of Cardiology
St. Francis Hospital
Roslyn, New York

Arnoud Kamman, MD
Surgical Resident
Department of Surgery
Ikazia Hospital Rotterdam
Rotterdam, the Netherlands

Samir R. Kapadia, MD
Professor of Medicine
Section Head, Interventional Cardiology
Director, Sones Cardiac Catheterization Laboratory
Cleveland, Ohio

Navin K. Kapur, MD
Associate Professor
Department of Medicine and Cardiology
Tufts Medical Center
Boston, Massachusetts

Karen M. Kim, MD
Department of Cardiac Surgery
Frankel Cardiovascular Center
University of Michigan
Ann Arbor, Michigan

Michael S. Kim, MD
Medical Director
Structural Heart & Valve Disease Program
Cardiovascular Institute of North Colorado
Banner Health
Greeley, Colorado

Aaron Kugelmass, MD
Professor
Department of Medicine
Univeristy of Massachusetts Medical School-Baystate
Medical Director
Heart and Vascular Program
Chief of Cardiology
Baystate Health System
Springfield, Massachusetts

Michael J. Landzberg, MD
Associate Professor of Medicine
Harvard Medical School
Boston, Massachusetts
Immediate-Past Director, Boston Adult Congenital Heart (BACH) Group
Department of Cardiology, Department of Medicine
Boston Children's Hospital and Brigham and Women's Hospital
Boston, Massachusetts

Matthew Liakos, MD
Stony Brook University Medical Center
Stony Brook, New York

Ruby Lo, MD
Assistant Professor
Vascular and Endovascular Surgery
Brown University
Providence, Rhode Island
Boston, Massachusetts

Calin V. Maniu, MD
Director
STEMI Program Lifebridge Health
Baltimore, Maryland

Claudia A. Martinez, MD
Associate Professor
Department of Medicine
University of Miami
Miami, Florida

Mauro Moscucci, MD, MBA
Chairman, Department of Medicine
Sinai Hospital of Baltimore
Baltimore, Maryland
Adjunct Professor of Medicine,
University of Michigan Health System
Physician Consultant
Joint Commission Resources
Baltimore, Maryland

Himanshu J. Patel, MD
Joe D. Morris Collegiate Professor
Section Head
Department of Cardiac Surgery
University of Michigan
Ann Arbor, Michigan

Jayendrakumar S. Patel, MD
Fellow
Department of Interventional Cardiology
Heart and Vascular Institute, Cleveland Clinic
Cleveland, Ohio

Tejas Patel, MD, DM, FACC, FSCAI, FESC
Professor
Department of Cardiology
Sheth V.S. General Hospital
Chairman & Chief Interventional Cardiologist
Apex Heart Institute
Ahmedabad, India

Robert N. Piana, MD
Professor of Medicine
Director, Adult Congenital Interventional Cardiology
Division of Cardiovascular Medicine
Vanderbilt University Medical Center
Nashville, Tennessee

Duane S. Pinto, MD, MPH
Harvard Medical Faculty Physicians (HMFP)
Beth Israel Deaconess Medical Center
Boston, Massachusetts

Diego Porras, MD
Assistant Professor
Department of Pediatrics
Harvard Medical School
Department of Cardiology
Boston Children's Hospital
Boston, Massachusetts

Robert A. Quaife, MD
Professor of Medicine and Radiology Director
Advanced Cardiac Imaging University of Colorado
Anschutz Medical Campus Aurora
Division of Cardiology
University of Colorado Denver
Aurora, Colorado

Michael Joseph Reardon, MD
Professor of Cardiothoracic Surgery
Allison Family Distinguished Chair of Cardiovascular Research
Department of Cardiovascular Surgery Associates
Houston Methodist Physician Specialty Group
Houston, Texas

Kiran V. Reddy, MD, FACC
Interventional Cardiologist
Division of Cardiology
St Francis Hospital
Roslyn, New York

Yogesh N.V. Reddy, MBBS, MSc
Advanced Heart Disease Failure Fellow
Division of Cardiovascular Diseases
Mayo Clinic
Rochester, Minnesota

Ross Michael Reul, MD
Attending Surgeon of Cardiovascular Surgery Associates
Department of Cardiovascular Surgery Associates
Houston Methodist Physician Specialty Group
Houston, Texas

Ada C. Stefanescu Schmidt, MD, MSc
Clinical and Research Fellow
Adult Congenital Heart Disease
Boston Children's Hospital
Harvard Adult Congenital Heart Disease Fellowship
Department of Cardiology
Boston, Massachusetts

Mehdi H. Shishehbor, DO, MPH, PhD
Clinical Assistant Professor of Medicine
Department of Cardiovascular Medicine
Director, Interventional Cardiovascular Center, University Hospitals
Heart & Vascular Institute
Cleveland Clinic
Cleveland, Ohio

Hector Tamez, MD
Co-director of Chronic Total Occlusion Projection
Instructor of Medicine
Division of Cardiology
Department of Medicine
Beth Israel Deaconess Medical Center
Boston, Massachusetts

Thomas M. Tu, MD
Director, Cardiac Catheterization Lab
Baptist Health Louisville
Interventional Cardiology
Department of Medicine
Baptist Hospital Medical Group
Louisville, Kentucky

Juan F. Viles-Gonzalez, MD, FACC, FAHA, FHRS
Associate Professor
Director, Cardiac Electrophysiology
Tulane University School of Medicine
Heart and Vascular Institute
New Orleans, Louisiana

David M. Williams, MD
Kyung J. Cho Professor of Radiology
Department of Radiology
Frankel Cardiovascular Center
University of Michigan
Ann Arbor, Michigan

Paul G. Yock, MD
Martha Meier Weiland Professor of Bioengineering and Medicine
Founding Director, Stanford Byers Center for Biodesign
Stanford, California

Hong Jun (Francisco) Yun, MD
Interventional Cardiology Fellow
Division of Cardiovascular Medicine
Department of Internal Medicine
University of Michigan
Ann Arbor, Michigan

chapter **1**

Integrated Imaging Modalities in the Cardiac Catheterization Laboratory

MICHAEL S. KIM, MD, and ROBERT A. QUAIFE, MD

INTRODUCTION

Over the last decade, there has been an exponential growth in the number of transcatheter therapies designed to treat both congenital and acquired structural heart disease (SHD) pathologies. Along with this growth have come major advances in image guidance including three-dimensional transesophageal echocardiography (3D TEE), cardiac computed tomographic angiography (CCTA), and magnetic resonance imaging and angiography (MRI/MRA). In contemporary practice, catheter-based treatments of various structural heart and valve diseases have become increasingly reliant on accurate preprocedural imaging assessment and intraprocedural guidance to maximize outcomes and minimize complications.[1] For example, CCTA has become the "gold standard" in aortic annulus analysis in preplanning for transcatheter aortic valve replacement (TAVR) procedures.[2,3] Similarly, 3D TEE has become a mainstay in both preprocedure evaluation and intraprocedural guidance for transcatheter mitral valve repair with the MitraClip device.[4,5]

A major challenge facing all SHD interventionalists and imaging specialists, however, centers on the importance of integrating efficiently multiple imaging modalities so as to prevent "sensory imaging overload." Oftentimes, many operators also struggle with "mentally translating" two-dimensional (2D) imaging sequences (eg, CCTA, 2D echocardiography) into accurate and useful 3D spatial images in their own minds to both effectively preplan and efficiently perform complex SHD procedures. To overcome these barriers, imaging manufacturers are actively developing new software tools that are designed to take the complexities of multimodality imaging integration out of the hands of the operators, while simultaneously giving back to the operator a simplified and efficient mechanism by which to manipulate and analyze the processed images.[6-8]

This chapter, through several clinical examples, will highlight how both high-quality preprocedure imaging and intraprocedural imaging using novel multimodality image integration tools can be effectively used to guide complex SHD interventions.

CASE 1 *Right Ventricular to Left Atrium Fistula Repair*

A 55-year-old male with a history of an endocardial cushion defect that was surgically repaired at age 7 years with a patch at the septum primum and inlet ventricular septal defect (VSD) was referred to evaluate and treat a residual right ventricular (RV) to left atrial (LA) fistula. He had a recent biventricular pacemaker/internal cardiac defibrillator (ICD) placed for asymptomatic complete heart block in the setting of left ventricular (LV) dysfunction. After device implantation, he began complaining of new visual symptoms (intermittent vision loss in his left eye) concerning for transient ischemic attacks (TIAs); a brain MRI could not be obtained owing the presence of his ICD. A transthoracic echocardiogram (TTE) was performed demonstrating a residual defect/fistula between the RV and LA with at least moderate right to left shunting following injection of agitated saline contrast (**FIGURE 1.1**; Video 1.1). Given the concern that the patient would be at risk for forming small thrombi on his ICD leads that both may have and could in the future embolize paradoxically, the decision was made to proceed with transcatheter closure of the residual fistula.

As part of his preprocedure evaluation, the patient underwent a CCTA to better elucidate the size and location of the fistula (**FIGURE 1.2**; Video 1.2). The CCTA demonstrated a clear communication between the RV and LA with a tract diameter of approximately 5 to 7 mm (depending on timing within the cardiac cycle) and a length of approximately 6 mm. Intraprocedure 3D TEE was used as image guidance (**FIGURE 1.3**). Using an antegrade approach (transvenous access with transseptal puncture and defect crossing from the LA), the patient underwent an uncomplicated fistula closure using a 6 × 6 Amplatzer Duct Occluder II device (**FIGURE 1.4**). Postprocedure TEE and TTE demonstrated no residual flow across the device. The patient was discharged on postprocedure day 1 and remains in good condition.

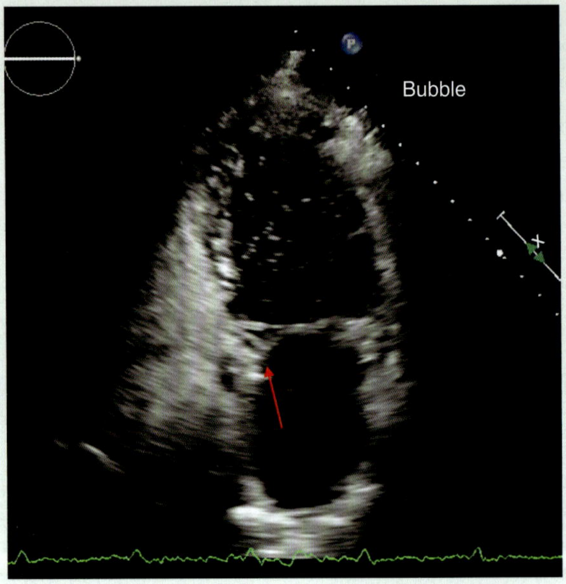

FIGURE 1.1 TTE agitated saline contrast ("bubble") study through a peripheral vein demonstrating a communication between the RV and LA (arrow) with right to left shunting.

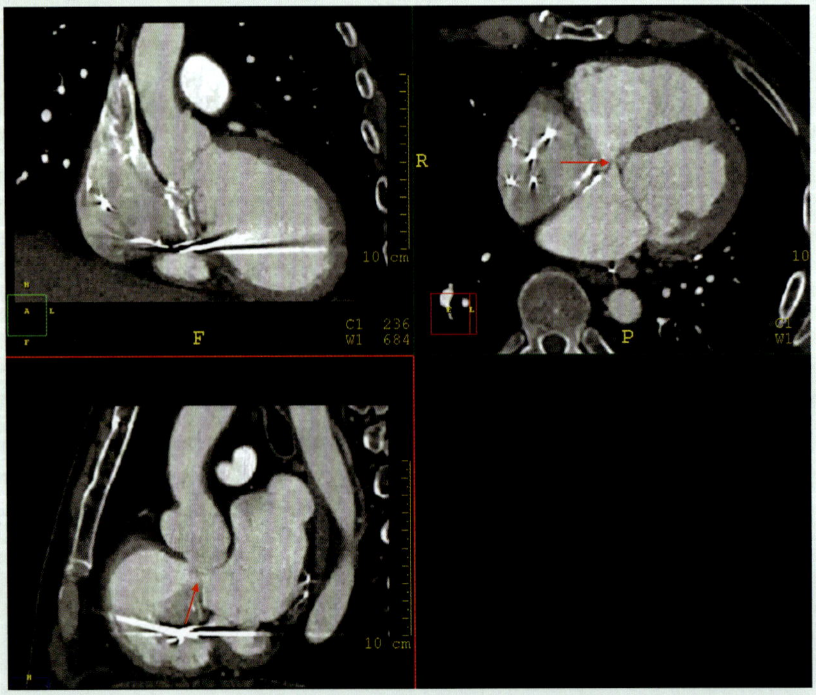

FIGURE 1.2 Multiplanar reconstruction of the CCTA demonstrating the fistula between the RV and LA (arrows) in orthogonal planes. The fistula was dynamic in nature and measured approximately 7 mm in diameter and 6 mm in length during ventricular systole.

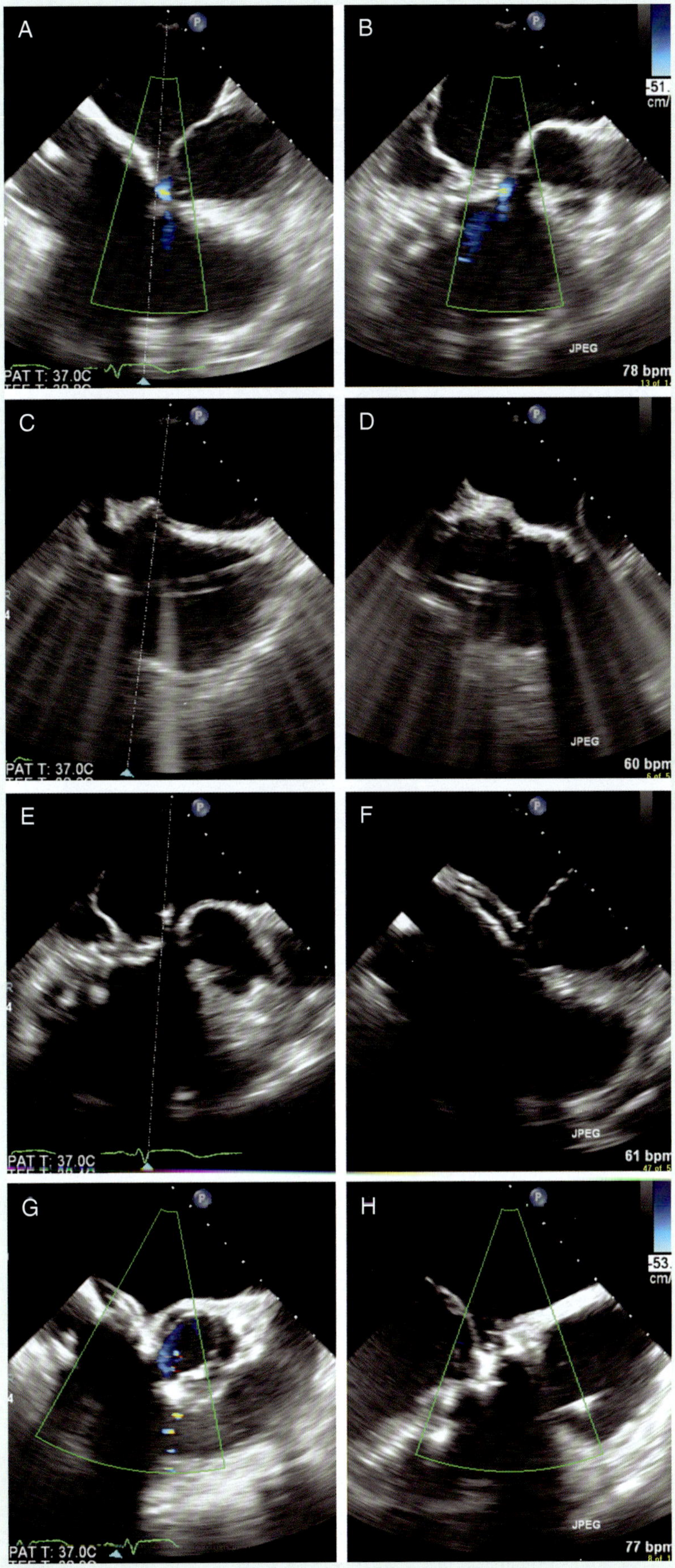

FIGURE 1.3 Intraprocedure TEE. **A and B**, 4 chamber and LV outflow tract view showing color flow between the LA and RV. **C and D**, Location of the transseptal puncture inferior (C) and posterior (D). **E and F**, Orientation of the steerable guide catheter directly into the location of the fistula from the LA. **G and H**, Occluder device across the fistula with absence of flow by color Doppler indicating complete closure.

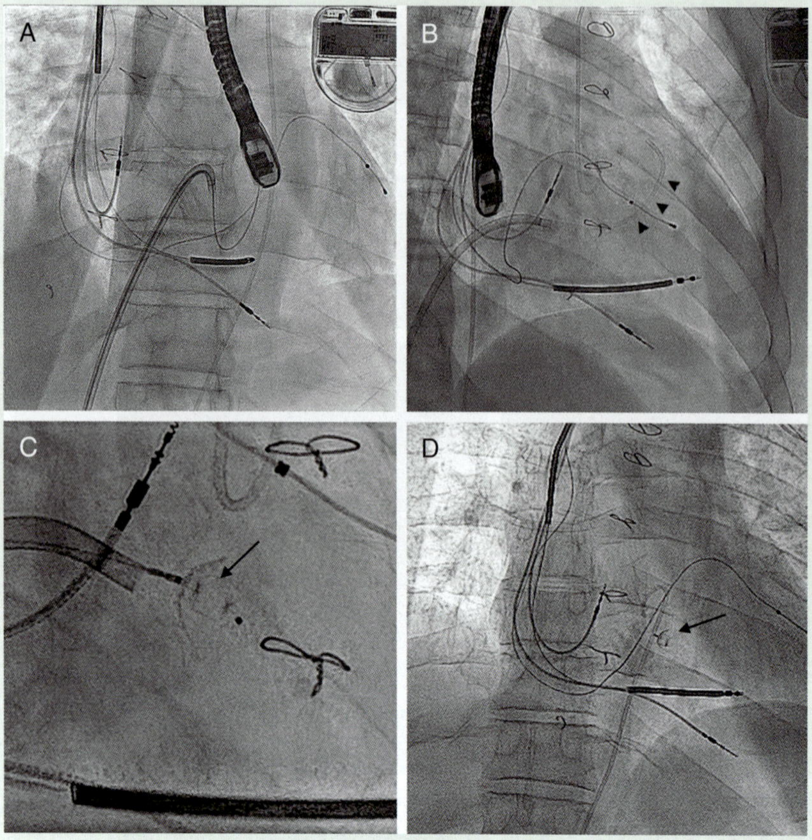

FIGURE 1.4 Fluoroscopic images of RV to LA fistula closure. **A**, With the steerable guide catheter (arrowheads, positioned guide catheter) pointed into the LA side of the fistula, a Magic Torque wire is advanced across the defect and out the LV outflow tract across the aortic valve into the ascending aorta (Ao). **B**, A 5 French diagnostic catheter is advanced over the wire into the ascending Ao, and the wire is removed. **C**, Amplatzer Duct Occluder II device (arrow, showing deployed device) is fully deployed across the fistula. **D**, Final angiography demonstrating stable placement of the occluder device.

CASE 2 *Prosthetic Mitral Paravalvular Leak Repair*

A 70-year-old female with a history of rheumatic heart disease underwent surgical mitral valve replacement with a 29 mm porcine bioprosthesis. Although her immediate postoperative course was uneventful, she presented several weeks after surgery with decompensated heart failure symptoms (New York Heart Association Class III-IV). A TTE and TEE confirmed the presence of a severe paravalvular leak located on the posterior aspect of the sewing ring. There was also evidence of mild hemolysis. A cardiothoracic surgeon was consulted who felt that a reoperation would put the patient at excessive risk given her current clinical state, and thus she was referred for transcatheter paravalvular leak (PVL) repair.

The patient underwent a preprocedure CCTA to evaluate the size and extent of the posterior PVL as well as assess for any additional defects (**FIGURE 1.5**). The CCTA clearly demonstrated the presence of a large, crescentic defect located on the posterior aspect of the bioprosthetic valve sewing ring. The defect measured approximately 10 mm in diameter at its widest segment and approximately 24 mm in total length. Intraprocedure 3D TEE coupled with novel live echo-fluoro image integration technology (EchoNavigator—Philips Healthcare, The Netherlands) was used for image guidance (**FIGURE 1.6**; **Video 1.3**). Using an antegrade approach, the patient underwent an uncomplicated PVL closure with implantation of a 14 and 12 mm Amplatzer Vascular Plug II device (St Jude Medical, Inc., St Paul, MN) across the large posterior PVL, resulting in complete eradication of the PVL (**FIGURE 1.7**; **Video 1.4**). The patient was discharged on postprocedure day 2 and remains in excellent clinical condition with NYHA Class I symptoms and no evidence of hemolysis.

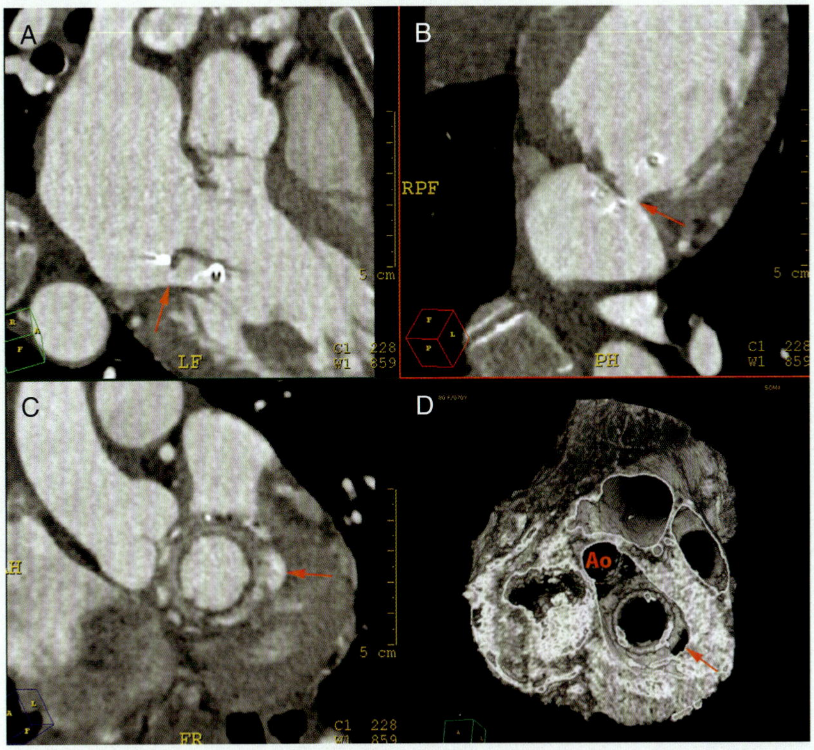

FIGURE 1.5 CCTA of posterior mitral paravalvular leak. **A-C**, 2D multiplanar reconstruction of the mitral annulus demonstrating a large paravalvular leak located on the posterior aspect of the sewing ring (arrows). **D**, 3D en face view of the prosthetic mitral valve localizing the size and extent of the posterior paravalvular leak (arrow) immediately opposite to the Ao.

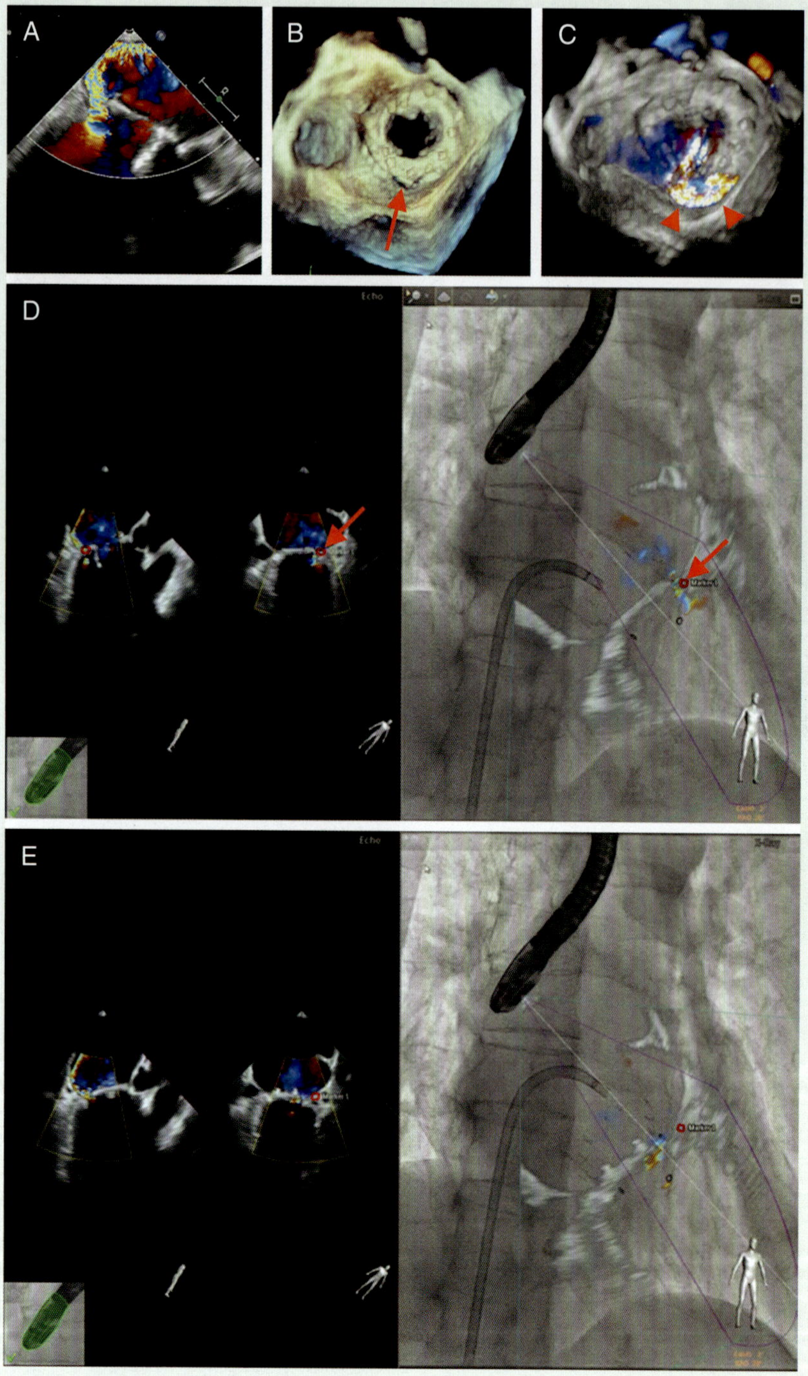

FIGURE 1.6 Intraprocedural TEE with live echo-fluoro image integration technology (EchoNavigator) to guide transcatheter mitral paravalvular leak repair. **A**, LV outflow tract view demonstrating severe paravalvular regurgitation located posteriorly on the sewing ring. **B**, 3D en face view of the prosthetic mitral valve demonstrating a crescentic defect located on the posterior aspect (6 o'clock) on the sewing ring (arrow). **C**, 3D en face view with color Doppler showing a crescentic leak originating from approximately 4 o'clock to 7 o'clock (arrowheads). **D**, Live echo-fluoro image integration technology with the PVL labeled with the red dot (arrows). The steerable guide catheter is located medial to the location of the PVL. **E**, Live echo-fluoro image integration showing that torqueing the steerable guide catheter posteriorly and slightly advancing it further into the LA aligns it directly above the location of the PVL.

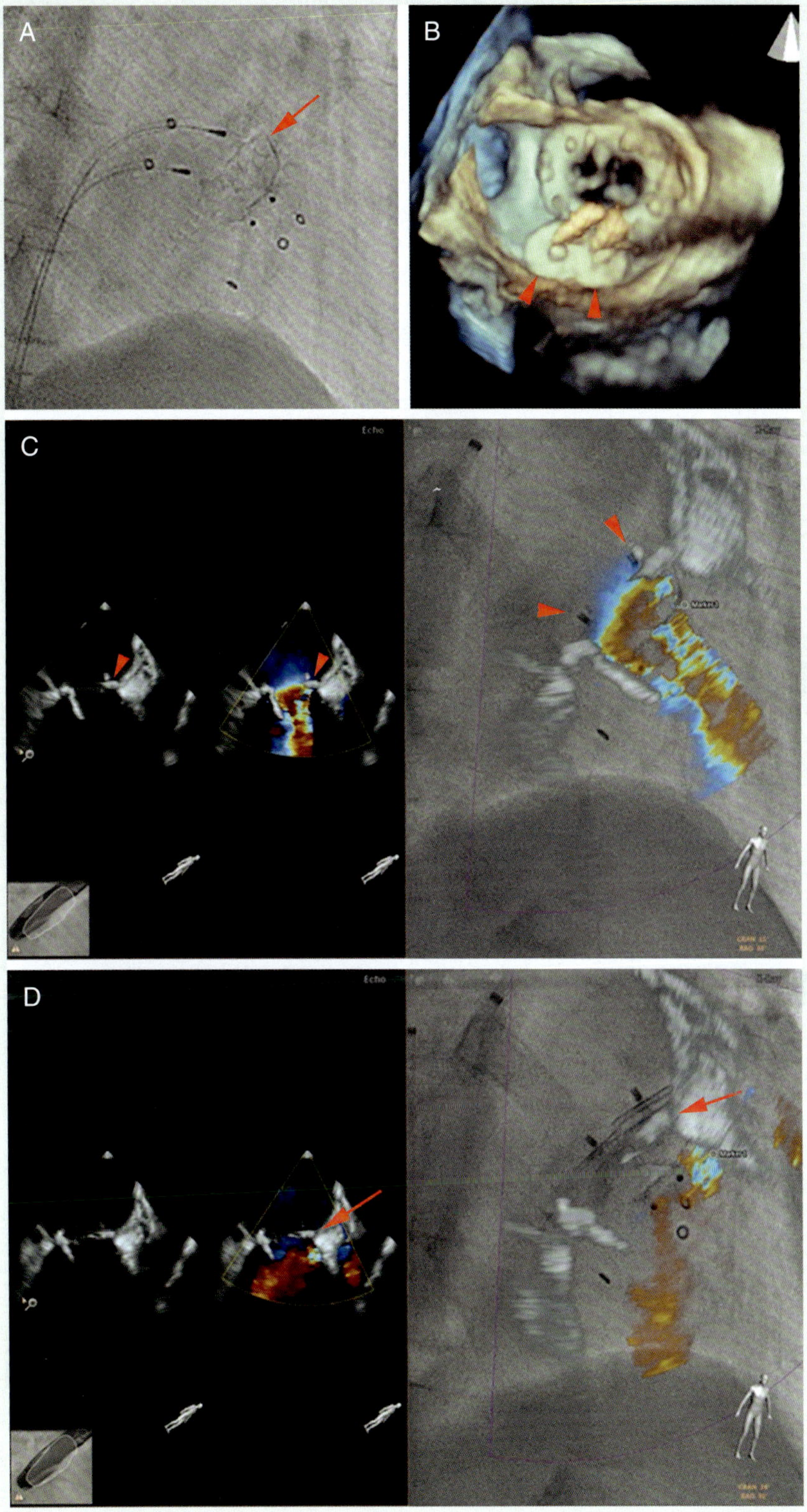

FIGURE 1.7 Intraprocedural TEE with live echo-fluoro image integration demonstrating eradication of the mitral paravalvular leak. **A**, Fluoroscopy showing 2 Amplatzer Vascular Plug II devices across the sewing ring (arrow) in the area of the paravalvular leak. **B**, 3D TEE view demonstrating the posterior location of the 2 vascular plug devices (arrowheads). **C and D**, Live echo-fluoro image integration technology demonstrating location of the vascular plug devices (arrowheads) and complete eradication of paravalvular leak with absence of color flow across the sewing ring (arrows).

CASE 3 *Left Ventricular Apical Pseudoaneurysm Repair*

A 75-year-old female with severe, symptomatic aortic stenosis who was deemed prohibitive risk for surgical aortic valve replacement owing to frailty, severe lung disease, and prior pericardiectomy in the 1980s for chronic pericarditis was referred for TAVR. She also had a history of severe peripheral arterial disease (PAD) with bilateral femoral-popliteal bypass surgery in the past. Given her severe PAD, she underwent attempted TAVR via a transapical approach. The procedure was aborted owing to severe bleeding during placement of the pledgeted sutures in the LV apex. The patient fortunately had an uneventful postoperative course. The procedure plan was then changed to attempt TAVR using a self-expanding transcatheter heart valve via a subclavian approach once she had recovered from her index procedure. A repeat CCTA performed to evaluate the suitability of using her left subclavian artery for access incidentally also detected the presence of a large, LV apical pseudoaneurysm (PSA) that had developed in the interim postoperative recovery period (**FIGURE 1.8**). The neck of the PSA measured 3 mm with the PSA body measuring 12 mm × 25 mm. Given the size of the PSA and the inherent risk of rupture, the decision was made to attempt transcatheter repair of the PSA concomitantly with the planned TAVR procedure.

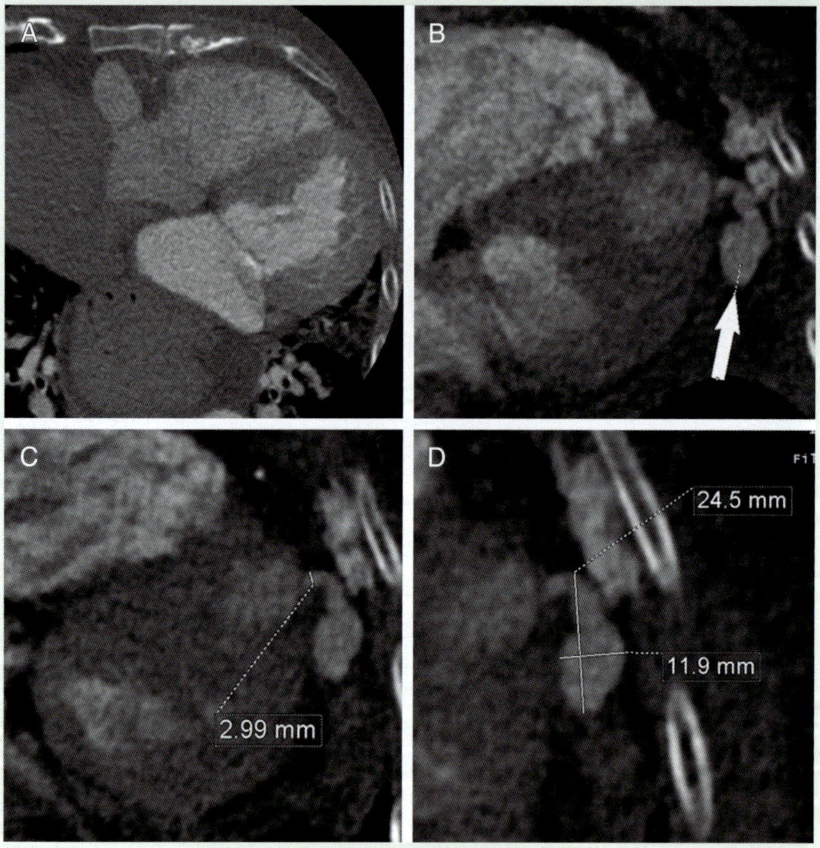

FIGURE 1.8 CCTA demonstrating the evolution of LV apical PSA. **A**, Baseline CCTA before attempted transapical TAVR. **B**, Repeat CCTA demonstrating the interval development of a new LV apical PSA (arrow, aneurysm chamber). **C and D**, Measurements of the PSA with a neck diameter of 3 mm and body dimensions of 12 mm × 25 mm.

Successful and uncomplicated TAVR via left subclavian access was performed, and a 29 mm Medtronic CoreValve transcatheter heart valve (Medtronic, Minneapolis, MN) was implanted. LV angiography performed post-TAVR confirmed the presence of a large LV apical PSA (**FIGURE 1.9**; **Video 1.5**). 3D TEE was then used as adjunctive imaging during the PSA repair (**FIGURE 1.10**). The patient underwent successful PSA repair using a 6 × 6 Amplatzer Duct Occluder II device (St Jude Medical, Inc., St Paul, MN) resulting in near resolution of flow into the PSA (**FIGURE 1.11**A and B; **Video 1.6**). The patient had an uncomplicated postoperative course and was discharged on postoperative day 5. A repeat CCTA performed approximately 3 months postprocedure demonstrated a sealed off PSA that had completely thrombosed with no residual flow into the defect.

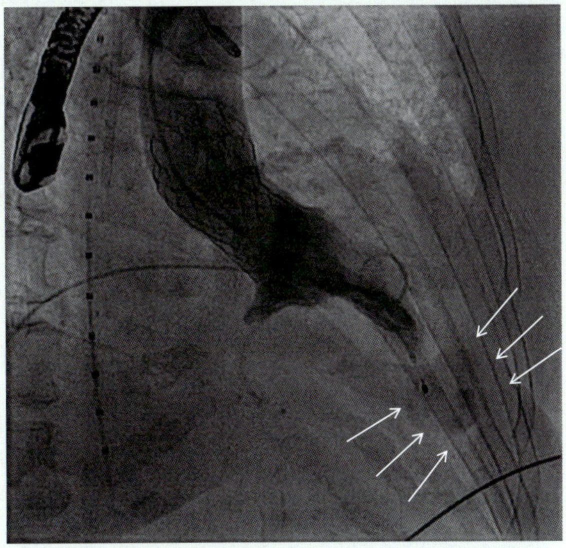

FIGURE 1.9 Baseline LV angiography following successful TAVR confirming the presence of a large LV apical PSA (arrows, pseudoaneurysm chamber).

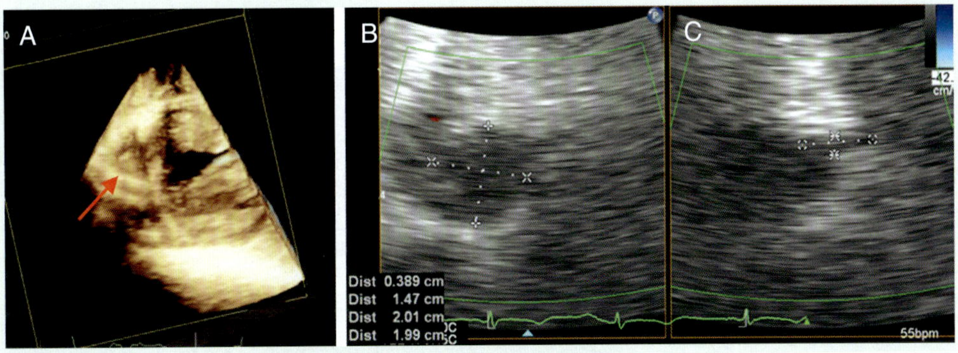

FIGURE 1.10 Intraprocedural TEE guidance of LV apical PSA repair. **A**, 3D TEE demonstrating location of the PSA at the LV apex (arrow, guide catheter at aneurysm os). **B and C**, 2D TEE (biplane TEE, os of pseudoaneurysm) measurements of the PSA confirming findings from prior CCTA.

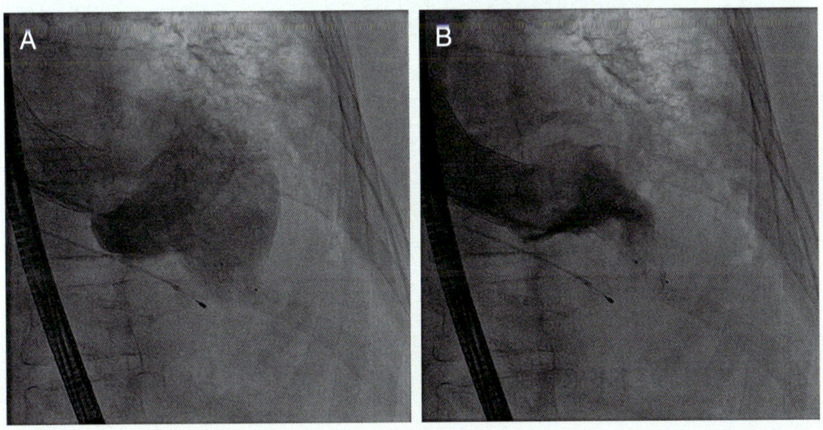

FIGURE 1.11 **A and B**, Diastolic and systolic left ventriculographic frames respectively, after deployment a 6 × 6 Amplatzer Duct Occluder II device (St Jude Medical, Inc.) showing closure of the PSA.

CASE 4 *Aortic Pseudoaneurysm Repair*

A 52-year-old male with a history of congenital heart disease with bicuspid pulmonic valve and congenital pulmonic stenosis underwent open valvotomy and repair of subvalvular stenosis as a child. This procedure was followed by a repeat sternotomy for critical aortic stenosis from a bicuspid aortic valve in adulthood at which time a 23 mm homograft was implanted in the aortic position with coronary reimplantation. He subsequently developed homograft failure with severe regurgitation. During his work-up for redo aortic valve replacement, he was noted to have a large PSA adjacent to the reimplanted right coronary ostium. He was deemed high surgical risk for both PSA repair with aortic valve replacement, and thus was referred for transcatheter device closure of the PSA to be followed by TAVR.

Fluoroscopy and 3D TEE were used for procedural guidance. In this particular case, the operators had difficulty engaging the PSA neck using fluoroscopy alone. Using live echo-fluoro image integration technology (EchoNavigator—Philips Healthcare, The Netherlands), the precise location of the PSA neck was clearly delineated and was easily engaged with a standard right coronary guide catheter (**FIGURE 1.12**; **Video 1.7**). Ultimately, a 12 mm Amplatzer Vascular Plug II device (St Jude Medical, Inc., St Paul, MN) was implanted resulting in near cessation of flow into the PSA (**FIGURE 1.13**B and D; **Video 1.8**). A repeat CCTA performed several months post closure confirmed absence of flow into the PSA with successful thrombosis of the PSA body (**FIGURE 1.13**A and C).

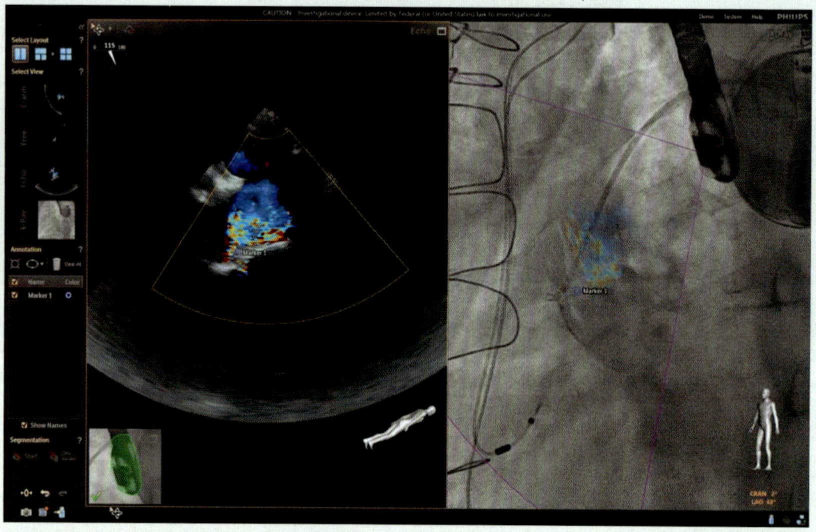

FIGURE 1.12 Echo-fluoro image integration showing the coregistered location of the PSA by both echocardiography and fluoroscopy (marker 1) thereby guiding manipulation of the guide catheter to selectively engage the neck of the PSA.

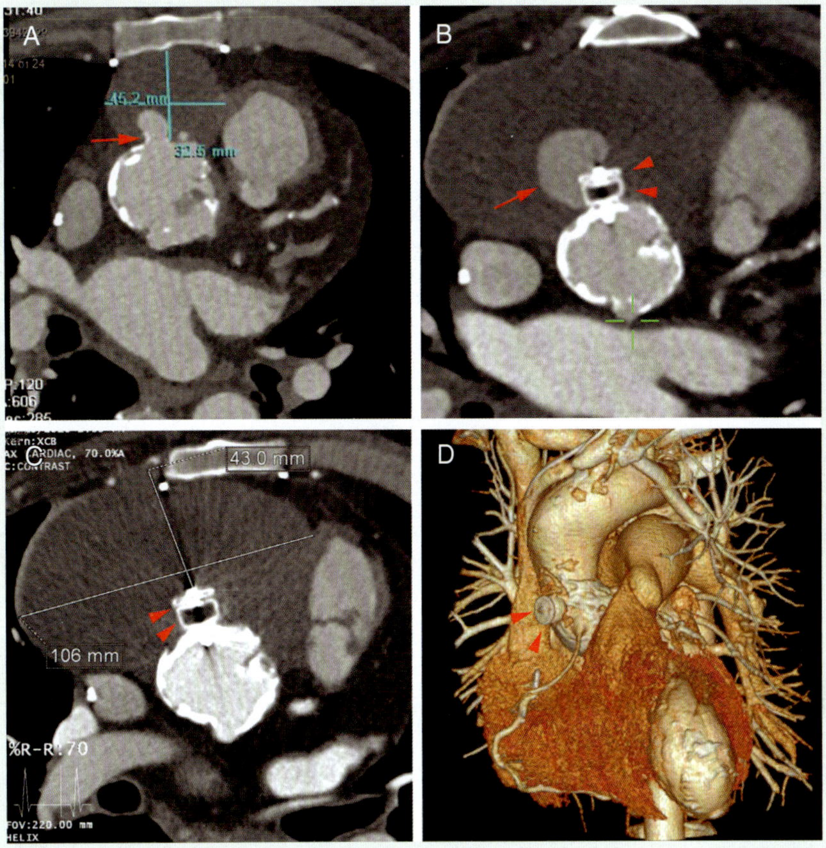

FIGURE 1.13 Interval CCTAs of aortic PSA. **A**, Baseline CCTA demonstrating a wide necked (arrow) PSA near the right coronary ostium. The PSA at baseline measured approximately 3 cm × 4.5 cm. **B**, CCTA immediately after successful transcatheter closure with an Amplatzer Vascular Plug II device (arrowheads, show center, aneurysm and aortic disks) with a small degree of residual flow into the PSA (arrow). At the time of closure, the PSA body had nearly tripled in size. **C**, Repeat CCTA performed several months after successful transcatheter closure demonstrating absence of residual flow and fully thrombosed PSA body. **D**, 3D reconstruction showing the close proximity of the vascular plug device (arrowheads) to the right coronary ostium (the large thrombosed PSA was removed from this picture).

CONCLUSION

Significant growth in transcatheter therapies for SHD has led to a concomitant evolution of imaging modalities used in both preprocedure planning and intraprocedural guidance. As highlighted in this chapter, careful selection of the most appropriate and effectual imaging modality for both preprocedure planning and intraprocedural guidance is of paramount importance to simplify the transcatheter therapy of very complex SHD pathologies. In addition, while the gap between high-quality imaging and the efficient integration of various imaging modalities in a cohesive and clinically useful manner remains considerable, the development of novel assimilation tools will continue to narrow this gap.

REFERENCES

1. Schoenhagen P, Numburi U, Halliburton SS, et al. Three-dimensional imaging in the context of minimally invasive and transcatheter cardiovascular interventions using multi-detector computed tomography: from pre-operative planning to intra-operative guidance. *Eur Heart J*. 2010;31:2727-2740.
2. Achenbach S, Delgado V, Hausleiter J, Schoenhagen P, Min JK, Leipsic JA. SCCT expert consensus document on computed tomography imaging before transcatheter aortic valve implantation (TAVI)/transcatheter aortic valve replacement (TAVR). *J Cardiovasc Comput Tomogr*. 2012;6:366-380.
3. Leipsic J, Gurvitch R, Labounty TM, et al. Multidetector computed tomography in transcatheter aortic valve implantation. *JACC Cardiovasc Imaging*. 2011;4:416-429.
4. Altiok E, Hamada S, Brehmer K, et al. Analysis of procedural effects of percutaneous edge-to-edge mitral valve repair by 2D and 3D echocardiography. *Circ Cardiovasc Imaging*. 2012;5:748-755.
5. Quaife RA, Salcedo EE, Carroll JD. Procedural guidance using advance imaging techniques for percutaneous edge-to-edge mitral valve repair. *Curr Cardiol Rep*. 2014;16:452.
6. Clegg SD, Chen SJ, Nijhof N, et al. Integrated 3D echo-x ray to optimize image guidance for structural heart intervention. *JACC Cardiovasc Imaging*. 2015;8:371-374.
7. Fagan TE, Truong UT, Jone PN, et al. Multimodality 3-dimensional image integration for congenital cardiac catheterization. *Methodist Debakey Cardiovasc J*. 2014;10:68-76.
8. Kim MS, Bracken J, Nijhof N, et al. Integrated 3D Echo-X-Ray navigation to predict optimal angiographic deployment projections for TAVR. *JACC Cardiovasc Imaging*. 2014;7:847-848.

chapter 2

Complications of Percutaneous Coronary Intervention

MAURO MOSCUCCI, MD, MBA

Advancements in technology have led to a significant increase in the safety of invasive diagnostic and therapeutic cardiovascular procedures. However, the recognition, management, and prevention of complications continue to be critical components of current practice of interventional cardiology. The objective of this chapter is to provide a visual resource that can be used for the identification and management of common and less common complications of percutaneous coronary intervention (PCI).

CORONARY ARTERY DISSECTION

Following the introduction of coronary stents, coronary artery dissection requiring emergency coronary bypass grafting has become a rare occurrence, with most series listing it at less than 0.2%.[1,2] That said, it is critical to recognize this complication even in the absence of abrupt closure, as early treatment improves vessel patency and patients' outcomes. Causes of iatrogenic coronary artery dissections include guiding catheter–induced dissection, spiral dissection following initial balloon dilatation, and stent edge dissection. The classic type "A-F" classification remains useful to describe the severity of luminal injury[3] (**Tables 2.1** and **2.2**). Thorough angiographic and IVUS evaluation and appropriate intervention can avoid progression and maintain vessel patency (**FIGURES 2.1-2.5**).

AORTIC AND GREAT VESSELS DISSECTION

In rare instances, aggressive guiding catheter manipulation or forceful contrast injection with a poorly engaged catheter can result in dissection of a sinus of Valsalva[4] or of a subclavian artery. Retrograde dissection involving the sinus of Valsalva and the ascending aorta is more frequent with interventions on the right coronary artery (81% of cases) and with the use of Amplatz guiding catheter. The classification of aortic dissection is shown in **Table 2.3**. Prompt recognition and assessment of the extent of the dissection and hemodynamic state should guide appropriate management with either conservative, percutaneous rescue, or surgical therapy. In general, management includes ostial stenting to seal the dissection in class I and II and surgery for extensive dissections (class III) associated with hemodynamic instability (**FIGURES 2.6-2.9**).

TABLE 2.1

Coronary Dissection Type and Suggested Interventions

Dissection Type	Interventions
Guide catheter dissection	Protect main branches Avoid repeat contrast injections until distal stent is placed Cover injured segment with stent Assess for propagation Consider switching to a different guiding catheter curve if unable to wire true lumen
Spiral dissection	Do not lose guide wire position If the guide wire position is lost, IVUS evaluation is performed to ensure that the true lumen is re-entered Wire main branches Stent distal edge first to minimize propagation Cover entire involved segment
Stent edge dissection	IVUS to assess stent deployment Consider stenting if tissue flap is apparent on IVUS or for any flow limitation Conservative management for small, localized dissections when additional stent is contraindicated

TABLE 2.2

Morphologic Classification of Coronary Dissection

Classification	Description
Type A	Minor radiolucent areas in the lumen without impairment of flow or persistent dye staining after contrast runoff
Type B	Luminal flap that is radiolucent and that runs parallel to the vessel wall with contrast injection but without impairment of flow or persistent dye staining after contrast runoff
Type C	Contrast appears outside of the vessel lumen as an "extraluminal cap." The staining appears even after contrast clears the lumen
Type D	Spiral radiolucent luminal filling defects. Often persistent staining after contrast clears from the vessel
Type E	New and persistent filling defects in the vessel lumen
Type F	Lesions that progress to impaired flow or total occlusion

Reproduced with permission from Moscucci M. *Complications of Cardiovascular Procedures: Risk Factors, Management and Bailout Techniques*. Philadelphia: Lippincott Williams and Wilkins; 2011.

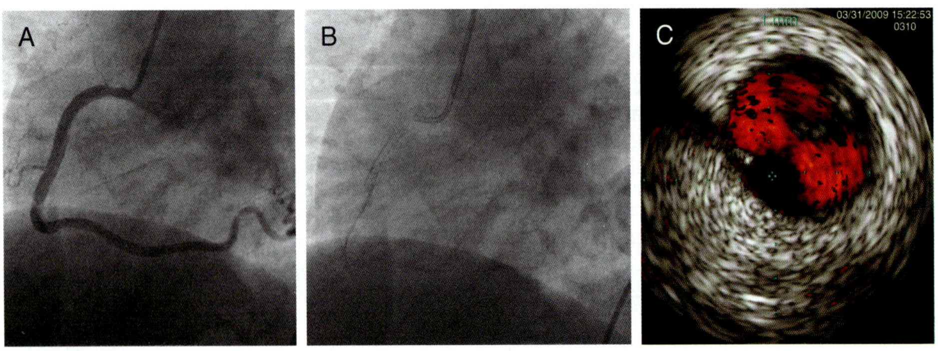

FIGURE 2.1 Angiographic appearance of a Type D spiral dissection, during and after contrast injection. IVUS images show the true and false lumen. **A**, A thin spiral dissection line can be visualized throughout the length of the vessel. **B**, False lumen staining becomes apparent after injection of contrast. **C**, IVUS demonstration of true and false lumen. It can be noticed that the IVUS catheter is located in the false lumen. Reproduced with permission from Moscucci M. *Complications of Cardiovascular Procedures: Risk Factors, Management and Bailout Techniques*. Philadelphia: Lippincott Williams and Wilkins; 2011.

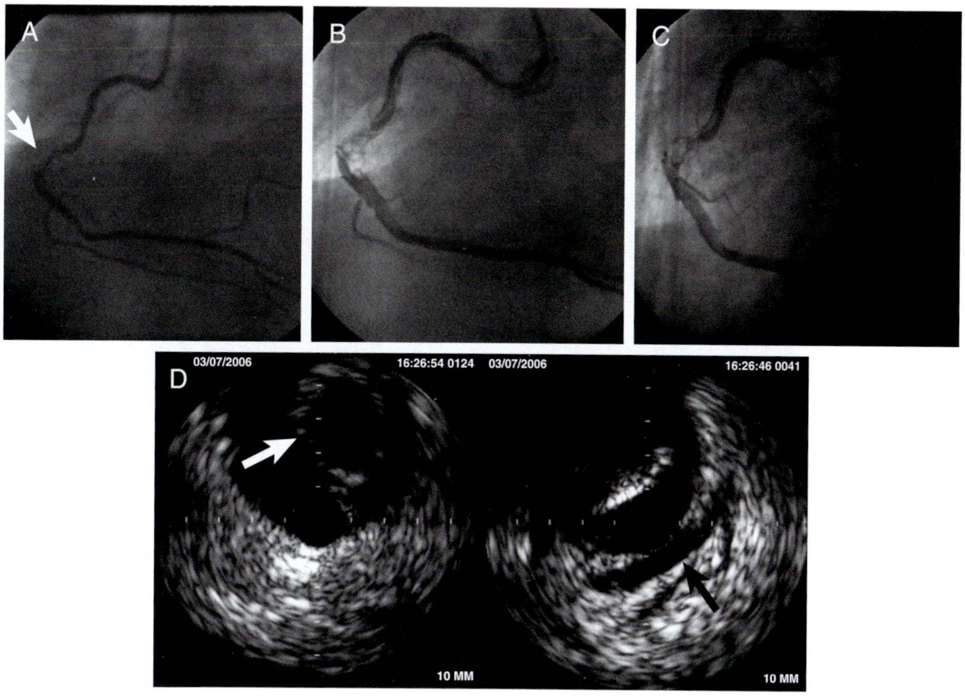

FIGURE 2.2 Spiral dissection caused by aggressive manipulation of a guiding catheter. **A**, Diagnostic right coronary contrast injection demonstrates a severe stenosis in the mid-vessel (arrow). **B**, Aggressive manipulation of an Amplatz guiding catheter caused a spiral dissection that extended throughout the length of the vessel. **C**, The true lumen could not be wired, despite exchanging the guiding catheter for a Judkins right shape. **D**, The round shape in the IVUS image to the left demonstrates that the wire and catheter were in the false lumen (white arrow). In the image to the right, the true lumen (white arrow) is compressed by the false lumen. Reproduced with permission from Moscucci M. *Complications of Cardiovascular Procedures: Risk Factors, Management and Bailout Techniques*. Philadelphia: Lippincott Williams and Wilkins; 2011.

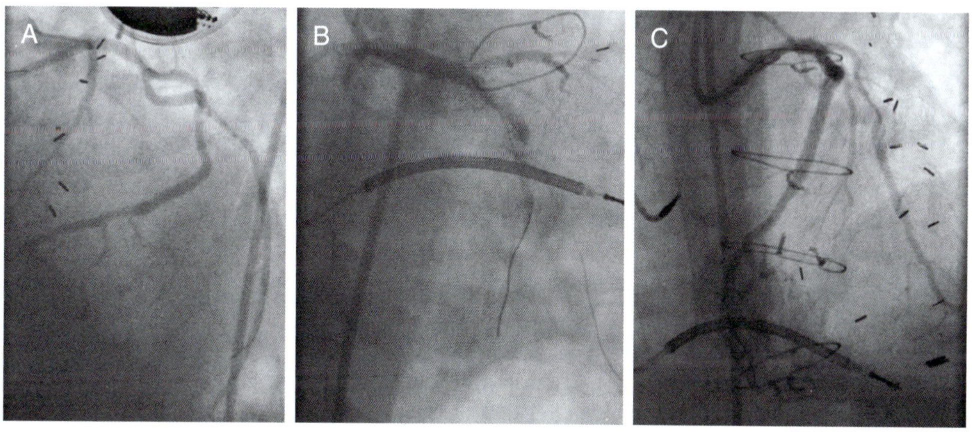

FIGURE 2.3 Guide catheter–induced coronary dissection and treatment with stent placement. **A**, Cranial left anterior oblique image showing the aggressive selective cannulation of the left circumflex coronary artery with an extra backup catheter. **B**, Occlusive dissection and contrast staining in the left circumflex in right anterior oblique. Note that the wire position was preserved throughout the case. **C**, Final result with complete restoration of flow after stent placement. Reproduced with permission from Moscucci M. *Complications of Cardiovascular Procedures: Risk Factors, Management and Bailout Techniques*. Philadelphia: Lippincott Williams and Wilkins; 2011.

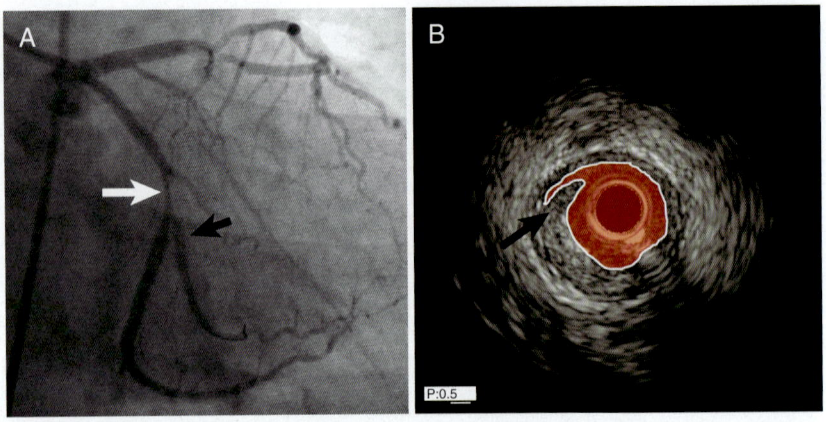

FIGURE 2.4 Stent edge dissection with intravascular ultrasound imaging. **A**, Narrowed segment (white arrow) in the main left circumflex that became apparent after placement of a stent in a moderate-sized second obtuse marginal branch (black arrow). **B**, Intravascular ultrasound demonstrated the presence of a proximal edge stent dissection (arrow) that was treated with placement of an additional stent. Reproduced with permission from Moscucci M. *Complications of Cardiovascular Procedures: Risk Factors, Management and Bailout Techniques*. Philadelphia: Lippincott Williams and Wilkins; 2011.

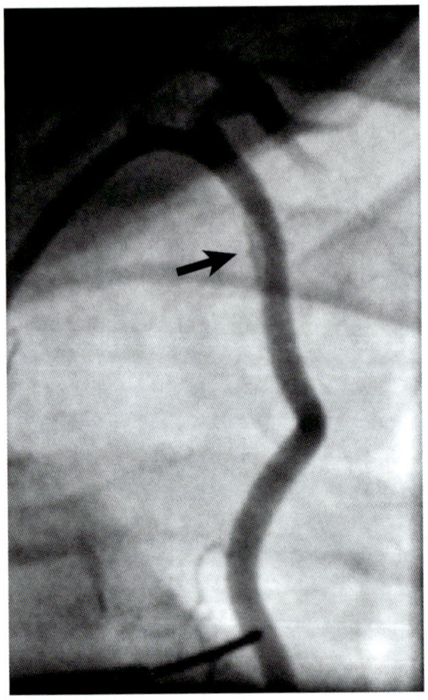

FIGURE 2.5 Proximal dissection of a left internal mammary artery caused by aggressive manipulation of a 0.035" guide wire (arrow). Reproduced with permission from Moscucci M. *Complications of Cardiovascular Procedures: Risk Factors, Management and Bailout Techniques*. Philadelphia: Lippincott Williams and Wilkins; 2011.

TABLE 2.3

Classification of Retrograde Dissection of Sinus of Valsalva and Ascending Aorta

Class I—Focal dissection restricted to ipsilateral cusp
Class II—Involving cusp, extending up the aorta <40 mm
Class III—Involving cusp, extending up the aorta >40 mm

Reproduced with permission from Moscucci M. *Complications of Cardiovascular Procedures: Risk Factors, Management and Bailout Techniques*. Philadelphia: Lippincott Williams and Wilkins; 2011.

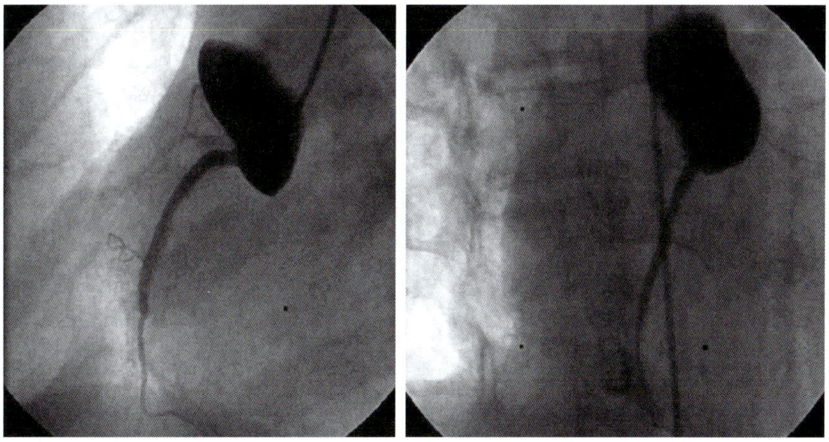

FIGURE 2.6 Guiding catheter dissection of the right coronary ostium extending into sinus of Valsalva and the aortic root. Orthogonal views obtained with biplane angiographic equipment, showing a large dissection of the right sinus of Valsalva. The patient presented with clinical instability including hypotension and severe chest pain and was immediately referred for surgical repair of the aortic root. Reproduced with permission from Moscucci M. *Complications of Cardiovascular Procedures: Risk Factors, Management and Bailout Techniques*. Philadelphia: Lippincott Williams and Wilkins; 2011.

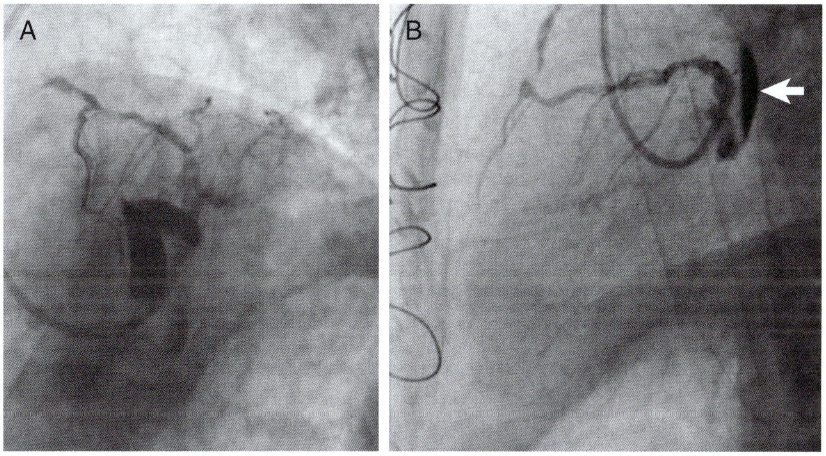

FIGURE 2.7 **A and B**, Left main dissection extending into the left coronary and noncoronary aortic cusps (arrow). Reproduced with permission from Moscucci M. *Complications of Cardiovascular Procedures: Risk Factors, Management and Bailout Techniques*. Philadelphia: Lippincott Williams and Wilkins; 2011.

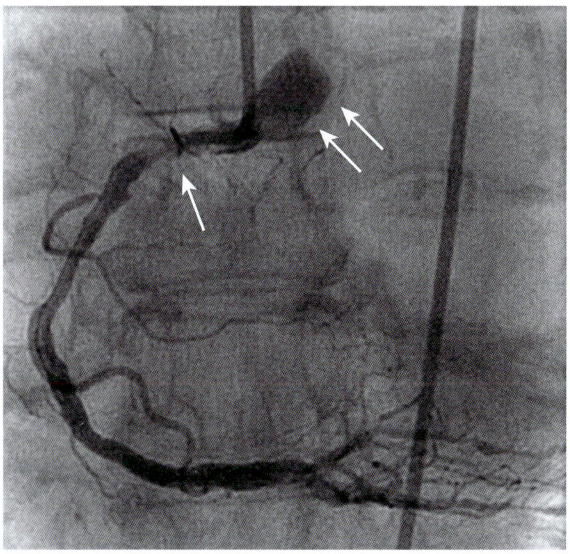

FIGURE 2.8 Guiding catheter dissection of the proximal right coronary artery and sinus of Valsalva. Coronary angiography showing a dissection in the proximal right coronary artery (single arrow) extending to the right sinus of Valsalva (double arrow). The dissection developed following engagement of the right coronary artery with an Amplatz guiding catheter during PCI of a mid–right coronary artery stenosis. It was managed by stenting the proximal right coronary artery segment through a JR4 guiding catheter.

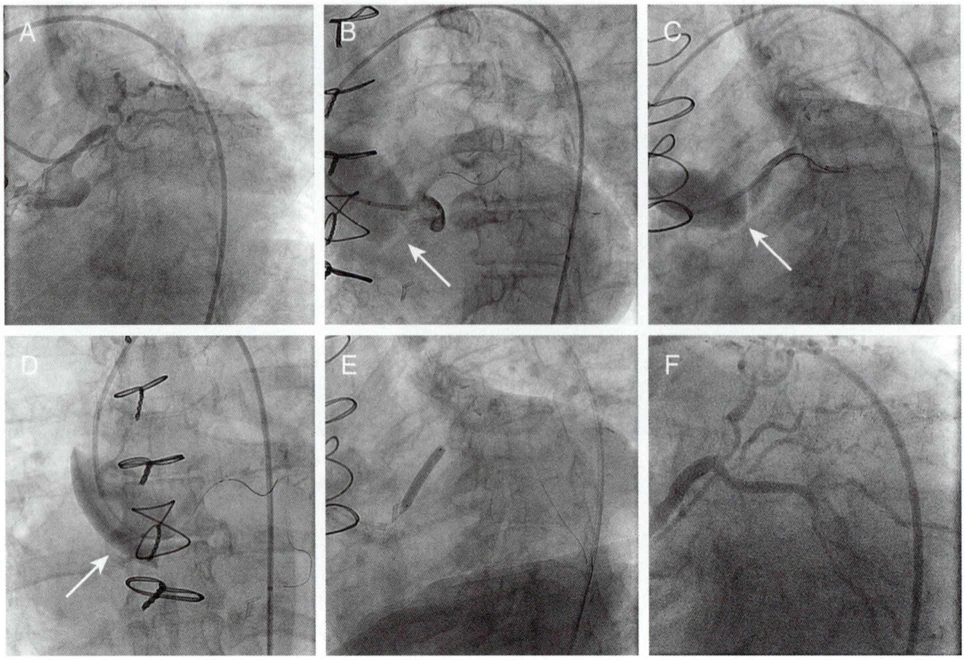

FIGURE 2.9 Left main dissection extending to the ascending aorta. **A**, Total occlusion of the left circumflex artery and of the left anterior descending artery in an 86-year-old patient presenting with NSTEMI. The left internal mammary artery graft to the LAD and the saphenous vein grafts to the obtuse marginal artery and to the PDA were patent. **B-D**, Following aggressive guiding catheter manipulation, there is an extensive dissection involving the left main coronary artery and the ascending aorta (white arrows). **E**, Deployment of a 3.5 mm × 20 mm stent in the left main coronary artery. **F**, Following stenting of the left main coronary artery, there is no further visualization of the aortic dissection, consistent with sealing of the dissection entry port.

CORONARY PERFORATION

Coronary perforation is a relatively uncommon complication of percutaneous coronary interventions. It can present with a spectrum of severity ranging from an extraluminal crater without extravasation of contrast to extravasation of contrast through a >1-mm exit hole leading to pericardial tamponade, or to a coronary-cameral fistula[5] (**Table 2.4**). While the introduction

TABLE 2.4

Ellis Classification of Coronary Artery Perforation

	Morphology	Clinical Sequelae
Type I	Extraluminal crater without extravasation	Almost always benign, treated effectively with stent placement
Type II	Pericardial or myocardial blush without contrast jet extravasation and without a >1-mm exit hole	Can result in late presentation of tamponade, requires close observation
Type III	Extravasation through a frank perforation with a ≥1-mm exit hole	High risk of tamponade, requires reversal of anticoagulation and immediate treatment
Type III—cavity spilling	Perforation into an anatomic chamber, such as coronary sinus, atria, or ventricles	Can often have a benign course, may result in fistulae formation, large perforation requires repair to avoid coronary steal

of covered stents and of coil embolization has provided interventional cardiologist with new tools for a nonsurgical management, coronary perforation continues to be associated with high morbidity and mortality, and it is responsible for up to 20% of cases referred for emergency bypass surgery. Thus, familiarity with its early recognition and emergency management are critical components of current interventional cardiology practice[6] (**FIGURES 2.10-2.19**).

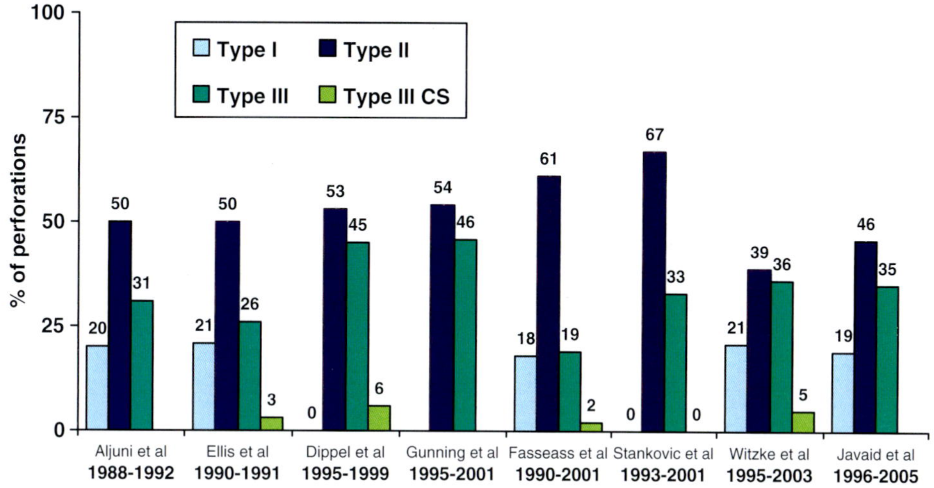

Different series demonstrated a low prevalence (20%) of Type I perforations, most likely related to under-reporting. Approximately 50% of the perforations were Type II and a third were Type III. Despite the different time periods, the distribution of the type of perforation did not show significant secular variation.

FIGURE 2.10 Type of perforation reported in different series.[5-12] Modified with permission from Moscucci M. *Complications of Cardiovascular Procedures: Risk Factors, Management and Bailout Techniques*. Philadelphia: Lippincott Williams and Wilkins; 2011.

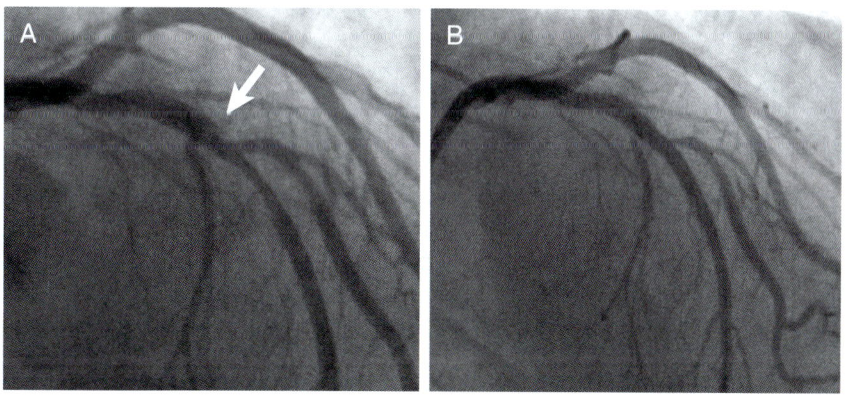

FIGURE 2.11 Type I coronary perforation. **A**, The arrow indicates an extraluminal crater after balloon angioplasty of a 90% lesion in the left anterior descending coronary artery. **B**, The perforation is completely sealed after stent placement. Reproduced with permission from Moscucci M. *Complications of Cardiovascular Procedures: Risk Factors, Management and Bailout Techniques*. Philadelphia: Lippincott Williams and Wilkins; 2011.

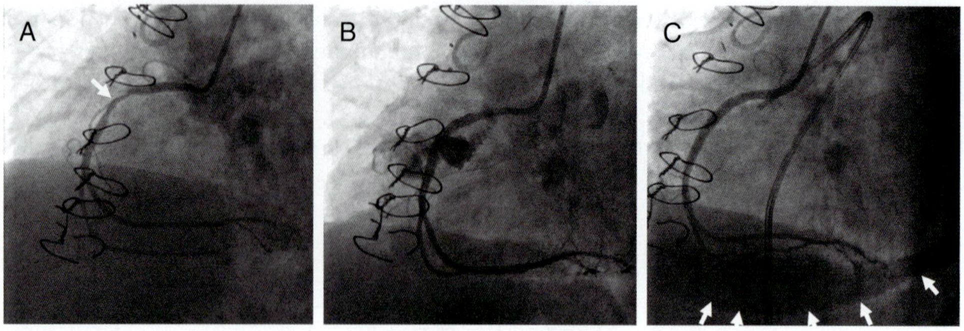

FIGURE 2.12 Type III perforation in a native right coronary artery causing tamponade. Right coronary perforation in an 82-year-old woman with a 75% lesion in the right coronary artery (white arrow) **(A)**. A 3.5 × 15 mm bare metal stent, which had a stent-to-artery ratio greater than 1.2, was directly deployed at the lesion causing a large Type III perforation with contrast extravasation into the pericardial space **(B)**. A JOMED covered stent was successfully inserted sealing the perforation **(C)**. The arrows in panel C indicate the presence of a substantial amount of contrast in the pericardial space. Reproduced with permission from Moscucci M. *Complications of Cardiovascular Procedures: Risk Factors, Management and Bailout Techniques*. Philadelphia: Lippincott Williams and Wilkins; 2011.

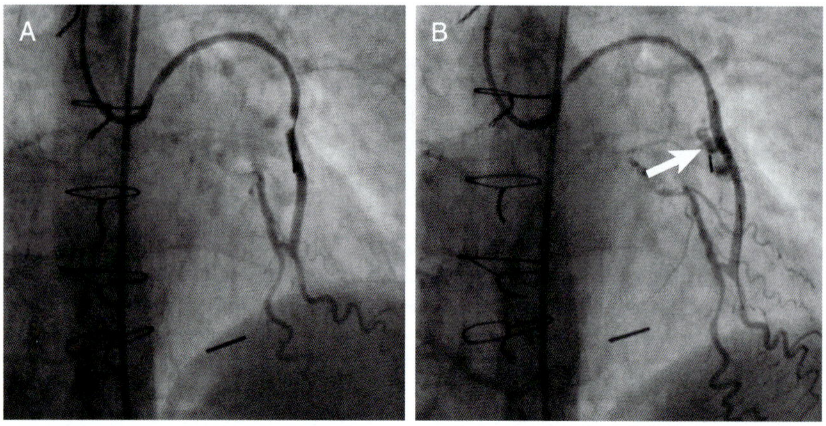

FIGURE 2.13 Mediastinal hemorrhage after direct stenting of a saphenous vein graft with a bare metal stent. **A**, Severe 95% stenosis in a saphenous vein graft to an obtuse marginal. **B**, After direct deployment of a bare metal stent, a Type III perforation causing mediastinal hemorrhage became apparent (arrow). The patient suffered profound hypotension and had to be intubated and started on inotropic support. Multiple attempts to deliver a JOMED covered stent were unsuccessful due to lack of guiding catheter support. The stent came off balloon, as it was being retrieved in the guiding catheter and finally embolized to the profunda femoral artery. In the end, the perforation was sealed with prolonged low-pressure balloon inflation. Reproduced with permission from Moscucci M. *Complications of Cardiovascular Procedures: Risk Factors, Management and Bailout Techniques*. Philadelphia: Lippincott Williams and Wilkins; 2011.

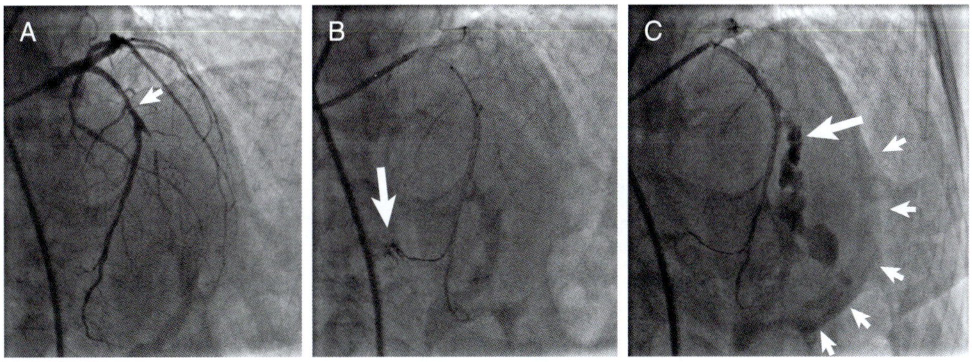

FIGURE 2.14 Type III cavity spilling and Type III perforations with tamponade. These are the angiographic images of a 76-year-old woman admitted through the emergency department with chest pain and left bundle branch block. There was a 95% lesion in the proximal-mid left anterior descending that was initially stented. **A**, A second stent was deemed necessary, as there was a significant residual stenosis proximal to the stented segment (arrow). **B**, A stent is being positioned in the proximal LAD. Notice the position of the wire in the septal perforator and contrast spilling in the right ventricle (arrow). **C**, After deployment of the stent, a large perforation was noticed at the origin of a diagonal branch (large arrow). The small arrows indicate the rapid accumulation of contrast in the pericardial space causing tamponade. The patient collapsed rapidly and was taken emergently to the operating room. The patient did not survive. Reproduced with permission from Moscucci M. *Complications of Cardiovascular Procedures: Risk Factors, Management and Bailout Techniques*. Philadelphia: Lippincott Williams and Wilkins; 2011.

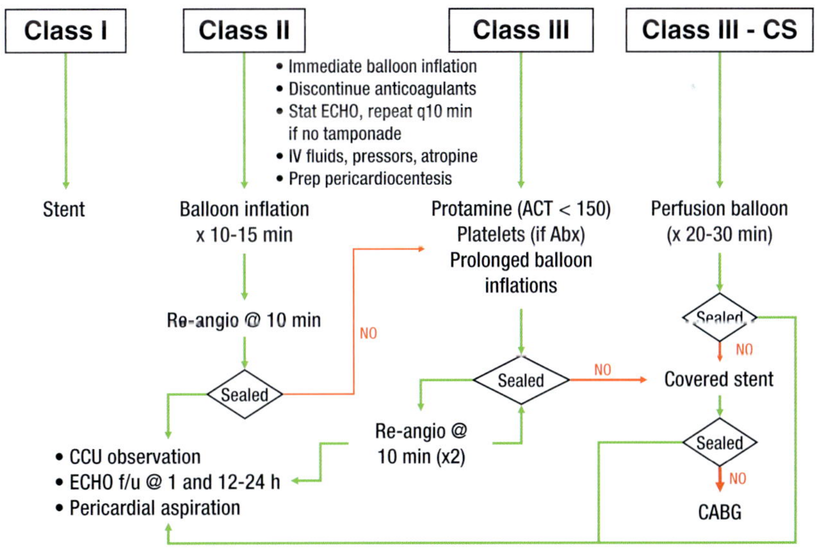

FIGURE 2.15 Algorithm for the management of coronary perforations. CS, cavity spilling; CABG, coronary artery bypass graft surgery. Modified from Dippel EJ, Kereiakes DJ, Tramuta DA, et al. Coronary perforation during percutaneous coronary intervention in the era of abciximab platelet glycoprotein IIb/IIIa blockade: an algorithm for percutaneous management. *Catheter Cardiovasc Interv*. 2001;52:279-286; Reproduced with permission from Moscucci M. *Complications of Cardiovascular Procedures: Risk Factors, Management and Bailout Techniques*. Philadelphia: Lippincott Williams and Wilkins; 2011.

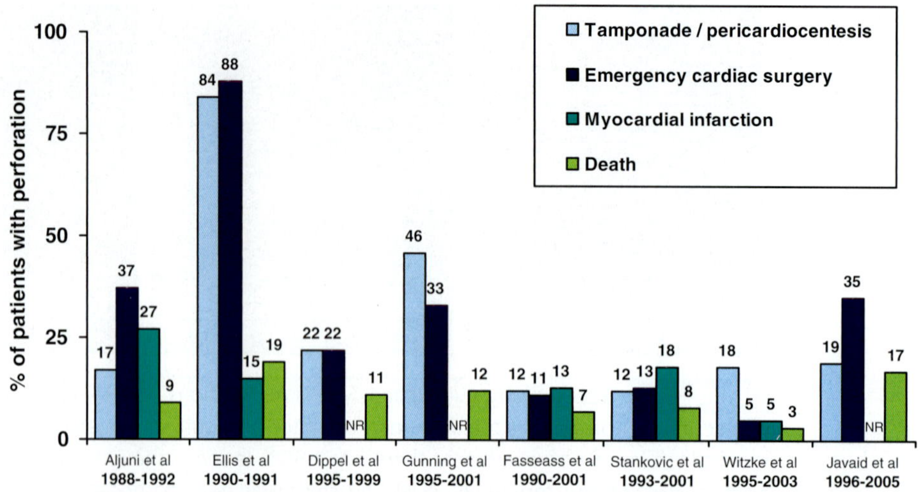

Reported case series demonstrated a disparate rates of tamponade/pericardiocentesis (12%-84%), emergency surgery (5%-88%), myocardial infarction (5%-27%), and death (3%-17%). In general lower rate of complications were noted in the more contemporary series.

FIGURE 2.16 Outcomes after perforation in different series.[5-12] Modified with permission from Moscucci M. *Complications of Cardiovascular Procedures: Risk Factors, Management and Bailout Techniques*. Philadelphia: Lippincott Williams and Wilkins; 2011.

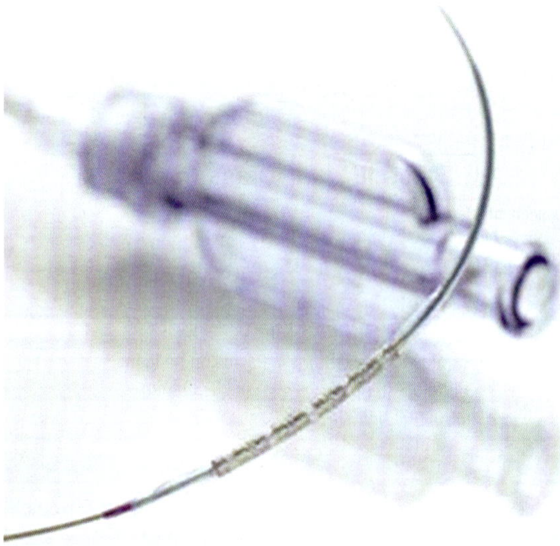

FIGURE 2.17 GRAFTMASTER RX stent (Abbott Vascular). The GRAFTMASTER RX stent has replaced the original "JOSTENT," and it is indicated for the treatment of free perforations in native coronary vessels or saphenous vein bypass grafts ≥2.75 mm in diameter. It consists of an ultrathin PTFE expandable layer sandwiched between 2 coaxial 316L stainless steel, slotted-tube, balloon-expandable stents. It is available in 6F compatible sizes with a diameter of 2.8, 3.5 and 4.0 mm, and 7F compatible sizes with a diameter of 4.5 and 4.8 mm. Courtesy of Abbott Laboratories. 100 Abbott Park Road. Abbott Park, Illinois 60064–350.

FIGURE 2.18 Aneugraft Dx (Amnis Therapeutics). The Aneugraft Dx is a single-layer coronary stent graft covered by equine pericardium. It consists of a 316L stainless steel metal stent covered by an equine pericardium cylinder. The bovine pericardium is sutured on the bare metal stent with a propylene suture. It is a low-profile stent that can be delivered through a 6F guiding catheter. Courtesy of Amnis Therapeutics Ltd., 22 Ha'ilan Street, P.O. Box 146, Or Akiva, 3060000 Israel. info@amnis.life.

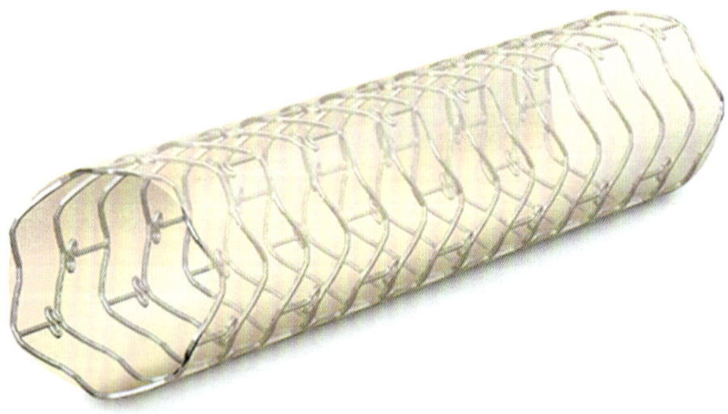

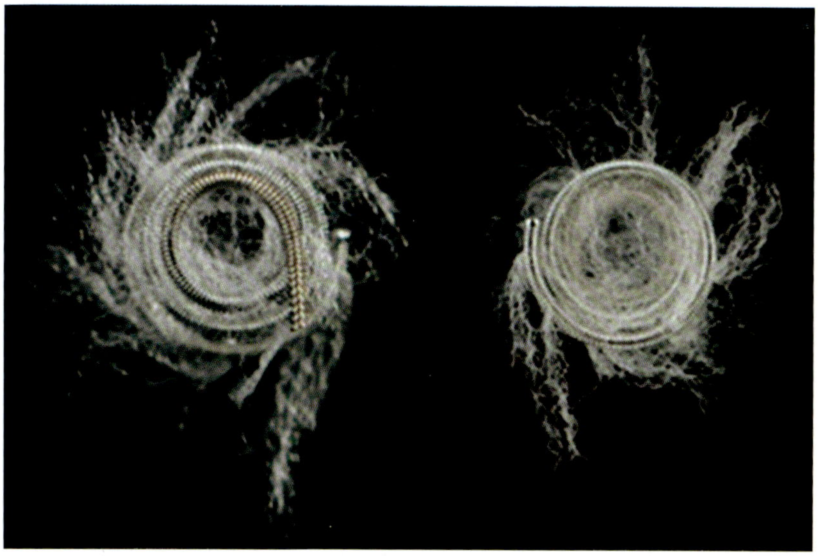

FIGURE 2.19 Tornado Platinum 0.018 Microcoil Configuration (Cook Medical) Coil embolization can be attempted when the amount of myocardium at risk is small and unlikely to result in significant myocardial dysfunction. The microcoils are loaded into a microcatheter and are advanced through the microcatheter by pushing a "coil-pushing wire." Given the stiffness of the system, the procedure requires careful guiding catheter technique for support and maintenance of distal catheter position. www.cookmedical.com/di/dataSheet.do?id=4162.

AIR EMBOLISM

Air embolism is a rare complication of coronary diagnostic and therapeutic procedures, and in theory, if meticulous technique is applied when flushing and exchanging catheters and during coronary angiography, it should never occur. Beyond inadequate preparation of the manifold and/or inadequate monitoring of the remaining amount of saline flushing and contrast in the manifold system, rapid removal of devices, by entraining air in the guiding catheter, can result in air embolization. While small air bubbles can be tolerated, larger bubbles can cause air lock leading to hypotension, pulseless electric activity, and/or ventricular fibrillation. Treatment includes 100% oxygen, mechanical aspiration if possible, saline flushing and defibrillation, and hemodynamic support as needed (**FIGURES 2.20** and **2.21**).

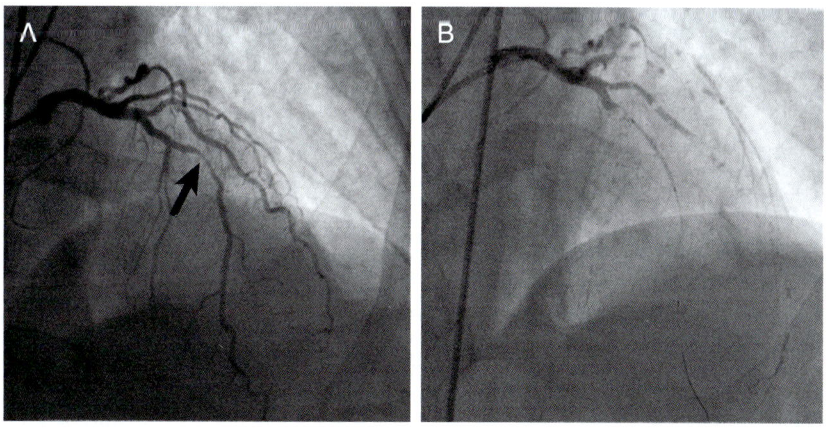

FIGURE 2.20 Diagnostic coronary angiography of the left anterior descending artery in the right anterior oblique cranial projection, showing **(A)** a severe mid–left anterior descending artery lesion (black arrow) and **(B)** several coronary intraluminal filling defects attributable to massive air embolism. Reproduced with permission from Prasad A, Banerjee S, Brilakis ES. Hemodynamic Consequences of Massive Coronary Air Embolism. *Circulation*. 2007;115:e51-e53.

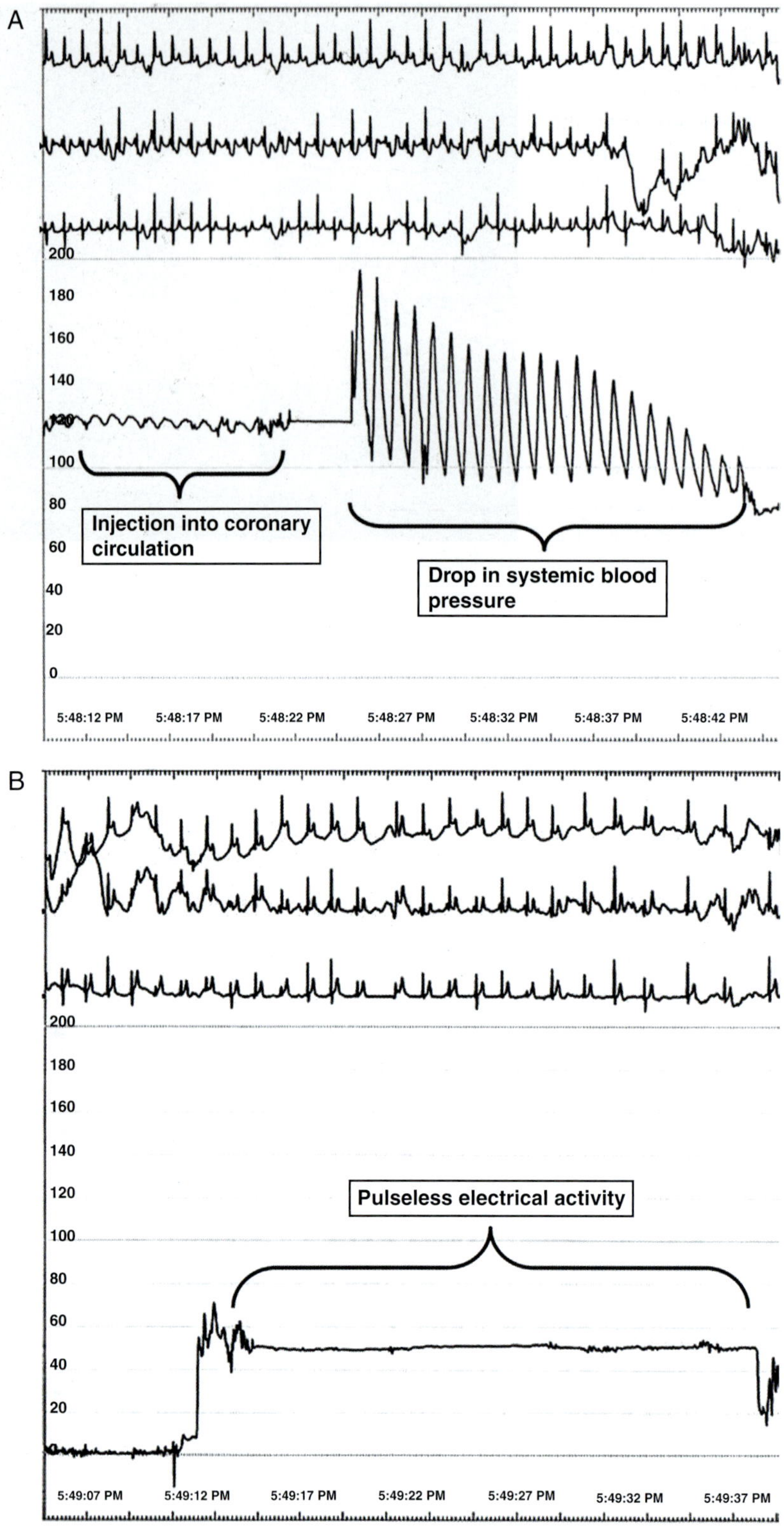

FIGURE 2.21 Electrocardiography and coronary guide used to obtain blood pressure immediately after air embolism **(A)** showing rapid development of hypotension, followed by the onset of pulseless electrical activity **(B)**. Reproduced with permission from Prasad A, Banerjee S, Brilakis ES. Hemodynamic Consequences of Massive Coronary Air Embolism. *Circulation*. 2007;115:e51-e53.

ARTERIAL ACCESS VASCULAR COMPLICATIONS

Arterial access vascular complications can be classified in 3 main domains: thrombotic, embolic, and hemorrhagic.

Thrombotic Complications

Thrombotic complications are more commonly seen in the pediatric population, although the growth of procedures for structural heart disease requiring large bore vascular access has resulted in an increased frequency also in the adult patients' population. Risk factors for thrombotic complications include large arterial sheaths, prolonged dwell time, prolonged compression after sheath removal, small or diseased common femoral arteries (females, severe peripheral arterial disease), and local dissection during arterial sheath site insertion.

They usually present with a painful white lower extremity and varying degrees of decreased sensorium and motor function.

Atheroembolism

Atheroembolism is a relatively rare complication of arterial vascular access, with a reported incidence around 0.08%. Patients with extensive atherosclerosis are at increased risk, and the clinical presentation depends on the location of the embolic source. When the embolic source is at the femoral artery access site, the clinical presentation usually includes symptoms and signs limited to the distal lower extremities, with manifestation ranging from livedo reticularis (**FIGURE 2.22**) to acrocyanosis and gangrene. When the source is in the aorta, the presentation can be with multisystem organ failure including renal failure, mesenteric ischemia, and pancreatitis, and it is associated with poor prognosis and a mortality rate as high as 80%.[13,14]

Hemorrhagic Complications

Despite advancement in technology, hemorrhagic complications continue to be an important cause of morbidity and mortality.[15-18] They include local access hematoma, pseudoaneurysm, free hemorrhage, and the rare but potentially fatal retroperitoneal hematoma. Identification of patients at increased risk, meticulous management of anticoagulation and of vascular access site, optimal vascular access technique, prompt recognition, and appropriate management are paramount for their prevention and management (**FIGURES 2.23-2.32**).

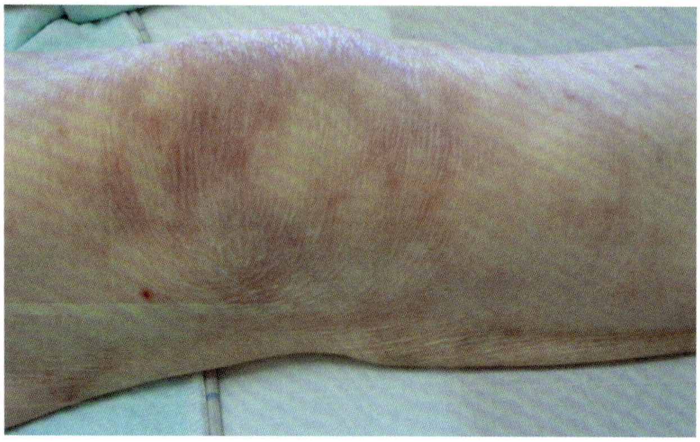

FIGURE 2.22 Livedo reticularis. The triad of leg and foot pain, intact peripheral pulses, and livedo reticularis is diagnostic of cholesterol embolism.[13] Reproduced with permission from Moscucci M. *Complications of Cardiovascular Procedures: Risk Factors, Management and Bailout Techniques.* Philadelphia: Lippincott Williams and Wilkins; 2011.

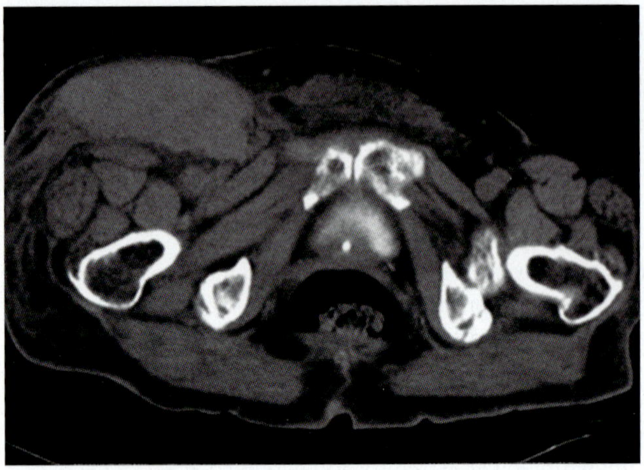

FIGURE 2.23 CT scan in a patient following the development of a femoral hematoma. There is no evidence of extension to the retroperitoneal space. Reproduced with permission from Moscucci M. *Complications of Cardiovascular Procedures: Risk Factors, Management and Bailout Techniques*. Philadelphia: Lippincott Williams and Wilkins; 2011.

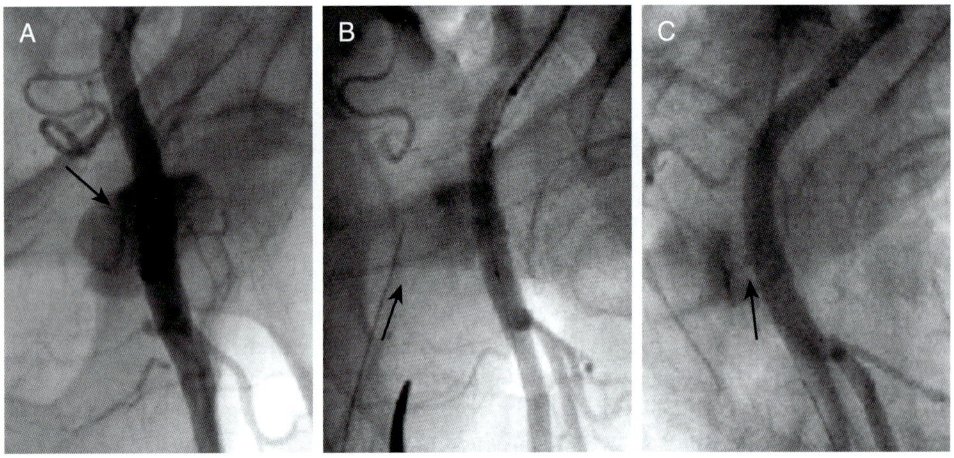

FIGURE 2.24 Femoral pseudoaneurysm. **A**, To evaluate a pulsatile mass in the left groin following a catheterization, crossover angiography was performed from the right groin showing a large pseudoaneurysm over the common femoral artery (arrow). **B**, An angioplasty balloon was positioned under the prior puncture site, as a needle (arrow) was advanced to puncture the pseudoaneurysm cavity confirmed by contrast injection. **C**, After occlusion of the common femoral by inflation of the angioplasty balloon, thrombin was injected through the needle into the pseudoaneurysm cavity, causing it to clot, as shown by the absence of further contrast flow into it on the postprocedure angiogram (arrow). Case provided courtesy of Dr Andrew Eisenhauer, Brigham and Women's Hospital; Reproduced from Donald S. *Baim, Grossman's Cardiac Catheterization, Angiography, and Intervention*. 7th ed. Philadelphia: Lippincott Williams & Wilkins; 2006.

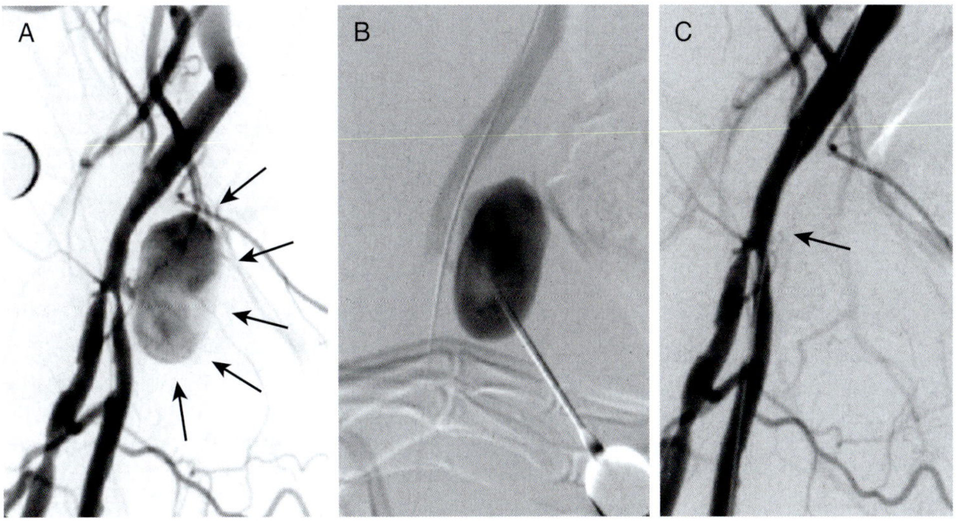

FIGURE 2.25 Angiographic appearance of a pseudoaneurysm sac (outlined by arrows). **A**, The hole in the artery is between the sac and the common femoral artery. **B**, Using road mapping and fluoroscopy, a needle is inserted percutaneously into the pseudoaneurysm sac. Once pulsatile flow is obtained, contrast is injected to confirm location, followed by very slow injection of thrombin one-tenth of a cubic centimeter at a time. **C**, Final angiography demonstrates closure of the hole in the common femoral artery and obliteration of the pseudoaneurysm (arrow). Reproduced from Donald S. *Baim, Grossman's Cardiac Catheterization, Angiography, and Intervention*. 7th ed. Philadelphia: Lippincott Williams & Wilkins; 2006.

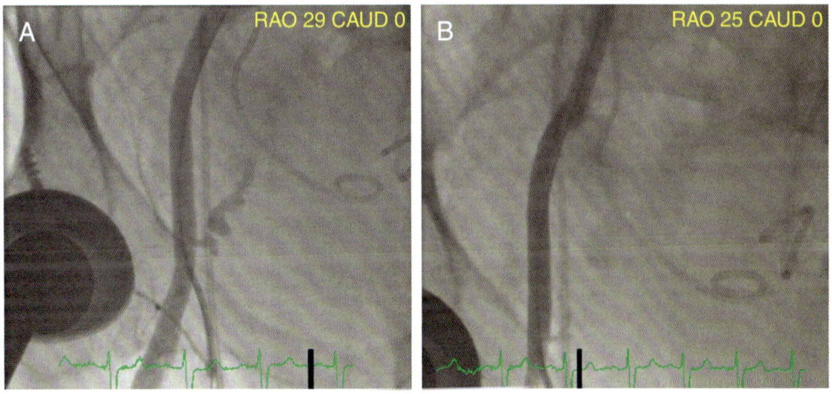

FIGURE 2.26 Angiography of the right femoral artery. **A**, The arterial sheath has been inserted above the inguinal ligament, and there is extravasation of contrast in the retroperitoneal space. **B**, Repeat angiography after deployment of a covered stent. There is no further extravasation of contrast in the retroperitoneal space. Reproduced with permission from Moscucci M. *Complications of Cardiovascular Procedures: Risk Factors, Management and Bailout Techniques*. Philadelphia: Lippincott Williams and Wilkins; 2011.

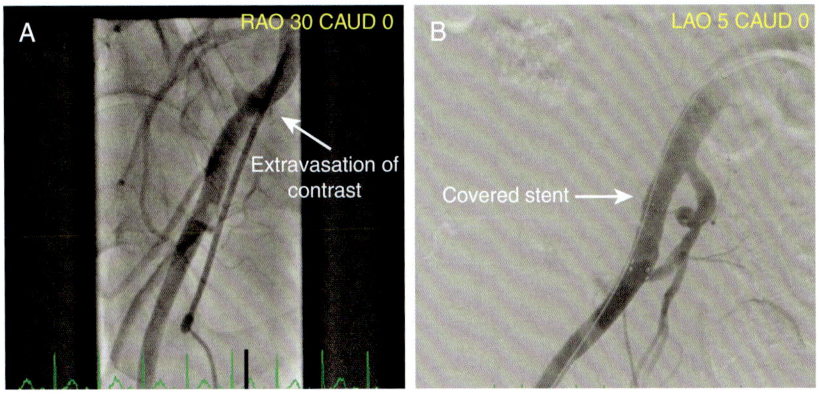

FIGURE 2.27 **A**, Angiography of the right femoral artery showing extravasation of contrast from the inferior epigastric artery. **B**, Repeat angiography following deployment of a covered stent. Reproduced with permission from Moscucci M. *Complications of Cardiovascular Procedures: Risk Factors, Management and Bailout Techniques*. Philadelphia: Lippincott Williams and Wilkins; 2011.

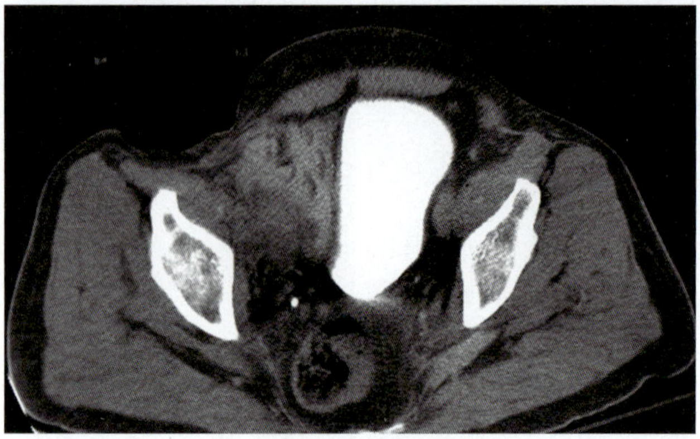

FIGURE 2.28 Pelvic CT scan showing a large retroperitoneal hematoma. Reproduced with permission from Moscucci M. *Complications of Cardiovascular Procedures: Risk Factors, Management and Bailout Techniques*. Philadelphia: Lippincott Williams and Wilkins; 2011.

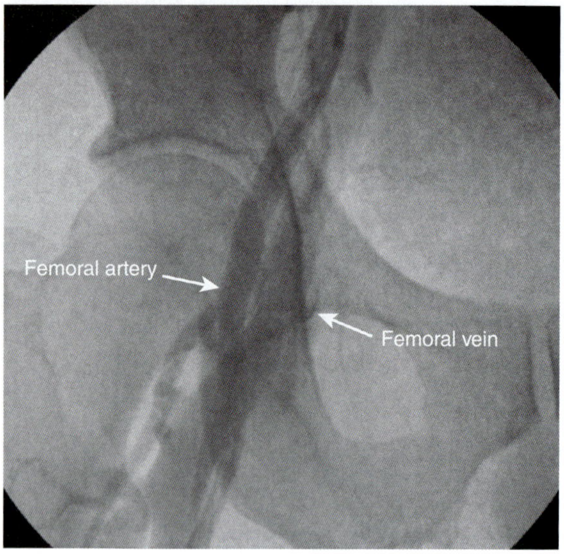

FIGURE 2.29 Femoral arteriovenous fistula. During angiography of the femoral artery, there is simultaneous visualization of the femoral vein. Reproduced with permission from Moscucci M. *Complications of Cardiovascular Procedures: Risk Factors, Management and Bailout Techniques*. Philadelphia: Lippincott Williams and Wilkins; 2011.

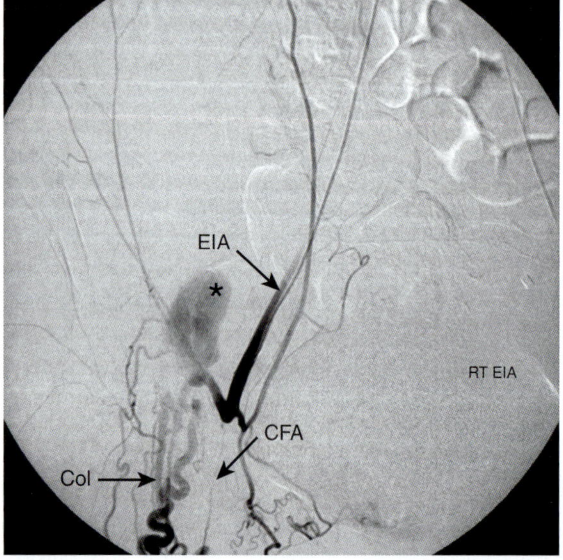

FIGURE 2.30 Retroperitoneal bleeding demonstrated by selective catheterization of the right internal and external iliac branches with contrast extravasation (*) around a prominent collateral (Col) running from the right distal external iliac artery (EIA) to the femoral bifurcation. CFA, chronic subtotal occlusion of the common femoral artery. Reproduced from Morris GM, O'Grady EA, Wynn GJ, Davis GK. Retroperitoneal hematoma after diagnostic coronary angiography caused by collateralization of a chronic common femoral artery occlusion secondary to childhood femoral cannulation. *Circ Cardiovasc Interv*. 2009;2:580-581.

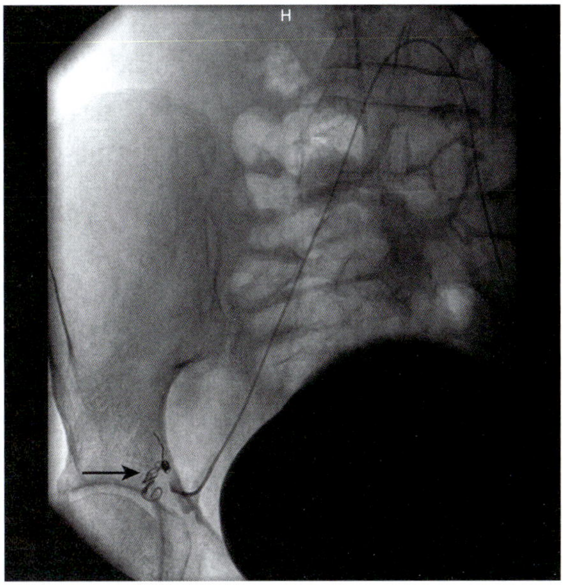

FIGURE 2.31 Treatment of bleeding point by coil embolization (arrow). Reproduced from Morris GM, O'Grady EA, Wynn GJ, Davis GK. Retroperitoneal hematoma after diagnostic coronary angiography caused by collateralization of a chronic common femoral artery occlusion secondary to childhood femoral cannulation. *Circ Cardiovasc Interv*. 2009;2:580-581.

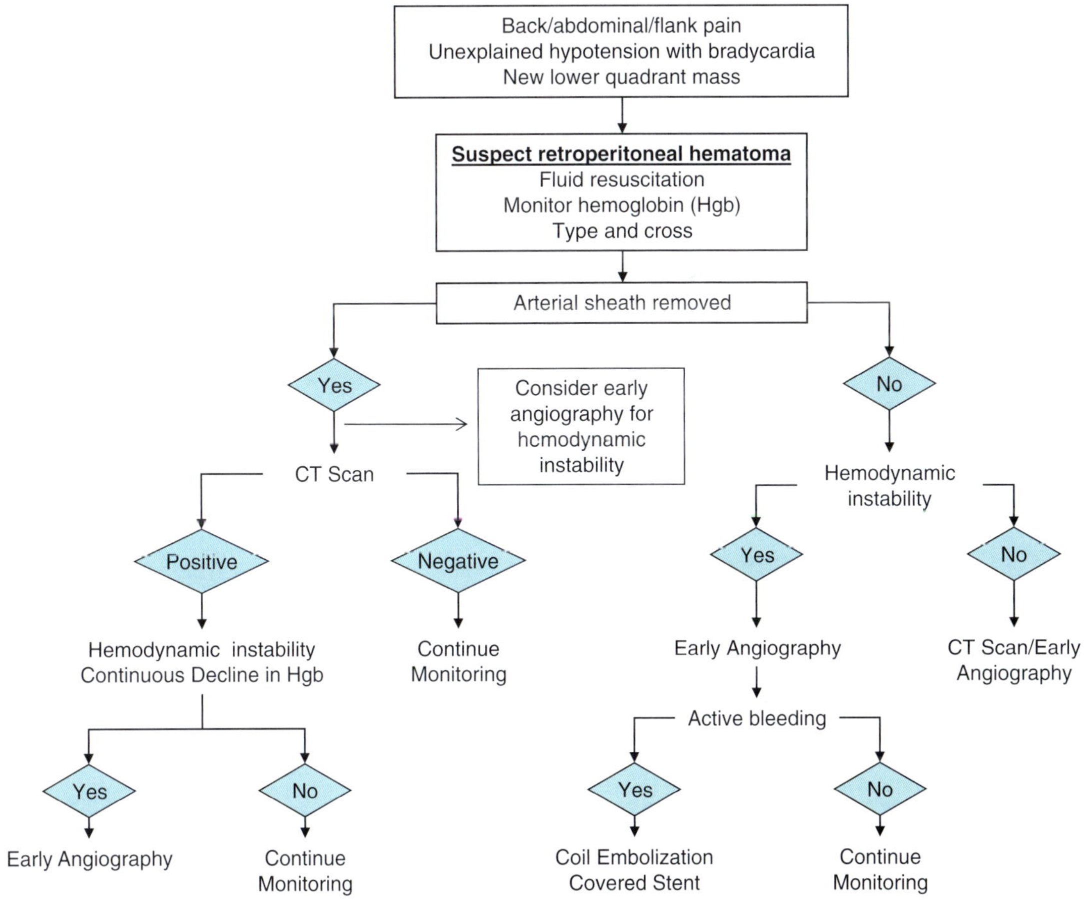

FIGURE 2.32 Suggested algorithm for the management of patients with suspected retroperitoneal hematoma. Reproduced with permission from Chetcuti SJ, Cohen GC, Moscucci M. Local arterial and venous vascular access site complication. In: Moscucci M, ed. *Complications of Cardiovascular Procedures: Incidence, Risk Factors and Bailout Techniques*. Philadelphia, PA: Lippincott Williams & Wilkins; 2011.

REFERENCES

1. Roy P, de Labriolle A, Hanna N, et al. Requirement for emergent coronary artery bypass surgery following percutaneous coronary intervention in the stent era. *Am J Cardiol.* 2009;103:950-953.
2. Yang EH, Gumina RJ, Lennon RJ, Holmes DR Jr, Rihal CS, Singh M. Emergency coronary artery bypass surgery for percutaneous coronary interventions: changes in the incidence, clinical characteristics, and indications from 1979 to 2003. *J Am Coll Cardiol.* 2005;46:2004-2009.
3. Huber MS, Mooney JF, Madison J, Mooney MR. Use of a morphologic classification to predict clinical outcome after dissection from coronary angioplasty. *Am J Cardiol.* 1991;68:467-471.
4. Dunning DW, Kahn JK, Hawkins ET, O'Neill WW. Iatrogenic coronary artery dissections extending into and involving the aortic root. *Catheter Cardiovasc Interv.* 2000;51:387-393.
5. Ellis SG, Ajluni S, Arnold AZ, et al. Increased coronary perforation in the new device era. Incidence, classification, management, and outcome. *Circulation.* 1994;90:2725-2730.
6. Dippel EJ, Kereiakes DJ, Tramuta DA, et al. Coronary perforation during percutaneous coronary intervention in the era of abciximab platelet glycoprotein IIb/IIIa blockade: an algorithm for percutaneous management. *Catheter Cardiovasc Interv.* 2001;52:279-286.
7. Ajluni SC, Glazier S, Blankenship L, O'Neill WW, Safian RD. Perforations after percutaneous coronary interventions: clinical, angiographic, and therapeutic observations. *Cathet Cardiovasc Diagn.* 1994;32:206-212.
8. Fasseas P, Orford JL, Panetta CJ, et al. Incidence, correlates, management, and clinical outcome of coronary perforation: analysis of 16,298 procedures. *Am Heart J.* 2004;147:140-145.
9. Gunning MG, Williams IL, Jewitt DE, Shah AM, Wainwright RJ, Thomas MR. Coronary artery perforation during percutaneous intervention: incidence and outcome. *Heart.* 2002;88:495-498.
10. Javaid A, Buch AN, Satler LF, et al. Management and outcomes of coronary artery perforation during percutaneous coronary intervention. *Am J Cardiol.* 2006;98:911-914.
11. Stankovic G, Orlic D, Corvaja N, et al. Incidence, predictors, in-hospital, and late outcomes of coronary artery perforations. *Am J Cardiol.* 2004;93:213-216.
12. Witzke CF, Martin-Herrero F, Clarke SC, Pomerantzev E, Palacios IF. The changing pattern of coronary perforation during percutaneous coronary intervention in the new device era. *J Invasive Cardiol.* 2004;16:257-301.
13. Falanga V, Fine MJ, Kapoor WN. The cutaneous manifestations of cholesterol crystal embolization. *Arch Dermatol.* 1986;122:1194-1198.
14. Fine MJ, Kapoor W, Falanga V. Cholesterol crystal embolization: a review of 221 cases in the English literature. *Angiology.* 1987;38:769-784.
15. Grossman PM, Gurm HS, McNamara R, et al. Percutaneous coronary intervention complications and guide catheter size: bigger is not better. *JACC.* 2009;2:636-644.
16. Kent KC, Moscucci M, Gallagher SG, DiMattia ST, Skillman JJ. Neuropathy after cardiac catheterization: incidence, clinical patterns, and long-term outcome. *J Vasc Surg.* 1994;19:1008-1013; discussion 1013-1004.
17. Kent KC, Moscucci M, Mansour KA, et al. Retroperitoneal hematoma after cardiac catheterization: prevalence, risk factors, and optimal management. *J Vasc Surg.* 1994;20:905-910; discussion 910-903.
18. Moscucci M, Mansour KA, Kent KC, et al. Peripheral vascular complications of directional coronary atherectomy and stenting: predictors, management, and outcome. *Am J Cardiol.* 1994;74:448-453.

chapter **3**

Percutaneous Vascular Access: Transfemoral, Transseptal, Apical, and Transcaval Approach

MICHAEL DAVID DYAL, MD, FACC and CLAUDIA A. MARTINEZ, MD

INTRODUCTION

Arterial and venous access are essential components of all cardiac catheterization procedures. Arterial access sites include the common femoral artery, the radial, ulnar, brachial, and the axillary arteries. In addition, the carotid artery,[1] the iliac, and the subclavian artery have been used for direct access to the ascending aorta. Vascular access site complications are common,[2] and intimate knowledge of vascular anatomy and proper technique are critical for a successful and safe procedure. In this chapter, we will review femoral access and closure, left-sided heart catheterization via the transseptal and transapical routes, and the recently introduced transcaval approach. For radial access and open cut down, the reader is referred to chapters 4 and 6.

FEMORAL ACCESS

The common femoral artery (CFA) has traditionally been used for percutaneous cardiac interventions.[3] Despite the adoption of radial artery access, CFA access remains the most commonly used approach for coronary and peripheral vascular procedures.[4] Furthermore, CFA access has been shown to have more favorable outcomes when compared with alternative access sites for transcatheter aortic valve replacement.[5] Vascular complications are increased significantly when arterial access is obtained below the common femoral artery bifurcation or above the inguinal ligament (external iliac artery).[6] Successful CFA access can be obtained in nearly all procedures with proper training and technique using multiple modalities including anatomic landmarks, fluoroscopic landmarks, and real-time ultrasound guidance (**FIGURES 3.1-3.8**, **Videos 3.1-3.3**).[7]

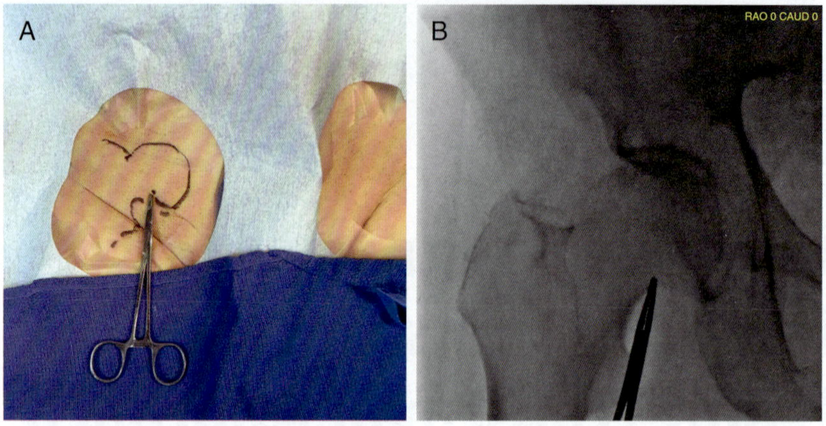

FIGURE 3.1 Femoral anatomic landmarks. **A**, Skin landmarks. **B**, Fluoroscopic landmarks with the aid of a hemostat.

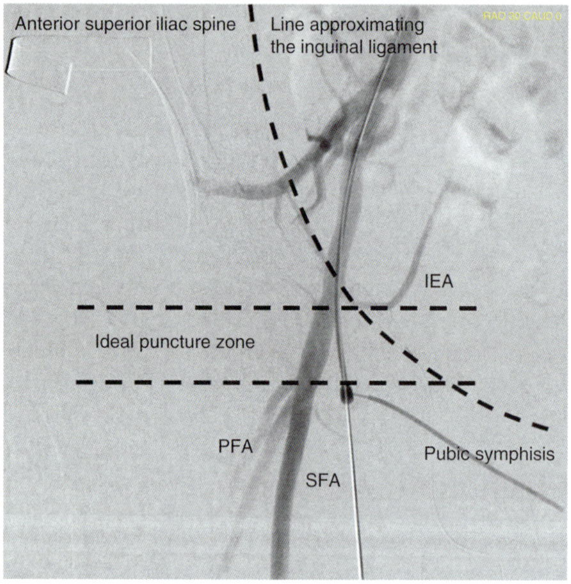

FIGURE 3.2 Femoral anatomy: Femoral angiogram with fluoroscopic and vascular landmarks illustrating the ideal puncture zone below the IEA and above the femoral bifurcation. CFA, common femoral artery; IEA, inferior epigastric artery; PFA, profunda femoris artery; SFA, superficial femoral artery.

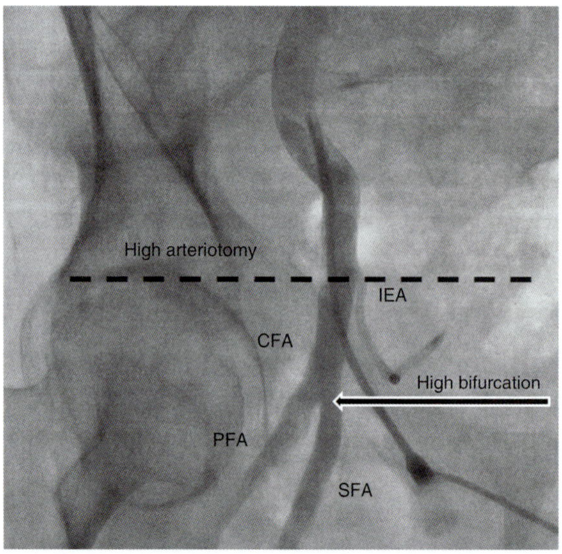

FIGURE 3.3 High bifurcation. The utility of ultrasound guidance is illustrated here. The very high femoral bifurcation leaves a very narrow window for common femoral artery puncture. Ultrasound guidance can help in preventing a low arteriotomy, while the fluoroscopic landmarks help in preventing a high arteriotomy.

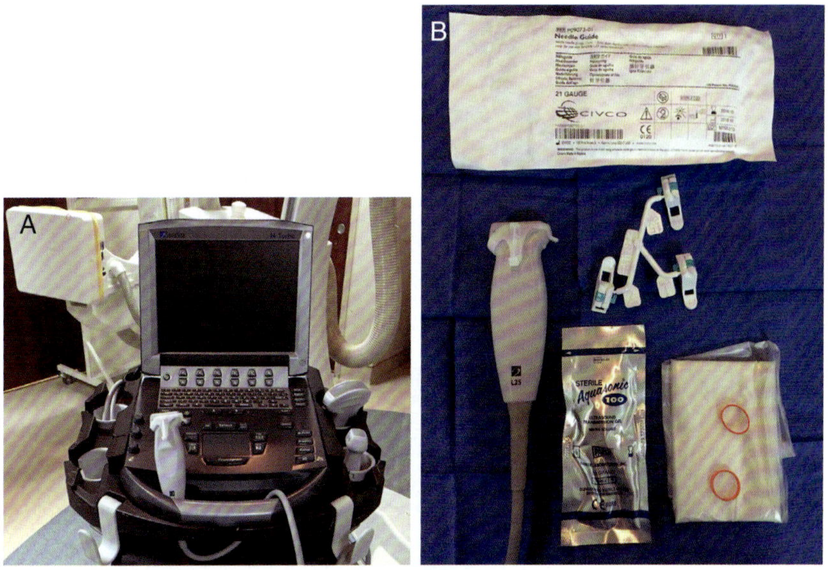

FIGURE 3.4 Ultrasound-guided femoral access. **A**, Sonosite ultrasound machine. **B**, Sonosite vascular probe with needle guide attachment, probe cover, sterile gel, and assorted needle guides.

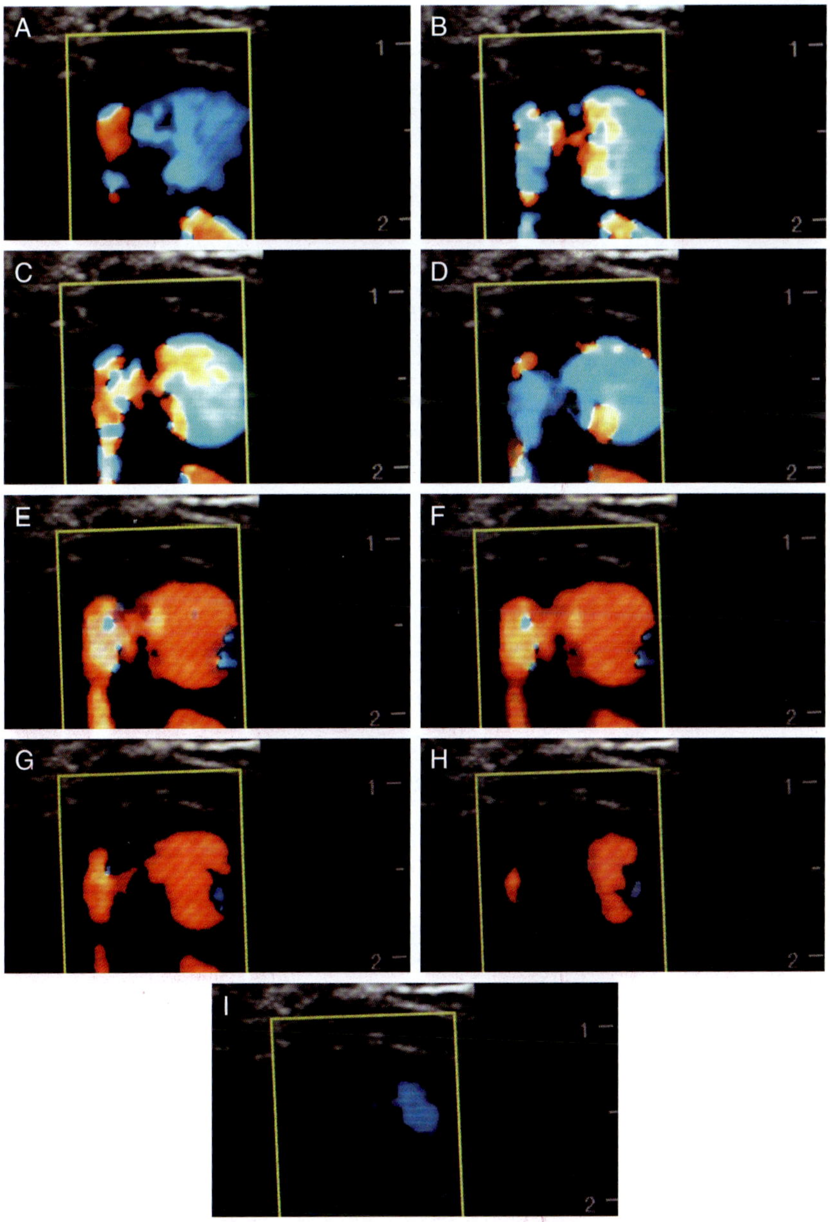

FIGURE 3.5 **A-I**, Pulsatile arterial blood flow seen on color Doppler. **A-F**, Systolic frames; **G-I**, diastolic frames.

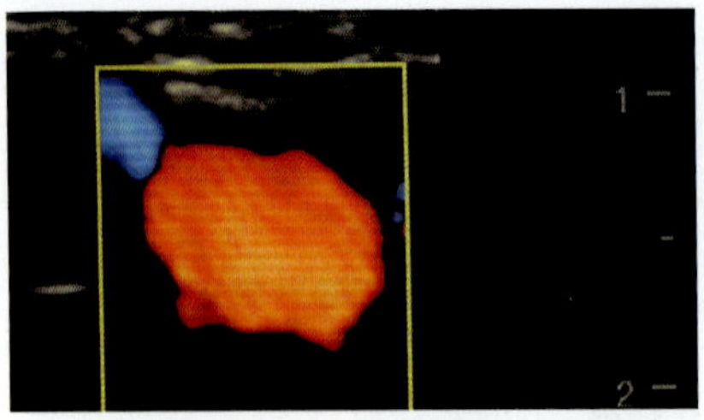

FIGURE 3.6 Continuous venous blood flow seen on color Doppler.

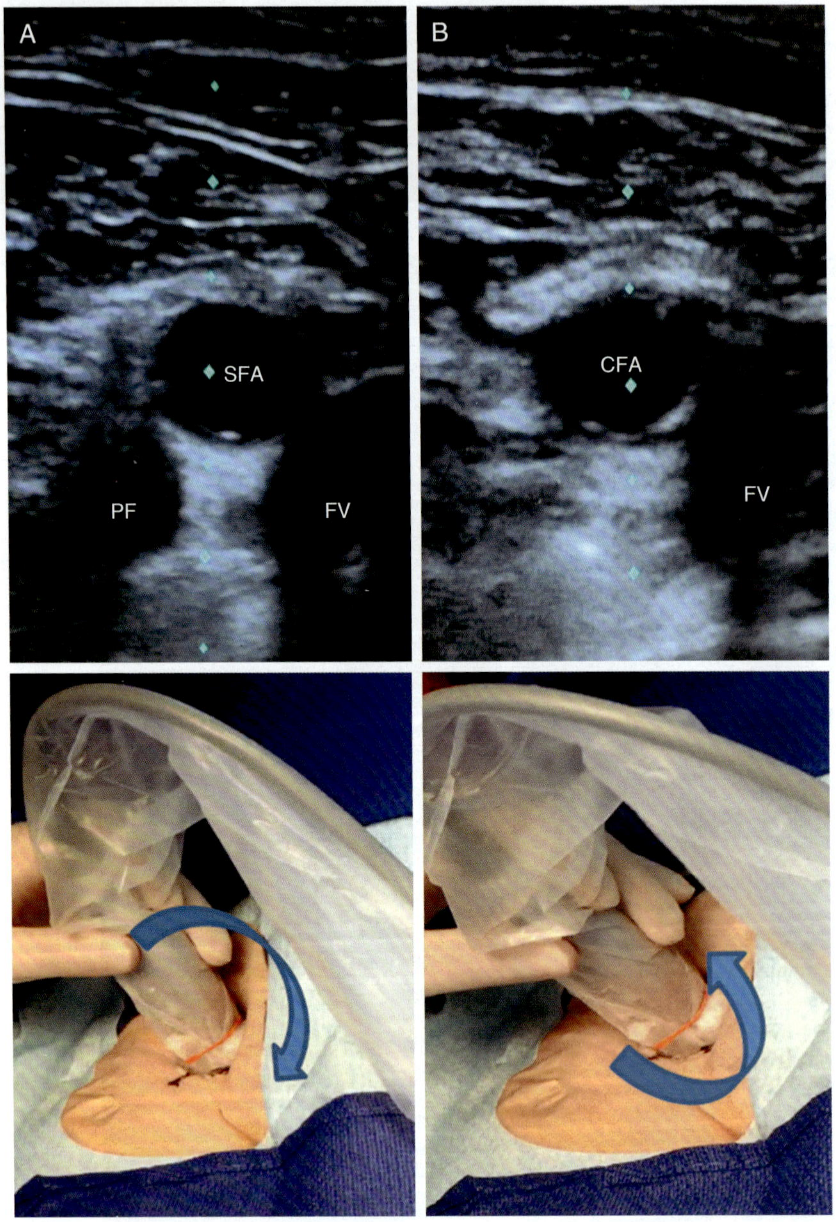

FIGURE 3.7 Ultrasound of the CFA and vein as the operator scans distally to illustrate the bifurcation into profunda femoris and the superficial femoral artery **(A)** then back proximally to the common femoral artery **(B)**. Ultrasound is used to ensure puncture proximal to the bifurcation and to avoid any large calcific femoral artery plaques. With ultrasound alone, there is a small risk of a high arterial puncture. Fluoroscopic landmarks and proper ultrasound technique can ensure CFA arteriotomy in the optimal location. The operator clearly identifies the CFA bifurcation. From here, the operator scans the vessel proximally with either a slight tilt or slide of the probe.

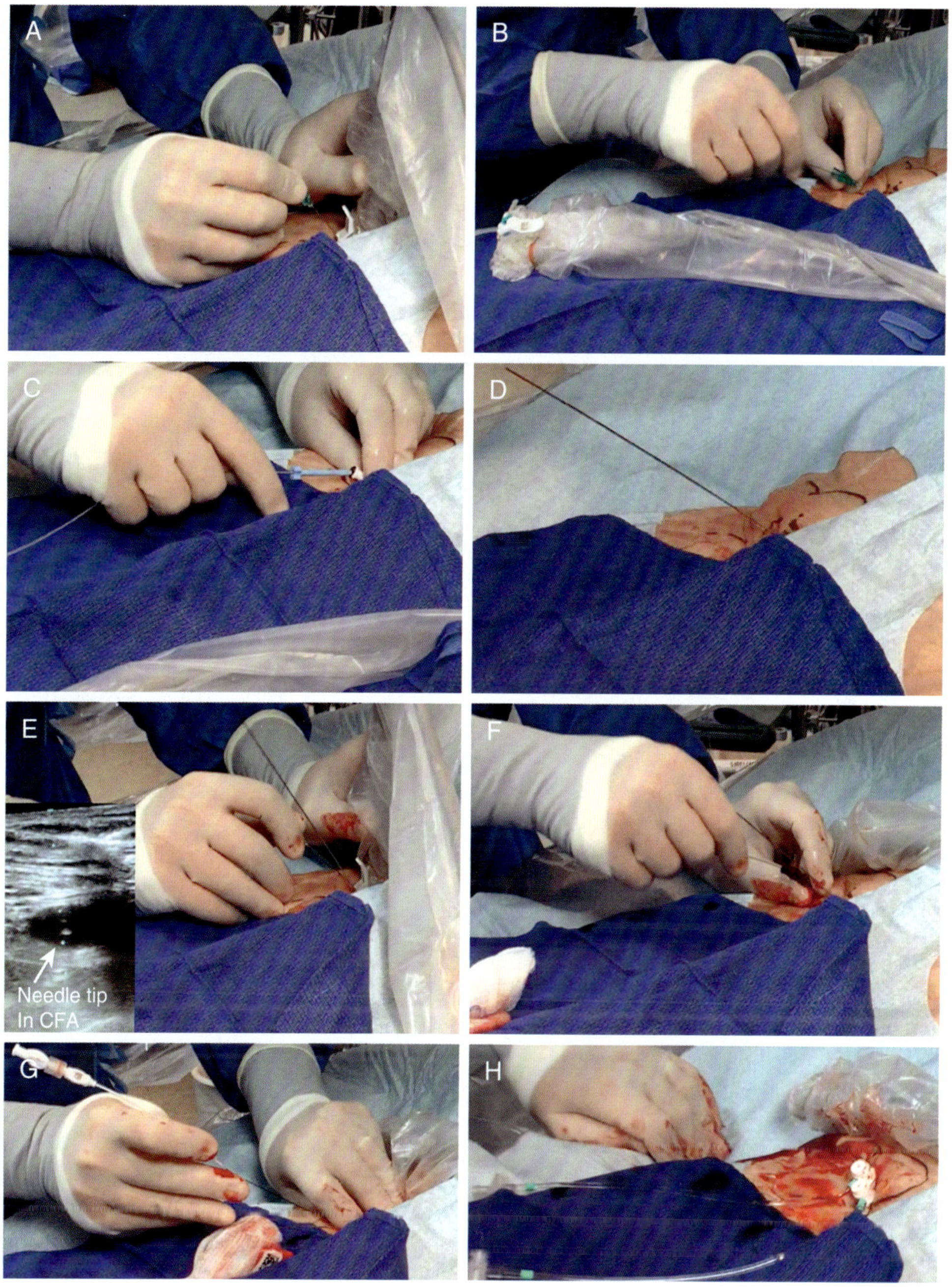

FIGURE 3.8 Arterial and venous access, basic technique. After identifying the skin and fluoroscopic landmarks, real-time ultrasound guidance with the assistance of a needle guide and micropuncture system is used for venous puncture **(A-C)**. A 0.035″ wire is left in the vein and the artery is also accessed using real-time ultrasound guidance **(D-F)**. A sheath is placed in the femoral artery and finally the venous sheath is inserted over the wire **(G-H)**.

LARGE BORE ACCESS AND PRECLOSURE

Femoral vascular complications increase relative to access sheath size.[2,6] The current era of interventional cardiology has been characterized by a surge in interventions for structural heart disease and in the use of percutaneous left ventricular assist devices requiring large bore arterial access. The importance of proper technique is even more critical for patient safety and procedural success. In the following section, we will discuss large bore access and closure techniques (**FIGURES 3.9** and **3.10**).

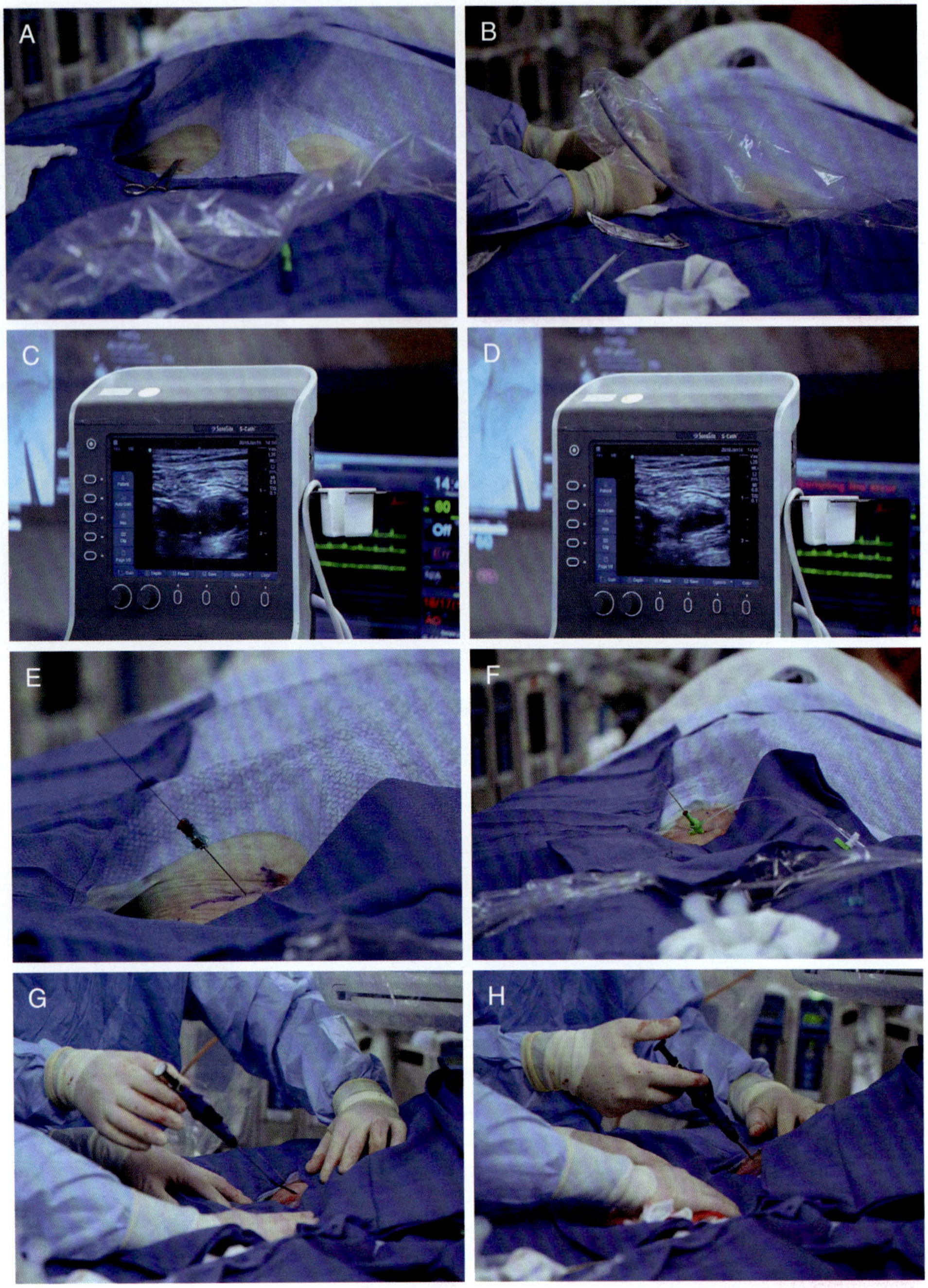

FIGURE 3.9 Preclosure technique. The anatomic land marks are identified and marked **(A)**. Under ultrasounds guidance, the common femoral artery, and the femoral vein are identified **(B-D)**. Vascular access is obtained using a micropuncture kit **(E-F)**. Once vascular access has been obtained, preclosure is performed using 2 Perclose Proglide devices. A skin nick is made with a scalpel, and the skin is dilated with a hemostat. A wire is advanced, and the sheath is exchanged for the first Perclose device **(G-I)**. This suture is deployed approximately in the 10 o'clock position, and the loose ends of the sutures are secured to the ipsilateral side with a hemostat. A guide wire is reinserted **(J and K),** and a second Perclose device is deployed approximately in the 2 o'clock position **(L-N)**. The loose end of the sutures are secured to the ipsilateral side, a wire is advanced through the second Proglide, which is then exchanged for an 8 FR sheath **(O)**. The 8 FR sheath will then be exchanged for the large bore sheath needed for the planned intervention.

Continued on following page

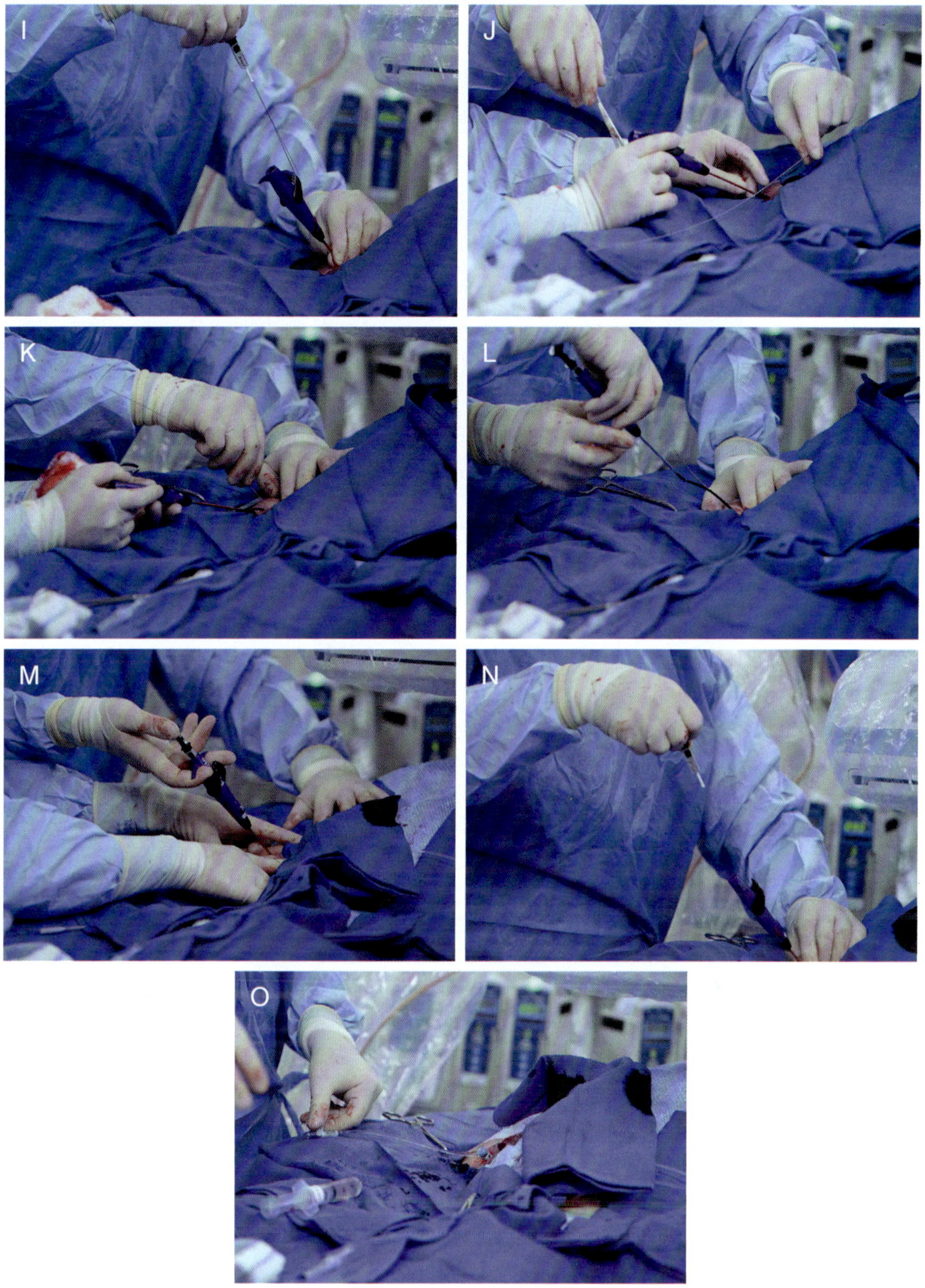

FIGURE 3.9 (Continued)

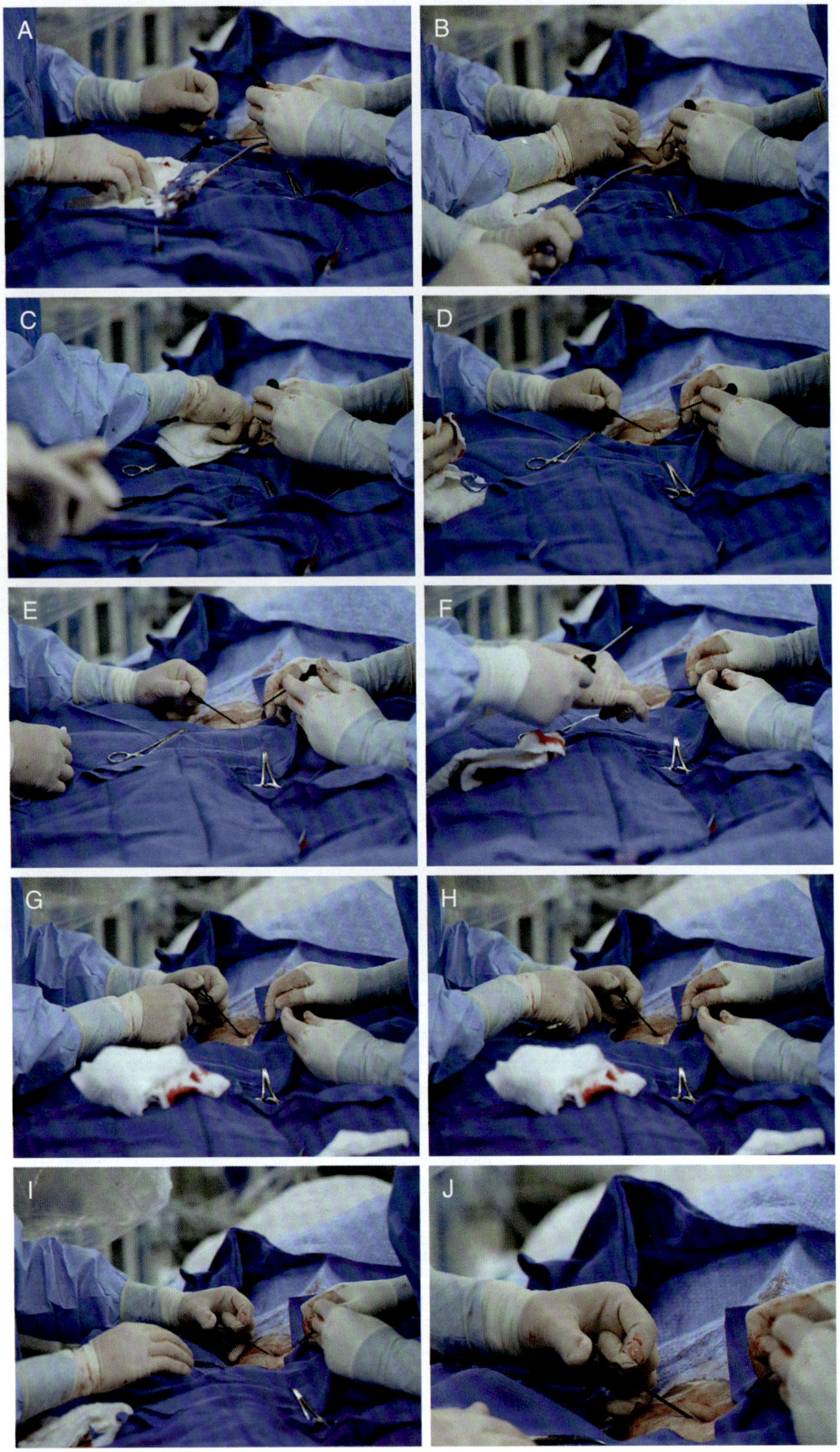

FIGURE 3.10 Final closure. After the planned intervention is completed, the sutures are secured in place to obtain hemostasis. In our laboratory, 3 operators work together. The first operator controls the suture and knot pusher, while the second and third operators remove the sheath over the wire and apply manual compression, respectively. A wire is placed through the large sheath into the aorta; we typically use a glide wire (theoretically there is less abrasion of the sutures). One person obtains proximal control of the arteriotomy by applying manual pressure as the sheath is removed over the wire. The first Perclose knot is pushed down to the femoral artery as the sheath is removed in simultaneous fashion. It is important to note that the wire is left in place leaving the option for deployment of a third Perclose or other device if hemostasis is not achieved or one of the sutures fails. The second knot is pushed down to the artery. Once hemostasis is achieved, the wire is removed and the knots are pushed down one final time before being locked and cut. Selective ileofemoral angiography is recommended postclosure **(A-J)**.

ACCESS TO THE LEFT-SIDED HEART

Owing to the growth of structural heart interventions in the mitral space, left atrial appendage exclusion, and catheter-based treatment of arrhythmias, transseptal access to the left atrium has seen resurgence (**FIGURES 3.11-3.14**).[8]

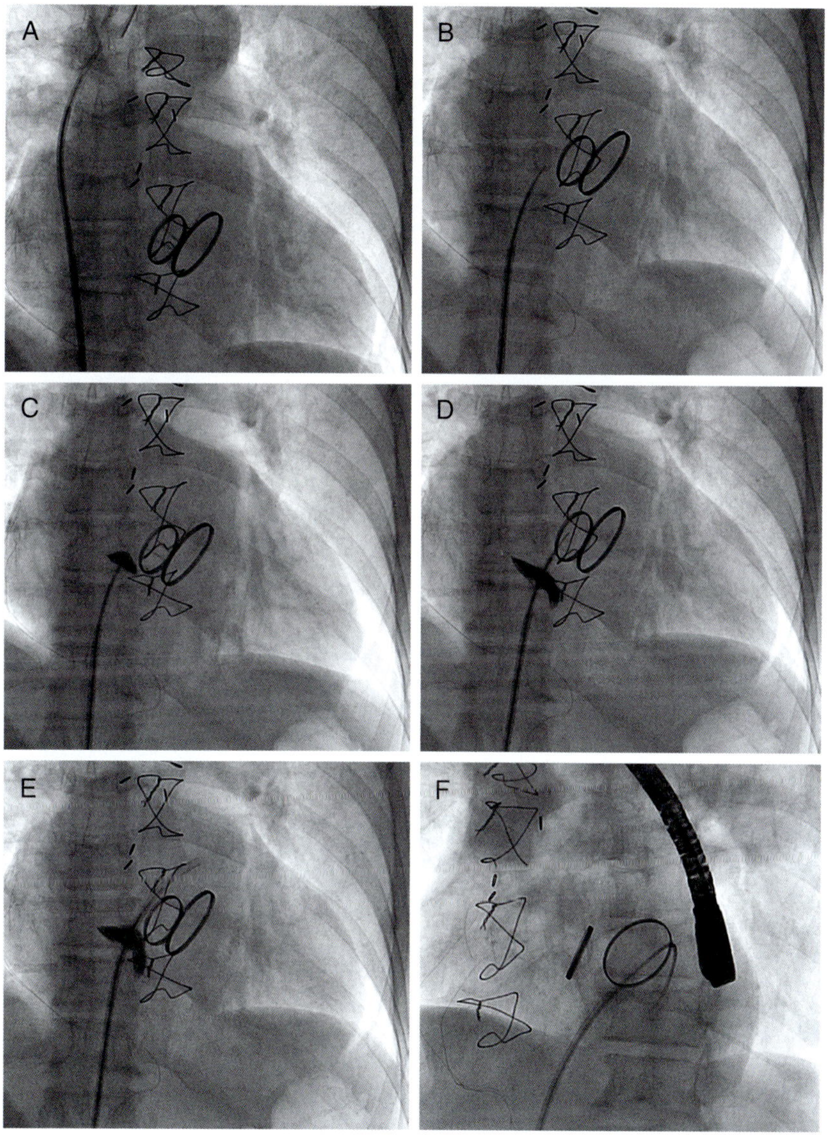

FIGURE 3.11 Transseptal puncture steps. Still frame images step by step of a transseptal puncture. **A,** Transseptal sheath, dilator, and needle in the superior vena cava in a patient with double metallic valve. **B**, Descent into the right atrium and engagement of the dilator tip into the fossa ovalis. **C**, Interatrial septum stain, tenting, and advancement of the needle into the left atrium. **D**, Needle and dilator in the left atrium across the interatrial septum. **E**, The sheath is advanced into the left atrium, and the dilator and needle are retracted into the sheath. **F**, A guide wire is advanced through the transseptal sheath to access the left ventricle. A transesophageal probe is noted posteriorly and the metallic aortic valve anteriorly.

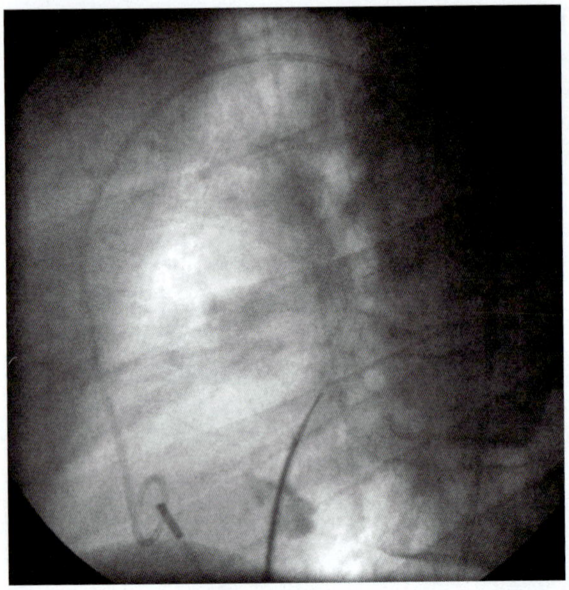

FIGURE 3.12 Still frame image of fluoroscopy in left anterior oblique projection, demonstrating transseptal needle pointing posterior toward the spine, pigtail anterior in ascending aorta, and intracardiac echo catheter in right atrium.

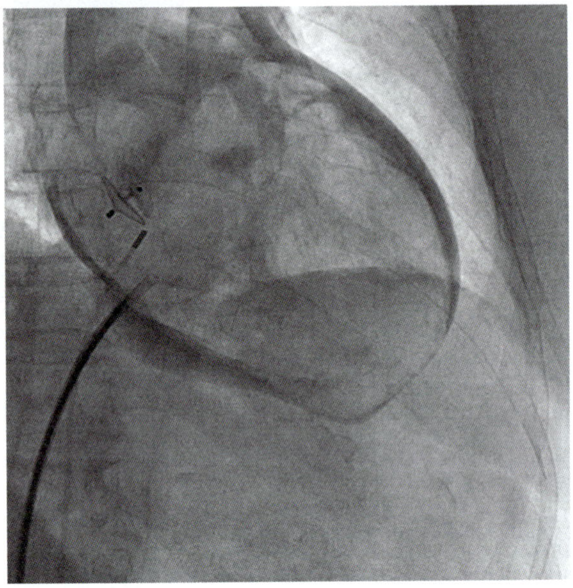

FIGURE 3.13 Pericardial effusion during transseptal puncture. Still frame image of a pericardial effusion by fluoroscopy from a transseptal sheath perforation of right atrium. Amplatzer device in right atrium; intracardiac echo catheter and transseptal sheath in right atrium. Courtesy of Dr Carlos Ruiz.

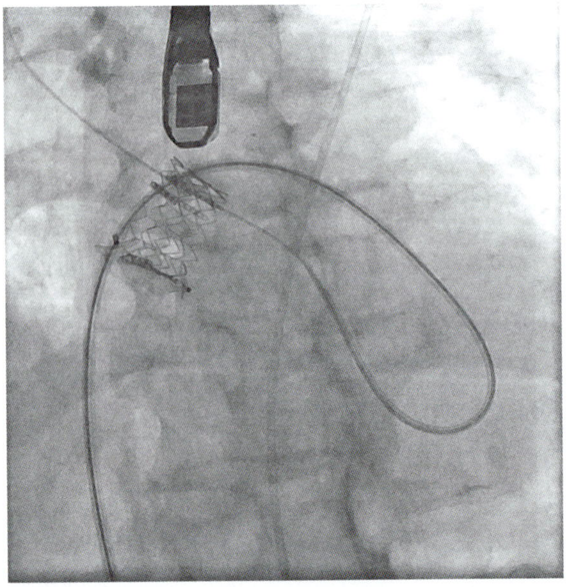

FIGURE 3.14 Transseptal access in a patient with transcatheter aortic valve. Still frame image of a transseptal access in a patient with a paravalvular leak of an Edwards Sapien transcatheter valve. The transseptal puncture was performed to obtain antegrade access to the ascending aorta via the paravalvular leak. There is an Amplatzer device occluding another paravalvular leak.

TRANSAPICAL ACCESS

While the need for direct transapical left-sided heart catheterization is today limited, there are still clinical scenarios and structural heart disease interventions that might require a direct transapical percutaneous approach (**FIGURES 3.15-3.18**).

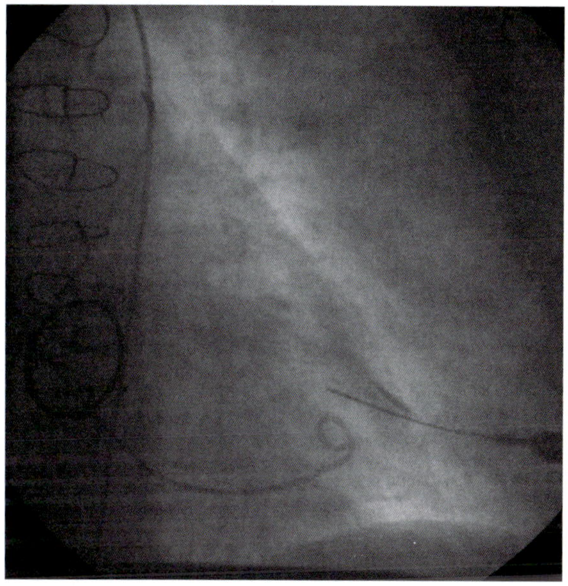

FIGURE 3.15 A pigtail has been advanced retrograde in the left ventricle and a 4 FR sheath has been advanced through a transapical approach.

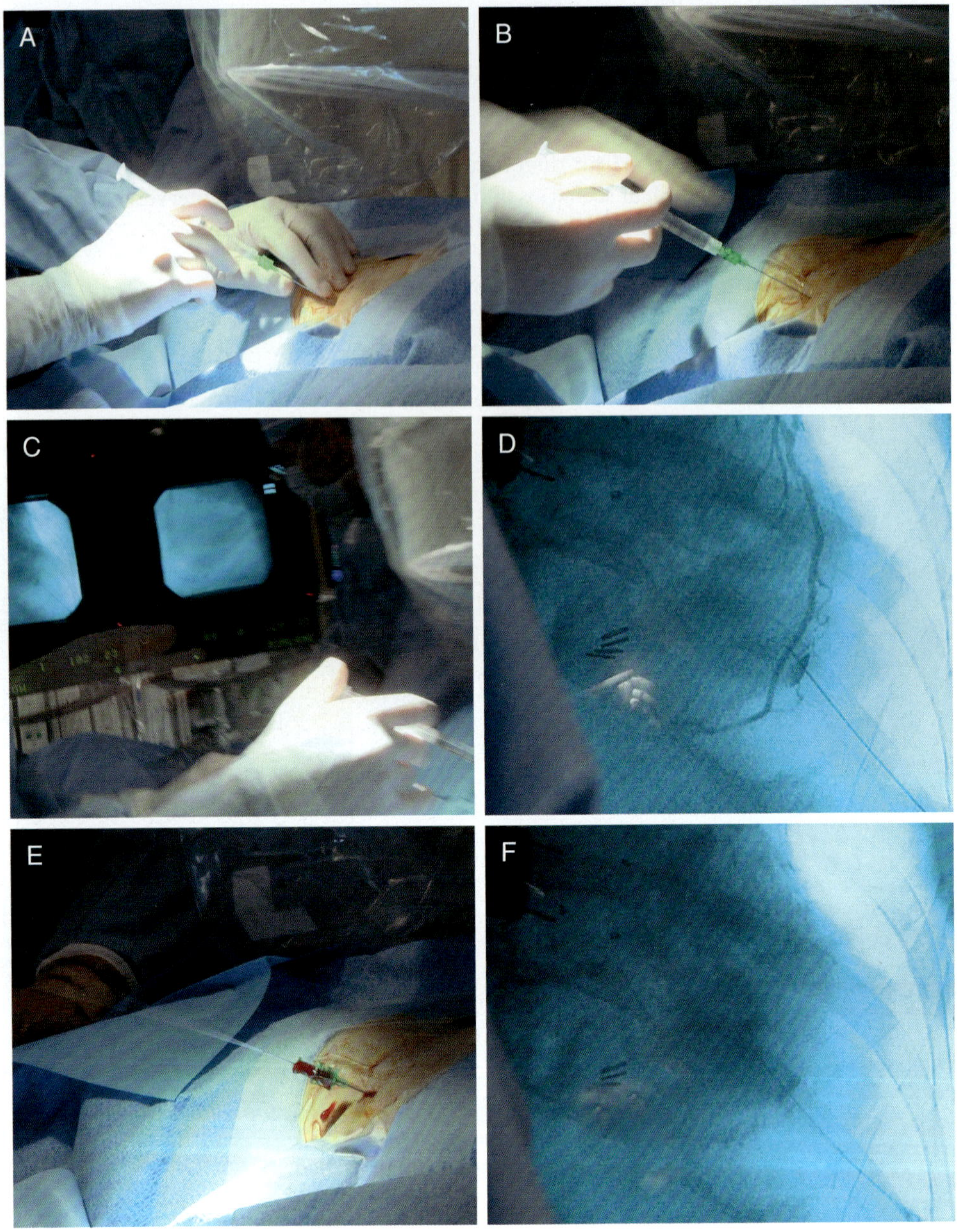

FIGURE 3.16 **A and B**, Micropuncture needle used to obtain percutaneous transapical access. **C**, Micropuncture needle with simultaneous fluoroscopic guidance. **D**, Simultaneous coronary angiography of the left anterior descending artery as the micropuncture needle is advanced in the left ventricular cavity. **E**, Micropuncture needle and wire with pulsatile movement from direct access in the left ventricular cavity. **F**, Contrast injection in the left ventricular cavity.

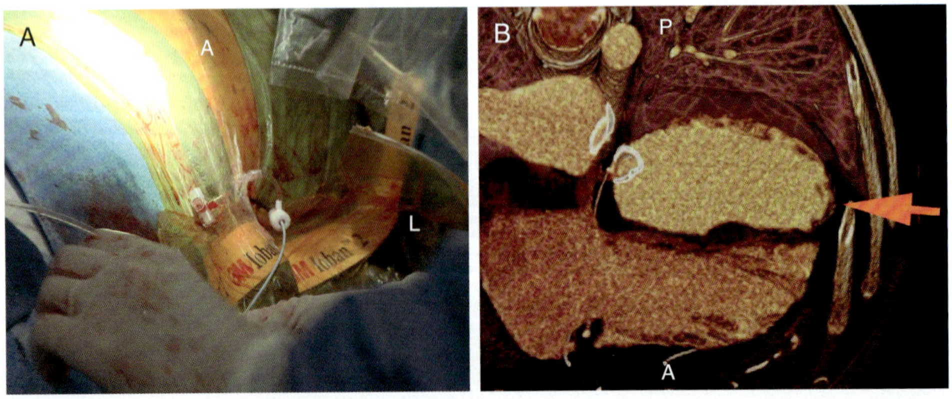

FIGURE 3.17 **A**, Still frame picture of a percutaneous transapical access in a patient with a laterally displaced left ventricle. **B**, Computed tomography image of displaced right and left ventricle laterally. A, anterior; L, lateral; P, posterior.

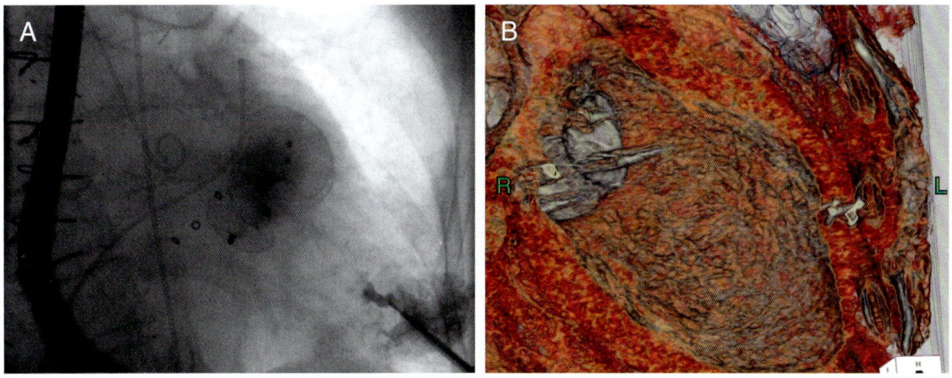

FIGURE 3.18 Percutaneous transapical access closure with a ventricular septal defect (VSD) device. **A**, Still frame fluoroscopic image of a percutaneous transapical access closure using a VSD Amplatzer device. **B**, Computed tomography image of the same patient, demonstrating anterior wall location of the VSD deployed, compared with the fluoroscopic image that suggested it was at the apex. Courtesy of Dr Carlos Ruiz.

TRANSCAVAL ACCESS

The transcaval access is a novel percutaneous vascular approach that has been introduced to allow large bore access for patients who have unfavorable transfemoral, transaortic, and transapical anatomy. So far, it has been used successfully in numerous transcatheter aortic valve replacement (TAVR) procedures (**FIGURES 3.19-3.23**).[9]

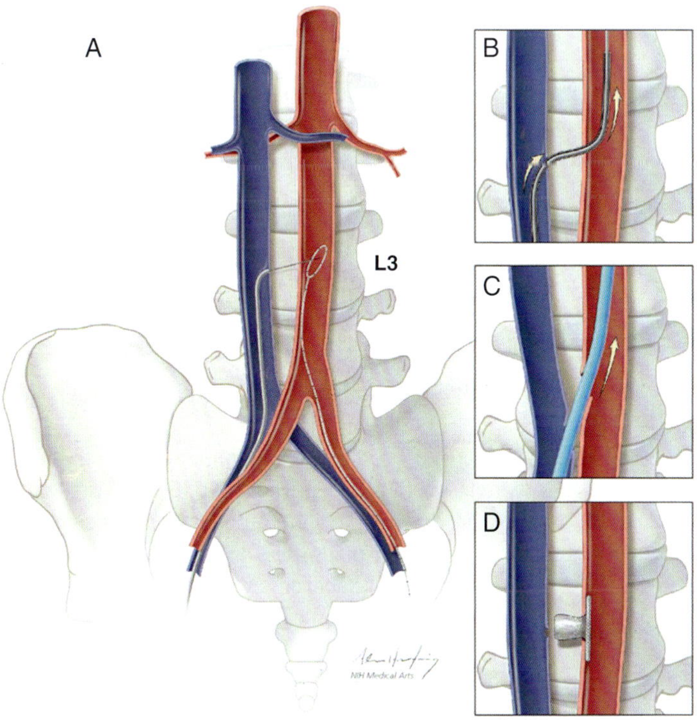

FIGURE 3.19 Transcaval access for TAVR. **A**, Transcaval access is obtained over an electrified guide wire directed from the inferior vena cava toward a snare in the abdominal aorta. **B**, After delivering a microcatheter to exchange for a stiff guide wire, **(C)** the transcatheter heart valve introducer sheath is advanced from the femoral vein into the abdominal aorta for conventional transfemoral retrograde TAVR. **D**, The aortocaval access site is closed with a nitinol cardiac occluder. Reproduced with permission from Greenbaum AB, Babaliaros VS, Chen MY, et al. Transcaval access and closure for transcatheter aortic valve replacement: a prospective investigation. *J Am Coll Cardiol*. 2017;69(5):511-521.

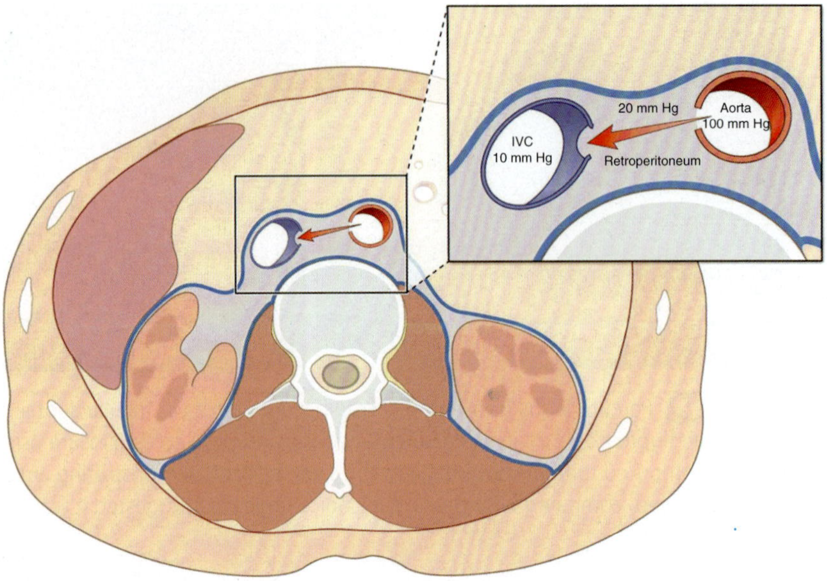

FIGURE 3.20 Proposed mechanism of hemodynamic stability after transcaval access using permeable nitinol occluder devices. Higher pressure in the relatively confined retroperitoneal space exceeds venous pressure (inset) and causes aortic blood to return to the venous circulation through a nearby hole in the inferior vena cava (IVC) (inset). The result is aortocaval fistula rather than hemodynamic collapse. Reproduced with permission from Greenbaum AB, Babaliaros VS, Chen MY, et al. Transcaval access and closure for transcatheter aortic valve replacement: a prospective investigation. *J Am Coll Cardiol*. 2017;69(5):511-521.

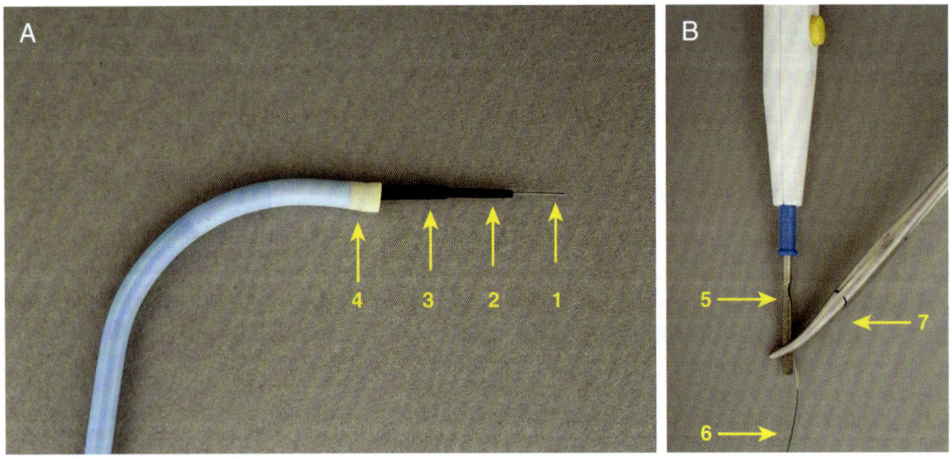

FIGURE 3.21 Crossing equipment. **A**, Coaxial crossing system consisting of (1) 0.014-inch guide wire inside of a (2) Piggyback 0.035-inch wire converter inside of a (3) braided microcatheter, inside of a (4) 55-cm guiding catheter. **B**, An electrosurgery pencil (5) is connected to the backend of the 0.014-inch guide wire (6) using a hemostatic forceps (7). Reproduced with permission from Greenbaum AB, Babaliaros VS, Chen MY, et al. Transcaval access and closure for transcatheter aortic valve replacement: a prospective investigation. *J Am Coll Cardiol*. 2017;69(5):511-521.

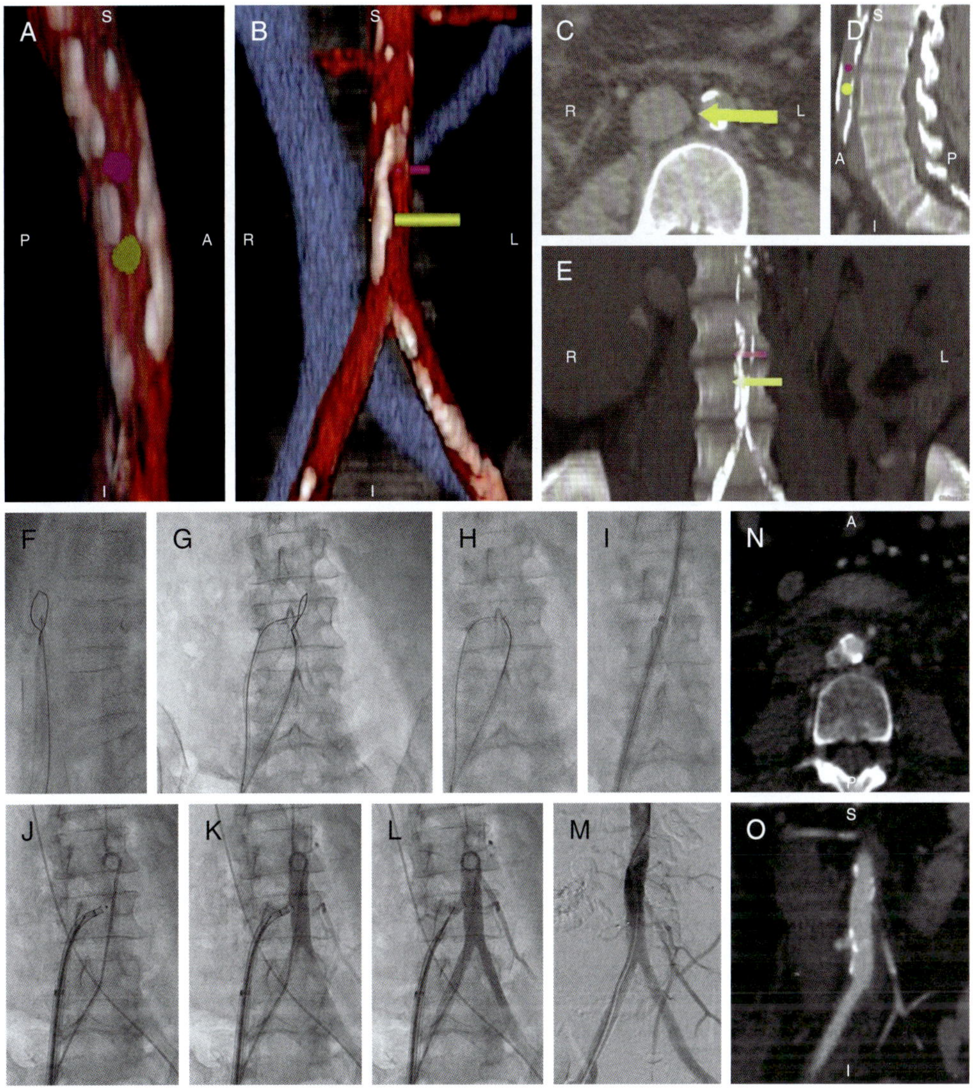

FIGURE 3.22 Representative transcaval TAVR procedure. **A-E**, A suitable target (yellow arrow) is identified on computed tomography (CT) and displaced in **(C)** axial reconstruction to show the crossing point (yellow arrow), **(D)** sagittal reconstruction to show the lumbar level, and **(E)** coronal thick-slab projection to simulate fluoroscopy. **F**, Under fluoroscopy, the transvenous crossing catheter is aligned with the aortic snare in a lateral projection; **(G)** the guide wire is electrified during advancement into the aorta and **(H)** then snared and exchanged for a stiff guide wire. **I**, The transcatheter heart valve (THV) sheath is advanced from the femoral vein into the aorta. **J-L**, After TAVR, a nitinol cardiac occluder device is positioned across the aortic wall. **M**, In this case, completion angiography shows complete occlusion of the aortocaval fistula. **N and O**, Predischarge CT shows the device in position with a small retroperitoneal hematoma and an occluded tract. An alternative target is depicted with a purple arrow. Reproduced with permission from Greenbaum AB, Babaliaros VS, Chen MY, et al. Transcaval access and closure for transcatheter aortic valve replacement: a prospective investigation. *J Am Coll Cardiol*. 2017;69(5):511-521.

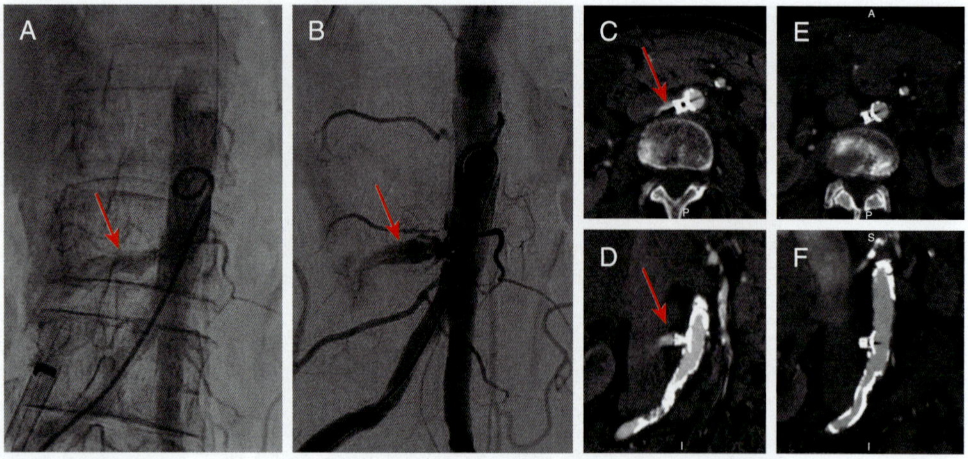

FIGURE 3.23 Unconstrained aortocaval shunt after inadvertent pull-through of a closure device. **A**, This angiogram was performed while preparing a new closure device. The blood pressure was not changed. The arrow points to the unrepaired aortocaval fistula. **B**, A fistula persists on the completion angiogram after a closure device was implanted. **C and D**, On predischarge computed tomography, there is no retroperitoneal hematoma, and the fistula is reduced but persistent. **E and F**, It is occluded on follow-up computed tomography. Reproduced with permission from Greenbaum AB, Babaliaros VS, Chen MY, et al. Transcaval access and closure for transcatheter aortic valve replacement: a prospective investigation. *J Am Coll Cardiol*. 2017;69(5):511-521.

REFERENCES

1. Mylotte D, Sudre A, Teiger E, et al. Transcarotid transcatheter aortic valve replacement. *J Am Coll Cardiol Intv*. 2016;9:472-480.
2. Applegate RJ, Sacrinty MT, Kutcher MA, et al. Trends in vascular complications after diagnostic cardiac catheterization and percutaneous coronary intervention via the femoral artery, 1998 to 2007. *J Am Coll Cardiol Intv*. 2008;1:317-326.
3. Gruentzig A. Transluminal dilatation of coronary-artery stenosis. *Lancet*. 1978;1:263.
4. Feldman DN, Swaminathan RV, Kaltenbach LA, et al. Adoption of radial access and comparison of outcomes to femoral access in percutaneous coronary intervention. *Circulation*. 2013;127:2295-2306.
5. Chandrasekhar J, Hibbert B, Ruel M, et al. Transfemoral vs non-transfemoral access for transcatheter aortic valve implantation: a systematic review and meta-analysis. *Can J Cardiol*. 2015;31(12):1427-1438.
6. Sherev DA, Shaw RE, Brent BN. Angiographic predictors of femoral access site complications: implication for planned percutaneous coronary intervention. *Catheter Cardiovasc Interv*. 2005;65(2):196-202.
7. Dyal M. TCT-410 arteriotomy location guided by fluoroscopy plus real-time ultrasound: in defense of the femoral approach. *J Am Coll Cardiol, suppl. S*. 2012;60(17):B117.
8. Ren JF, Marchlinski FE. Training methodology for transseptal catheterization should incorporate difficult anatomic conditions and the use of intracardiac echocardiographic imaging. *J Am Coll Cardiol*. 2012;59:291-292.
9. Greenbaum AB, Babaliaros VC, Chen MY, et al. Transcaval access and closure for transcatheter aortic valve replacement: a prospective investigation. *J Am Coll Cardiol*. 2017;69(5):511-521.

chapter **4**

Radial Artery Approach

CARLOS ENRIQUE ALFONSO, MD, TEJAS PATEL, MD, DM, FACC, FSCAI, FESC , and MAURICIO G. COHEN, MD, FACC, FSCAI

INTRODUCTION

Transradial access (TRA) for cardiac catheterization, angiography, and intervention has well-documented advantages over the transfemoral approach.[1] Mastering TRA requires the development of complementary skills including precise radial artery puncture, prevention and management of radial artery spasm, a thorough understanding of the vascular anatomy of the arm and associated variants, catheter manipulation for selective coronary cannulation, and maximization of support during percutaneous coronary interventions (PCI).[2] In this chapter, we will review unique aspects of TRA. We will also provide tips-and-tricks on how to manage common and not-so-common difficulties encountered during TRA.

CATHETERIZATION LABORATORY SETUP, PATIENT EVALUATION, AND PREPARATION

A dedicated radial catheterization laboratory requires a team effort. Education of the catheterization laboratory staff is critical to ensure that every staff member is well versed in procedural requirements. The procedure setup is relatively simple. Use of an arm board is helpful to enhance patient's comfort and to facilitate the task of the physician performing the procedure (**FIGURE 4.1**). Previously, tests to evaluate the hand collateral circulation such as the Allen test and modified Barbeau test were suggested before TRA[3] (**FIGURE 4.2**). However, given the extensive collateral circulation, the low rate of radial artery occlusion (RAO), and the extremely rare incidence of ischemic complications, TRA catheterization can be safely performed even in borderline cases, and these tests are no longer considered necessary.[4] While the right radial artery ergonomically works best with the configuration of most catheterization laboratories (**FIGURE 4.3**), the setup for left TRA is just as easy (**FIGURE 4.4**). Left TRA is the preferred approach in various circumstances including the following: (1) the presence of a left internal mammary graft; (2) elderly, short, or female patients in whom tortuous anatomy is anticipated; and (3) the need for lower extremity angiography or intervention, especially in taller patients, because it is shorter and straighter to reach the lower extremity circulation.[11]

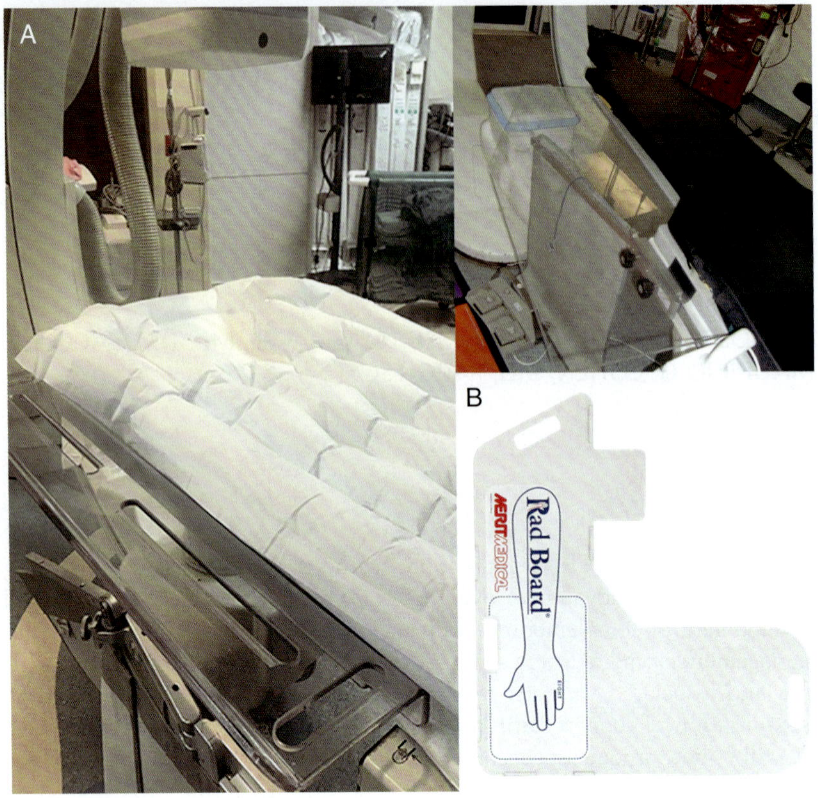

FIGURE 4.1 Catheterization laboratory setup and patient preparation. **A**, Arm board. Arm boards are designed to keep the arm in a relaxed and comfortable position, while also providing the operator with an extension of the working space. **B**, Equipment and hardware. Equipment for TRA includes dedicated sheaths and guide wires. Various hydrophilic sheaths are available for TRA access.

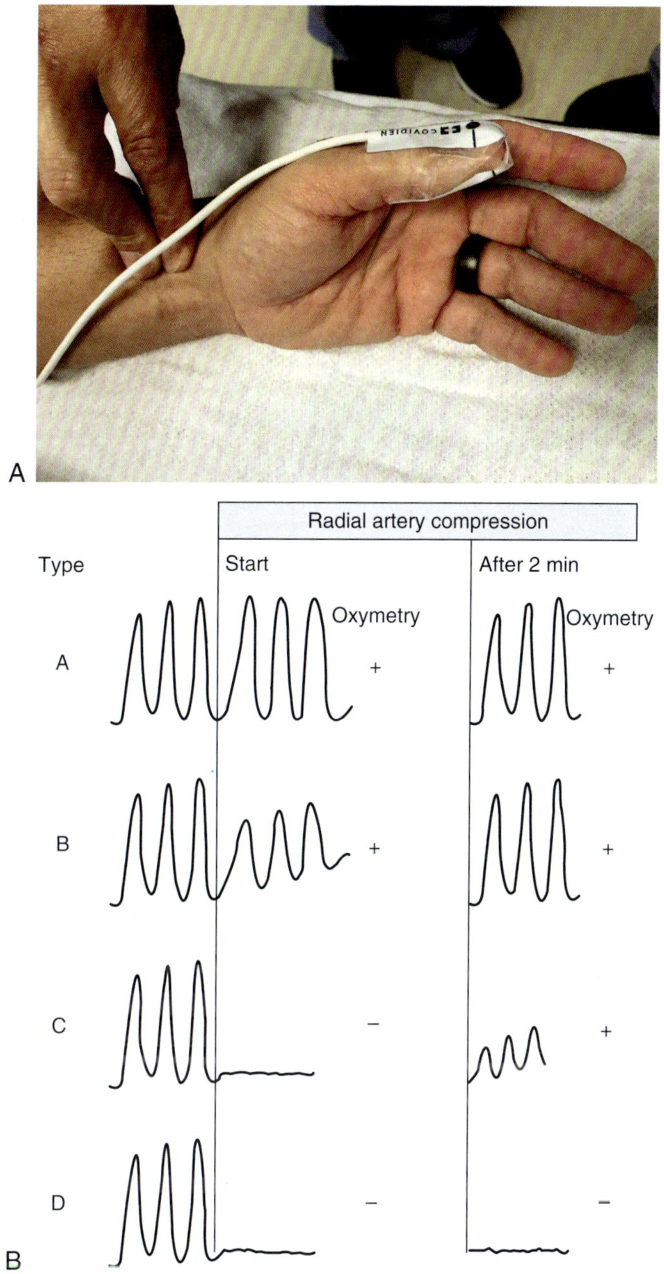

FIGURE 4.2 Patient evaluation—modified Allen test (MAT) and modified Barbeau. **A**, The MAT has been suggested to evaluate patent hand collateral circulation.[5] The MAT measures the time needed for maximal palmar blush after release of the ulnar artery compression with occlusive pressure of the radial artery. **B**, The Barbeau test evaluates the patency of the hand collateral arteries with combined plethysmography (PL) and pulse oximetry (OX). PL readings during radial artery compression are divided into 4 types: A, no damping; B, slight damping of pulse tracing; C, loss followed by recovery; and D, no recovery of pulse tracing within 2 min. The type D response is excluded from radial access, and it is found in a minority (1.5%) of patients. Preprocedural ultrasound evaluation of the diameter of the radial and ulnar arteries is useful to anticipate difficulties, especially in patients who may need complex intervention requiring 7F access. In certain circumstances the ulnar artery is larger and may be preferred over the radial artery for access.

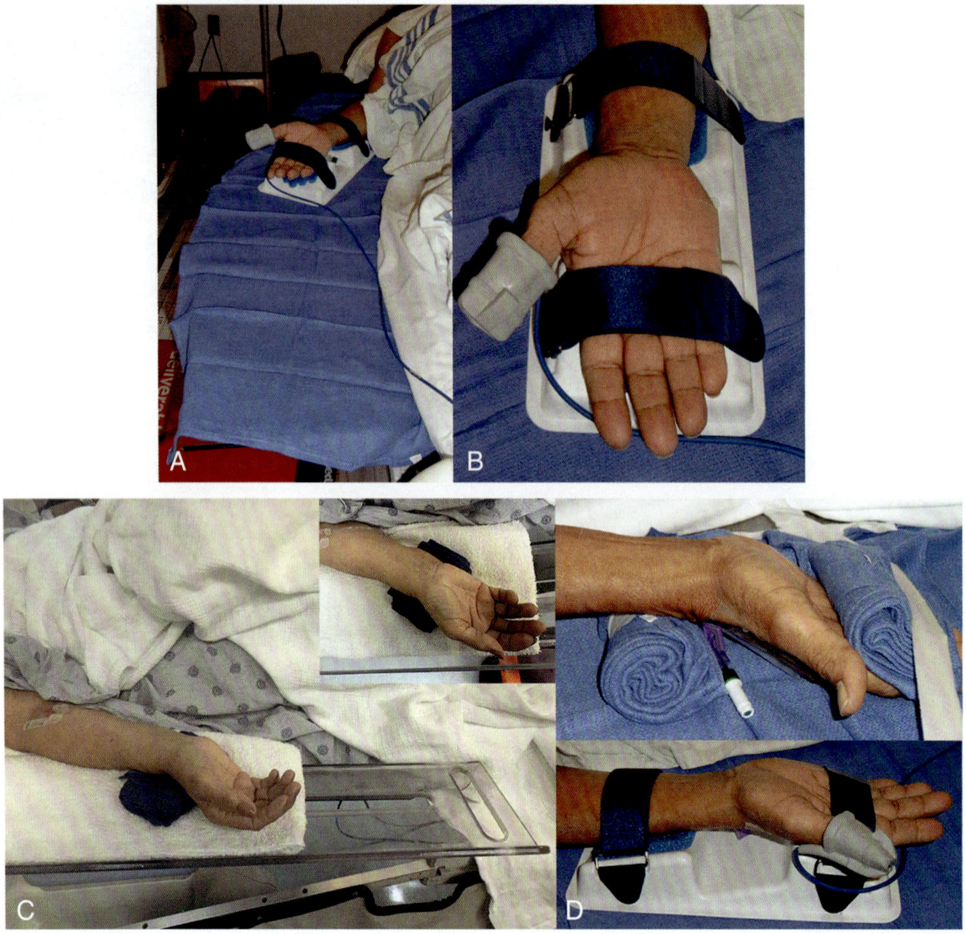

FIGURE 4.3 Right radial artery setup. An ergonomically efficient TRA setup in the catheterization laboratory includes the use of an arm board, positioning the arm, use of the board to maintain position of the wrist, and a pulse oximeter placed on the thumb to monitor OX throughout case (**A and B**). Preparation requires comfortably positioning the arm, hyperextension of the wrist, and use of towels placed directly under the dorsum of the everted and hyperextended wrist (**C**). Alternatively, a dedicated TRA wrist support can be used to hyperextend the wrist (**D**).

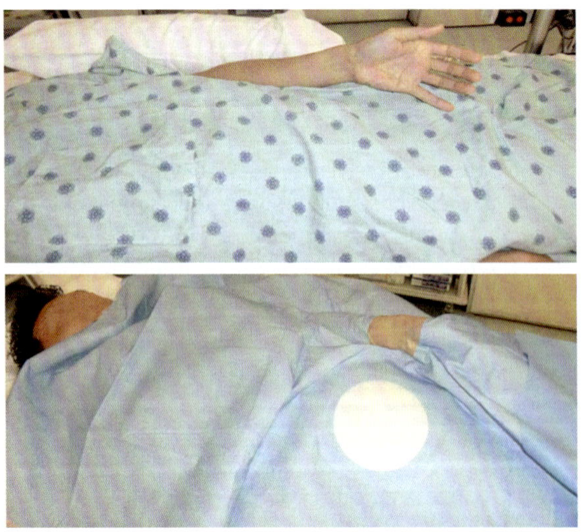

FIGURE 4.4 Left radial artery access setup. During Left TRA, the left forearm can be brought over the midline and placed on top of the left groin

ARTERIAL ACCESS

It is important to understand the vascular anatomy of the wrist, arm, and forearm (**FIGURE 4.5**). The radial artery lies between the tendons of the brachioradialis and flexor carpi radialis over the prominence of the radius. The artery can be accessed with either an anterior wall puncture or a through-and-through back wall puncture (**FIGURE 4.6**). Vascular ultrasound can be helpful[6] (**FIGURE 4.7**), and alternatively, ulnar access (**FIGURE 4.8**) and radial artery access in the anatomic snuffbox have been recently described (**FIGURE 4.9**). This last approach is particularly convenient for left TRA.

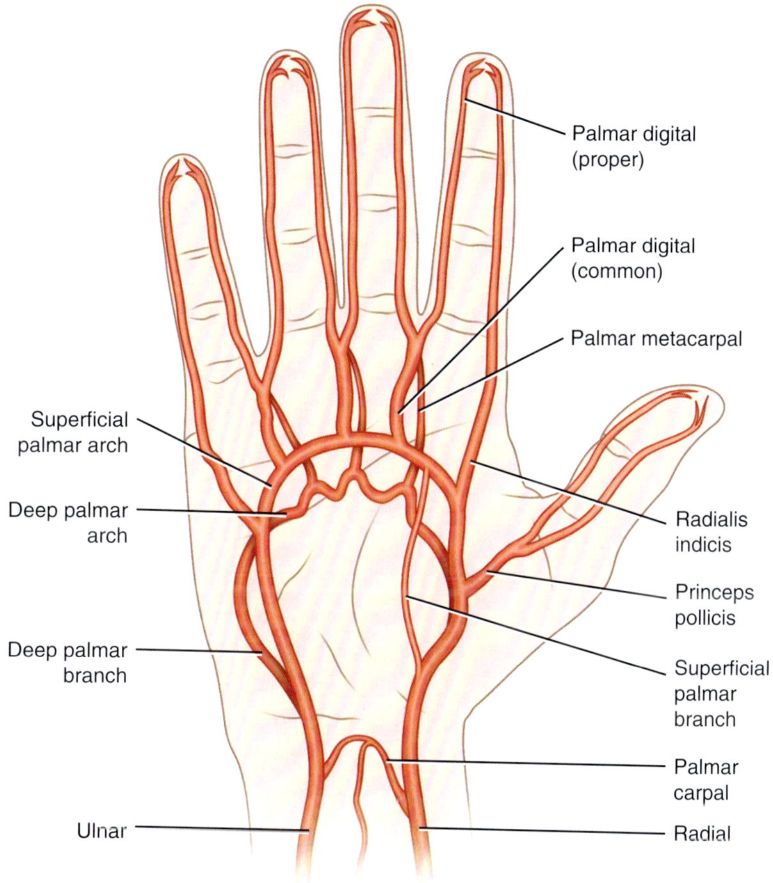

FIGURE 4.5 Arterial circulation of the wrist and hand. The radial and ulnar artery normally supply the hand via the palmar arch.

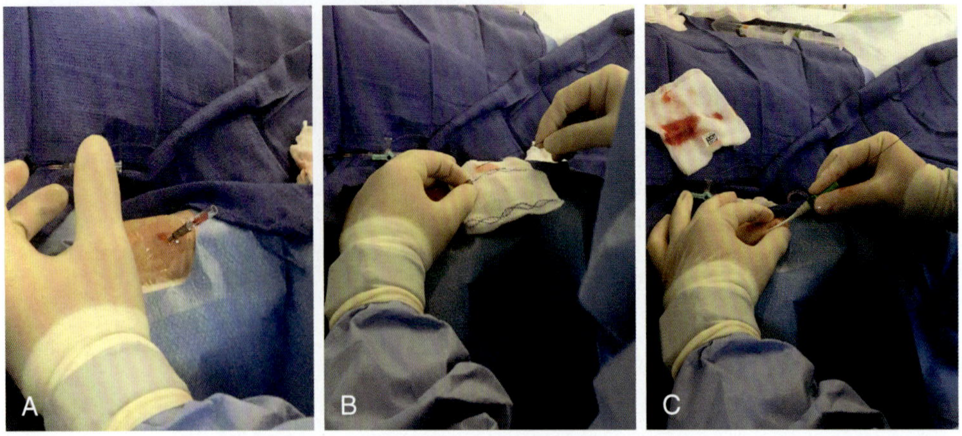

FIGURE 4.6 Radial artery puncture technique. The ideal puncture site is 2-3 cm, proximal to the flexor retinaculum. A small amount of lidocaine is given (1 mL) using a 25-gauge needle. The radial pulse is palpated with the index and middle fingers of the operator left hand. The needle or angiocatheter is advanced along the pulsations at an angle of 30 to 45°. Once backflow is obtained, the needle is advanced further to puncture the posterior wall (**A**). The needle is removed, and the cannula is slowly pulled back at an angle of 10-20° until free backflow of blood is observed indicating intraluminal position. At this point the guide wire is inserted and advanced into the radial artery, ensuring that it is free and not pushing against resistance (**B**). Once the guide wire has been sufficiently advanced, the arterial sheath can be introduced keeping it lubricated with saline solution while advancing at a shallow angle (**C**). A vasodilator cocktail is administered through the side port of the arterial sheath. Mixing the vasodilator cocktail with blood by aspirating and then pushing forward through the syringe can decrease burning sensation in the patient's forearm. A transparent film dressing (ie, Tegaderm) can be placed over the sheath to secure it in place.

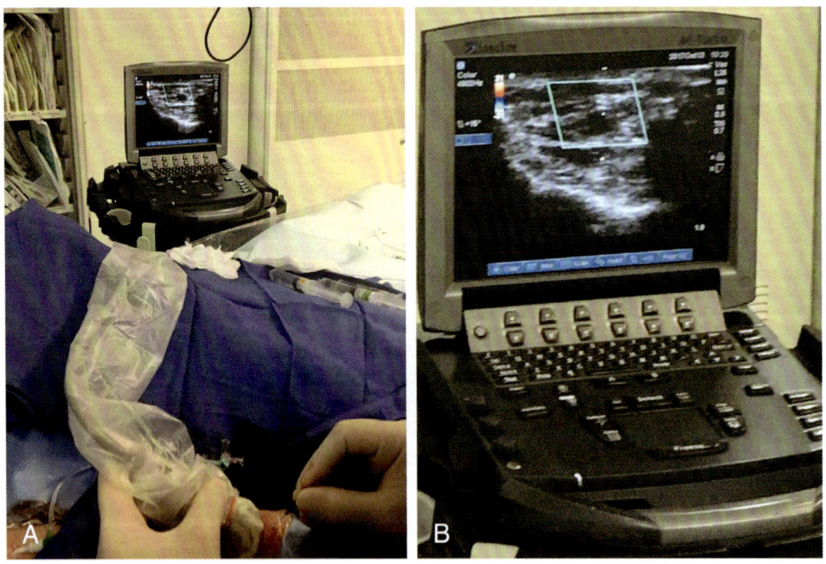

FIGURE 4.7 Vascular ultrasound to guide radial artery access.[6] Ultrasound guidance can facilitate TRA and ulnar access. If ultrasound is used, the artery is positioned immediately below the transducer (**A**) and the depth is minimized, and while color Doppler can be used to confirm identification of the artery (**B**), the arterial puncture should be done under regular ultrasound guidance, which maximizes the quality of the image.

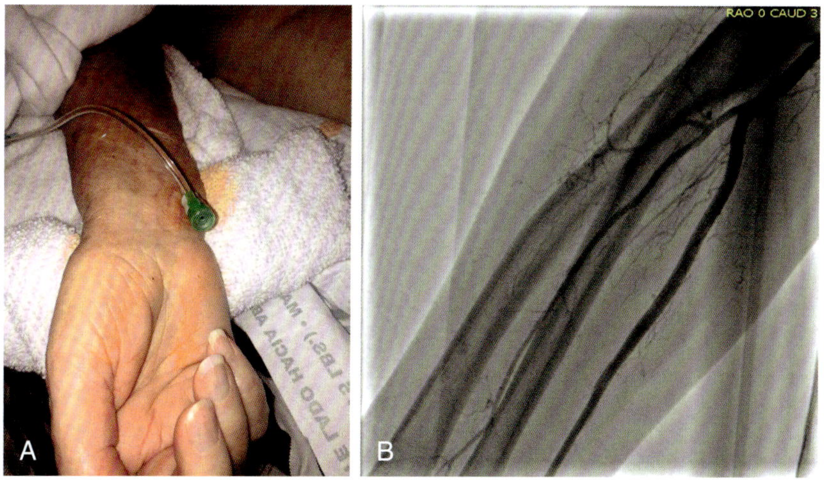

FIGURE 4.8 Ulnar artery access. Ulnar artery access may be used in cases of radial access failure owing to small or absent radials (**A and B**). The ulnar artery is actually larger than the radial artery, and the success rate with this access is greater than 90%. Methods for obtaining access, complications, and postprocedure management are similar to radial access.[15] Patent hemostasis is obtained using a hemostasis band, which can be placed in an opposite direction on the wrist and centered on the ulnar artery.

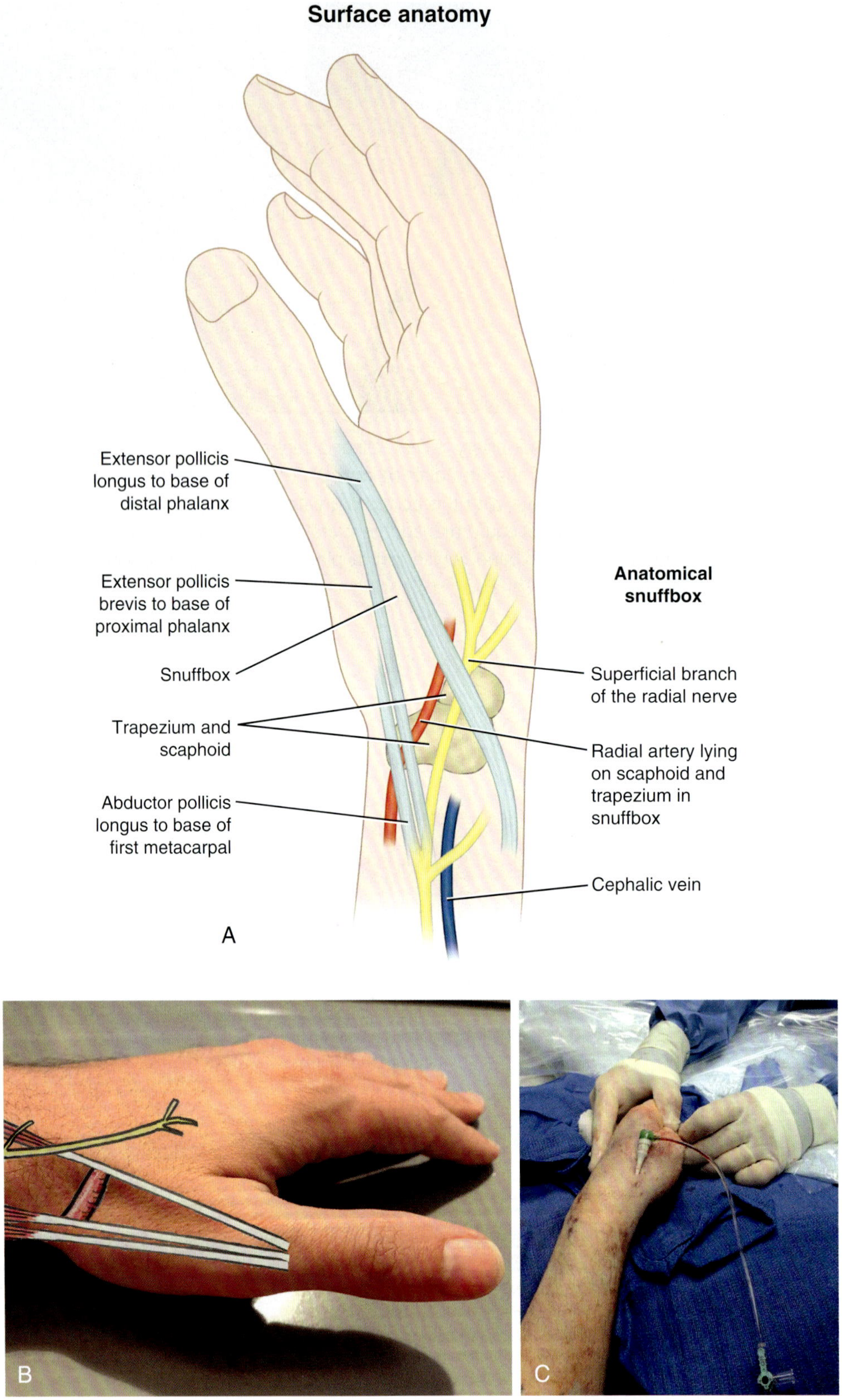

FIGURE 4.9 Dorsal radial artery "snuffbox" access. Radial artery access can also be obtained on the dorsal aspect of the hand in the anatomical "snuffbox," which is defined by the extensor pollicis longus tendon on the medial (ulnar) border and the tendons of the extensor pollicis brevis and the abductor pollicis longus on the lateral (radial) border (**A-C**). Snuffbox access can facilitate natural positioning of the wrist, particularly for left radial artery access cases. Hemostasis in snuffbox access can be obtained by using a pressure dressing (a 4 × 4 gauze firmly applied, then wrapped) (**D**) or standard hemostatic bands (**E and F**). Courtesy of Giselle Baquero, MD.

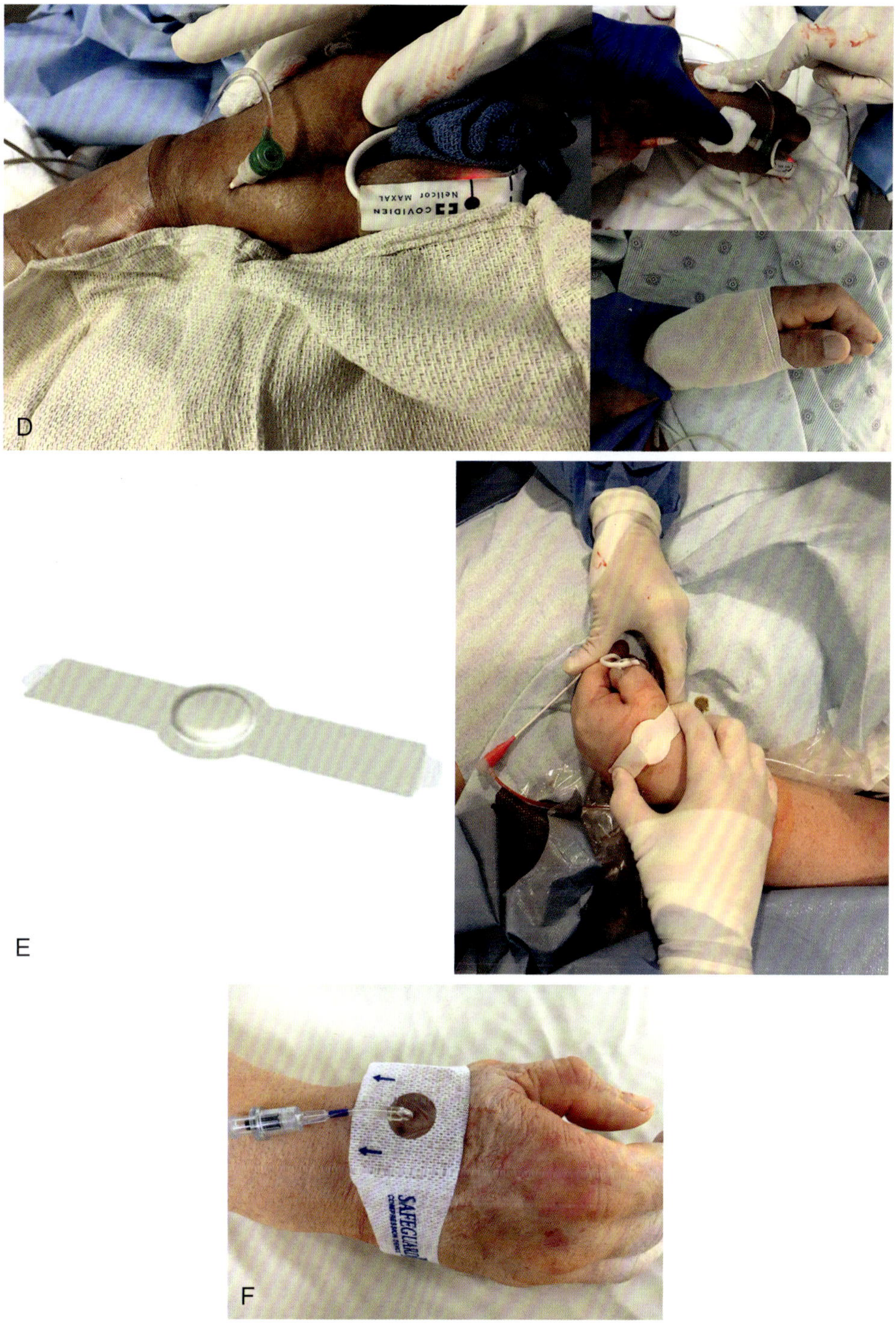

FIGURE 4.9 (Continued)

RIGHT-SIDED HEART CATHETERIZATION

Right-sided heart catheterization can be performed via the arm veins.[7-9] For certain patients, this may be the preferred approach. The bleeding risk is minimized for patients that are coagulopathic, such as end-stage liver disease patients, and the brachial vein access for right-sided heart catheterization can also overcome the need to halt anticoagulation, as the venous system is easily compressible in the antecubital fossa.[10] Having the nurse place a heparin lock in the forearm, which can then be used in the catheterization laboratory to exchange for venous sheath, can save time and improves catheterization laboratory efficiency. Contraindications to brachial vein approach include obstruction to radial drainage, breast surgery, trauma, and superior vena cava (SVC) disease. Caution should be exercised in patients with prior brachial cutdown, arrhythmia devices, or no visible veins. See **FIGURES 4.10-4.12.**

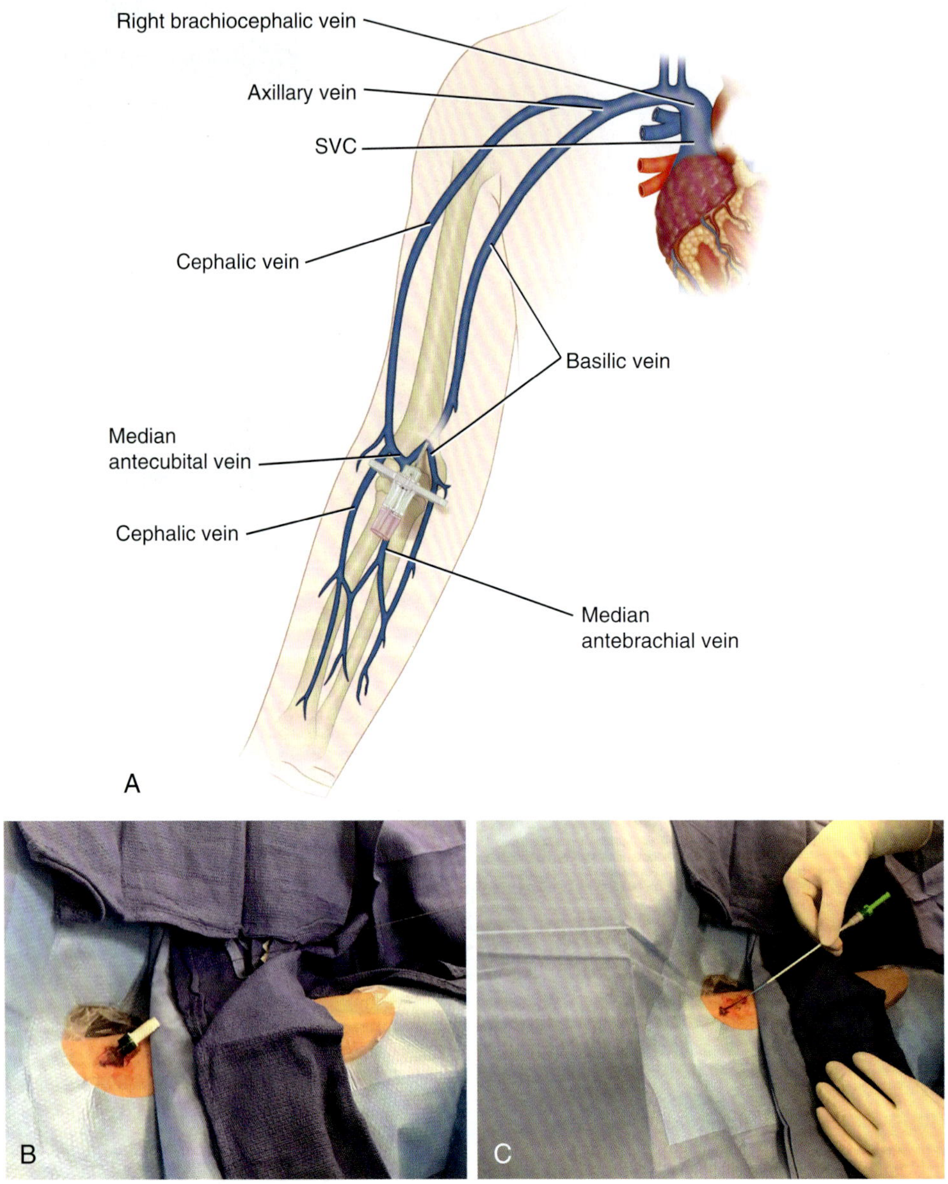

FIGURE 4.10 Right-sided heart catheterization from the brachiocephalic veins. **A**, Venous circulation of the arm. **B**, Venous access can be obtained by nurses in the preprocedural holding area, using a 20-gauge or larger lumen angiocath that is then heparin-locked. **C**, In the cardiac catheterization laboratory, the angiocath is exchanged for a venous access sheath over a wire. **D**, 5-French sheaths are typically used in the venous system with 110-120 cm balloon-tipped catheters. **E** and **F**, The catheter is advanced through the brachiocephalic vein. **G**, A 0.014" coronary guide wire can also be used to help navigate the brachiocephalic vein.

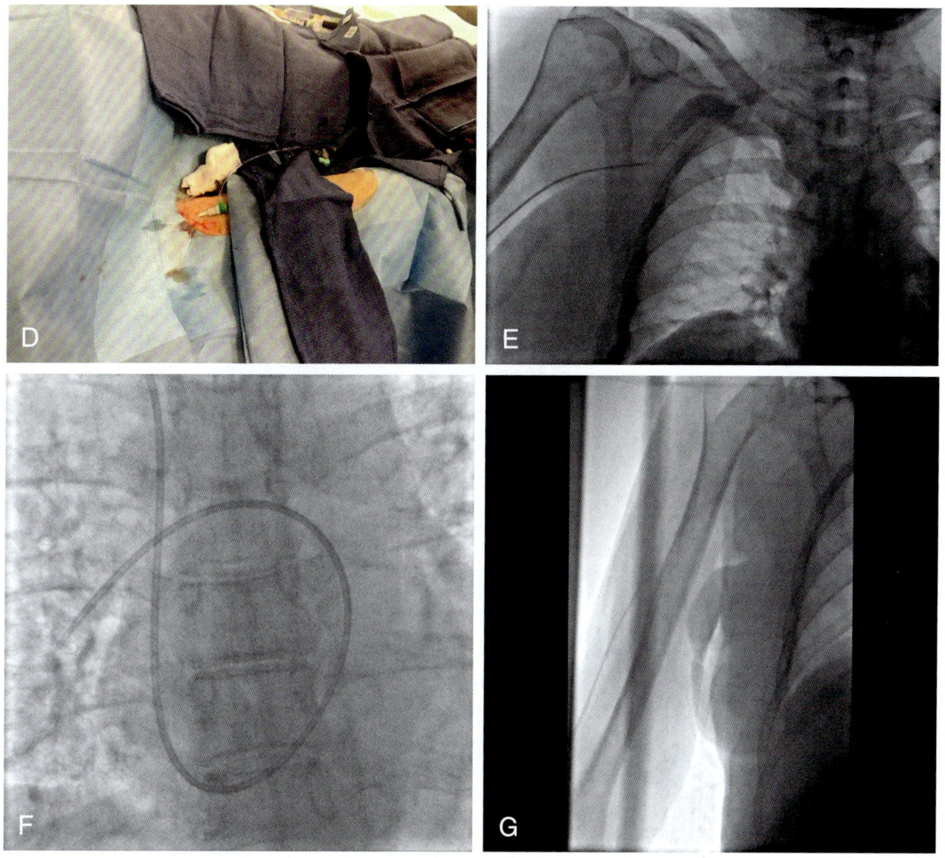

FIGURE 4.10 (Continued)

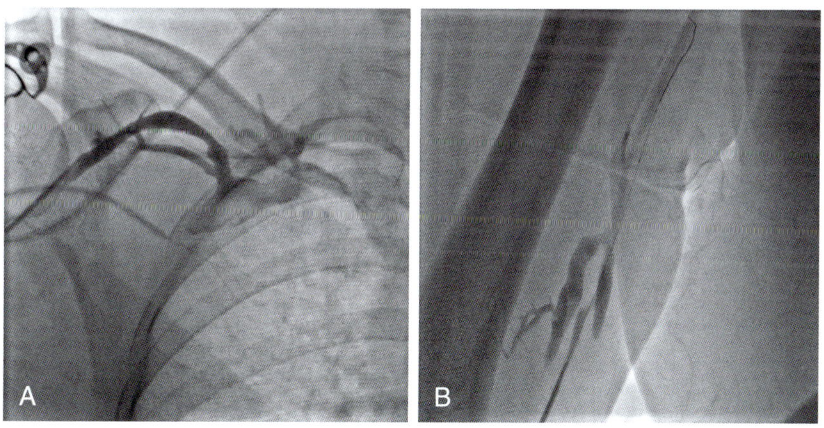

FIGURE 4.11 Antecubital venous circulation. The low-pressure antecubital venous circulation has marked anatomic variability with collaterals and redundant passages, but in general, the radial veins join either the cephalic or basilica vein whereas the medial ulnar veins continue as the basilica vein. The veins are relatively distensible, and venous spasm is rare but possible, in which case nitrates are recommended. Ideally, the operator gains access to the basilic vein medially located in the arm. However, in many occasions, the angiocath is placed in the cephalic vein. The cephalic vein joins the axillary vein at a straight angle or T-junction, which defines the start of the subclavian and central venous system (**A**). Technical issues in navigating this anatomy can be addressed by using a 0.014" coronary guide wire (**B**).

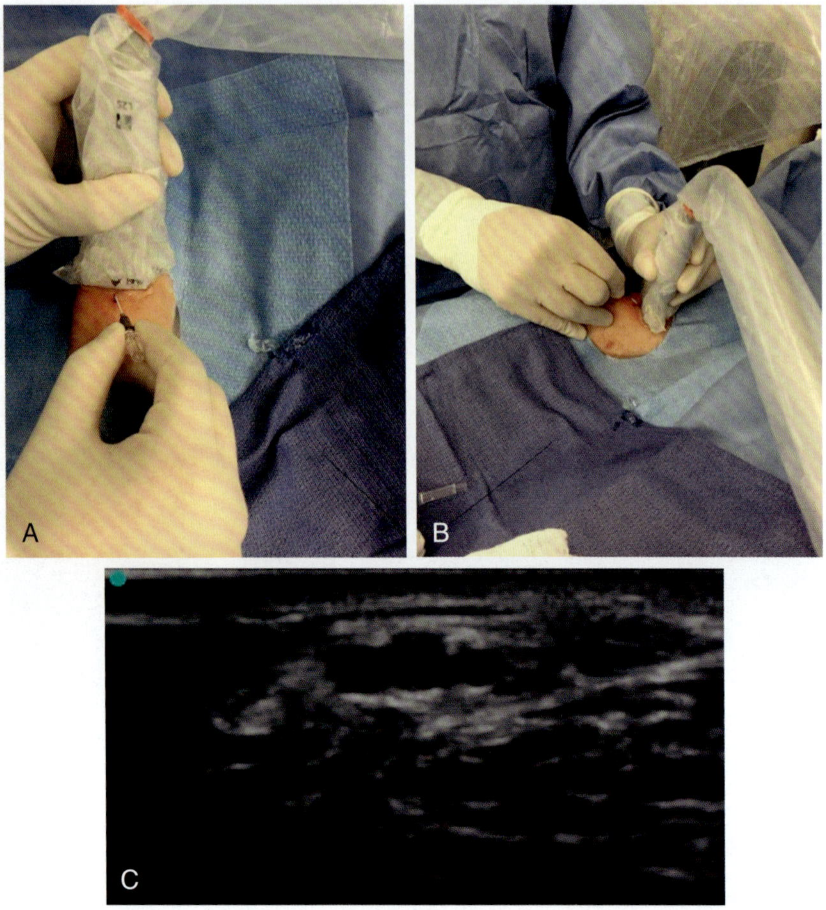

FIGURE 4.12 Ultrasound guided venous access. **A and B**, Ultrasound guidance can also facilitate venous access for antecubital approach. Ultrasound imaging can differentiate the (**C**) venous circulation from arterial circulation to avoid arterial puncture. The veins are more compressible, are thin walled, and have less pulsatile and more continuous flow by color Doppler.

Postprocedure

See FIGURE 4.13.

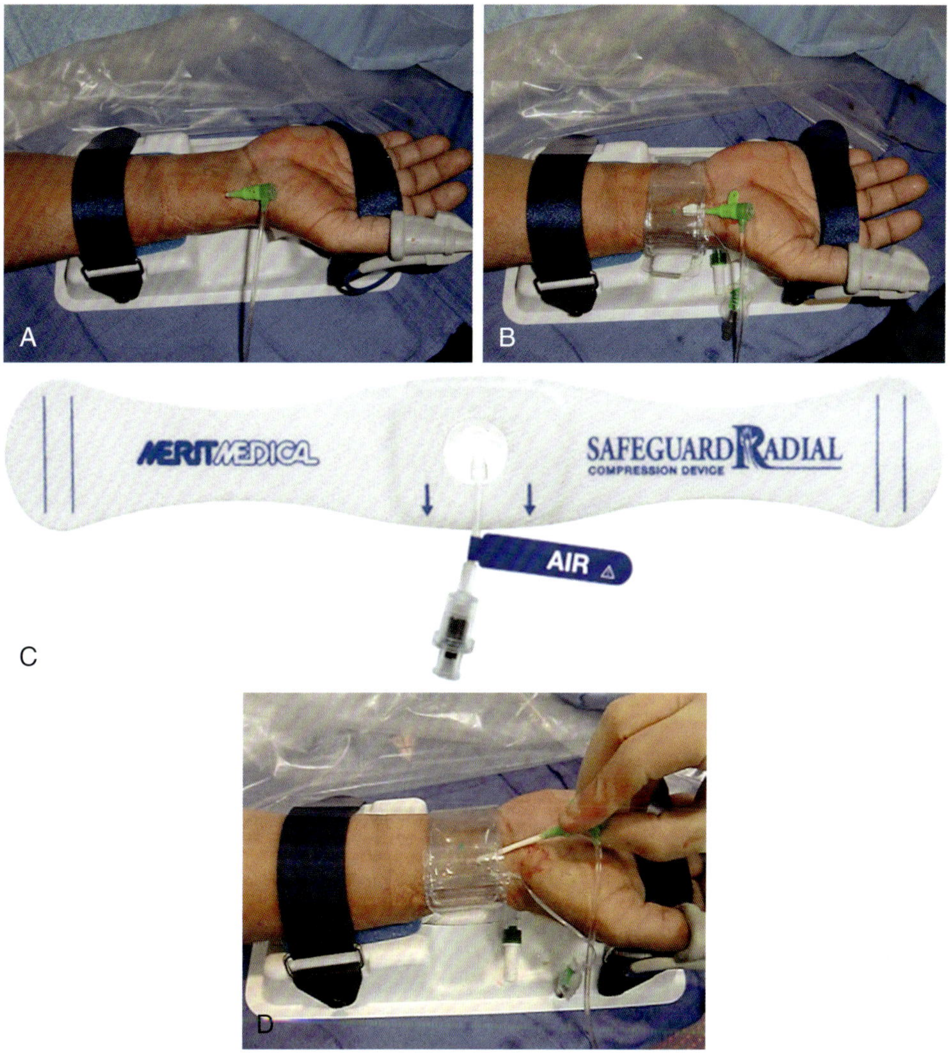

FIGURE 4.13 Sheath removal and hemostasis. Sheath removal is performed in the cardiac catheterization laboratory immediately after the procedure (**A**). Additional vasodilator cocktail can be administered for vasospasm. **B** and **C**, An air bladder hemostasis band or other similar devices can be used to compress the arterial entry site. Patent hemostasis has been demonstrated to minimize the risk of RAO.[12-14] To obtain patent hemostasis, compression is applied via the band to stop bleeding, and then the hemostatic pressure is adjusted to maintain hemostasis without complete occlusive pressure, therefore preserving radial artery patency (**D**). Radial patency is monitored every 15 min using a reverse Barbeau test with PL and OX, and the pressure device is removed after 2 h or less.

VASCULAR ANATOMY

See **FIGURES 4.14-4.16**.

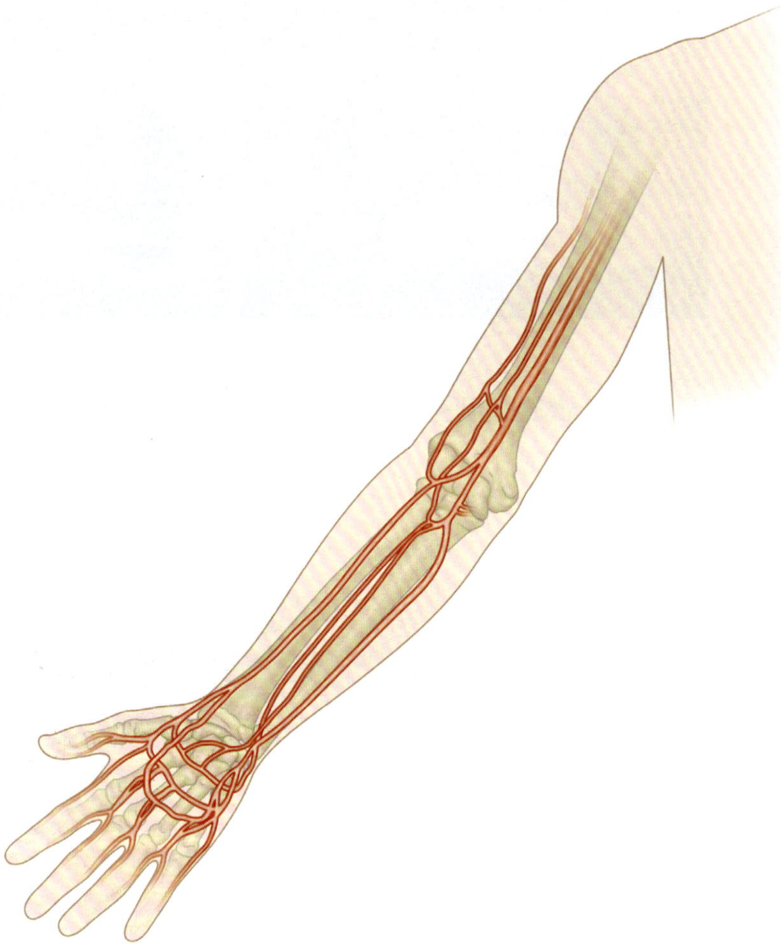

FIGURE 4.14 Anatomy of the brachial and radial arteries. Normal branching pattern of the forearm circulation in which the brachial artery branches into the radial and ulnar branches.

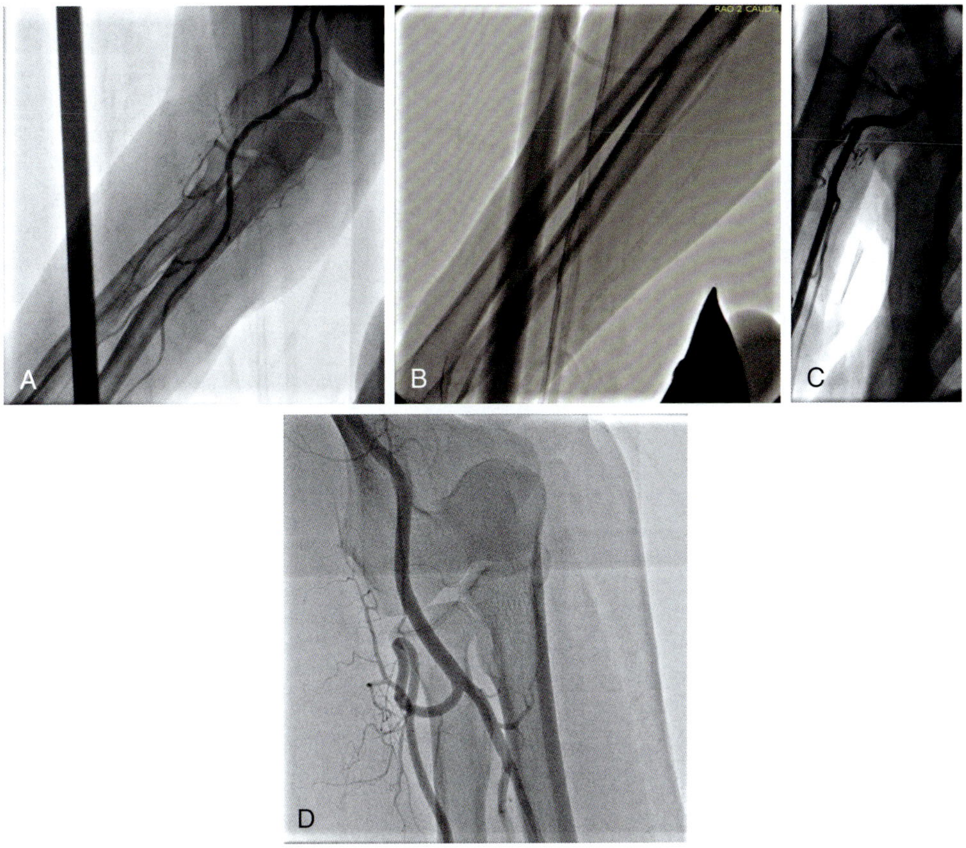

FIGURE 4.15 Difficulties with TRA. **A**, Radial artery spasm. Arterial spasm can limit the ability to perform TRA. It can be minimized with the administration of various spasmolytic cocktails including calcium channel blockers and/or nitroglycerin. In cases of refractory spasm, hot towels applied to the arm causing vasodilation, or a regional anesthesia block can be used as alternatives. **B**, Calcification and atherosclerosis. Extreme arterial calcification is occasionally noted, as in this case demonstrating Mönckeberg arteriosclerosis in the ulnar artery of a patient with end-stage renal disease. Radial anomalies remain one of the primary reasons for procedural failure and include the following[16]: (**C**) high origin of the radial artery from the brachial artery, the most commonly encountered variant which may occasionally limit TRA; (**D**) radial loops and tortuosity.

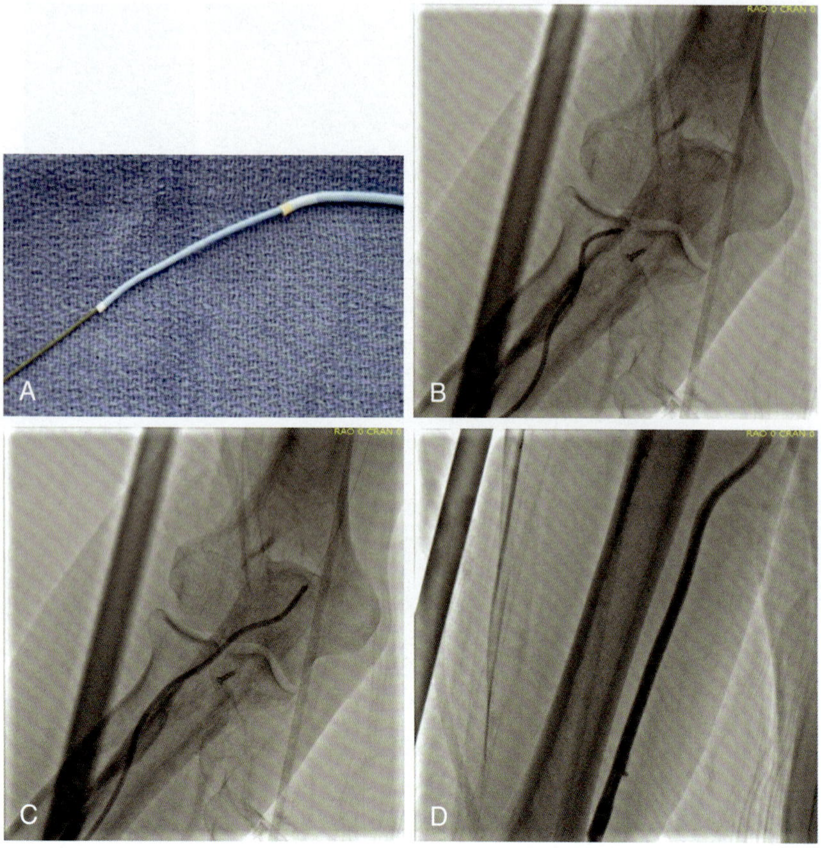

FIGURE 4.16 Techniques to navi-gate vascular anatomy. There are various techniques to overcome challenges due to unusual vascular anatomy: (**A**) the "Mother-and-Child" technique. Using a catheter within a catheter technique can facilitate passage of the equipment to the aortic arch for TRA. Shown here is a 5 Fr diagnostic catheter insider a 7 Fr guide over a 0.035" guide wire;[24] (**B-D**) alternatively, the technique of "balloon-assisted tracking of a catheter" can be used to navigate radial artery loops and tortuosity.[25] In this technique, a 0.014" floppy-tip wire is used to cross the lesion. An angioplasty balloon catheter is then inflated and extruded 4 to 5 mm outside the tip of the catheter, and the whole system is advanced as a unit. (A 1.5 mm, 2.0 mm, or 2.5 mm balloon is used for 5, 6, or 7 Fr catheters, respectively).

TRA INTERVENTIONS

TRA is feasible for the majority of interventions in the coronaries as well as peripheral vascular arteries. With the continued downsizing of equipment, the majority of interventional procedures and techniques can be accomplished through 6 Fr guide catheters. Complex coronary interventions including atherectomy, bifurcation lesion with simultaneous stent placement, vein graft interventions, and chronic total occlusions (CTO) are also feasible. See **FIGURES 4.17-4.21**.

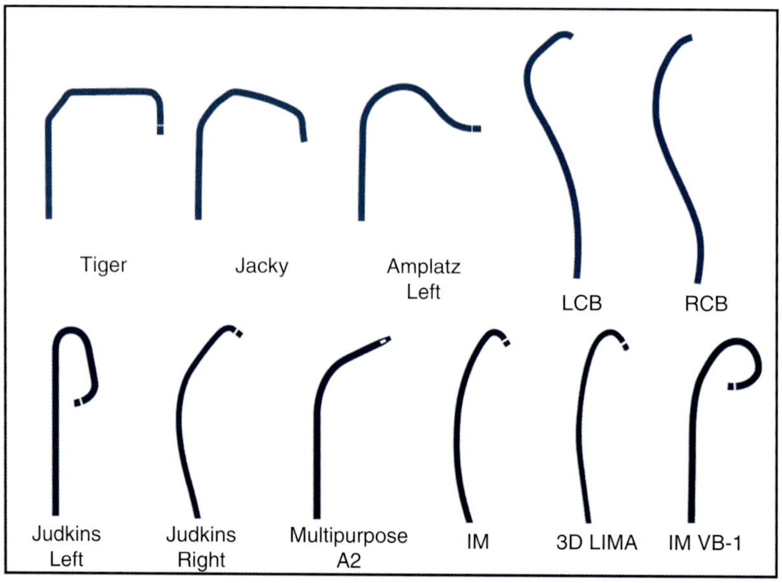

FIGURE 4.17 TRA guide catheter selection. There are various guide catheter shapes available, and the standard guide catheters work just as well for TRA interventions. For diagnostic coronary angiograms in addition to the standard curves, there are unique universal catheters, such as the Tiger and Jacky catheters, specifically dedicated for TRA, which can be used to engage both coronaries. Standard coronary guide catheters work well for coronary interventions.

FIGURE 4.18 TRA for complex coronary anatomy. **A**, This case of severe complex coronary disease illustrates that TRA is feasible for even the most complex anatomical cases. **B**, Atherectomy—rotational, orbital, and laser atherectomy are all possible via TRA using 6 Fr access. A 1.25, 1.5, and 1.75 mm burr will fit through certain 6 Fr guides. For larger rotational atherectomy burrs, the sheath can be upsized to a 7 Fr to accommodate up to a 2.0 mm burr. **C**, Bifurcations lesions can also be addressed, and standard bifurcation techniques can be used with (**D**) excellent angiographic results.

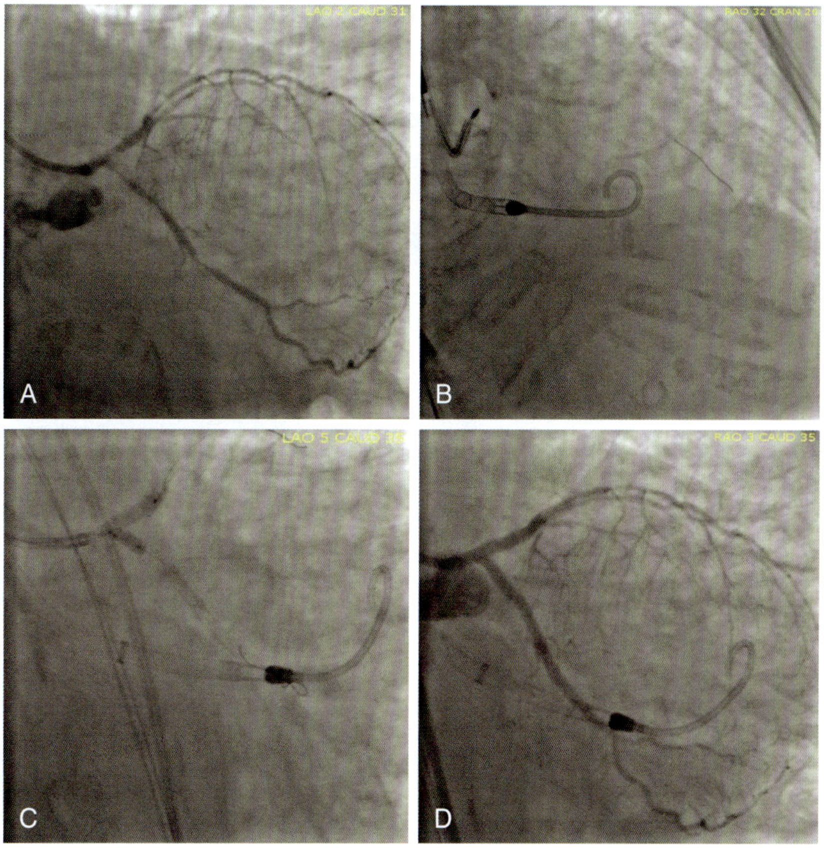

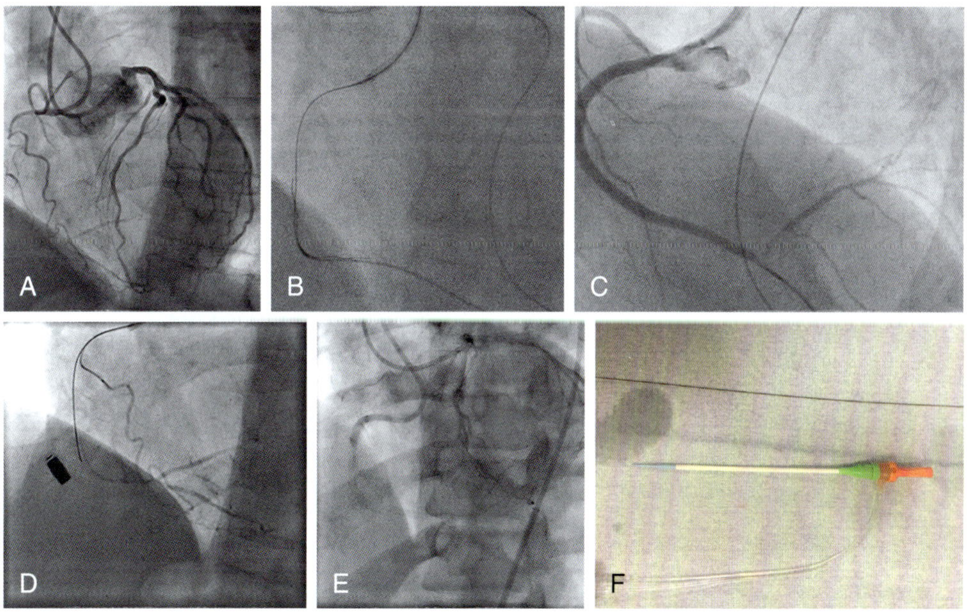

FIGURE 4.19 TRA for CTO. An increasing number of CTO interventions can be performed using a TRA approach, as in this case (**A-C**) where a bilateral radial approach was used to successfully open a long right coronary artery CTO using the "reverse controlled antegrade and retrograde subintimal tracking" technique (reverse CART) in a patient with Leriche syndrome. A minimum 7 Fr guide is usually required for CTO interventions to facilitate passage of equipment including (**D**) microcatheters for collateral imaging, dissection reentry equipment, retrograde procedures, snares, and other devices. **E**, An alternative to bilateral radial artery access is to use 1 radial and 1 femoral access point. Guide-extension devices such as the GuideLiner or Guidezilla can be used for increased support. Options for larger sheaths include using a 7 slender sheath (**F**), going sheathless, or sheathless catheters such as Eucath.

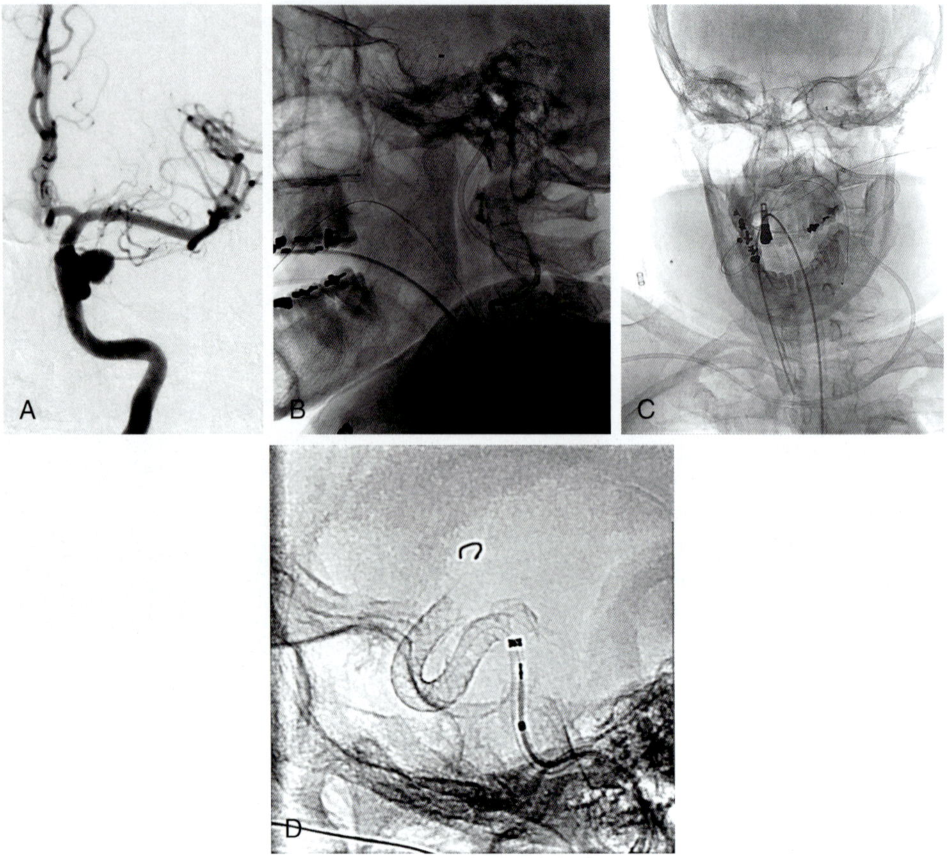

FIGURE 4.20 Cerebral interventions. TRA can be used for carotid and intracerebral interventions.[17] This figure illustrates a patient with a type 3 aortic arch and a left ophthalmic artery aneurysm (**A**). A 6 F Envoy catheter was used for placement of a flow diverting stent to embolize the intracranial arterial aneurysm (**B-D**). Courtesy of Priyank Khandelwal, MD and Dileep R. Yavagal, MD, Department of Neurosurgery, University of Miami Miller School Of Medicine.

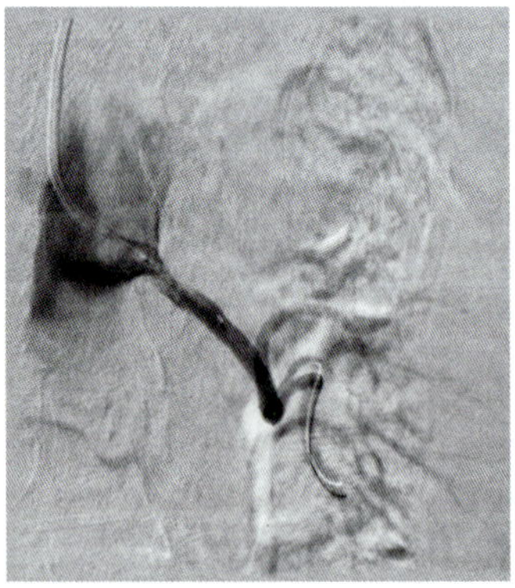

FIGURE 4.21 Peripheral interventions. TRA access can also be used for infradiaphragmatic peripheral interventions including renal artery stenosis, iliac artery lesions, and femoral interventions.[23] While femoral lesions can be treated with a TRA approach, some limitations do exist, as the deployment of a large long sheath in the descending aorta may be more difficult and cumbersome due to aortic arch curvature, subclavian and innominate tortuosity, and radial artery spasm. For more distal disease of the lower extremity, especially in taller patients, left radial access can be considered because it shortens the length and is straighter. The longest shaft length on the stents remain a limiting factor, and without longer shaft balloons, the most distal peripheral vascular disease such as below-the-knee disease is currently impossible to access via TRA.

Complications and Management

Despite an overall favorable safety profile, there are still several potential complications associated with TRA interventions. The majority of complications is not specific to TRA and is a risk of any cardiac catheterization procedure. Of note, there is no difference in the risk of cerebrovascular accident (CVA) with TRA compared with femoral cardiac catheterization. RAO is a complication specific to the TRA approach. It can occur in 5% to 10% of cases, and it usually manifests as a loss of the radial pulse. It can be confirmed by ultrasound, it is usually asymptomatic, and it often resolves over time within 1 to 2 months. The risk of RAO can be minimized with the administration of routine anticoagulation, using patent hemostasis technique, avoiding prolonged compression time (>2 hours) and using catheters with a diameter less than the radial artery. Bleeding complications can be reduced by using a weight-adjusted anticoagulation strategy of 50 U/kg to a max of 5000 U of heparin as supported by the adjusted weight anticoagulation for radial approach in elective coronarography (AWARE) trial. Hand ischemia is extremely rare, and it is more commonly due to brachial artery injury or distal embolization. Other access site complications include hematoma, pseudoaneurysm, arteriovenous (AV) fistulas, and noninfectious granulomas. See **FIGURES 4.22-4.30**.

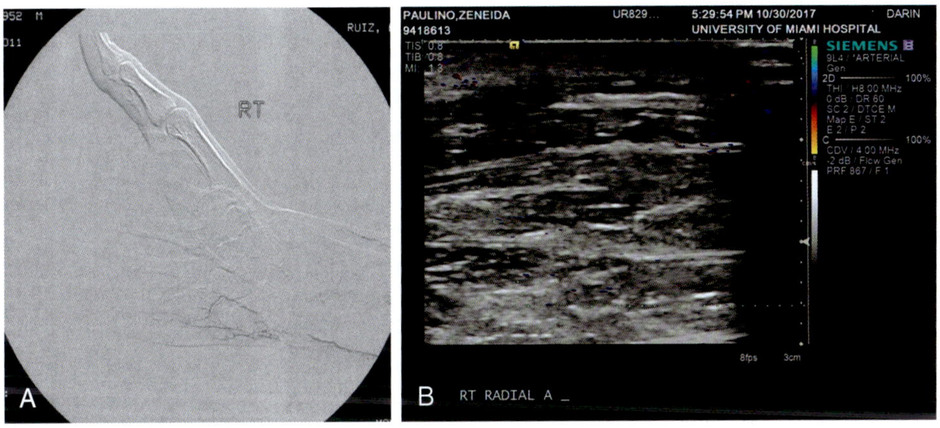

FIGURE 4.22 RAO. RAO occurs in ~5% of cases, it is often asymptomatic, and it can be diagnosed either angiographically (**A**) or by ultrasound (**B**). RAO can be minimized with routine use of anticoagulation.[26]

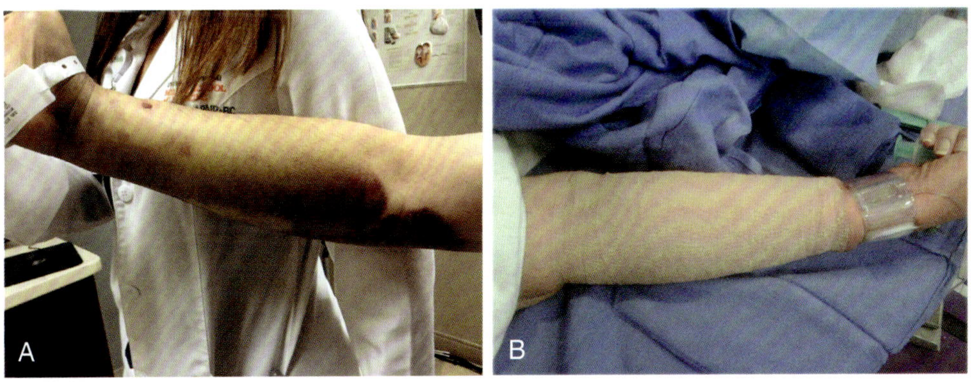

FIGURE 4.23 Forearm hematoma. Forearm bleeding and/or hematoma should be suspected if forearm pain and/or firmness are noted (**A**). Early recognition and continuous monitoring for compartment syndrome are key.[20] Immediate compression should be applied to the site, and an elastic band can be used (**B**).

EASY Hematoma Classification after Transradial/Ulnar PCI

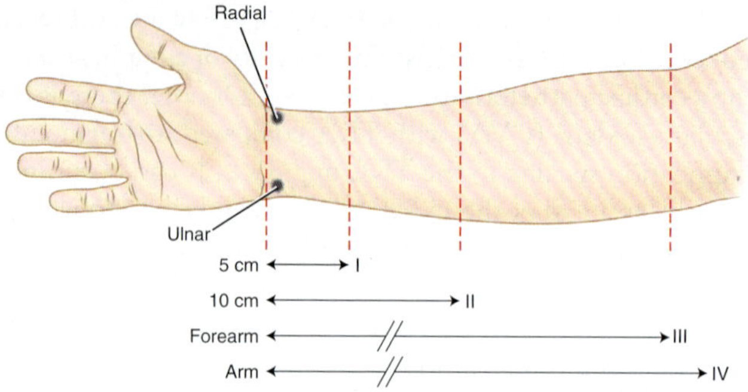

Grade	I	II	III	IV	V
Incidence	≤5%	<3%	<2%	≤0.1%	<0.01%
Definition	Local hematoma, superficial	Hematoma with moderate muscular infiltration	Forearm hematoma and muscular infiltration, below the elbow	Hematoma and muscular infiltration extending above the elbow	Ischemic threat (compartment syndrome)
Treatment	Analgesia Additional bracelet Local ice	Analgesia Additional bracelet Local ice	Analgesia Additional bracelet Local ice Inflated BPcuff	Analgesia Additional bracelet Local ice Inflated BPcuff	Consider surgery
Notes		Inform physician	Inform physician	Inform physician	STAT call to physician
Remarks	• Control blood pressure (BP) (importance of pain management) • Consider interruption of any anticoagulation and/or antiplatelet infusion • Follow forearm and arm diameters to evaluate requirement for additional bracelet and/or BP cuff inflation • Additional bracelet(s) can be placed alongside artery anatomy • Ice cubes in a plastic bag or washcloth are placed on the hematoma • Finger O_2 saturation can be monitored during inflated blood pressure cuff • To inflate blood pressure cuff, select a pressure of 20 mmHg <systolic pressure and deflate every 15 min • After bracelet removal, use "Velpeau bandage" around forearm/arm for a few hours to maintain mild positive pressure				

FIGURE 4.24 Classification of forearm hematoma. For grade I-III hematomas, treatment can be largely limited to analgesia and use of local ice. An additional hemostatic bracelet placed proximally to the initial device can be used to limit expansion of the hematoma. In grade V hematomas, the threat of ischemia and/or compartment syndrome warrants surgical evaluation and possible intervention. Redrawn from Bertrand OF. Acute forearm muscle swelling post transradial catheterization and compartment syndrome: prevention is better than treatment!. *Catheterization Cardiovasc Interv*. 2010;75:366-368.

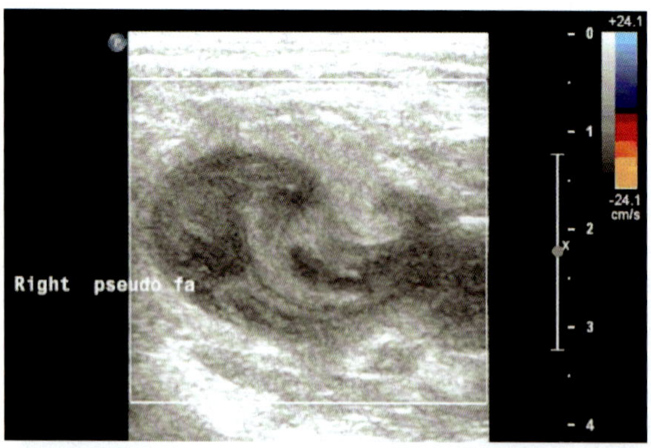

FIGURE 4.25 Pseudoaneurysm.

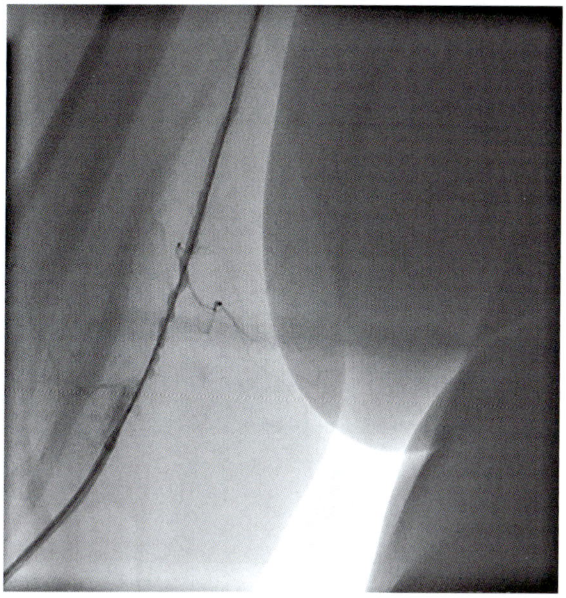

FIGURE 4.26 Perforation. Perforation is characterized by extravasation of contrast in the forearm. It can often be managed conservatively. It is very important to keep the wire in the vessel and proceed with the procedure. The catheter in the radial artery can seal the perforation and prevent further extravasation of blood into the forearm.

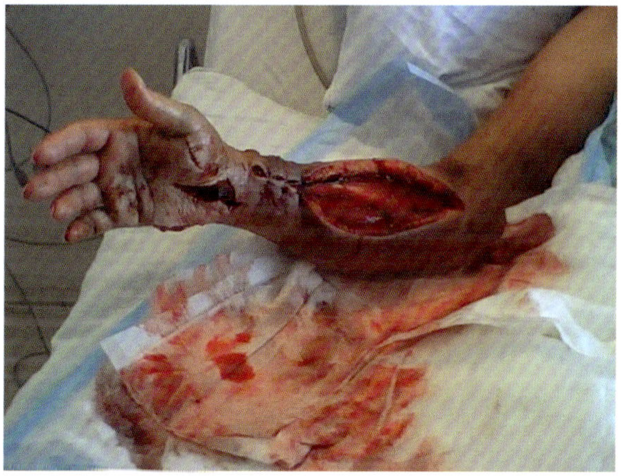

FIGURE 4.27 Compartment syndrome of forearm.[19]

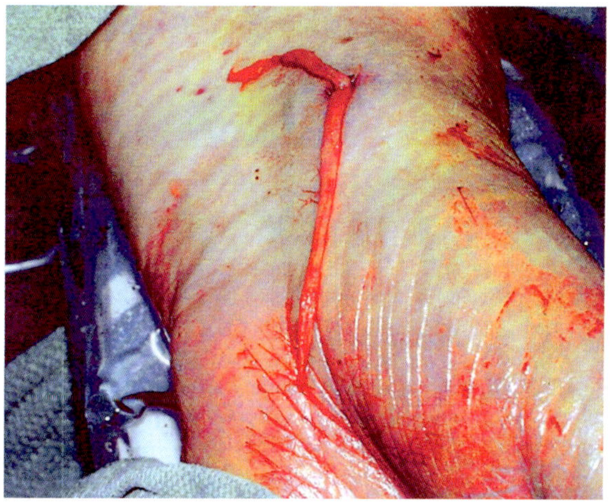

FIGURE 4.28 Radial artery eversion during sheath removal. Radial artery eversion is an extremely rare complication, with only 1 case reported in the literature. With the use of hydrophilic coated sheaths, this event is unlikely to occur. From Dieters RS, Akef A, Wolff M. Eversion endarterectomy complicating radial artery access for left heart catheterization. *Catheter Cardiovasc Interv*. 2003;58(4):478-480.

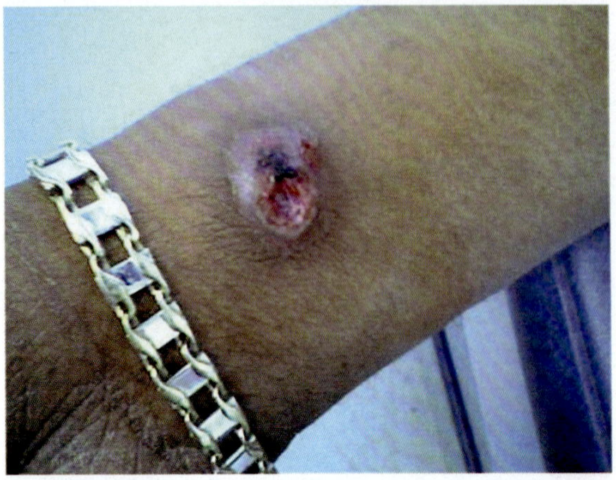

FIGURE 4.29 Noninfectious, sterile abscess/granuloma formation. Sterile abscesses have been reported as a reaction to the hydrophilic coating of certain sheaths. With improvements in equipment, sterile abscesses or granulomas occur very rarely.[21,22]

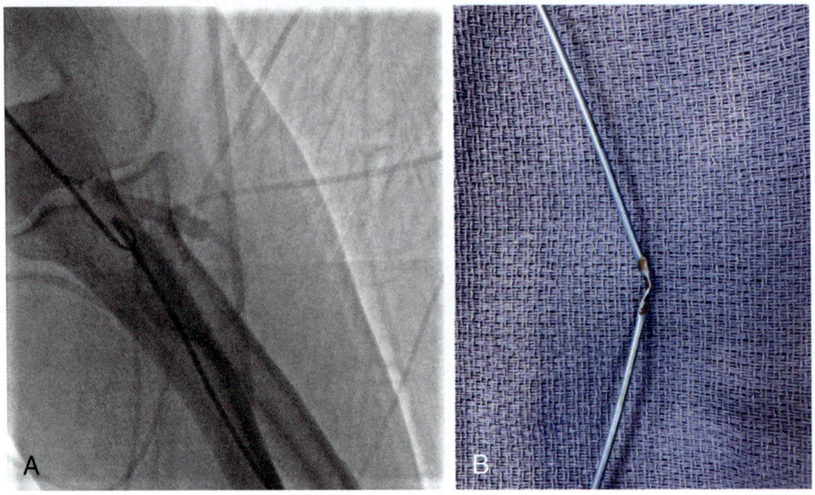

FIGURE 4.30 Guide catheter kinking. Guide catheter kinking can occur with excessive manipulation and torqueing. Catheter kinking can result in serious consequences because of catheter entrapment or rupture. In many instances, catheter kinking can be managed by slow pullback and counter torqueing of the catheter and advancement of a 0.035" wire. Applying pressure to the brachial artery above the kink or the use of a blood pressure cuff to anchor while pulling back slowly under fluoroscopic guidance can facilitate withdrawal of the catheter. If this technique does not work, secondary access should be obtained to snare the tip of the guide. With the tip secured, gentle rotation can be applied to unwind and then pullback the catheter (**B**).

REFERENCES

1. Cohen MG, Alfonso C. Starting a transradial vascular access program in the cardiac catheterization laboratory. *J Invasive Cardiol.* 2009;21(suppl A 8):11A-17A.
2. Patel T, Shah S, Pancholy S. *Patel's Atlas of Transradial Intervention: The Basics and Beyond.* 2012. HMP Communications.
3. Valgimigli M, Campo G, Penzo C, Tebaldi M, Biscaglia S, Ferrari R; RADAR Investigators. Transradial coronary catheterization and intervention across the whole spectrum of Allen test results. *J Am Coll Cardiol.* 2014;63(18):1833-1841.
4. Bertrand OF, Carey PC, Gilchrist IC. Allen or No allen that is the question! *JACC (J Am Coll Cardiol).* 2014;63(18):1842-1844.
5. Barbeau GR, Arsenault F, Dugas L, Simard S, Larivière MM. Evaluation of the ulnopalmar arterial arches with pulse oximetry and plethysmography: comparison with the Allen's test in 1010 patients. *Am Heart J.* 2004;147(3):489-493.
6. Seto A, Roberts JS, Abu-Fadel MS, et al. Real-time ultrasound guidance facilitates transradial access: RAUST (radial artery access with ultrasound trial). *JACC Cardiovasc Interv.* 2015;8(2):283-291.
7. *Forssmann Klinische Wochenschrift.* 1929;8(45)2085-2087.
8. Gilchrist IC, Moyer CD, Gascho JA. Transradial right and left heart catheterizations: a comparison to traditional femoral approach. *Catheter Cardiovasc Interv.* 2006;67:585-588.

9. Pancholy SB, Sweeney J. A technique to access difficult to find upper extremity veins for right heart catheterization: the levogram technique. *Catheter Cardiovasc Interv*. 2011;78(5):809-812.
10. Jacobs E, Singh V, Damluji A, et al. Safety of transradial cardiac catheterization in patients with end-stage liver disease. *Catheter Cardiovasc Interv*. 2014;83:360-366.
11. Spaulding C, Lefèvre T, Funck F, et al. Left radial approach for coronary angiography: results of a prospective study. *Cathet Cardiovasc Diagn*. 1996;39(4):365-370.
12. Pancholy S, Coppola J, Patel T, Roke-Thomas M. Prevention of radial artery occlusion- patent hemostasis evaluation trial (PROPHET study): a randomized comparison of traditional versus patency documented hemostasis after transradial catheterization. *Catheter Cardiovasc Interv*. 2008;72:335-340.
13. Rao SV. Observations from a transradial registry: our remedies oft in ourselves do lie. *JACC Cardiovasc Interv*. 2012;5(1):36-43.
14. Schiano P, Barbou F, Chenilleau MC , Louembe J, Monsegu J. Adjusted weight anticoagulation for radial approach in elective coronarography: the AWARE coronarography study. *EuroIntervention*. 2010;6(2):247-250.
15. Hahalis G, Tsigkas G, Xanthopoulou I, et al. Transulnar compared with transradial artery approach as a default strategy for coronary procedures: a randomized trial. The Transulnar or Transradial Instead of Coronary Transfemoral Angiographies Study (the AURA of ARTEMIS Study). *Circ Cardiovasc Interv*. 2013;6:252-261.
16. Lo TS, Nolan J, Fountzopoulos E, et al. Radial artery anomaly and its influence on transradial coronary procedural outcome. *Heart*. 2009;95:410-415.
17. Snelling BM, Sur S, Shah SS, Marlow MM, Cohen MG, Peterson EC. Transradial access: lessons learned from cardiology. *J Neurointerv Surg*. 2018;10(5):487-492.
18. Dieter RS, Akef A, Wolff M. Eversion endarterectomy complicating radial artery access for left heart catheterization. *Catheter Cardiovasc Interv*. 2003;58:478-480.
19. Bertrand OF. Acute forearm muscle swelling post transradial catheterization and compartment syndrome: prevention is better than treatment!. *Catheter Cardiovasc Interv*. 2010;75(3):366-368.
20. Tizon-Marcos H, Barbeau G. Incidence of compartment syndrome of the arm in large series of transradial approach for coronary procedures. *J Interv Cardiol*. 2008;21(5):380-384.
21. Swaminathan R, Wong S. Radial access site inflammatory reaction to recently available hydrophilic-coated sheath. *Catheter Cardiovasc Interv*. 2011;77(7):1050-1053.
22. Zellner C, Ports T, Yeghiazarians Y, et al. Sterile radial artery granuloma after transradial procedures: a unique and avoidable complication. *Catheter Cardiovasc Interv*. 2010;76(5):673-676.
23. Patel T, Shah S, Pancholy S, et al. Utility of transradial approach for peripheral vascular interventions. *J Invasive Cardiol*. 2015;27(6):277-282.
24. Patel T, Shah S, Pancholy S. "Combo" technique for the use of 7F guide catheter system during transradial approach. *Catheter Cardiovasc Interv*. 2015;86(6):1033-1040.
25. Patel T, Shah S, Pancholy S, Rao S, Bertrand OF, Kwan T. Balloon-assisted tracking: a must know technique to overcome difficult anatomy during transradial approach. *Catheter Cardiovasc Interv*. 2014;83(2).
26. Rashid M, Kwok CS, Pancholy S, et al. Radial artery occlusion after transradial interventions: a systematic review and meta-analysis. *J Am Heart Assoc*. 2016;5.

chapter 5

Cutdown Approach: Femoral, Axillary, Direct Aortic, and Transapical

ROSS MICHAEL REUL, MD, PHILIP L. AUYANG, MD, and
MICHAEL JOSEPH REARDON, MD

INTRODUCTION

The development of catheter-based treatment for structural heart disease and the limitations of percutaneous femoral artery access for large bore catheters have led to a recent growth in the use of alternative access sites. In this chapter, we describe the cutdown approach for femoral, axillary, direct aortic, and transapical access. For a description of percutaneous left ventricular apical and transcaval access the reader is referred to chapter 3.

FEMORAL ARTERY ACCESS (VIDEO 5.1)

The common femoral artery (CFA) is localized with ultrasound, and the site is marked on the skin. A 3-cm vertical incision is made on the skin just above the inguinal crease with a scalpel (FIGURE 5.1), the subcutaneous tissue is divided with electrocautery, and the inguinal ligament is exposed. A soft tissue retractor is used for lateral-medial retraction, and a handheld retractor is used to retract the inguinal ligament cranially (FIGURE 5.2). The CFA is localized by palpating the pulse, by feeling for a calcified artery, or with the sterile ultrasound probe. The fascia lata is incised vertically, and the CFA is exposed along its anterior surface (FIGURE 5.3). The artery is palpated to identify the optimum location for arterial access. Preferably, the anterior surface at the access site is free of calcified plaque, and there is a soft portion of the artery for clamping for control proximal and distal to the proposed arteriotomy. The distal external iliac artery (EIA), CFA, superficial femoral artery (SFA), and profunda femoris artery (PFA) can be exposed through this incision. The preferred access site is via the CFA, at or just cranial to the bifurcation of the SFA and PFA. The soft tissue is dissected away from the artery circumferentially cranial to the access site and an umbilical tape is passed around the CFA with a right angle clamp (FIGURE 5.4). The common femoral vein is medial to the CFA, the femoral nerve is lateral, and these are avoided by dissecting directly on the surface of the arteries. The SFA and PFA are dissected free, and umbilical tapes are passed around the SFA and PFA for distal vascular control. The profunda femoris vein courses between the SFA and PFA at the bifurcation and can be avoided with careful dissection but may be ligated if necessary.

If the CFA is severely calcified, the inguinal ligament can be elevated with the retractor or partially divided to expose the EIA more proximally. Care is taken to identify and preserve the medial and lateral collateral arteries, and these can be controlled with vessel loops if more proximal access is needed. A vein branch crosses anterior to the distal EIA just cranial to the inguinal ligament and should be ligated and divided if more proximal control is needed. The soft tissue is circumferentially dissected away from the artery above and below the access site and encircled with umbilical tapes for vascular control to allow proximal and distal clamping of the artery for repair of the arteriotomy site if a soft area of the artery can be identified for clamping.

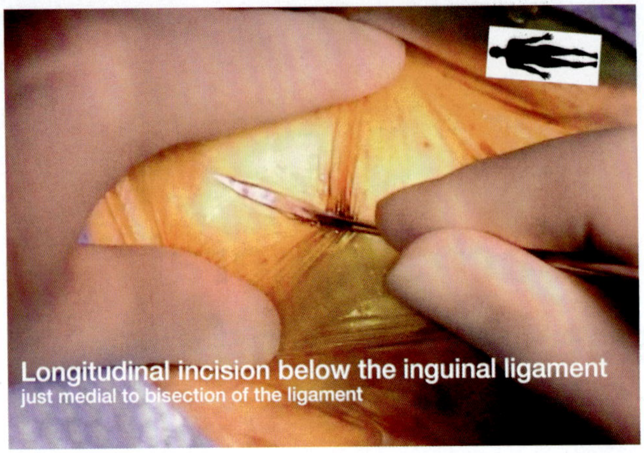

FIGURE 5.1 Femoral artery access. After localization of the CFA with ultrasound, a 3-cm vertical incision is made on the skin just above the inguinal crease with a scalpel, the subcutaneous tissue is divided with electrocautery, and the inguinal ligament is exposed.

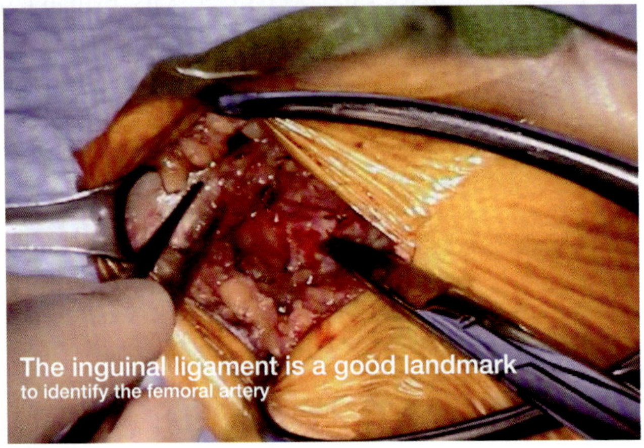

FIGURE 5.2 Soft tissue retractor for lateral-medial retraction and handheld retractor used to retract the inguinal ligament cranially.

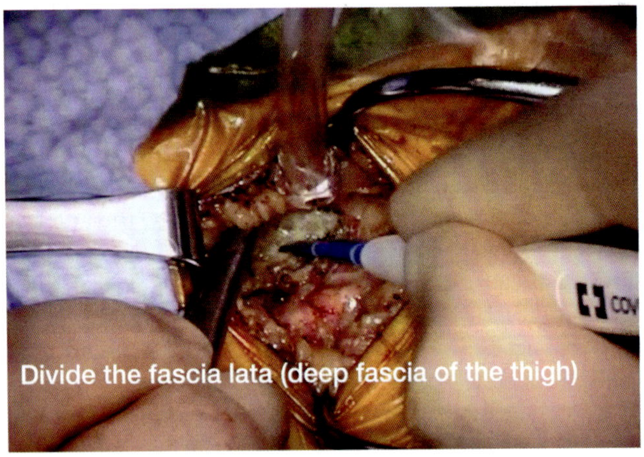

FIGURE 5.3 After localization of the CFA by palpation, the fascia lata is incised vertically and the CFA is exposed along its anterior surface.

If the CFA and EIA are severely calcified and there is not an adequate location for clamping, a purse-string 5-0 Prolene suture can be used to control and close the arteriotomy site. The purse-string suture is placed in the soft area of the anterior artery before access and must be wider than the diameter of the sheath to be used (FIGURE 5.5).

The artery lumen is accessed with a needle directly, and the guide wire is advanced and the needle removed. The artery is sequentially dilated over the wire, and the catheter is placed and anchored to the skin. At the completion of the endovascular procedure, the sheath is removed and the arteriotomy is closed. If a purse-string suture was placed before the arterial access, the sheath and wire are removed and the purse-string suture is tied to close the arteriotomy (FIGURE 5.6). If the artery is soft enough to clamp, the SFA and PFA are each occluded with a vascular clamp and gentle traction is placed on the umbilical tape proximal to the arteriotomy.

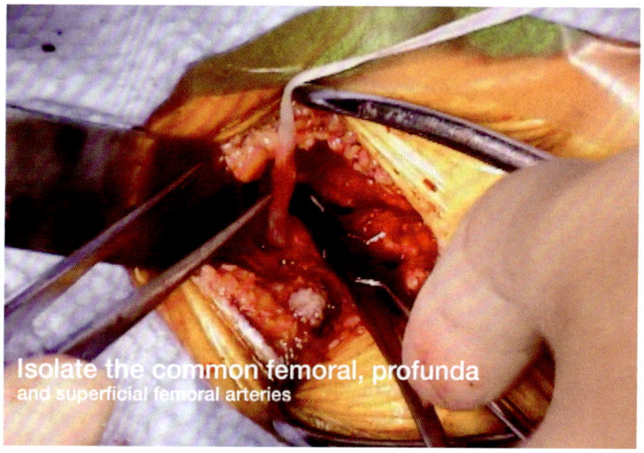

FIGURE 5.4 The soft tissue is dissected away from the artery circumferentially cranial to the access site, and an umbilical tape is passed around the CFA with a right angle clamp. The common femoral vein is medial to the CFA, and the femoral nerve is lateral; these are avoided by dissecting directly on the surface of the arteries.

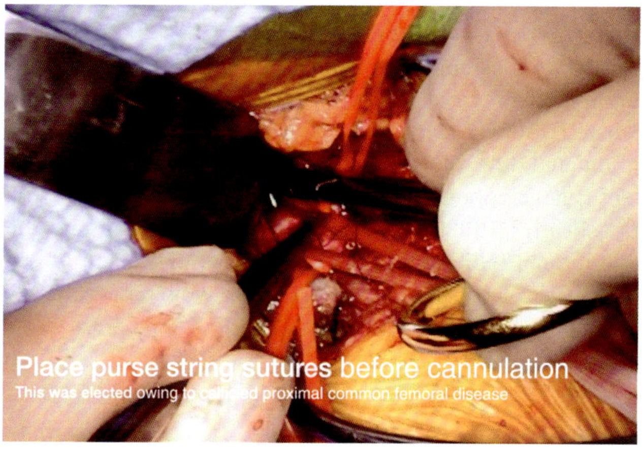

FIGURE 5.5 If the CFA and EIA are severely calcified and there is not an adequate location for clamping, a purse-string 5-0 Prolene suture can be used to control and close the arteriotomy site. The purse-string suture is placed in the soft area of the anterior artery before access and must be wider than the diameter of the sheath to be used.

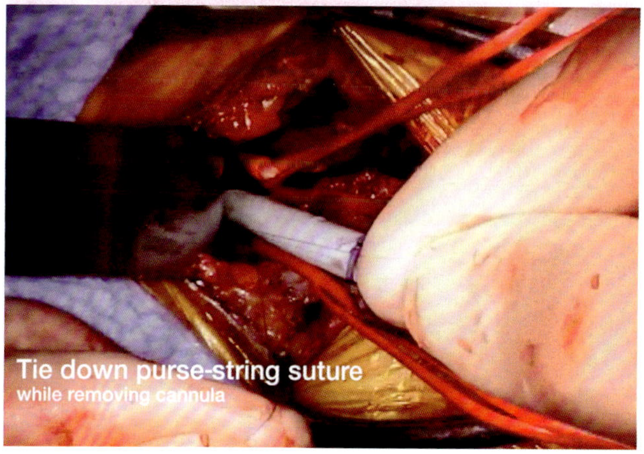

FIGURE 5.6 The sheath and wire are removed, and the purse-string suture is tied to close the arteriotomy.

The catheter is gently withdrawn from the artery, and a vascular clamp is used to occlude the artery proximal to the arteriotomy. The edges of the access site in the artery are debrided as necessary to approximate all 3 layers of the artery. The arteriotomy is then closed directly with 5-0 Prolene sutures in an interrupted or running fashion, everting the edges of the arteriotomy for endothelial-to-endothelial approximation. The vascular clamps are each flashed to flush any thrombus or debris from the artery and de-air the vessels, and the knots are tied. The clamps are removed, restoring distal flow. The quality of the anastomosis is evaluated with Doppler of the distal vessels and arteriography if needed.

Protamine sulfate is given to reverse the heparin. Hemostasis is ensured. The fascia is approximated with running 2-0 absorbable sutures. The subcutaneous tissue is closed with running 2-0 absorbable sutures. The subdermal and subcuticular tissues are then closed with absorbable sutures, and dry sterile dressings are applied.

AXILLARY ARTERY ACCESS (VIDEO 5.2)

A 3- to 4-cm incision is made with a knife 3 cm caudal and parallel to the clavicle, medial to the deltopectoral groove (**FIGURE 5.7**). The incision is carried down through the subcutaneous fat, and the pectoralis major muscle is identified. The pectoralis major muscle is divided along its fibers and retracted (**FIGURE 5.8**). The axillary artery pulse is palpated to guide the direction of the dissection. The soft tissue between the pectoralis muscles is divided, exposing the pectoralis minor muscle. The pectoralis minor muscle may be divided partially or completely (**FIGURE 5.9**) or left intact and retracted laterally. The axillary vein is superficial and caudal to the artery. The clavipectoral fascia is divided along the superior edge of the axillary vein exposing the axillary artery (**FIGURE 5.10**). The brachial plexus is usually located cranial and deep to the axillary artery and care must be taken to avoid the branches of the brachial plexus. The axillary artery is bluntly dissected free of the surrounding soft tissue and encircled with vessel loops. The thoracoacromial artery, and its branches are usually preserved and controlled with a vessel loop but can be divided if obstructing the exposure (**FIGURE 5.11**).

Most often, the artery can be cannulated directly using Seldinger technique to accommodate up to a 20 FR sheath if the artery is large enough. After the procedure is completed, the axillary artery is clamped distal to the sheath (**FIGURE 5.12**). The sheath is removed, and the artery is clamped proximal to the arteriotomy (**FIGURE 5.13**). The arteriotomy is then closed transversely with running or interrupted 5-0 Prolene sutures, taking care to avoid narrowing the artery.

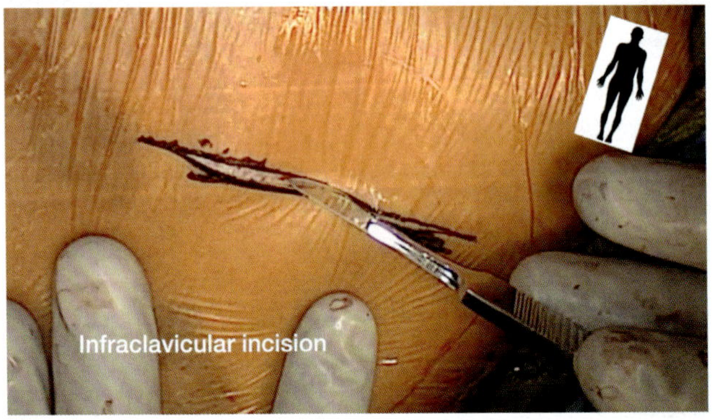

FIGURE 5.7 For axillary artery access, a 3- to 4-cm incision is made with a knife 3 cm caudal and parallel to the clavicle, medial to the deltopectoral groove.

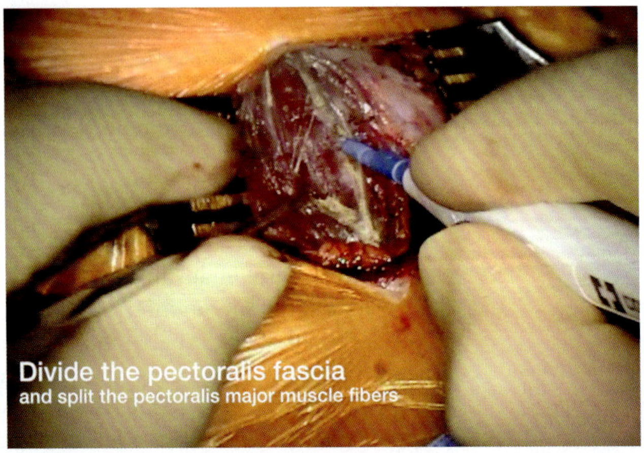

FIGURE 5.8 The incision is carried down through the subcutaneous fat, and the pectoralis major muscle is identified. The pectoralis major muscle is divided along its fibers and retracted.

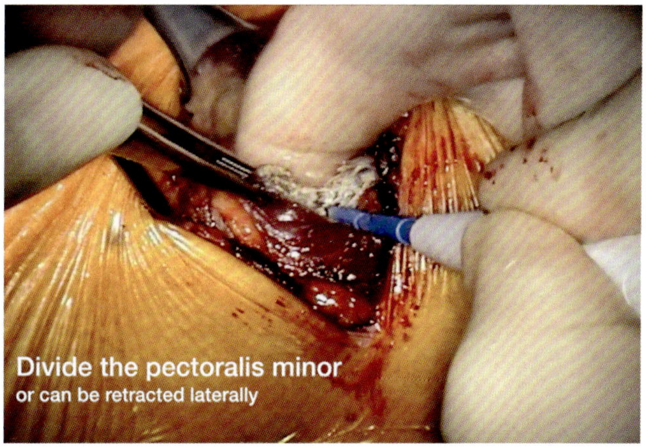

FIGURE 5.9 The axillary artery pulse is palpated to guide the direction of the dissection. The soft tissue between the pectoralis muscles is divided, exposing the pectoralis minor muscle. The pectoralis minor muscle may be divided partially or completely or left intact and retracted laterally.

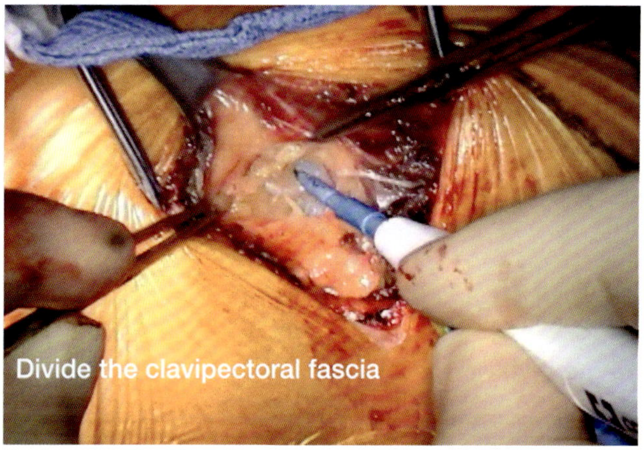

FIGURE 5.10 The clavipectoral fascia is divided along the superior edge of the axillary vein exposing the axillary artery.

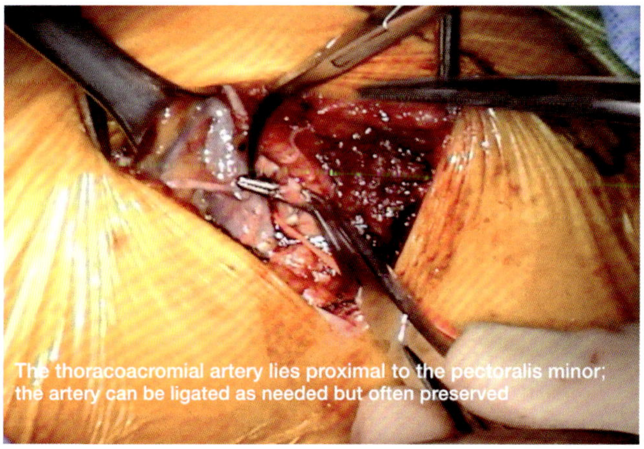

FIGURE 5.11 The axillary artery is bluntly dissected free of the surrounding soft tissue and encircled with vessel loops. The thoracoacromial artery and its branches are usually preserved and controlled with a vessel loop but can be divided if obstructing the exposure.

The axillary artery may be thin-walled, and sewing a Dacron graft to the axillary artery sometimes can simplify cannulation. If a graft is used, heparin 1 mg/kg is given. The axillary artery is clamped proximally and distally. A transverse arteriotomy is made on the anterior artery. An 8 to 10 mm Dacron graft is anastomosed to the arteriotomy in an end-to-side fashion with running 5-0 Prolene suture. The graft is clamped, the arterial clamps are removed, and hemostasis is assured. The sheath is placed directly into the distal end of the graft, and the graft and sheath are carefully de-aired. After completion of the procedure, the graft is clamped a few mm distal to the anastomosis and divided 2 to 3 mm from the clamp. The graft is closed with 5-0 Prolene sutures in a double running fashion, and the clamp is removed.

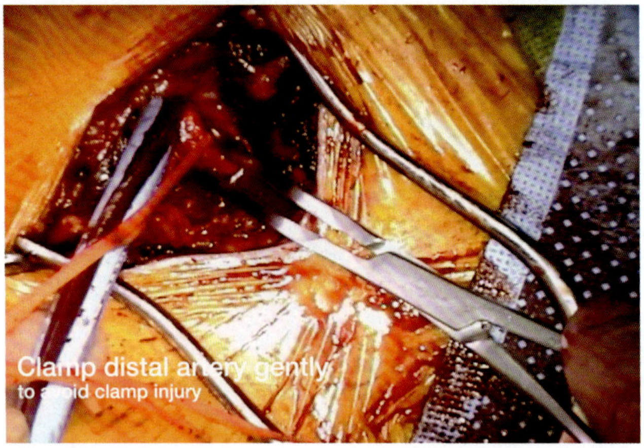

FIGURE 5.12 After the procedure is completed, the axillary artery is clamped distal to the sheath.

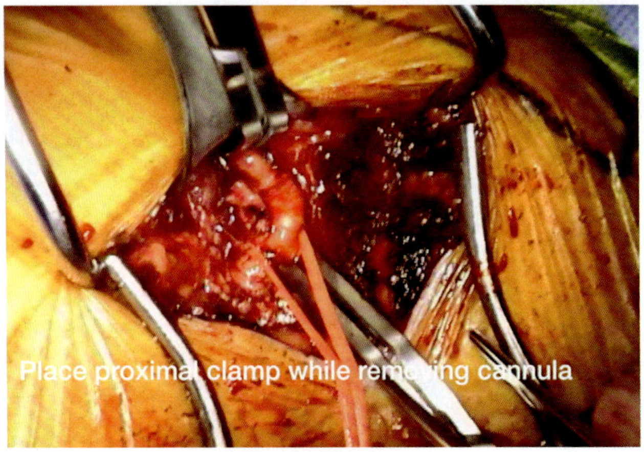

FIGURE 5.13 The sheath is removed, and the artery is clamped proximal to the arteriotomy. The arteriotomy is then closed transversely with running or interrupted 5-0 Prolene sutures, taking care to avoid narrowing the artery.

Hemostasis is ensured, and the distal pulse is evaluated. The pectoralis major muscle fascia is approximated with 2-0 absorbable sutures. The subcutaneous fat is approximated with running 2-0 absorbable suture. The skin is closed with running 4-0 absorbable suture in a subcuticular fashion.

DIRECT AORTIC ACCESS VIA UPPER MINISTERNOTOMY (VIDEO 5.3)

The aorta can be accessed directly when other more distal approaches are not appropriate. Preoperative computed tomography (CT) scan is used to evaluate the aorta for calcification and angulation as well as measurements of distance from the entry site to the aortic annulus. An upper ministernotomy is the most direct surgical approach, but a right anterior minithoracotomy can also be used. General endotracheal anesthesia is required. The midline over the sternum is marked from the sternal notch to the tip of the xiphoid process. The first 4 right interspaces are palpated and marked at the junction with the sternum. A 4-cm incision is made over the upper sternum in the midline from 2 cm below the sternal notch to the level of the third intercostal space. The subcutaneous tissue is divided over the top of the sternal notch. The incision is extended down the midline of the sternum to the level of the third rib. Landmarks used to define the midline include palpating the sternal notch and the edges of the sternum at each interspace. The decussations of the insertion of the pectoralis major muscles can also guide you to the midline but may be variable. A hemostat is used to mark the right edge of the sternum in the third interspace.

The upper sternum is divided from the sternal notch to the third interspace and angled to the right into the right third interspace taking care to avoid the internal mammary artery and veins (**FIGURE 5.14**). The sternum is opened with a small sternal retractor. The periosteum is

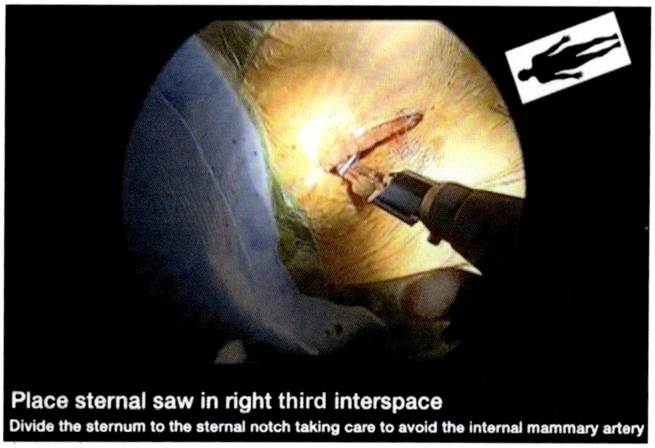

FIGURE 5.14 Upper ministernotomy for direct aortic surgical approach. The sternum midline is identified using, as landmarks, the sternal notch and the edges of the sternum at each intercostal space. A 4-cm incision is made over the upper sternum in the midline from 2 cm below the sternal notch to the level of the third intercostal space. The subcutaneous tissue is divided over the top of the sternal notch. The incision is extended down the midline of the sternum to the level of the third rib. The upper sternum is divided from the sternal notch to the third interspace and angled to the right into the right third interspace taking care to avoid the internal mammary artery and veins.

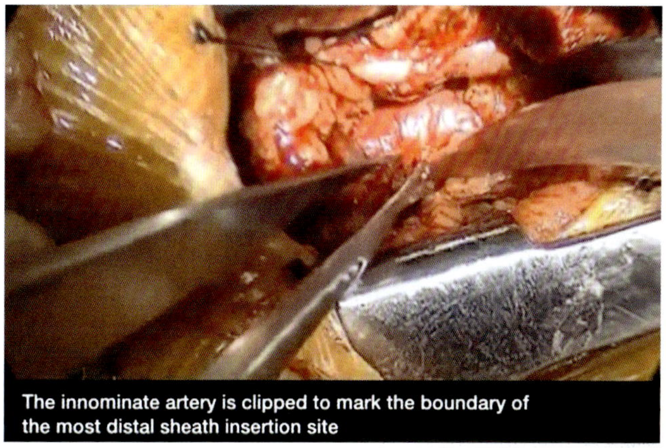

FIGURE 5.15 The sternum is opened with a small sternal retractor. The periosteum is cauterized for hemostasis. The thymus is divided in the midline up to the innominate vein. The pericardium is divided in the midline, and the edges of the pericardium are sutured to the presternal fascia to pull the ascending aorta anteriorly, closer to the level of the sternum. The base of the innominate artery is marked with a clip to determine the most distal site of appropriate access fluoroscopically.

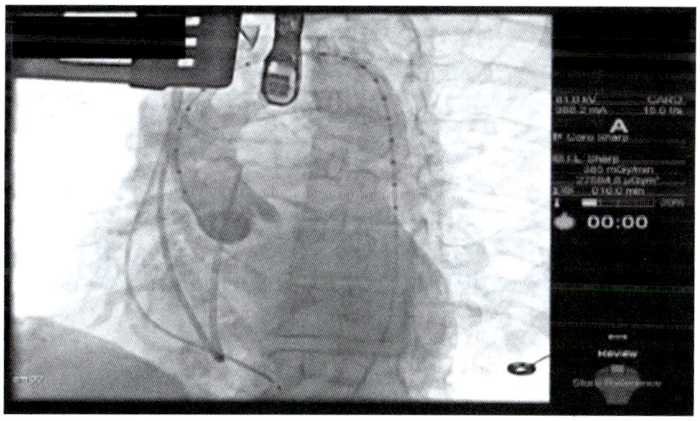

FIGURE 5.16 Marker pigtail catheter placed into the noncoronary sinus of the aorta via separate access in the femoral artery.

cauterized for hemostasis. The thymus is divided in the midline up to the innominate vein. The pericardium is divided in the midline, and the edges of the pericardium are sutured to the presternal fascia to pull the ascending aorta anteriorly, closer to the level of the sternum. The base of the innominate artery is marked with a clip to determine the most distal site of appropriate access fluoroscopically (**FIGURE 5.15**). A marker pigtail catheter is placed into the noncoronary sinus of the aorta via separate access in the femoral artery (**FIGURE 5.16**), in the left radial or brachial artery, or directly in the ascending aorta.

The site of entry in the distal ascending aorta is marked with an ink dot at a site determined by the preoperative CT, by intraoperative angiography, and using external landmarks to achieve the optimum angle of the delivery system to the aortic annulus. A purse-string suture is placed around the marked entry site large enough to allow insertion of the delivery sheath. A needle is inserted into the ascending aorta in the center of the purse string (**FIGURE 5.17**). A J-wire is inserted via the needle into the aortic root, and the needle is replaced with a 6 FR

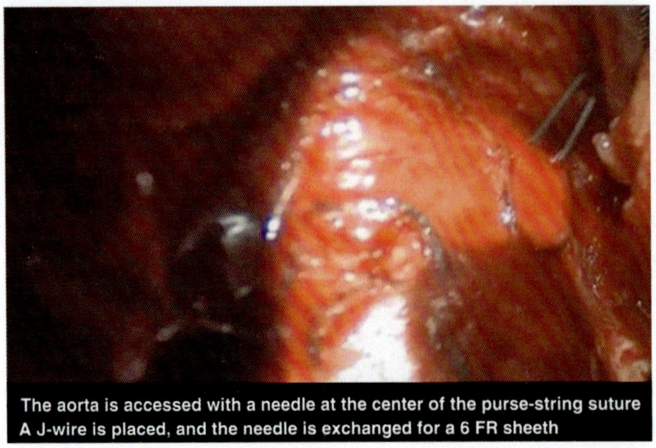

FIGURE 5.17 A purse-string suture has been placed around the marked entry site, and a needle is inserted into the ascending aorta in the center of the purse string. A J-wire is then inserted through the needle into the aortic root, and the needle is replaced with a 6 FR sheath.

sheath. A catheter is placed through the sheath, and a soft straight wire is used to cross the aortic valve into the left ventricle (LV). A pigtail catheter is inserted into the LV. The pigtail catheter is replaced with a precurved Safari or Lunderquist wire. The aorta is sequentially dilated, and the working sheath is placed into the ascending aorta over the wire.

After completion of the procedure, the sheath is removed and the purse-string sutures are tied without clamping the aorta. The thymus is closed over the aorta, and a chest tube is placed in the mediastinum. Hemostasis is ensured. The sternum is closed with stainless steel wires. The presternal muscle fascia is closed with 0 absorbable sutures in a running fashion. The subcutaneous, subdermal, and subcuticular layers are approximated separately with absorbable sutures.

TRANSAPICAL LEFT VENTRICULAR ACCESS (VIDEO 5.4)

The apex of the LV can be approached via a left anterolateral minithoracotomy. This access can be used for transcatheter aortic valve replacement (TAVR), transcatheter mitral valve replacement (TMVR), valve-in-valve procedures on bioprosthetic valves in the aortic or mitral positions, or transcatheter closure of prosthetic paravalvular leaks. The best intercostal space level to approach the apex can be variable. The preoperative CT scan can be used for measurements and identification of external landmarks to enter the appropriate interspace, usually the fifth or sixth left interspace. Fluoroscopy can also be used with a hemostat clamp to mark the level of the apex. A 5 cm incision is made below the left mammary fold medial to the nipple (**FIGURE 5.18**). The incision is taken down through the subcutaneous tissue to the pectoralis major muscle fascia. The interspace to be entered is palpated, and the pectoralis major muscle is divided with electrocautery over the interspace. The intercostal muscle is divided along the superior edge of

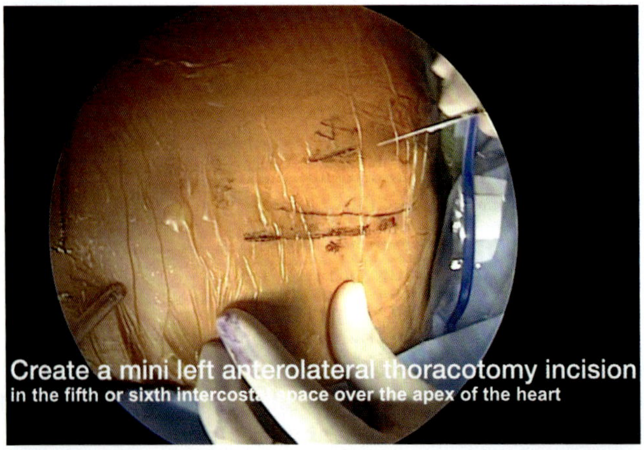

FIGURE 5.18 The apex of the LV can be approached via a left anterolateral minithoracotomy. The best intercostal space level to approach the apex can be variable. The preoperative CT scan can be used for measurements and identification of external landmarks to enter the appropriate interspace, usually the fifth or sixth left interspace. Fluoroscopy can also be used with a hemostat clamp to mark the level of the apex. A 5-cm incision is made below the left mammary fold medial to the nipple.

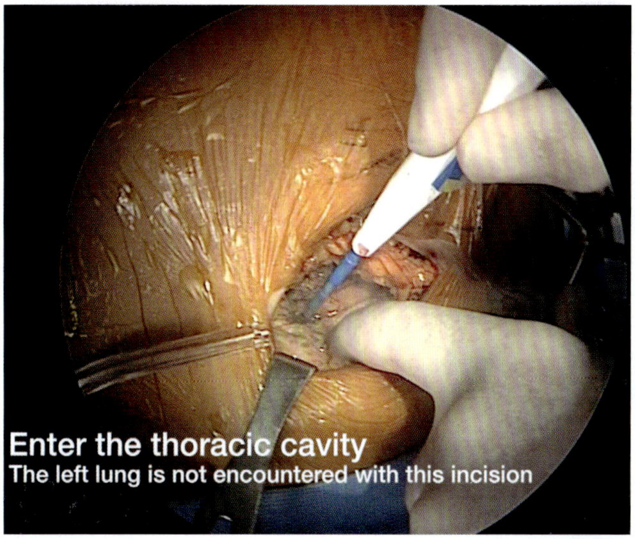

FIGURE 5.19 The intercostal muscle is divided along the superior edge of the rib, and the pleura is entered and divided.

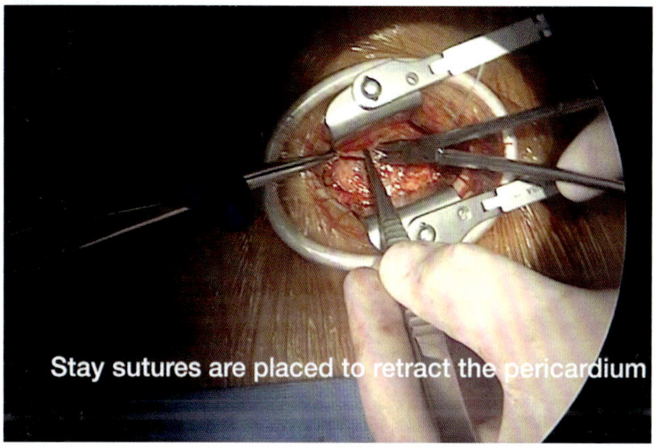

FIGURE 5.20 The epipericardial fat is divided exposing the pericardium. The pericardium is divided and retracted with stay sutures.

the rib. The pleura is entered and divided (**FIGURE 5.19**). A soft tissue retractor is inserted. The epipericardial fat is divided exposing the pericardium. The pericardium is divided and retracted with stay sutures (**FIGURE 5.20**). The exposed LV is evaluated, and the area of entry is determined 2 cm cranial and lateral to the true apex. This area should be lateral to the left anterior descending coronary artery and medial to the first diagonal branch if it reaches the apex. Using transesophageal echocardiography, the appropriate site of entry can be determined by depressing the LV gently with a finger during diastole (**FIGURE 5.21**). The optimal entry site is marked with an ink dot.

Two interlocking purse-string sutures are placed around the entry site wider than the size of the access sheath (**FIGURE 5.22**). We use 2-0 Prolene sutures reinforced with Teflon felt pledgets. Care must be taken to place the needle deeply enough in the myocardium to support the closure while avoiding extension into the LV chamber, which can result in hematoma formation. Tourniquets are placed on the sutures and can be tightened if the access site leaks around the sheath. The access needle is inserted through the wall of the LV (**FIGURE 5.23**), and a guide wire is inserted into the LV chamber and through the aortic valve into the aorta, guided by fluoroscopy. The needle is removed, and the sheath is gently inserted across the LV muscle over the guide wire.

After completion of the procedure, the sheath is removed and the purse-string sutures are tied to close the ventriculotomy. Rapid pacing can be used to decrease the LV pressure while removing the sheath and tying the knots. Hemostasis is ensured. The epipericardial fat can be closed over the LV closure to avoid direct contact between the ventricular repair and the exposed ribs. A chest tube is placed in the left pleural space through a separate skin incision.

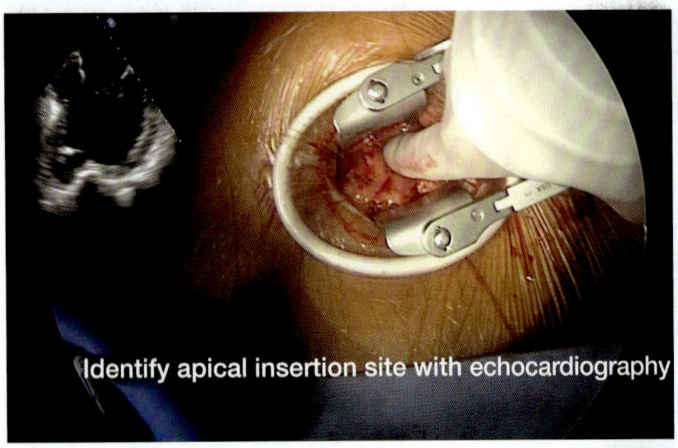

FIGURE 5.21 Identification of the appropriate site of entry using transesophageal echocardiography by depressing the LV gently with a finger during diastole.

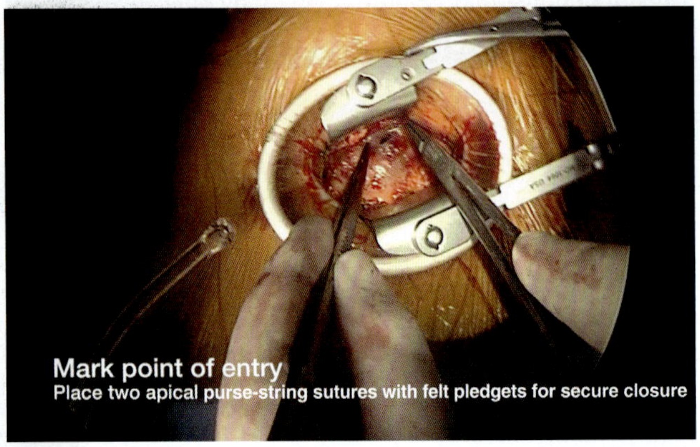

FIGURE 5.22 Two interlocking purse-string sutures reinforced with Teflon felt are placed around the entry site wider than the size of the access sheath. Care must be taken to place the needle deeply enough in the myocardium to support the closure while avoiding extension into the LV chamber, which can result in hematoma formation.

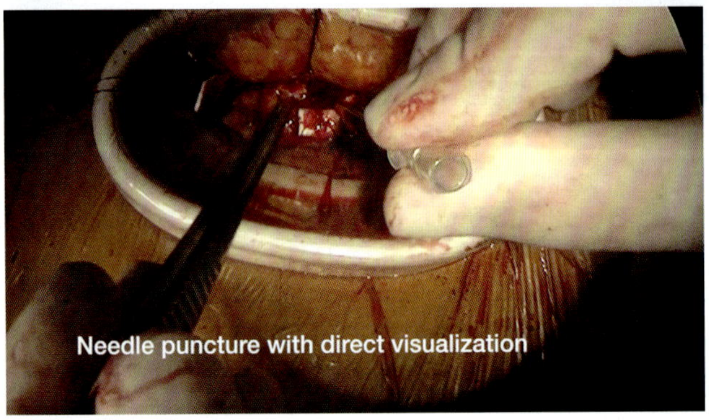

FIGURE 5.23 Insertion of the access needle through the wall of the LV under direct visualization. A guide wire is then inserted into the LV chamber and through the aortic valve into the aorta, guided by fluoroscopy. The needle is removed, and the sheath is gently inserted across the LV muscle over the guide wire.

Hemostasis of the ribs and intercostal vessels and muscle must be verified. The ribs are approximated with #1 braided absorbable sutures placed through the inferior rib and around the superior rib to avoid the intercostal nerves. The pectoralis muscle fascia is closed with running 2-0 absorbable sutures. The subcutaneous tissue, subdermal layer, and subcuticular tissue are closed in layers with absorbable sutures.

chapter 6

Catheterization in Childhood and Adult Congenital Heart Disease

ADA C. STEFANESCU SCHMIDT, MD, MSC, SAMUEL L. CASELLA, MD, MPH, MICHAEL J. LANDZBERG, MD, and DIEGO PORRAS, MD

Catheterization of children and adults with congenital heart disease brings together the breadth of physiology and disease of multiple interacting and, at times, interconnecting vascular beds, abnormal cardiac chambers and loading conditions, individualized surgical repairs, and both adaptive and maladaptive changes in supporting organ systems. Few aspects of medicine display such dynamic pathology over the entirety of patients' lifetimes. The congenital heart disease catheterizer must rely on an in-depth knowledge of congenital heart lesions and natural disease course, personalized history, review of and alignment with patient and family goals, detailed review of past surgical and catheterization-based procedures, status of vascular access sites, and familiarity with changing physiology and comorbid medical conditions that have potential to influence procedural and life outcomes.

This chapter, reviewing common cardiac and vascular interventions performed on children and adults with congenital heart disease, is subdivided so as to focus on individualized lesions and to allow the reader greater knowledge and ability to partner in congenital heart disease care. In bulleted fashion, each section reviews indications, technique, outcomes, and risks of particular procedures, together with representative images, illustrative patient case examples and references.

RIGHT VENTRICULAR OUTFLOW TRACT AND PULMONARY VALVE INTERVENTIONS

Hemodynamic Assessment

- Pressure gradient across the stenotic valve or conduit is assessed before the procedure with echocardiography (transthoracic echocardiogram [TTE]), with the mean gradient by echo usually being a close correlate of the peak-to-peak (maximum instantaneous) gradient during catheterization.
- Severe pulmonic stenosis is classified as a mean gradient >35 mm Hg and peak gradient >64 mm Hg (peak velocity >4 m/s).
- Moderate pulmonic stenosis is classified as a peak gradient of 36 to 64 mm Hg (peak velocity 3-4 m/s).
- Mild pulmonic stenosis is classified as a peak gradient of <36 (peak velocity <3 m/s).

Indications and Risks of Intervention[1,2a,b]

- Symptoms of heart failure, exercise limitation, and cyanosis from interatrial right-to-left communication, thought to be caused by the moderate or severe pulmonary regurgitation or stenosis.
- Asymptomatic severe pulmonic stenosis.

- Asymptomatic severe pulmonary regurgitation with progressive dilation of the right ventricle (RV) should prompt further clinical workup to assess symptoms more closely, such as a cardiopulmonary exercise test, and consideration of transcatheter pulmonary valve replacement in selected patients.
- Evaluation of supravalvar and branch pulmonary stenosis (PS), as well as pulmonary hypertension, should be performed when considering right ventricular outflow tract (RVOT) or pulmonary valve interventions, as they may be contributing to or be the predominant cause of symptoms.

Balloon Pulmonary Valvuloplasty

Background and Indications[1]

- First described by Kan et al in 1982 in an 8 year old male with valvar PS[3]
- Valvar PS with an echocardiographic maximum instantaneous gradient > 40 mm Hg
- Critical PS with cyanosis and/or ductal dependency
- Severe PS with RV dysfunction
- May be considered as a temporary palliation in high-risk patients with tetralogy of Fallot (TOF) (prematurity or comorbid conditions)
- Contraindicated in patients with pulmonary atresia with intact ventricular septum (PA/IVS) and RV-dependent coronary circulation

Risks

- Generally considered a safe procedure.
- Perforation of the valve annulus or right ventricular outflow tract (RVOT) has been reported and is generally avoided with a balloon diameter to annulus ratio of 1.4:1.
- Damage to the tricuspid valve apparatus is avoided with initial passage through the valve with a balloon end-hole catheter.

Procedure[4]

- Routine hemodynamics are obtained with attention to the pulmonary valve gradient after pullback from the main pulmonary artery (MPA).
- A right ventricular angiogram is obtained with cranial angulation on the posterior-anterior (PA) camera and straight lateral projection.
- The pulmonary valve annulus is measured in systole and an appropriately sized balloon is selected based on this measurement, usually 120% of the annulus diameter.
- An exchange wire is placed in a distal PA, and the balloon is advanced across the pulmonary valve.
- The balloon is inflated by hand with attention to the level of the waist that is completely resolved at maximal inflation.
- The patient is allowed to recover, after which the balloon is reinflated to ensure that there is not a residual waist.
- The balloon is deflated and removed from the body, after which a gradient is repeated.
- A right ventricular angiogram is performed at the end of the case to rule out subvalvar obstruction or damage to the RVOT or MPA (**FIGURES 6.1** and **6.2**).

Short- and Long-Term Results

- Initial studies showed an average reduction in the transvalvar gradient by 61% or 43 mm Hg immediately following BPV, with 25% of patient having gradients of ≤15 mm Hg and 8% of patients having gradients >30 mm Hg.[5]
- Predictors of unfavorable outcome include more severe initial obstruction and pulmonary valve dysplasia.
- Long-term follow-up is limited; however, studies have shown an 84% to 94% and 84% freedom from intervention at 2 and 10 years, respectively.[6,7]
- More recent data have shown a 70% to 80% incidence of pulmonary regurgitation in late follow-up of patients who underwent balloon pulmonary valvuloplasty (BPV).[6]

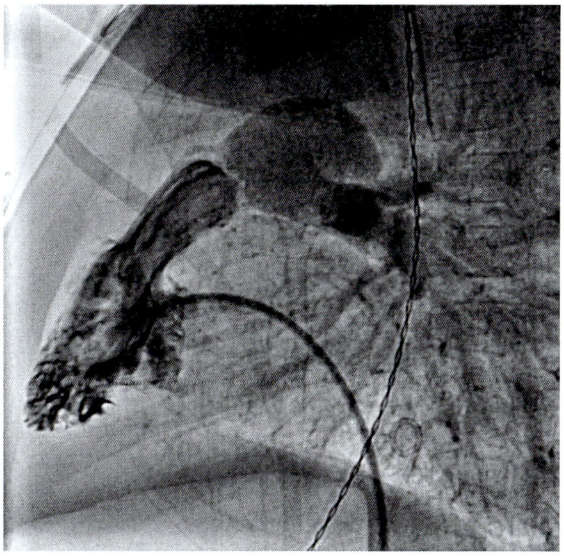

FIGURE 6.1 Antegrade right ventriculogram in the lateral projection shows valvar PS with slightly thickened and doming leaflets. The subvalvar and supravalvar regions are unobstructed.

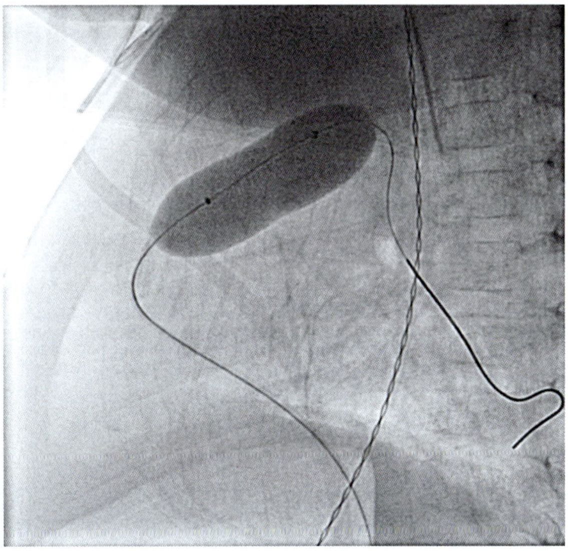

FIGURE 6.2 Lateral projection of a 12 mm × 2 cm Tyshak II balloon (B. Braun Medical Inc., Bethlehem, PA) inflated by hand with a mild residual waist at the level of the valve annulus and maximal balloon diameter of 12 mm (balloon to annulus ration of 1.2:1).

CASE 1 *Representative Cineangiography Loops*

A 14-month-old female with valvar PS followed as an outpatient with subsequent increase in the gradient by echocardiography prompting referral for catheterization. A preoperative echocardiogram showed severe valvar PS with a maximum instantaneous gradient of 80 to 90 mm Hg and mean gradient of 45 to 55 mm Hg and a patent foramen ovale (PFO) with bidirectional flow. Initial hemodynamics revealed a normal cardiac index of 4.1 L/min/m^2 and systemic RV systolic pressure of 66 mm Hg with a 55 mm Hg peak-to-peak gradient across the pulmonary valve with no gradient from the main pulmonary artery (PA) to the branch pulmonary arteries. A right ventriculogram confirmed the diagnosis of valvar PS with a pulmonary valve annulus measuring 10 mm (**FIGURE 6.3**; **Videos 6.1** and **6.2**). A 12 mm × 2 cm Tyshak II balloon was subsequently inflated by hand with relief of a discrete waist located at the valve leaflet tips and maximal balloon diameter of 12 mm (balloon to annulus ratio of 1.2:1) (**FIGURES 6.4** and **6.5**; **Videos 6.3** and **6.4**). Following dilation, the gradient decreased to 15 mm Hg with an RV systolic pressure of 37 mm Hg.

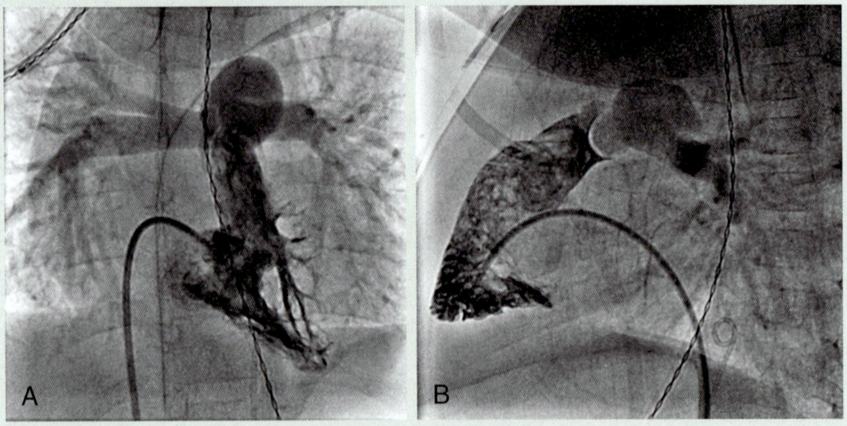

FIGURE 6.3 A, Frontal and (B) lateral projection of a right ventriculogram in a patient with valvar PS. Straight lateral projection usually clearly delineates the valve annulus as demonstrated in this image.

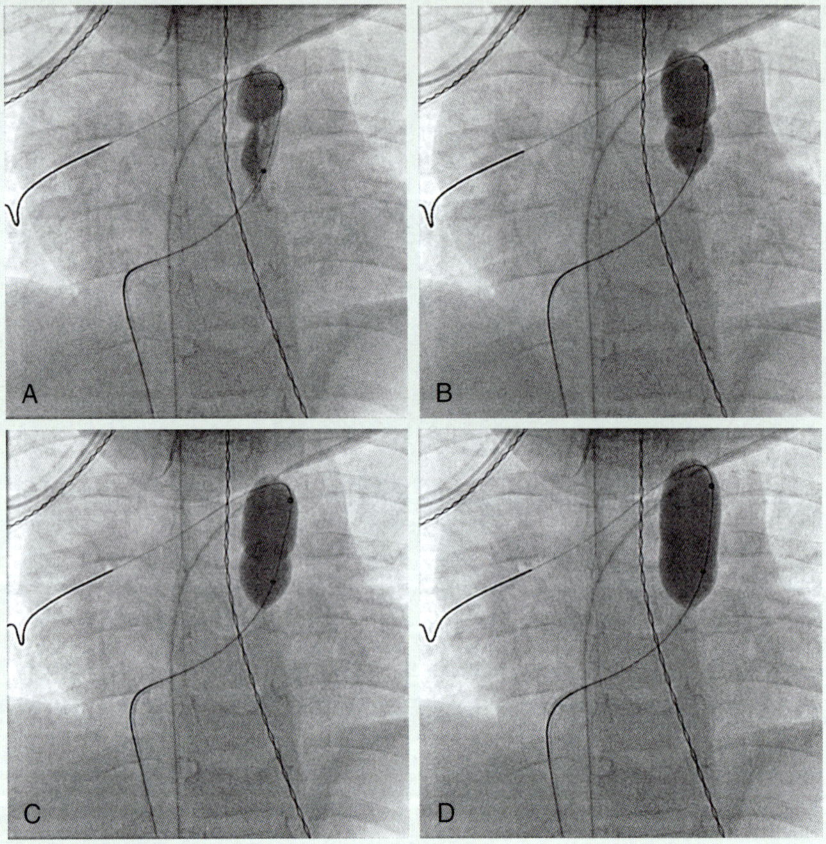

FIGURE 6.4 A-D, A 0.018" moderately stiff, exchange length guide wire (ThruWay Wire, Boston Scientific, Marlborough, MA) is positioned in the RPA after which a 12 mm × 2 cm Tyshak II (B. Braun Medical Inc., Bethlehem, PA) is positioned across the pulmonary valve and inflated by hand with relief of a discrete waist at the valve leaflet tips and maximal balloon diameter of 12 mm (balloon to annulus ration of 1.2:1).

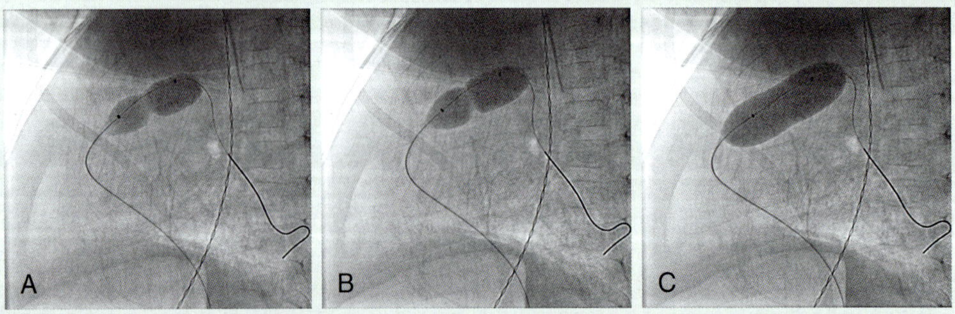

FIGURE 6.5 A-C, Lateral projection of a pulmonary balloon valvuloplasty with relief of a discrete waist at the valve leaflet tips.

Right Ventricle to Pulmonary Artery Conduit Interventions

Indications and Risks of Intervention

- Symptomatic patients with discrete obstructions with >50% stenosis or peak gradient >50 mm Hg or mean gradient >30 mm Hg.
- Asymptomatic patients with a bioprosthetic pulmonary valve with peak gradient >50 mm Hg.
- Preprocedural imaging can help elucidate the main etiology for conduit or bioprosthetic valve stenosis; focal lesions are more amenable.

Transcatheter Pulmonary Valve Interventions

Indications and Risks of Intervention

- The Melody (Medtronic, Minneapolis, MN) and Sapien XT (Edwards Lifesciences, Irvine, CA) are FDA-approved for treatment of stenotic or regurgitant RV to PA conduit or bioprosthetic PVR.
- Off-label use of the Melody valve in native RVOT (usually in patients with PS and a smaller native RVOT) has been reported.
- Off-label use of the Sapien valves has been reported for treatment of native RVOT that are too large for Melody implantation.

Key Aspects of Intervention

- Preprocedural imaging with computed tomography (CT) or magnetic resonance imaging (MRI) is often used to determine RVOT/annular size and candidacy for valve implantation, as well as distance from the valve implantation site to the PA bifurcation, and size of the PAs. 3D rotational angiography can also be performed (**FIGURES 6.6** and **6.7**; Video 6.5).
- Access is usually obtained from the femoral vein, although subclavian, jugular, or transhepatic access can also be used.
- A Swan-Ganz catheter is used to perform hemodynamic assessment and to establish position in the distal PA of a Super Stiff wire.
- Angiography is performed in the main PA to assess size of the RVOT landing zone and morphology of the branch PAs.
- The size and compliance of the conduit and pulmonary valve annulus are tested by serial inflation of a low-pressure balloon (**FIGURE 6.8**A and B).

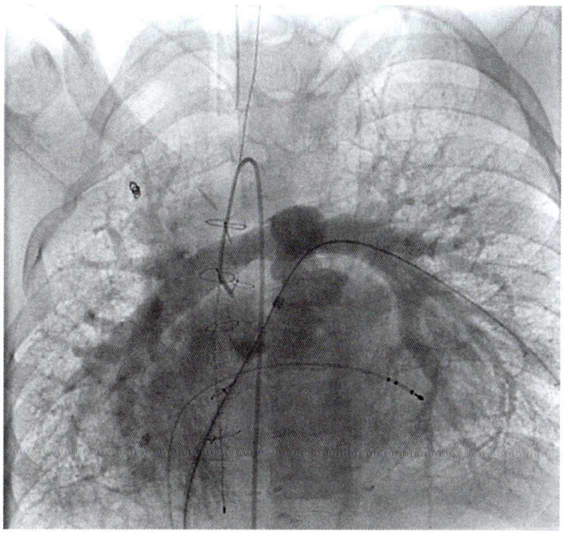

FIGURE 6.6 Preprocedural imaging with CT or MRI is often used to determine RVOT/annular size and candidacy for valve implantation, as well as distance from the valve implantation site to the PA bifurcation, and size of the PA. 3D rotational angiography can also be performed.

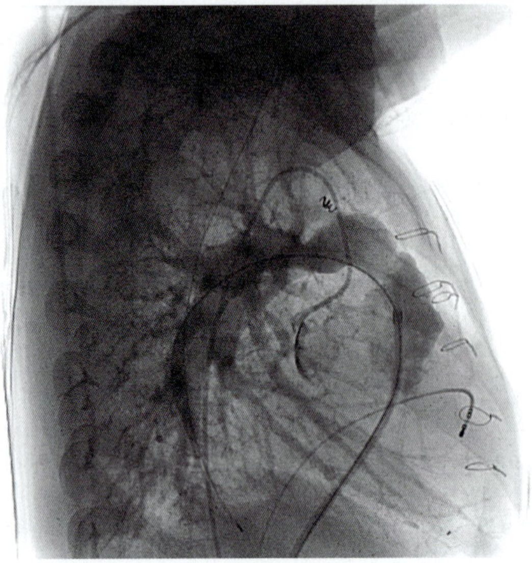

FIGURE 6.7 3D rotation angiography to demonstrate RVOT, pulmonary valve, main PA, and branch PA anatomy. Additional angulated imaging can typically optimize visualization of precise mechanism, anatomy, and measurements associated with obstruction.

- Coronary compression testing is performed by inflating a balloon to target diameter in the RVOT and doing a root aortogram with a pigtail catheter, in both anteroposterior (AP) and lateral projections. Alternatively, selective coronary angiography can be performed during balloon inflation (**FIGURE 6.9**; **Video 6.6**).
- Once a decision is made to proceed with valve implantation, prestenting is usually performed with a bare-metal stent. A covered stent can be used if there is evidence of conduit tear during the predilation (**FIGURES 6.10** and **6.11**; **Videos 6.7 and 6.8**).

Short- and Long-Term Results

- Postprocedural hospitalization length is shorter, but other early clinical outcomes appear similar between TPVR and surgical PVR in a recent single-center propensity-matched comparison.[8]
- The short- and mid-term results from the Melody trials have reported good longevity of the valve, although 25% of patients required reintervention at 4 years in the early Melody experience, in particular in patients who did not have prestenting and developed Melody stent fracture leading to stenosis.[9,10]
- New York Heart Association (NYHA) class improves in most symptomatic patients after TPVR, with improvements lasting up to 6 years in the Melody IDE trial.[9]
- Despite short-term improvement in PR fraction and indexed right ventricular end-diastolic volume (RVEDVi), observational studies suggest progression of PR and increase in ventricular size starting 2 years after intervention in some patients.[11-13]
- The reported incidence of Melody valve endocarditis is 3% per year[14,15]; it appears higher, although is better tracked and reported through prospective registries and clinical trials than

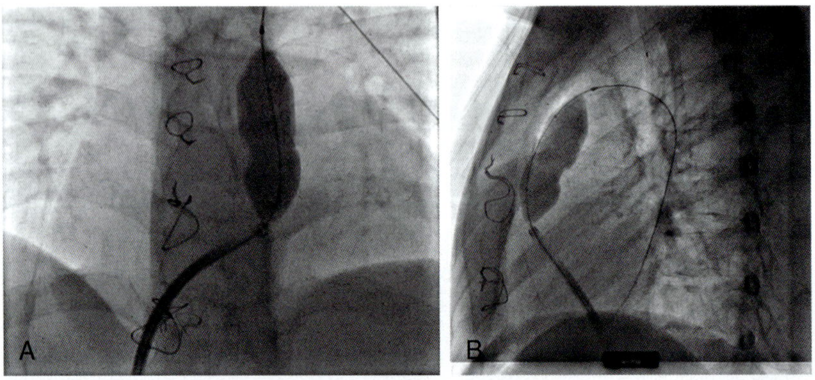

FIGURE 6.8 A and B, Balloon sizing in a patient with a stenotic bioprosthetic valve in an RV-PA conduit. The RV and its outflow are often best visualized from lateral projections, although associations with the branch pulmonary arteries or with surgical attachment from the RV to a conduit can oftentimes be best imaged and assessed with additional angulation.

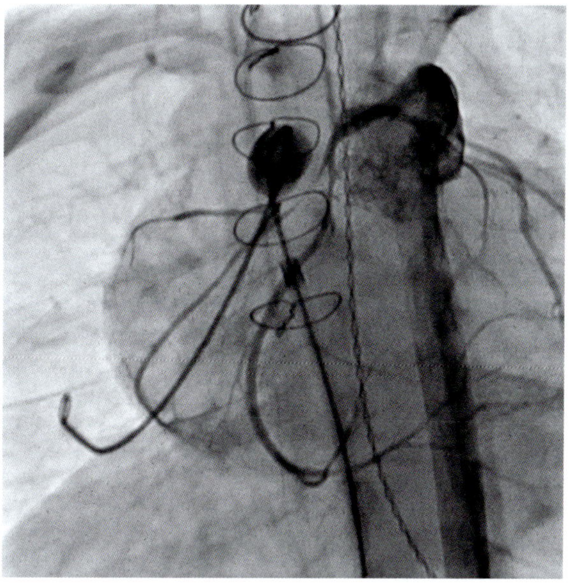

FIGURE 6.9 Compression of the RCA during balloon inflation of in an RV-PA conduit, in a patient with TOF and a single coronary origin.

the incidence based on case reports and retrospective studies of surgical PVR. Patient selection, differential ascertainment, as well as biomechanical factors that influence flow dynamics through the valve are being further studied.

Subvalvar and Supravalvar Pulmonary Stenosis

- Subvalvar PS is usually due to malposition or hypertrophy of the infundibular muscle. Balloon dilation rarely has a lasting effect and is not recommended.
- Supravalvar PS at the site of prior surgical intervention can be treated with balloon dilation. There is often recoil and recurrent stenosis after balloon dilation; longer lasting results can be obtained with stenting in the lesions that are distal enough to the pulmonary valve.

Peripheral Pulmonary Stenosis Interventions

Indications and Risks of Intervention

- Consequences of branch PS are not only increased RV afterload but also lack of circulation and growth of affected lung segments, as well as overcirculation to the unaffected pulmonary arteries.
- Branch PS with >50% stenosis and RVSP > 50 mm Hg and/or symptoms of heart failure.[2a,b]
- Symptoms related to decreased pulmonary blood flow, abnormal differential perfusion (<35% in 1 lung), and elevated RVSP (between 1/2 and 3/4 of systemic blood pressure).[1]
- There is an increasing experience with PA balloon angioplasty in patients with chronic thromboembolic pulmonary hypertension who are not candidates for surgical embolectomy.[16]

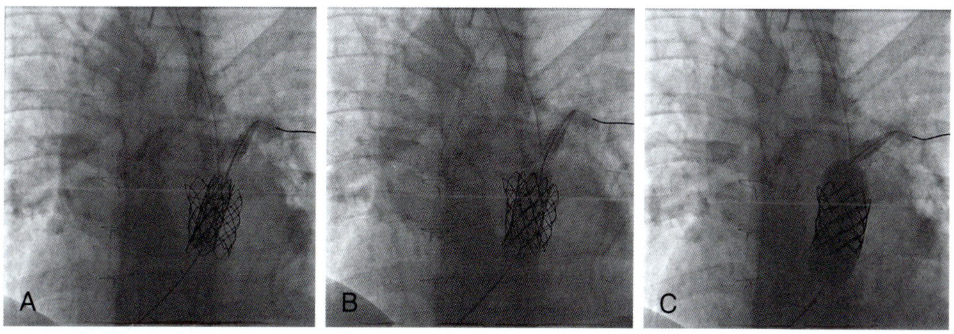

FIGURE 6.10 A-C, Deployment of transcatheter valve (Melody) within a prestented conduit.

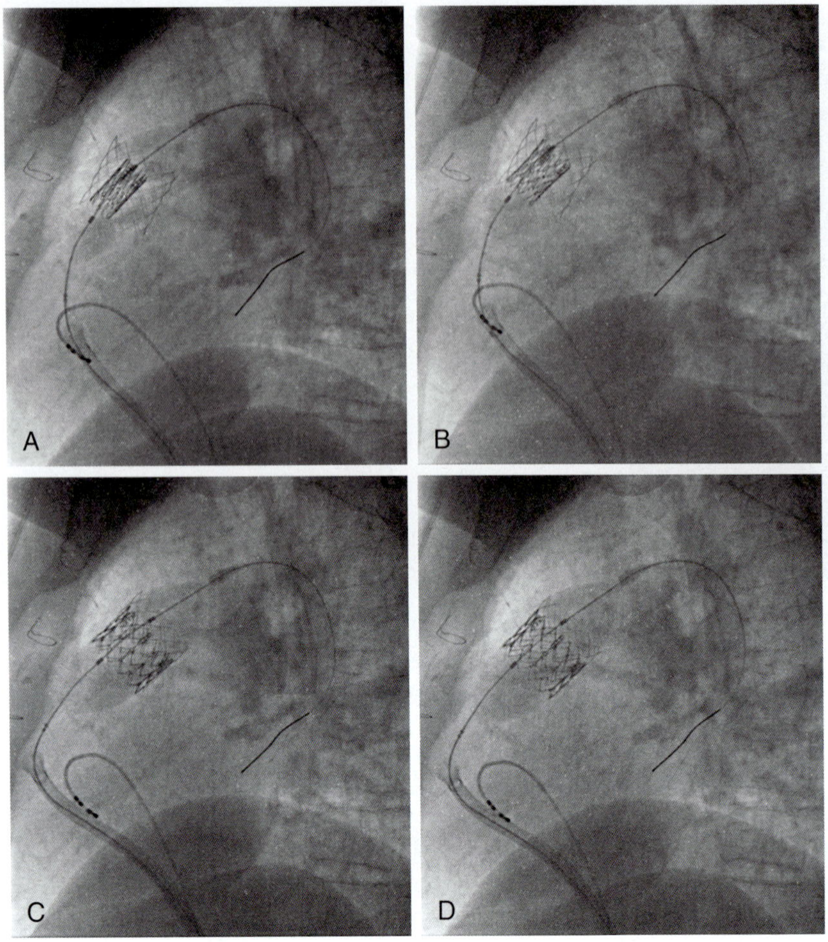

FIGURE 6.11 A-D, Deployment of transcatheter valve (Sapien XT) within a prestented RVOT.

Key Aspects of Intervention

- Venous access and hemodynamics are performed as described above. Access to the right PA may be easier from the left subclavian or internal jugular approach.
- Injection in the central PA allows estimation of blood flow to each lung segment, as well as caliber of distal vessels (**FIGURE 6.12**).

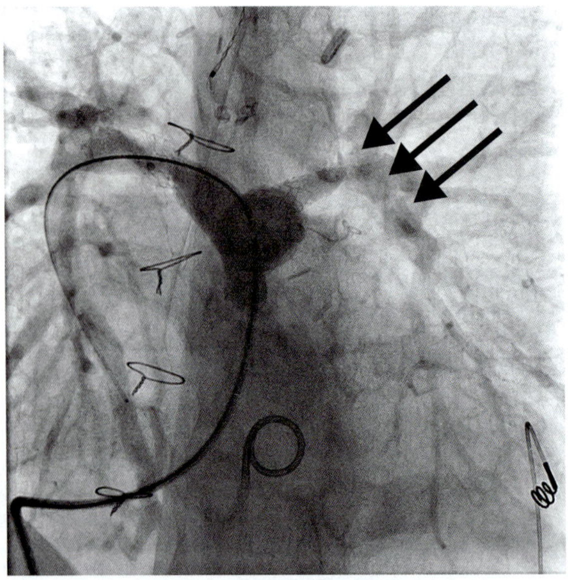

FIGURE 6.12 Angiography in the main PA demonstrating relatively hypoplastic left PA and more focal proximal branch stenosis (full arrow) distal to a previously placed stent and in-stent stenosis within the proximal branch of the right PA.

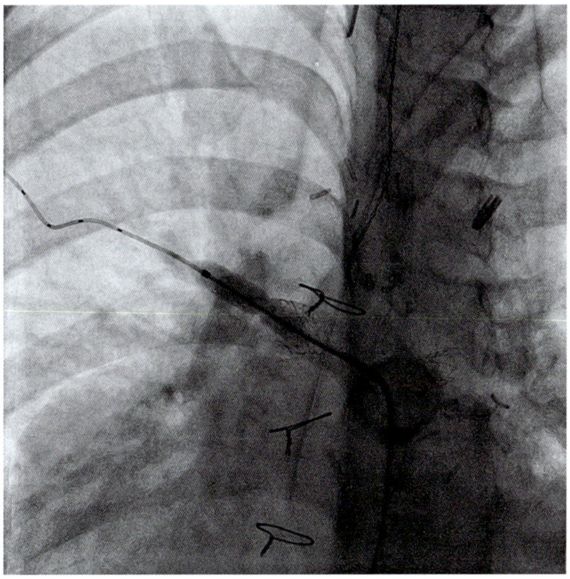

FIGURE 6.13 Balloon angioplasty of stenosis in the distal portion of previously placed right PA stent. Guide wire location is often chosen to optimize stability of balloon dilation catheter, as well as to provide access into a more distal vessel that has sufficient diameter to optimally seat the dilation balloon.

- The end-hole catheter used for angiography and measurement of pressure gradient is exchanged over the wire for a balloon catheter. Wire position is maintained in a distal PA.
- A high-pressure balloon with diameter not more than that of the adjacent normal vessel is used to dilate the stenotic area.
- Cutting balloons may be used for lesions that are difficult to dilate, especially if planning stent implantation (**FIGURE 6.13**).

Short- and Long-Term Results

- In older children, who have completed their growth, and in adults, stents are favored, especially in more proximal segments of the PAs (that will demonstrate more recoil after balloon angioplasty).
- PA dissection, either due to wire trauma or at the site of balloon angioplasty, hemothorax, and hemoptysis are rare procedural complications. Reperfusion pulmonary edema and lung injury are more common and were reported in 22% of patients in 1 institutional series.[17]
- Stent fracture, PA aneurysm formation, and restenosis have been reported in follow-up,[18,19] with restenosis seen in 15% of patients in early series.[20] The incidence of unplanned reintervention varies based on the severity of disease and age at intervention, with the majority of children <5 years of age with multiple stenoses requiring percutaneous reintervention.[19]

INTERVENTIONS FOR PULMONARY VEIN STENOSIS

Hemodynamic Assessment

- The degree of obstruction is usually best assessed angiographically, as low gradients can still cause hemodynamic sequelae and clinically important flow disturbances in the low-pressure, parallel constructed, pulmonary venous system.
- As isolated pulmonary vein (PV) stenosis will lead to decreased pulmonary arterial flow in only a lung segment and may not affect RV systolic pressures until late in the course of disease, a high degree of suspicion is needed. In children, the most common causes are after surgical manipulation (such as repair of anomalous pulmonary venous return or lung transplantation), idiopathic stenosis (which tends to affect multiple veins and cause more severe pulmonary hypertension), and extrinsic compression, while in adults the most common cause is scarring after a PV isolation/ablation for atrial fibrillation (occurring in 3% of patients, up to 40% in early series[21]), as well as occasional fibrotic diseases of the mediastinum.
- Isolated gradients may occur and can be estimated by measurement of the difference between the pulmonary capillary wedge pressure (PCWP) and systemic ventricular end-diastolic pressure (EDP) (assuming no other obstructions at the level of the atrium or mitral valve). Flow imbalance can be identified by nuclear lung scintigraphy or MRI.

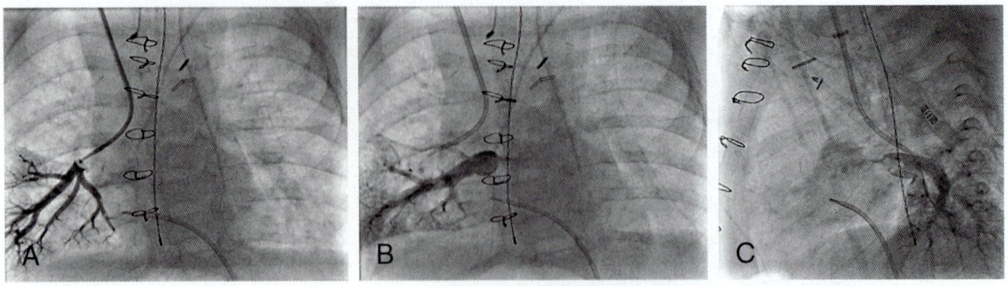

FIGURE 6.14 Patient with D-looped transposition of the great arteries, pulmonary atresia, atrioventricular canal defect, and total anomalous pulmonary venous return who underwent a bidirectional Glenn shunt and repair of venous return to the left atrium; (A) injection in the right lower segmental PA. B and C, Anteroposterior and lateral views venous return phase showing stenosis of the right lower PV at the site of surgical anastomosis, with pre-stenotic dilation.

Indications for Intervention

- Angiographic stenosis ≥50%
- Gradient > 3 to 5 mm Hg
- Flow imbalance coupled with otherwise unexplained symptomatology or RV or PA hypertension

Key Aspects of Intervention

- Angiographic evaluation of PV stenosis is most easily performed by (1) an injection in a segmental PA through the tip of a Swan-Ganz catheter, with the balloon inflated to prevent mixing, and follow-through to pulmonary venous phase, (2) direct access of the left atrium, and (3) angiography within the affected PV (**FIGURE 6.14**).
- Access into the left atrium is usually obtained by transseptal puncture, via existing atrial septal defect (ASD), or transbaffle puncture. Crossing through a PFO may direct catheters inferiorly and makes manipulation more difficult.
- Angioplasty alone has a higher risk of restenosis but is the procedure of choice in infants and children who risk outgrowing their initial stent and if a repeat surgical procedure is considered (**FIGURE 6.15A**-C).[1]

Short- and Long-Term Results

- Procedural complications, especially in small children, have been reported in up to 25% of patients, with clinically evident systemic embolization in 3% of patients.[22]
- Restenosis is common in children, in particular for congenital PV stenosis,[23] with 75% of children needing repeat intervention by 12 months after intervention. Treatment with systemic antineoplastic agents has been described as a way to reduce restenosis.[24]
- Angioplasty in adults with iatrogenic PV stenosis has better long-term results, with restenosis rates <30%, in particular if the final diameter of the stent is ≥10 mm.[1,25] Use of coronary drug-eluting stents in adults with iatrogenic PV stenosis has been reported to be associated with a higher restenosis rate than large diameter (≥8 mm) peripheral bare-metal stents.[26]

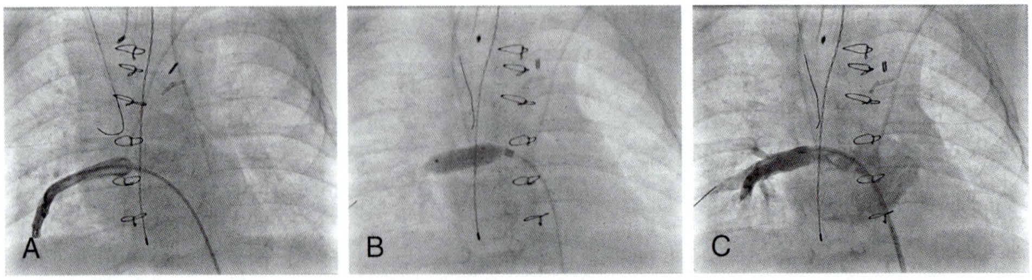

FIGURE 6.15 Retrograde venogram into the stenosed right lower PV (A). Access obtained through the inferior vena cava (IVC), right atrium, and large ASD into the left atrium. Serial balloon dilations were performed (B), and postangioplasty venogram showed improvement in the degree of stenosis (C).

SHUNT CREATION

Balloon Atrial Septostomy

Background and Indications

- First performed by Rashkind and Miller on a neonate with dextro transposition of the great arteries in 1966.[27]
- Cyanotic heart disease is the most common indication (ie, transposition of the great arteries) with insufficient mixing of systemic and pulmonary venous blood.[1]
- The septum is deliberately torn, effectively enlarging the interatrial communication, allowing for improved mixing of pulmonary venous and systemic venous blood.
- Complicating lesions include a bowing or aneurysmal atrial septum, juxtaposed atrial appendages, and patients with a left subclavian vein to coronary sinus.

Risks

- Generally well tolerated with adverse events limited to case reports.
- Confirmation of balloon location via echocardiography or angiography avoids inadvertent injury to the mitral valve apparatus or cardiac rupture.[27]
- Balloon rupture and embolization.[28]
- Inability to deflate the balloon after septostomy.[29,30]
- Current debate about possible subclinical cerebrovascular injury with the most recent literature has found no significant association related to balloon atrial septostomy (BAS).[31-35]

Procedure

- Usually performed at bedside unless complicated septal anatomy or associated lesions.
- Venous access is usually sufficient and obtained via the umbilical or femoral vein.
- Heparinization is obtained at the treating provider's discretion.
- A septostomy balloon is advanced across the PFO or ASD.
- The balloon is filled with a predetermined amount of saline.
- Echocardiography confirms appropriate position of the balloon in the left atrium, clear of the PVs, left atrial appendage, or mitral valve apparatus.
- The balloon is pulled across the atrial septum with a rapid "jerking" motion with the provider's hand anchored against the table until it crosses the septum to the right atrium after which it is deflated.
- Echocardiography assesses the size of the ASD and excludes mitral regurgitation or pericardial effusion.
- The patient's saturations usually increase rapidly.
- May repeat several times with incrementally increasing balloon sizes until an effective atrial communication is created.
- Hemostasis is obtained and a trial at discontinuing prostaglandin administration may be attempted while the patient is monitored before surgical intervention.[4]

Short- and Long-Term Results

- BAS is usually a successful procedure and results in an abrupt increase in systemic arterial saturation in most patients with reports of absolute increases in the SaO_2 of 25% to 30% allowing for stabilization of the patient and discontinuation of prostaglandins in some patients before surgical repair (**FIGURES 6.16** and **6.17**).[27,36,37]

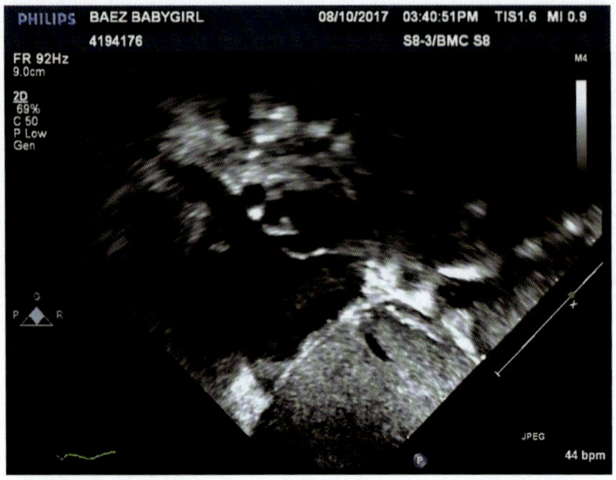

FIGURE 6.16 Subcostal short-axis imaging of the atrial septum shows a PFO bowing into the RA before BAS.

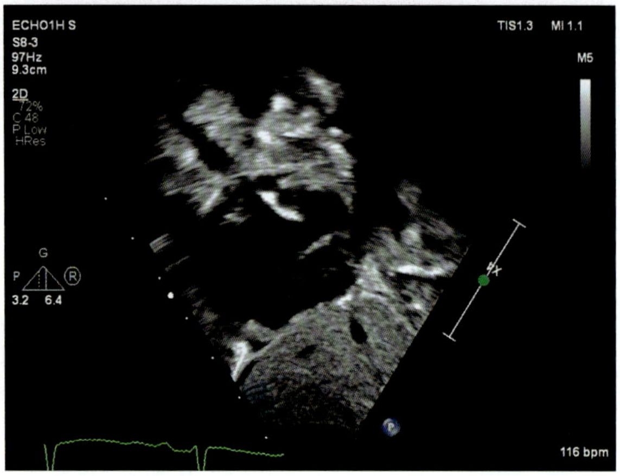

FIGURE 6.17 Following BAS there is a large atrial communication with a flail septum primum, which was intentionally torn during the BAS.

CASE 2 *Cineangiography Loops*

Newborn, 3.63 kg, full-term female transferred from a referring hospital with postnatally diagnosed D-looped transposition of the great arteries. Intubated in the delivery room and started on PGE with improvement of saturations to the low 80s. On arrival to the CICU an echocardiogram confirmed the diagnosis and identified a small PFO with accelerated left to right flow (**FIGURE 6.18**; **Video 6.9**). A BAS was subsequently requested owing to concern for LA hypertension and inadequate atrial mixing. A bedside BAS was performed via the umbilical vein with 4 attempts (**FIGURES 6.19** and **6.20**; **Videos 6.10 and 6.11**). Following the BAS the atrial communication appeared unrestrictive, measuring up to 6 mm (**FIGURE 6.21**; **Video 6.12**), and saturations rose to 97% to 99% with 30% FiO_2. The patient subsequently underwent complete repair with an arterial switch operation, repair of the atrial septum, and patent ductus arteriosus (PDA) ligation 4 days later.

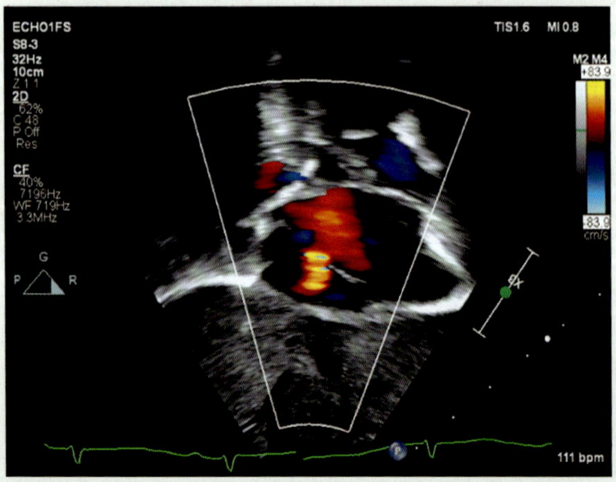

FIGURE 6.18 Subcostal long-axis projection of a PFO with accelerated left to right flow in a patient with D-looped transposition of the great arteries.

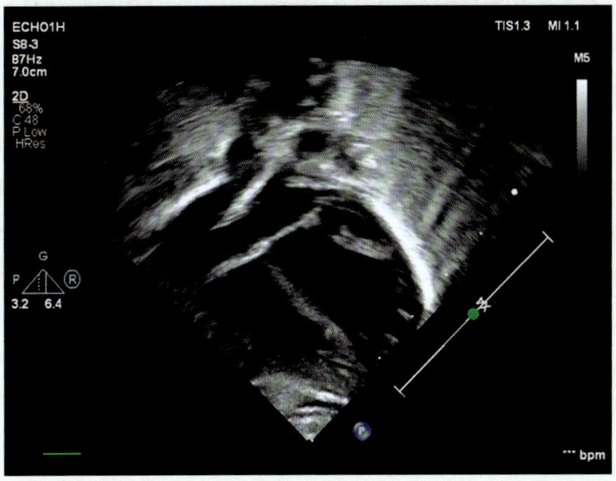

FIGURE 6.19 An atrioseptostomy catheter (B. Braun Medical, Inc., Bethlehem, PA) is advanced over a 0.018″ wire, across the PFO, into the left atrium with position confirmed by echocardiography.

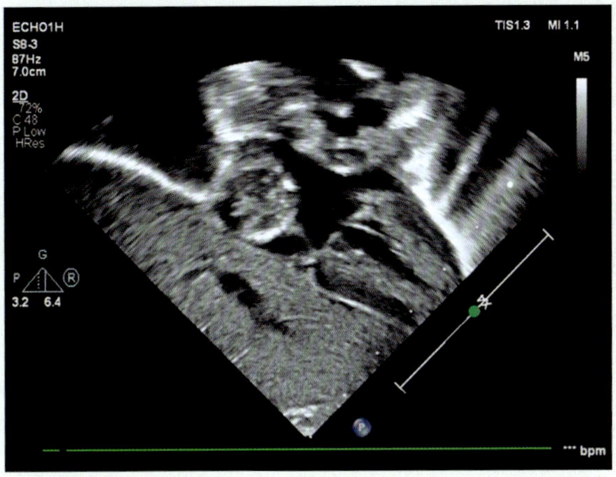

FIGURE 6.20 The balloon is inflated with the appropriate amount of contrast (2 cc in this example, diameter 14 mm) during which echocardiography confirms clearance of the mitral valve or PVs. After inflation, the balloon is rapidly pulled across the atrial septum as illustrated in the above image, after which the balloon is deflated in the RA.

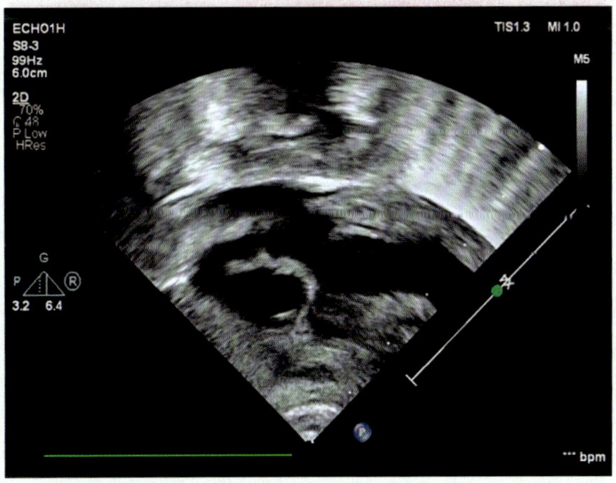

FIGURE 6.21 Following BAS the ASD is noticeably larger with a visible torn flap of septum primum.

STENTING OF A DUCTUS ARTERIOSUS

Background

- First described by Gibbs et al 1992.[38]
- An effective temporary palliation for some neonates with insufficient pulmonary blood flow with avoidance of the morbidity associated with a surgical palliative shunt.
- The need for reintervention due to restenosis, usually secondary to ductal tissue ingrowth, remains high.[38-42]

Indications[1]

- Infants with ductal dependent cyanotic heart disease (ie, pulmonary atresia with intact ventricular septum).
- Infants with cyanotic heart disease and >1 source of pulmonary blood flow (ie, critical PS).
- Previously been limited to patients with so-called simple ducts (<2 turns); however, current experience has shown success with more complicated ducts.

Risks

- Acute ductal spasm or dissection is the most feared complication.
- Techniques are available to overcome such circumstances.[43]
- Prostaglandin as well as extracorporeal membrane oxygenation and/or surgical shunt placement must be immediately available, as this may result in a surgical emergency.
- Stent malposition or embolization may occur.
- At the time of surgical correction or palliation, the stent may present a challenge for the surgeon, especially when it protrudes significantly into the aorta or the branch pulmonary arteries, and may add time to the operation and time on bypass or circulatory arrest.

Procedure

- Performed antegrade (femoral vein) or retrograde (femoral, axillary or carotid artery).
- Prostaglandin therapy is discontinued before the procedure, allowing for ductal constriction.
- Prostaglandin therapy should not be reinstituted after stent placement because this may result in-stent embolization.
- A floppy-tipped hydrophilic wire is carefully guided through the duct with care to avoid forceful manipulation, as this may result in ductal spasm or dissection.
- A flexible coronary stent (3.5-4 mm in full-term infants and 3 mm in premature or growth-restricted infants) is deployed across the PDA.
- The entire length of the duct is covered to avoid early restenosis.
- Some centers have used drug-eluting (sirolimus or rapamycin) stents, which may decrease the rate of in-stent restenosis.[43-45]
- Angiography confirms adequate coverage of the entire duct.
- Hemodynamics are repeated with attention to the PA pressure and arterial saturation.
- May require additional stent delivery or postdilation in the event of persistent cyanosis or inadequate coverage (**FIGURES 6.22** and **6.23**).

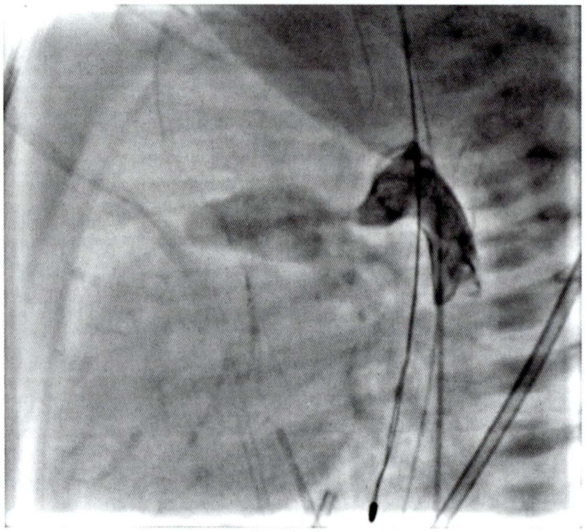

FIGURE 6.22 Retrograde injection in the distal aortic arch shows a conical PDA with left to right flow and restriction of the PA insertion of the duct to approximately 2.5 mm.

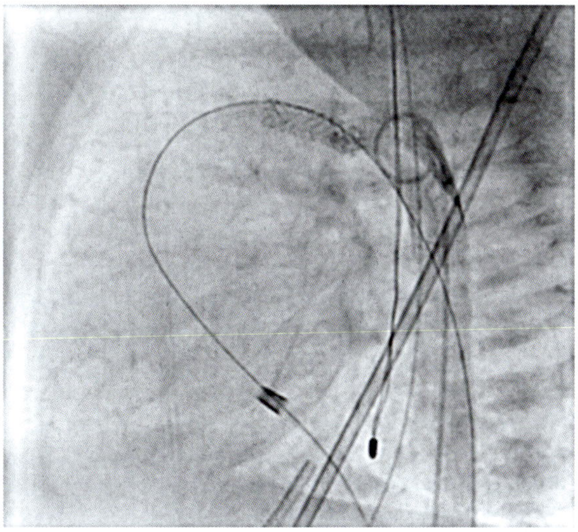

FIGURE 6.23 Retrograde injection in the distal aortic arch following stent placement with a 4 × 12 Rebel coronary stent (Boston Scientific, Marlborough, MA).

Short- and Long-Term Results

- Procedural success rates have been reported above 90% in single center studies.[40,42,46]
- Shown to reduce blood product transfusion rates, ICU length of stay, hospital length of stay, and days on mechanical ventilation as compared with surgical shunts.[47,48]
- Serious procedural complications occur in 9% to 23% of patients in some series, including access sites complications, ductal spasm, or acute PDA thrombosis requiring emergency ECMO and/or surgery, stroke, and excessive pulmonary blood flow leading to low systemic output and necrotizing enterocolitis or other complications.[42,46]
- Neointimal proliferation of the ductal stent is considered the rule rather than the exception.
- Favorable occurrence in patients with only a temporary need for additional pulmonary blood flow (ie, PA/IVS with eventual biventricular circulation).
- Single ventricle patients have an increased likelihood of reintervention, as high as 40% before their first surgical palliation.[46,49]

CASE 3 *Cineangiography Loops*

A 7-day-old 2.4-kg male transferred from a referring institution with postnatally diagnosed critical PS. An initial echocardiogram confirmed the diagnosis of critical PS with valvar and subvalvar PS, a hypoplastic pulmonary valve annulus measuring 4.5 mm (Z-score -2.3), normally sized main and branch pulmonary arteries, moderately hypoplastic tricuspid annulus (Z-score -2.2), PFO with predominately right to left flow, and large PDA with continuous left to right flow.

He was initially managed with prostaglandin E and at 4 days of life underwent catheterization where he underwent pulmonary valve dilation up to a 5 mm balloon with a residual gradient of 25 mm Hg across the pulmonary valve owing to subvalvar PS. The diameter of the PDA was quite large (5.5 mm), so ductal stenting was deferred.

The patient recovered in the cardiac ICU following this procedure, and prostaglandin E was discontinued with saturations consistently in the 80s with transient drops to the 70s in room air. Given his persistently low saturations and hypoplastic tricuspid valve, he was referred for ductal stenting at 7 days of life. Access was obtained in the femoral artery and vein, and angiography revealed a restrictive tubular PDA measuring 2.5 mm at the PA insertion and 12 mm in length (**FIGURE 6.22**; **Video 6.13**). A 3 × 12 mm Rebel coronary stent was subsequently delivered across the PDA via antegrade approach with a resultant diameter of 3.3 mm (**FIGURES 6.24A-D** and **6.25**; **Videos 6.13-6.18**). The child was ultimately discharged 10 days later with saturations in the mid-to upper 80s. He was clinically well following this procedure with good growth and development and at 3 months underwent a biventricular repair with a transannular RVOT patch, RV muscle bundle resection, tricuspid valvuloplasty, stent removal, and PDA ligation.

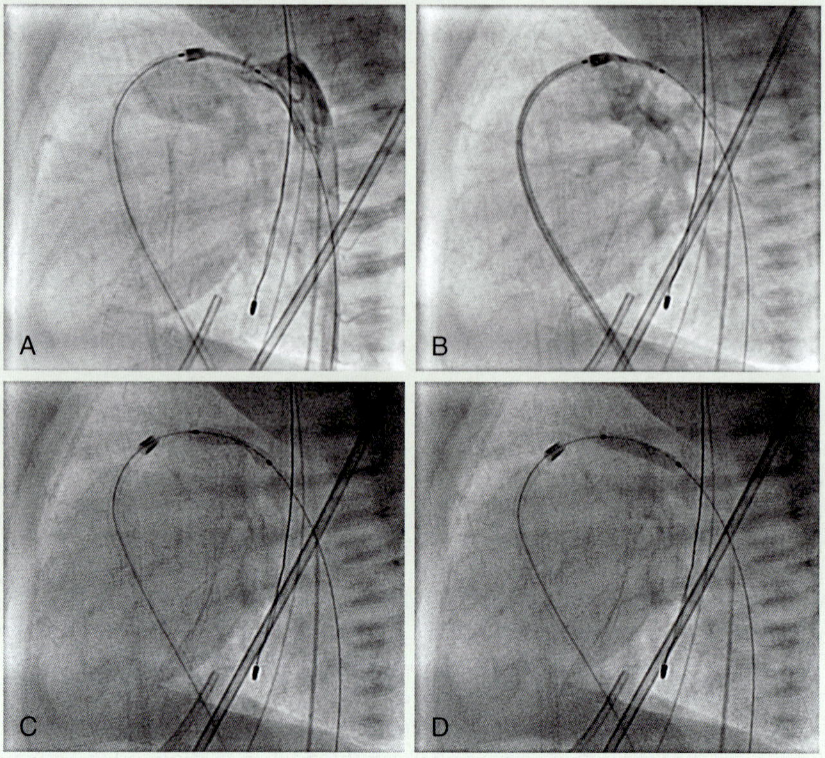

FIGURE 6.24 A Rebel coronary stent (Boston Scientific, Marlborough, MA) is positioned across the PDA. A, Retrograde injection through the pigtail catheter confirms the location of the stent in relation to the aortic and pulmonary insertions of the PDA. B, Antegrade injection through the long sheath confirms the position of the ductal stent in relation to the PA insertion of the PDA. C and D, The PDA stent is flared, then fully inflated across the PDA.

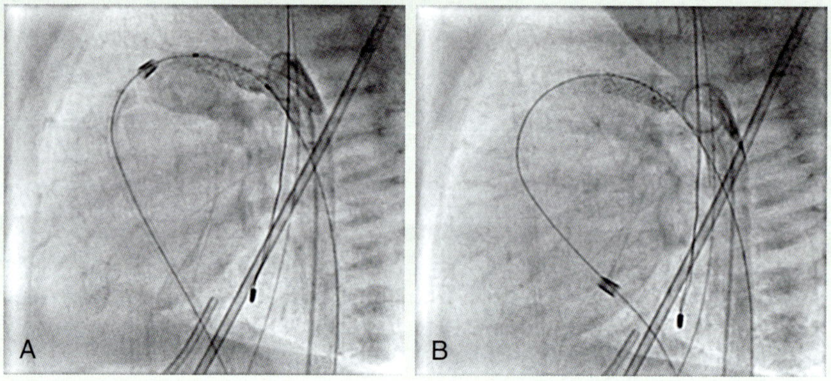

FIGURE 6.25 A, Retrograde injection with a pigtail catheter confirming stent position following inflation, while the guide wire and balloon remain in place. B, Retrograde injection with the pigtail catheter confirming stent position following removal of the balloon and before removal of the guide wire.

CLOSURE OF INTERATRIAL COMMUNICATIONS

Atrial Septal Defects, Patent Foramen Ovale Closure

Hemodynamic Assessment

- The ratio of pulmonary to systemic blood flow (Qp:Qs) is calculated by obtaining saturations in the superior vena cava (SVC), right or left PA, the aorta (Ao), and the PVs. Qp:Qs = (Ao-SVC)/(PA-PV). A Qp:Qs of 2 or greater in children, or Qp:Qs of 1.5 or greater in adults, is typically considered hemodynamically significant, although this assessment can vary depending on the clinical circumstances.
- Shunting across an ASD is determined by ventricular compliance properties, not by pressure differential, as a very large ASD, by definition, will equalize the pressures in both atria. The net shunt in patients with an isolated ASD is therefore left to right, as the left ventricle is less compliant than the RV. In conditions associated with restrictive RV physiology, such as advanced pulmonary hypertension and certain repaired right-sided heart congenital lesions, the net shunt is actually right to left.

Indications[1,2a,b]

- In the current era, the primary indication for ASD closure is RV volume overload. In general, echocardiographic and/or MRI data are used to make this determination. Most patients with RV volume overload will have a measured Qp:Qs > 2, and patients with a Qp:Qs < 1.5 are not generally thought to have a significant shunt.
- Symptoms, such as exercise intolerance, generally occur with large, long-standing shunts and are also an indication for intervention.
- Cryptogenic stroke or transient ischemic attack (TIA) is suspected to be due to paradoxical embolization of a venous thrombus through the ASD.
- In children, the presence of a right to left shunt in a patient with a pacemaker or device in the right atrium, who thus may be at increased risk of developing device thrombosis and embolization through the ASD leading to a systemic embolus.
- In adults, documented orthodeoxia-platypnea is an indication for percutaneous closure.
- Right to left shunt causing symptomatic cyanosis, in the subgroup of patients who do not have obstruction of flow through the lungs and will be able to maintain their cardiac output after closure of the ASD.
- Management of ASD in adults with more than mild elevation of pulmonary vascular resistance should include expertise in both adult congenital heart disease (ACHD) and pulmonary vascular disease, as ASD closure may worsen symptoms (pulmonary systolic pressure >=50% systemic, or pulmonary vascular resistance >= 30% of systemic vascular resistance).
- Indications for closure of PFO are not well defined, as data in randomized clinical trials have suggested but not consistently proven benefit compared with anticoagulation.[50-54] PFO closure may be considered in selected patients with a cryptogenic stroke and either a large PFO or atrial septal aneurysm (with 10 mm excursion of the septum),[53] if a complete workup does not reveal another reversible cause for stroke. Of note, atrial arrhythmias appear to be more common in the short-term period after PFO device closure, which can therefore put patients at risk of a cardioembolic event.

Key Aspects of Intervention

- With current technology, only secundum ASD are amenable to transcatheter closure; sinus venosus, coronary sinus, or primum ASD do not have circumferential rims to allow safe placement of current devices.
- Currently approved devices in the United States can close defects up to 38 mm, as long as there is enough distance from the edge of the device to other cardiac structures (adequate rims). Preprocedural assessment of maximal defect size and minimal rim size is usually performed by transesophageal echocardiogram (TEE)[55]
- Intraprocedural imaging with echocardiographic imaging (TEE or intracardiac echocardiogram, ICE) is used to guide the procedure. It helps reduce radiation exposure, confirm size of defect and characterize the rims of the defect and the proximity of other intracardiac structures (FIGURE 6.26).

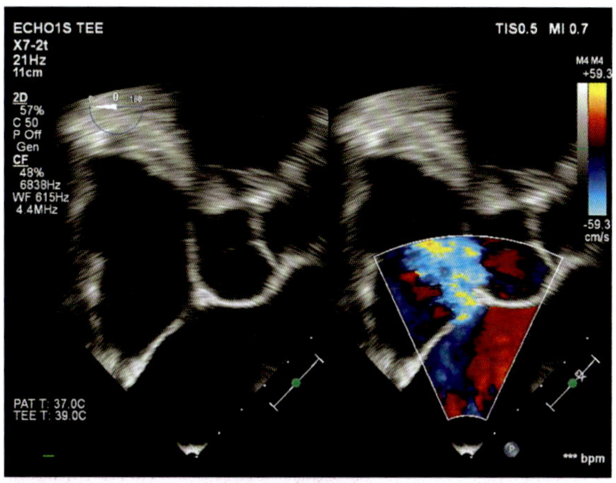

FIGURE 6.26 TEE images of ASD before closure. A 4 mm rim of retroaortic tissue is blurred by color flow Doppler imaging.

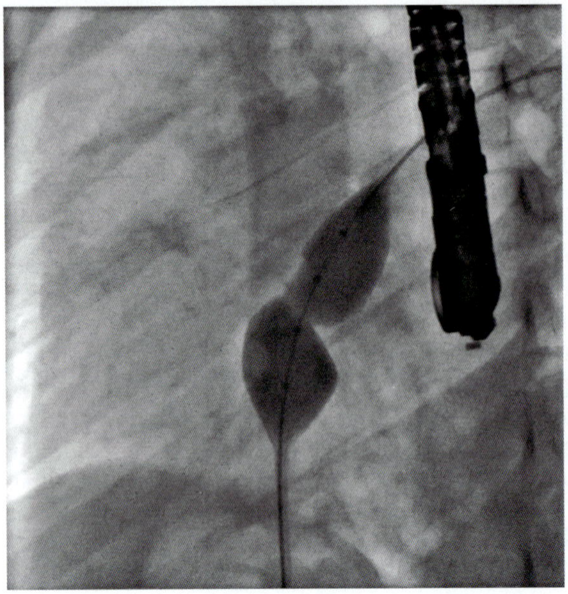

FIGURE 6.27 ASD balloon sizing. Note that for atrial defect closure considerations, the atrial septum is typically well profiled in LAO cranial or caudal angulation.

- Balloon sizing of the defect is performed to determine the "stretch size" of the defect, which will determine the size of the device used. It also helps exclude additional defects that may have been missed (**FIGURES 6.27** and **6.28**).
- Once the stretch size is determined, a device can be chosen and delivered under echocardiographic guidance.
- Once the device is delivered, adequate placement and lack of interference with valve function or venous return (pulmonary or systemic veins) can be confirmed before final release of the device.
- There are multiple devices currently available for ASD device closure. The most commonly used devices, and the only devices with FDA approval currently in the United States, are the Amplatzer septal occluder (St Jude Medical, St Paul, MN) and the Gore septal occluder (W.L. Gore and Associates, Inc, Flagstaff, AZ) (**FIGURES 6.29-6.32**; **Videos 6.19-6.22**).

Short- and Long-Term Results

- The short- and long-term results of ASD device closure are excellent, with over 98% complete closure rate at 1 year in most studies.[56,57]
- Procedural risks include device migration or malposition, access site complications, and heart block.
- Long-term complications such as device infection, thrombosis, and erosion are extremely rare. Device erosion has been reported in approximately 0.1% of patients undergoing device closure with devices made exclusively with Nitinol mesh, such as the Amplatzer septal

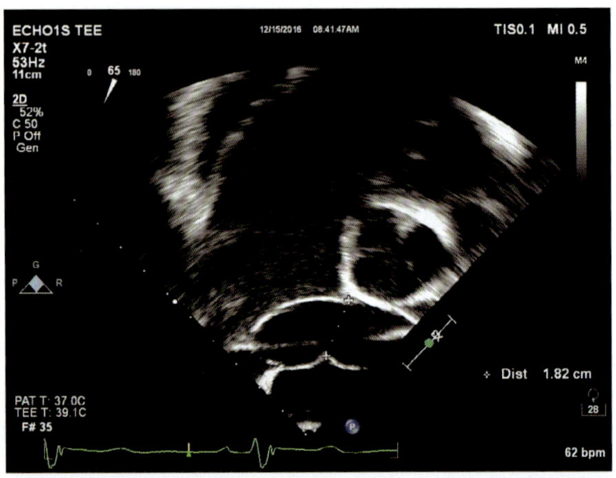

FIGURE 6.28 Balloon sizing on TEE. Measure is made along the plane of the atrial septum. Note how balloon sizing can obliterate adjacent atrial septal tissue; care should be taken to inflate only until interatrial flow has ceased, minimizing balloon overextension.

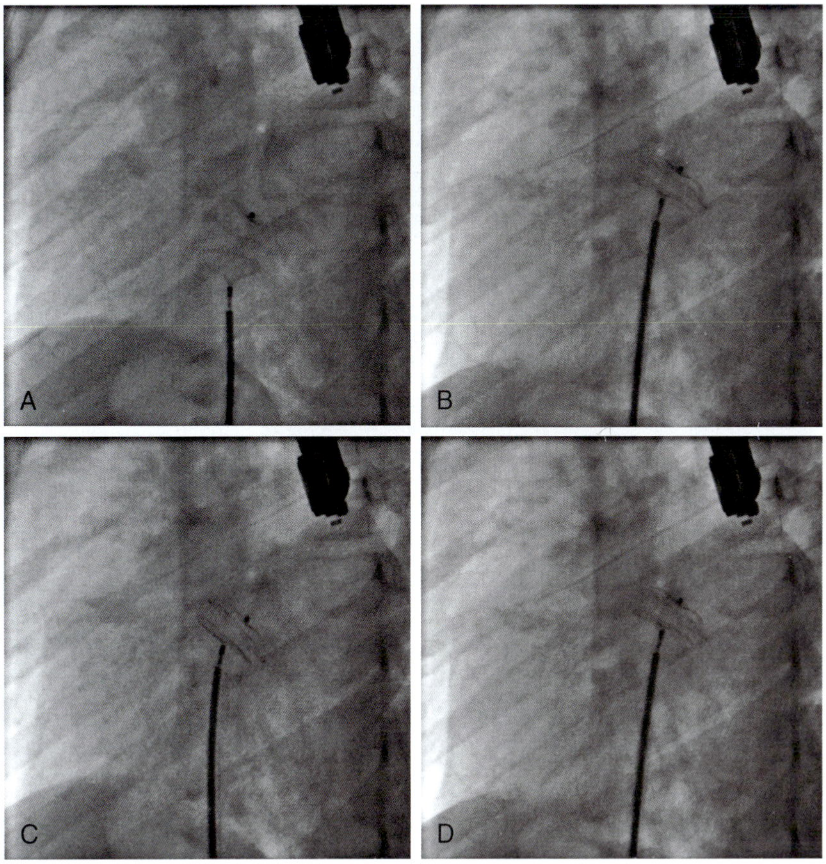

FIGURE 6.29 A-D, ASD closure device (Amplatzer) before release. Before release, it is critical to ensure that the ASD closure device is appropriately anchored to the atrial septum rims. This can be achieved by applying a to-and-fro force on the delivery cable.

occluder. In these patients, the device eroded through the roof of the atrium, into the pericardial space and/or the aortic root, producing acute hemopericardium. This is a rare, but potentially catastrophic complication. Currently, studies are ongoing to identify risk factors for this complication. It is worth mentioning that this kind of complication has not been reported with other types of devices with different design.

- Atrial arrhythmias (atrial flutter and fibrillation, most commonly) can occur despite closure of the defect and should be evaluated in follow-up.

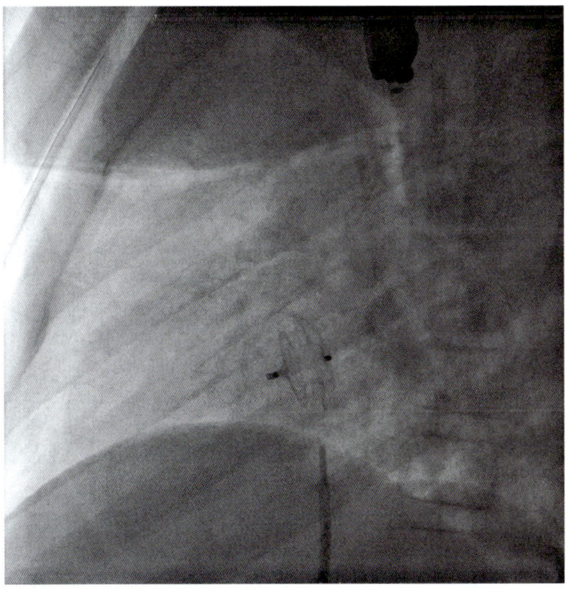

FIGURE 6.30 ASD closure device after release from the delivery cable.

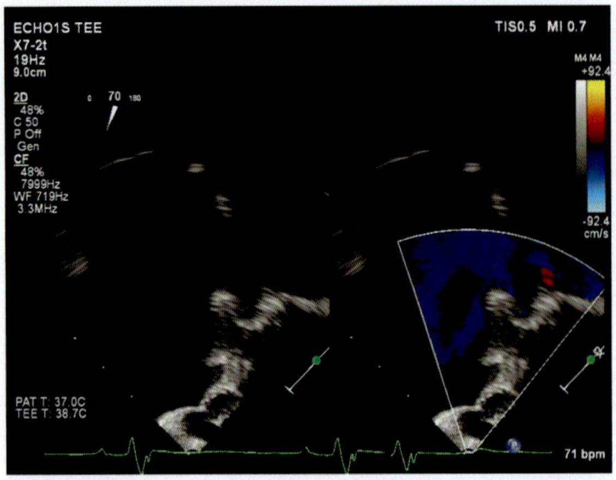

FIGURE 6.31 ASD closure device before release, as visualized by TEE. Note difficulty in visualizing atrial tissue caught between the discs of the closure device; care should be taken to visualize appropriate seating before device release.

Closure of Fontan Fenestrations or Baffle Leaks

Indications[1]

- Reduction of right to left shunts causing systemic desaturation associated with symptoms.
- Reduction of risk of paradoxical emboli, especially in patients with a large Fontan chamber, slow flow, atrial leads, or previous thrombi.

Key Aspects of Intervention

- The risks of the procedure and technique used depend on pulmonary pressures[58] and the material of the baffle (atrial tissue in intracardiac Fontan, or synthetic material in extracardiac baffles, which can become very calcified).
- The fenestration is crossed with a wire from the venous side. A low-pressure balloon is then used to occlude the fenestration for 10 to 20 minutes. Hemodynamics are measured at the end of the observation time, to ensure that there is no significant elevation in Fontan pressures and that systemic saturations do improve.
- TEE or ICE can be useful to determine which device is best suited for the anatomy. Fontan fenestrations are generally created with a 4 to 5 mm punch in the operating room and can be closed with an atrial septal occluder, while baffle leaks can have a more complex anatomy.

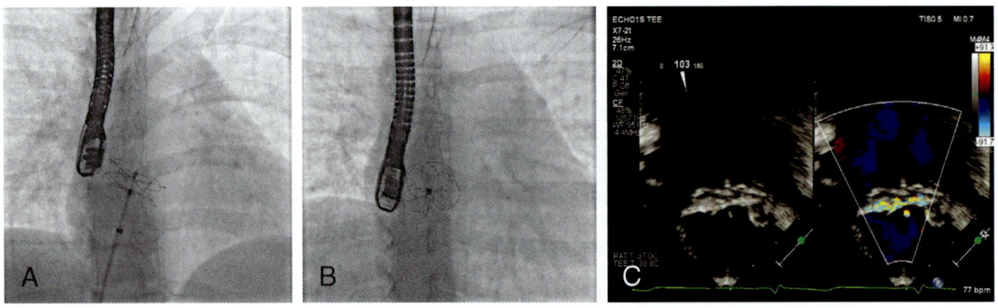

FIGURE 6.32 A and B, ASD closure device (GORE® CARDIOFORM® Septal Occluder) before and after release, in anterioposterior (AP) orientation. Note the change in orientation of the occluder after release from the catheter. C, ASD closure device after release, in 2D and with color Doppler on TEE. Note device flattening on both sides of the atrial septum and atrial septal tissue between the device discs. No interatrial passage of color Doppler flow is noted, although in many cases can be visualized until the device fully scars/endothelializes.

CLOSURE OF VENTRICULAR SEPTAL DEFECTS

Background

- Percutaneous ventricular septal defect (VSD) closure was first reported by Lock et al in 1987 in 6 patients using a Rashkind double umbrella closure device.[59]
- In the United States, the Amplatzer muscular VSD occluder, introduced in 1999, is the only FDA-approved device for closure of muscular VSDs.
- In the United States, there is currently no approved device for closure of perimembranous VSDs owing to a 6% incidence of bundle branch block and 3% incidence of complete heart block requiring permanent pacemaker placement in the US phase I trial[60]. More recent follow-up of the European registry showed a 5% incidence of complete AV block with closure of perimembranous VSDs versus 0.8% in muscular VSDs.[61]

Devices

- The Amplatzer muscular VSD occluder is a nitinol device composed of 2 flat discs, 8 mm larger in diameter than the central stalk, which is available in sizes from 4 to 18 mm and delivered through sheaths measuring 6 to 9 F.

Indications[1]

- In adults, Qp:Qs of at least 1.5:1, without pulmonary hypertension (Class I), as well as endocarditis attributed to the VSD (Class IIb).
- Hemodynamically significant muscular VSDs.
- Weight ≥5 kg.
- >4 mm of distance from the semilunar or atrioventricular valves.
- May consider periventricular approach in patients weighing <5 kg. In patients weighing less than 5 kg or unfavorable anatomy, a periventricular hybrid approach may be considered.

Risks

- Conduction disturbance ranging from first degree block to bundle branch block or complete heart block
- Device embolization
- Atrioventricular or semilunar valve regurgitation
- Hemolysis
- Cerebrovascular accident

Procedure

- Hemodynamic assessment including Qp:Qs, PVR, and ventricular EDP.
- Antegrade approach is preferred in small patients.
- Access via the internal jugular vein is preferred for the antegrade approach given the acute angle of the cardiac apex.
- Transesophageal or intracardiac echo are recommended to confirm device position and absence of associated valvar incompetence.
- An arteriovenous loop is recommended for device delivery.
- Following advancement of the sheath, the arteriovenous loop is removed from the body and the device is advanced to the tip of the sheath.
- Appropriately sized occluder (1-2 mm larger than the largest diameter of the defect) is advanced into the sheath.
- The distal disc is deployed in the appropriate chamber (LV if antegrade; RV if retrograde).
- The disc is pulled against the ventricular septum. Echo confirms clearance of the AV valve at this time.
- The proximal disk is deployed.
- Angiogram confirms appropriate placement.
- Device is released, and sheath is removed from the body (**FIGURES 6.33** and **6.34**).

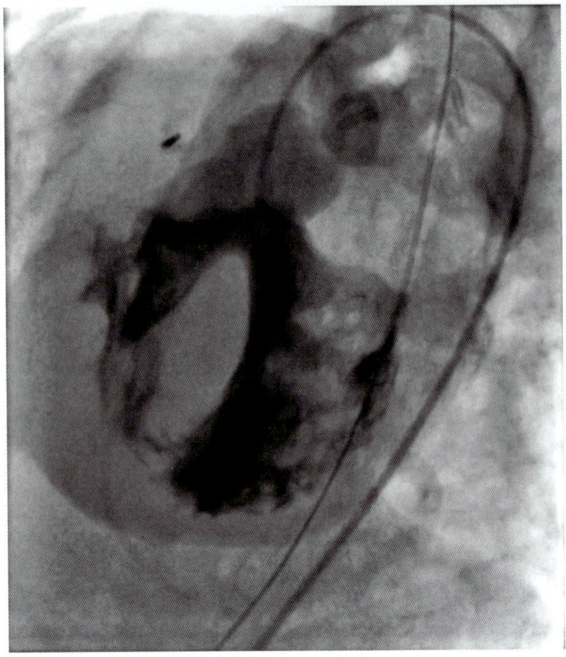

FIGURE 6.33 Retrograde LV injection (70° LAO, 28° cranial) shows a large conoventricular VSD and complex apical muscular VSD.

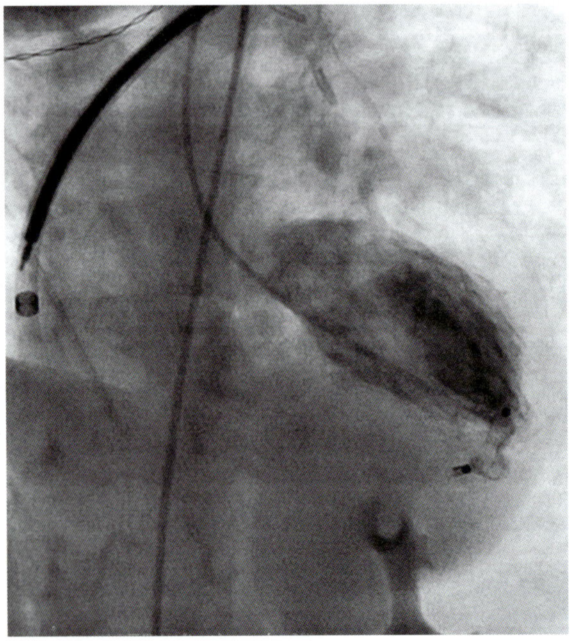

FIGURE 6.34 Retrograde LV injection (8° RAO, 39° cranial) following placement of a 4 mm Amplatzer VSD occluder shows trivial residual flow across the apical muscular VSDs.

CASE 4 *Representative Cineangiography Loops*

A 2-year-old, 8.2-kg male born at 31 weeks' gestational age with a large conoventricular VSD, PDA, and ASD with multiple comorbidities including duodenal atresia, malrotation, and bilateral inguinal hernias. Given his small size, multiple defects, and comorbidities, he underwent PA banding and PDA closure at 4 weeks of age. He was clinically well following this procedure with good growth and development and subsequently presented for VSD repair. After discussion with his surgeon, it was felt that he may benefit from transcatheter closure of the apical VSDs before closure of the conoventricular VSD given that there were multiple defects, which were located in the ventricular apex. He subsequently underwent catheterization, which revealed a well-placed PA band with a systemic RV pressure and Qp:Qs of 0.8. Angiography revealed a large, unrestrictive conoventricular VSD, small anterior muscular defect, and moderate apical muscular VSD measuring 3 to 4 mm using a balloon end-hole catheter to size the defect (**FIGURE 6.35**A and B; **Videos 6.23 and 6.24**). The VSD was subsequently crossed after which the arterial wire was snared, creating an arteriovenous loop (**FIGURE 6.36**; **Video 6.25**). A 4 mm Amplatzer VSD occluder was subsequently deployed via an antegrade approach with trivial residual flow across the defect (**FIGURE 6.37A**-D; **Videos 6.26-6.29**). He subsequently underwent surgical closure of the conoventricular VSD and a residual anterior muscular VSD.

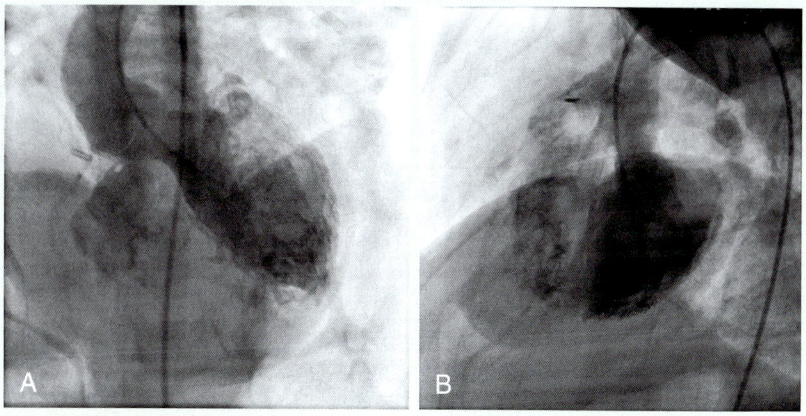

FIGURE 6.35 A, Retrograde LV injection in AP projection with 47° cranial angulation showing a large conoventricular VSD and a complex apical muscular VSD. B, Retrograde LV injection in the lateral projection (70° LAO, 28° cranial).

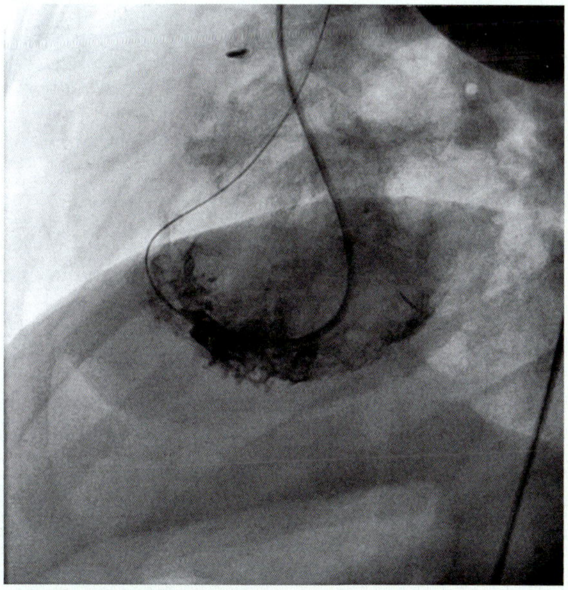

FIGURE 6.36 The VSD has been crossed. The arterial relay wire has been snared creating an arteriovenous loop.

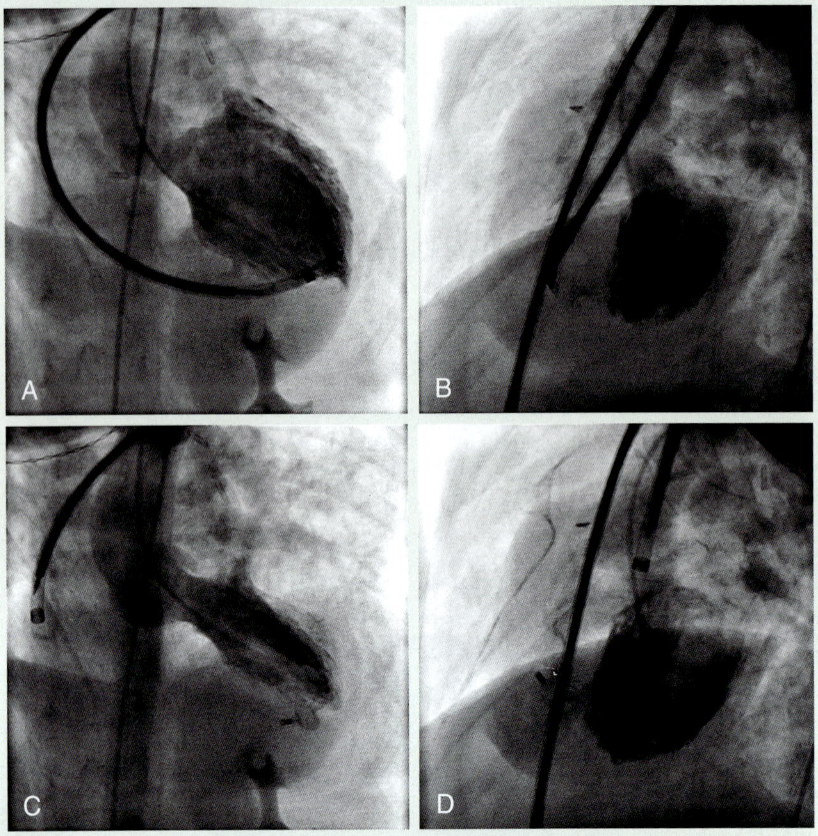

FIGURE 6.37 A, A long sheath is advanced from the left subclavian vein across the VSD into the LV, after which the guide wire is removed and the Amplatzer muscular VSD occluder (St. Jude Medical, St. Paul, MN) is delivered to the tip of the sheath. The distal disc is deployed in the LV apex after which the sheath is pulled back, opposing the RA disc against the ventricular septum. Retrograde left ventriculogram confirms the location of the VSD device in relation to the VSD, ventricular septum, and mitral valve apparatus. B, The RV disk is deployed and a retrograde left ventriculogram again confirms the placement of the device across the VSD. C and D, The device is released, and a left ventriculogram confirms the device location and assesses for residual VSDs. In this case, there is a mild amount of flow through the device (a usual findings) as well as residual left to right flow through the residual anterior muscular and conoventricular VSDs.

PATENT DUCTUS ARTERIOSUS CLOSURE

Preprocedural Assessment

- Although O_2 saturation assessment has been recommended, true measure of shunt amount (Qp:Qs) and pulmonary vascular resistance (PVR) require accurate measure of pulmonary blood flow (Qp), which is not possible, as shunt flow is preferentially into 1 PA, and adequate mixing of the shunted blood sample is not possible given the lack of a chamber distal to the shunt.
- Theoretically, combination of temporally related pressure assessment at catheterization and measure of total pulmonary blood flow and differential blood flow to each lung, obtained by MRI, could allow for precise measure of PVR.
- Flow through a PDA is left to right through all phases of the cardiac cycle (in the absence of severe pulmonary arterial hypertension); a PDA may have greater hemodynamic consequence than a similarly sized ASD or VSD.
- PDA are commonly described by their angiographic appearance as once of 5 types.

Indications and Risks of Intervention[1,2a,b]

- Significant left to right shunt with evidence of left atrial and/or ventricular enlargement/ overload thought to be due to the PDA or pulmonary hypertension (PA systolic pressure ≥ ½ systemic, or PVR ≥ 1/3 SVR).
- History of endarteritis.
- Controversial indication in asymptomatic children and adults to reduce the potential for future endarteritis.
- In children, distinction has been made between audible and inaudible PDA, with closure recommended for the former regardless of symptoms. With improved imaging techniques, in particular assessment of LV size and function, that distinction maybe clinically relevant.
- PDA closure is contraindicated in patients with pulmonary hypertension and a net right to left shunt, with PA systolic pressure >2/3 systemic or PVR >2/3 SVR.

Key Aspects of Intervention

- Intraprocedural imaging with TEE or ICE is needed to confirm the size of defect and adequate placement of the closure device before final deployment.
- Device types
  - Amplazer PDA occluder (St Jude Medical, St Paul, MN)
  - Amplazer vascular plug
  - Coils can be used for small PDAs, usually in infants or small children (up to 10% in a large series of patients weighing under 6 kg).[62]
  - Sizing
  - Angiography in the aorta just proximal to the PDA is performed with a pigtail catheter, in multiple views to determine the anatomy and largest diameter. Preprocedural imaging, such as CT, MRI or TEE, or rotational angiography during the procedure, can be used to identify ideal angles (FIGURE 6.38).
  - The Amplazer ductal occluder is composed of 2 discs; the largest is designed to be positioned in the aortic side of the PDA. The chosen device should have a pulmonary (smaller) disc that is at least 2 mm larger than the smallest diameter of the PDA.
- The PDA can be cannulated in an antegrade (venous femoral access, PA to aorta) or retrograde fashion (arterial femoral access, aorta to PA).

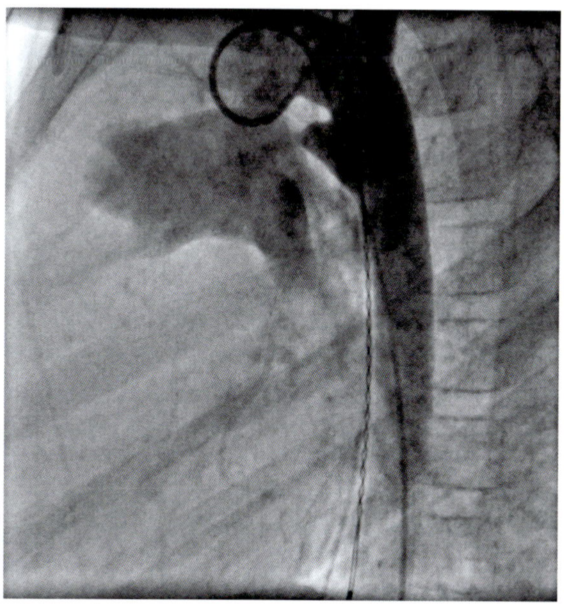

FIGURE 6.38 Lateral aortogram demonstrating shunt through PDA.

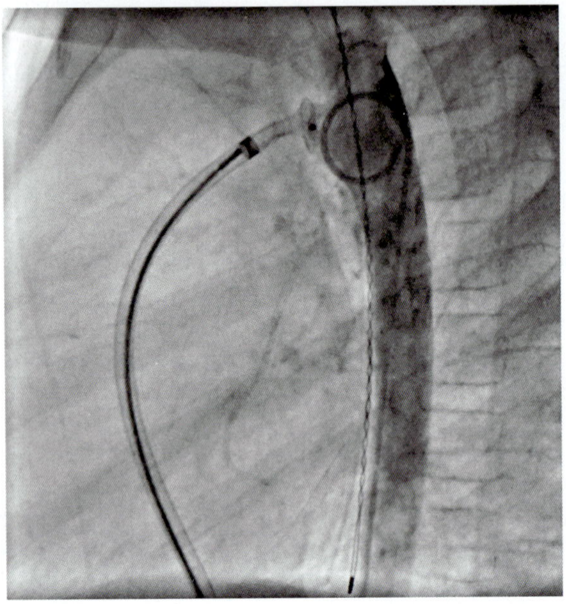

FIGURE 6.39 Amplatzer ductal occluder placed from PA across defect, partially deployed.

- Device placement is usually performed from the PA. If an antegrade approach is used, a multipurpose catheter and floppy wire are used to cross the PDA, and the catheter is advanced in the descending aorta. The wire is then exchanged for a stiff wire, over which the sheath and device are positioned (FIGURE 6.39).
- A repeat angiogram is performed 10 minutes after device deployment, to evaluate residual shunt (FIGURES 6.40 and 6.41).

Short- and Long-Term Results

- Procedural success in adolescents and adults is reported in ≥97% of cases, with angiographic or echocardiographic demonstration of occlusion ranging from 76% during the procedure to 99.7% at 1 year, after device endothelialization.[63,64]
- In children <6 kg, there is a lower incidence of procedural success (94.7%), with device embolization requiring retrieval occurring in 2.4% in a large observational study.[62]

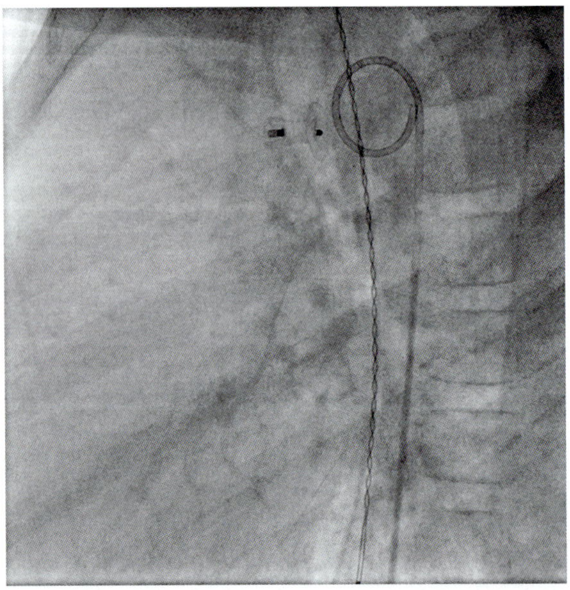

FIGURE 6.40 Amplatzerductal occluder after release.

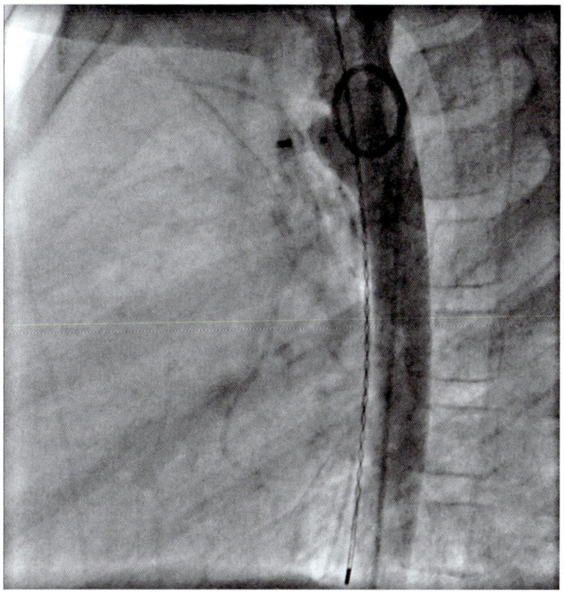

FIGURE 6.41 Lateral aortogram demonstrating patency of PDA after deployment of closure device.

CLOSURE OF EXTRACARDIAC SHUNTS

Assessment

- Extracardiac shunts can be categorized by their main symptoms.
  - Cyanosis: right to left shunts
    - Venovenous collaterals (from systemic veins to PVs or veins leading to pulmonary venous atrium, thus bypassing the lungs). Tend to develop most commonly in patients with a palliation of venous return connected to the higher resistance pulmonary arterial circuit, necessitating systemic venous pressure to be greater than pulmonary venous pressure.
    - Arteriovenous malformation (AVMs) in the lungs, between pulmonary arterioles (before alveoli) to pulmonary venules, therefore bypassing the oxygenated alveoli. These can either be of "macro" (large enough to visualize at angiography) or "micro" (rapid transit time through lungs, appearing, at times, similar to a miliary pattern) in nature (**FIGURE 6.42**).
  - Volume overload: left to right shunts
    - Systemic arteriovenous fistulas
      - Volume load for both ventricles.
      - Rarely congenital, more often due to trauma, or iatrogenic (such as after arterial and venous access for catheterization).
      - Coronary AV fistulas can also cause ischemia due to steal away from the downstream coronary tree.
    - Aortopulmonary collaterals (APCs; from aorta or its branches to branches of the pulmonary arterial tree). They are most commonly seen in patients with cyanotic heart disease and, in particular, in patients with a palliated single ventricle circulation.
    - PDA
    - Extrapulmonary arteriovenous malformations

Indications for Intervention[1]

- Symptomatic cyanosis
- Hemoptysis
- Ventricular enlargement without another identifiable cause
- High-output heart failure, pulmonary overcirculation, pleural effusions, or protein-losing enteropathy
- Systemic embolic events (in the setting of large pulmonary arteriovenous fistulas)

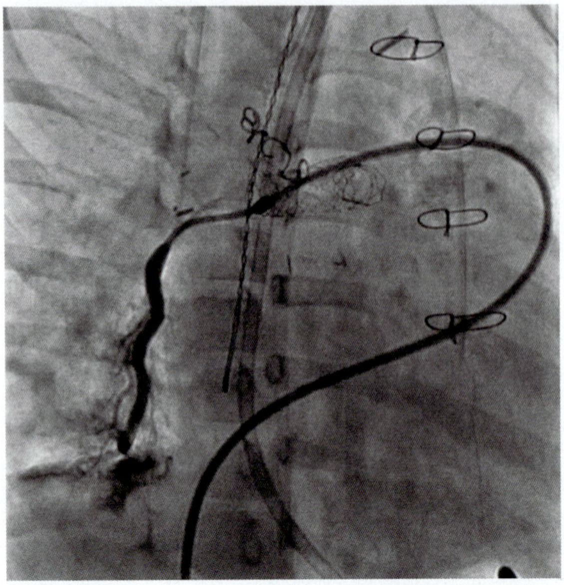

FIGURE 6.42 Selection angiography in a pulmonary arterial branch demonstrating AVM.

Key Aspects of Intervention

- Collaterals are identified by selective angiography in the most common vessels of origin, such as the subclavian arteries and veins, as well as an aortogram.
- Coils are most commonly used, chosen to have a diameter 1-2 mm larger than the target vessel.
- Coils are usually implanted at the most distal portion of target vessel that also allows for occlusion at the narrowest point in the target vessel (often at a kink, turn, or bifurcation). The vessel is filled as much as feasible with additional coils, so as to reduce potential for formation or progression of additional bridging collaterals.
- The guide catheter is positioned distal to the chosen site. The selected coil is inserted in the catheter and pushed to the tip of the catheter by a straight wire. The first loop is deployed by slight withdrawal of the guide catheter as well as push by the wire. The rest of the coil is then released either by pulling back on the guide catheter or by pushing with the guide wire.
- The Amplatzer vascular plugs (St. Jude Medical, St Paul, MN), made of self-expanding nitinol mesh, are available in 3 to 22 mm diameter and 3 shapes.
- Microspheres and gelfoam can be used to embolize smaller vessels (**FIGURE 6.43A**-C).

Short- and Long-Term Results

- Success of the procedure is >92%[65-67] and mostly depends on the stability of the guide catheter and ability to reach the target vessel.
- Vessel injury, bleeding, and distal embolization are possible complications.
- Endocarditis at the site of the coil is a very rare complication.

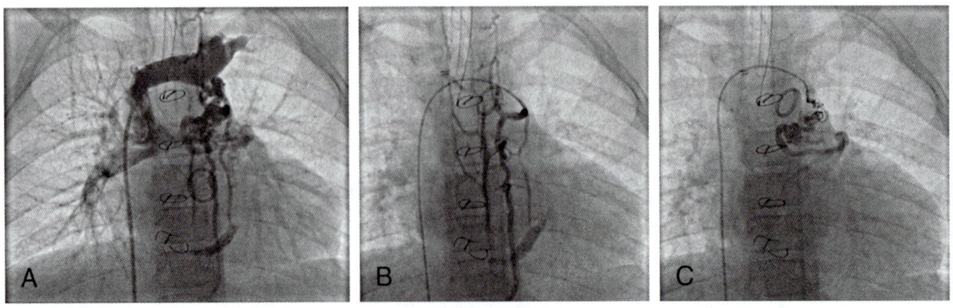

FIGURE 6.43 Network of venovenous collaterals from the innominate vein, including a branch to the coronary sinus, in a patient with pulmonary atresia and intact ventricular septum after a Fontan operation. A, Nonselective injection in upper limb of Fontan pathway. B, Selective injection inside collateral. C, Immediately after coiling; some residual may be seen.

AORTIC INTERVENTIONS

Coarctation of the Aorta

Hemodynamic Assessment

- Includes assessment of possible consequences of coarctation (CoA), such as elevated LV filling pressures (LVEDP or PCWP measurement); if high, consider RHC to assess RV and PA pressures.
- Measurement of gradient across the stenosis is traditionally reported as the peak-to-peak gradient, which is the difference between the peak systolic pressure proximal and distal to the obstruction during the same beat or 2 beats that are temporally as close as possible. There are 3 main methods of obtaining the peak-to-peak gradient.
  - Pullback method: simply pulling a pigtail or similar catheter back from proximal to distal to the area of obstruction.
  - Simultaneous pressures measurements with a catheter proximal and distal to the obstruction. This can be done with 2 separate catheters or by using a long sheath of at least 1 French-size larger than the pigtail or multipurpose catheter. Using this method, the long sheath and the catheter are placed in the transverse arch (proximal to the obstruction), and pressures are recorded simultaneously to show that the transducers are well calibrated. The long sheath is then pulled back "over" the catheter so that its tip is slowly pulled across the area of stenosis into the thoracic aorta, showing simultaneous pressures above and below the obstruction.
  - Simultaneous pressures using the standing wave: this method involves using the short sheath placed in the femoral artery and a smaller catheter proximal to the obstruction. Because the femoral artery pressure is usually higher than the thoracic aorta pressure (due to amplification from pressure waves reflected from the peripheral vasculature), a "standing wave" must be calculated first to avoid underestimating the pressure gradient. The standing wave is the difference between the systolic pressure in the thoracic aorta and the systolic pressure in the femoral artery. This standing wave is then added to the peak-to-peak gradient obtained with simultaneous measurements proximal to the obstruction and at the femoral artery. For example, if the systolic pressure in the thoracic aorta is 110 mm Hg and the systolic pressure in the femoral artery is 120 mm Hg, then the standing wave is 10 mm Hg. In this example, if the simultaneous pressure measurement in the transverse arch and the femoral artery is 150 and 120 mm Hg, the peak-to-peak gradient would be 40 mm Hg ([150-120] + 10).

Indications for intervention are based on consensus opinion and some data derived from nonrandomized studies. They include the following:

- Peak-to-peak gradient >20 mm Hg[1, 2a,b]
- Lower threshold of 10 mm Hg is sometimes used in patients with a single ventricle or presence of collaterals which may lead to lower measured gradient or heart failure without another identified cause.
  - The 2018 ACC/AHA guidelines for management of adults with congenital heart disease now recommend intervention for hypertension and severe CoA (defined as echo mean gradient >20 mm Hg, upper to lower extremity peak systolic BP gradient >20 mm Hg, or gradient >10 mm Hg with decreased LV function, or aortic regurgitation, or significant collateral flow) and anatomic narrowing.
  - Claudication symptoms and elevation in gradient with exercise (measured by ankle: brachial pressure index) are expanding indications

Key Aspects of Intervention

- In a single plane laboratory, the usual angiographic angle that is most useful for the initial angiography is the straight lateral view or sometimes an LAO projection (generally between 55 and 70° LAO). In a dual plane laboratory, the AP camera can be moved to an extreme caudal with 20 to 35° RAO. These views usually give good visualization of lesions in the distal arch or isthmus, but adjustments must be made for more complex lesions.

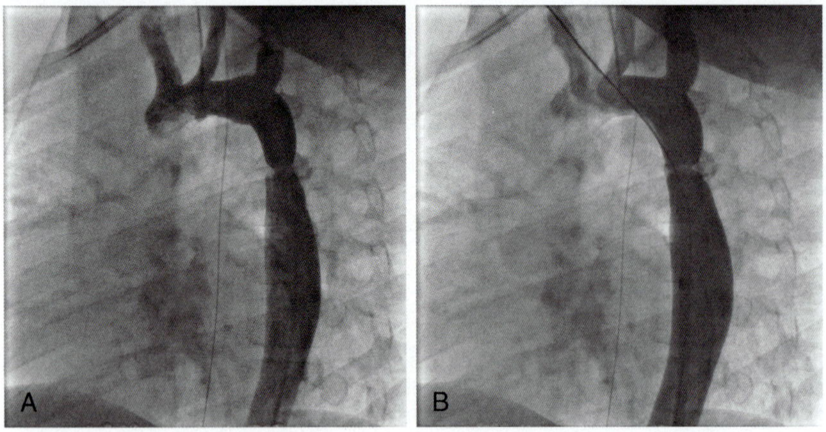

FIGURE 6.44 Angiogram of ringlike stenosis distal to origin of the left subclavian artery before (A) and after balloon dilation (B). Stent-free dilation leaves what is often viewed as a "less pleasing" immediate visual result, although in the setting of gradient relief, subsequent healing typically results in more optimal vessel appearance.

- Another technique to optimize the angiographic views is to place a pigtail catheter in the ascending aorta and then move the AP camera RAO until the part of the pigtail in the ascending aorta is perfectly aligned with the part of the pigtail in the descending aorta. The lateral camera is then made orthogonal to the AP camera. This ensures that the lateral camera is aligned perpendicular to the long axis of the aortic arch. Finally, the AP camera is brought to an extreme caudal orientation (approximately 30° caudal) and kept at the same degree of RAO. This ensures that the ascending aorta, transverse arch, and isthmus are not overlying each other and the angiogram will give a good "frontal" view of the isthmus (**FIGURE 6.44**A and B).
  - Once the angiogram has been obtained, the following measurements are performed:
    - Minimal luminal diameter
    - Diameter of the "normal aorta" above the obstruction
    - Diameter of the "normal aorta" below the obstruction

  The smaller of the latter 2 diameters will be used as the "normal aorta adjacent to the CoA", which helps guide balloon size choices (see below).

- 3D rotational angiography can be useful, especially in complex cases, when the arch is tortuous or when the obstruction involves the origin of the left subclavian artery (or that of an aberrant right subclavian artery). Use of preprocedural imaging (such as magnetic resonance angiography [MRA] or gated computed tomography angiography [CTA]) can be helpful to define 3D anatomy in advance of the procedure and decide on optimal fluoroscopy angle. The 3D data-sets can also be fused with the fluoroscopy images, which helps guide the procedure and may help reduce radiation and contrast use during the procedure (**FIGURE 6.45**A and B).
- Balloon angioplasty
  - Can be performed in native CoA, as a reintervention after initial surgical repair or prior stenting or as a predilation and/or compliance testing before planned stenting.
  - Rapid pacing during inflation is generally not required.
  - Initial choice of balloon is typically 80% to 90% of the diameter of the "normal" aorta adjacent to the obstruction, as long as it does not exceed 2 to 3× the narrowest luminal diameter.
  - Once the balloon is inflated, the waist on the balloon is examined by the operator before resolution of the waist. The ideal waist should be about 85% of the expanded part of the balloon. If the waist is tighter than 85%, the balloon is taken down and replaced with a smaller balloon, until the appropriate size balloon is identified. If the waist is above 85% of the expanded balloon, then the waist is resolved. This process is repeated until the obstruction is resolved, a therapeutic tear is seen on angiography, or a complication occurs. The balloon should not exceed 110% of the diameter of the normal aorta adjacent to the CoA.
  - Angiography should be performed after each balloon inflation to evaluate the result of the intervention and to confirm there have been no vascular tears or complications.
- Stenting
  - Performed as primary stenting, stenting after predilation and therapeutic tear, and stenting as rescue when a complication of balloon angioplasty occurs.

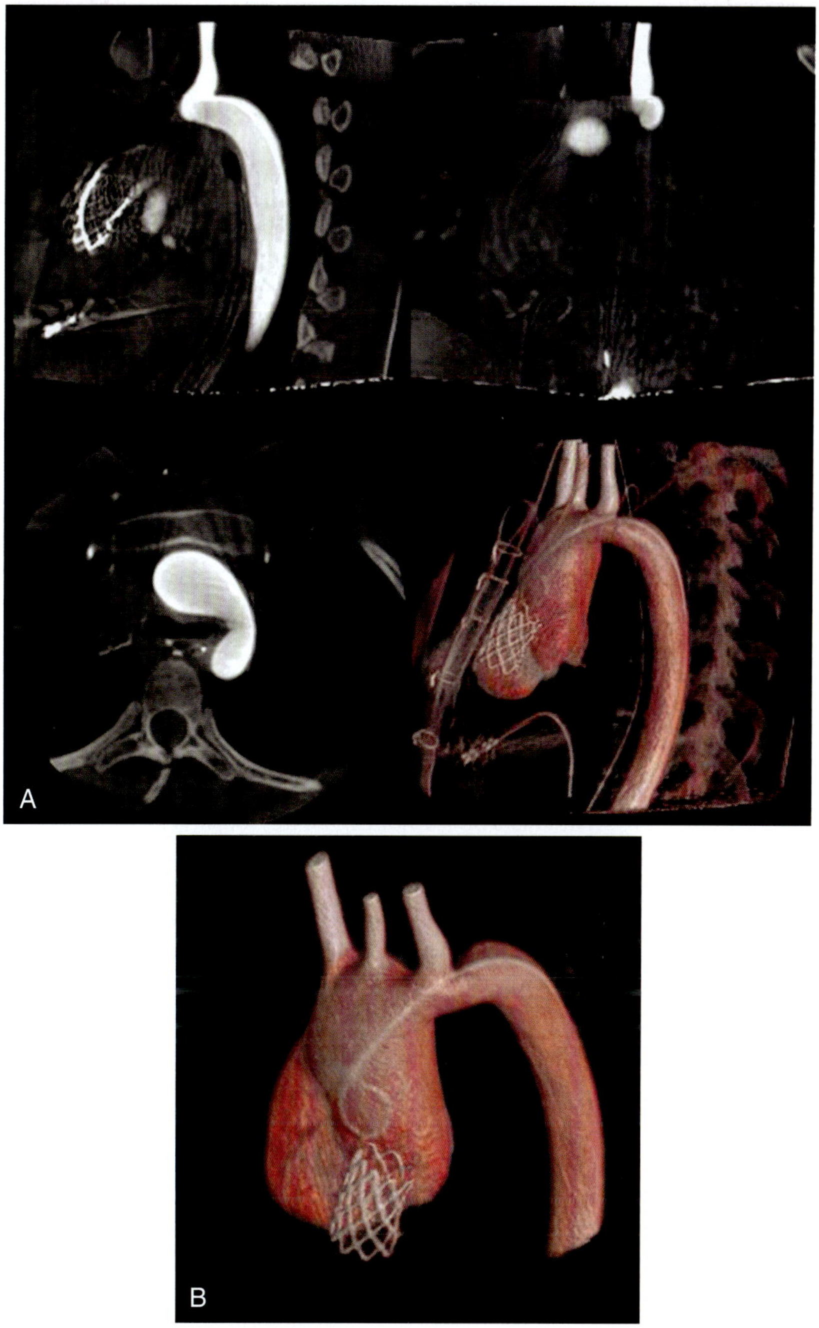

FIGURE 6.45 A and B, CTA and 3D reconstruction of a complex coarctation in a patient who had a Damus-Kaye-Stansel operation for hypoplastic left heart syndrome (anastomosis of the hypoplastic ascending aorta and the main PA, creating an ascending aorta with a "double-barrel" inverted "Y" appearance). Dilation and stenting of the hypoplastic proximal native aorta is uncommon; anatomic considerations were facilitated by use of 3D CTA reconstruction.

- Primary stenting refers to stenting the lesion without predilation. Sometimes a balloon is inflated across the lesion to size the lesion and to test the compliance, but this is done in a way that avoids therapeutic tears. This technique is preferred over balloon angioplasty alone or followed by stenting after a therapeutic tear in older children and adults in the majority of centers, as it is thought to have a lower incidence of aortic wall complications, including aneurysm formation in the long-term.[68] Stenting is also preferred in patients with longer segment of CoA and is the intervention of choice in patients with recurrent CoA after a previous balloon angioplasty.
- Bare-metal or covered stents can be used; the latter is preferred if there is a high risk of vessel injury or dissection, such as patients with severe CoA, prior aortic injury, aortopathy associated with higher risk of dissection, and older age, leading to less compliant aortic wall.[69,70] Stents should be available to the operator even if only balloon angioplasty is planned, in case it causes a dissection that needs to be treated with a stent.
- Goal for final stent diameter is to approximate size of most "normal" nearby aorta (**FIGURES 6.46** and **6.47**A, B; **Videos 6.30 and 6.31**).

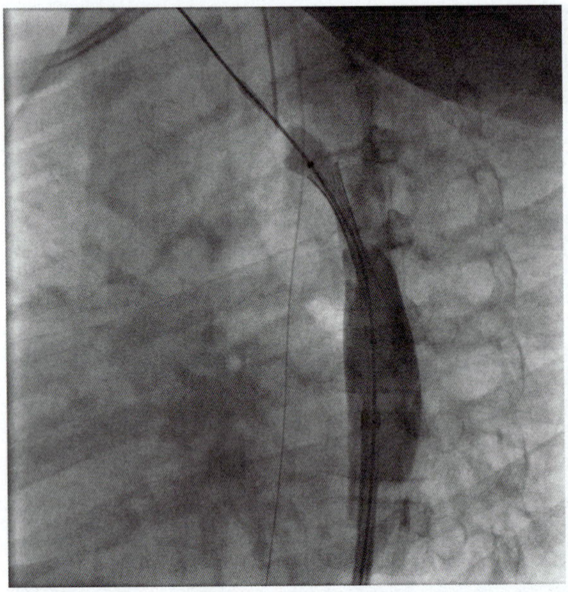

FIGURE 6.46 Angiogram in the descending aorta during early inflation of the balloon on which the stent is mounted, to confirm position of the stent across the stenosis. Angiogram can be performed via large covering sheath or via a second angiographic catheter placed from the radial artery.

Short- and Long-Term Results

- Balloon angioplasty alone in native CoA has high acute success rates (ranging from 80% to 100%[71-74]), but restenosis is common, especially in infants,[75] so it is usually only performed in patients who are not candidates for surgery.[1]
- Observational series and randomized trials of stent types report high degree (>95%) of procedural success.[68,76,77]
- Early procedural complications include access-site injury as well as aortic wall complications (dissection, rupture, and/or aneurysm/pseudoaneurysm formation). Aortic wall complications are reported to occur in approximately 4% of patients.[68] Technical complications such as stent migration or malposition can occur in up to 5% of patients in some series.[68] Long-term complications include dissection, aneurysm formation, and stent restenosis, which occur in 3% to 10% of patients, although the incidence of these complications may decrease in the current era.[68]

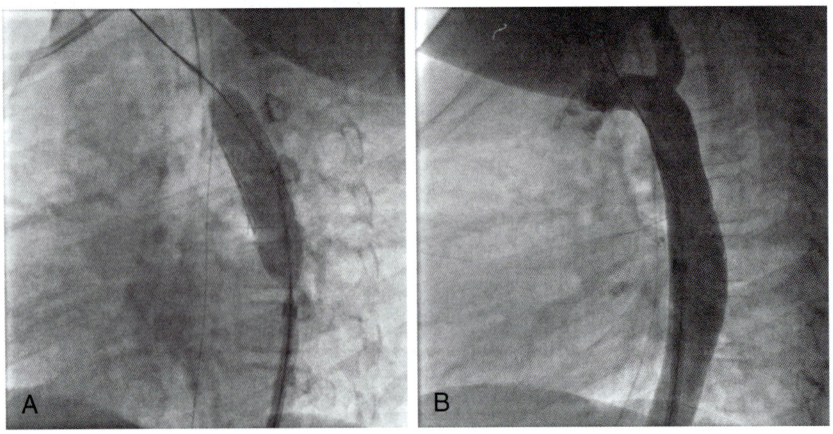

FIGURE 6.47 A and B, Stent deployment and final aortogram. Proximal guide wire positioning is chosen to allow greatest expansion of dilation balloon and stent parallel to the native aortic walls, with as unobstructed balloon expansion as possible. Typically, distal stent margins are not acutely flared to oppose more dilated poststenotic aneurysmal descending aorta; subsequent imaging after healing often demonstrates lack of such gap between distal stent and aorta.

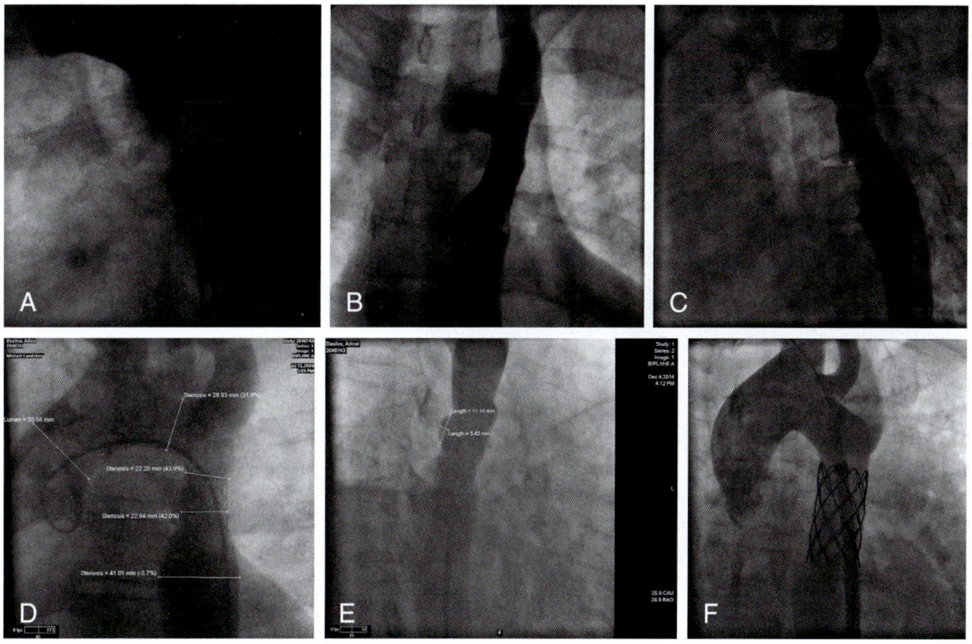

FIGURE 6.48 Severe coarctation s/p stenting in childhood (A and B) with original minimal diameter 3-4 mm; given severity of initial lesion, stenting to full aortic size at first setting, without graded dilations over multiple procedures, may have contributed to acute dissection or future aneurysm risk. Aneurysm distal to the stent was diagnosed 10 y later (C, D, and E), for which a covered stent (F) was implanted.

- Unplanned reinterventions for restenosis or aneurysm formation are reported in 5% of children at a mean of 1.7 years and 18% to 22% of children and adults followed for a mean of 5 years. Nearly all reinterventions are done percutaneously (balloon angioplasty with or without stent placement).
- Long-term implications of stent placement in the aorta and how this may affect vascular health and myocardial work are unknown (**FIGURE 6.48A**-F; Video 6.32).

Midaortic Syndrome

Background

- Midaortic syndrome is a term used to describe the syndrome of patients with obstructive lesions of the midaorta.
- Etiologies include idiopathic, thrombotic lesions, inflammatory disorders (Takaysu arteritis), and genetic disorders (neurofibromatosis-1, Williams syndrome, Alagille syndrome).

Indications

- There are no consensus guidelines at the present time.
- Reasonable indications would include systemic hypertension refractory to medical therapy and/or evidence of end-organ damage including renal dysfunction, congestive heart failure, or cerebrovascular accident.

Risks

- Small case series have reported a procedural mortality of 0% to 2%.[78-81]
- Acute vascular injury including tears or aneurysm formation.
  - Patients with NF-1 are at higher risk for vascular complications.
  - Patients with Takayasu arteritis and elevated inflammatory markers may be at increased risk of complications.
  - Younger age is associated with increased risk of complications.

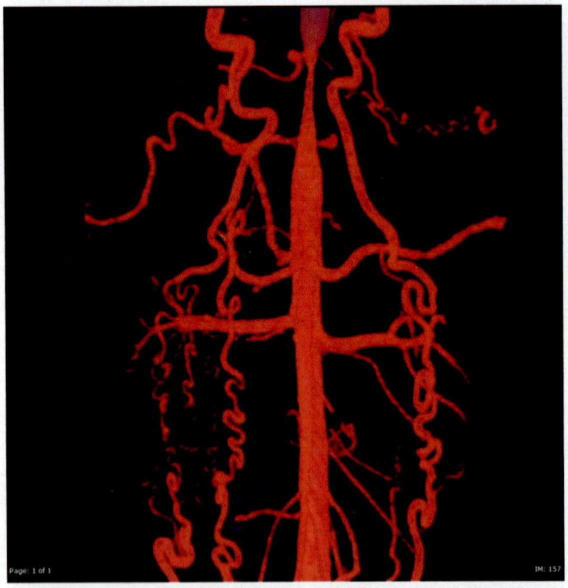

FIGURE 6.49 CTA of a patient with long-segment abdominal coarctation, which is located at the level of the diaphragm, cephalad to the origin of the celiac trunk. There is robust collateralization via the bilateral internal mammary arteries owing to long-standing obstruction.

Procedure

- Highly variable depending on the location, length, severity, and number of lesions.
- May require a combination of transcatheter and surgical interventions.
- Selective angiography is obtained of the associated lesions. 3D angiography and/or preoperative MRA of CTA provides invaluable information for complex interventions.
- Concordant use of intravascular ultrasound may provide useful information in regard to the lesion diameter as well as evidence of vessel wall inflammation.
- A combination of balloon angioplasty and/or endovascular stenting is used depending on the lesion severity and the age of the patient. Covered stents or vascular endografts should be available in the event of vascular rupture or aneurysm formation.
- There are currently no guidelines for the recommended ratio of the balloon to the luminal diameter of the lesion; however, some groups have adopted an approach of intentional underexpansion of stents in highly stenotic lesions with subsequent dilations 2 to 3 months later as a staged approach to avoid complications such as vascular tears or aneurysm formation (**FIGURES 6.49** and **6.50**).

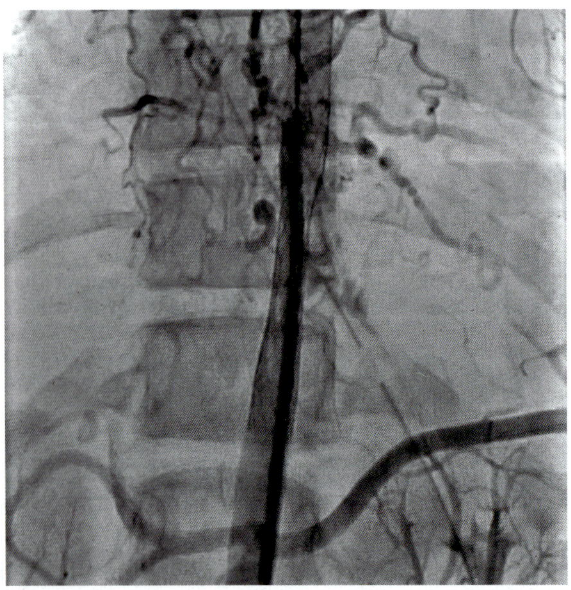

FIGURE 6.50 Injection in the descending thoracic aorta following stent placement shows improved caliber of the coarctation segment. The stent was intentionally underexpanded with an hourglass appearance and will be further dilated at a later date in an attempt to avoid aneurysm formation.

Short- and Long-Term Outcomes

- Acute successful relief of obstruction in most cases.
- In the largest reported cohort of patients with MAS, there was a 58% and 33% freedom from reintervention at 1 and 5 years, respectively.[80]
- Aneurysm formation, at the site of dilation or spontaneous formation remote to the area of intervention, remains frequent, occurring in 20% to 25% of patients.[79,80]
- A combination of surgical and catheter-based interventions led to a 96% and 90% survival at 1 and 15 years, respectively.

CASE 5 *Cineangiography Loops*

A 12-year-old, 37-kg, female was incidentally noted to be hypertensive at an urgent care visit for an upper respiratory infection. Subsequent evaluation revealed diminished lower extremity pulses, and an echocardiogram was suggestive of coarctation of the aorta. CTA subsequently revealed severe coarctation of the aorta approximately 15 mm above the celiac trunk, measuring approximately 11 mm in length with a luminal diameter of 3 mm. She was referred for a second opinion, and given the discrete nature of the coarctation segment and its proximity with a good amount of distance from the splanchnic vessels, we decided to pursue transcatheter intervention with primary stenting of the lesion. Given the frequent association with vascular tears and/or aneurysm formation, we elected to perform this as a staged procedure with intentional underexpansion of the stent with a plan to return in 2 to 3 months for gradual expansion of the stent to the appropriate size.

Initial hemodynamics revealed a normal LVEDP of 10 mm Hg with no gradient across the aortic valve or aortic arch. There was a 70 mm Hg peak-to-peak gradient from the proximal descending thoracic aorta to the abdominal aorta. Angiography demonstrated severe narrowing of the descending thoracic aorta as previously described. Intravascular ultrasound subsequently demonstrated that the mechanism of narrowing was due to homogenous concentric thickening of the intima/media of the vessel (**FIGURES 6.51-6.53**; **Videos 6.33-6.35**).

A 59 mm Genesis XD stent was placed over a 9 mm × 6 cm Cordis Powerflex balloon, which was expanded by hand with approximation of the distal and proximal ends of the stent against the vessel wall and with persistent narrowing of the midstent (**FIGURES 6.54** and **6.55**; **Videos 6.36 and 6.37**). The middle of the stent was subsequently dilated with a 6 m × 4 cm Conquest Balloon to 10 atm, expanding the mid portion of the stent (**FIGURES 6.56** and **6.57**; **Videos 6.38 and 6.39**). The gradient decreased to 29 mm Hg following this intervention. The patient returned to the catheterization laboratory 3 months later at which time the stent was further dilated up to an 8 mm balloon with a 15 mm Hg residual gradient.

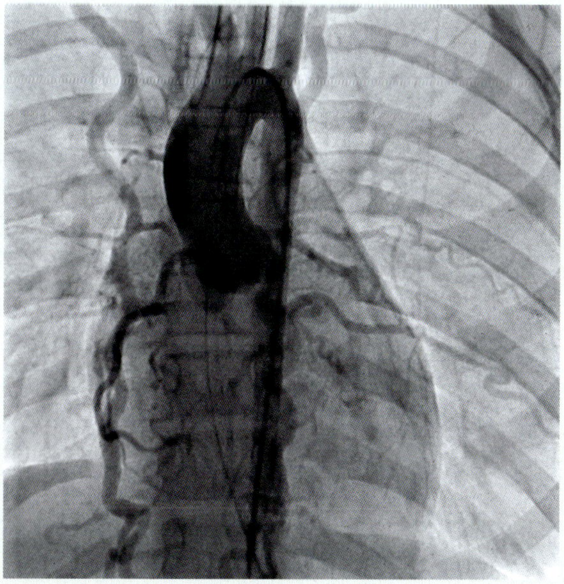

FIGURE 6.51 Aortogram shows no arch obstruction with severely dilated internal mammary and lateral thoracic arteries, suggestive of collateralization due to downstream obstruction.

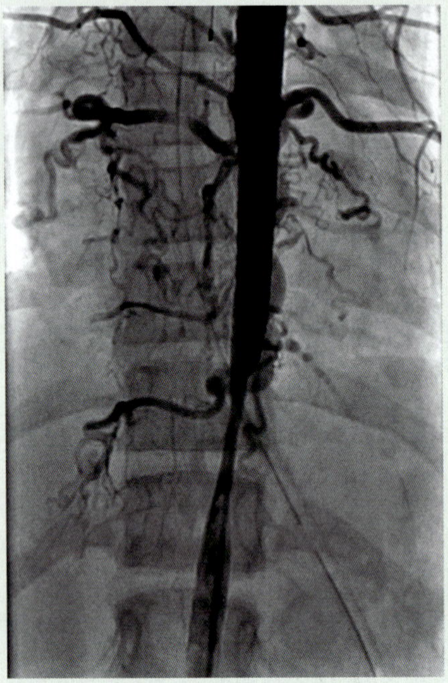

FIGURE 6.52 Injection in the descending thoracic aorta shows a long-segment coarctation in the AP projection at the level of the diaphragm, immediately superior to the celiac trunk, with collateralization of the splanchnic and thoracic vessels.

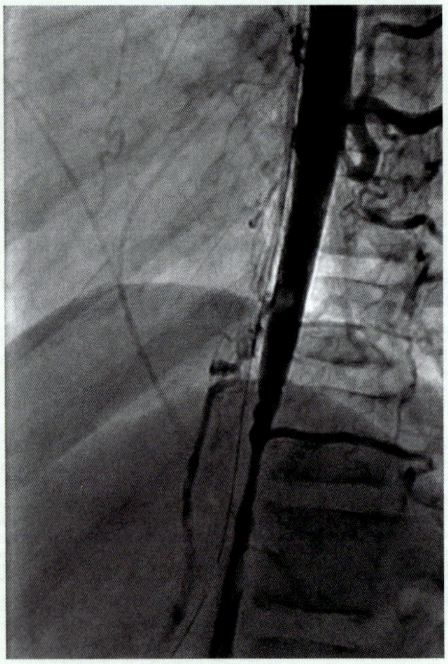

FIGURE 6.53 Injection in the descending thoracic aorta shows a long-segment coarctation in the lateral projection at the level of the diaphragm, immediately superior to the celiac trunk, with collateralization of the splanchnic and thoracic vessels.

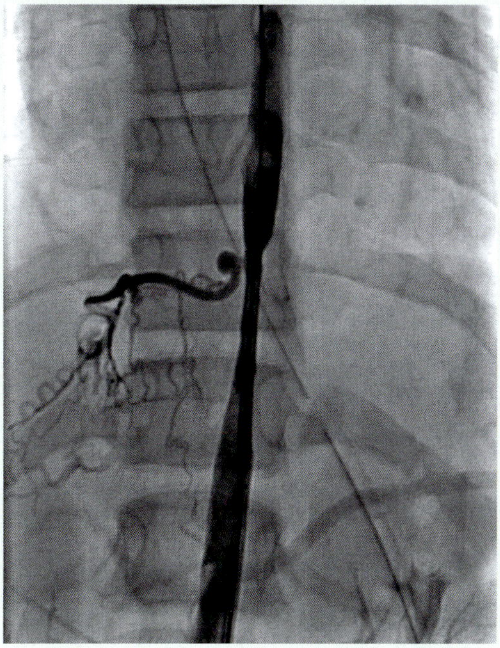

FIGURE 6.54 A stent is positioned across the coarctation segment, partially uncovered, and flared distally. Injection through the long sheath confirms the stent's location in relation to the coarctation as well as the splanchnic vessels.

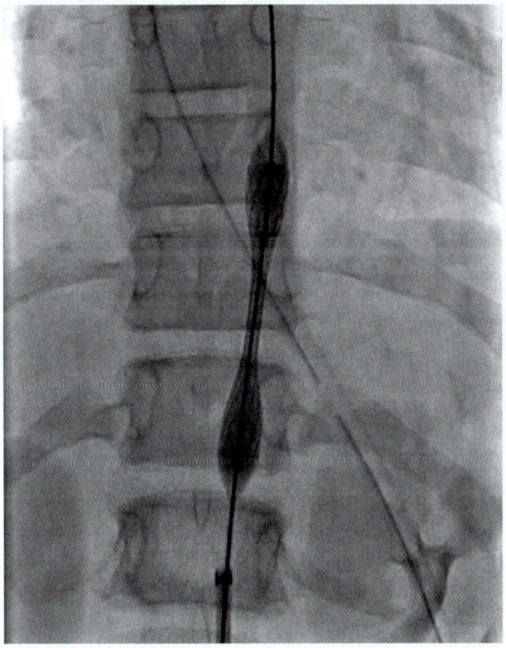

FIGURE 6.55 The stent is uncovered and inflated by hand with flaring of the distal and proximal ends of the stent, intentionally leaving a central stenosis, which is not resolved.

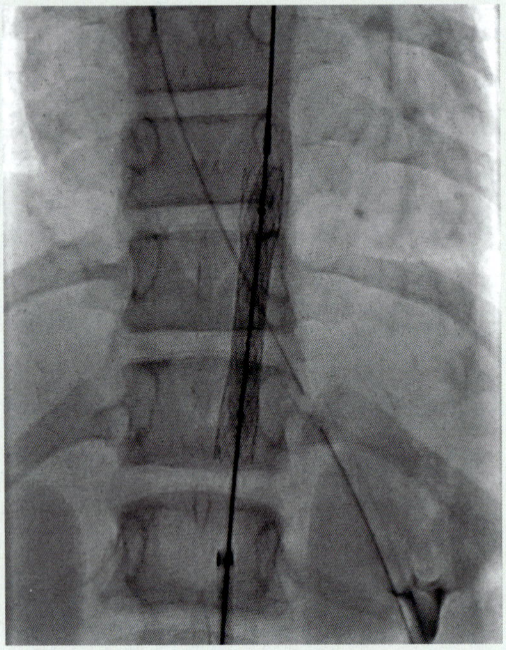

FIGURE 6.56 The central portion of the stent is dilated with a 6 mm balloon, partially resolving the central stenosis.

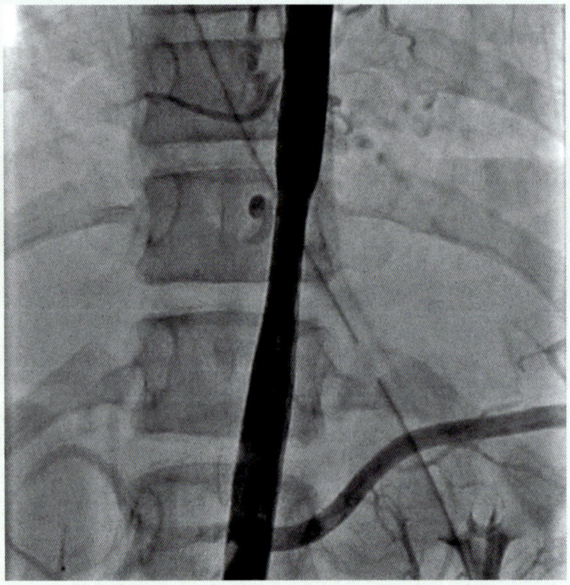

FIGURE 6.57 Injection following dilation of the stent shows improvement of the central stenosis. The proximal and distal stent is well opposed to the vessel wall and has not jailed the celiac artery. There is reduced flow through the collateral arteries, consistent with improved flow across the stenotic segment.

REFERENCES

1. Feltes TF, Bacha E, Beekman RH III, et al. Indications for cardiac catheterization and intervention in pediatric cardiac disease: a scientific statement from the American Heart Association. *Circulation*. 2011;123:2607-2652.

2a. Warnes CA, Williams RG, Bashore TM, et al. ACC/AHA 2008 guidelines for the management of adults with congenital heart disease: a report of the American College of Cardiology/American Heart Association Task Force on Practice Guidelines (Writing Committee to Develop Guidelines on the Management of Adults With Congenital Heart Disease). *Circulation*. 2008;118:e714-e833.

2b. Stout KK, Daniels CJ, Aboulhosn JA, et al. AHA/ACC 2018 Guideline for the management of adults With congenital heart disease: a report of the American College of Cardiology/American Heart Association Task Force on Clinical Practice Guidelines. J Am Coll Cardiol. 2018.

3. Kan JS, White RI Jr, Mitchell SE, Gardner TJ. Percutaneous balloon valvuloplasty: a new method for treating congenital pulmonary-valve stenosis. *N Engl J Med*. 1982;307:540-542.

4. *Congenital Heart Disease: The Catheterization Manual*. Boston, MA: Springer; 2009.

5. Stanger P, Cassidy SC, Girod DA, Kan JS, Lababidi Z, Shapiro SR. Balloon pulmonary valvuloplasty: results of the valvuloplasty and angioplasty of congenital anomalies registry. *Am J Cardiol.* 1990;65:775-783.
6. Rao PS, Galal O, Patnana M, Buck SH, Wilson AD. Results of three to 10 year follow up of balloon dilatation of the pulmonary valve. *Heart.* 1998;80:591-595.
7. McCrindle BW. Independent predictors of long-term results after balloon pulmonary valvuloplasty. Valvuloplasty and angioplasty of congenital anomalies (VACA) registry investigators. *Circulation.* 1994;89:1751-1759.
8. Steinberg ZL, Jones TK, Verrier E, Stout KK, Krieger EV, Karamlou T. Early outcomes in patients undergoing transcatheter versus surgical pulmonary valve replacement. *Heart.* 2017;103:1455-60.
9. Cheatham JP, Hellenbrand WE, Zahn EM, et al. Clinical and hemodynamic outcomes up to 7 years after transcatheter pulmonary valve replacement in the US melody valve investigational device exemption trial. *Circulation.* 2015;131:1960-1970.
10. Butera G, Milanesi O, Spadoni I, et al. Melody transcatheter pulmonary valve implantation. Results from the registry of the Italian Society of Pediatric Cardiology. *Cathet Cardiovasc Interv.* 2013;81:310-316.
11. Oosterhof T, van Straten A, Vliegen HW, et al. Preoperative thresholds for pulmonary valve replacement in patients with corrected tetralogy of fallot using cardiovascular magnetic resonance. *Circulation.* 2007;116:545-551.
12. Lee C, Kim YM, Lee C-H, et al. Outcomes of pulmonary valve replacement in 170 patients with chronic pulmonary regurgitation after relief of right ventricular outflow tract obstruction: implications for optimal timing of pulmonary valve replacement. *J Am Coll Cardiol.* 2012;60:1005-1014.
13. Hallbergson A, Gauvreau K, Powell AJ, Geva T. Right ventricular remodeling after pulmonary valve replacement: early gains, late losses. *Ann Thorac Surg.* 2015;99:660-666.
14. McElhinney DB, Benson LN, Eicken A, Kreutzer J, Padera RF, Zahn EM. Infective endocarditis after transcatheter pulmonary valve replacement using the Melody valve: combined results of 3 prospective North American and European studies. *Circ Cardiovasc Interv.* 2013;6:292-300.
15. Hascoet S, Mauri L, Claude C, et al. Infective endocarditis risk after percutaneous pulmonary valve implantation with the melody and sapien valves. *JACC Cardiovasc Interv.* 2017;10:510-517.
16. Ogawa A, Satoh T, Fukuda T, et al. Balloon pulmonary angioplasty for chronic thromboembolic pulmonary hypertension: results of a multicenter registry. *Circ Cardiovasc Qual Outcomes.* 2017;10.
17. Yacouby S, Meador M, Mossad E. Lung reperfusion injury in patients after balloon angioplasty for pulmonary artery stenosis. *J Cardiothorac Vasc Anesth.* 2014;28:502-505.
18. Law MA, Shamszad P, Nugent AW, et al. Pulmonary artery stents: long-term follow-up. *Catheter Cardiovasc Interv.* 2010;75:757-764.
19. Cunningham JW, McElhinney DB, Gauvreau K, et al. Outcomes after primary transcatheter therapy in infants and young children with severe bilateral peripheral pulmonary artery stenosis. *Circ Cardiovasc Interv.* 2013;6:460-467.
20. Rothman A, Perry SB, Keane JF, Lock JE. Early results and follow-up of balloon angioplasty for branch pulmonary artery stenoses. *J Am Coll Cardiol.* 1990;15:1109-1117.
21. Fender EA, Packer DL, Holmes DR Jr. Pulmonary vein stenosis after atrial fibrillation ablation. *EuroIntervention.* 2016;12(suppl X):X31-X34.
22. Esch JJ, Porras D, Bergersen L, Jenkins KJ, Marshall AC. Systemic embolic complications of pulmonary vein angioplasty in children. *Pediatr Cardiol.* 2015;36:1357-1362.
23. Peng LF, Lock JE, Nugent AW, Jenkins KJ, McElhinney DB. Comparison of conventional and cutting balloon angioplasty for congenital and postoperative pulmonary vein stenosis in infants and young children. *Catheter Cardiovasc Interv.* 2010;75:1084-1090.
24. Rehman M, Jenkins KJ, Juraszek AL, et al. A prospective phase ii trial of vinblastine and methotrexate in multivessel intraluminal pulmonary vein stenosis in infants and children. *Congenit Heart Dis.* 2011;6:608-623.
25. Prieto LR, Schoenhagen P, Arruda MJ, Natale A, Worley SE. Comparison of stent versus balloon angioplasty for pulmonary vein stenosis complicating pulmonary vein isolation. *J Cardiovasc Electrophysiol.* 2008;19:673-678.
26. Fink T, Schluter M, Heeger CH, et al. Pulmonary vein stenosis or occlusion after catheter ablation of atrial fibrillation: long-term comparison of drug-eluting versus large bare metal stents. *Europace.* 2017. doi:10.1093/europace/eux291.
27. Rashkind WJ, Miller WW. Transposition of the great arteries. Results of palliation by balloon atrioseptostomy in thirty-one infants. *Circulation.* 1968;38:453-462.
28. Vogel JH. Balloon embolization during atrial septostomy. *Circulation.* 1970;42:155-156.
29. Williams GD, Ahrend TR, Dungan WT. An unusual complication of balloon-catheter atrial septostomy. *Ann Thorac Surg.* 1970;10:556-559.
30. Ellison RC, Plauth WH Jr, Gazzaniga AB, Fyler DC. Inability to deflate catheter balloon: a complication of balloon atrial septostomy. *J Pediatr.* 1970;76:604-606.
31. Applegate SE, Lim DS. Incidence of stroke in patients with d-transposition of the great arteries that undergo balloon atrial septostomy in the University Healthsystem Consortium Clinical Data Base/Resource Manager. *Catheter Cardiovasc Interv.* 2010;76:129-131.
32. Beca J, Gunn J, Coleman L, et al. Pre-operative brain injury in newborn infants with transposition of the great arteries occurs at rates similar to other complex congenital heart disease and is not related to balloon atrial septostomy. *J Am Coll Cardiol.* 2009;53:1807-1811.
33. McQuillen PS, Hamrick SE, Perez MJ, et al. Balloon atrial septostomy is associated with preoperative stroke in neonates with transposition of the great arteries. *Circulation.* 2006;113:280-285.
34. Petit CJ, Rome JJ, Wernovsky G, et al. Preoperative brain injury in transposition of the great arteries is associated with oxygenation and time to surgery, not balloon atrial septostomy. *Circulation.* 2009;119:709-716.
35. Polito A, Ricci Z, Fragasso T, Cogo PE. Balloon atrial septostomy and pre-operative brain injury in neonates with transposition of the great arteries: a systematic review and a meta-analysis. *Cardiol Young.* 2012;22:1-7.
36. Baker EJ, Allan LD, Tynan MJ, Jones OD, Joseph MC, Deverall PB. Balloon atrial septostomy in the neonatal intensive care unit. *Br Heart J.* 1984;51:377-378.
37. Zellers TM, Dixon K, Moake L, Wright J, Ramaciotti C. Bedside balloon atrial septostomy is safe, efficacious, and cost-effective compared with septostomy performed in the cardiac catheterization laboratory. *Am J Cardiol.* 2002;89:613-615.
38. Gibbs JL, Rothman MT, Rees MR, Parsons JM, Blackburn ME, Ruiz CE. Stenting of the arterial duct: a new approach to palliation for pulmonary atresia. *Br Heart J.* 1992;67:240-245.
39. Alwi M, Choo KK, Latiff HA, Kandavello G, Samion H, Mulyadi MD. Initial results and medium-term follow-up of stent implantation of patent ductus arteriosus in duct-dependent pulmonary circulation. *J Am Coll Cardiol.* 2004;44:438-445.
40. Mallula K, Vaughn G, El-Said H, Lamberti JJ, Moore JW. Comparison of ductal stenting versus surgical shunts for palliation of patients with pulmonary atresia and intact ventricular septum. *Catheter Cardiovasc Interv.* 2015;85:1196-1202.

41. McMullan DM, Permut LC, Jones TK, Johnston TA, Rubio AE. Modified blalock-taussig shunt versus ductal stenting for palliation of cardiac lesions with inadequate pulmonary blood flow. *J Thorac Cardiovasc Surg*. 2014;147:397-401.
42. Udink Ten Cate FE, Sreeram N, Hamza H, Agha H, Rosenthal E, Qureshi SA. Stenting the arterial duct in neonates and infants with congenital heart disease and duct-dependent pulmonary blood flow: a multicenter experience of an evolving therapy over 18 years. *Catheter Cardiovasc Interv*. 2013;82:E233-E243.
43. Roggen M, Rega F, Gewillig M. Short-cut under pressure: stenting the tortuous neonatal duct involves induced spasm. *JACC Cardiovasc Interv*. 2012;5:e25-e26.
44. Lee KJ, Hinek A, Chaturvedi RR, et al. Rapamycin-eluting stents in the arterial duct: experimental observations in the pig model. *Circulation*. 2009;119:2078-2085.
45. Lee KJ, Seto W, Benson L, Chaturvedi RR. Pharmacokinetics of sirolimus-eluting stents implanted in the neonatal arterial duct. *Circ Cardiovasc Interv*. 2015;8.
46. Santoro G, Gaio G, Giugno L, et al. Ten-years, single-center experience with arterial duct stenting in duct-dependent pulmonary circulation: early results, learning-curve changes, and mid-term outcome. *Catheter Cardiovasc Interv*. 2015;86:249-257.
47. Bentham JR, Zava NK, Harrison WJ, et al. Duct stenting versus modified blalock-taussig shunt in neonates with duct-dependent pulmonary blood flow: associations with clinical outcomes in a multicenter national study. *Circulation*. 2018;137:581-588.
48. Glatz AC, Petit CJ, Goldstein BH, et al. Comparison between patent ductus arteriosus stent and modified blalock-taussig shunt as palliation for infants with ductal-dependent pulmonary blood flow: insights from the congenital catheterization research collaborative. *Circulation*. 2018;137:589-601.
49. Sivakumar K, Bhagyavathy A, Coelho R, Satish R, Krishnan P. Longevity of neonatal ductal stenting for congenital heart diseases with duct-dependent pulmonary circulation. *Congenit Heart Dis*. 2012;7:526-533.
50. Meier B, Kalesan B, Mattle HP, et al. Percutaneous closure of patent foramen ovale in cryptogenic embolism. *N Engl J Med*. 2013;368:1083-1091.
51. Furlan AJ, Reisman M, Massaro J, et al. Closure or medical therapy for cryptogenic stroke with patent foramen ovale. *N Engl J Med*. 2012;366:991-999.
52. Carroll JD, Saver JL, Thaler DE, et al. Closure of patent foramen ovale versus medical therapy after cryptogenic stroke. *N Engl J Med*. 2013;368:1092-1100.
53. Mas JL, Derumeaux G, Guillon B, et al. Patent foramen ovale closure or anticoagulation vs. antiplatelets after stroke. *N Engl J Med*. 2017;377:1011-1021.
54. Saver JL, Carroll JD, Thaler DE, et al. Long-term outcomes of patent foramen ovale closure or medical therapy after stroke. *N Engl J Med*. 2017;377:1022-1032.
55. Silvestry FE, Cohen MS, Armsby LB, et al. Guidelines for the echocardiographic assessment of atrial septal defect and patent foramen ovale: from the American Society of Echocardiography and Society for Cardiac Angiography and Interventions. *J Am Soc Echocardiogr*. 2015;28:910-958.
56. Turner DR, Owada CY, Sang CJ Jr, Khan M, Lim DS. Closure of secundum atrial septal defects with the amplatzer septal occluder: a prospective, multicenter, post-approval study. *Circ Cardiovasc Interv*. 2017;10.
57. Javois AJ, Rome JJ, Jones TK, et al. Results of the U.S. Food and Drug Administration continued access clinical trial of the GORE HELEX septal occluder for secundum atrial septal defect. *JACC Cardiovasc Interv*. 2014;7:905-912.
58. Pihkala J, Yazaki S, Mehta R, et al. Feasibility and clinical impact of transcatheter closure of interatrial communications after a fenestrated Fontan procedure: medium-term outcomes. *Catheter Cardiovasc Interv*. 2007;69:1007-1014.
59. Lock JE, Block PC, McKay RG, Baim DS, Keane JF. Transcatheter closure of ventricular septal defects. *Circulation*. 1988;78:361-368.
60. Fu YC, Bass J, Amin Z, et al. Transcatheter closure of perimembranous ventricular septal defects using the new Amplatzer membranous VSD occluder: results of the U.S. Phase I trial. *J Am Coll Cardiol*. 2006;47:319-325.
61. Carminati M, Butera G, Chessa M, et al. Transcatheter closure of congenital ventricular septal defects: results of the European Registry. *Eur Heart J*. 2007;28:2361-2368.
62. Backes CH, Kennedy KF, Locke M, et al. Transcatheter occlusion of the patent ductus arteriosus in 747 infants <6 kg: insights from the NCDR IMPACT registry. *JACC Cardiovasc Interv*. 2017;10:1729-1737.
63. Pass RH, Hijazi Z, Hsu DT, Lewis V, Hellenbrand WE. Multicenter USA amplatzer patent ductus arteriosus occlusion device trial: initial and one-year results. *J Am Coll Cardiol*. 2004;44:513-519.
64. Wang JK, Wu MH, Hwang JJ, Chiang FT, Lin MT, Lue HC. Transcatheter closure of moderate to large patent ductus arteriosus with the amplatzer duct occluder. *Catheter Cardiovasc Interv*. 2007;69:572-578.
65. Pereira-da-Silva T, Martins JD, de Sousa L, et al. Percutaneous occlusion of vascular malformations in pediatric and adult patients: 20-year experience of a single center. *Catheter Cardiovasc Interv*. 2016;87:E62-E68.
66. Barwad P, Ramakrishnan S, Kothari SS, et al. Amplatzer vascular plugs in congenital cardiovascular malformations. *Ann Pediatr Cardiol*. 2013;6:132-140.
67. Hill SL, Hijazi ZM, Hellenbrand WE, Cheatham JP. Evaluation of the amplatzer vascular plug for embolization of peripheral vascular malformations associated with congenital heart disease. *Catheter Cardiovasc Interv*. 2006;67:113-119.
68. Forbes TJ, Garekar S, Amin Z, et al. Procedural results and acute complications in stenting native and recurrent coarctation of the aorta in patients over 4 years of age: a multi-institutional study. *Catheter Cardiovasc Interv*. 2007;70:276-285.
69. Taggart NW, Minahan M, Cabalka AK, Cetta F, Usmani K, Ringel RE. Immediate outcomes of covered stent placement for treatment or prevention of aortic wall injury associated with coarctation of the aorta (COAST II). *JACC Cardiovasc Interv*. 2016;9:484-493.
70. Sohrabi B, Jamshidi P, Yaghoubi A, et al. Comparison between covered and bare cheatham-platinum stents for endovascular treatment of patients with native post-ductal aortic coarctation: immediate and intermediate-term results. *JACC Cardiovasc Interv*. 2014;7:416-423.
71. McCrindle BW, Jones TK, Morrow WR, et al. Acute results of balloon angioplasty of native coarctation versus recurrent aortic obstruction are equivalent. Valvuloplasty and Angioplasty of Congenital Anomalies (VACA) Registry Investigators. *J Am Coll Cardiol*. 1996;28:1810-1817.
72. Porras D, Brown DW, Marshall AC, Del Nido P, Bacha EA, McElhinney DB. Factors associated with subsequent arch reintervention after initial balloon aortoplasty in patients with norwood procedure and arch obstruction. *J Am Coll Cardiol*. 2011;58:868-876.
73. Forbes TJ, Kim DW, Du W, et al. Comparison of surgical, stent, and balloon angioplasty treatment of native coarctation of the aorta an observational study by the CCISC (Congenital Cardiovascular Interventional Study Consortium). *J Am Coll Cardiol*. 2011;58:2664-2674.

74. Fletcher SE, Nihill MR, Grifka RG, O'Laughlin MP, Mullins CE. Balloon angioplasty of native coarctation of the aorta: midterm follow-up and prognostic factors. *J Am Coll Cardiol.* 1995;25:730-734.
75. Fruh S, Knirsch W, Dodge-Khatami A, Dave H, Pretre R, Kretschmar O. Comparison of surgical and interventional therapy of native and recurrent aortic coarctation regarding different age groups during childhood. *Eur J Cardio Thorac Surg.* 2011;39:898-904.
76. Ringel RE, Vincent J, Jenkins KJ, et al. Acute outcome of stent therapy for coarctation of the aorta: results of the coarctation of the aorta stent trial. *Catheter Cardiovasc Interv.* 2013;82:503-510.
77. Meadows J, Minahan M, McElhinney DB, McEnaney K, Ringel R. Intermediate outcomes in the prospective, multicenter coarctation of the aorta stent trial (coast). *Circulation.* 2015;131:1656-1664.
78. Rao SA, Mandalam KR, Rao VR, et al. Takayasu arteritis: initial and long-term follow-up in 16 patients after percutaneous transluminal angioplasty of the descending thoracic and abdominal aorta. *Radiology.* 1993;189:173-179.
79. Siwik ES, Perry SB, Lock JE. Endovascular stent implantation in patients with stenotic aortoarteriopathies: early and medium-term results. *Catheter Cardiovasc Interv.* 2003;59:380-386.
80. Porras D, Stein DR, Ferguson MA, et al. Midaortic syndrome: 30 years of experience with medical, endovascular and surgical management. *Pediatr Nephrol.* 2013;28:2023-2033.
81. Sharma S, Bahl VK, Saxena A, Kothari SS, Talwar KK, Rajani M. Stenosis in the aorta caused by non-specific aortitis: results of treatment by percutaneous stent placement. *Clin Radiol.* 1999;54:46-50.

chapter 7

Pressure Measurements

MAURO MOSCUCCI, MD, MBA, and CALIN V. MANIU, MD

INTRODUCTION

The beginning of invasive hemodynamics can be traced back to the early 1700s, when Rev. Stephen Hales measured the blood pressure of a horse by inserting a brass rod in the femoral artery (FA), and observing a column of blood rising into a 9 foot glass tube connected to the rod.[1,2] He was surprised to see that the horse barely moved and appeared to be well afterward. Stephen Hales later proceeded to define what we know today as cardiac output, by measuring the amount of blood going through the heart in 1 minute. About a century later, in 1844, the first invasive cardiac catheterization was performed by Claude Bernard. Again, the subject was a horse, and both the right and left ventricles were entered by retrograde approach from the jugular vein and from the carotid artery. In 1861, Chauveau and Marey published their work regarding the cardiac cycle and their discovery that ventricular systole and apical beat are simultaneous. In addition, they were able to measure simultaneously left ventricular (LV) and central aortic (Ao) pressure. Over the following century, the field of cardiac catheterization continued to expand.[2] In 1929, Werner Forssmann performed the first right-sided heart catheterization of a human heart on himself[3] (**FIGURE 7.1**), and in 1931, he proceeded to demonstrate that it was possible to inject contrast material in the human heart.[4] In the same year, O'Klein in Prague measured cardiac output in man according to Fick principle.[5] Further progress ensued with the pioneering work of Cournand and Richards, who performed cardiac catheterization in many clinical conditions including hypertension, circulatory shock, and chronic lung disease.[6-17] As Cournand elegantly said in his Nobel Prize acceptance speech, the cardiac catheter was "only the key that opened the lock".[18] However, the lock that was open has been critical in understanding the pathophysiology of many cardiovascular conditions.[2]

While the past 2 decades have been characterized by an expansion of noninvasive assessment of cardiac function, with the development of the new field of catheter-based interventions for structural heart disease, invasive hemodynamic assessment remains a mainstay of cardiac catheterization and interventional cardiology. The objective of this chapter is to provide a brief review of classic hemodynamic measurements and tracings.

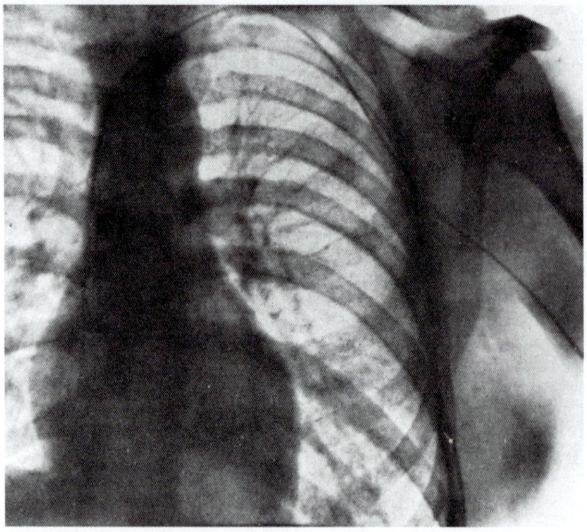

FIGURE 7.1 The first documented cardiac catheterization. At the age of 25 years, while receiving clinical instruction in surgery at Eberswalde, Werner Forssmann passed a catheter 65 cm through one of his left antecubital veins until its tip entered the right atrium (RA). He then walked to the radiology department where this roentgenogram was taken. Reproduced with permission from *Klin Wochenschr.* 1929;8:2085. Berlin, Heidelberg, New York: Springer-Verlag.

PRESSURE WAVEFORMS

As shown in **FIGURES 7.2-7.5** the pressure waveform is the summation of forward pressure, forward flow waves, and reflected waves.[19-22] Various conditions can affect the magnitude of reflected waves. For example, pressure reflections decrease during the strain phase of the Valsalva maneuver and increase during the release phase.[23] They decrease in the setting of hypovolemia and in response to vasodilators, while they are higher in patients with hypertension, heart failure,[20] and aortic or iliofemoral obstruction.[24] The interaction between forward flow waves, forward pressure, reflected waves, and the time needed for pressure and flow waves to travel in the arterial tree will result in different timing and shape of the arterial waveform at different sites of the arterial tree[19,22,25] (**FIGURES 7.4-7.6**).

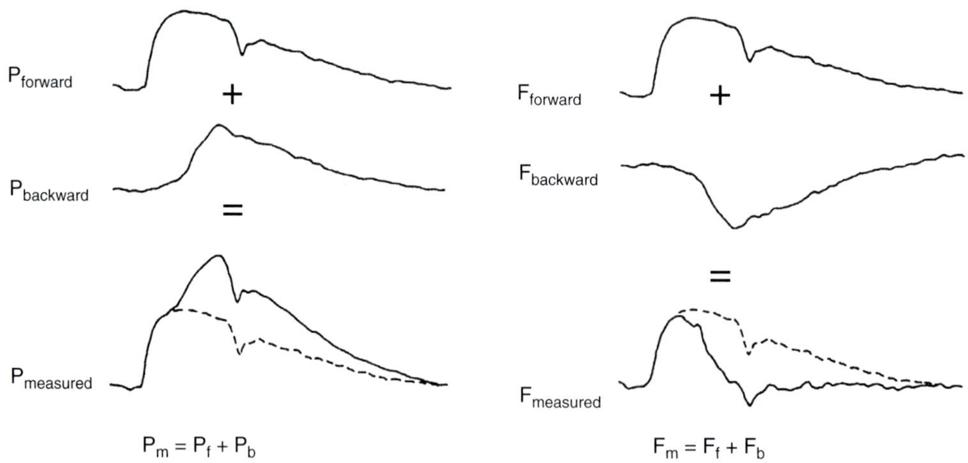

FIGURE 7.2 Central Ao pressure (P) and flow (F) measured in a patient during cardiac catheterization. Computer-derived forward and backward pressure and flow components are shown individually. Their sum results in the measured waves. (See text for discussion.) From Murgo JP, Westerhof N, Giolma JP, et al. Manipulation of ascending aortic pressure and flow wave reflections with Valsalva maneuver: relationship to input impedance. *Circulation*. 1981;63:122, with permission.

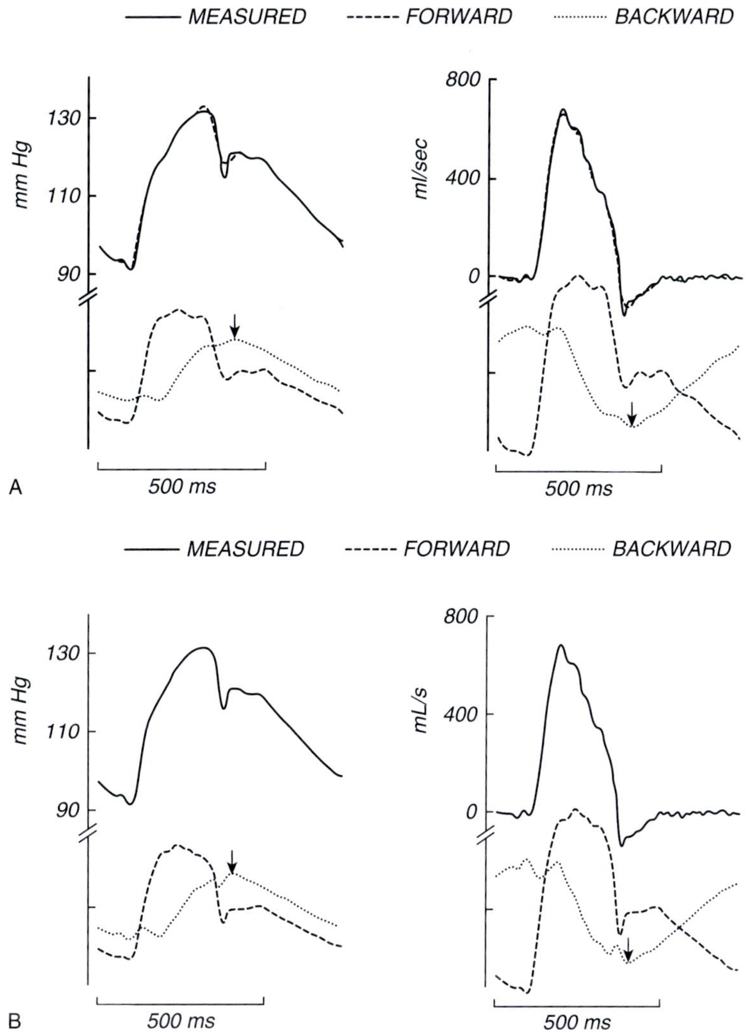

FIGURE 7.3 Representative ascending Ao pressure and velocity signals from normal subject at rest. The upper panels (A) are the measured pressure (left) and flow (right) pulses, and the lower panels depict the composite forward and reflected components. The superimposed dashed line in the upper panels represents the inverse Fourier transformed composite wave (derived from frequency domain analysis). Arrow indicates peak of backward wave. B, the time domain method of measured wave (upper panels) decomposition yields forward and reflected components (lower panels) in close agreement with the frequency domain method illustrated in panel A Reproduced with permission from Laskey WK, Kussmaul WG. Arterial wave reflection in heart failure. *Circulation*. 1987;75:711-722.

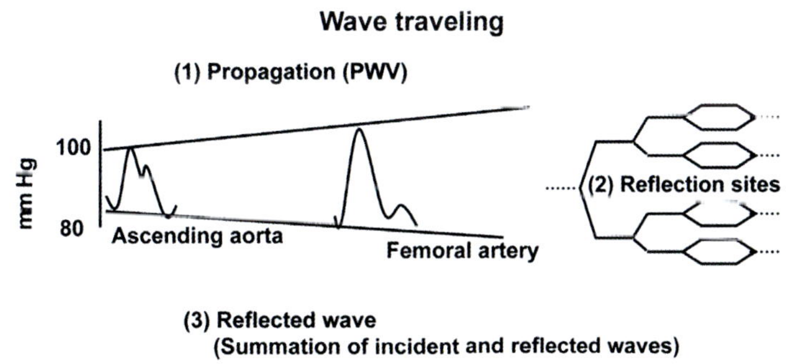

FIGURE 7.4 Pressure wave traveling along the arterial tree, involving the following: (1) propagation of the incident wave at a given speed (pulse wave velocity—PWV), (2) wave reflection at arteriolar sites, and (3) backward (reflected) pressure wave, which summates with incident wave, giving the Ao blood pressure (BP) curve. Note that, as a consequence of arterial stiffness and wave reflections, systolic blood pressure (SBP) and pulse pressure (PP) are higher in central than in peripheral arteries. Under drug treatment, PWV is reduced as a consequence of decrease in pressure distension; reflection coefficients are reduced as a consequence of reduced wall on lumen ratio of arterioles (under ACEI); such changes lead to reduction of central SBP and PP through change in the amplitude and timing of reflected pressure wave. (1) represents an oversimplified description of wave reflections. Numerous textbooks may depict reflected waves with more precision. ACEI, Angiotensin converting enzyme inhibitors. Reproduced with permission from Safar ME. Mechanism(s) of systolic blood pressure reduction and drug therapy in hypertension. *Hypertension*. 2007;50:167-171.

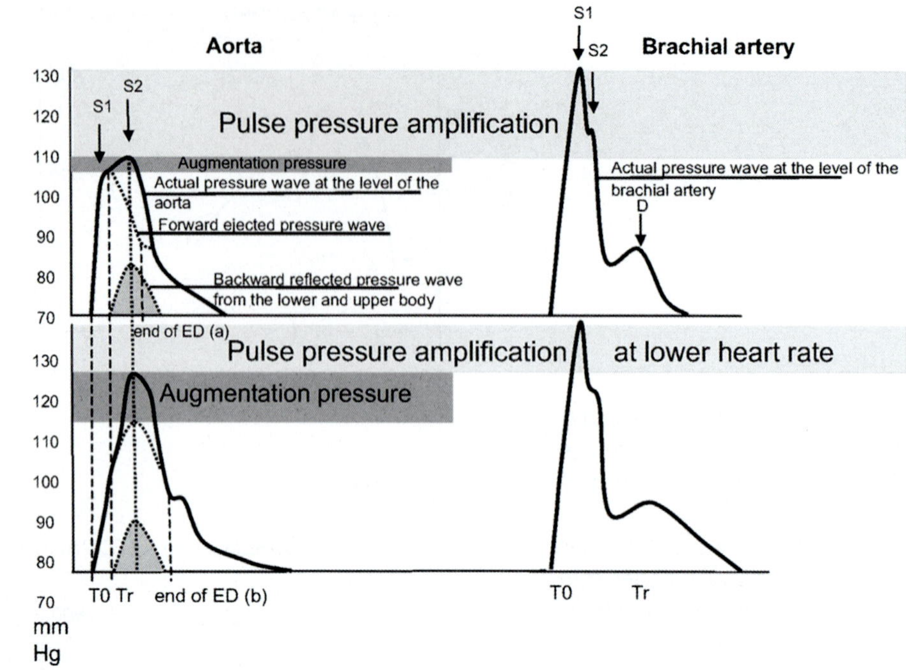

FIGURE 7.5 Schematic representation of (1) the morphological differences of the pulse wave (PW) between the aorta and the brachial artery in young healthy subjects (upper panel) and (2) the effect of heart rate (upper panel vs lower panel) on SBP augmentation and PW amplification, for the same reflected pressure wave and similar pulse height of the forward ejected pressure wave (modified from Safar et al). Aortic S1 indicates first systolic peak attributed to the forward wave; aortic S2, second late systolic peak attributable to the augmentation by the reflected pressure wave; brachial S2, systolic peak attributable to the reflected wave from the upper limb; D, accentuated diastolic wave attributable to the delayed arrival of the reflected wave from the lower body; ED, ejection duration; T0, onset of the forward ejected wave; Tr, time to return at the aorta of the backward reflected wave from the T0. Reproduced with permission from Avolio AP, Van Bortel LM, Boutouyrie P, et al. Role of pulse pressure amplification in arterial hypertension: experts' opinion and review of the data. *Hypertension*. 2009;54:375-383.

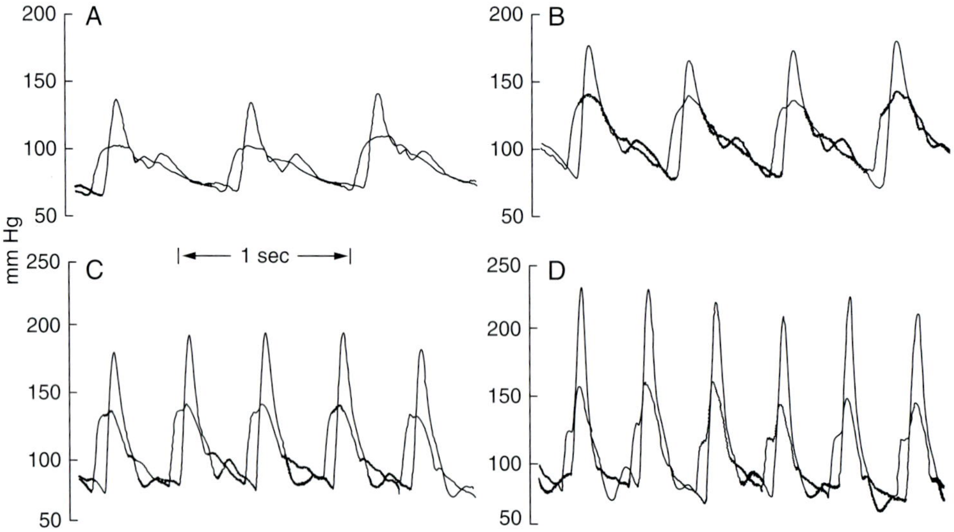

FIGURE 7.6 Simultaneous recording of aortic and radial artery pressure waves during rest (A), 28.2 (B), 47.2 (C), and 70% (D) of maximal oxygen uptake in a subject. Tracings were taken at the peaks of slow pressure oscillation and show the relationship of these extreme peripheral values to the severity of exercise. Reproduced with permission from Rowell LB, Brengelmann GL, Blackmon JR, Bruce RA, Murray JA. Disparities between aortic and peripheral pulse pressures induced by upright exercise and vasomotor changes in man. *Circulation*. 1968;37:954-964.

Ventricular Pressure

The ventricular pressure waveform can be divided into 4 major phases: isovolumic contraction, ejection, isovolumic relaxation, and diastolic filling. With the beginning of ventricular systole and closure of the atrioventricular mitral valve, intraventricular pressure rises without a change in volume (isovolumic contraction) until opening of the aortic valve. On opening of the aortic valve, ventricular ejection begins and continues until closure of the semilunar valve. This phase is followed by isovolumic relaxation, during which LV pressure decreases progressively without a change in volume. At the end of this phase, the atrioventricular valve opens and rapid filling begins. As relaxation continues during rapid filling, the ventricular diastolic pressure continues to fall. After the minimum pressure is reached, ventricular filling results in a progressive increase of LV diastolic pressures, followed by a positive wave corresponding to the atrial contribution to the ventricular filling[26](**FIGURES 7.7-7.9**). Diastasis corresponds to a specific phase of diastole between rapid filling and atrial contraction, during which the progressive rise in LV diastolic pressure is not accompanied by a significant increase in volume.

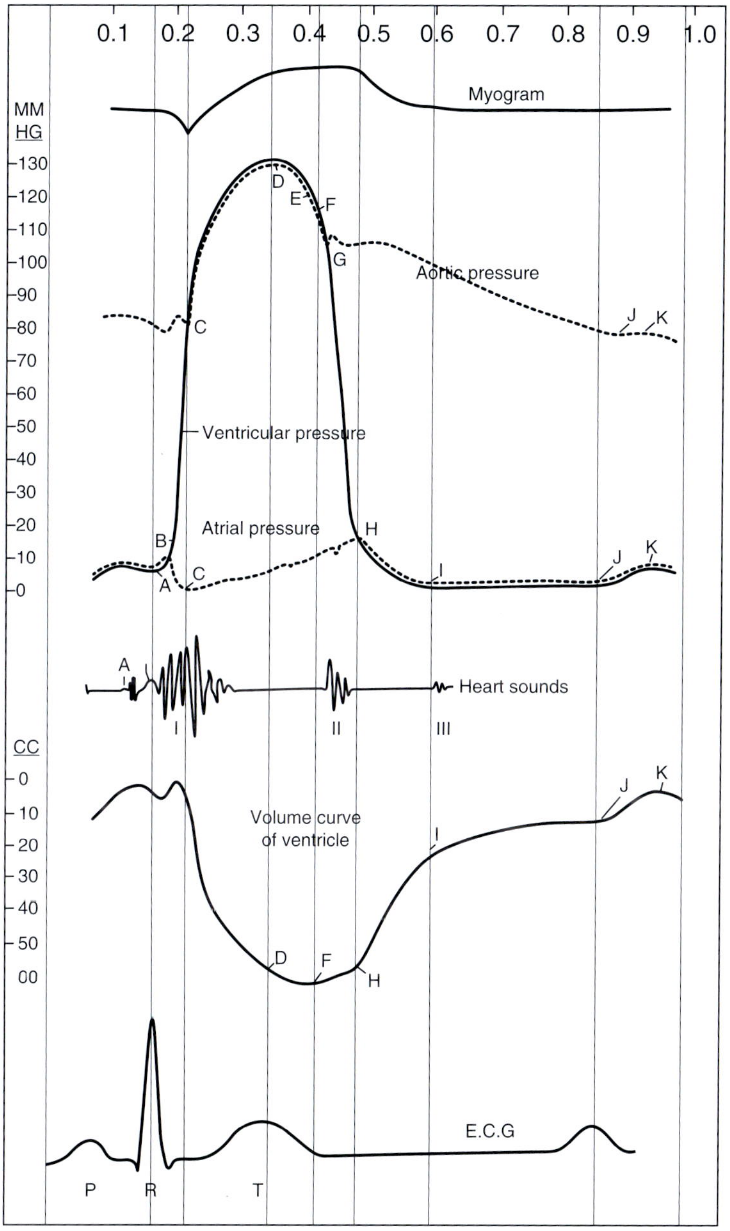

FIGURE 7.7 Classic Wiggers Diagram illustrating the dynamic, mechanical, acoustic, and electrical events during a cardiac cycle. As described by Wiggers in his landmark lecture: "*According to this scheme, mechanical systole begins with the rise of pressure at A and ends with the release of tension in all muscle units at F (Figure 7.3). It is divided into phases of isometric contraction (A-C), maximum ejection (C-D) and reduced ejection (D-F). The subsequent period of diastole is divided into phases of protodiastole, representing the time required for closure of the semilunar valves (F-G), isometric relaxation (G-H), rapid ventricular filling (H-I), diastasis (I-J), and filling by atrial contraction (J-K)*". Reproduced with permission from Wiggers CJ. The Henry Jackson memorial lecture dynamics of ventricular contraction under abnormal conditions. *Circulation.* March 1952;V.

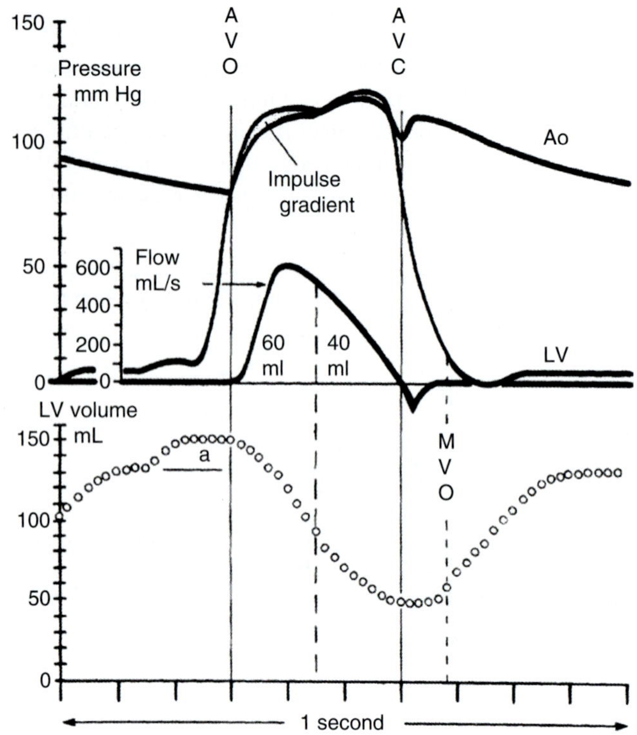

FIGURE 7.8 Wiggers diagram illustrating the impulse gradient in a normal ventricle and corresponding changes in volumes. LV and Ao pressure, aortic flow, and volumetric relationship are displayed. Vertical lines indicate aortic valve opening (AVO) and aortic valve closure (AVC) and encompass the systolic ejection period. Dashed lines indicate the midpoint of systole and mitral valve opening (MVO). a = atrial contribution to ventricular filling Reproduced with permission from Criley JM, Siegel RJ. *Circulation*. 1985;72:1148-1154.

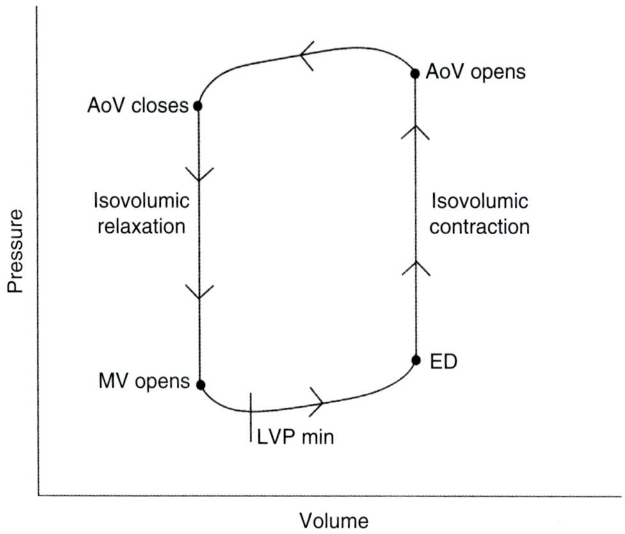

FIGURE 7.9 Pressure-volume loop. In addition to the Wiggers diagram, pressure-volume changes during the cardiac cycle can be illustrated with a pressure-volume loop. AoV, aortic valve; LVP min, left ventricular pressure minimal; MV, mitral valve; ED, end diastole.

Aortic Pressure

As outlined above, the Ao pressure waveform is the result of the interaction between the forward wave during ejection, reflected waves, and aortic compliance (**FIGURES 7.2** and **7.3**). During ejection, there are to 2 distinct slopes in the aortic waveform; an initial steep slope corresponding to rapid ejection is followed by a shallow slope, corresponding to delayed ejection. The initial steep increase after opening of the aortic valve is followed by a peak and then by a decline to the dicrotic notch, which corresponds to closure of the aortic valve and end of ejection (**FIGURES 7.7** and **7.8**).

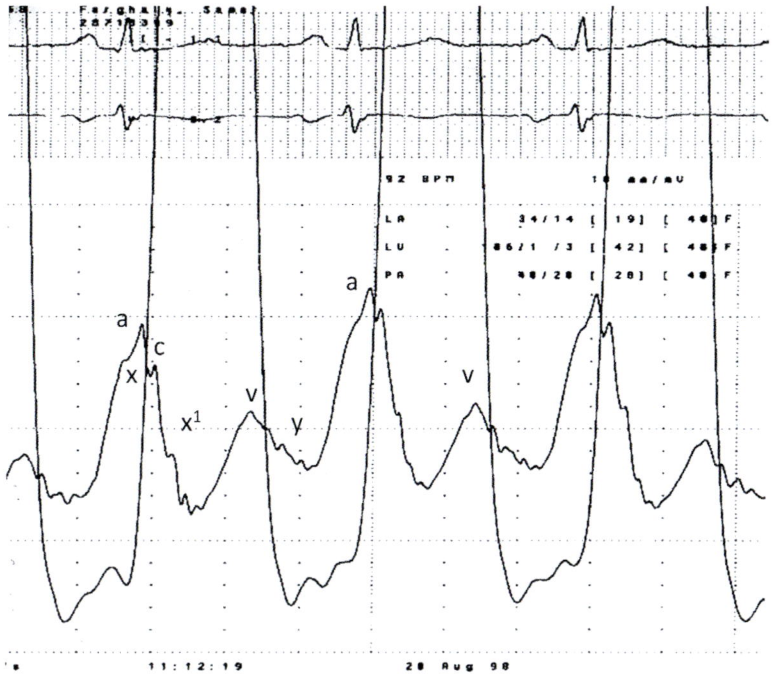

FIGURE 7.10 Simultaneous LA and LV pressure recording in a patient with mitral stenosis. See text for the description of the components of the atrial pressure waveform. Reproduced with permission from Moscucci M, ed. *Grossman & Baim's Cardiac Catheterization, Angiography and Intervention*. 8th ed. Philadelphia: Lippincott Williams and Wilkins; 2014.

Atrial Pressure

The atrial pressure waveform includes 3 positive waves, the *a*, c, and *v* waves, and 3 negative waves or descents, the *x*, *x*1, and *y* descent. In sequence, atrial contraction (a wave) is followed by atrial relaxation (x descent). Following atrial relaxation, closure and bulging of the atrioventricular valve during ventricular systole lead to the c wave. The c wave is followed by the x1 descent, which is the result of continuous atrial relaxation and the descent of the atrioventricular valve annulus during ventricular systole. Venus return to the atrium while the atrioventricular valve is closed leads to a progressive increase in atrial pressure (*v* wave), which is then followed by the *y* descent after opening of the atrioventricular valve and rapid empting of the atrium (**FIGURE 7.10**). The development of constrictive or tamponade physiology results in characteristic changes in the atrial pressure waveform, which are illustrated in details in chapter 8.

Pulmonary Artery Wedge Pressure

The pulmonary artery (PA) wedge pressure is obtained by advancing a balloon-tipped end-hole catheter to a distal branch of the PA. Non–balloon-tipped catheters such as Cournand catheter or a multipurpose catheter can also be used, although, being stiffer, they increase the risk of perforation. By occluding with the balloon the distal branch of the PA, forward flow is blocked and the pulmonary capillary bed distal to the balloon, the corresponding pulmonary veins (PVs), the left atrium (LA), the open mitral valve, and the LV become an unrestricted vascular bed during diastole. Pressure changes in the LA will be transmitted to the transducer distal to the balloon (**FIGURE 7.11**). Thus, the pulmonary capillary wedge waveform is similar to the LA waveform, with a time delay of 0.02 to 0.08 seconds (**FIGURE 7.12**). It is critical to ensure adequate wedge position by observing the pressure waveform and by obtaining an oxygen saturation in wedge position, which should be above 95%.[27] **FIGURE 7.13** shows pressure waveform contours of adequate and inadequate wedge positions.[27] It should be noted that motion of the tip of a catheter within the heart and great vessels accelerates the fluid contained within the catheter and can occasionally lead to superimposed waves of up to ±10 mm Hg.[24] These catheter whip artifacts are particularly common in tracings from the PAs and might be difficult to avoid (**FIGURES 7.14** and **7.27**).

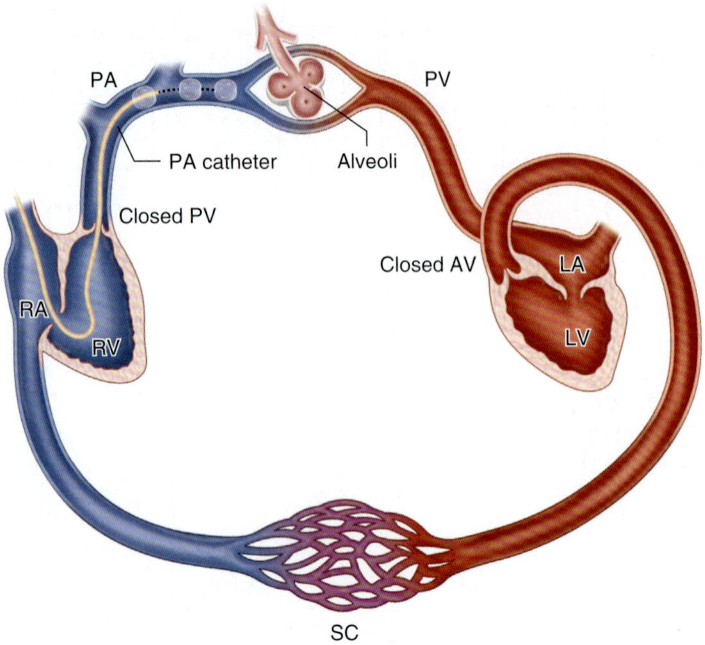

FIGURE 7.11 Schematic representation of the pulmonary and systemic circulation during PA catheterization and balloon inflation in diastole. There is an unrestricted vascular bed spanning from the distal PA (distal to the transducer) to the pulmonary circulation, the PVs, the LA, and the LV. AV, aortic valve; RV, right ventricle; SC, systemic circulation.

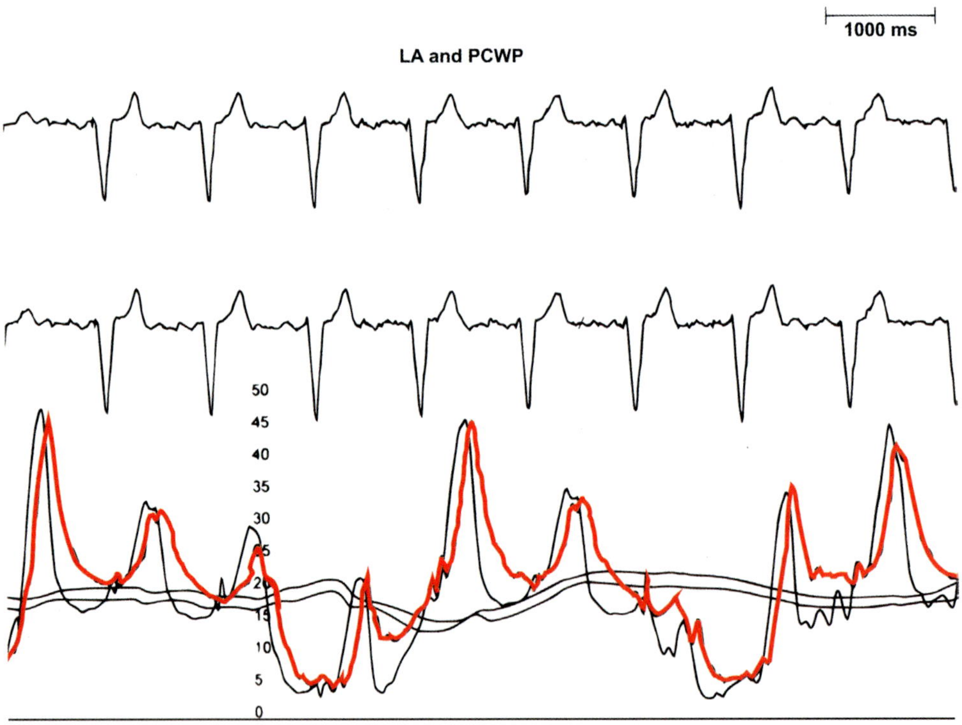

FIGURE 7.12 Simultaneous LA and pulmonary capillary wedge pressure (PCWP) measurements in a patient with a bioprosthetic mitral valve. Note the time delay of the PCWP tracing (in red) as well as prominent V waves and overall elevated pressures.

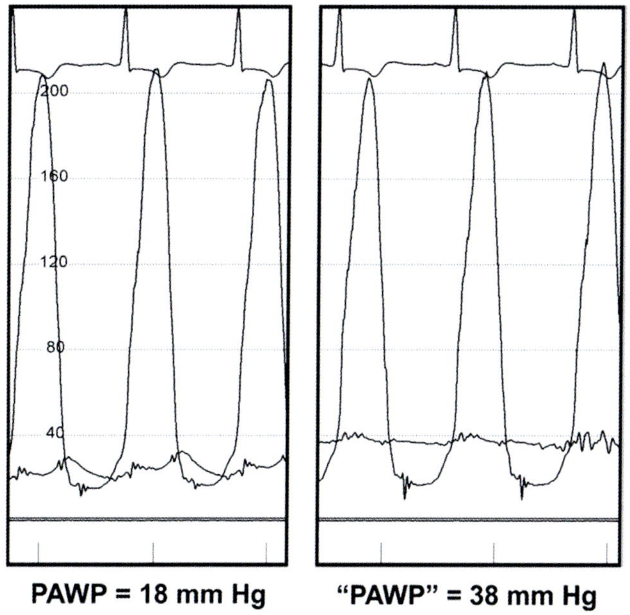

FIGURE 7.13 The PAWP must be obtained meticulously during cardiac catheterization, optimally performed with a large-bore end-hole catheter. Confirmation of the PAWP examining the pressure contour for respiratory variation and a >95% saturation is recommended to ensure an accurate pressure measurement. Left, PAWP was taken with a large-bore 7F balloon wedge catheter with a 98% saturation confirmation. There is appropriate respiratory variation and a proper contour of the PAWP. Right, The attempt at PAWP was done with a small lumen thermodilution catheter. This most likely represents a damped PA pressure. Confirmation by saturation was not performed. Reproduced with permission from Nishimura RA, Carabello BA. Hemodynamics in the Cardiac Catheterization Laboratory of the 21st Century. *Circulation*. 2012;125:2138-2150.

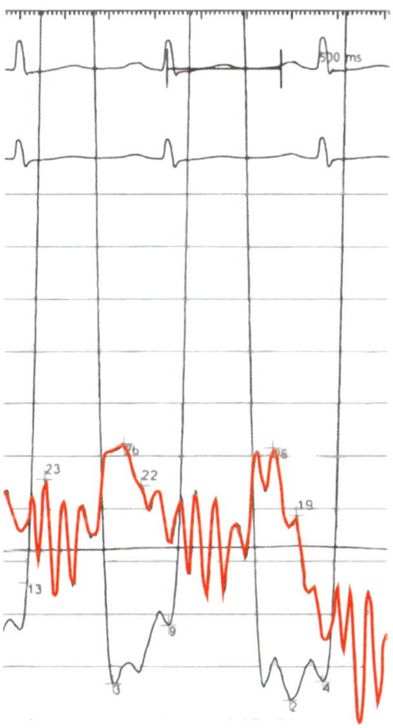

FIGURE 7.14 PAWP during nipride infusion in a patient with severe mitral regurgitation. Note the multiple superimposed waves secondary to catheter whip artefact.

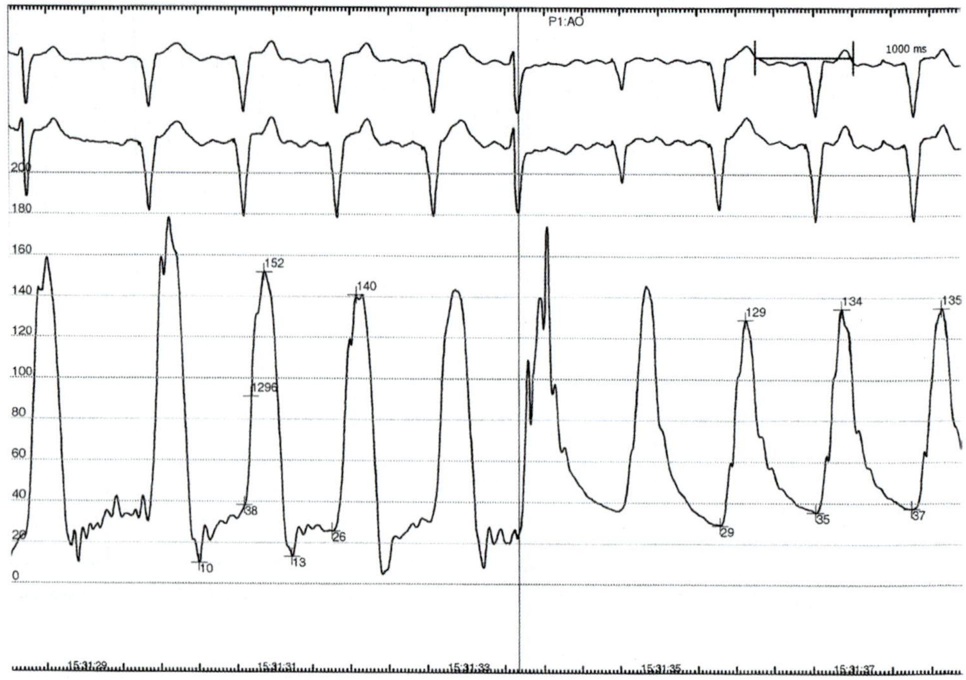

FIGURE 7.15 Severe aortic regurgitation. Catheter pullback across the left ventricular outflow tract (LVOT) into the ascending aorta. The aortic diastolic pressure is between 29 mm Hg and 37 mm Hg, and it matches the LV end diastolic pressure. The waveform and measurements are consistent with severe aortic regurgitation.

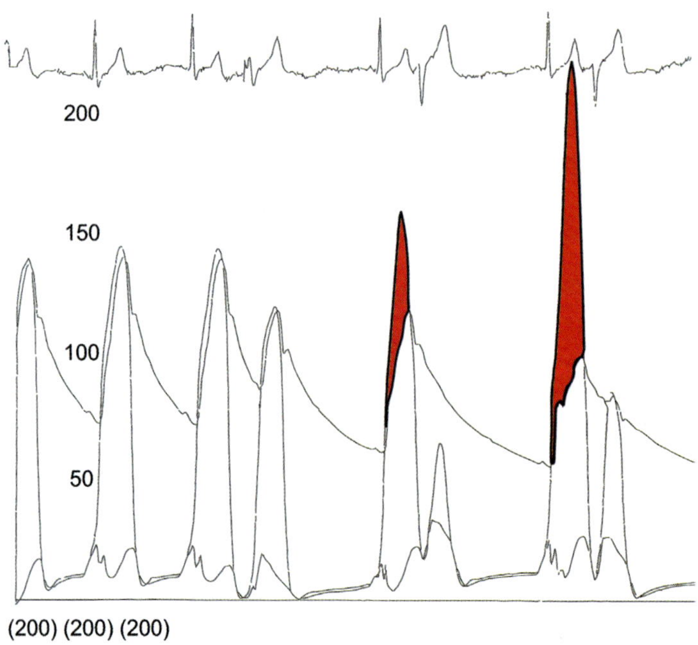

FIGURE 7.16 Hypertrophic cardiomyopathy. Simultaneous left ventricular and aortic pressure measured in a patient with hypertrophic cardiomyopathy (HCM). Note the typical "Brockenbrough-Braunwald-Morrow sign", represented by a marked increase in LVOT gradient accompanied by a reduction in aortic pressure following a premature beat. The postextrasystolic potentiation following the premature beat leads to an increase in dynamic obstruction and resultant reduction in stroke volume and pulse pressure.

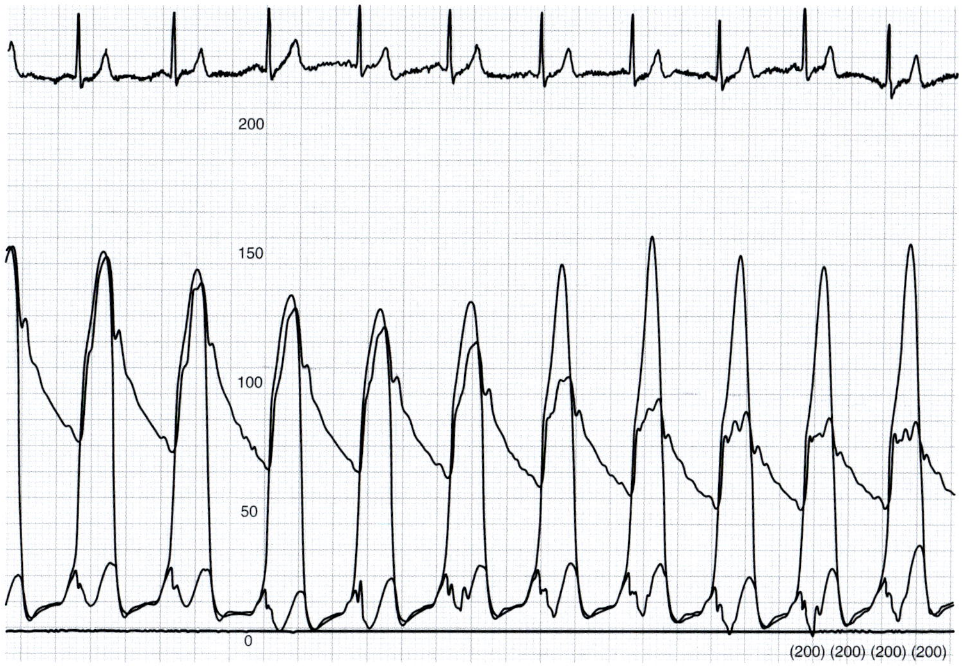

FIGURE 7.17 HCM. Baseline hemodynamic measurements at rest and during amyl nitrate challenge. Note the marked increase in LVOT gradient during amyl nitrate challenge.

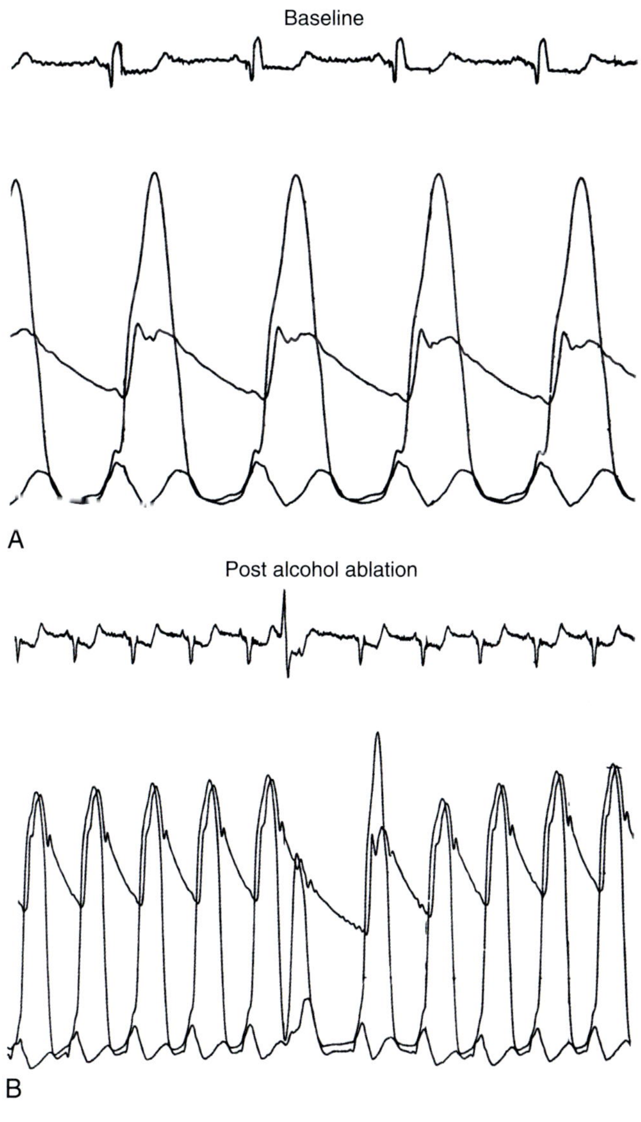

FIGURE 7.18 HCM. Hemodynamic tracings obtained immediately before (A) and after (B) alcohol septal ablation from a patient with HCM. Before septal ablation, the patient had undergone echocardiographic evaluation, which revealed a resting gradient of 64 mmHg, increasing to 81 mmHg with the Valsalva maneuver, and to 104 mmHg with amyl nitrate. Follow-up evaluation 3 months post alcohol septal ablation revealed a resting gradient of 6 mm Hg, increasing to 23 mm Hg with amyl nitrate.

PRESSURE TRACINGS IN VALVULAR AND NONVALVULAR HEART DISEASE

FIGURES 7.15-7.34 illustrate hemodynamic tracings in valvular and nonvalvular heart disease. The figure legends describe salient components of each case and findings. We hope that our readers will find them useful as an aid to rapid recognition of abnormal findings in the cardiac catheterization laboratory.

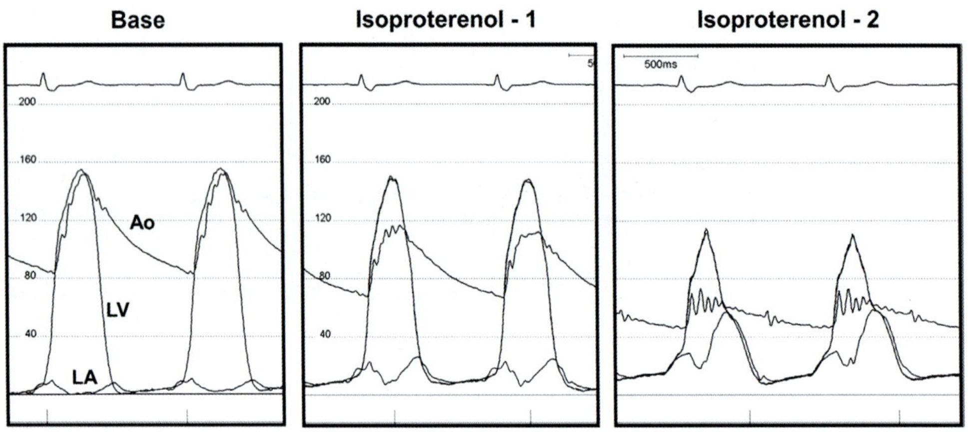

FIGURE 7.19 HCM. Patients with HCM may have labile LVOT gradients. If septal reduction therapy is to be considered, there must be a gradient of >50 mm Hg either at rest or during provocation. Exercise would be the optimal physiological mechanism to provoke a labile obstruction but is difficult in the catheterization laboratory. Isoproterenol infusion is an excellent method to simulate exercise by stimulating both B1 and B2 receptors. Left, There is no LV outflow gradient at rest. Middle, With initial infusion of isoproterenol, there is a 40-mm Hg gradient across the LVOT. Right, With a greater infusion of isoproterenol, there is a 65-mm Hg LV outflow gradient. Ao indicates central aortic. Reproduced with permission from Nishimura RA, Carabello BA. Hemodynamics in the cardiac catheterization laboratory of the 21st century. *Circulation*. 2012;125:2138-2150.

FIGURE 7.20 A visual assessment of the contour of the Ao and LV pressures is important during cardiac catheterization. Left, Patients with fixed obstruction (either valvular stenosis or fixed subvalvular stenosis) will demonstrate a parvus and a tardus in the upstroke of the aortic pressure, beginning at the time of aortic valve opening. Right, In patients with a dynamic obstruction (such as that found in HCM), the aortic pressure will rise rapidly at the onset of aortic valve opening and then develop a spike-and-dome contour as the obstruction occurs in late systole. The LV pressure also has a late peak because of the mechanism of this dynamic obstruction. Reproduced with permission from Nishimura RA, Carabello BA. Hemodynamics in the cardiac catheterization laboratory of the 21st century. *Circulation*. 2012;125:2138-2150.

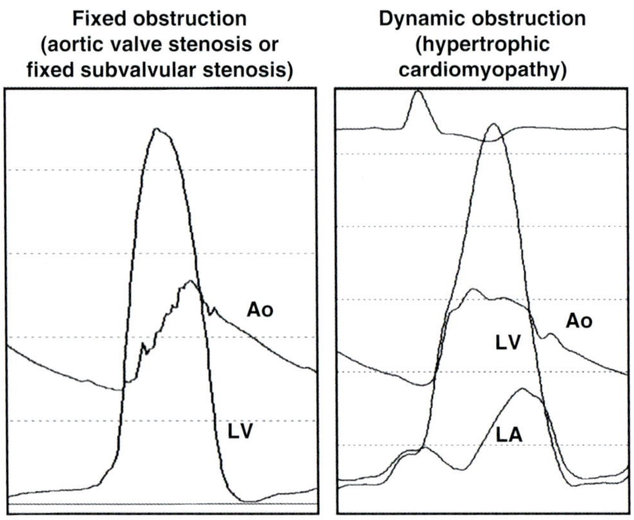

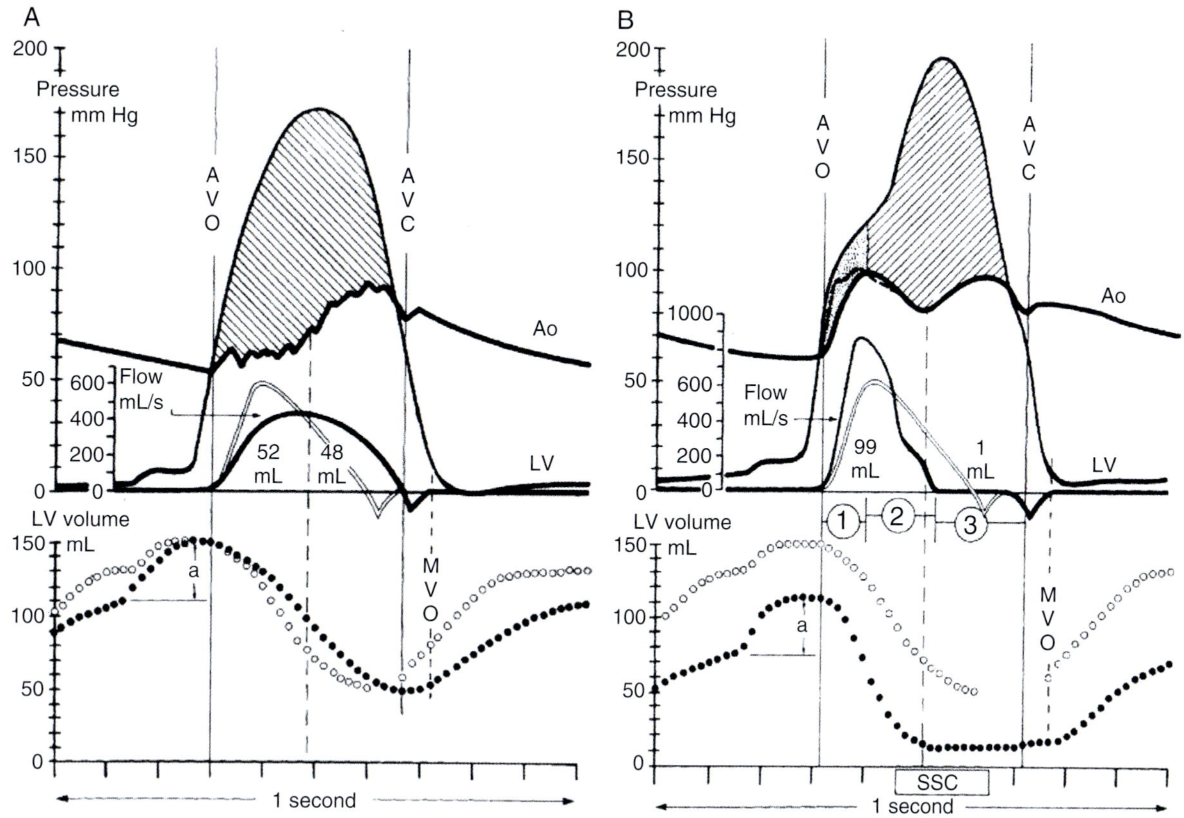

FIGURE 7.21 A, Discrete obstructive gradient in aortic stenosis. The format is similar to that of **FIGURE 7.8.** Normal contours for aortic flow and instantaneous volume curves are depicted in open lines and circles for comparison. B, Dynamic gradient in HCM. The contour depicted by a dashed line following aortic valve opening represents LVOT pressure. See text for explanation of phases (encircled numbers). SSC, onset and duration of systolic anterior motion (SAM)-septal contact; LV and Ao pressure, aortic flow, and volumetric relationship are displayed. Vertical lines indicate AVO and AVC and encompass the systolic ejection period. Dashed lines indicate the midpoint of systole and MVO. a, atrial contribution to ventricular filling. Adapted with permission from Criley JM, Siegel RJ. Has 'obstruction' hindered our understanding of hypertrophic cardiomyopathy? *Circulation*. 1985;72:1148-1154.

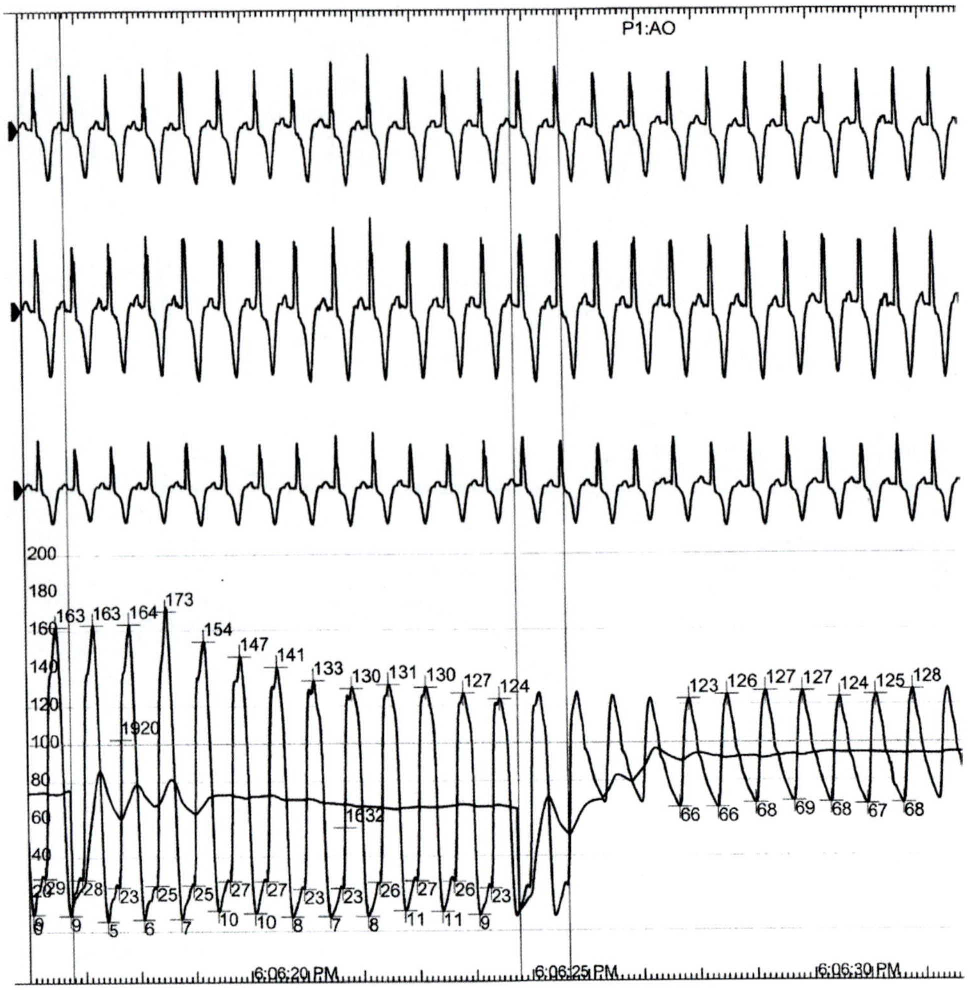

FIGURE 7.22 Pullback of an end-hole catheter across the LVOT in a patient with Takotsubo cardiomyopathy. Note the pressure gradient due to dynamic LVOT obstruction as the catheter is pulled back across the LV.

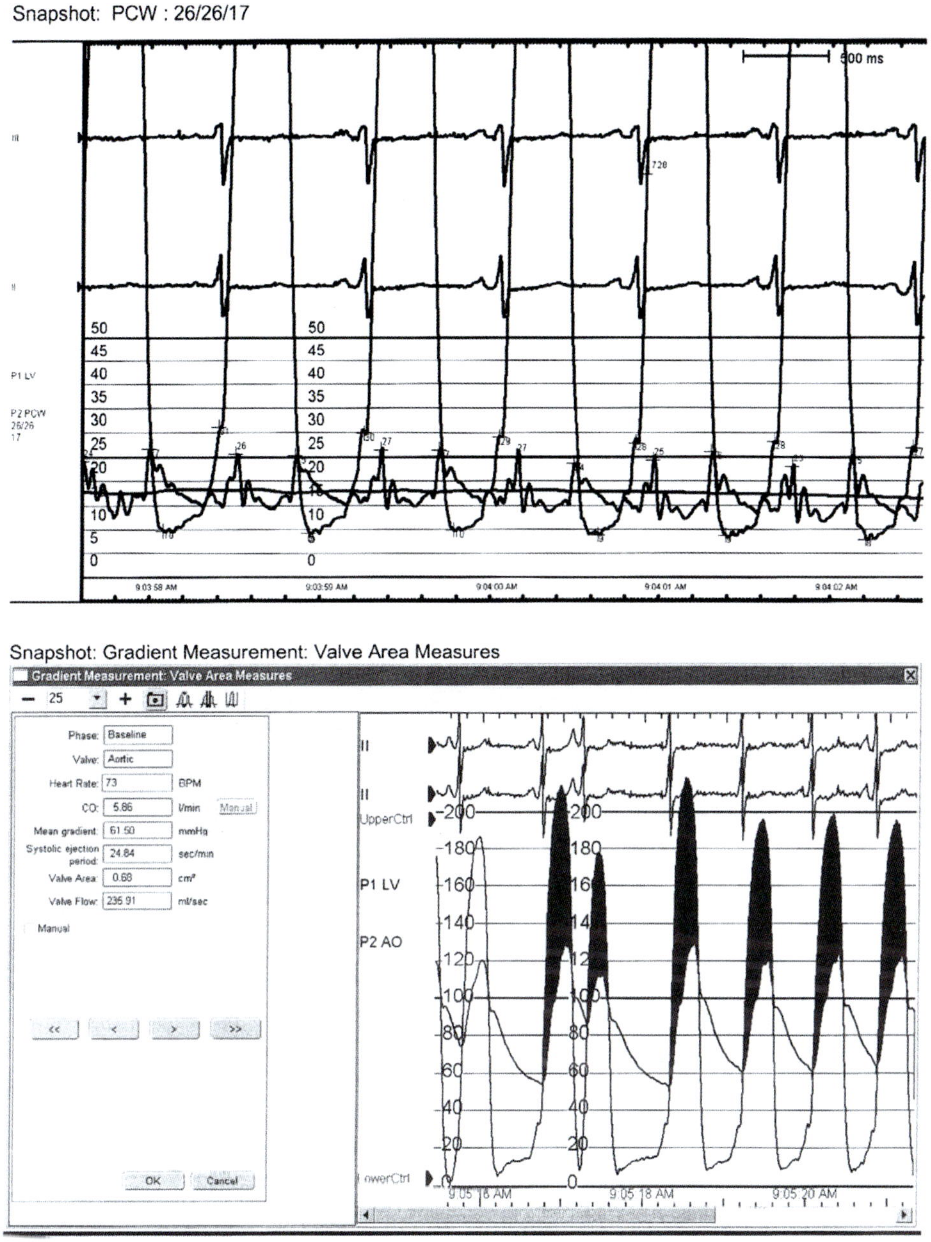

FIGURE 7.23 Hemodynamic tracings from a patient with severe aortic stenosis. Note the pressure waveform immediately after the premature beat (lower panel). Contrary to what is shown in **FIGURE 7.16**, the postpremature beat is characterized by an increase in both LV and Ao pressure, rather than by an increase in gradient associated with a decrease in Ao pressure. This finding can help in differentiating valvular aortic stenosis from LVOT obstruction. Top panel shows LV and PCWP.

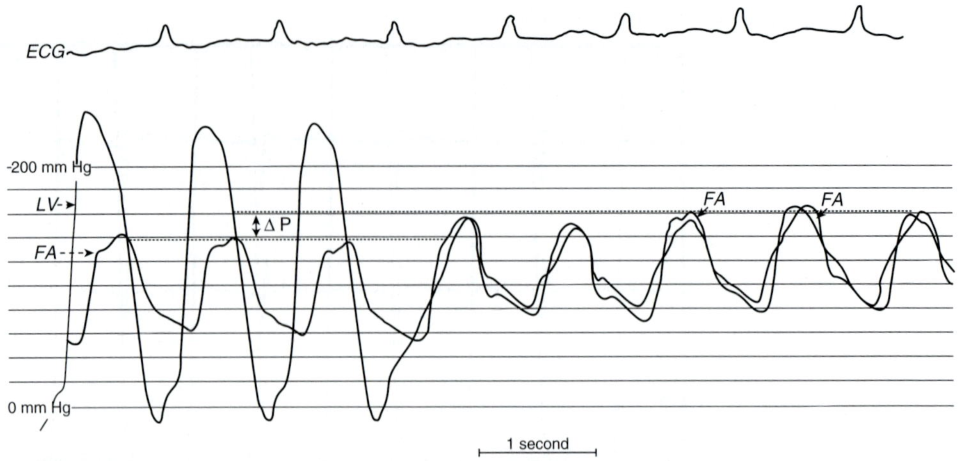

FIGURE 7.24 Carabello sign. LV and FA pressure tracings in a patient with severe aortic stenosis (aortic valve area 0.4 cm^2). During pullback of the retrograde catheter from LV to ascending aorta, the peak systolic FA pressure can be seen to increase (ΔP) by approximately 20 mm Hg. This sign is seen only in patients with aortic valve areas <0.6 cm^2. The mechanism of this phenomenon is believed to be partial obstruction of an already narrowed aortic orifice by the retrograde catheter and relief of this obstruction with catheter withdrawal. Reproduced with permission from Carabello BA, Barry WH, Grossman W. Changes in arterial pressure during left heart pullback in patients with aortic stenosis. *Am J Cardiol*. 1979;44:424.

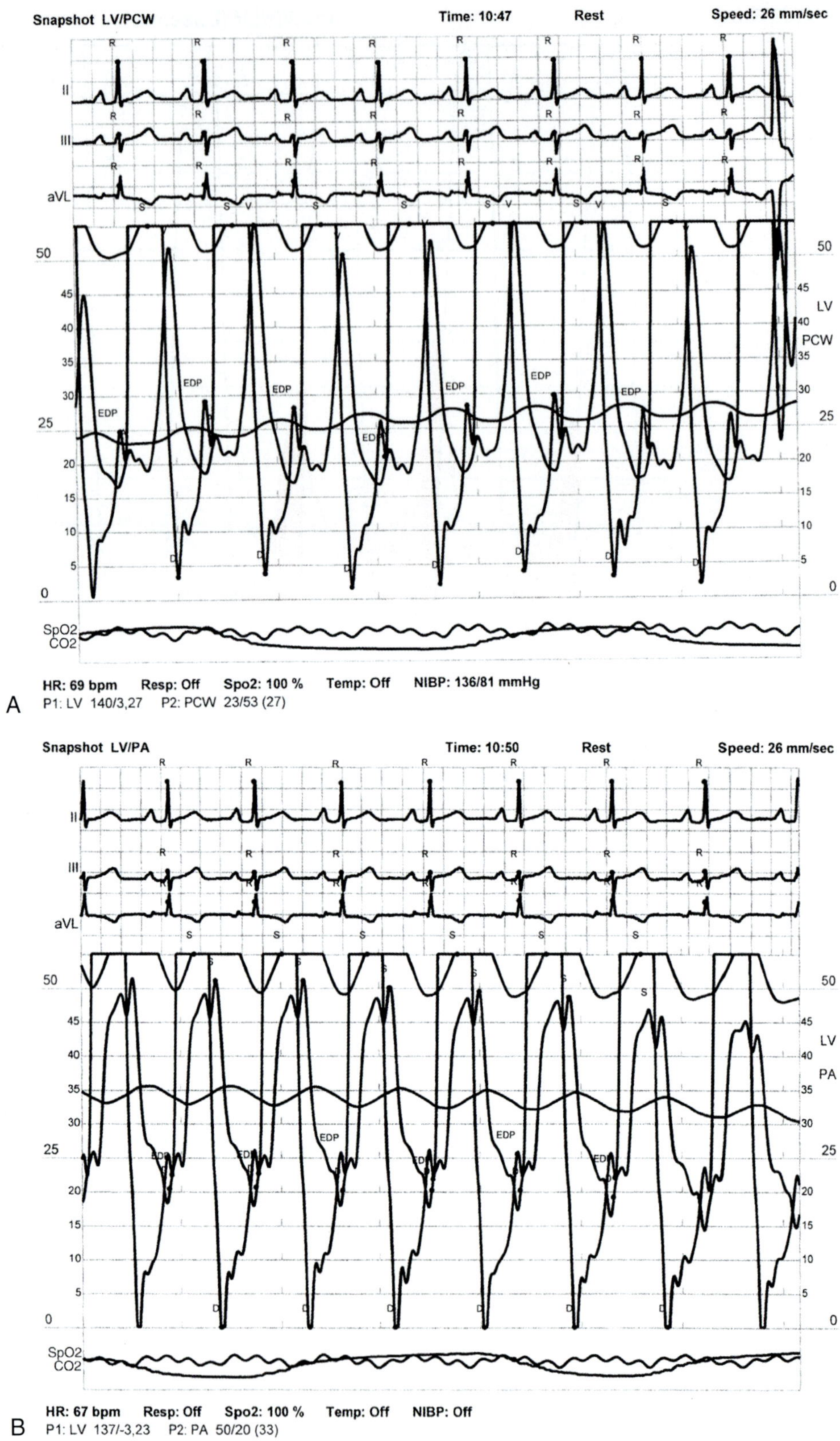

FIGURE 7.25 Severe mitral regurgitation. Hemodynamic tracings from a patient with severe mitral regurgitation. Panel A shows the PCWP with "giant" V waves. Panel B shows the PA pressure. Note the double peak of the PA pressure tracing. The second positive wave is a manifestation of the V wave transmitted retrograde through the pulmonary vasculature, and it can be seen in the setting of severe mitral regurgitation.

PCWP/LV (baseline)

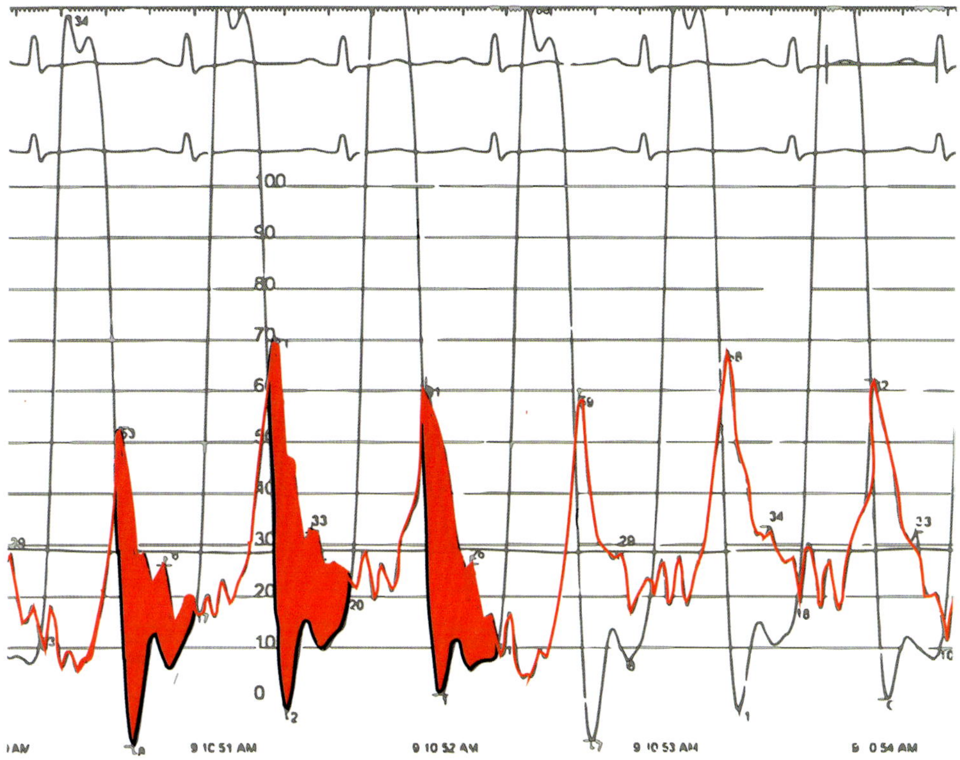

FIGURE 7.26 Severe mitral regurgitation. Hemodynamic tracings from a patient with severe mitral regurgitation. Note the elevated LA pressure and the giant V waves.

PCWP/LV (nipride)

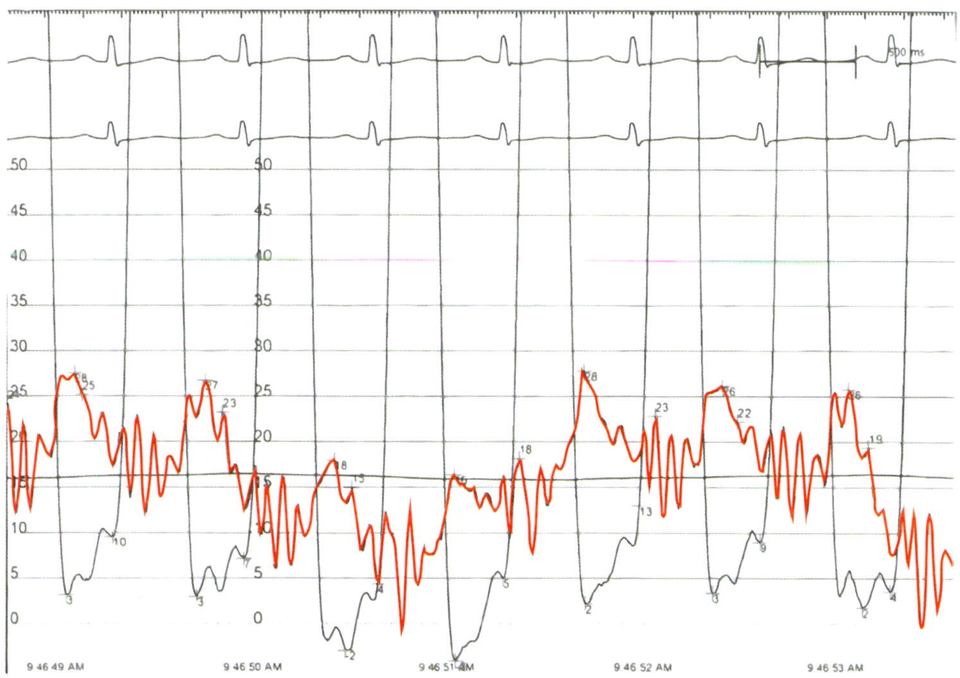

FIGURE 7.27 Hemodynamic tracing obtained during nipride infusion from the same patient shown in FIGURE 7.26. There is a marked reduction in PCWP. The prominent V waves shown in FIGURE 7.26 are no longer evident. Pharmacological manipulation with vasodilators, positive inotropic agents, or volume loading during cardiac catheterization has a critical role in the evaluation of valvular and nonvalvular hemodynamic parameters and in estimating the potential response to surgical or catheter-based interventions.

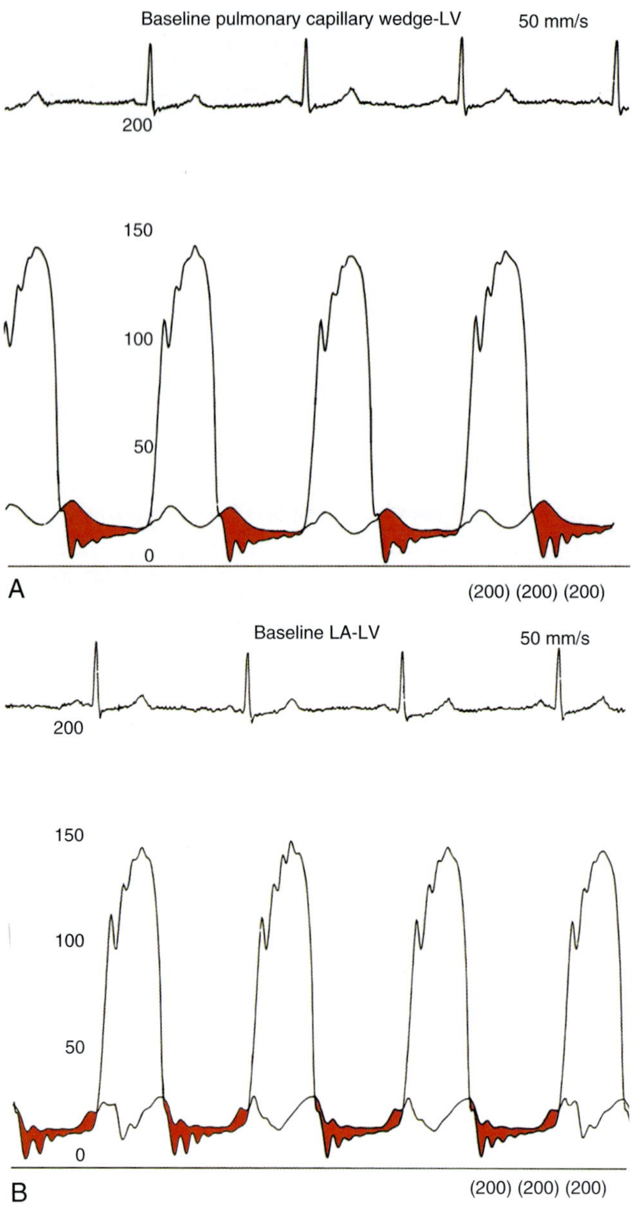

FIGURE 7.28 Mitral stenosis. Baseline gradient measurements in a patient with mitral stenosis. Panel A shows pulmonary capillary wedge to LV gradient, while panel B shows LA pressure to LV gradient obtained through a transseptal approach. As also shown in **FIGURE 7.31**, pulmonary capillary wedge to LV gradient tends to overestimate the true gradient across the mitral valve.

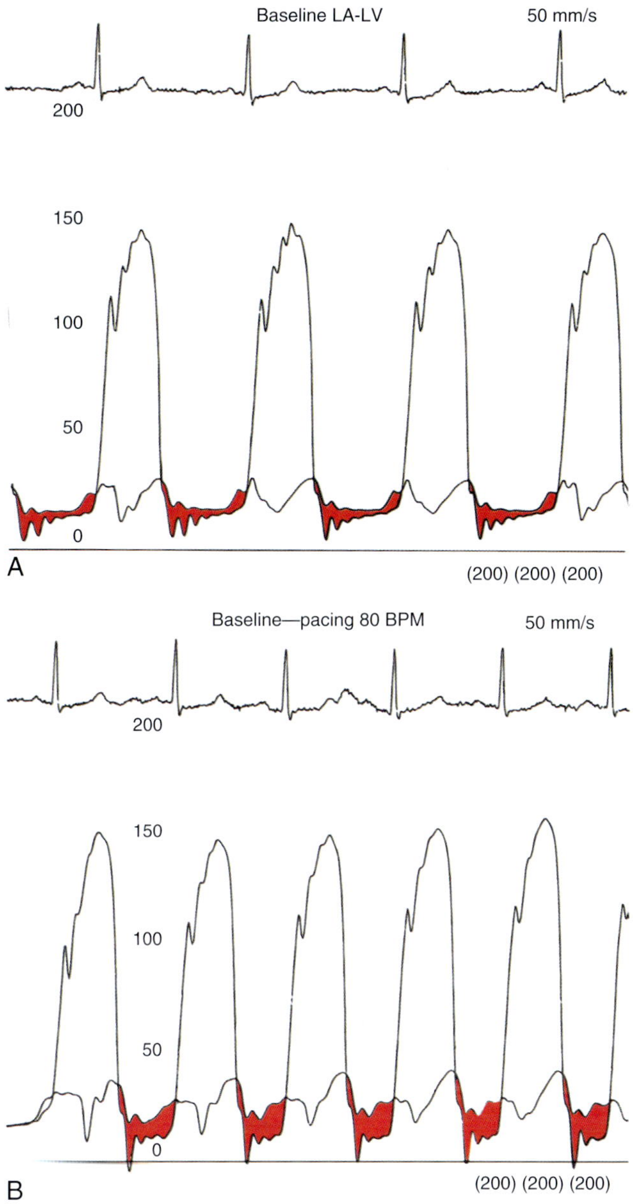

FIGURE 7.29 Mitral stenosis. Baseline hemodynamic measurements obtained before balloon mitral valvuloplasty at rest (A) and during atrial pacing at a rate of 80 BPM (B). Note the significant increase in gradient during pacing, consistent with the rate dependency of transmitral gradient. Please note that panel A is the same as panel B in **FIGURE 7.28**, and it has been used in this figure for ease of direct visual comparison. Evaluation of patients with mitral stenosis with either exercise of atrial pacing might be critical in the determination of the true severity of stenosis when the baseline gradient might be low.

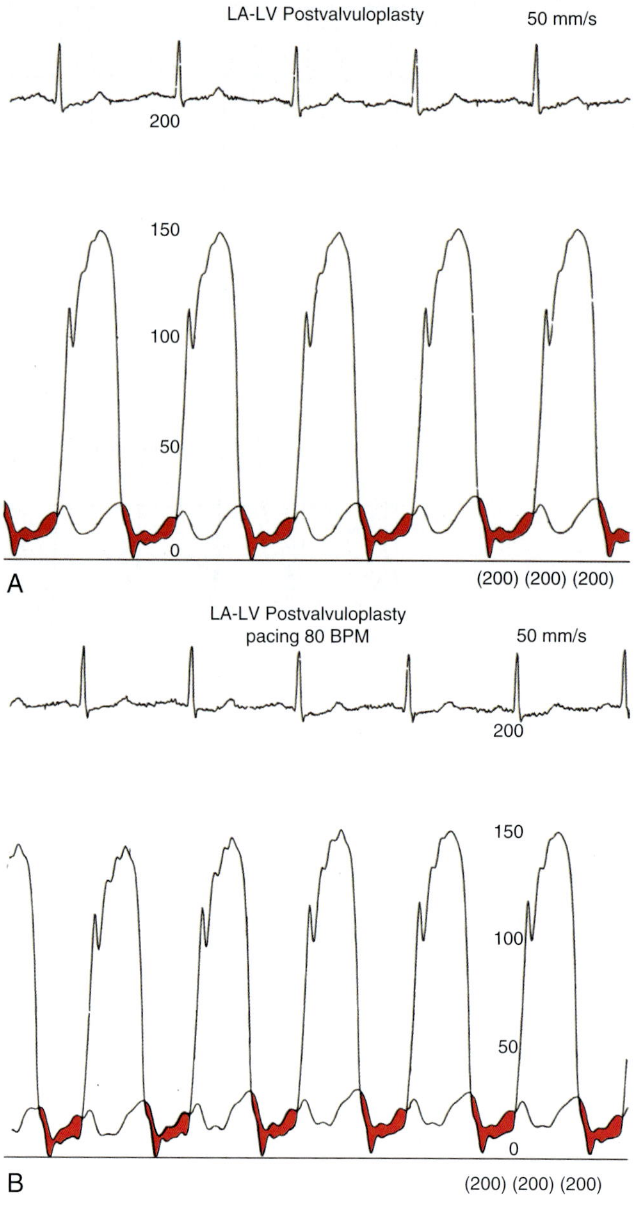

FIGURE 7.30 Mitral stenosis. Repeat hemodynamic measurements after mitral balloon valvuloplasty at baseline (A) and during atrial pacing (B) in the same patient shown in **FIGURE 7.28** and **7.29**. Note the significantly lower gradient during atrial pacing when compared with **FIGURE 7.29**.

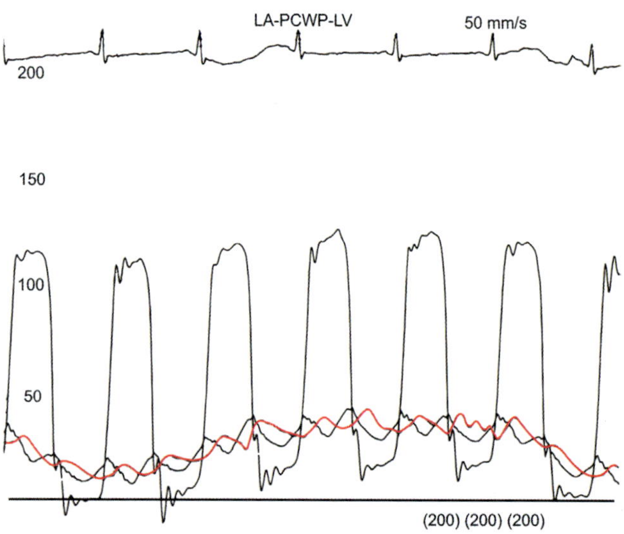

FIGURE 7.31 Simultaneous LA and PCWP measurements in a patient with mitral stenosis. Note the time delay of the PCWP tracing (in red). In addition, when compared with LA pressure, the use of PCWP might result in overestimating the severity of mitral stenosis.

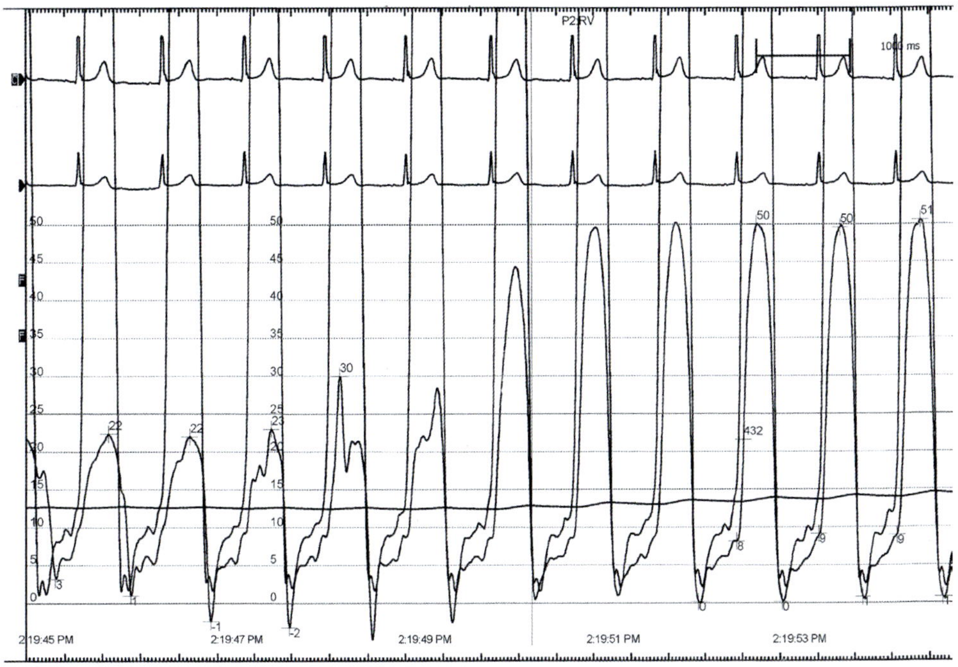

FIGURE 7.32 RV outflow tract obstruction. Pullback of a right-sided heart catheter from the RV outflow track to the RV inflow tract. Note the significant pressure gradient when the catheter is withdrawn in the RV inflow tract.

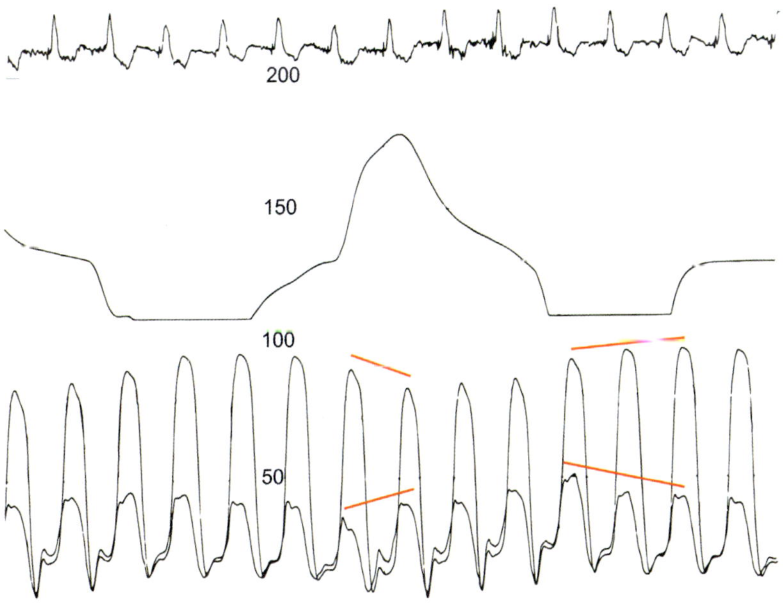

FIGURE 7.33 Constrictive physiology. Ventricular interdependence (or discordance) in a patient with constrictive pericarditis. During inspiration, as RV pressure increases, the LV pressure decreases.

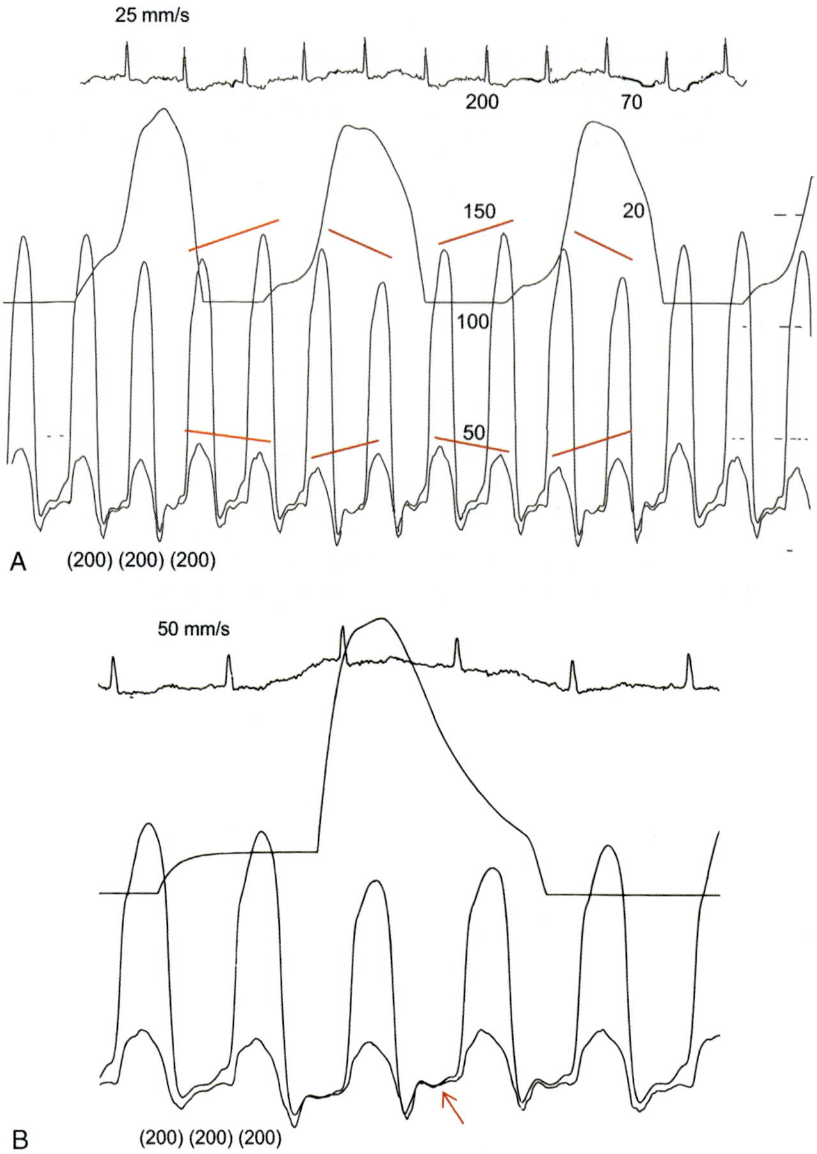

FIGURE 7.34 Constrictive physiology. A, Ventricular interdependence (or discordance) in another patient with constrictive pericarditis. As in the case illustrated in **FIGURE 7.33**, during inspiration RV pressure increases and LV pressure decreases. B, Note also the equalization of end diastolic pressures and the brisk rise in ventricular pressure after rapid filling, resulting in a "square root" or "dip and plateau" sign. Hemodynamic measurements evaluating constrictive versus restrictive physiology should be obtained with simultaneous recording of the respiratory cycle and after volume loading if filling pressures are low. In addition, to highlight respirophasic variations and diastolic pressure contours, assessment of ventricular interdependence (constrictive physiology) or concordance (restrictive physiology) should be performed both at low and high sweep speeds.

REFERENCES

1. Statical Essays: Containing Haemastatics: or, an Account of Some Hydraulic and Hydrostatical Experiments Made on the Blood and Blood-Vessels of Animals. To Which Is Added, and Appendix, With an Index to Both Vs Vol. II. 3rd ed. v 2 of 2- Stephen Hales. 1733.
2. Moscucci M. Cardiac catheterization history and current practice standards. In: Moscucci M, ed. *Grossman & Baim's Cardiac Catheterization, Angiography and Intervention*. Philadelphia: Wolters Kluwer; 2014.
3. Forssmann W. Die Sondierung des rechten Herzens. *Klin Wochenschr*. 1929;8:2085.
4. Forssmann W. *Experiments on Myself; Memoirs of a Surgeon in Germany*. New York: St. Martin's Press; 1974.
5. Klein O. Zur Bestimmung des zerkulatorischen minutens Volumen nach dem Fickschen Prinzip. *Munch Med Wochenschr*. 1930;77:1311.
6. Cournand A. Cardiac catheterization; development of the technique, its contributions to experimental medicine, and its initial applications in man. *Acta Med Scand Suppl*. 1975;579:3-32.
7. Cournand A, Riley RL, Breed ES, et al. Measurement of cardiac output in man using the technique of catheterization of the right auricle or ventricle. *J Clin Invest*. 1945;24(1):106-116.
8. Cournand AF. Pulmonary circulation; its control in man, with some remarks on methodology. *Am Heart J*. 1957;54(2):172-181.
9. Cournand AF. Presentation of the Kober Medal for 1970 to Dickinson W. Richards. *Trans Assoc Am Phys*. 1970;83:36-42.
10. Cournand AF. Dickinson Woodruff Richards: 1895-1973. A survey of his contributions to the physiology and physiopathology of respiration in man. *Am J Med*. 1974;57(3):312-328.
11. Richards DW. The circulation in traumatic shock in man. *Bull N Y Acad Med*. 1944;20(7):363-393.
12. Richards DW Jr. Observations on the dynamics of the systemic circulation in man. *Bull N Y Acad Med*. 1946;22(12):630-646.
13. Richards DW Jr. Contributions of right heart catheterization to the physiology of congestive heart failure. *Am J Med*. 1947;3(4):434-446.
14. Richards DW Jr. Dynamics of congestive heart failure. *Am J Med*. 1949;6(6):772-780.
15. Richards DW. Cardiac failure. *Bull N Y Acad Med*. 1950;26(6):384-394.
16. Richards DW. Right heart catheterization; its contributions to physiology and medicine. *Science*. 1957;125(3259):1181-1185.
17. Richards DW . Cardiac catheterization; its uses in medicine and surgery. In: *Seminar Report*. Merck Sharp & Dohme; 1958;3(2):9-12 passim.
18. Cournand AF. Nobel lecture, December 11, 1956. In: *Nobel Lectures, Physiology and Medicine 1942–1962*. Amsterdam: Elsevier; 1964:529.
19. Avolio AP, Van Bortel LM, Boutouyrie P, et al. Role of pulse pressure amplification in arterial hypertension: experts' opinion and review of the data. *Hypertension*. 2009;54(2):375-383.
20. Laskey WK, Kussmaul WG. Arterial wave reflection in heart failure. *Circulation*. 1987;75(4):711-722.
21. Murgo JP, Westerhof N, Giolma JP, Altobelli SA. Manipulation of ascending aortic pressure and flow wave reflections with the valsalva maneuver: relationship to input impedance. *Circulation*. 1981;63(1):122-132.
22. Safar ME. Mechanism(s) of systolic blood pressure reduction and drug therapy in hypertension. *Hypertension*. 2007;50(1):167-171.
23. Murgo JP, Westerhof N, Giolma JP, Altobelli SA. Aortic input impedance in normal man: relationship to pressure wave forms. *Circulation*. 1980;62(1):105-116.
24. Moscucci M, Grossman W. Pressure measurement. In: Moscucci M, ed. *Grossman & Baim's Cardiac Cathetrization, Angiography and Intervention*. Philadelphia: Wolters Kluwer; 2014:223-244.
25. Rowell LB, Brengelmann GL, Blackmon JR, Bruce RA, Murray JA. Disparities between aortic and peripheral pulse pressures induced by upright exercise and vasomotor changes in man. *Circulation*. 1968;37(6):954-964.
26. Wiggers CJ. Dynamics of ventricular contraction under abnormal conditions. *Circulation*. 1952;5(3):321-348.
27. Nishimura RA, Carabello BA. Hemodynamics in the cardiac catheterization laboratory of the 21st century. *Circulation*. 2012;125(17):2138-2150.
28. Criley JM, Siegel RJ. Has 'obstruction' hindered our understanding of hypertrophic cardiomyopathy? *Circulation*. 1985;72(6):1148-1154.

chapter **8**

Hemodynamics of Tamponade, Constrictive, and Restrictive Physiology

YOGESH N. V. REDDY, MBBS, MSc, MAURO MOSCUCCI, MD, MBA, and
BARRY A. BORLAUG, MD

INTRODUCTION

The pericardium is a fluid-filled sac composed of 2 layers: the visceral and parietal pericardium. Normally there is around 20 to 40 cc of fluid in the pericardial sac, which serves to lubricate the heart and minimize friction during mechanical work. The pericardium also serves to couple left- and right-sided ventricular stroke volume, such that a respiratory or positional increase in stroke volume from the right ventricle is associated with a compensatory decrease in stroke volume from the left. This ventricular interdependence, however, is exaggerated in pathological states associated with poor operating compliance of the pericardial unit, such as abnormal fluid accumulation in the pericardial sac (tamponade) or stiffening of the pericardial membrane (constriction) (**FIGURE 8.1**).

TAMPONADE PHYSIOLOGY

Pericardial fluid accumulation exaggerates ventricular interdependence and limits ventricular preload through enhanced pericardial restraint. Left ventricular (LV) end diastolic volume (preload) is directly proportional to left ventricular transmural filling pressure (LV diastolic pressure – pericardial pressure). Therefore an increase in pericardial pressure from accumulation of pericardial fluid can compromise LV filling, leading to hypotension and clinical tamponade. Increased pericardial pressure can also directly compress the right ventricle (which is at lower pressure) impeding right ventricular filling additionally compromising cardiac output and left ventricular preload (**FIGURES 8.2-8.7**).

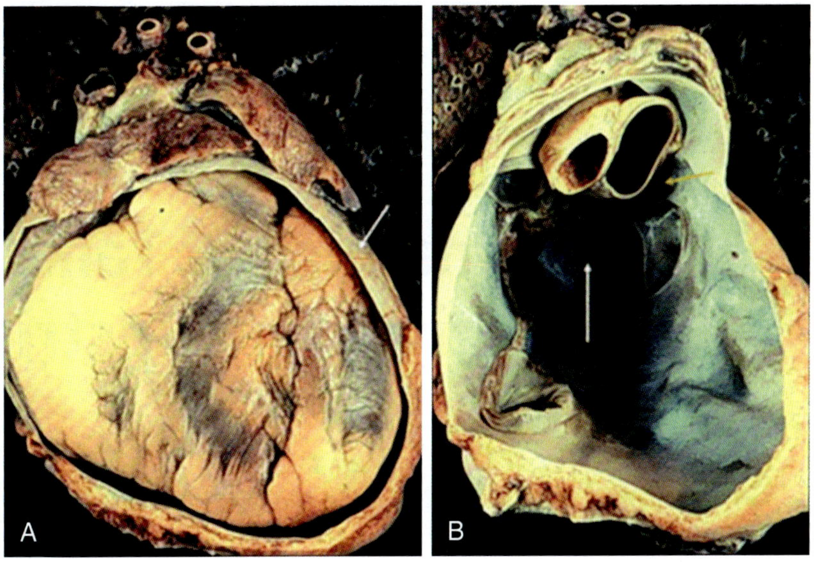

FIGURE 8.1 Pericardial anatomy. Anatomy of the pericardium in the epicardial space. The left panel (A) shows a "window" of the parietal pericardium (arrow) cut away. Note the extensive epicardial fat adhered to the visceral pericardium. The right panel (B) has the heart removed, showing the visceral pericardium posteriorly and around the great vessels. The white arrow points to the oblique sinus and the yellow arrow to the transverse sinus. Reprinted with permission from Lachman N, Syed FF, Habib A, et al. Correlative anatomy for the electrophysiologist, Part I: the pericardial space, oblique sinus, transverse sinus. *J Cardiovasc Electrophysiol*. 2010;21(12):1421-1426.

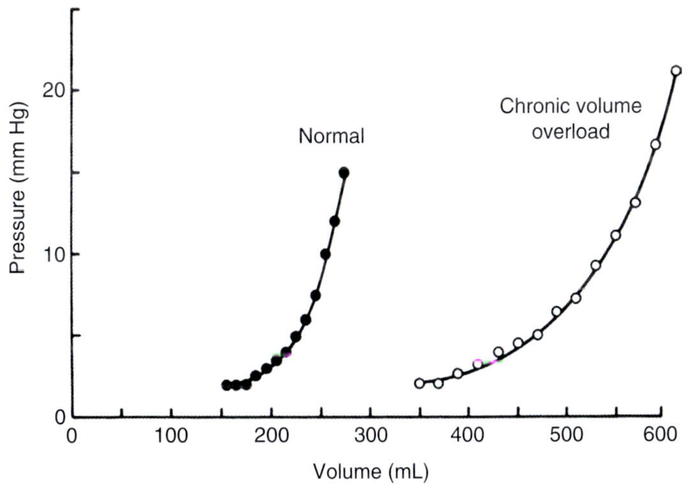

FIGURE 8.2 Pericardial pressure-volume relationship in response to acute and chronic pericardial effusion or volume load. Pericardial pressure-volume relationship in a normal dog (left) and chronic volume loaded dog (right). The pericardial compliance adaptation (right) with rightward shift of the pressure-volume relationship in response to chronic volume load allows even large pericardial effusions to be tolerated hemodynamically without tamponade if they develop slowly. However, in the acute setting, the rapid accumulation of smaller amounts of pericardial fluid can lead to a rapid rise in pericardial pressure (left) and clinical tamponade. Adapted from Freeman GL, LeWinter MM. Pericardial adaptations during chronic cardiac dilation in dogs. *Circ Res*. 1984;54:294-300; Little WC, Freeman GL. Pericardial disease. *Circulation*. 2006;113(12):1622-1632; *Circulation*. 2007;115(15):e406.

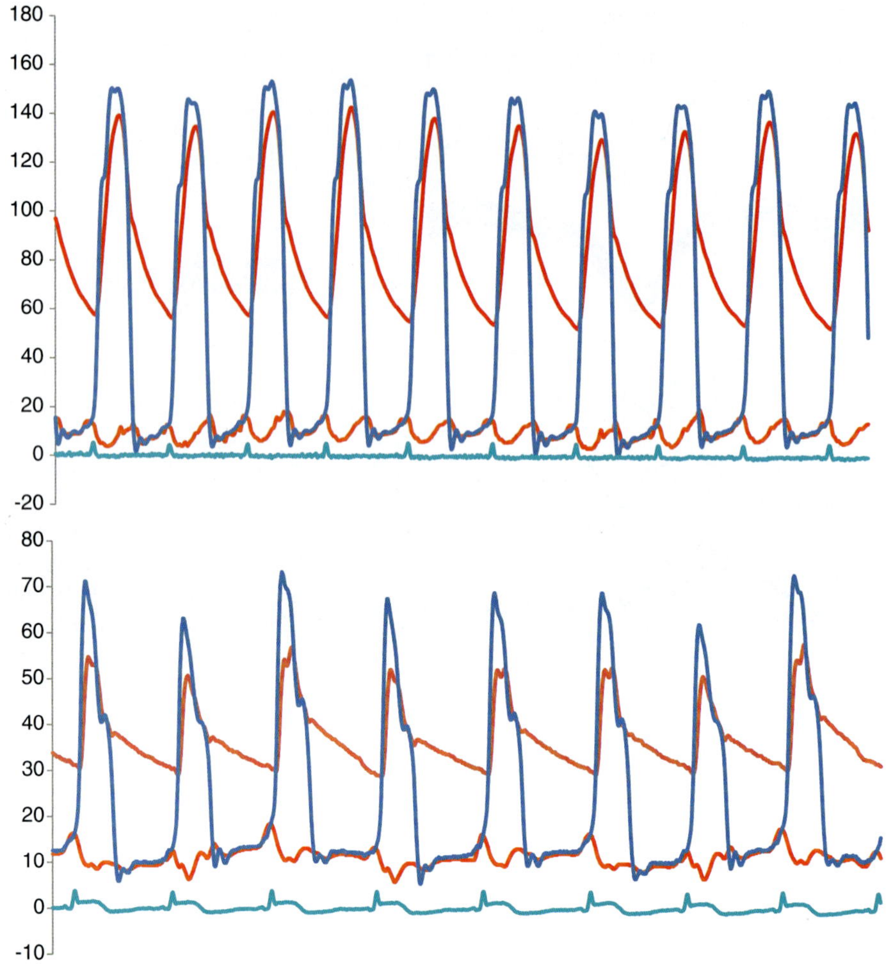

FIGURE 8.3 Hemodynamic tracings in cardiac tamponade. This patient underwent evaluation for dyspnea on exertion in the setting of suspected aortic prosthetic stenosis with transseptal heart catheterization to evaluate the aortic pressure gradient. Top panel shows aortic pressure, left ventricular (LV) pressure, and left atrial pressure demonstrating mildly elevated LV end diastolic pressure with minimal aortic pressure gradient and normal left atrial pressure tracing. During the catheterization, hypotension developed abruptly with systolic blood pressures declining from 140 to 50 mm Hg along with ST elevation on the ECG leads (bottom panel). There was evidence of pulsus paradoxus along with elevation of left atrial pressure and loss of the y descent consistent with pericardial tamponade. Echocardiogram confirmed a new pericardial effusion, which was emergently drained with resolution of hypotension.

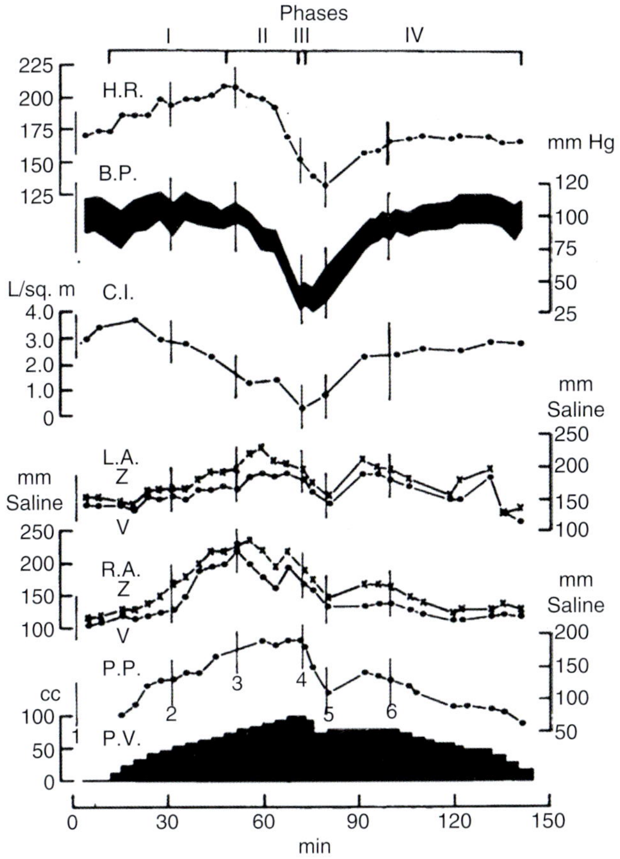

FIGURE 8.4 Stages of tamponade. Changes in heart rate (HR), mean blood pressure (BP), cardiac index (CI), left atrial pressure (LA), right atrial pressure (RA), and pericardial pressure (PP) with infusion of increasing pericardial volume (PV). Phases I, II, and III represent increasing hypotension with a decrease in CI and increase in right and left atrial pressures corresponding to rising pericardial pressures. In phase I, HR increases to compensate for declining stroke volume in an attempt to maintain cardiac output. In phase II, HR, BP and CI begin to decline with further rise in pericardial pressure. Phase III represents a preterminal phase requiring intermittent small pericardial fluid drainage to keep the dog alive and is associated with declining HR. Phase IV represents hemodynamic improvement following pericardiocentesis. Reprinted with permission from Nerlich WE. Determinants of impairment of cardiac filling during progressive pericardial effusion. *Circulation*. 1951;3(3):377-383.

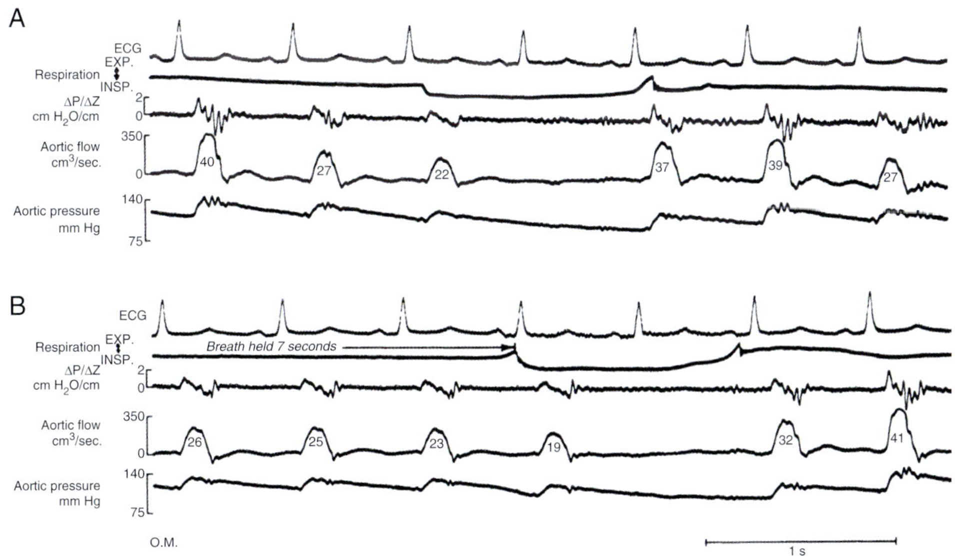

FIGURE 8.5 Pulsus paradoxus. The aortic pressure tracing, aortic blood flow, and ratio of pressure change to flow change (ΔP/ΔV) are demonstrated along with numeric stroke volume (mL) underneath each aortic flow curve in a patient with cardiac tamponade. The top curve demonstrates the absence of aortic flow and pressure pulse with inspiration (pulsus paradoxus) due to exaggerated ventricular interdependence and ineffective LV filling with inspiration. The bottom curve demonstrates the same after prolonged expiratory hold followed by inspiration. Reprinted with permission from Ruskin J, Bache RJ, Rembert JC, Greenfield JC Jr. Pressure-flow studies in man: effect of respiration on left ventricular stroke volume. *Circulation*. 1973;48(1):79-85.

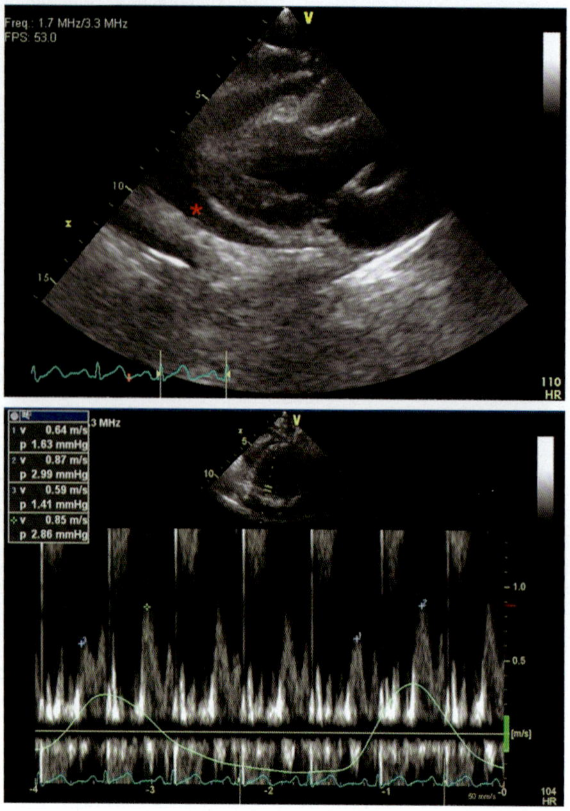

FIGURE 8.6 Echocardiographic findings in cardiac tamponade. A young female with metastatic lung cancer presented with hypotension and shortness of breath. The top panel shows the parasternal long axis view demonstrating a circumferential pericardial effusion (*). The lower panel shows significant respiratory variation in mitral inflow velocity consistent with intrathoracic intracavitary dissociation and exaggerated ventricular interdependence in the setting of tamponade.

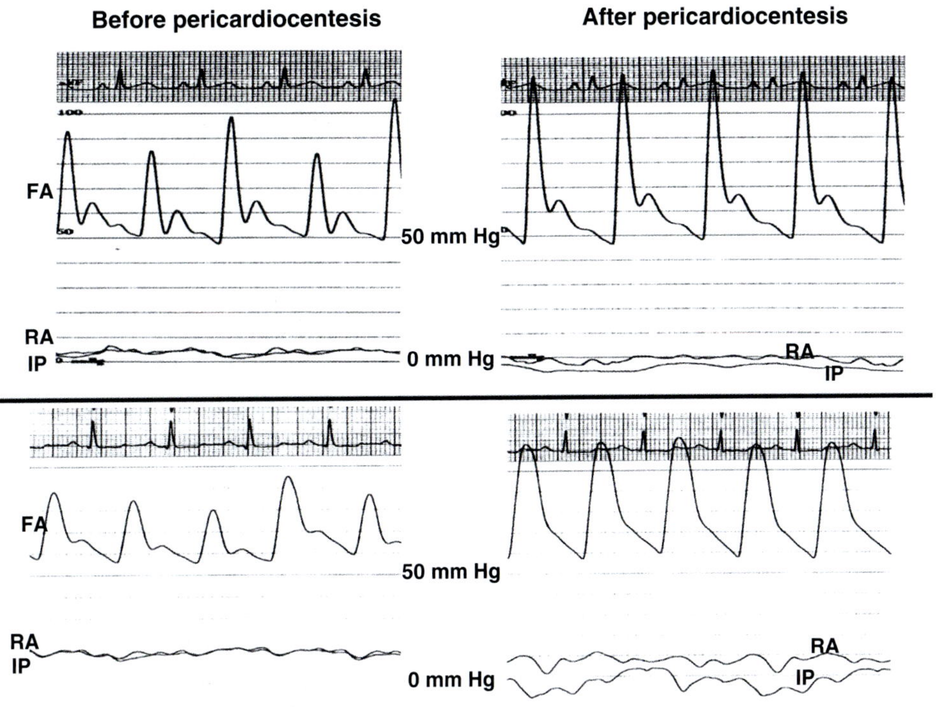

FIGURE 8.7 Low-pressure cardiac tamponade. The top panel shows right atrial and pericardial pressure with low-pressure tamponade. There is pulsus paradoxus that resolves with improvement in blood pressure after pericardiocentesis despite the low right atrial and pericardial pressure. Classic tamponade is shown at the bottom with a higher pericardial pressure that resolves after pericardiocentesis. The postdrainage right atrial pressure is higher than in low-pressure tamponade, and the hemodynamic benefit obtained from drainage is often greater. FA, femoral artery pressure; RA, right atrial pressure; IP, intrapericardial pressure. Cardiac tamponade represents the extreme spectrum of hemodynamic embarrassment caused by a pericardial effusion. The hemodynamics of a significant pericardial effusion exist over a spectrum, however, and in the presence of hypovolemia, a lower pressure in the pericardial space can cause clinical symptoms, the so called low-pressure tamponade. In the classic paper by Sagrista-Sauleda et al, low-pressure tamponade was defined as a pericardial pressure <7 mm Hg, with a postpericardiocentesis right atrial pressure <4 mm Hg. Typical tamponade patients had a pericardial pressure >7 mm Hg with a postpericardiocentesis right atrial pressure >4 mm Hg. Clinical findings may be more subtle than full blown tamponade with frequent absence of jugular venous distension due to the hypovolemic state and less prominent pulsus paradoxus. However, these patients demonstrate an improvement in right atrial transmural pressure and cardiac index after pericardiocentesis proving that they have hemodynamically significant pericardial effusions. Reprinted with permission from Sagristà-Sauleda J, Angel J, Sambola A, Alguersuari J, Permanyer-Miralda G, Soler-Soler J. Low-pressure cardiac tamponade: clinical and hemodynamic profile. *Circulation*. 2006;114(9):945-952. Epub August 21, 2006.

CONSTRICTIVE PERICARDITIS

Even in the absence of pericardial fluid accumulation, inflammatory thickening of the pericardial membrane can lead to poor operating compliance of the pericardium. This can exacerbate pericardial restraint leading to decreased cardiac output and increased intracardiac pressures, with resultant fluid retention and systemic congestion. As opposed to tamponade, symptoms and clinical presentation are more chronic in constrictive pericarditis. Key findings by catheterization include ventricular interdependence and equalization of diastolic pressures due to enhanced pericardial restraint (**FIGURES 8.8-8.23**).

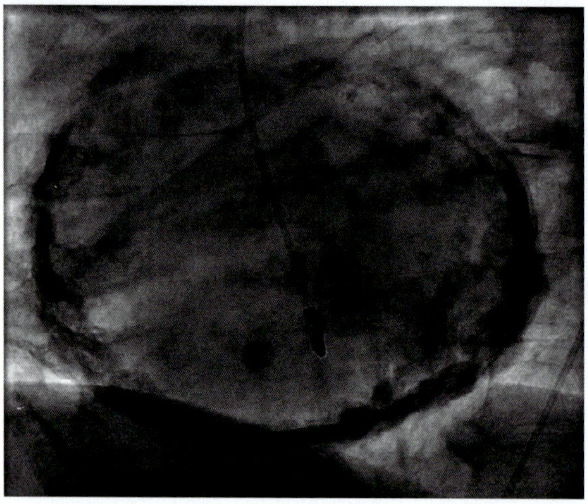

FIGURE 8.8 Pericardial calcification. Ventriculogram showing heavily calcified pericardium in constrictive pericarditis. This can be appreciated on fluoroscopy or by X-ray and is suggestive of underlying constriction in the presence of elevated jugular venous pressure with prominent y descents. Reprinted with permission from Sharif D, Radzievsky N, Rosenschein U. Images in cardiovascular medicine. Recurrent pericardial constriction: vibrations of the knock, the calcific shield, and the evoked constrictive physiology. *Circulation*. 2008;118(16):1685-1688.

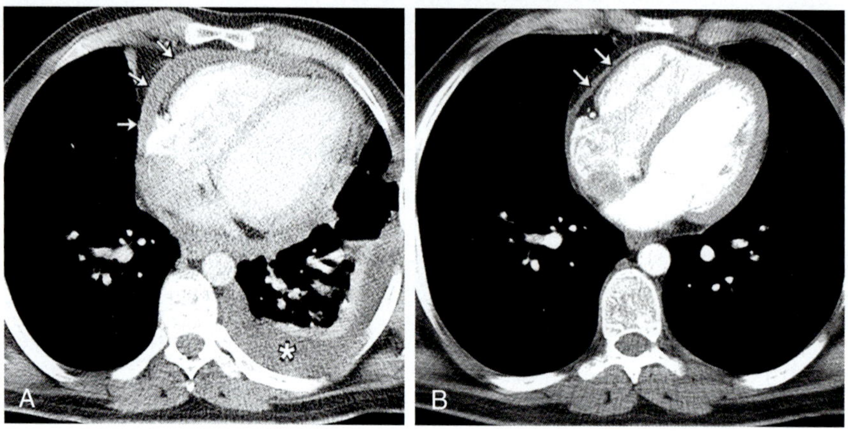

FIGURE 8.9 CT showing pericardial thickening. A, CT scan showing inflammatory pericardial thickening (15 mm) (arrows) with a left pleural effusion (asterisk) in a patients with clinical constrictive pericarditis. B, Anti-inflammatory therapy led to a dramatic decrease in pericardial thickness to 3 mm (arrows) with resolution of constrictive hemodynamics. However, it is important to remember that constriction can still occur in the absence of pericardial thickening (18% in a Mayo Clinic Series of surgically proven constriction had normal pericardial thickness [<2 mm]) Reproduced from Tom CW, Oh JK. Images in cardiovascular medicine. A case of transient constrictive pericarditis. *Circulation*. 2005;111(21):e364; Reprinted with permission from Talreja DR, Edwards WD, Danielson GK, et al. Constrictive pericarditis in 26 patients with histologically normal pericardial thickness. *Circulation*. 2003;108(15):1852-1857.

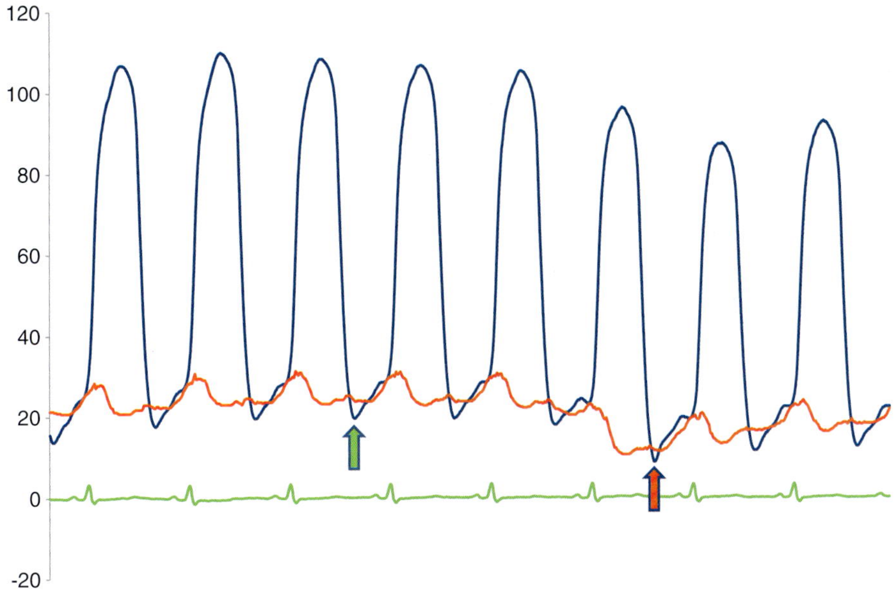

FIGURE 8.10 Simultaneous pulmonary capillary wedge and left ventricular catheterization tracings demonstrating intrathoracic-intracardiac dissociation. In constrictive pericarditis, the thickened pericardium causes relative insulation of the heart from intrathoracic pressure changes, leading to proportionally larger respiratory changes in pulmonary capillary wedge (PCWP) (intrathoracic pressure outside the pericardium in the pulmonary veins) than LV diastolic pressure (intrathoracic pressure inside the pericardium). With inspiration (red arrow), there is a decrease in PCWP that is greater than the drop in LV diastolic pressure leading to a narrowing of the PCWP-LV diastolic pressure gradient. With expiration (green arrow), opposite changes are seen leading to a widening of the PCWP-LV diastolic gradient. This change in PCWP-LV diastolic gradients (which drives LV filling) is one of the major mechanisms underlying ventricular interdependence, respiratory variation in mitral inflow velocity by Doppler, and pulsus paradoxus in constrictive pericarditis.

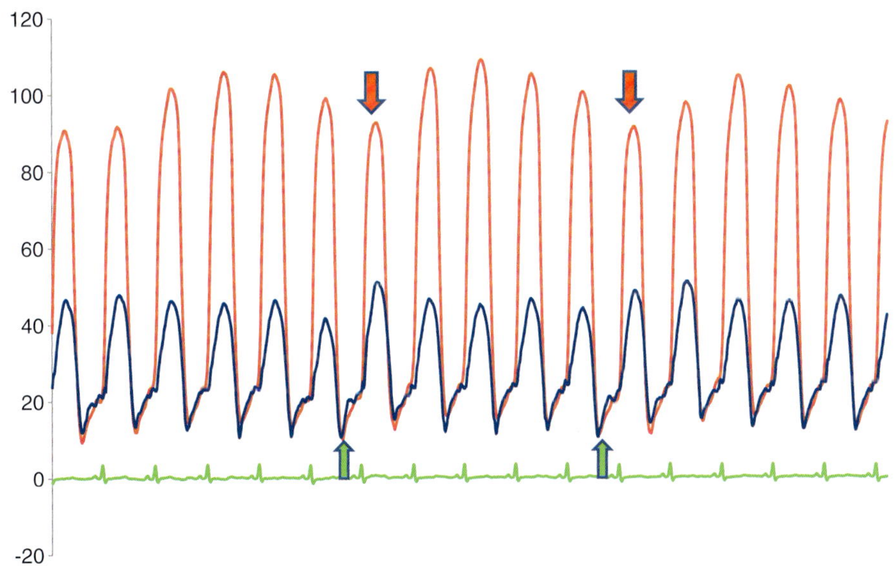

FIGURE 8.11 Simultaneous left and right heart catheterization in a patient with constrictive pericarditis. Note the elevated left and right ventricular diastolic pressures with a square root sign and near equalization of diastolic pressures. With inspiration (green arrow), there is a decrease in left ventricular (LV) systolic pressure with a simultaneous increase in right ventricular (RV) pressure (red arrow), indicative of ventricular interdependence. Inspiration is marked by maximal negative early diastolic pressure (green arrow) and is accompanied by an increase in venous return to the RV coupled with a decrease in driving pressure for LV filling through a decreased pulmonary vein to LV gradient (see previous figure). This results in increased RV stroke volume and decreased LV stroke volume with inspiration, which results in an increase in the RV pressure contour with reciprocal LV contour changes due to exaggerated ventricular interdependence. This may also result in pulsus paradoxus (red arrows). Conventional criteria for constriction were also present with LV-RV end diastolic pressure <5 mm Hg, RV end diastolic pressure >1/3 of RV systolic pressure, and pulmonary artery systolic pressure <55 mm Hg.

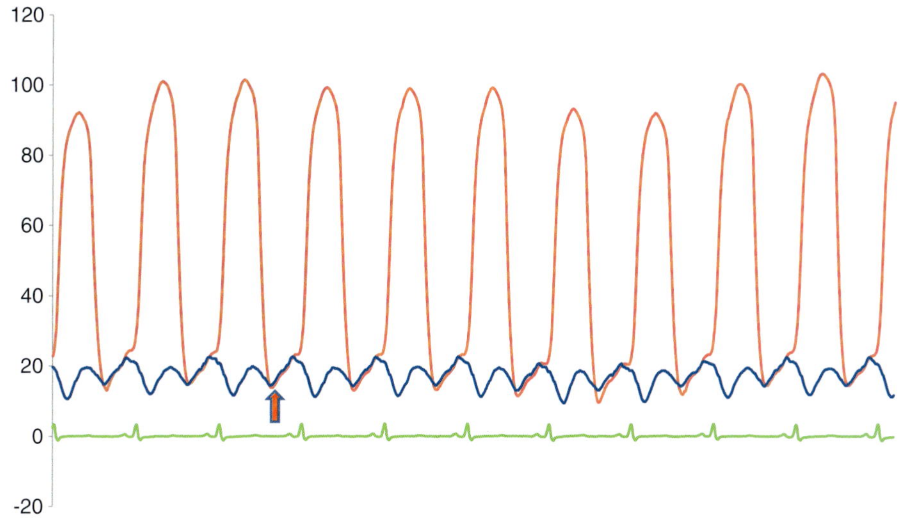

FIGURE 8.12 Simultaneous right atrial (RA) and left ventricular (LV) pressure tracing in constrictive pericarditis. Note the elevated RA pressure with prominent y descents (red arrow). The mean RA pressure fails to drop with inspiration (positive Kussmaul sign). Left ventricular end diastolic pressure is elevated with a rapid filling wave (square root sign). There is equalization of right atrial and LV diastolic pressures, which suggests that pericardial restraint, as opposed to underlying myocardial disease, is the underlying cause of the elevated LV diastolic pressures.

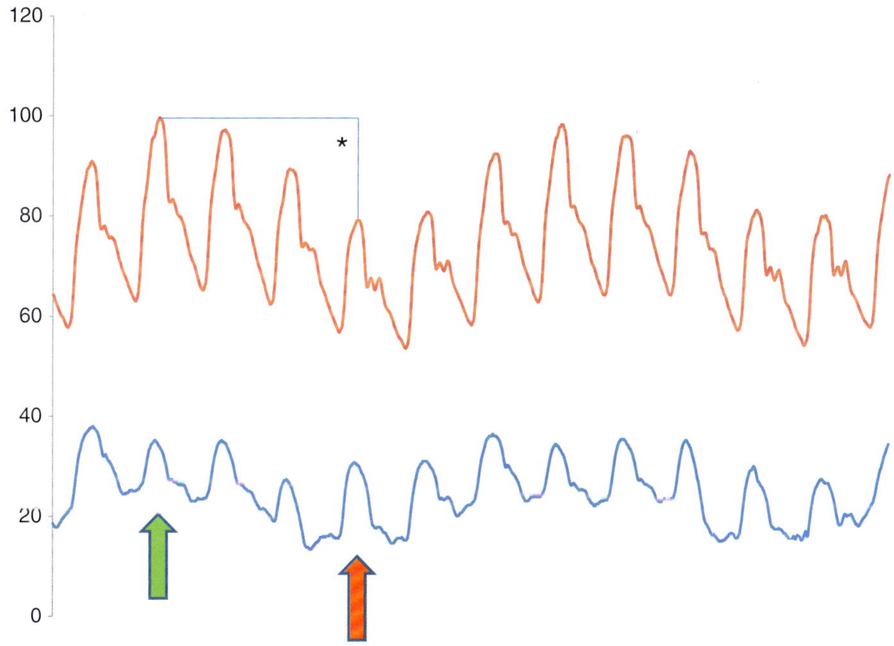

FIGURE 8.13 Simultaneous aorta and pulmonary artery tracings in constrictive pericarditis. Similar to left and right ventricular tracings, simultaneous aorta and pulmonary artery tracings reflect ventricular stroke volume changes with respiration due to ventricular interdependence. With expiration (green arrow), there is a decrease in RV stroke volume reflected by a decrease in RV systolic pressure and RV ejection time (time from onset of ventricular systolic waveform to the dicrotic notch from pulmonary valve closure), with opposite changes seen in the aortic tracing, namely an increase in aortic systolic pressure and an increase in aortic ejection time. The opposite is seen with inspiration, along with the presence of pulsus paradoxus (*).

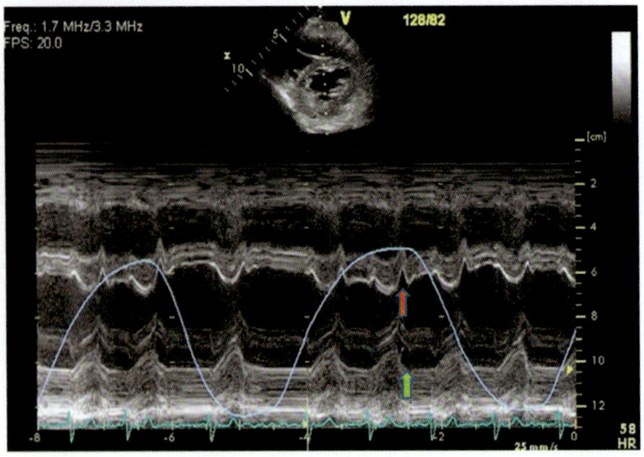

FIGURE 8.14 M mode in constrictive pericarditis. Rapid ventricular filling results in sudden cessation of flow in early to mid diastole with flattening of the posterior left ventricular wall (the M mode equivalent of the square root sign) (green arrow). With the high temporal resolution with M mode echocardiography, abnormal septal bounce (red arrow) can be appreciated with an initial anterior septal motion followed by a rapid posterior motion in early to mid diastole, which is more prominent with inspiration. Note also the respiratory septal motion with septal motion toward the right ventricle with expiration and toward the left ventricle with inspiration.

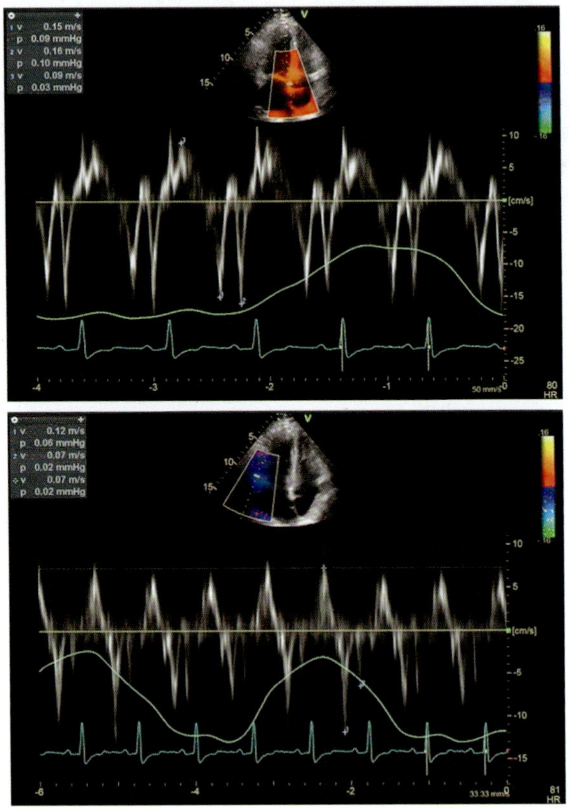

FIGURE 8.15 Tissue Doppler of the medial (top) and lateral (bottom) annulus in constrictive pericarditis. Despite signs of systemic congestion and heart failure, the presence of a normal e′ velocity >0.08 m/s (tissue doppler velocity of relaxation in early diastole) implies normal myocardial relaxation and essentially excludes restrictive cardiomyopathy. In constriction, the lateral e′ velocity is often abnormally lower than the septal e′ velocity (the opposite is seen in healthy controls). This has been called annulus reversus and is due to tethering of the lateral myocardial wall from constrictive pericarditis.

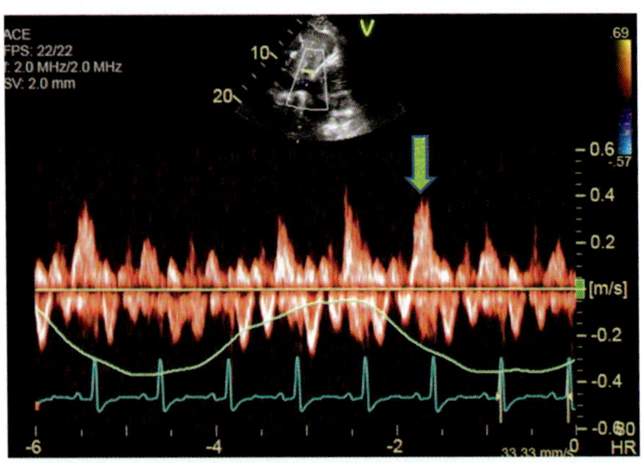

FIGURE 8.16 Hepatic vein Doppler in constrictive pericarditis. Expiration results in an increase in hepatic vein reversal velocity (green arrow) with a decrease in diastolic forward flow in expiration. This arises owing to ventricular interdependence and impaired compliance of the right ventricle with expiration due to expiratory movement of the ventricular septum into the RV, which compromises RV chamber size, effective operating compliance, and forward filling in diastole. If flow reversals are more prominent with inspiration, restrictive cardiomyopathy is more likely present.

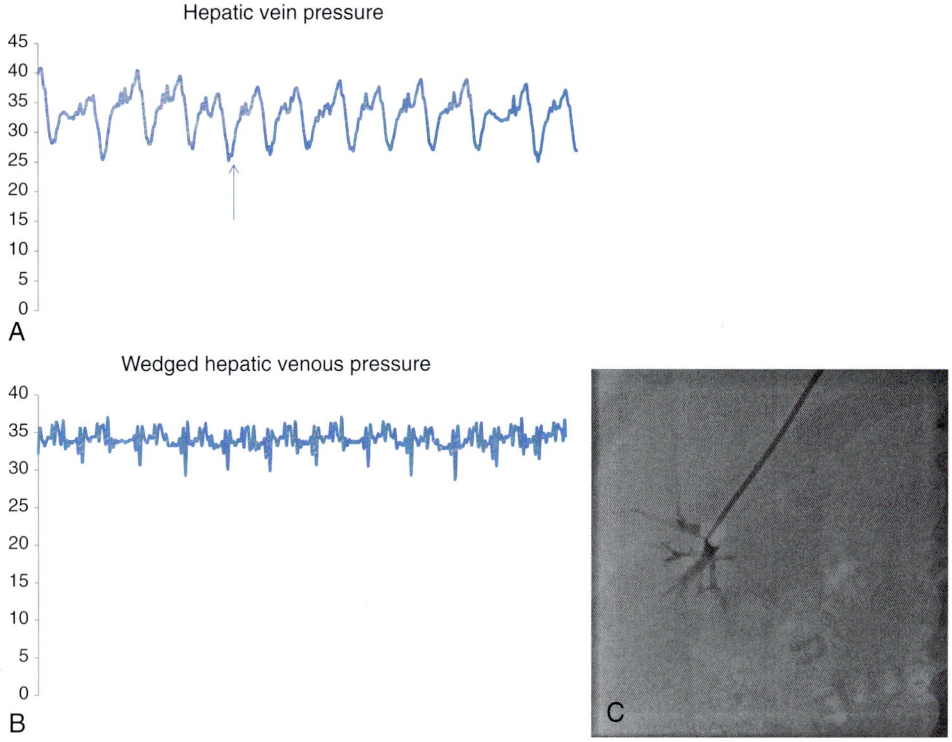

FIGURE 8.17 Assessment of liver dysfunction in constrictive pericarditis during cardiac catheterization. Patients with constriction often present with liver dysfunction from chronic congestion, which complicates assessment of operative risk. Assessment for primary liver disease versus passive congestion is therefore helpful before surgery and can be accomplished by cardiac catheterization to determine the hepatic wedge pressure. A, shows the free hepatic vein pressure obtained through placement of a balloon wedge catheter in the hepatic vein. Note that the tracing appears similar to the right atrial pressure tracing in constriction with elevated pressures (33 mm Hg) with prominent y descents (arrow). B, shows the wedged hepatic venous pressure obtained from balloon inflation and wedging the catheter in smaller hepatic venules to provide an estimate of sinusoidal pressure. Here the hepatic wedge pressure is also 34 mm Hg providing a hepatic wedge to free hepatic vein gradient of 1 mm Hg (abnormal >7-10 mm Hg). This provides confirmation that the elevated portal pressures are due to cardiac venous congestion from constriction and not due to intrinsic liver disease. C, Injection of a few mL of contrast while the balloon is inflated can confirm the hepatic wedge position. Reprinted with permission from Bosch J, Abraldes JG, Berzigotti A, García-Pagan JC. The clinical use of HVPG measurements in chronic liver disease. *Nat Rev Gastroenterol Hepatol*. 2009;6(10):573-582. doi:10.1038/nrgastro.2009.149. Epub September 1, 2009.

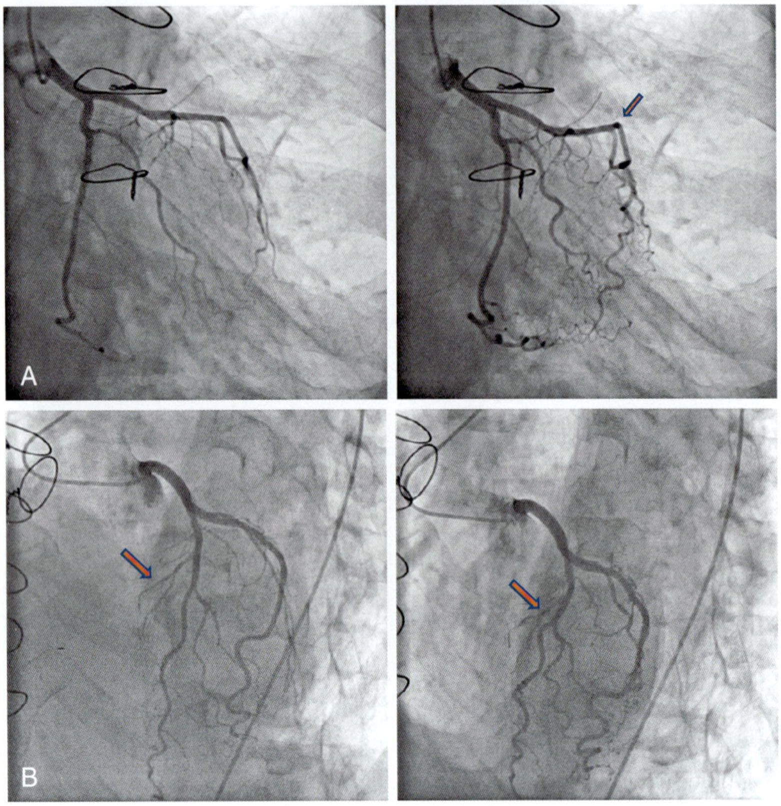

FIGURE 8.18 A, Coronary angiography in constrictive pericarditis demonstrating coronary artery fixation in the left anterior descending artery in the right anterior oblique caudal view. Red arrow points to hinge point where the coronary artery is fixed to the pericardium (see supplementary Video A). B, Left anterior oblique cranial view with respiration demonstrating abnormal beat-to-beat as well as respiratory septal motion in the septal perforators (see supplementary Video B). Red arrow points to change in septal coronary artery position with expiration (left figure) and inspiration (right figure). There is also beat-to-beat abnormal septal motion seen in the septal contrast blush as well as in the septal perforator better appreciated in the supplementary Video B.

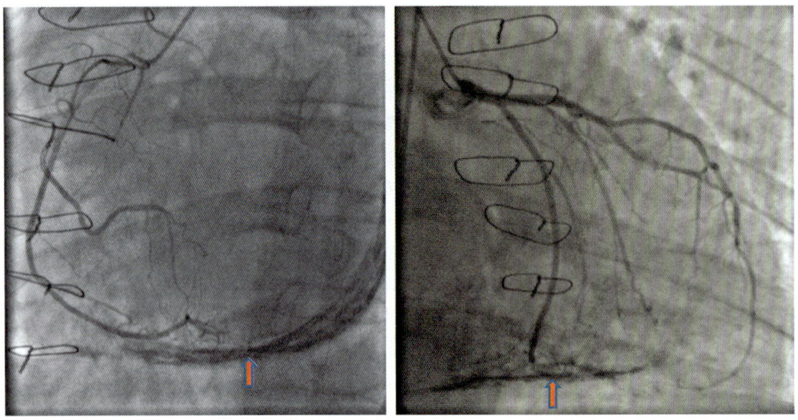

FIGURE 8.19 Fluoroscopy in calcific constrictive pericarditis on injection of right (left panel) and left (right panel) coronary arteries. Severe pericardial calcification noted along the inferior heart wall (red arrows) during coronary angiography in a patient with constrictive pericarditis. X-ray imaging or fluoroscopy at the time of cardiac catheterization can detect pericardial calcifications, which strongly support an underlying diagnosis of constrictive pericarditis.

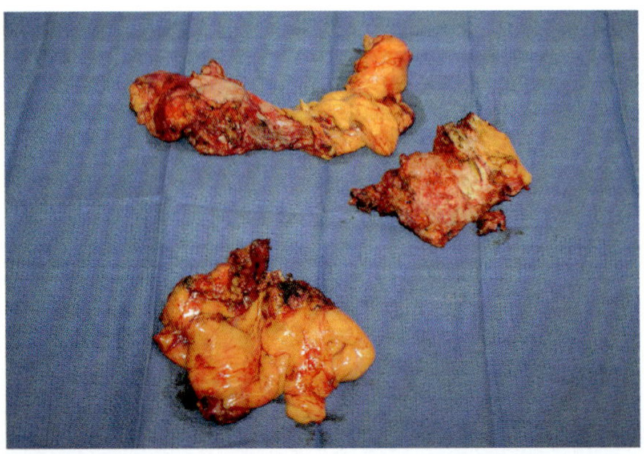

FIGURE 8.20 Thickened calcified pericardium after resection for constrictive pericarditis in the same patient as prior angiogram. The patient had undergone surgery 20 years prior for aortic valve replacement of a bicuspid aortic valve. He subsequently developed worsening ascites, dyspnea, and peripheral edema and was found to have severe constrictive pericarditis with a pulmonary capillary wedge pressure of 35 mm Hg and a right atrial pressure of 33 mm Hg before surgery.

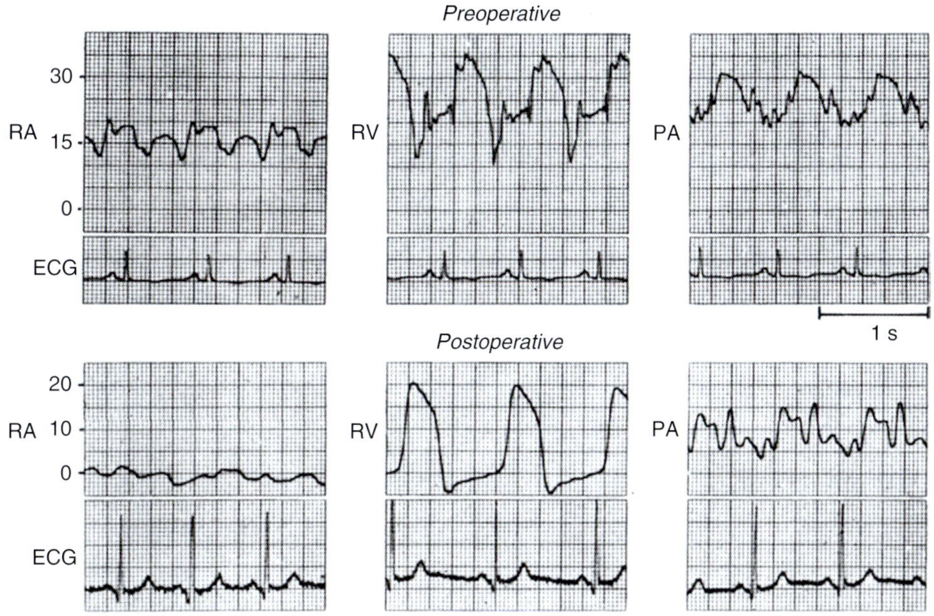

FIGURE 8.21 Hemodynamics after pericardiectomy. Top three panels demonstrate preoperative right atrial (RA), right ventricular (RV), and pulmonary artery (PA) tracings consistent with constrictive pericarditis. There are prominent y descents in the RA tracing, square root sign with elevated RV end diastolic pressure and mildly elevated pulmonary artery pressures. Bottom three panels show corresponding changes in the same patient after pericardiectomy. RA pressure has decreased dramatically and a prominent y descent is no longer seen. Also RV end diastolic pressure has decreased and there is no longer a square root sign, and mean PA pressure has decreased to normal. Reprinted with permission from Kloster FE, Crislip RL, Bristow JD, Herr RH, Ritzmann LW, Griswold HE.Hemodynamic studies following pericardiectomy for constrictive pericarditis. *Circulation*. 1965;32(3):415-424.

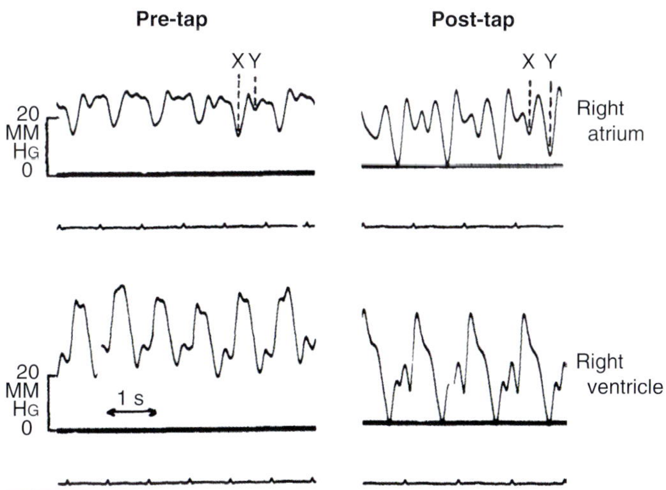

FIGURE 8.22 Right atrial and ventricular pressure in effusive-constrictive pericarditis. Right atrial and right ventricular pressure tracings before (left) and after (right) pericardiocentesis in a patient with effusive-constrictive pericarditis. Initially, in the presence of the pericardial effusion, blunting of the y descent is seen (left upper) consistent with tamponade physiology. After pericardiocentesis (right), there is a drop in right ventricular pressure and a mild drop in right atrial pressure. However, right atrial pressure remains elevated and the y descent becomes prominent along with the appearance of a rapid filling pattern in the right ventricular tracing (square root sign), consistent with underlying superimposed constriction. Reprinted with permission from Hancock EW. Subacute effusive-constrictive pericarditis. *Circulation*. 1971;43(2):183-192.

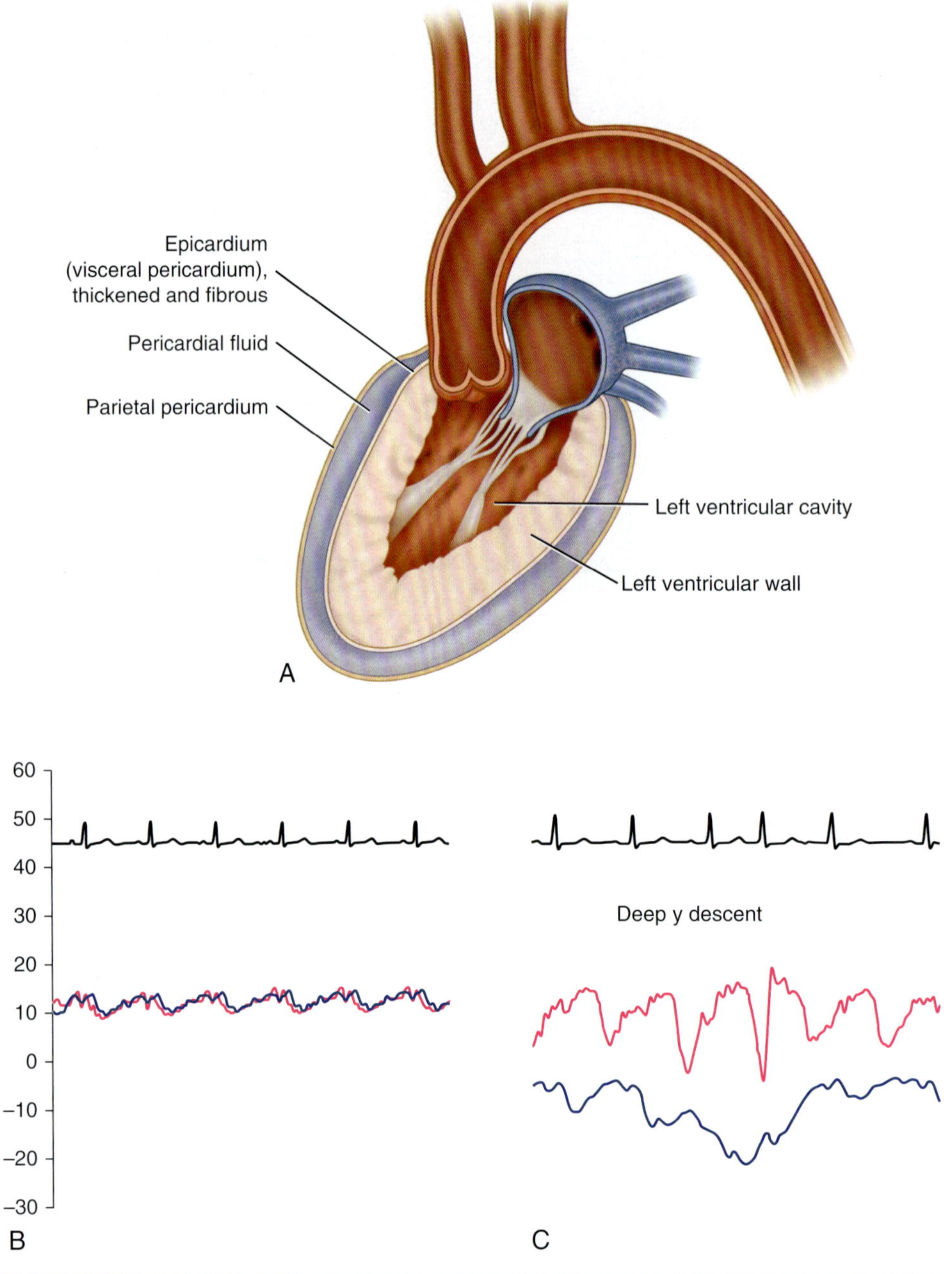

FIGURE 8.23 Effusive-constrictive pericarditis. The presence of pericardial fluid causes tamponade, and a thickened visceral pericardium (epicardium) causes constriction (A). Pressure tracing findings in effusive-constrictive pericarditis. Before pericardiocentesis (B), findings are consistent with tamponade with mild elevation in right atrial pressures (pink), equalization of right filling, and intrapericardial pressures (blue). Postpericardiocentesis (C), there is normalization of intrapericardial pressures but right atrial pressures remain elevated. Note the development of deep y descents after drainage of the pericardial effusion. B and C, Reproduced with permission from Miranda WR, Oh JK. Effusive-constrictive pericarditis. *Cardiol Clin*. 2017;35:551-558.

RESTRICTIVE CARDIOMYOPATHY

Myocardial disease and restrictive cardiomyopathy can simulate many of the clinical findings of constrictive pericarditis including systemic congestion, elevated jugular venous pressure, and dyspnea on exertion. However, this is primarily due to diastolic reserve limitations in restrictive cardiomyopathy, and careful evaluation including echocardiography and invasive catheterization are often required to differentiate this from constriction. The absence of ventricular interdependence or intrathoracic-intracardiac dissociation, along with the presence of significant elevation in left-sided filling pressures and mean pulmonary artery pressure, suggests underlying myocardial restrictive disease. Tricuspid regurgitation can complicate the evaluation and often requires a right ventriculogram to differentiate between severe tricuspid regurgitation and restrictive cardiomyopathy (**FIGURES 8.24-8.33**).

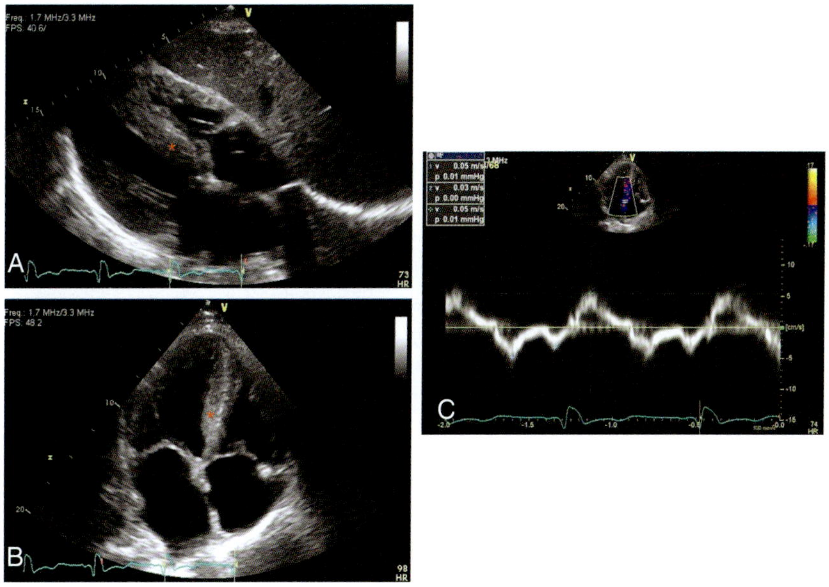

FIGURE 8.24 Echocardiographic findings in restrictive cardiomyopathy from cardiac amyloidosis. A and B, show left ventricular wall thickening (*) with severe biatrial enlargement consistent with restrictive cardiomyopathy. C, shows significantly decreased septal e' tissue Doppler relaxation velocities, consistent with impaired myocardial relaxation and intrinsic myocardial disease, in contrast to the preserved e' velocity seen in constrictive pericarditis.

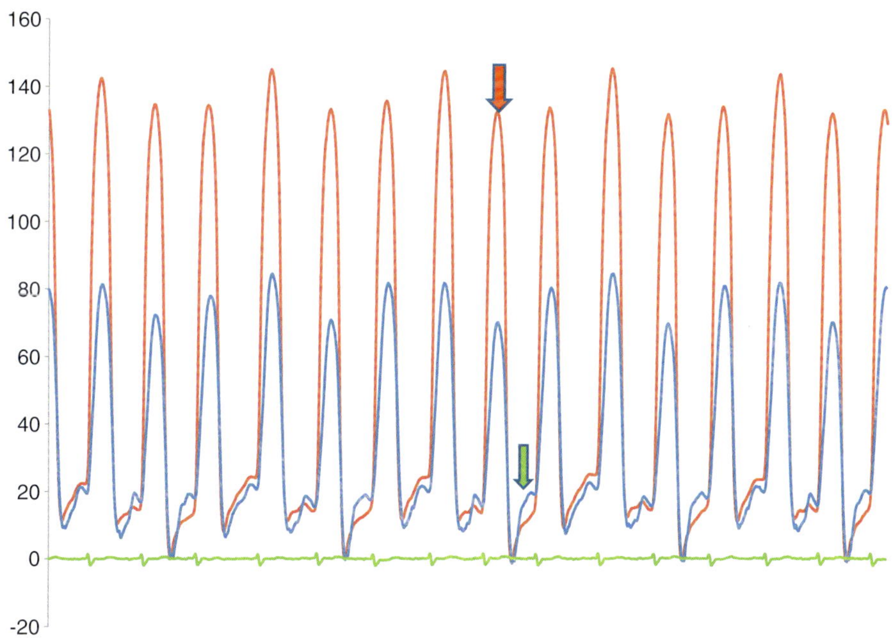

FIGURE 8.25 Simultaneous left and right heart catheterization in restrictive cardiomyopathy. Right and left ventricular end diastolic pressures are significantly elevated with elevated right ventricular (RV) systolic pressure consistent with pulmonary hypertension. With inspiration, there is concordant decrease of left and right ventricular systolic pressure changes consistent with myocardial restrictive (red arrow) disease as opposed to constrictive pericarditis. With inspiration and increased RV preload, there is a more prominent rapid filling wave along with an increase in RV diastolic pressure above LV diastolic pressure suggestive of greater RV than LV myocardial diastolic dysfunction with poor operating compliance of the right ventricle (green arrow). The elevated RV systolic pressure >55 mm Hg and the RV end diastolic pressure <1/3 of the RV systolic pressure are consistent with underlying restriction.

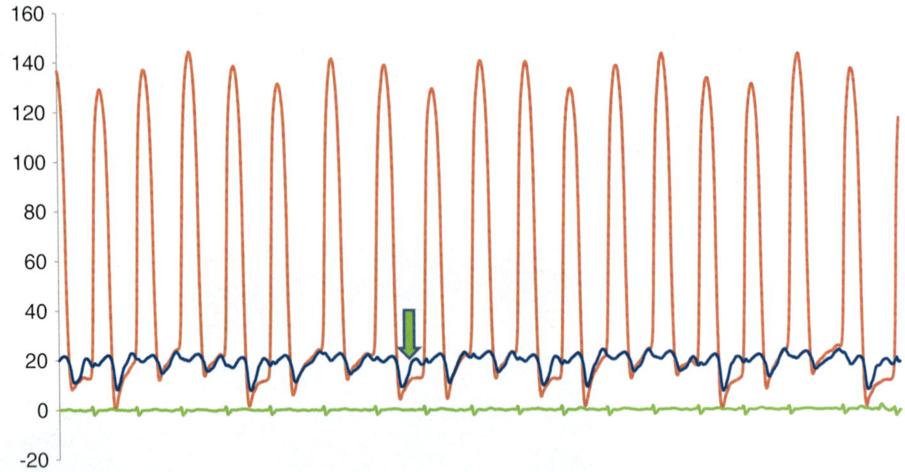

FIGURE 8.26 Simultaneous left ventricular and right atrial pressure tracing in restrictive cardiomyopathy. Right atrial pressure is elevated, but there is no equalization of right atrial and LV diastolic pressures (green arrow), which argues against pericardial restraint. The y descents appear more prominently with inspiration owing to poor baseline operating compliance of the right ventricle, which causes early rapid filling and rapid equalization with the increased preload associated with inspiration.

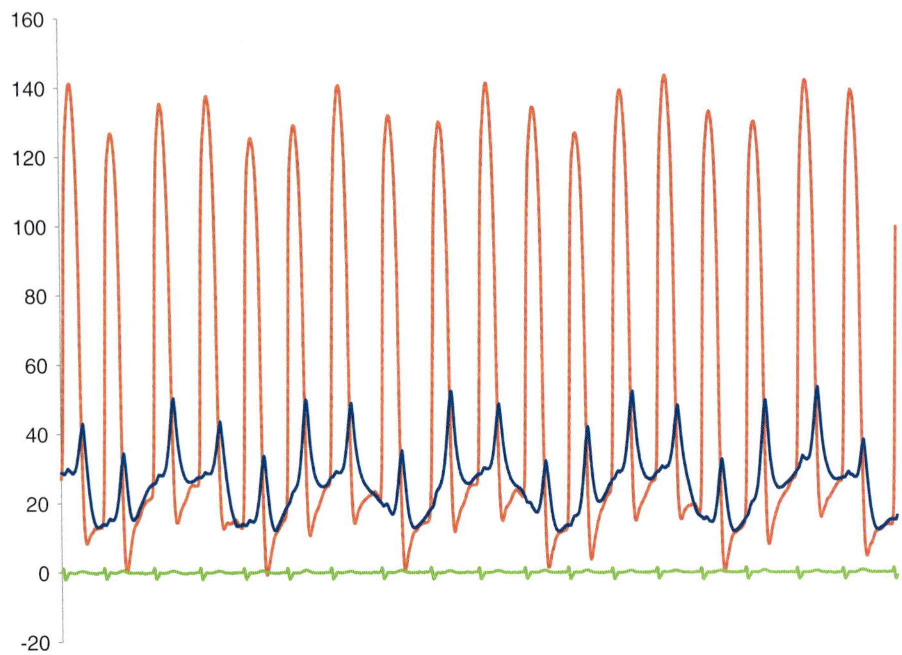

FIGURE 8.27 Simultaneous pulmonary capillary wedge (PCWP) and left ventricular (LV) pressure tracing in restrictive cardiomyopathy. The PCWP was severely elevated with prominent v waves. Left ventriculogram showed no evidence of mitral regurgitation, so the prominent v waves were from poor operating compliance of the left atrium. There was no evidence of intrathoracic-intracavitary dissociation, and the PCWP-LV diastolic pressure gradient remained fairly constant throughout respiration all supportive of underlying restrictive cardiomyopathy.

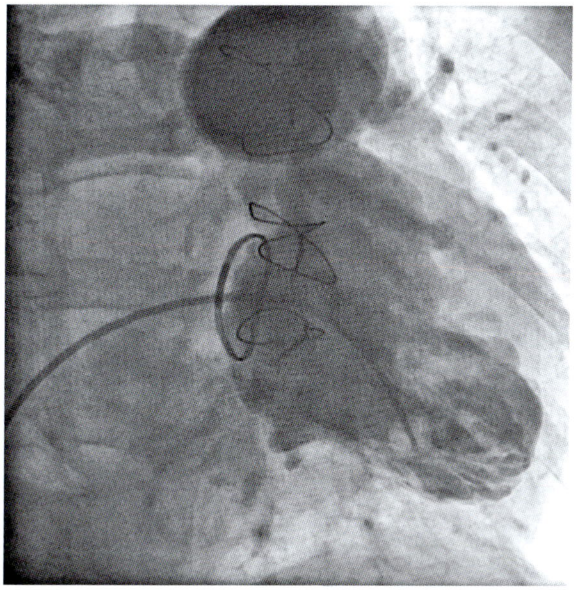

FIGURE 8.28 Right ventriculogram to assess for tricuspid regurgitation in the setting of underlying restrictive cardiomyopathy and demonstrating mild or 1+ tricuspid regurgitation across a previous tricuspid valve repair that is functioning normally.

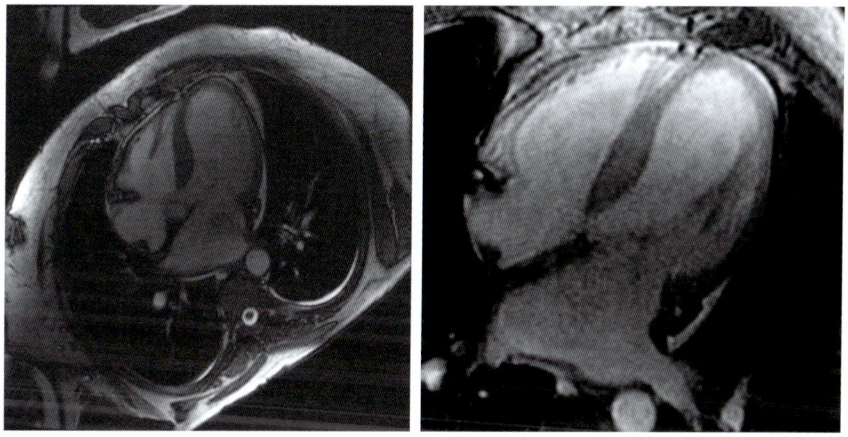

FIGURE 8.29 MRI in restrictive cardiomyopathy in a patient with cardiac amyloidosis (left panel, zoomed on right panel). Note the thickened walls with severely enlarged left atrium.

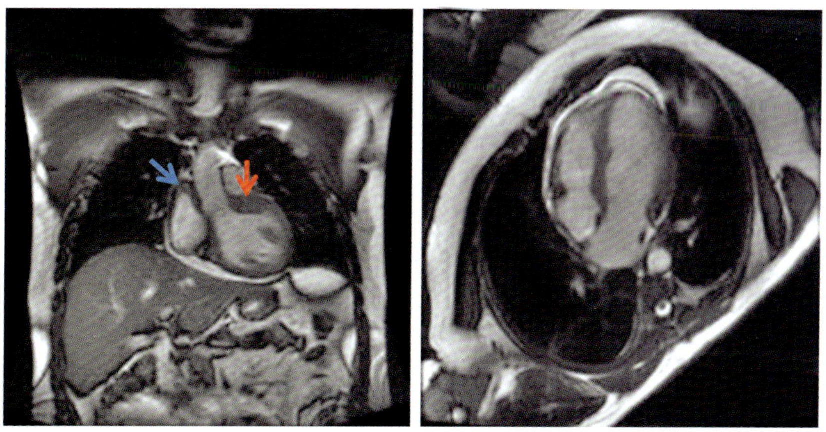

FIGURE 8.30 MRI in restrictive cardiomyopathy in a patient with cardiac sarcoidosis. Left image, Coronal cine fiesta imaging, still frame view obtained in ventricular diastole. Note thickening of the anterior LV (red arrow) and RA (blue arrow). Right image, 4-chamber fiesta imaging obtained during ventricular diastole with moderate left atrial enlargement and right atrial enlargement due to restrictive physiology. Cardiac biopsy demonstrated noncaseating granulomas consistent with cardiac sarcoidosis.

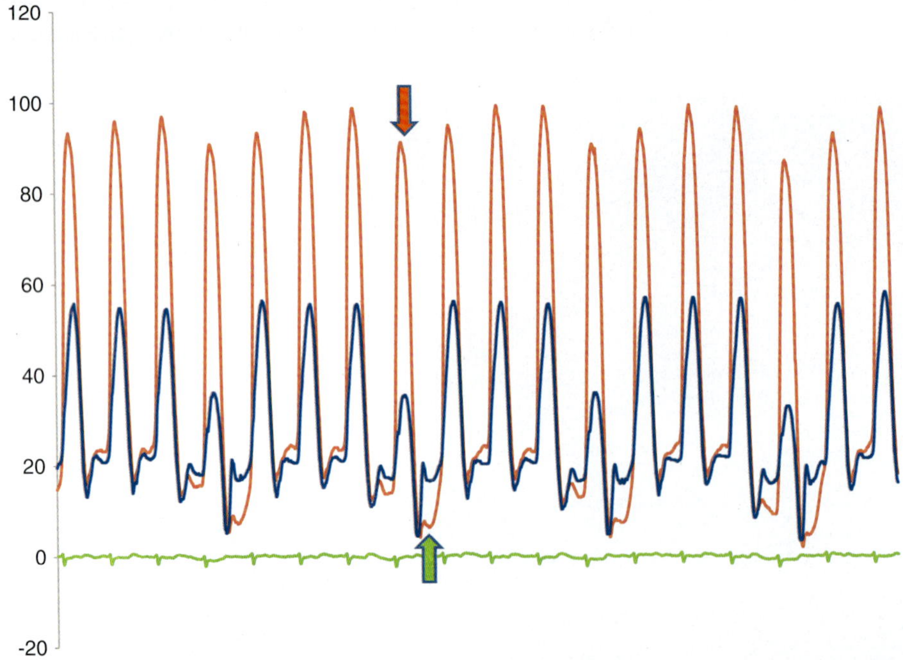

FIGURE 8.31 Simultaneous left and right ventricular catheterization tracings in severe tricuspid regurgitation with underlying restrictive cardiomyopathy. The left and right ventricular end diastolic pressures are elevated with early rapid ventricular filling. There is no ventricular interdependence and with inspiration there are concordant negative changes in right and left ventricular systolic pressures (red arrow). Furthermore, with inspiration, there is a dramatic elevation in right ventricular diastolic pressures above the left indicative of restrictive myocardial filling and inability to accommodate increased venous return to the right ventricle (green arrow). This can occur with both right-sided myocardial restrictive disease and significant tricuspid regurgitation with underlying right ventricular noncompliance. A right ventriculogram can help differentiate between restriction and tricuspid regurgitation in equivocal cases. In this case an RV gram demonstrated 4+ tricuspid regurgitation indicating that tricuspid regurgitation was the major abnormality and the elevated left-sided filling pressures were partially from relative pericardial restraint in addition to an underlying myocardial restrictive process.

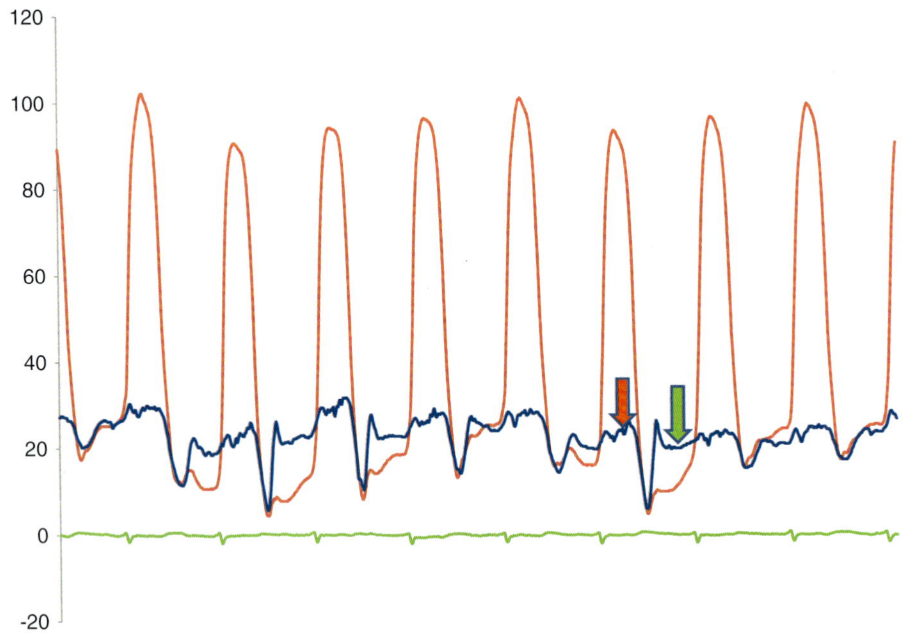

FIGURE 8.32 Continued from previous. Simultaneous right atrial and LV pressure in severe tricuspid regurgitation. Simultaneous left ventricular and right atrial tracing demonstrating elevated right atrial pressure with a prominent c-v wave (red arrow) and positive Kussmaul sign from severe tricuspid regurgitation (TR). There is ventricularization of the RA tracing particularly with inspiration indicative of severe TR and a common right ventricular and right atrial pressure chamber. The rapid filling wave in the right ventricle with inspiration from the previous tracing is reflected back to the RA (green arrow).

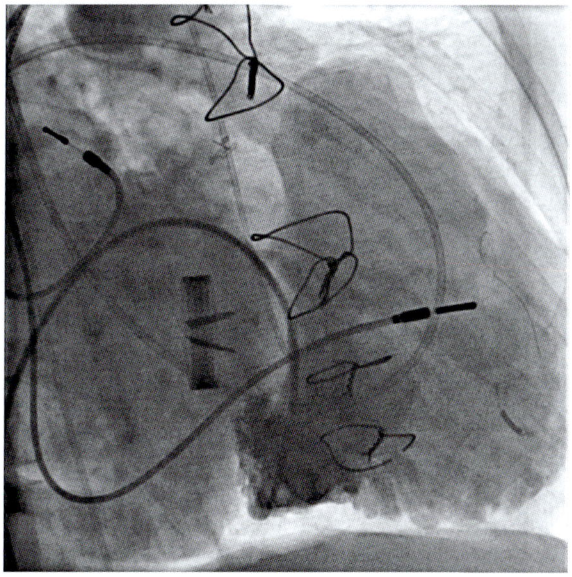

FIGURE 8.33 Right ventriculogram demonstrating severe tricuspid regurgitation. Right anterior oblique view of the RV gram demonstrates 4+ tricuspid regurgitation in the setting of a severely enlarged right atrium. There is a normally functioning mitral prosthesis.

chapter 9

Pitfalls in the Evaluation of Hemodynamic Data

MAURO MOSCUCCI, MD, MBA

INTRODUCTION

Potential sources of error in the recording and/or interpretation of hemodynamic data include inappropriate positioning, balancing and calibration of transducers, equipment failure, displacement, inappropriate placement and inadequate flushing of the recording catheter, and failure to recognize the role of loading conditions during acquisition of hemodynamic data. As a complement to Chapters 7 and 8, this chapter will review common pitfalls in the recording and evaluation of hemodynamic data (**FIGURES 9.1-9.16**).

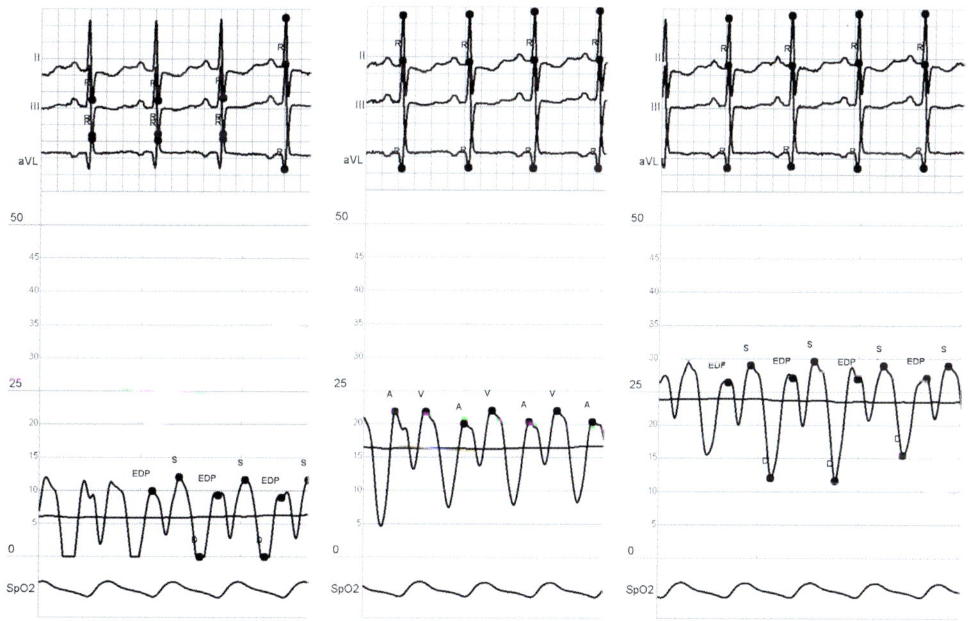

A B C

FIGURE 9.1 A-C, Three sets of right atrial pressures in a patient with severe aortic stenosis and radiation-induced pericardial disease s/p pericardiectomy. The panels reveal normal, moderately elevated, and severely elevated right atrial pressures, all recorded on a 5 mm Hg scale. The tracings were taken a few seconds apart, with the transducers positioned above, at, and below the level of the patient's heart. Failure to compulsively align the transducer with the level of the patient's heart produces substantial error in hemodynamic recordings. Note the steep Y descent, which falsely appears to have an excursion below zero in the tracing at left (A). Reproduced with permission from Turi ZG. Pitfalls in the evaluation of hemodynamic data. In: Moscucci M, ed. *Grossman & Baim's Cardiac Catheterization Angiography and Intervention*. Philadelphia: Lippincott Williams and Wilkins; 2014.

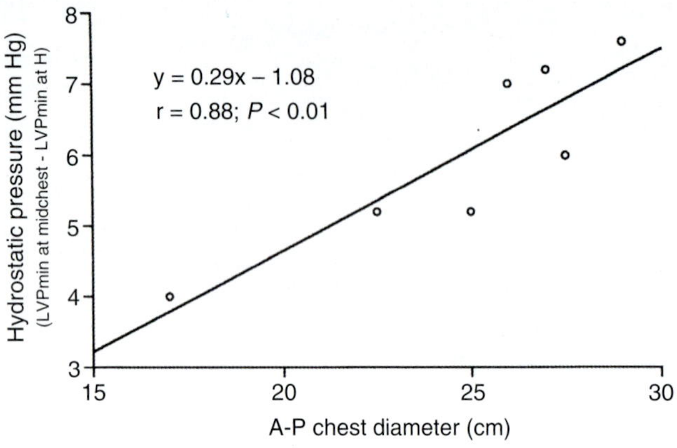

FIGURE 9.2 Graph showing minimum left ventricular pressure (LVPmin) measurement error due to hydrostatic pressure influences attributable to a midchest reference position as a function of patient anterior-posterior (A-P) chest thickness. H indicates measurement taken at the uppermost blood level in the left ventricle. Reproduced with permission from Courtois M, Fattal PG, Kovács SJ Jr, Tiefenbrunn AJ, Ludbrook PA. Anatomically and physiologically based reference level for measurement of intracardiac pressures. *Circulation*. 1995;92:1994-2000.

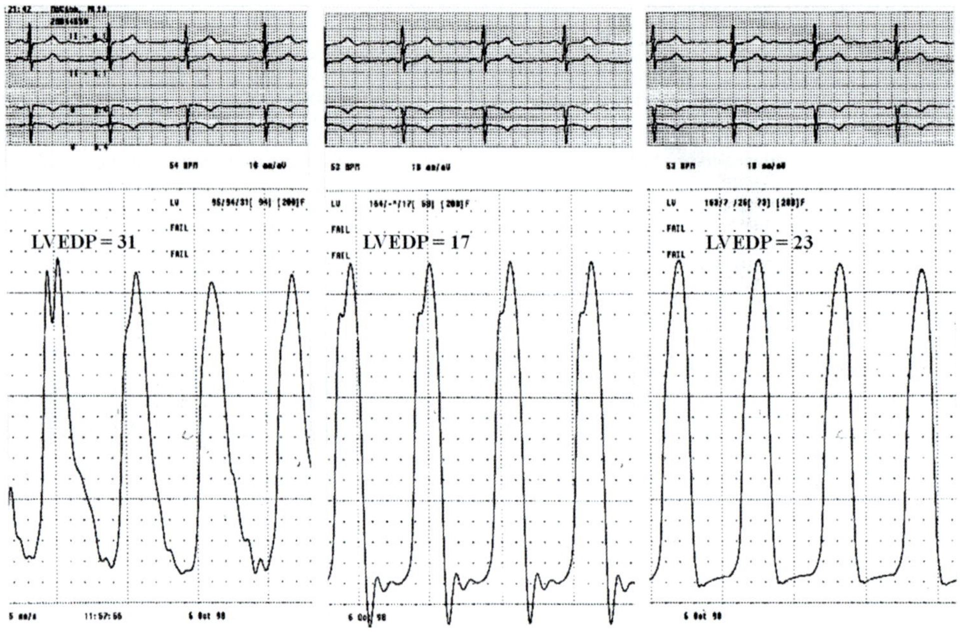

FIGURE 9.3 Pitfalls in measurements of the left ventricular diastolic pressure. All measurements were obtained in the same patient. Left panel: The left ventricular end diastolic pressure is markedly elevated, and there is an abnormal contour of the pressure waveform. The abnormal contour and elevation of left ventricular diastolic pressure is due to inappropriate position of the left ventricular pigtail catheter, with a side hole in the ascending aorta. Middle panel: There is an early diastolic overshoot, which is due to an air bubble in the system (ringing effect). Right panel: Normal tracing after repositioning and flushing the catheter. Reproduced with permission from Moscucci M, Grossman W. Pressure measurements. In: Moscucci M, ed. *Grossman & Baim's Cardiac Catheterization Angiography and Intervention*. Philadelphia: Lippincott Williams and Wilkins; 2014.

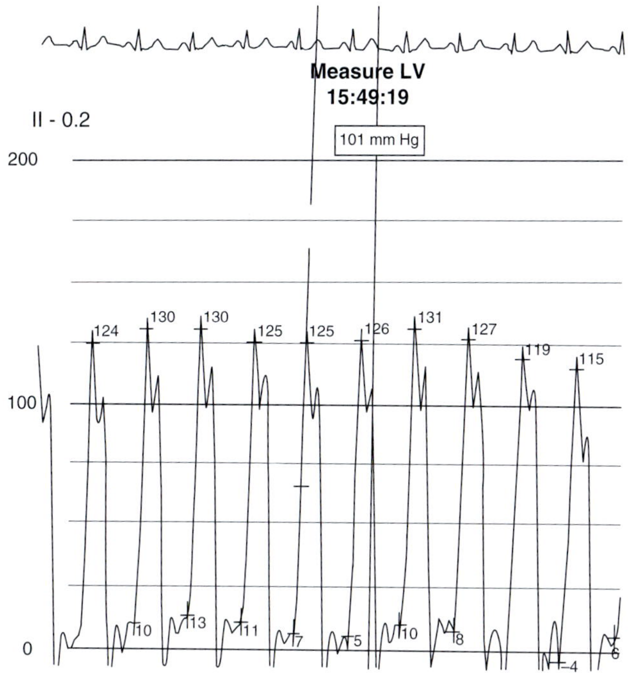

FIGURE 9.4 Left ventricular pressure tracing. Note the high spike of the left ventricular upstroke and the large negative overshoot wave in the left ventricular pressure downstroke. This artifact is to do an air bubble in the pressure line. The pressure bubble is rapidly accelerated and decelerated in the fluid-filled catheter, with a resulting movement of the fluid column back and forth in the catheter and a ringing effect.

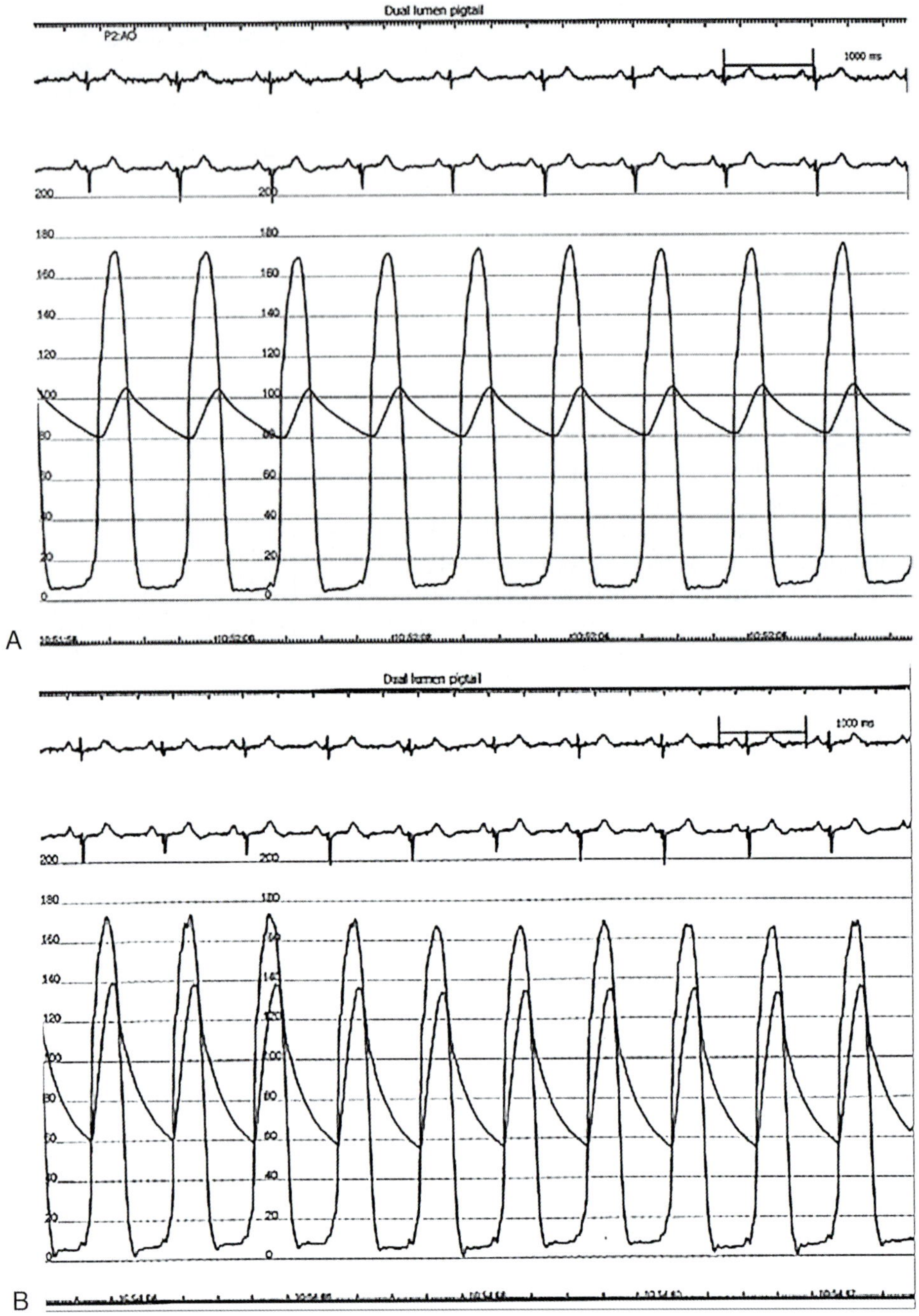

FIGURE 9.5 Evaluation of aortic stenosis. A, Note the damped appearance of the aortic pressure tracing with a significant gradient suggestive of severe aortic stenosis. B, This tracing was obtained in the same patient 1 min later. The only intervention that was made was to flash the catheter that had a clot.

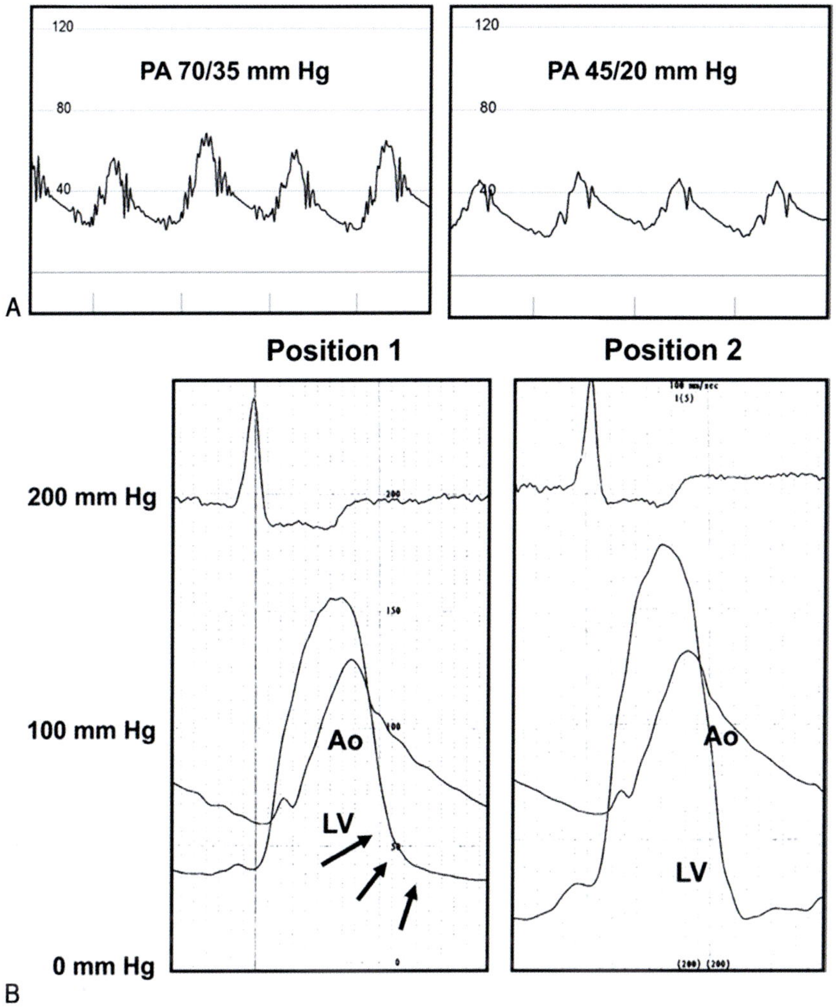

FIGURE 9.6 It is necessary to assess pressure contours continually throughout the catheterization procedure to identify pressure artifacts that may occur and lead to erroneous pressure measurements. A, The initial pulmonary artery (PA) pressure in this patient undergoing evaluation of pulmonary hypertension is 70/35 mm Hg (left). However, during the procedure, it was noted that the pulmonary artery pressure fell to 45/20 mm Hg in the absence of any other hemodynamic changes (right). This was due to the formation of a small thrombus in the small distal lumen of a thermodilution catheter. This pressure artifact should be avoided by meticulous technique, which includes constant monitoring of the pressure contour and intermittent frequent flushing of the lumen with heparinized saline. Using larger-bore catheters may be necessary to overcome this problem if damping of pressures continues despite the use of these techniques. B, In this patient with aortic stenosis, there is a pigtail catheter in the left ventricle (LV) and a separate catheter in the ascending aorta (Ao). In position 1, the contour of the left ventricular pressure is abnormal, with a marked delay in the fall of pressure during early diastole. This is due to some of the multiple side holes in the pigtail catheter straddling the aortic valve, resulting in a fusion of left ventricular and aortic pressure. Because the abnormal contour is recognized, the catheter is placed further distally so that all recording holes are in the left ventricle, as shown in position 2. Reproduced with permission from Nishimura RA, Carabello BA. Hemodynamics in the cardiac catheterization laboratory of the 21st century. *Circulation*. 2012;125:2138-2150.

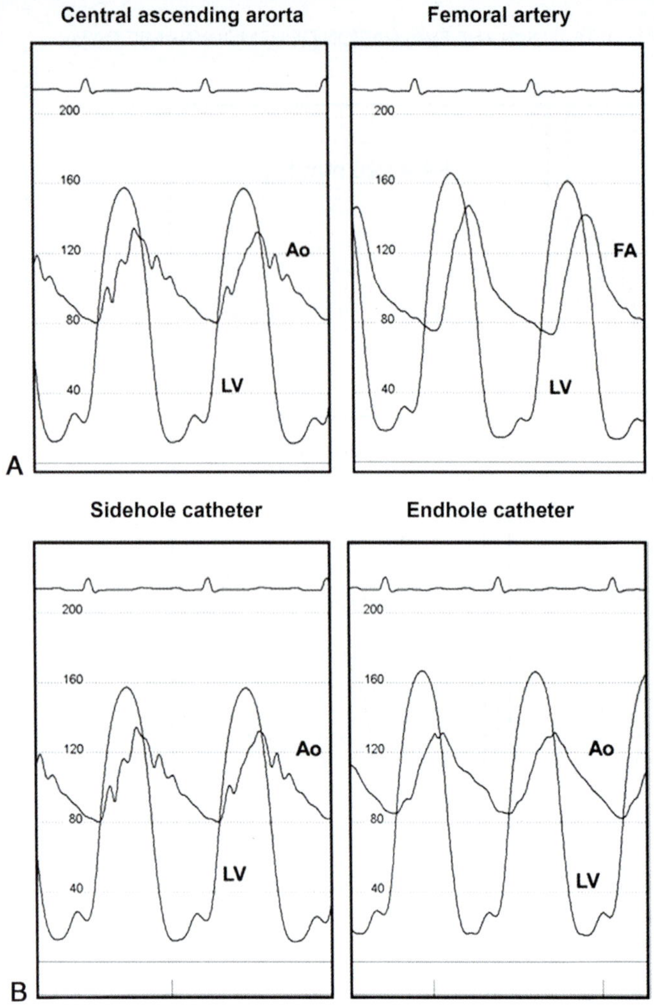

FIGURE 9.7 The optimal method to measure the transaortic gradient in a patient with aortic stenosis is a simultaneous left ventricular (LV) pressure and central aortic (Ao) pressure with side-hole catheters. Shown are examples in which alternative methods are used to obtain the pressures, which produce erroneous results. A, The simultaneous left ventricular and femoral artery (FA) pressures should not be used to measure the aortic valve gradient because peripheral amplification may cause a false decrease in gradient, and peripheral artery stenosis may cause a false increase in gradient. There is also a temporal delay when a femoral artery pressure is used that will affect the calculation of the mean gradient. In this patient, the use of a femoral artery pressure would significantly underestimate the peak-to-peak gradient as a result of peripheral amplification of the pressure. B, In the measurement of left ventricular and aortic pressures, catheters with side holes should be used because damping can occur with an end-hole catheter (ie, coronary artery catheters). Shown is the typical damping that may occur in the aortic pressure when an end-hole catheter (right) is used compared with a side-hole catheter (left). Reproduced with permission from Nishimura RA, Carabello BA. Hemodynamics in the cardiac catheterization laboratory of the 21st century. *Circulation*. 2012;125:2138-2150.

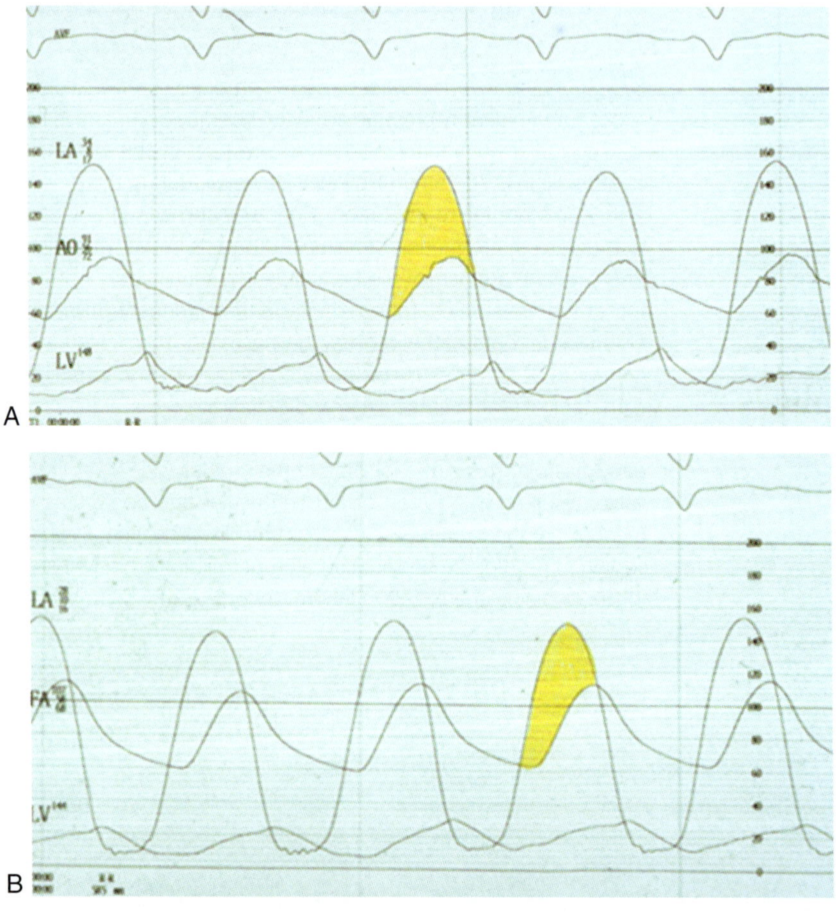

FIGURE 9.8 Left ventricular (LV) versus central aortic pressure (A) and LV versus femoral artery pressure (B). The tracings were recorded a few seconds apart. Note the dramatically higher gradient in A with classic features of severe aortic stenosis. In contrast, tracing B shows lower peak-to-peak gradient and much higher aortic dP/dt and pulse pressure. Using femoral artery pressure as a proxy for central aortic pressure can result in substantial underestimation of the severity of aortic stenosis. Reproduced with permission from Turi ZG. Pitfalls in the evaluation of hemodynamic data. In: Moscucci M, ed. *Grossman & Baim's Cardiac Catheterization Angiography and Intervention*. Philadelphia: Lippincott Williams and Wilkins; 2014.

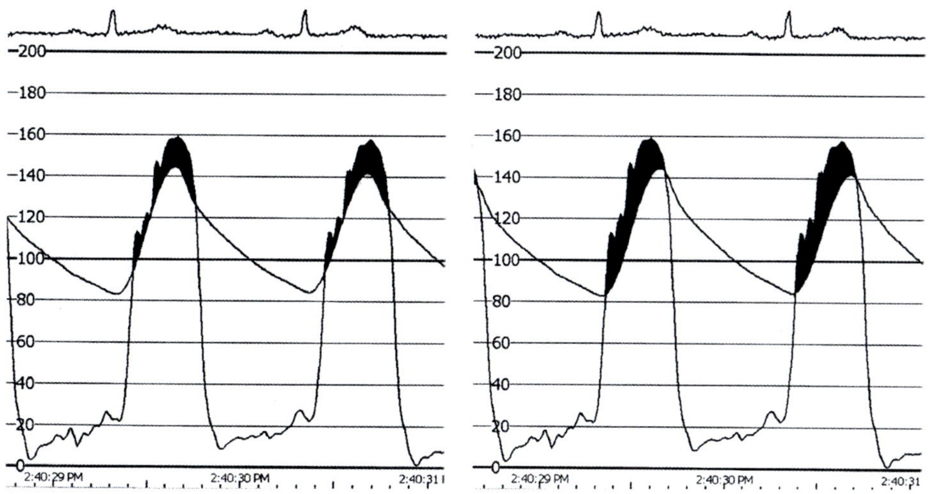

FIGURE 9.9 Inappropriate phase shift is seen in the image on the left (A). The software used by the cath lab assumed incorrectly that systemic pressure was being recorded at the level of the femoral/external iliac artery. The aortic pressure tracing was then moved forward in time, creating the artifact seen, which depicts systemic pressure rise occurring prior to left ventricular contraction, a physiologic impossibility (in the absence of certain types of cardiac assist devices that would have a quite different signature). The gradient on the left was reported as 11 mm Hg and the calculated aortic valve area as 1.7 cm^2. On the right (B), with elimination of the phase shift, the correct gradient is now reported as 20 mm Hg and the valve area as 1.3 cm^2. Courtesy of Dr John Hirshfeld, University of Pennsylvania. Reproduced with permission from Turi ZG. Pitfalls in the evaluation of hemodynamic data. In: Moscucci M, ed. *Grossman & Baim's Cardiac Catheterization Angiography and Intervention*. Philadelphia: Lippincott Williams and Wilkins; 2014.

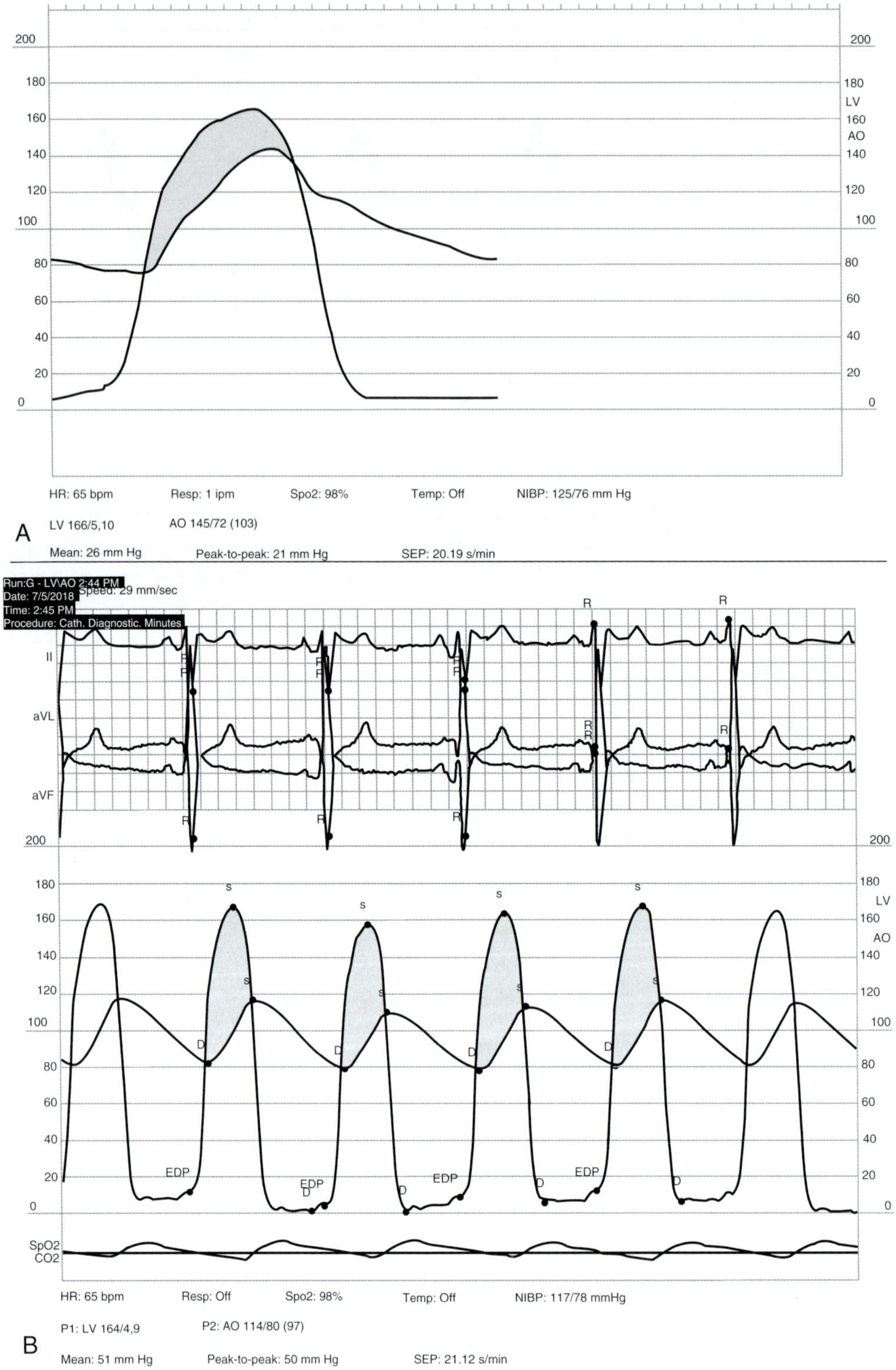

FIGURE 9.10 A, Transaortic gradient as measured by the computer on a single beat following pull-back of the pigtail catheter across the aortic valve. The computer takes one beat representative of left ventricular systolic pressure and overimposes the aortic pressure tracing from a different cardiac cycle for the determination of transvalvular gradient. Note the misalignment of the pressure tracings. The process does not take into account beat-to-beat variability in pulse pressure, as the 2 tracings are not simultaneous. B, shows the true gradient across the aortic valve measured using a dual lumen catheter. Note that in B, the non invasive blood pressure (NIBP) matches the invasive pressure, while in A it is lower than the pressure measured on a single beat. The difference between A and B is less likely to be due to an artifact similar to the one illustrated in **FIGURE 9.5**, which in this case can be ruled out given that the dual lumen catheter was appropriately flushed multiple times. The patient underwent at a later stage Transcatheter Aortic Valve Replacement.

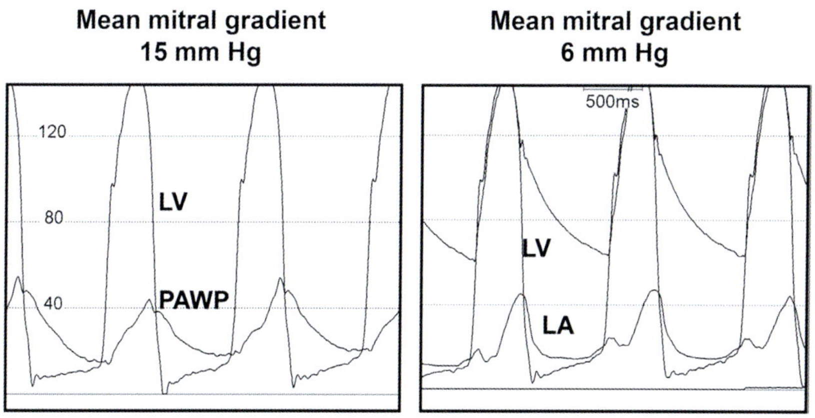

FIGURE 9.11 Measurement of the transmitral gradient by cardiac catheterization is frequently made with a simultaneous pulmonary artery wedge pressure (PAWP) and left ventricular (LV) pressure. However, as a result of the delay in transmission of the change in pressure contour and a phase shift, the gradient using a pulmonary artery wedge pressure will frequently overestimate the true transmitral gradient. Left, Simultaneous left ventricular and pulmonary artery wedge pressure in a patient with mitral stenosis. The measured mean gradient is 15 mm Hg. Right, In the same patient, the transmitral gradient is measured with a left ventricular and direct left atrial (LA) pressure. The true mean transmitral gradient is only 6 mm Hg. Reproduced with permission from Nishimura RA, Carabello BA. Hemodynamics in the cardiac catheterization laboratory of the 21st century. *Circulation*. 2012;125:2138-2150.

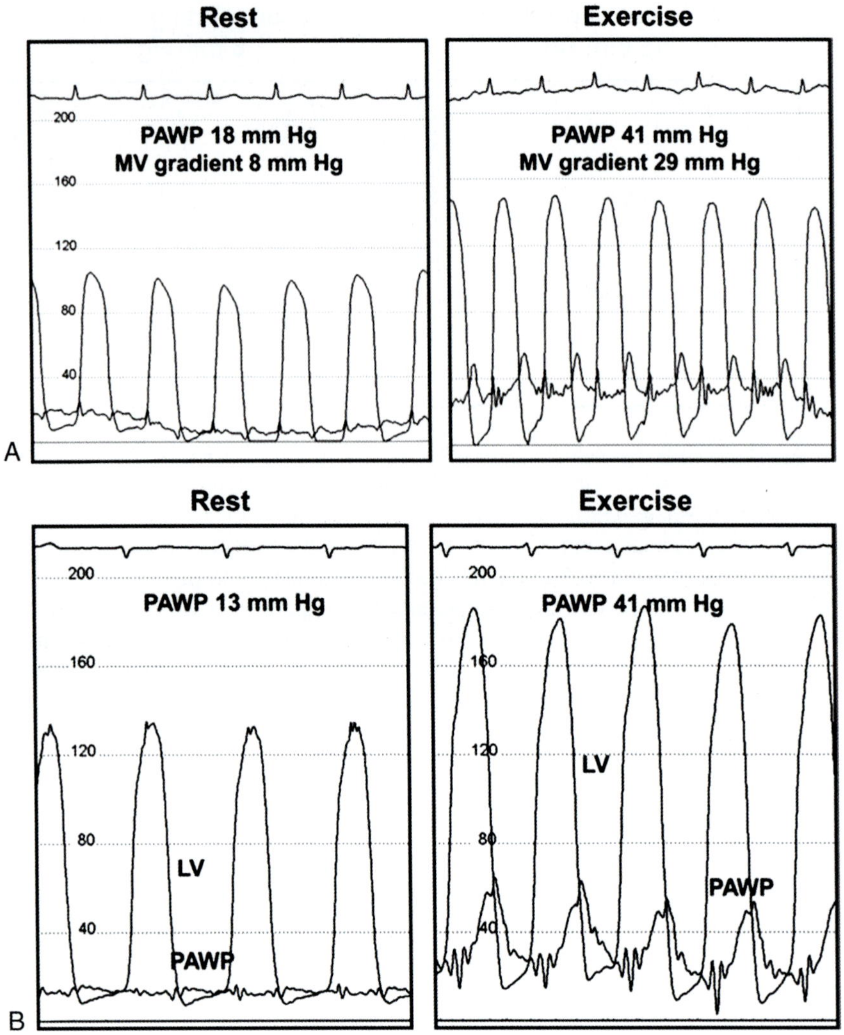

FIGURE 9.12 Exercise is frequently helpful in the cardiac catheterization laboratory to determine the cause of dyspnea in patients who do not have marked abnormalities of pressures in the resting state. A, In this patient with mitral stenosis, the mean resting gradient was only 8 mm Hg and the pulmonary artery wedge pressure (PAWP) was only 18 mm Hg. This patient had significant symptoms out of proportion to the resting hemodynamics. With supine bicycle exercise, the mean gradient rose to 29 mm Hg and the PAWP rose to 41 mm Hg, indicating that the mitral stenosis was hemodynamically significant causing the severe symptoms. B, This patient had no significant valve disease, normal left ventricular (LV) systolic function, but significant dyspnea on exertion. In the resting state, the PAWP was only 13 mm Hg. However, at a low level of supine bicycle exercise, there was a marked increase in PAWP to 41 mm Hg with a large V wave. There was not significant mitral regurgitation by simultaneous echocardiography, indicating that these symptoms were due to noncompliance of the left atrium and left ventricle. MV indicates mitral valve. Reproduced with permission from Nishimura RA, Carabello BA. Hemodynamics in the cardiac catheterization laboratory of the 21st century. *Circulation*. 2012;125:2138-2150.

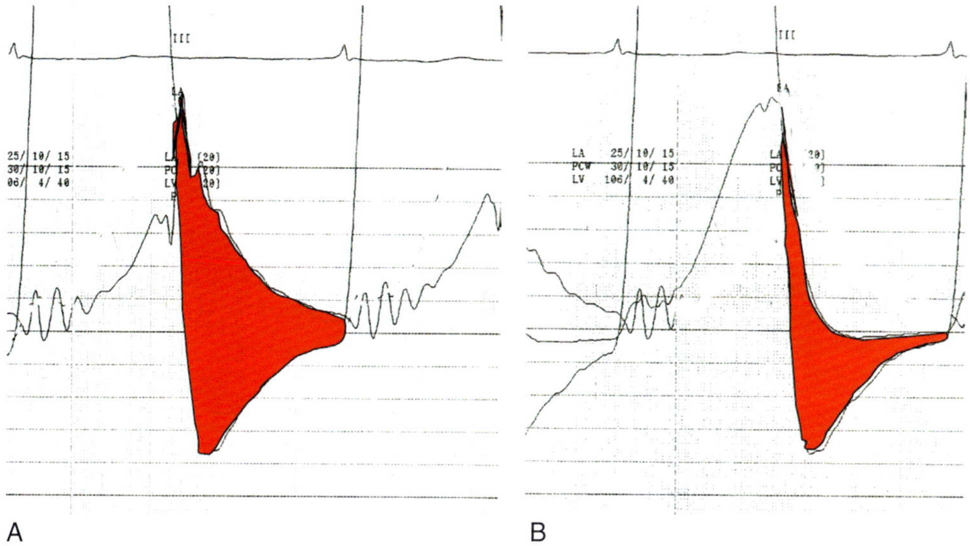

FIGURE 9.13 This patient was referred for percutaneous balloon mitral valvuloplasty based on echocardiographic findings of severe mitral stenosis and mild mitral insufficiency. The tall V wave and diastasis at late cycle in the left ventricle versus wedge tracing (A) are suspicious for severe mitral insufficiency and mild mitral stenosis, respectively. Left ventricle versus left atrial pressure (B) show early decompression of the left atrium consistent with mild mitral stenosis. The patient in fact had severe mitral insufficiency as her primary mitral valve pathology. Note the exaggerated gradient across the mitral valve in A consistent with recording left atrial decompression across the high-resistance pulmonary arteriolar bed. Reproduced with permission from Turi ZG. Pitfalls in the evaluation of hemodynamic data. In: Moscucci M, ed. *Grossman & Baim's Cardiac Catheterization Angiography and Intervention*. Philadelphia: Lippincott Williams and Wilkins; 2014.

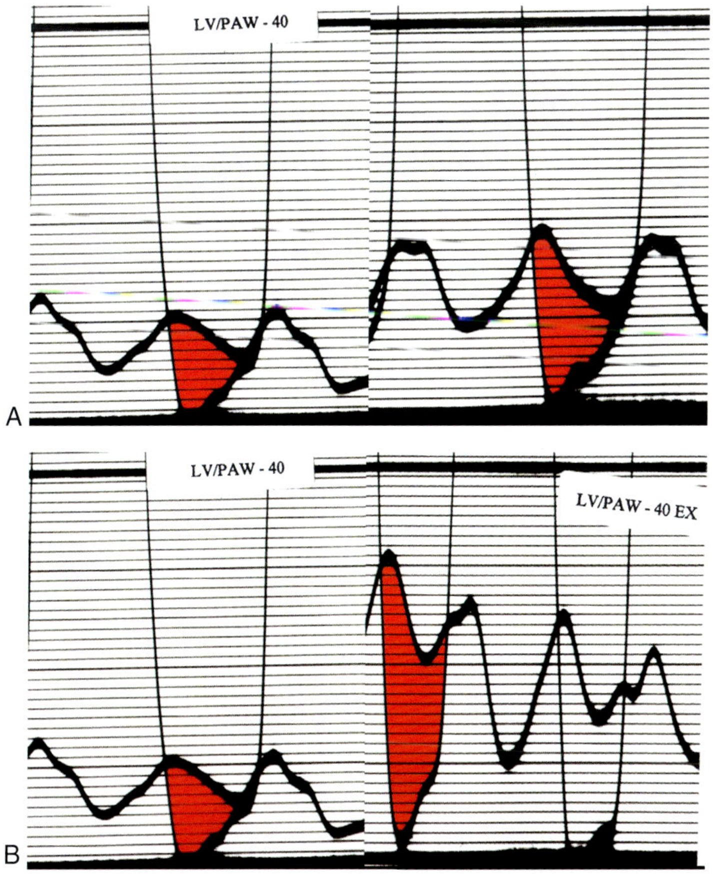

FIGURE 9.14 Response to 100 cc saline (A) and to arm exercise (B) in a patient undergoing cardiac catheterization in the late afternoon after having been NPO overnight. In the setting of a compliant left atrium, dehydration can result in substantial underestimation of the severity of mitral stenosis; the gradient on the right side of panel A has approximately doubled. Because of the disproportionate fall in diastolic filling period with increasing heart rate, and the effect of increasing flow across the valve with exercise, even relatively modest exertion can have a substantial effect on the gradient, which roughly tripled in the right side of panel B. See text for discussion. LV, left ventricle; PAW, pulmonary artery wedge pressure; EX, exercise. Reproduced with permission from Turi ZG. Pitfalls in the evaluation of hemodynamic data. In: Moscucci M, ed. *Grossman & Baim's Cardiac Catheterization Angiography and Intervention*. Philadelphia: Lippincott Williams and Wilkins; 2014).

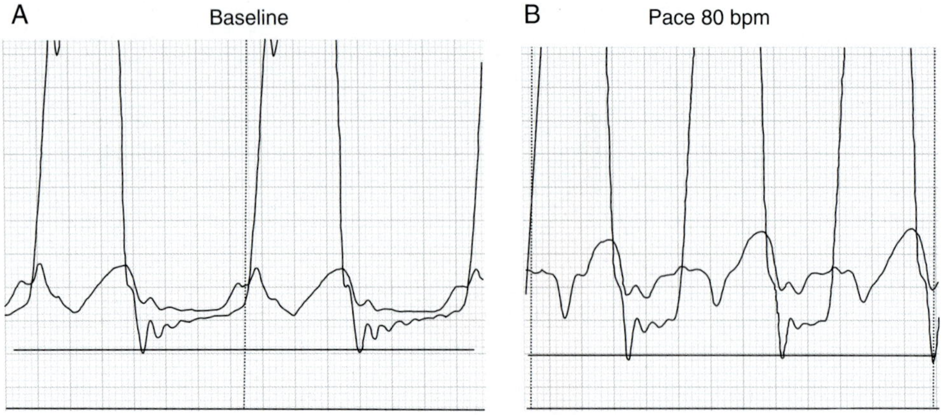

FIGURE 9.15 Effect of atrial pacing on mitral valve gradient in a patient with mitral stenosis. A, Baseline—At rest, there is no significant gradient. B, Atrial pacing at a rate of 80 bpm. The gradient increases significantly. The patient was managed with successful mitral balloon valvuloplasty.

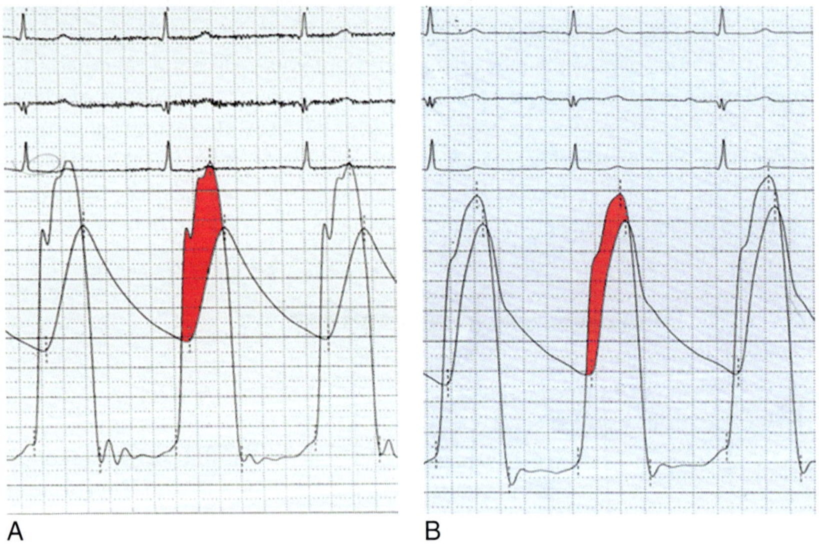

FIGURE 9.16 Left ventricular versus aortic pressure taken a few minutes apart. Note the dramatic difference in dP/dt and gradient. This patient had aortic sclerosis, not stenosis, with a small gradient. The pressures were recorded through a 6 French dual lumen catheter—the aortic pressure lumen is extremely small and damps easily from flow stasis and platelet sludging (A). Flushing the catheter resulted in resolution of most of the gradient (B). Reproduced with permission from Turi ZG. Pitfalls in the evaluation of hemodynamic data. In: Moscucci M, ed. *Grossman & Baim's Cardiac Catheterization Angiography and Intervention*. Philadelphia: Lippincott Williams and Wilkins; 2014.

chapter **10**

Coronary Angiography and Cardiac Ventriculography

ROBERT N. PIANA, MD, AARON KUGELMASS, MD, and MAURO MOSCUCCI, MD, MBA

INTRODUCTION

Diagnostic angiography begins with vascular access. Typically, this is achieved via the radial artery or common femoral artery, and less commonly through the brachial artery. The patient's vascular anatomy should be fully understood and assessed before attempting arterial access. For femoral access, the assessment may include palpation of the femoral, dorsalis pedis, and posterior tibial pulses; auscultation for femoral bruits, inspection for surgical scars to suggest prior vascular surgery, and a review of records to understand prior vascular interventions or surgery. For radial access, the radial and ulnar pulses are assessed, dialysis fistulae are noted, and an Allen test is typically performed to ensure adequate hand perfusion should the radial artery occlusion occur (5% to 10% of cases). In addition to these measures, ultrasound is increasingly used to guide vascular access and femoral artery angiography should be performed as a routine in preparation for vascular closure devices deployment (**FIGURE 10.1**).

Catheter advancement from the access site to the heart requires careful attention to stenosis, tortuosity, calcification, and vascular anomalies. From the radial access, the operator utilizes both fluoroscopy and tactile feedback during catheter advancement to recognize a "radial loop," accessory radial artery, or a true high origin of the radial artery from the upper segment of the brachial artery (**FIGURE 10.2**). Such anomalies may require crossing with coronary guide wires, downsizing of the catheter system, or potentially abandoning the approach for an alternative access. Exquisite attention to these vascular anomalies can help prevent painful severe radial artery spasm, dissection, or even perforation. As radial patients are generally anticoagulated, such complications can result in significant hematoma or even compartment syndromes.

Particularly in elderly patients, the right subclavian and brachiocephalic arteries may be quite tortuous, in some cases forming nearly a 360° loop. A hydrophilic guide wire can generally be negotiated successfully through such a loop. Deep inspiration can then help reduce the loop, allowing the catheter to be advanced to the ascending aorta (**FIGURE 10.3**).

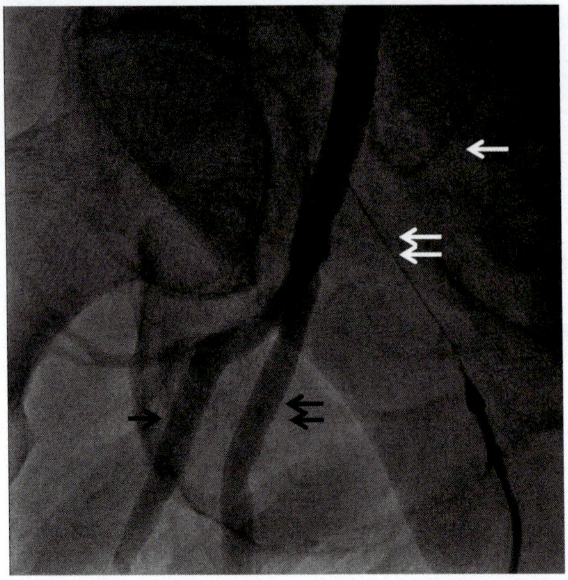

FIGURE 10.1 Angiography performed in RAO projection through the inner dilator of a micropuncture sheath (double white arrows) in the right common femoral artery. Also noted are the superficial epigastric artery (single white arrow), profunda femoral artery (single black arrow), and superficial femoral artery (double black arrows). Sheath placement above the femoral bifurcation and below the inguinal ligament reduces the likelihood of retroperitoneal bleeding from a high puncture, pseudoaneurysm from a low puncture in the profunda or superficial femoral artery and optimizes the opportunity to utilize a femoral closure device.

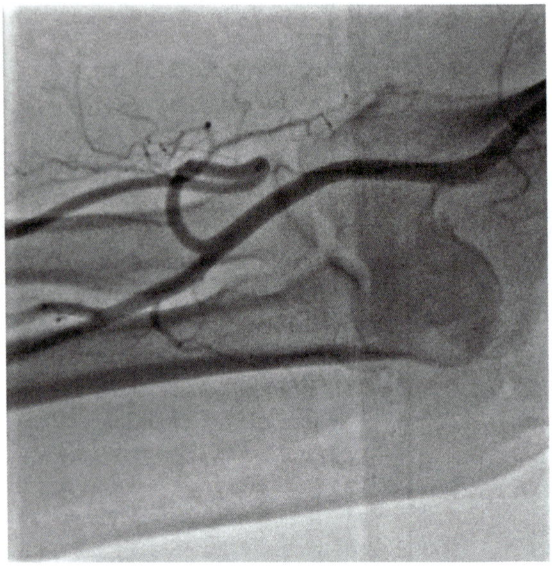

FIGURE 10.2 Radial artery loop.

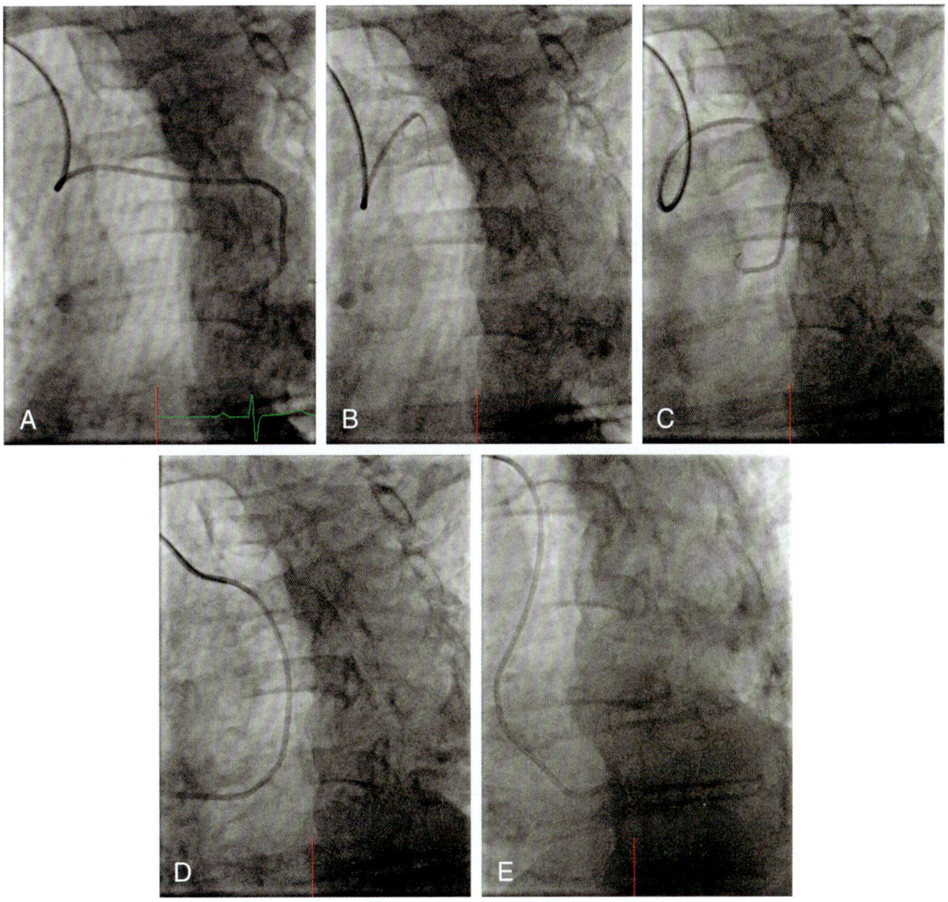

FIGURE 10.3 **A,** Tiger 4 Catheter with tip in proximal descending aorta. Note the loop in the right subclavian-innominate artery. **B,** Catheter withdrawn somewhat in attempt to access ascending aorta (AA), but loop becomes even more pronounced. **C,** Careful torqueing over the wire points catheter tip toward the AA. **D**, Deep inspiration reduces the vascular loop and allows the guide wire to be passed into the AA over which the catheter is advanced. **E,** Catheter now in the aortic root.

CORONARY ANGIOGRAPHIC VIEWS

Coronary angiography utilizes a combination of right to left and cranial to caudal angulations to optimize imaging of the coronary arteries. Specific views optimize visualization of specific coronary artery segments (**FIGURE 10.4**).

Body habitus may limit angulation of the imaging system, and sternal wires, pacemakers/defibrillators, and other implanted devices can obscure lesions. Vessel overlap can be challenging as well. Integrating information from fluoroscopy to assess for calcification and prior stents, multiple angiographic views, the pattern and speed of contrast flow and washout, and the pressure waveforms from the catheter tip is essential to maximizing the coronary assessment (**FIGURES 10.5-10.10**).

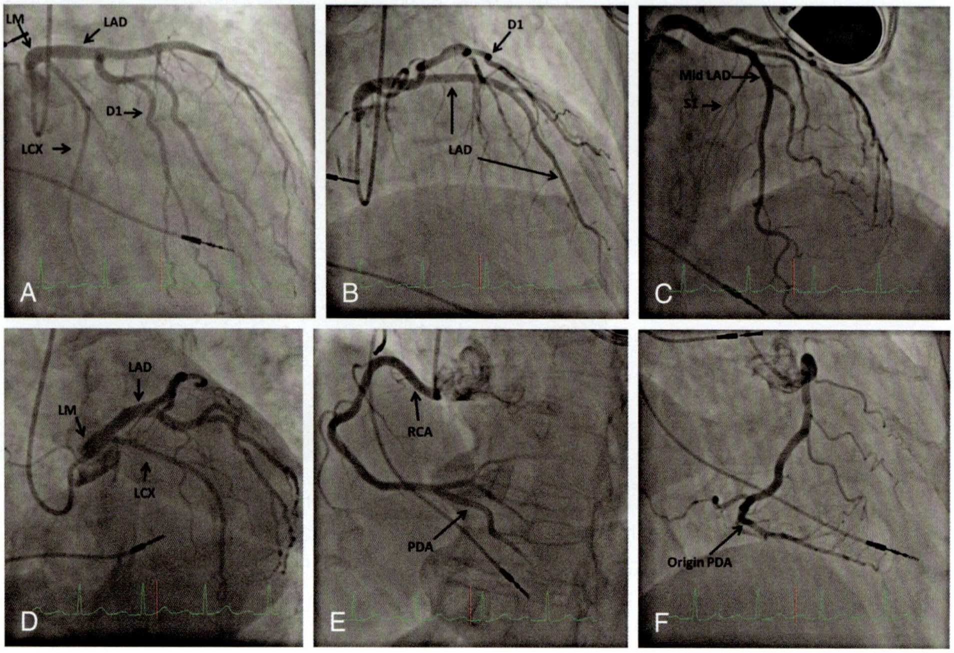

FIGURE 10.4 **A,** RAO Caudal projection of the left coronary artery. This view is used to visualize the left main (LM), proximal left anterior descending (LAD), and proximal circumflex (LCX) arteries. Note brisk contrast reflux from the LM, reflecting adequate contrast injection to assess for an ostial lesion. A broad flush of contrast reflux and the absence of damping/ventricularization of the catheter tip pressure both help in excluding a significant ostial left main stenosis. A large branching first diagonal artery is noted (D1). **B,** RAO Cranial projection of the left coronary artery. This view is used to visualize the mid- and distal LAD without overlap of septal or diagonal branches. In this case, however, the large branching D1 does overlap the mid-LAD. Steeper RAO angulation may eliminate this, or this segment may be better seen in LAO cranial (4C). **C,** LAO Cranial projection of the left coronary artery. This view is used to visualize the mid- and distal LAD in an orthogonal projection. Note that the mid-LAD just after the first septal (S1), which was obscured by D1 in the RAO Cranial (4B), is now clearly seen without obstruction. **D,** LAO Caudal projection of the left coronary artery. This view is used to visualize the LM and proximal LCX. **E,** LAO cranial projection of the right coronary artery RCA. This view is used to visualize the distal RCA and its bifurcation into the posterior descending (PDA) and posterolateral arteries. Note pacemaker wire that can obscure lesion assessment. In this example, angulation is adjusted to avoid overlap with the PDA origin. **F,** RAO projection of the right coronary artery RCA. This view is used to visualize midportion of the RCA and the body of the PDA, and in some cases it can demonstrate the origin of the PDA well, as in this example.

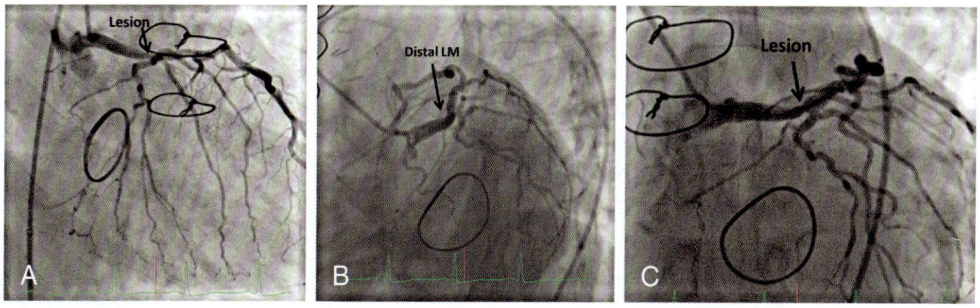

FIGURE 10.5 **A,** RAO Caudal projection of the left coronary artery. Distal LM lesion partially obscured by a sternal wire. **B,** LAO Caudal projection of the left coronary artery. Even at 40 LAO/40 Caudal the distal left main cannot be visualized owing to overlap. **C,** Shallow LAO with shallow cranial elongates the left main and allows visualization of a napkin ring distal left main lesion.

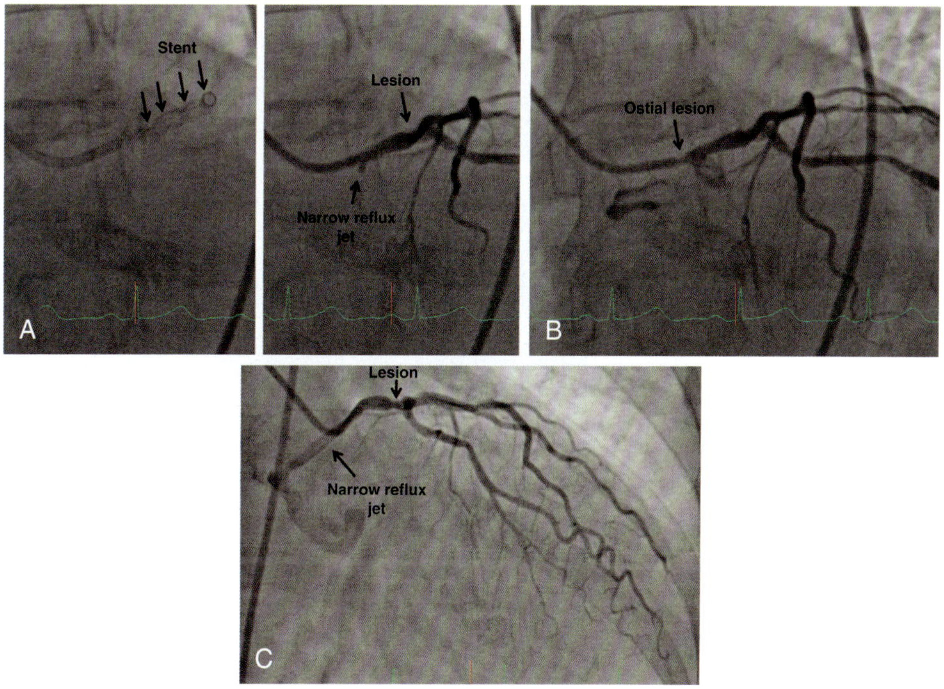

FIGURE 10.6 **A,** Left panel shows shallow LAO Caudal fluoroscopic view of the left main. A prior stent in the very proximal LAD appears to extent back into the distal LM. Right panel shows distal left main stenosis at the proximal stent edge. Note the narrow reflux of contrast from the ostial LM, suggesting ostial LM disease as well. In fact there was ventricularization of catheter pressure. **B,** Catheter pulled back slightly reveals ostial LM lesion. **C,** RAO Caudal projection of the left coronary artery. Distal LM lesion clearly seen with a narrow jet of contrast reflux, consistent with the ostial left main stenosis.

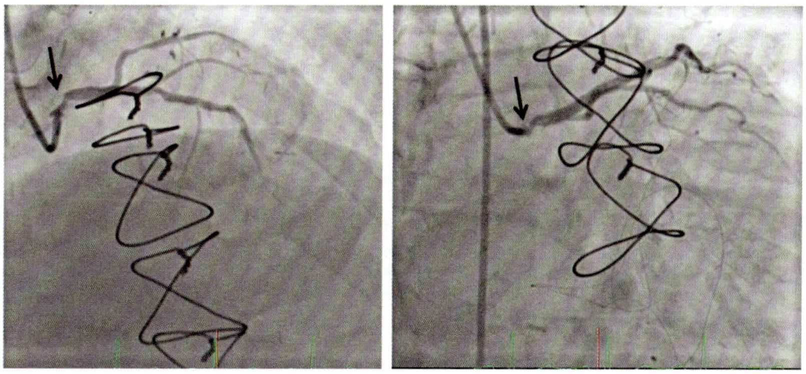

FIGURE 10.7 Two views of an ostial left main stenosis. Minimal contrast reflux is noted. There was damping of catheter pressure with engagement of the left main.

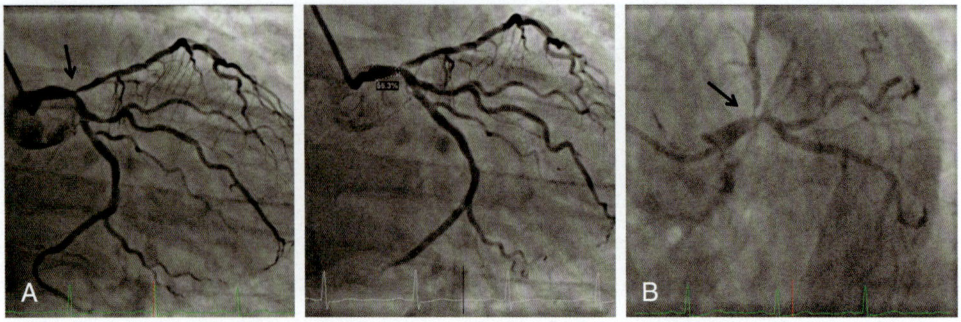

FIGURE 10.8 **A,** Left panel shows (arrow) distal LM tapering and severe ostial LAD lesion. Right panel shows quantitative angiography assessment of distal LM stenosis. **B,** Steep LAO Caudal projection now shows the ostial LAD stenosis (arrow) is critical.

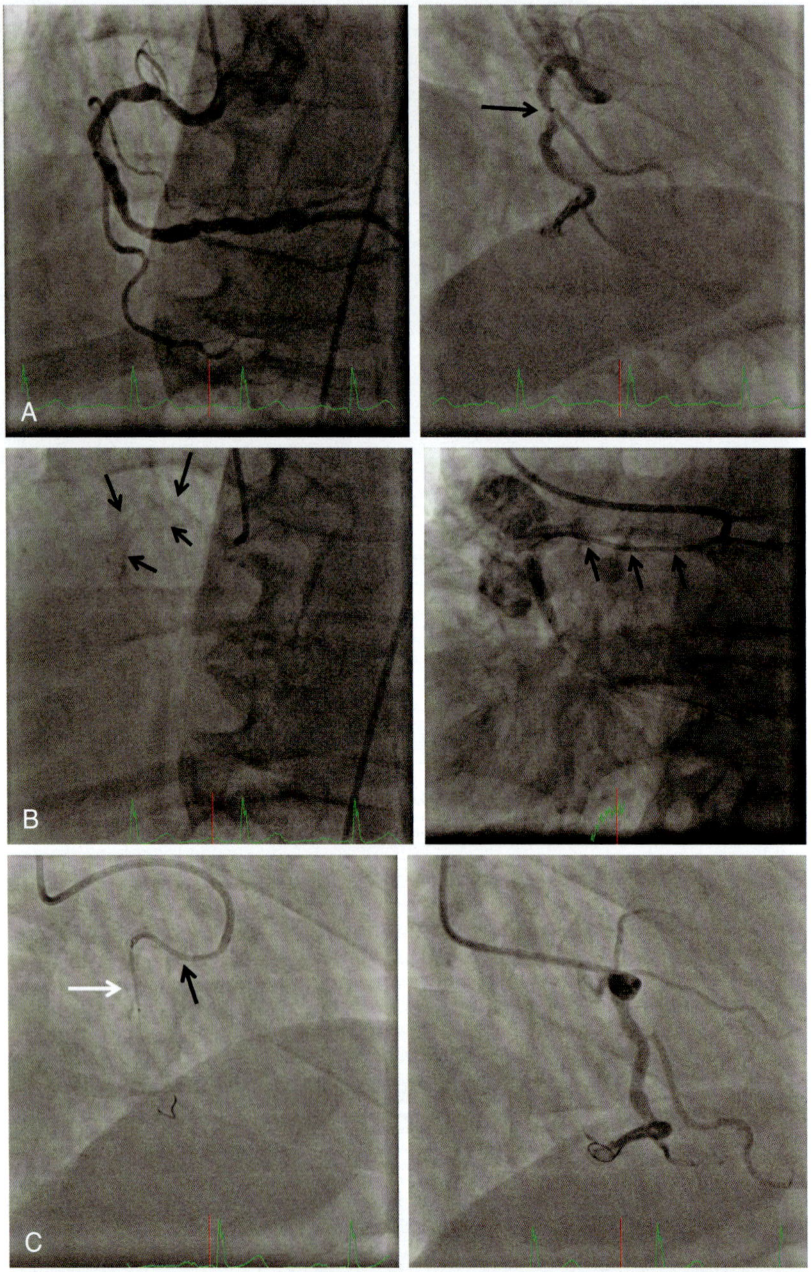

FIGURE 10.9 **A,** Left panel: LAO view of the RCA shows moderate diffuse disease. A "shepherd's staff" anatomy of the proximal RCA is noted. In the RAO projection a critical mid-RCA lesion (arrow) is now revealed (right panel). **B,** Left panel: Diffuse calcification (arrows) is noted in the proximal RCA. Along with the "shepherd's staff" anatomy of the proximal RCA, this information suggests stent delivery may be challenging. Ablative procedures such as rotational atherectomy would be considered. Right panel: After unsuccessful attempts with other guides, a 6 French 3DRC guide and a Guideliner (arrows) were used to deliver a balloon to the lesion site. Adequate balloon expansion is seen indicating this is a dilatable lesion. **C,** Left panel: Guideliner (black arrow) positioned in the proximal RCA provides additional support to the guide for successful stent delivery (white arrow). Right panel: mid-RCA lesion is now successfully stented.

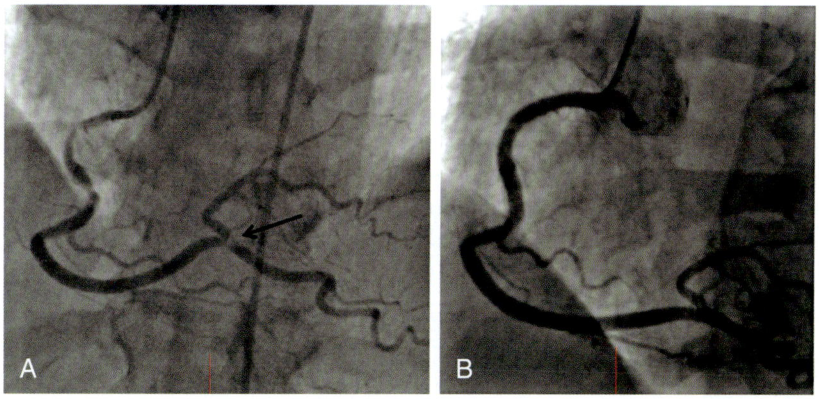

FIGURE 10.10 **A,** LAO Cranial view of the right coronary artery opens up a critical bifurcation lesion (arrow) in the distal RCA-origin PDA-origin posterolateral. This lesion was not seen in straight LAO or in the RAO. **B,** LAO Cranial view of the right coronary artery following successful stenting.

Although angiography remains the gold standard for imaging of the coronary arteries, it is not a physiologic assessment. In addition to multiple angiographic parameters, physiologic assessment may be needed to determine if a specific lesion is likely to be a source of ischemia (**FIGURES 10.11** and **10.12**).

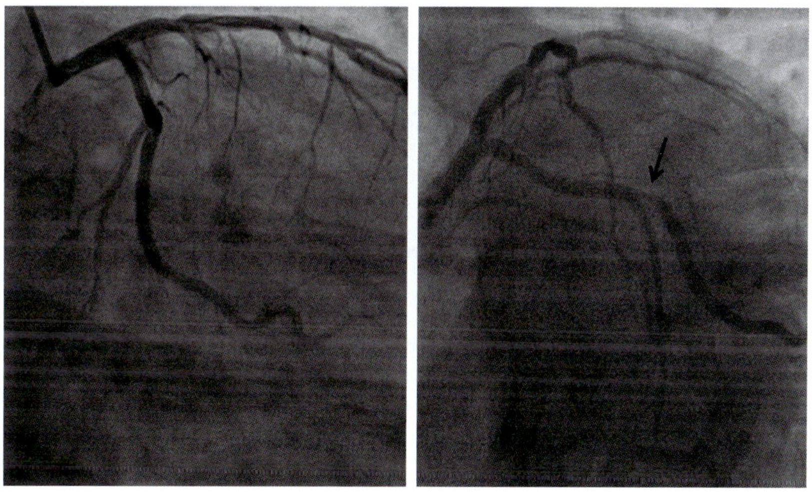

FIGURE 10.11 Left panel, RAO Caudal projection shows no significant stenosis in the LCX. Right panel, LAO Caudal projection now reveals a moderately severe stenosis (arrow) in the origin of the first marginal. Fractional flow reserve (FFR) was 0.93 consistent with a nonhemodynamically significant lesion.

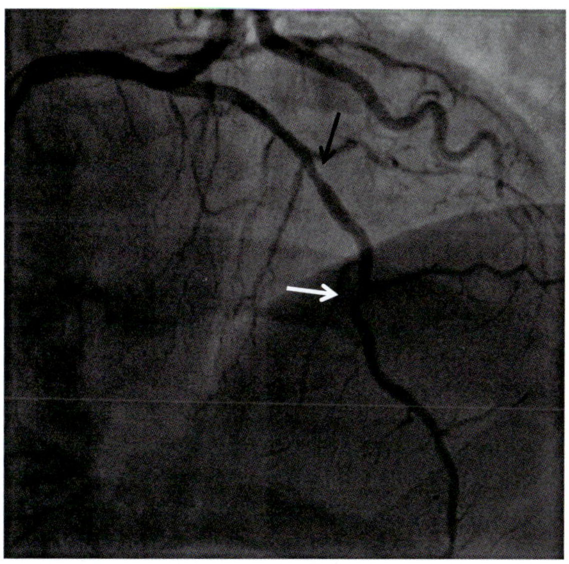

FIGURE 10.12 RAO Cranial projection of the LAD shows a moderate stenosis in the mid-LAD (black arrow) and a moderate stenosis in the junction of the mid and distal LAD (white arrow). While the mid-LAD lesion appears moderate angiographically, FFR just below this lesion was 0.80, consistent with a hemodynamically significant lesion.

Revascularization of chronic total occlusions (CTOs) is now common utilizing advances in wire technology, microcatheters, and combinations of antegrade and retrograde approaches. To assess patients' candidacy for such advanced CTO interventions appropriately, the angiographer must carefully interrogate occlusions and collateral flow. This may involve low-magnification views to allow visualization of both the donor vessel and the recipient vessel without panning. Prolonged imaging runs are used to ensure complete filling of collaterals. When appropriate, simultaneous injection of both the left and right coronary may be utilized to visualize antegrade and retrograde flow to the occluded vessel (**FIGURE 10.13**).

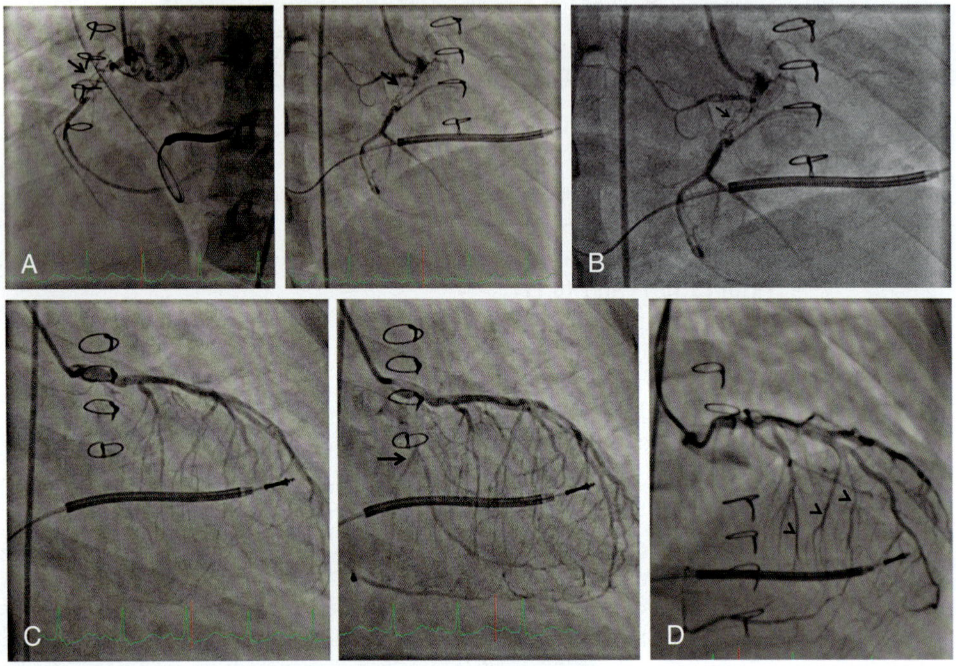

FIGURE 10.13 **A,** Coronary angiography of a patient who is status post cardiac transplantation and stenting of the mid-LAD. LAO (left panel) and RAO (right panel) projections demonstrate a chronic total occlusion of the proximal RCA with the distal vessel filling by bridging collaterals (arrow). **B,** Magnified RAO view of the bridging collaterals (arrow). **C,** RAO Caudal projection of the left coronary in the same patient. Left panel shows total occlusion of the LCX. Right panel shows retrograde filling of the LCX via left to left collaterals (arrow). **D,** In the same patient views are obtained to assess collateral circulation to the distal RCA. RAO cranial view of the left coronary is shown. Rich septal collaterals (arrowheads) are seen filling the PDA.

BYPASS ANGIOGRAPHY

Bypass graft angiography utilizes the same techniques as native coronary angiography, but it often requires different diagnostic catheters. It also may affect the choice of vascular access. The left internal mammary graft (LIMA) is difficult to engage from the right radial access, and left radial access or femoral access is generally utilized in these cases. If proper engagement of the mammary artery cannot be achieved, a nonselective injection can be performed with a blood pressure cuff inflated on the arm in an attempt to divert as much contrast as possible down the mammary artery. Radial artery bypass grafts are susceptible to vasospasm, and liberal use of intra-arterial vasodilators may be beneficial. Attention to graft markers and vascular clips may help identify the origin and course of a graft. As most patients do not have graft markers, and catheters may not successfully engage flush occluded grafts or grafts positioned in unusual locations, native coronary injections should be studied carefully for competitive flow to help confirm patency or occlusion of a graft. Supravalvular aortography can also be used to identify graft origins when standard techniques are unsuccessful in engaging them. Once the origin is identified, the operator is better equipped to select a catheter that will reach the origin successfully. Specific angiographic views help visualize the origin, body, and distal anastomosis of various grafts (**FIGURES 10.14-10.22**).

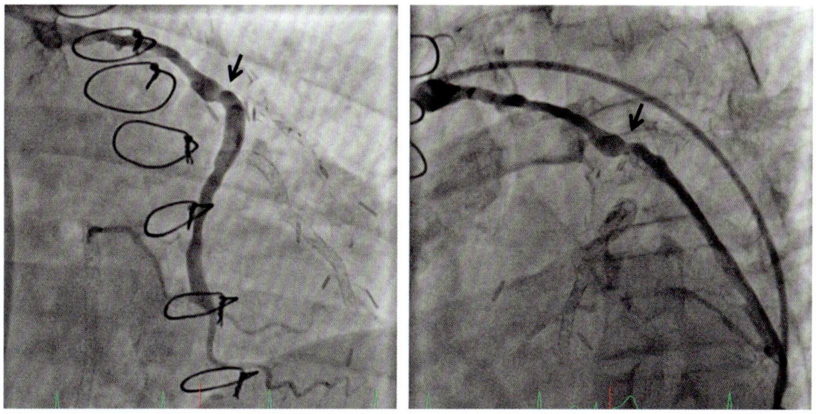

FIGURE 10.14 Left panel, RAO view of saphenous vein graft (SVG) to an obtuse marginal artery. The RAO view is useful to show the origin of the graft off the aorta and the subtended marginal. However, the lesions (arrow) in the mid-body of the graft can be obscured. Right panel, LAO view of the graft. The LAO view elongates the midportion of the graft and demonstrates only a mild stenosis (arrow) at the potential lesion site.

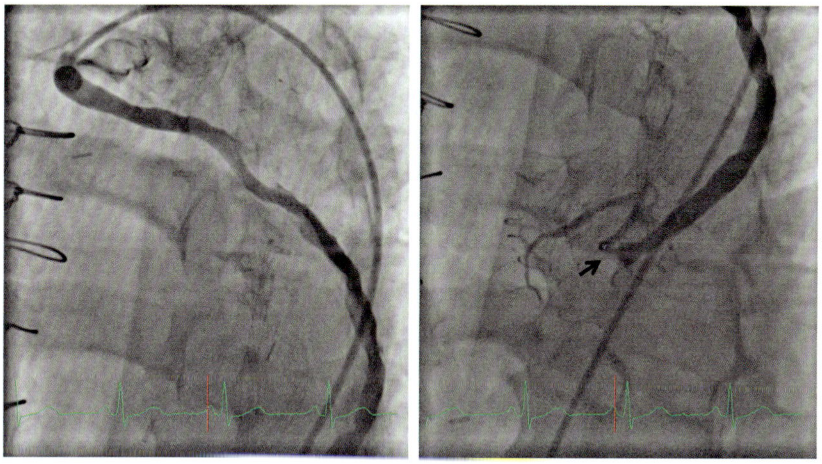

FIGURE 10.15 Left panel, LAO view of a diffusely degenerated SVG to a left posterolateral branch. Right panel, LAO Cranial view of the graft lays out the distal anastomosis (arrow).

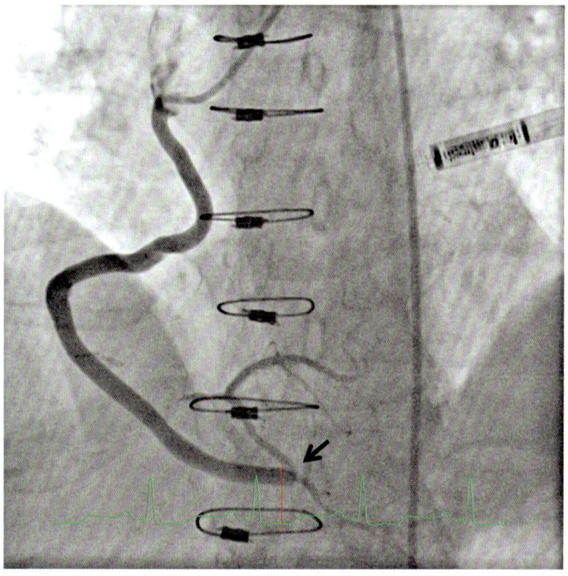

FIGURE 10.16 LAO Cranial view of the SVG to the PDA lays out the distal anastomosis (arrow). There is graft-target mismatch in terms of vessel caliber, but no stenosis.

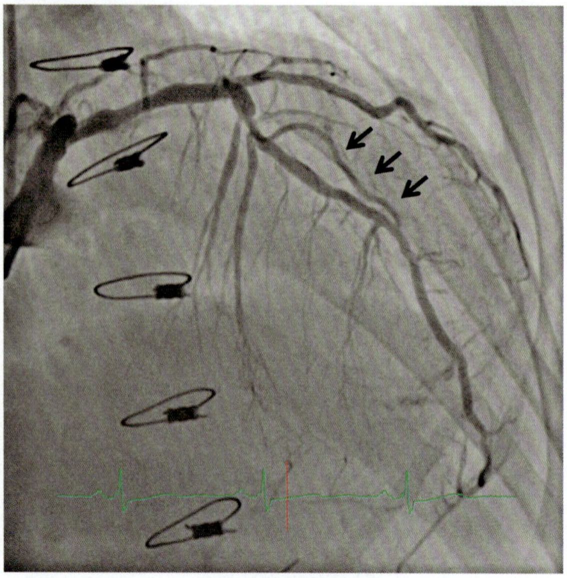

FIGURE 10.17 RAO Cranial view of the left coronary. There is retrograde filling (arrows) of the LIMA. This can be seen if the LIMA is compromised proximally. This may also be seen with a widely patent LIMA, but the contrast in the LIMA generally washes out rapidly owing to brisk antegrade flow of unopacified blood down the LIMA.

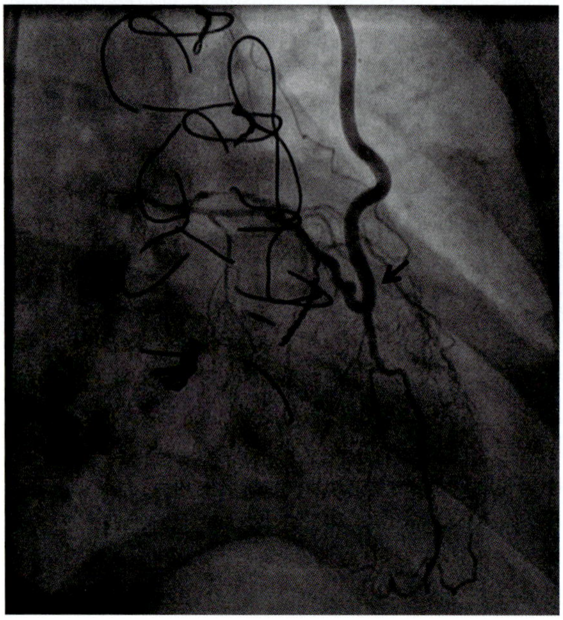

FIGURE 10.18 RAO Cranial view of LIMA injection showing a widely patent distal anastomosis. Contrast fills the distal LAD and also fills retrograde up the LAD, allowing assessment of the proximal and mid-LAD.

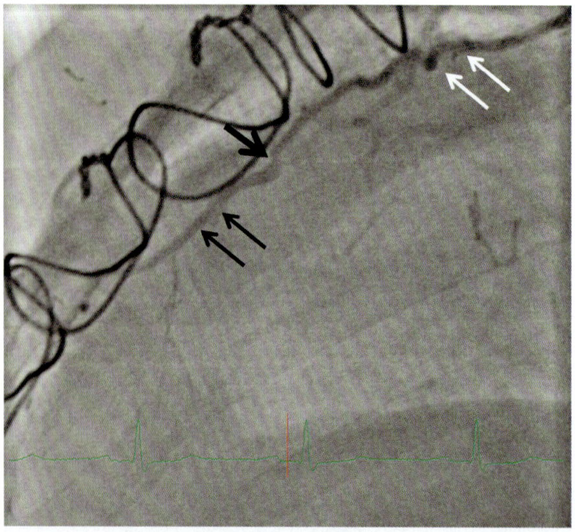

FIGURE 10.19 Lateral view of the LIMA distal anastomosis (thick black arrow). This view can often be invaluable in assessing the severity of a distal anastomotic lesion that cannot be clarified in other views. LAD (black arrows). LIMA body (white arrows).

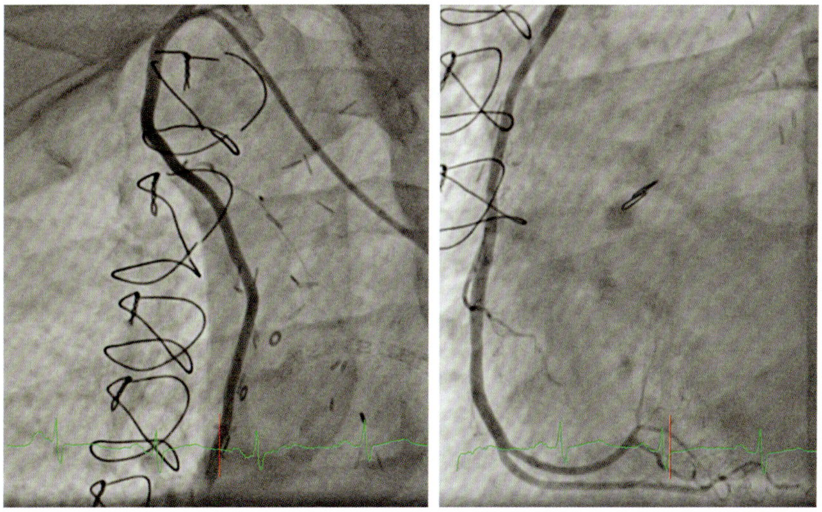

FIGURE 10.20 LAO view of a right internal mammary artery (RIMA) graft to the PDA. Left panel, Proximal portion of the RIMA. Right panel, Distal portion of the RIMA, distal anastomosis, and subtended PDA.

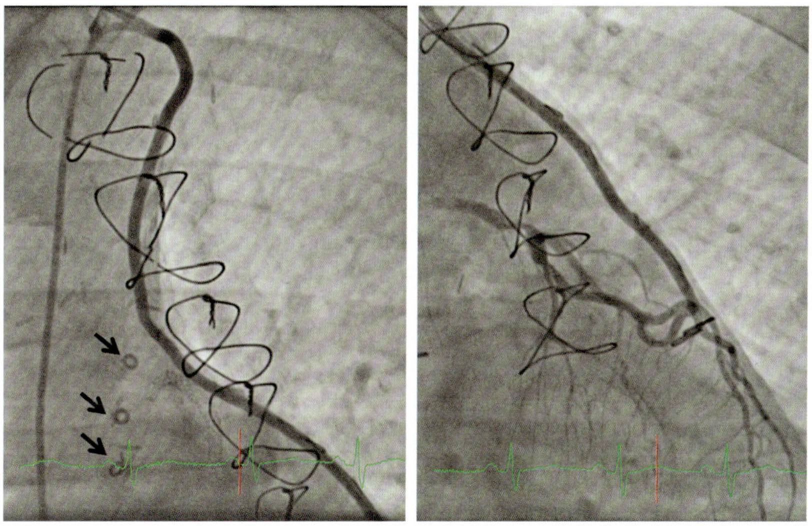

FIGURE 10.21 RAO view of a LIMA to LAD. Left panel: Proximal portion of the LIMA. Right panel: Distal portion of the LIMA, distal anastomosis, and subtended LAD. Vein graft markers are noted (arrows).

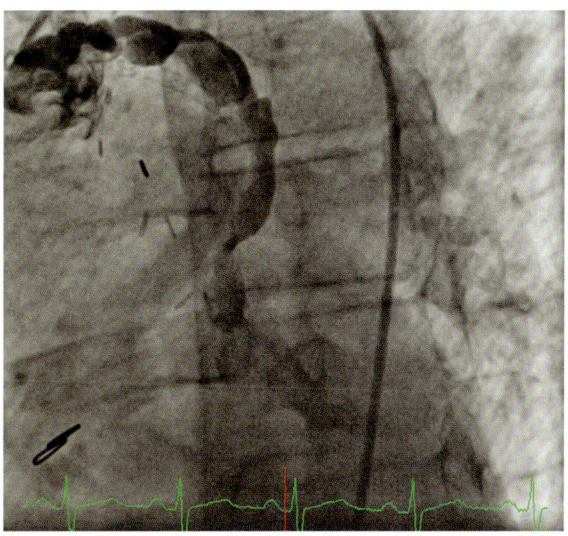

FIGURE 10.22 LAO view of SVG. There is severe ectasia and degeneration of the SVG. Intervention on an SVG with this morphology is fraught with complications, including distal embolization and "no-reflow."

CARDIAC VENTRICULOGRAPHY

Diagnostic catheterization usually includes left ventriculography. Typically this is done in the right anterior oblique (RAO) projection to assess the anterior, apical, and inferior walls. When the posterior wall needs to be assessed, as in the case of myocardial infarction due to LCX occlusion, or when a ventricular septal defect is suspected, the left anterior oblique (LAO) projection is utilized. Membranous ventricular septal defects are best visualized using an LAO cranial projection. In addition to wall motion, the ventriculogram evaluates for mitral regurgitation, and it can be diagnostic in the identification of congenital or acquired structural heart disease conditions such as congenital or post–myocardial infarction ventricular septal defects, pseudoaneurisms, ventricular diverticula, and left ventricular noncompaction (**FIGURES 10.23-10.30**). In addition, during left ventriculography attention should also be directed to the ascending aorta, to identify abnormalities that might suggest or demonstrate an acute aortic dissection in the setting of new onset severe chest pain (**FIGURE 10.31**).

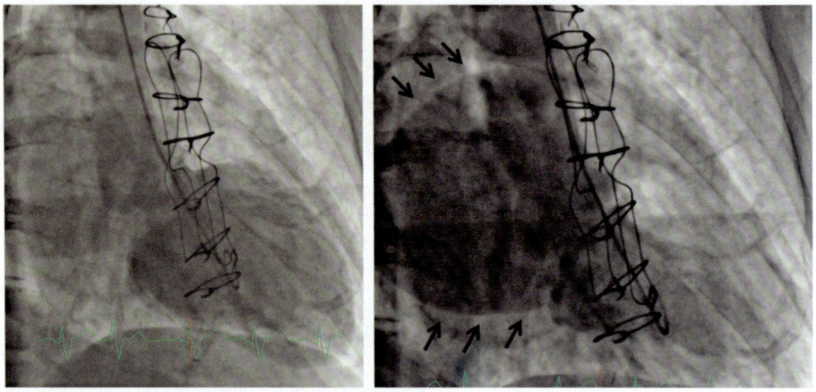

FIGURE 10.23 Severe mitral regurgitation. Left panel, Left ventricle in diastole. Right panel, Left ventricle in systole. Severe mitral regurgitation is noted. The dilated left atrium is outlined by arrows. In severe mitral regurgitation there may also be filling of the pulmonary veins during ventriculography.

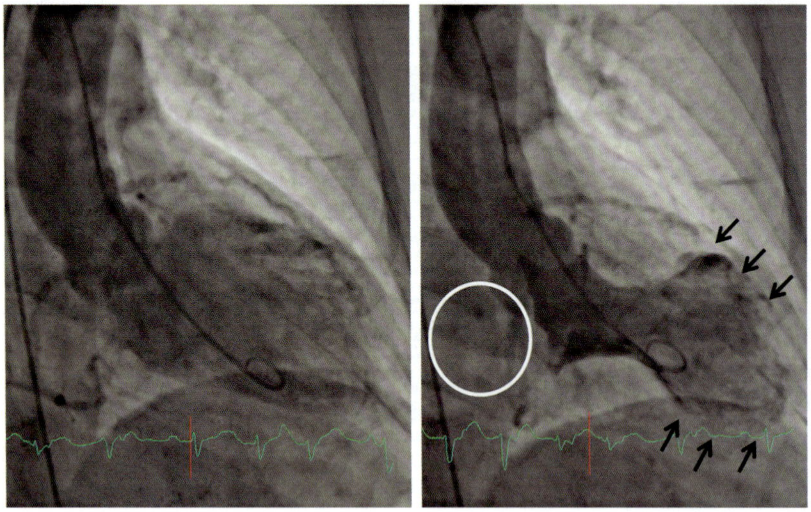

FIGURE 10.24 Stress-induced cardiomyopathy. Left panel, Left ventricle in diastole. Right panel, Left ventricle in systole. No mitral regurgitation is seen (white circle identifies the left atrium above the mitral valve plane where contrast would be seen with mitral regurgitation). The classic pattern of stress induced cardiomyopathy is seen, with vigorous contraction of the bases of the ventricle and akinesis/dyskinesis of the entire distal anterior wall, distal inferior wall, and apex (arrows).

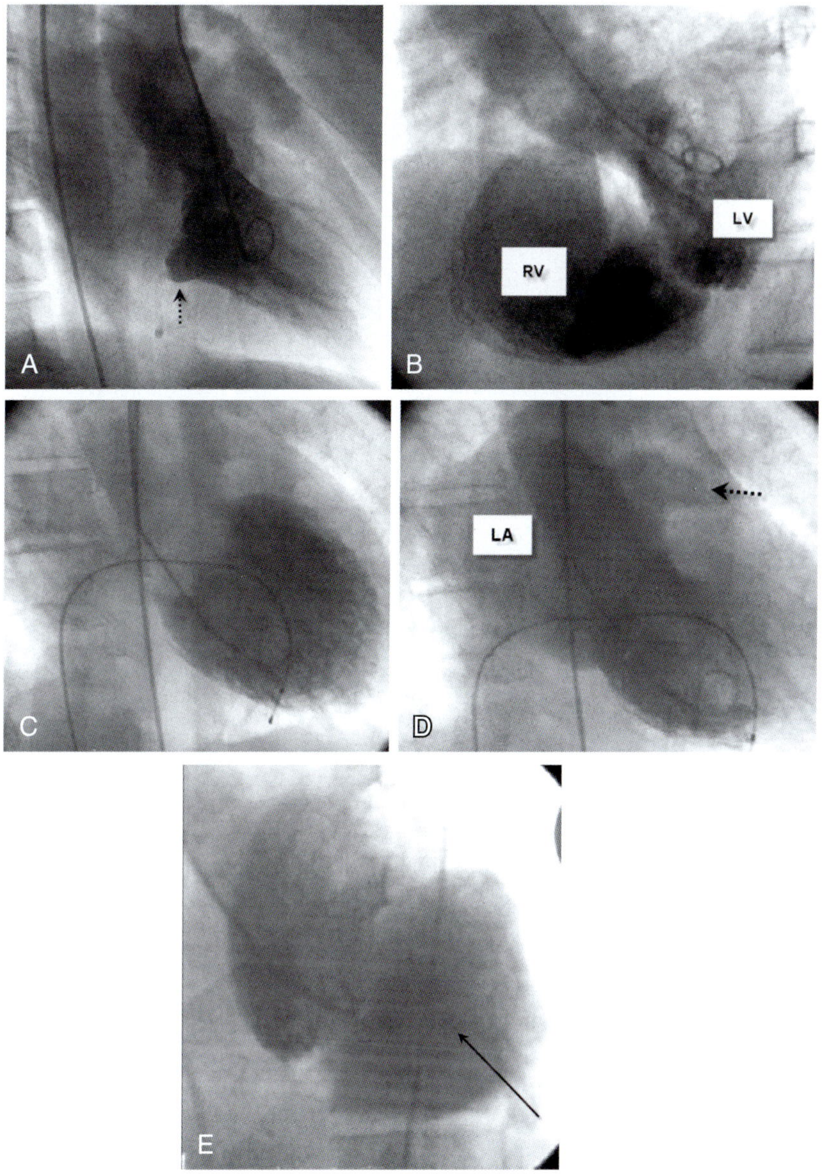

FIGURE 10.25 Various pathologies seen on left ventriculography. **A,** Mitral valve prolapse, with prolapse of a thickened posterior leaflet behind the fornix (dotted arrow) and mitral regurgitation in the RAO projection. **B,** Ventricular septal defect 3 d post inferior myocardial infarction owing to single-vessel right coronary occlusion, with contrast crossing from left to right ventricles in the LAO-cranial projection. **C** and **D,** Papillary muscle rupture 5 d post inferior myocardial infarction (diastolic and systolic frame, respectively, showing dense contrast filling the left atrium and left atrial appendage; dotted arrow). **E,** Pseudoaneurysm (contained myocardial rupture, arrow) seen several weeks following a lateral wall myocardial infarction owing to single-vessel circumflex marginal disease. Reproduced with permission from Moscucci M, Hendel RC. Cardiac ventriculography. In: *Grossman and Baim's Cardiac Catheterization, Angiography and Intervention*. 8th ed. Philadelphia, PA: Wolters Kluwer–Lippincott Williams & Wilkins; 2014.

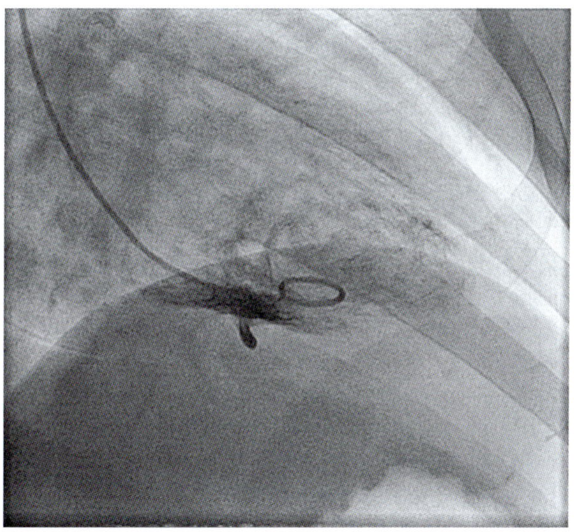

FIGURE 10.26 Incidental finding of left ventricular diverticulum of the inferior wall during left ventriculography. Left ventricular diverticula are rare congenital abnormalities resulting in outpouching of the ventricular wall. They might have an apical or nonapical location. Nonapical diverticula are usually isolated defects, whereas apical diverticula are associated with other midline thoracoabdominal defects and cardiac malformations.

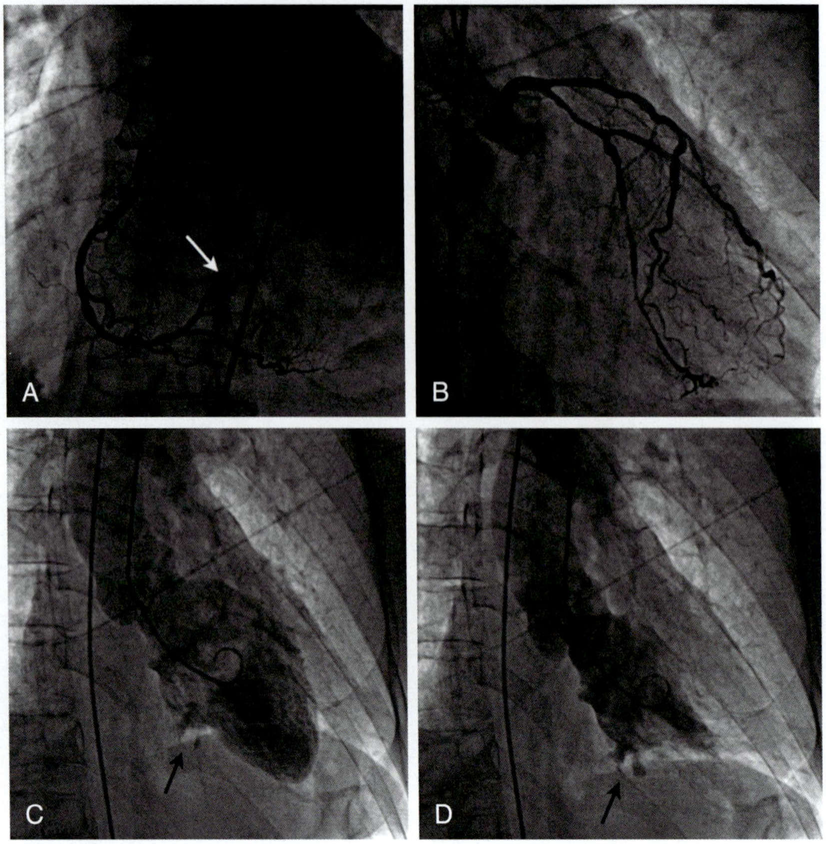

FIGURE 10.27 Rarely, the appearance of a left ventricular diverticulum might be the manifestation of myocardial necrosis and of the development of a dissecting intramural hematoma. Panels A through D show coronary angiography and left ventriculography in a patient presenting with acute worsening chest pain 5 d after the onset of substernal chest pain. Invasive angiography showed an abrupt occlusion of a right posterolateral branch (**A;** white arrow) and diffuse nonocclusive stenoses in all 3 epicardial coronary arteries (**A** and **B**). Ventriculography in a right anterior oblique projection showed a dyskinetic basal inferior wall with 2 craters of contrast extending outside the contour of the contrast-filled left ventricular cavity (**C** and **D;** black arrows). Reproduced with permission from Wilson JR, Marshall RJ, Shanbhag SM, et al. Multimodality imaging of a dissecting intramyocardial hematoma extending into the left atrial wall following myocardial infarction. *Circulation*. 2012;126:e339-e341.

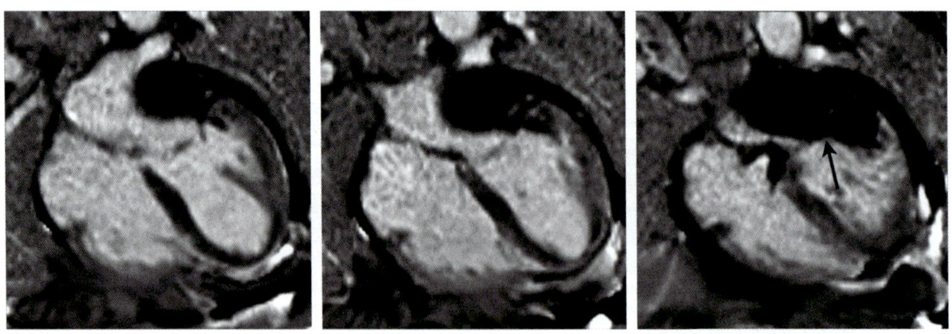

FIGURE 10.28 MRI perfusion imaging with gadolinium contrast in the same patient described in **FIGURE 10.27**. There is an intramyocardial hematoma extending from the inferolateral wall through the mitral annulus into the left atrial wall. Single-shot, inversion recovery, steady-state, free precession images were obtained in a parallel 4-chamber orientation 3 min after administration of gadolinium contrast. The left image was at a level slightly below the aortic root; subsequent images (middle, right) moved toward the diaphragm. They demonstrated an intramyocardial hematoma extending from the basal and midinferolateral walls into the posterolateral left atrial wall beneath the mitral valve annulus (arrow). Reproduced with permission from Wilson JR, Marshall RJ, Shanbhag SM, et al. Multimodality imaging of a dissecting intramyocardial hematoma extending into the left atrial wall following myocardial infarction. *Circulation*. 2012;126:e339-e341.

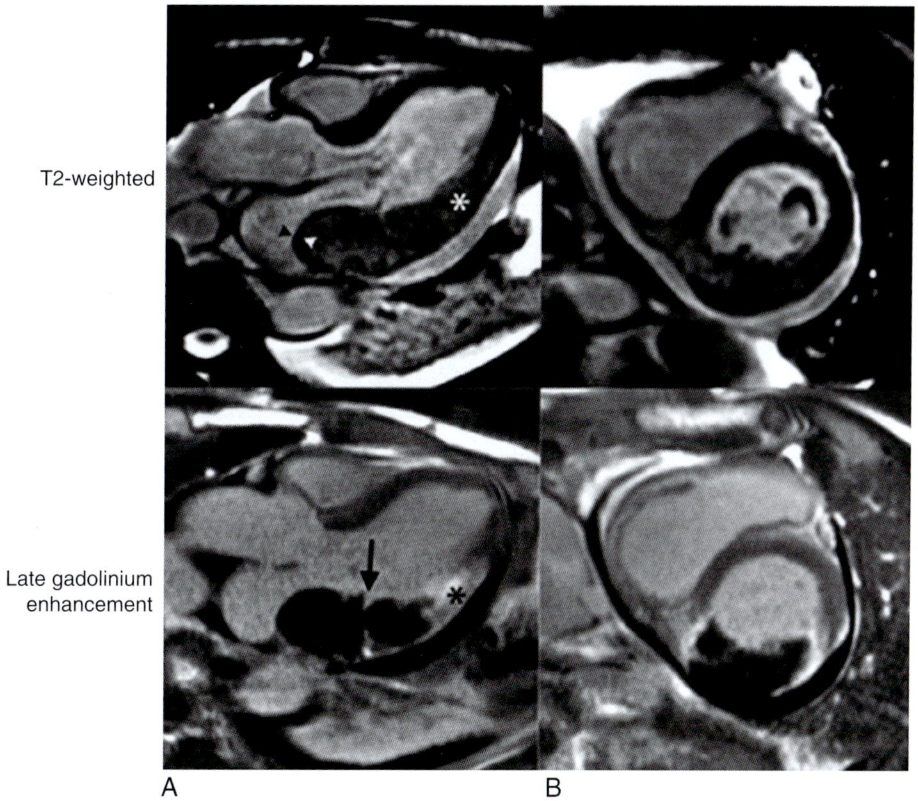

FIGURE 10.29 The intramyocardial hematoma was constrained inferiorly by visceral pericardium (pseudoaneurysm) and posteriorly by the left atrial wall. Bright-blood T2-weighted images and late gadolinium enhancement images were obtained in the 3-chamber **(A)** and short-axis **(B)** orientations, corresponding to the parasternal views in **FIGURE 10.28.** The left atrial wall was seen as a dark line separating the hematoma from the left atrial blood pool on the 3-chamber T2-weighted image (arrowheads). The short-axis images demonstrated that the intramyocardial hematoma had not ruptured into the pericardial space but appeared to be directly adjacent to it, contained by the visceral pericardium. The 3-chamber late gadolinium enhancement image showed the intramyocardial hematoma on both sides of the atrioventricular groove (arrow). Myocardium surrounding the intramyocardial hematoma was transmurally infarcted on late gadolinium enhancement images, with edema demonstrated on T2-weighted images (asterisks). Reproduced with permission from Wilson JR, Marshall RJ, Shanbhag SM, et al. Multimodality imaging of a dissecting intramyocardial hematoma extending into the left atrial wall following myocardial infarction. *Circulation*. 2012;126:e339-e341.

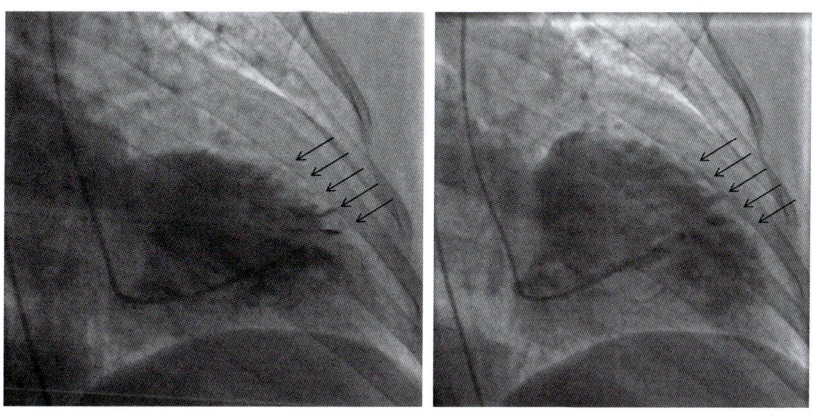

FIGURE 10.30 Left ventricular noncompaction. Left ventricular angiography: dilated left ventricle with prominent trabeculae and deep intertrabecular recesses (left: diastole; right: systole) and severely depressed left ventricular function. Reproduced with permission from Brunetti ND, Centola A, Campanale EG, et al. Combined finding of left ventricular non-compaction and dilated cardiomyopathy. *J Clinic Experiment Cardiol*. 2010;1:113.

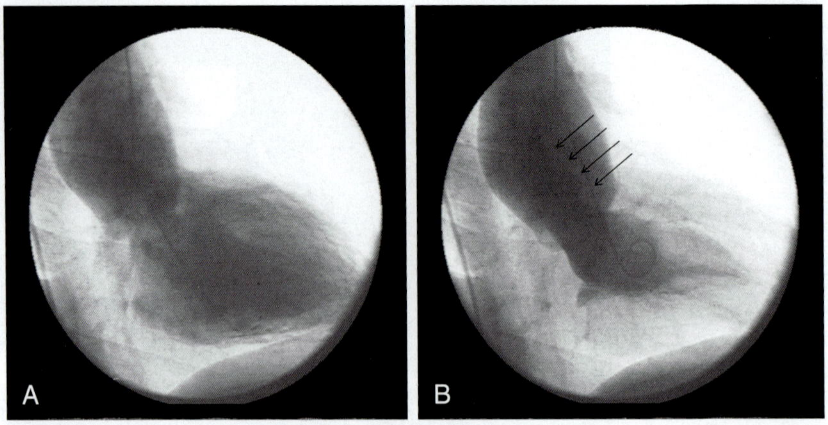

FIGURE 10.31 Left ventriculography and aortography in a patient presenting with severe acute chest pain and referred for emergency cardiac catheterization. **A,** Diastolic frame. Note the marked dilatation of the ascending aorta. **B,** Systolic frame. Note the uneven opacification of the sinotubular junction and of the aorta, suggestive of a double lumen. The patient presented with a type A aortic dissection complicated by acute aortic regurgitation, pericardial effusion, and tamponade physiology.

chapter **11**

Coronary Anomalies

MAURO MOSCUCCI, MD, MBA

INTRODUCTION

Coronary anomalies can be defined as any anomaly of a coronary artery in origination and course, termination, and intrinsic characteristics.[1] According to this definition, they can be classified into 3 major groups and subcategories (**Tables 11.1-11.3**).

The reported prevalence of coronary anomalies across different case series has varied between 0.2% and 5.6%.[2-19] Different definitions, variability in the populations studied and diagnostic methods used, and differences in criteria for inclusion or exclusion of the type of anomaly can explain this variability. It is currently agreed by several investigators that of all the coronary anomalies, the group of anomalous origin of coronary artery from the opposite sinus of Valsalva is responsible for most cases of sudden death.[5,20-26] In addition, anomalies of termination can be associated with chronic volume overload leading to heart failure, or to ischemia secondary to a "steal" phenomenon. The objective of this chapter is to provide a visual review of coronary anomalies, with a focus on the identification of coronary anomalies that might be associated with an increased risk of adverse outcomes.

ANOMALIES OF ORIGINATION AND COURSE

FIGURES 11.1 and **11.2** provide an overview of the relationship between the coronary tree, the great vessels, and cardiac chambers. Taking into account these relationships and a "normal anatomy," the group of coronary anomalies of origination and course can therefore include multiple categories with different clinical significance (**Table 11.1**). For example, while an absent left main trunk with split origination of the left coronary artery or an anomalous location of the coronary and ostium within the aortic root or near the proper aortic sinus of Valsalva are anomalies which are rarely associated with adverse outcomes or symptoms, it is currently agreed that the anomalous origin of the coronary artery from the opposite sinus of Valsalva (anomalous coronary artery from the opposite sinus—ACAOS) with interarterial course (**FIGURES 11.3** and **11.4**),[17,18] and in particular the variant with " intramural" course in which the coronary artery course is through the media of the aorta (ACAOS/IAC) (**FIGURE 11.5**)[27,28] are variants of coronary anomalies that can be associated with ischemia and an increased risk of sudden death in young people.[17,20,21,26] A recent study evaluating the use of MRI screening in a general population of adolescents has shown a prevalence of high-risk ACAOS as high as 0.44% (0.11% L-ACAOS-IAC and 0.32% R-ACAOS).[29]

TABLE 11.1

Anomalies of Origination and Course

1. Absent left main trunk (split origination of LCA)
2. Anomalous location of coronary ostium within aortic root or near proper aortic sinus of Valsalva (for each artery)
   a. High
   b. Low
   c. Commissural
3. Anomalous location of coronary ostium outside normal "coronary" aortic sinuses
   a. Right posterior aortic sinus
   b. Ascending aorta, with anomalous course
      1. Intramural (ACAOS)
      2. Extramural
   c. Left ventricle
   d. Right ventricle
   e. Pulmonary artery. Variants:
      1. LCA arising from posterior-facing sinus (ALCAPA)
      2. Cx arising from posterior-facing sinus
      3. LAD arising from posterior-facing sinus
      4. RCA arising from anterior-right-facing sinus
      5. Ectopic location (outside facing sinuses) of any coronary artery from pulmonary artery
         a. From anterior left sinus
         b. From pulmonary trunk
         c. From pulmonary branch
   f. Aortic arch
   g. Innominate artery
   h. Right carotid artery
   i. Internal mammary artery
   j. Bronchial artery
   k. Subclavian artery
   l. Descending thoracic aorta
4. Anomalous origination of coronary ostium from opposite, facing "coronary" sinus (which may involve joint origination or adjacent double ostia). Variants:
   a. RCA arising from left anterior sinus, with anomalous course
      1. Posterior atrioventricular groove[a] or retrocardiac
      2. Retroaortic[a]
      3. Between aorta and pulmonary artery,[a] preaortic, intramural (aortic), or ACAOS
      4. Intraseptal[a]
      5. Anterior to pulmonary outflow[a] or precardiac
      6. Posteroanterior interventricular groove[a]
   b. LAD arising from right anterior sinus, with anomalous course
      1. Between aorta and pulmonary artery, preaortic, intramural (aortic), or ACAOS
      2. Intraseptal
      3. Anterior to pulmonary outflow or precardiac
      4. Posteroanterior interventricular groove
   c. Cx arising from right anterior sinus, with anomalous course
      1. Posterior atrioventricular groove
      2. Retroaortic
   d. LCA arising from right anterior sinus, with anomalous course
      1. Posterior atrioventricular groove[a] or retrocardiac
      2. Retroaortic
      3. Between aorta and pulmonary artery,[a] preaortic, intramural (aortic), or ACAOS
      4. Intraseptal
      5. Anterior to pulmonary outflow[a] or precardiac
      6. Posteroanterior interventricular groove[a]
   e. LCA arising from the "noncoronary" sinus, with anomalous course
      1. Intramural (ACAOS)
      2. Extramural
5. Single coronary artery

[a]If a single, common ostium is present, the pattern is considered to represent "single coronary artery".

ACAOS, anomalous origin of a coronary artery from the opposite sinus of Valsalva, with intramural course; ALCAPA, anomalous origin of the left coronary artery from the Pulmonary artery; Cx, Circumflex; LAD, Left anterior descending coronary artery; LCA, left coronary artery; RCA, right coronary artery.

Reproduced with permission from Angelini P, Monge G. Coronary anomalies. In: Moscucci M, ed. *Grossman & Baim's Cardiac Catheterization Angiography and Intervention*. Philadelphia: Lippincott Williams and Wilkins; 2014.

TABLE 11.2

Anomalies of Intrinsic Coronary Arterial Anatomy

1. Congenital ostial stenosis or atresia (LCA, LAD, RCA, Cx)
2. Coronary ostial dimple
3. Coronary ectasia or aneurysm
4. Absent coronary artery
5. Coronary hypoplasia
6. Intramural coronary artery (myocardial bridge)
7. Subendocardial coronary course
8. Coronary crossing
9. Anomalous origination of posterior descending branch or septal penetrating branch
10. Absent PD or split RCA
    a. Proximal + distal PDs, arising from separate RCA sources
    b. Proximal PD arising from RCA, distal PD arising from LAD
    c. Proximal PD arising from RCA, distal PD arising from Cx
11. Absent or split LAD
    a. Large first septal branch and small distal LAD
    b. Double LAD
12. Ectopic origination of the first septal branch

PD, Posterior descending branch.
Reproduced with permission from Angelini P, Monge G. Coronary anomalies. In: Moscucci M, ed. *Grossman & Baim's Cardiac Catheterization Angiography and Intervention*. Philadelphia: Lippincott Williams and Wilkins; 2014.

TABLE 11.3

Anomalies of Coronary Termination

1. Decreased number of arteriolar/capillary ramifications (hypothetical)
2. Fistulas from RCA, LCA, or infundibular artery to:
    a. Right ventricle
    b. Right atrium
    c. Coronary sinus
    d. Superior vena cava
    e. Pulmonary artery
    f. Pulmonary vein
    g. Left atrium
    h. Left ventricle
    i. Multiple microfistulas draining into one or both ventricles

Reproduced with permission from Angelini P, Monge G. Coronary anomalies. In: Moscucci M, ed. *Grossman & Baim's Cardiac Catheterization Angiography and Intervention*. Philadelphia: Lippincott Williams and Wilkins; 2014.

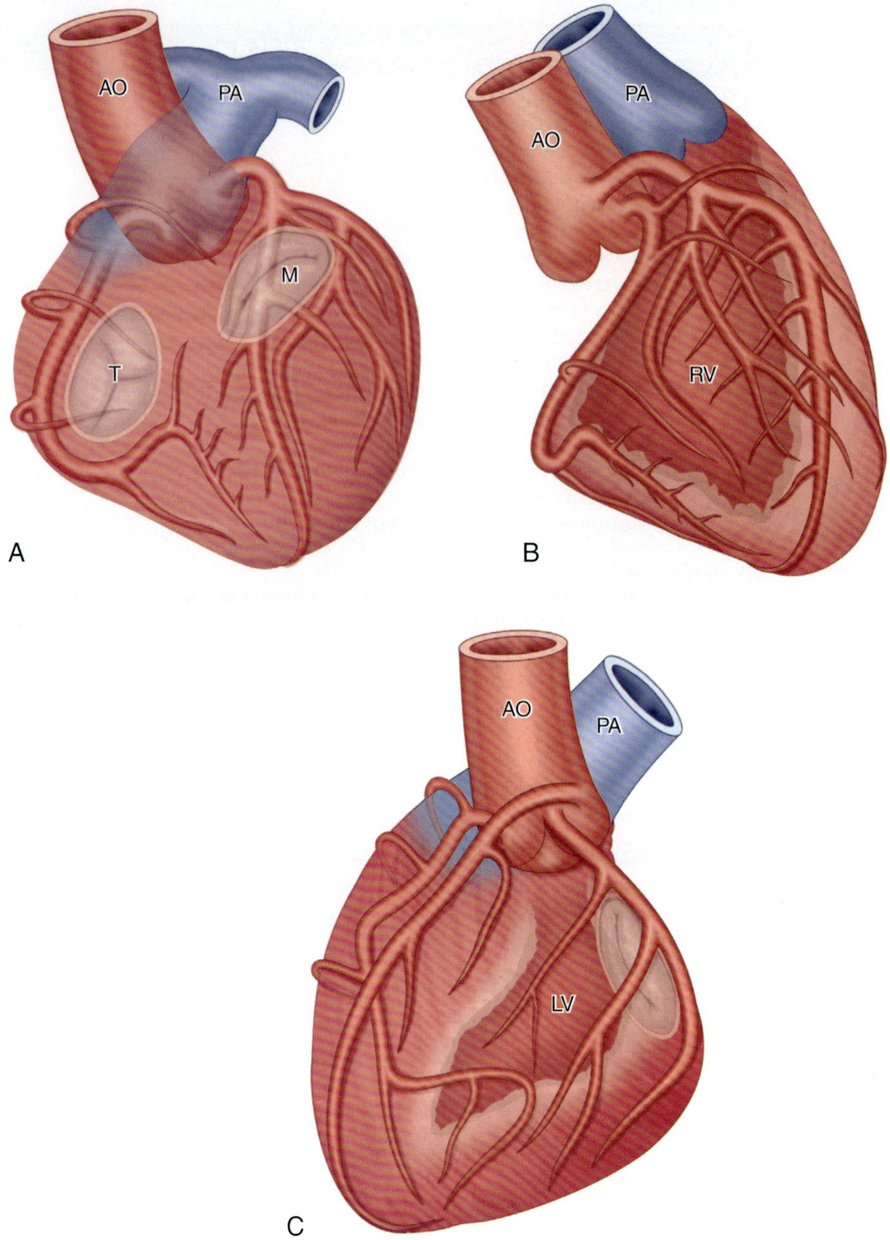

FIGURE 11.1 Relationship between coronary arteries and cardiac structures as seen in the frontal (A), right anterior oblique (B), and left anterior oblique projections (C). AO, aorta; LV, left ventricle; M, mitral valve; PA, pulmonary artery; RV, right ventricle; M, mitral valve; PA, pulmonary artery; RP, right ventricle; T, tricuspid valve. Reproduced with permission from Angelini P, ed. Coronary Artery Anomalies. Philadelphia: Lippincott Williams & Wilkins. Copyright 1999.

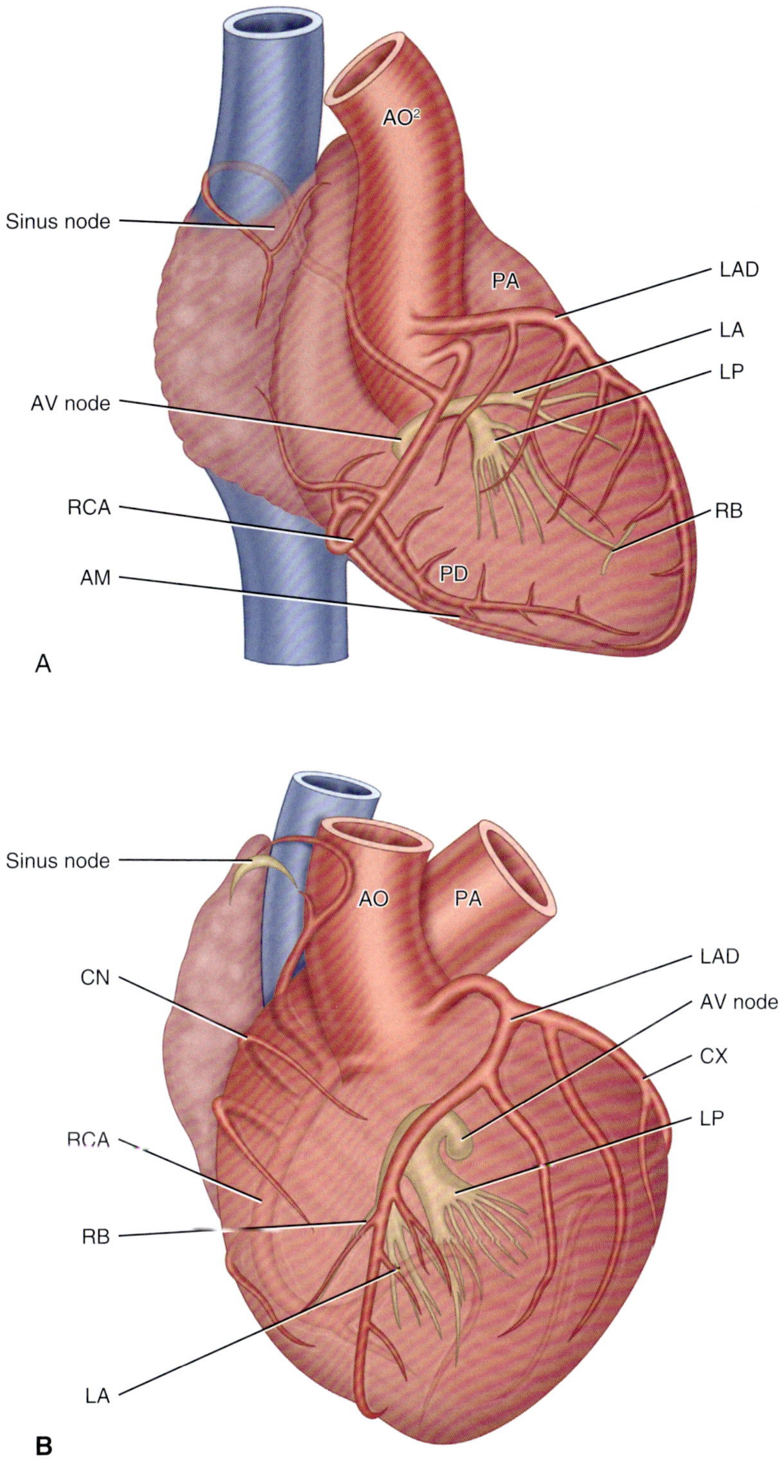

FIGURE 11.2 Right (A) and left (B) anterior oblique views of the main coronary branches and related cardiac structures. AM, acute marginal artery; Ao, aorta; AV, atrioventricular; CN, conal branch; Cx, circumflex artery; LA, left anterior fascicle of the left bundle branch; LAD, left anterior descending artery; LP, left posterior fascicle of the left bundle branch; PD, posterior descending branch; PA, pulmonary artery; RB, right bundle; RCA, right coronary artery; SN, sinus node. Reproduced with permission from Angelini P, ed. Coronary Artery Anomalies. Philadelphia: Lippincott Williams & Wilkins. Copyright 1999.

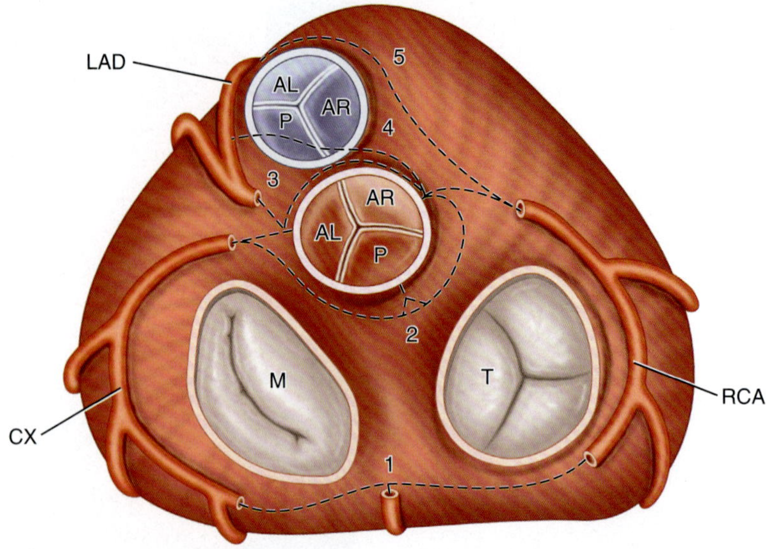

FIGURE 11.3 Conceptual diagram that shows most of the possible paths (1 through 5) by which the RCA, left anterior descending artery (LAD), and circumflex artery (Cx) can potentially connect with the opposite coronary cusps. Paths: 1, Retrocardiac; 2, retroaortic; 3, preaortic, or between the aorta and pulmonary artery; 4, intraseptal (supracristal); 5, prepulmonary (precardiac). The aortic and pulmonary cusps are labeled according to their position in space: AL indicates antero-left; AR, antero-right; P, posterior; M, mitral valve; and T, tricuspid valve. Reproduced with permission from Angelini P. Coronary artery anomalies: an entity in search of an identity. *Circulation*. 2007;115: 1296-1305.

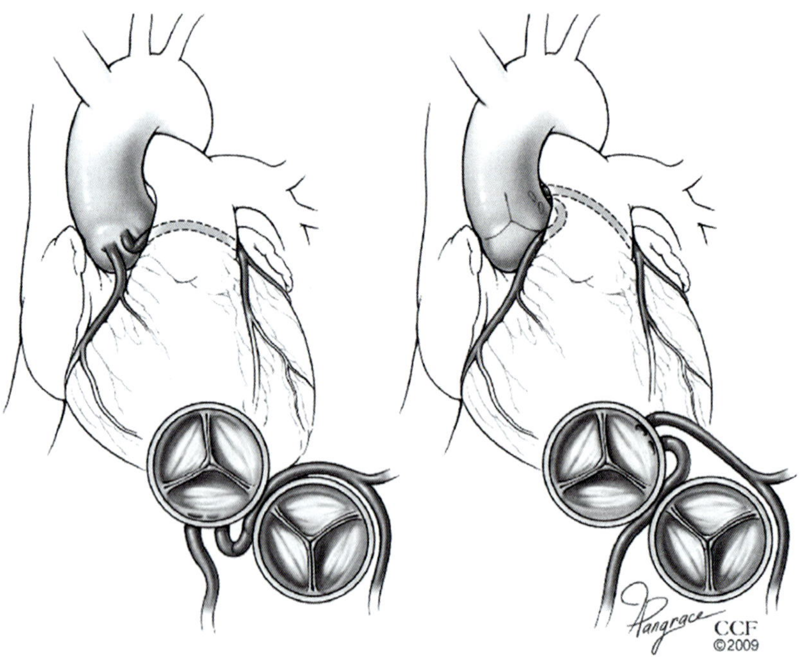

FIGURE 11.4 Illustration of an ALCA-R passing between the aorta and the pulmonary artery (left) and ARCA-L passing between the aorta and the pulmonary artery (right). Reproduced with permission from Krasuski RA, Magyar D, Hart S, et al. Long term outcomes and impact of surgery on adults with coronary arteries originating from the opposite coronary cusp. *Circulation*. 2011;123:154-162.

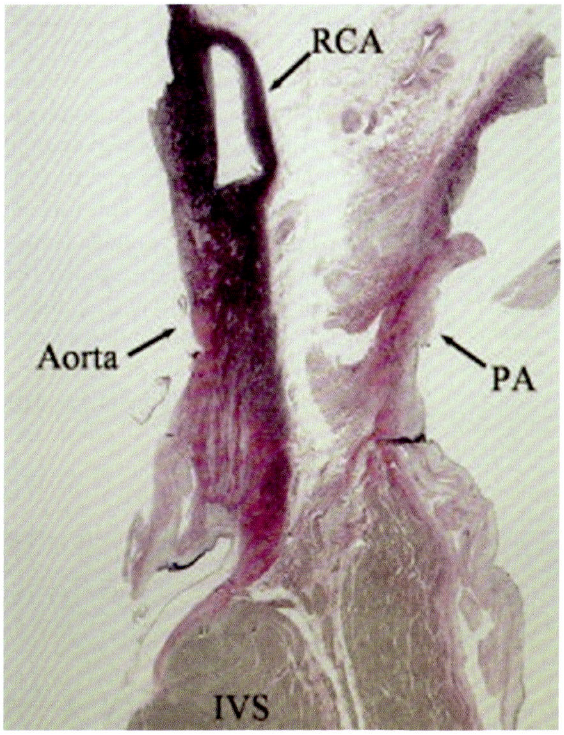

FIGURE 11.5 Histologic cross section of the anterior wall of the aorta and the posterior wall of the pulmonary artery at the level of the aortopulmonary "septum" (ie, the closest site between the 2), showing the critical autopsy findings in an athlete with R-ACAOS that resulted in his sudden death. Note that the space between the aorta and the pulmonary artery is not where the ectopic artery lies; rather, the artery passes within the media of the aorta, where it becomes laterally compressed (intramural). Reproduced with permission from Angelini P. Coronary artery anomalies—current clinical issues: definitions, classification, incidence, clinical relevance, and treatment guidelines. *Tex Heart Inst J.* 2002;29:271-278.

TABLE 11.4

Differential Angiographic Features in Cases of Preaortic (Intramural, L-ACAOS) and Infundibular (Intraseptal) Varieties of Ectopic Origin of the Left Coronary Artery From the Right Sinus of Valsalva

Feature	Intramural	Intraseptal
Retroaortic course in RAO projection	No	No
Initial course in RAO projection	Preaortic/superior (around aortic root)	Anterior-inferior
First branch off left main	Distal LAD/Cx splitting	First septal branch off mid left main
Left main systolic narrowing	Not usually recognized by angiography; if present, it is at proximal 1 cm (lateral compression)	Frequent, at distal left main (mild concentric myocardial bridge effect)
Distal left main location	Normal (next to left sinus)	LM connects with mid-LAD

Reproduced with permission from Angelini P, Monge G. Coronary anomalies. In: Moscucci M, ed. *Grossman & Baim's Cardiac Catheterization Angiography and Intervention*. Philadelphia: Lippincott Williams and Wilkins; 2014.
Cx, circumflex; LAD, left anterior descending coronary artery; RAO, right anterior oblique.

The identification of coronary anomalies and delineation of their course with standard coronary angiography can be challenging. As shown in **Table 11.4**, characteristics than can help in differentiating between the intramural course and the more benign intraseptal course of a left ACAOS include the course in right anterior oblique (RAO) projection, the type of first branch from the left main, the presence or absence of left main systolic narrowing, and the location of the distal left main (**FIGURES 11.6-11.11**).[30] In addition, to assessing these characteristics, in the past the challenge of appropriately identifying the course of ACAOS used to be approached by performing coronary angiography in multiple projections with catheters inserted in the left ventricle, right ventricle, the pulmonary artery, and the ascending aorta to facilitate the evaluation of the relationship between the anomalous course of the coronary artery, the cardiac chambers, and the great vessels. The introduction of CT angiography and cardiac magnetic resonance imaging (MRI) has provided new modalities for the proper evaluation of anomalous course and is today part of the standard of care (**FIGURES 11.12-11.15**).[5,31] In addition, the use of intravascular ultrasound imaging and of optical coherence tomography has provided new insights regarding the pathophysiology of ACAOS and the potential mechanism behind the development of ischemia and sudden death.[5] These imaging modalities and additional imaging obtained during surgery (**FIGURES 11.16-11.19**) have shown that the potential mechanisms leading to the

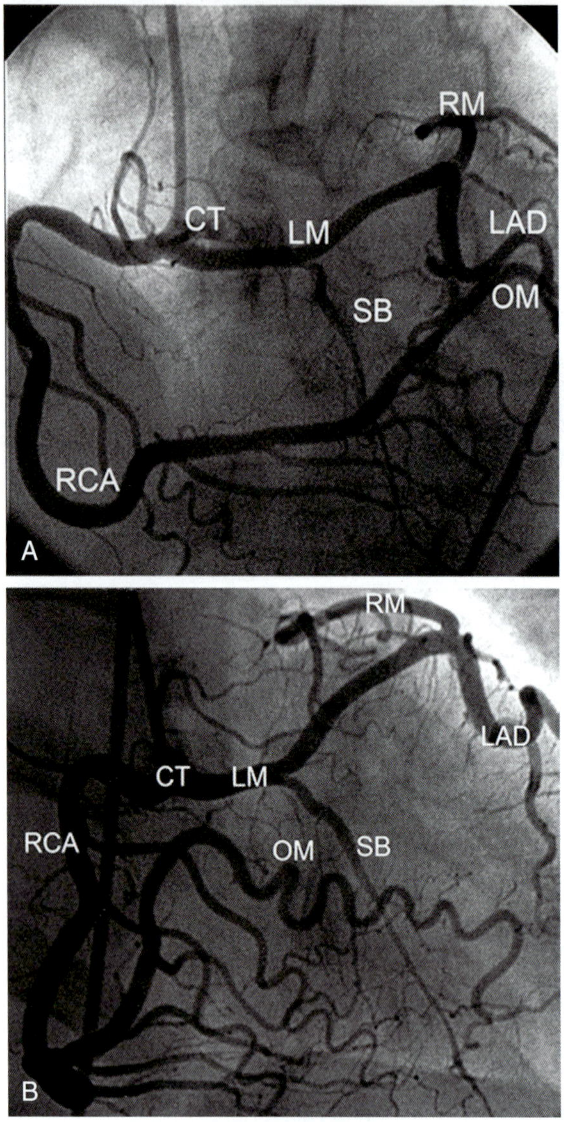

FIGURE 11.6 Angiograms from a 52-year-old man, in the left anterior oblique cranial (A) and right anterior oblique (B) projections. The patient had atypical chest pain and borderline nuclear stress test results. In these views, the whole coronary system is visualized from a single ostium, located at the right sinus. The right coronary artery (RCA) splits off from a short common trunk (CT) and continues into a terminal obtuse marginal branch (OM). The left main trunk (LM) crosses to the left off the CT, and courses intraseptally to give off a large septal branch (SB). The left coronary artery ends in the left anterior descending (LAD) and ramus (RM) branches. This is a case of clinically benign single coronary artery, which should more properly be called single coronary ostium because all the coronary arteries are present, although they are anomalous in their origin and course. Reproduced with permission from Angelini P. Coronary artery anomalies. *Circulation*. 2007;115:1296-1305.

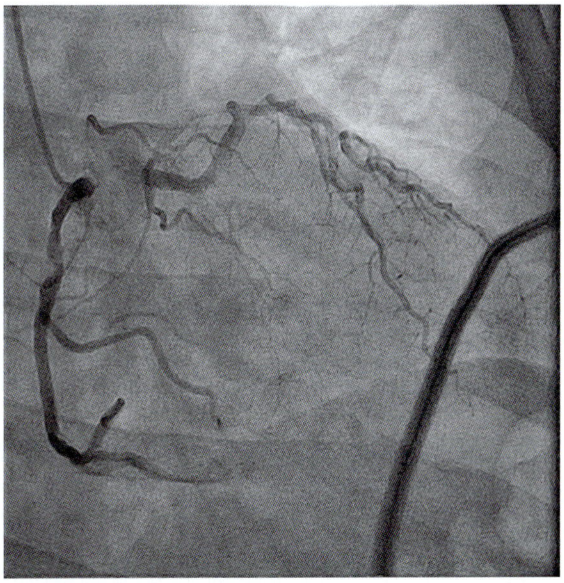

FIGURE 11.7 Angiogram from a 55-year-old man with a past medical history significant for systemic hypertension, hyperlipidemia, and type II diabetes presenting with progressive exertional and rest angina. His initial evaluation was consistent with an acute coronary syndrome and NSTEMI, as supported by elevation of serum troponin. Coronary angiography showed a significant stenosis in the proximal right coronary artery with haziness suggestive of either plaque rupture or thrombus, and an anomalous left coronary artery originating from the right coronary sinus.

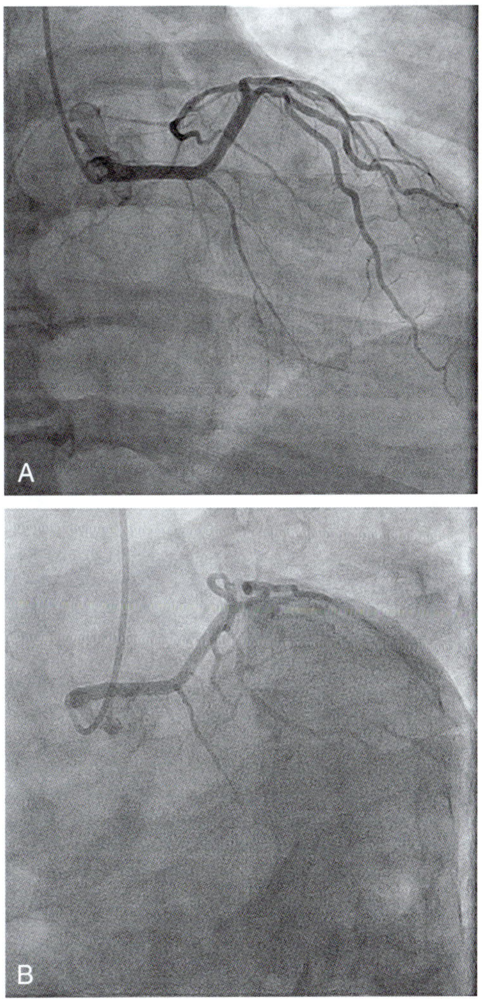

FIGURE 11.8 A and B, Selective left coronary angiography in right anterior oblique (RAO) view (A) and left anterior oblique (LAO) caudal view (B) in the case described in FIGURE 11.7. The anomalous coronary artery appears to have an intraseptal course based on the criteria listed in Table 11.4. In the RAO projection, the left main coronary artery has anterior-inferior course, the first branch of the left main coronary artery is a septal perforator the branch, and the left main coronary artery connects with the mid left anterior descending artery.

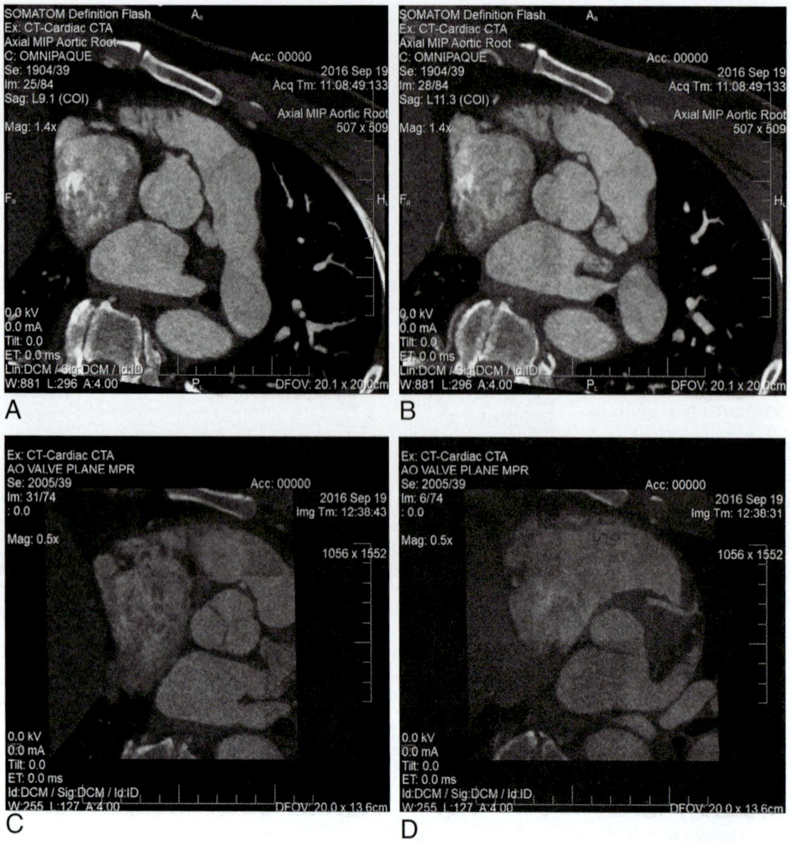

FIGURE 11.9 A-D, CT angiography confirmed the intraseptal course of the left main coronary artery suggested by the coronary angiography illustrated in **FIGURE 11.8**.

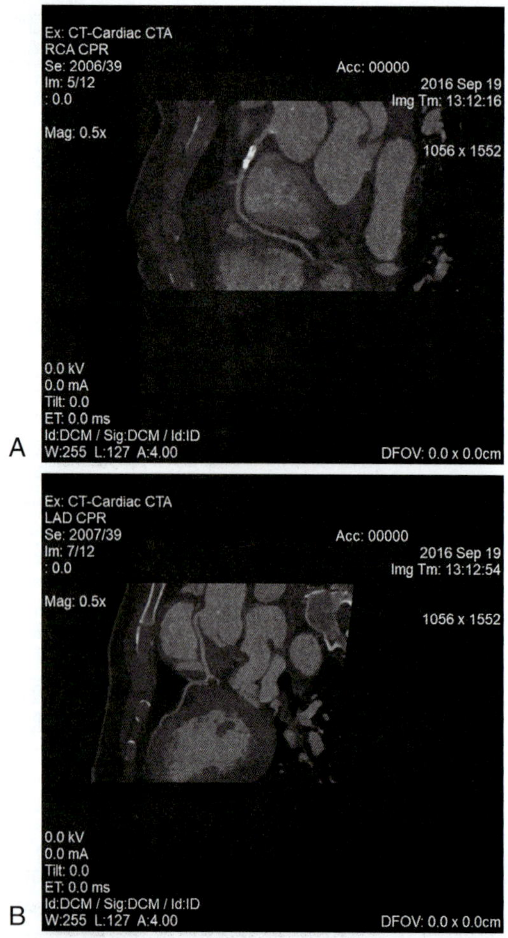

FIGURE 11.10 A, Right coronary artery. B, Left anterior descending artery with anomalous origin from the right coronary sinus of Valsalva in the case described in **FIGURE 11.7**. Please note the bright appearance of a stent implanted in the right coronary artery.

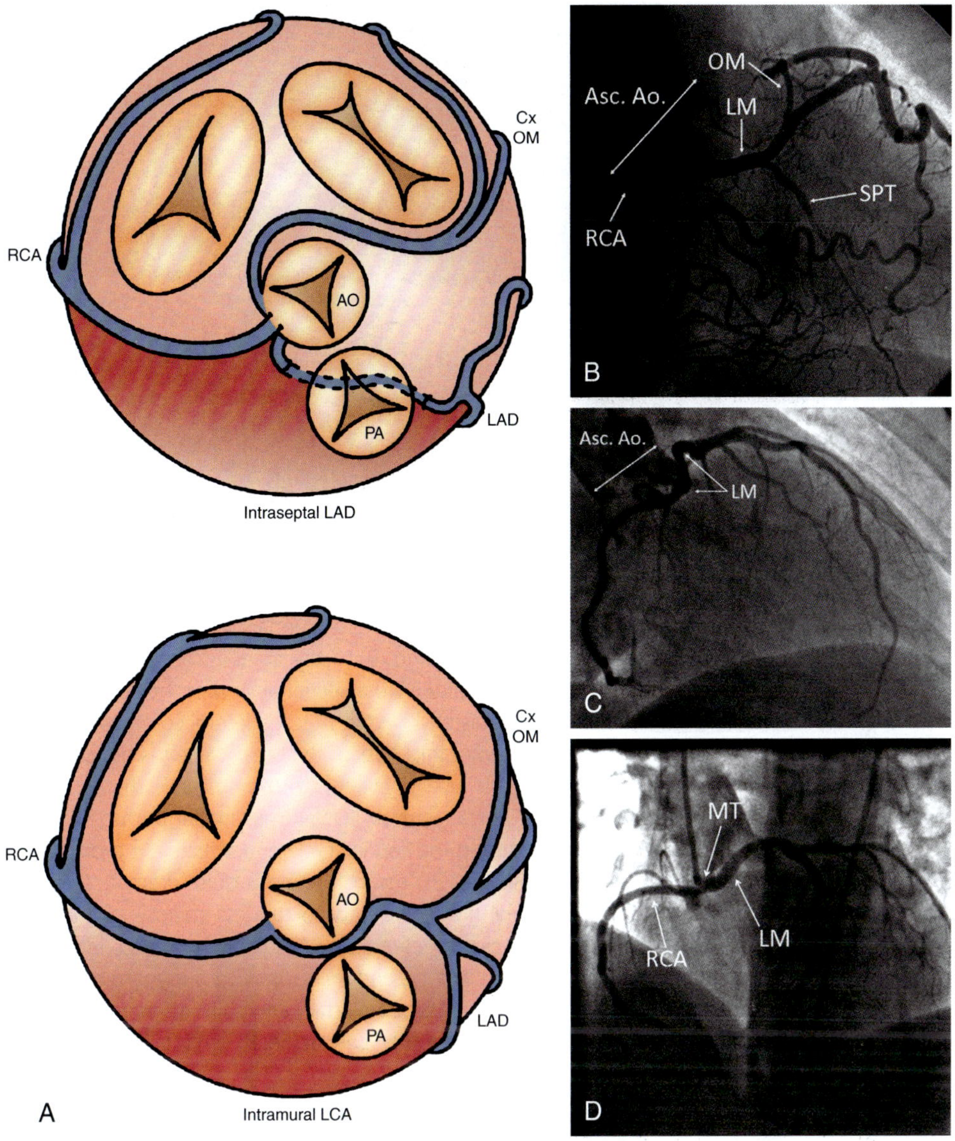

FIGURE 11.11 A-C, Diagrammatic representation of the abnormal proximal courses of ectopic left coronary arteries in 2 similar cases: the intraseptal, infundibular variant (diagram in A, with typical angiograms in B), and the intramural, preaortic variant (diagram in A, typical angiogram in C and D) Only the intramural case (ACAOS) has intrinsic ischemic potential. In B (intraseptal) and C (intramural), the 2 variants are shown in the same right anterior oblique projection; note that the intramural variant features a course stuck to the anterior border of the aorta (the one on the right side of the aorta, AO, in this view), and it is tilted upward. In the opposite case, the intraseptal variant is directed inferiorly and anteriorly in this projection, as it provides a characteristic first branch that is clearly a septal branch (SPT) (B). In the intraseptal case, the distal left main reaches the epicardial surface of the heart at the proximal left anterior descending. D, The left anterior oblique projection, in the intramural variety, shows the same uphill course as in C, with a "halo" that suggests an intramural course, just below the sinotubular junction. MT: mixed, short common trunk, joining the origins of the RCA and the LCA. Reproduced with permission fromAngelini P, Monge J. Coronary anomalies. In: Moscucci M, ed. *Grossman & Baim's Cardiac Catheterization Angiography and Intervention*. Philadelphia: Lippincott Williams and Wilkins; 2014:335-353.

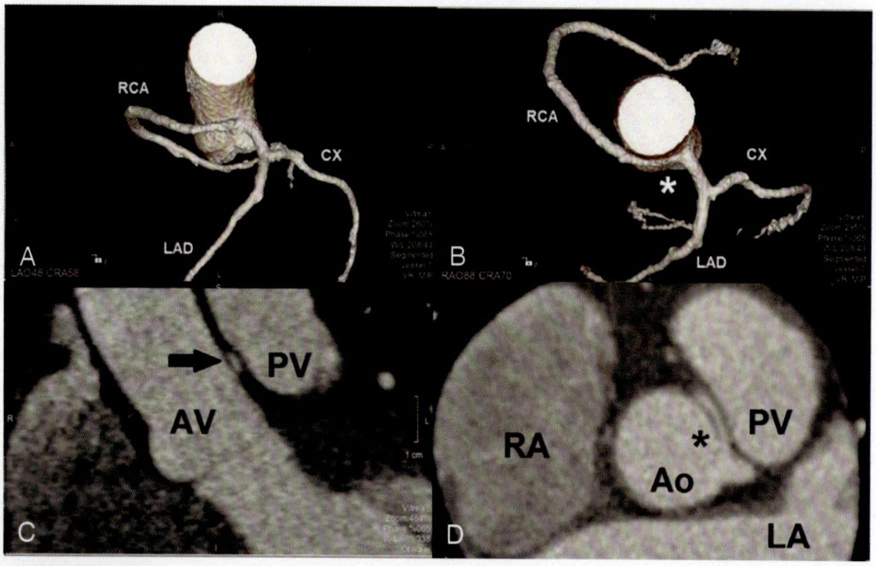

FIGURE 11.12 Computed coronary tomographic angiogram of the heart (3-dimensional [3D] reconstruction), in a case of anomalous right coronary artery (RCA) arising from the opposite sinus (R-ACAOS). A, in the frontal view and (B) in the cranial frontal view. Additionally, in tomographic source imaging, right anterior oblique cross-sectional view of the aorto/pulmonary septum (C), at the crossing of the ectopic artery (asterisk). Note that the lateral compression of the RCA is obvious only in view C; unfortunately, the wall thickness of the great vessels is not seen in this rendition. D, Cross section of the aortic root at the level of the RCA proximal trunk: the artery travels from the left sinus to the right in front of the aorta (asterisk). Only intravascular ultrasonography is able to clarify that lateral compression varies during the cardiac cycle and affects the proximal segment because of the intramural course. Note also that 3D reconstruction is quite dramatic in showing the ectopic origin of the RCA (A), but a cranial tilt is necessary to suggest stenosis of this segment (B). Ao indicates aorta; AV, aortic valve; CX, circumflex artery; LA, left atrium; LAD, left anterior descending artery; PV, pulmonary valve; RA, right atrium; and RCA, right coronary artery. Reproduced with permission from Angelini P. Novel imaging of coronary artery anomalies to assess their prevalence, the causes of clinical symptoms, and the risk of sudden cardiac death. *Circ Cardiovasc Imaging*. 2014;7:747-754.

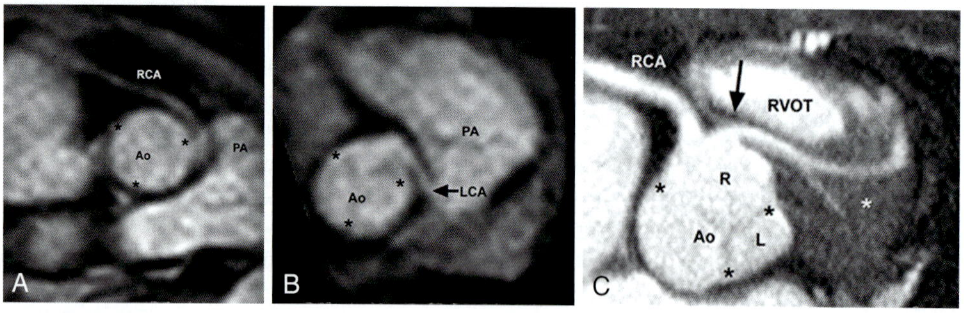

FIGURE 11.13 Screening cardiovascular magnetic resonance images of 3 typical coronary artery anomalies, which can be high-risk cardiovascular conditions, especially in athletes. The black asterisks indicate the 3 aortic valve commissures. A, Anomalous origin of the right coronary artery (RCA) from the left sinus of Valsalva, with a preaortic, interarterial course (right anomalous coronary artery arising from the opposite sinus). Ao indicates aorta; and PA, pulmonary artery. B, Anomalous origin of the left coronary artery (LCA; arrow) from the right sinus of Valsalva, with an interarterial course at the level of the aortic and pulmonary valves. C, Anomalous origin of the LCA from the right sinus of Valsalva, with an infundibular course, which is usually benign (also called an intraseptal course). Ao indicates aortic root; RCA, right coronary artery; and RVOT, right ventricular outflow tract. The white asterisk indicates ventricular septal myocardium. L indicates left sinus of Valsalva; and R, right sinus of Valsalva. Reproduced with permission from Angelini P. Novel imaging of coronary artery anomalies to assess their prevalence, the causes of clinical symptoms, and the risk of sudden cardiac death. *Circ Cardiovasc Imaging*. 2014;7:747-754.

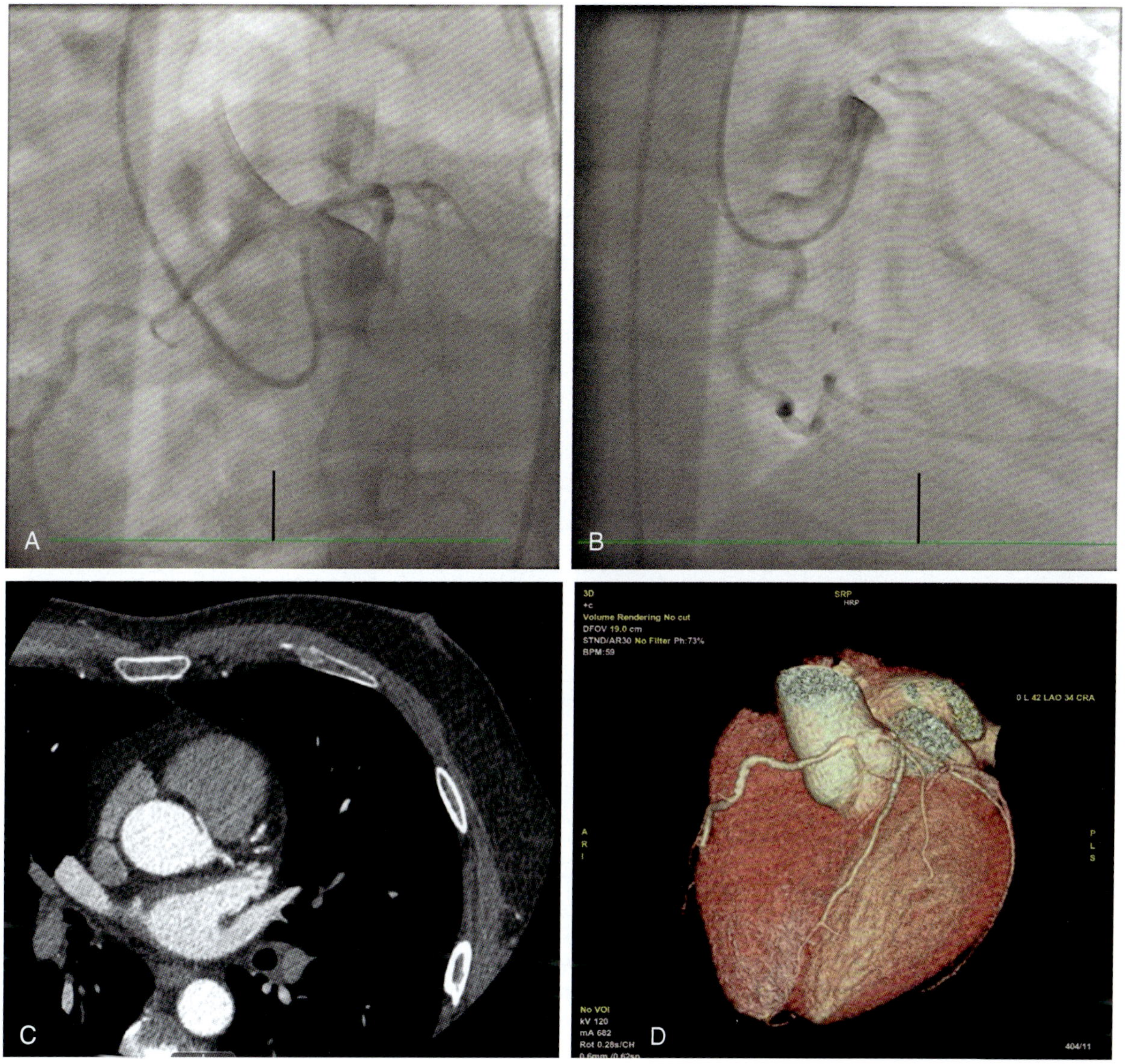

FIGURE 11.14 A-C, Anomalous origin of the right coronary artery from the left sinus of Valsalva in (A) left anterior oblique (LAO) view and (B) right anterior oblique (RAO) view. The artery is poorly visualized through nonselective angiography. C, CT angiography showing the anomalous origin of the RCA from the left sinus of Valsalva. D, Volume rendering reconstruction.

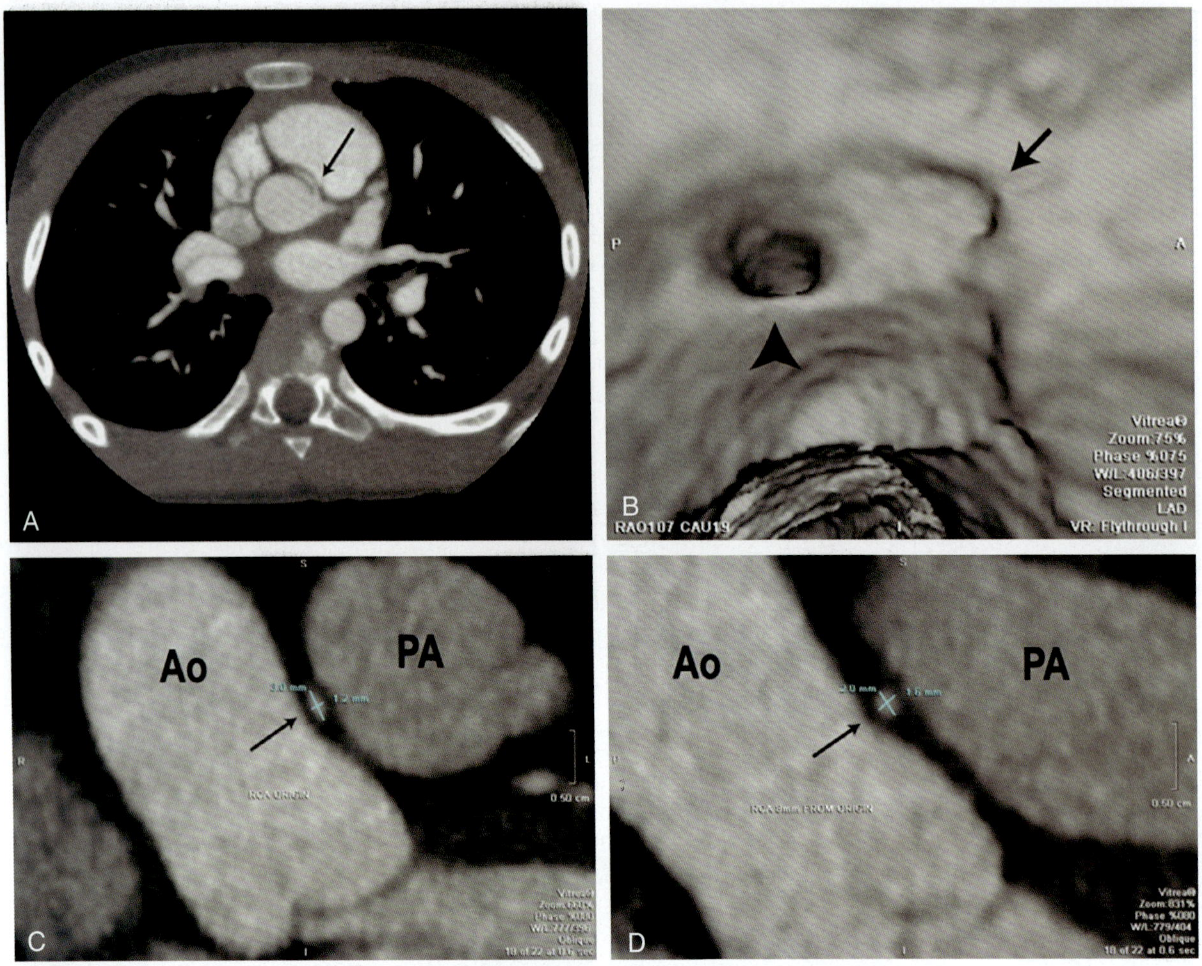

FIGURE 11.15 CTA imaging in anomalous aortic origin of a coronary artery (AAOCA). A, An anomalous right coronary artery (ARCA, arrow) arising from the left sinus of Valsalva and traveling intramurally and interarterially. B, A virtual angioscopy that demonstrates a normal left coronary ostium (arrowhead) and an abnormal, small, and slitlike ostium of the right coronary (arrow) arising just above and to the left of the intercoronary commissure of the aortic valve. C and D, A transverse cut of an anomalous right coronary artery (arrow) demonstrates an oval morphology close to its origin (likely due to intramurality) and a normal round morphology 8 mm from its origin. Intramurality is determined by quantification of the density of the tissue around the coronary (presence or absence of pericoronary fat between the coronary and the aorta) and the shape of the coronary artery. Ao, aorta; PA, pulmonary artery; RCA, right coronary artery. © 2014 Texas Children's Hospital; reprinted with permission; Reproduced with permission from Mery CM, Lawrence SM, Krishnamurthy R, et al. Anomalous aortic origin of a coronary artery: toward a standardized approach. *Semin Thoracic Surg.* 2014;26:110-122.

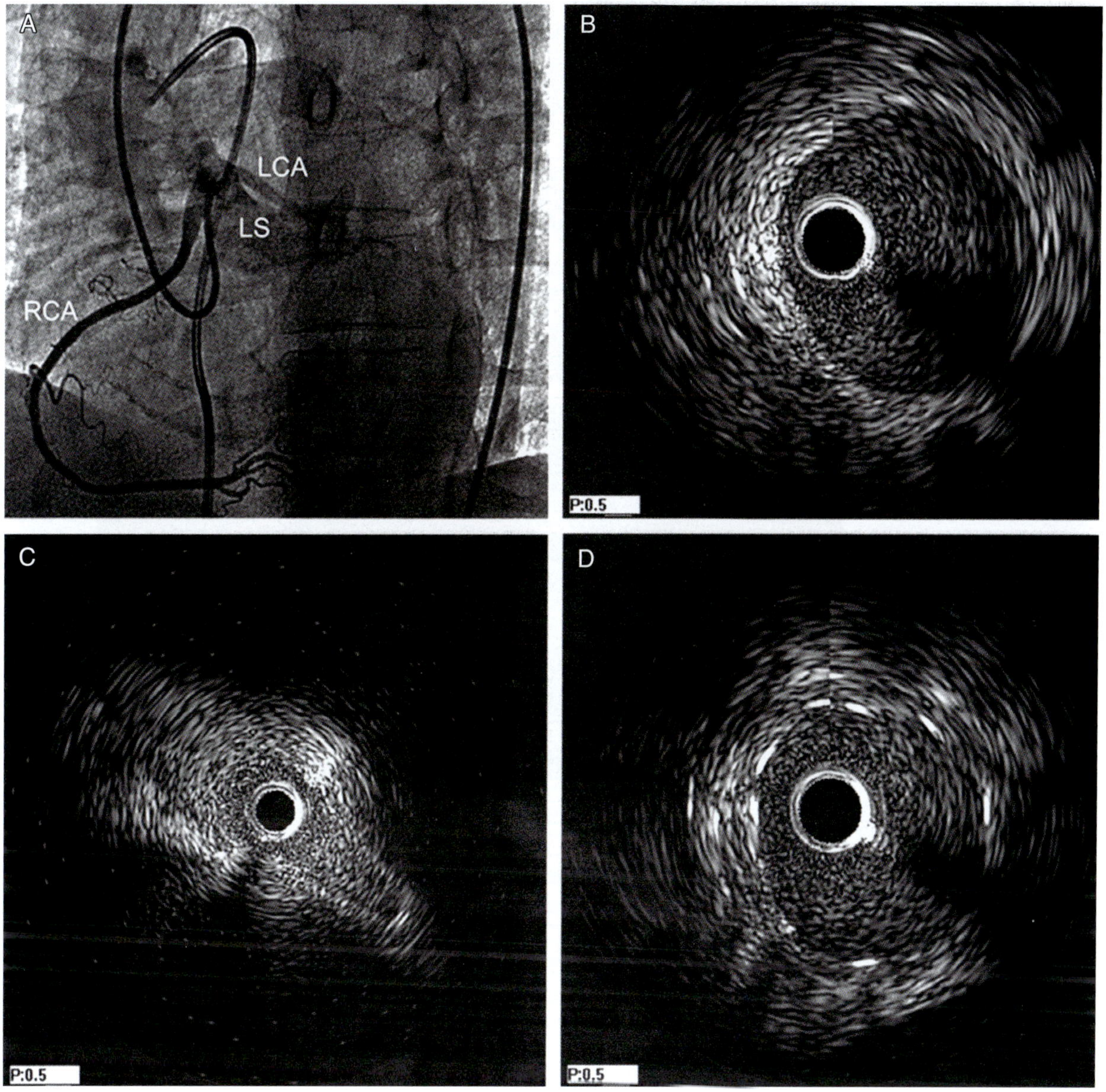

FIGURE 11.16 Images obtained from a 42-year-old man with severe angina of recent onset, who had recently developed hypertension. A, Selective angiogram of the RCA in the left anterior oblique projection. In this view, the proximal course appears wider than the more distal vessel, and it originates next to the LCA (which is also ectopic), high above the left aortic sinus (LS). B, IVUS image of the distal RCA. The cross-sectional area is 10.8 mm^2, and the shape is circular. C, IVUS image of the proximal segment of the RCA, whose lumen is severely compressed laterally (minimal diameter, 1.5 mm; maximal diameter, 3.8 mm; cross-sectional area, 4.2 mm^2; area stenosis, 61%). The LCA had also milder ostial stenosis. D, IVUS of the proximal RCA after stent angioplasty (3.5 × 12 mm; postdilated at 18 atm). The shape has become round, and the area has expanded to match that of the distal normal vessel. Reproduced with permission from Angelini P. Coronary artery anomalies. *Circulation*. 2007;115:1296-1305.

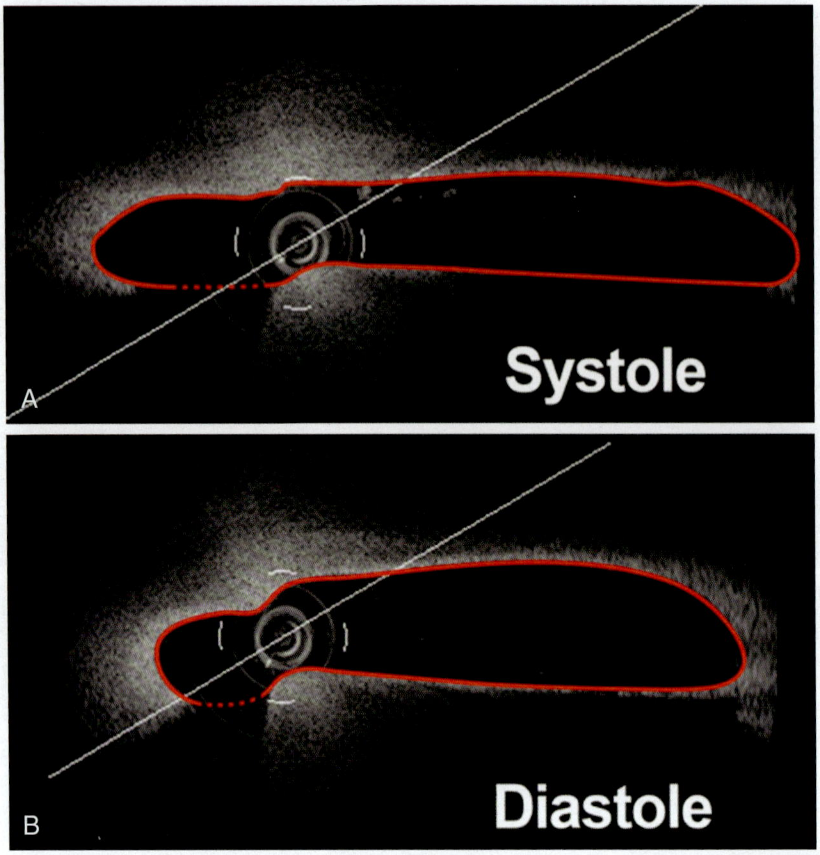

FIGURE 11.17 Optical coherence tomographic (OCT) images in systole (A) and diastole (B), showing the much improved definition of the intravascular anatomy afforded by OCT. Potentially, instantaneous changes in the severity of stenosis during simulated exercise could be much more easily quantified by OCT than by intravascular ultrasound. The probe marks (circle) show the calibration in the images (diameter = 0.9 mm). In both A and B, the interrupted line indicates the beginning of the slitlike orifice of the right coronary artery (the C sign typical of tangential origin). Reproduced with permission from Angelini P. Novel imaging of coronary artery anomalies to assess their prevalence, the causes of clinical symptoms, and the risk of sudden cardiac death. *Circ Cardiovasc Imaging*. 2014;7:747-754.

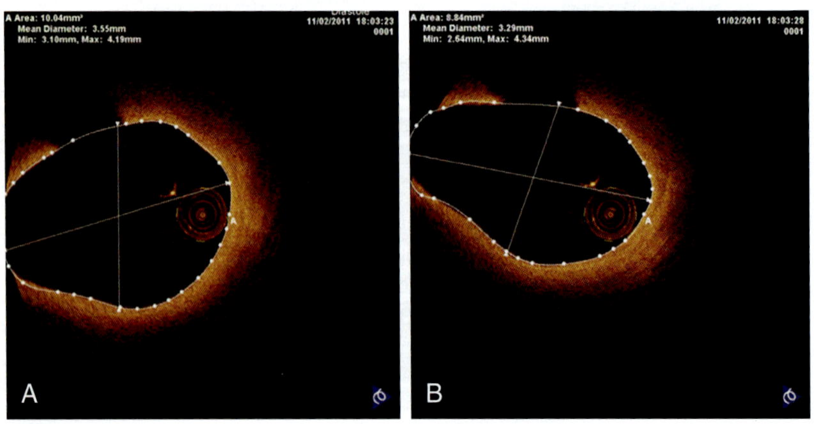

FIGURE 11.18 OCT imaging in systole (A) and diastole (B) in a case of mild stenosis of the intramural segment in a case of R-ACAOS (of the lowest severity ever seen in our practice). The mean degree of stenosis was 30% (mild). Reproduced with permission from Angelini P, Monge J. Coronary anomalies. In: Moscucci M, ed. *Grossman & Baim's Cardiac Catheterization Angiography and Intervention*. Philadelphia: Lippincott Williams and Wilkins; 2014.

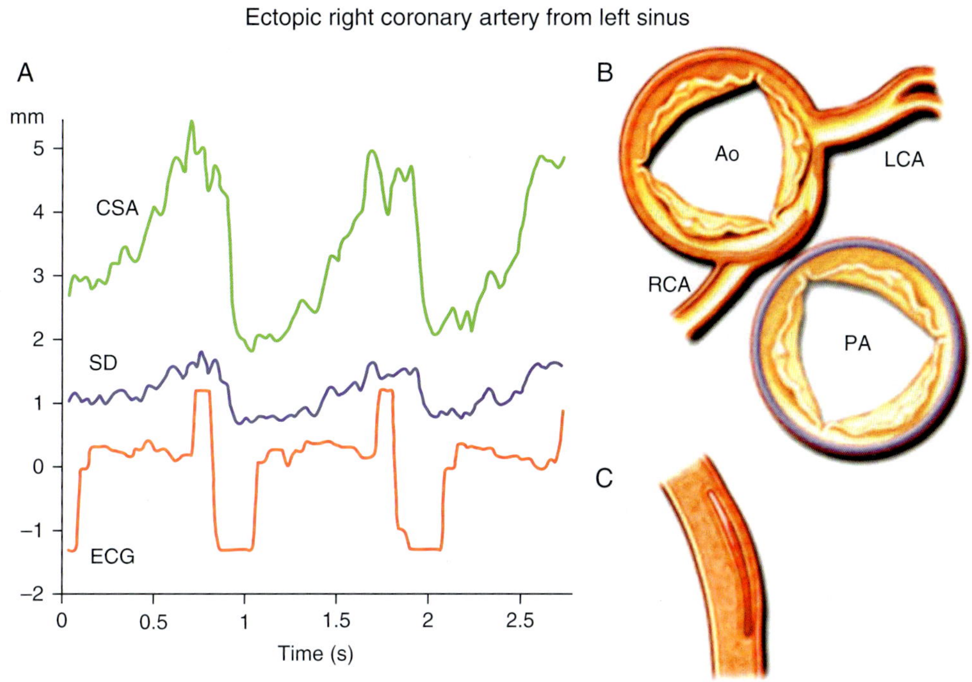

FIGURE 11.19 Instantaneous stenosis during the whole cardiac cycle in anomalous origin of the right coronary artery (RCA) from the opposite sinus of Valsalva. Systolic expansion of the aortic root leads to significant worsening of lateral compression, as indicated by the chart (A; left), which shows the variation in the cross-sectional area (CSA; blue line) during the cardiac cycle; the CSA increases from 2.3 to 5.1 mm^2 in diastole, whereas the short diameter (SD) of the intramural RCA (green line) increases from 0.8 to 1.5 mm. This is an example of severe functional stenosis. The chart readings were obtained by calculating each parameter of intramural stenosis in instantaneous intravascular ultrasonography (30 frames per second). The red line represents the ECG. B, Top right: Schematic cartoon illustrating the mechanism of stenosis. C, Bottom right: Cartoon showing a cross-sectional systolic frame of the intramural course. The 3 panels move synchronously. Reproduced with permission from Angelini P. Novel imaging of coronary artery anomalies to assess their prevalence, the causes of clinical symptoms, and the risk of sudden cardiac death. *Circ Cardiovasc Imaging*. 2014;7:747-754.

development of ischemia can include compression during the cardiac cycle (**FIGURES 11.19** and **11.20**), compression of the intramural segment of the artery, coronary spasm,[27] and/or an anomalous takeoff of the vessel leading to a slitlike origin of the native coronary artery (**FIGURES 11.15**, **11.21**, and **11.22**). Thus, it has been recently advocated to include intravascular ultrasound imaging or optical coherence tomography in the evaluation of ACAOS.[27] **FIGURES 11.23-11.26** illustrate additional variants of ACAOS, including the benign and common form of left circumflex ACAOS (**FIGURE 11.26**), whereas **FIGURES 11.27-11.29** illustrate 2 unusual cases of anomalous left coronary artery from the pulmonary artery (ALCAPA) with symptoms presenting in late adulthood.

As of today, the role of surgery in the management of ACAOS is to prevent ischemia and to reduce the risk of sudden death. Surgical interventions will vary according to the type of anomaly, the course of the coronary artery, and the associated pathology (**FIGURES 11.30** and **11.31**).[17,32]

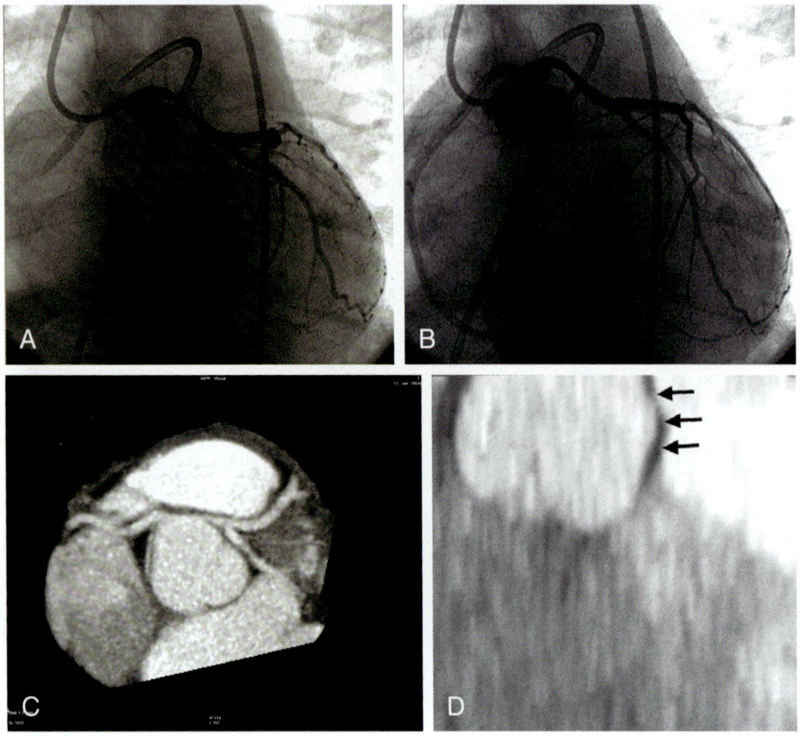

FIGURE 11.20 Angiographic images of L-ACAOS in systole (A) and diastole (B). A, The left main trunk shows the appearance of phasic narrowing relative to (B). C, CTA in the same case showing ectopic origin of the left coronary artery adjacent to the normally situated right coronary artery. D, Sagittal cross-section of the aortic root, showing a compressed left main (arrows) between the aorta and the pulmonary artery. Adapted with permission from Angelini P, Monge J. Coronary anomalies. In: Moscucci M, ed. *Grossman & Baim's Cardiac Catheterization Angiography and Intervention*. Philadelphia: Lippincott Williams and Wilkins; 2014.

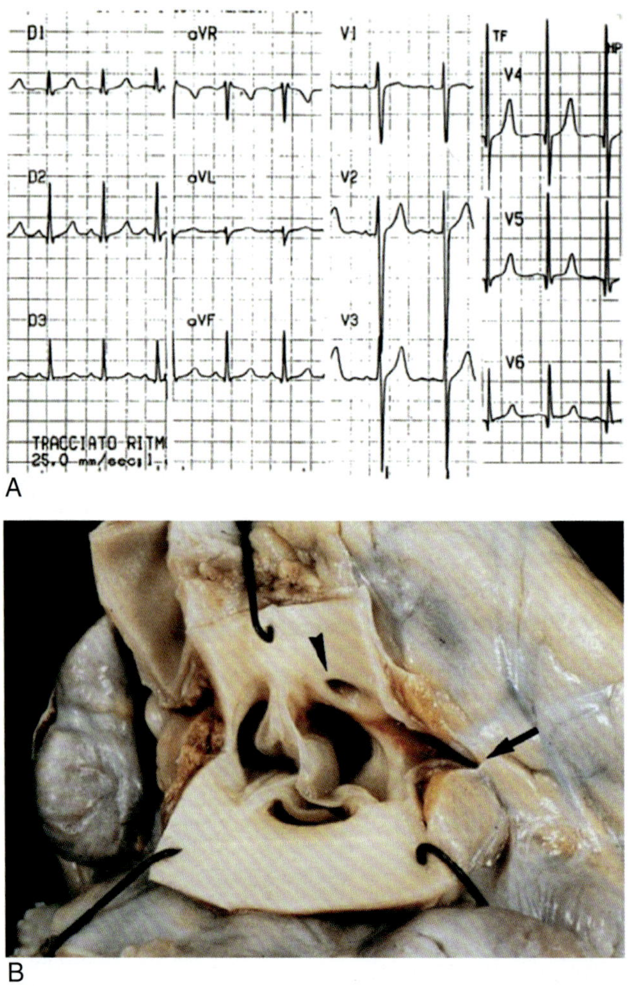

FIGURE 11.21 A 15-year-old male Italian soccer player with a history of exertional syncope 1 y before death who died suddenly while running during the second half of a game. A, A 12-lead ECG performed 10 mo before death, as part of routine preparticipation screening, is within normal limits. B, View of the aortic root; RCA arises normally from the right aortic sinus (arrow), and the LMCA arises anomalously from the right sinus with an acute angle takeoff producing a slitlike lumen (arrowhead). Reproduced with permission from Basso C, Maron BJ, Corrado D, Thiene G. Clinical profile of congenital coronary artery anomalies with origin from the wrong aortic sinus leading to sudden death in young competitive athletes. *J Am Coll Cardiol*. 2000;35:1493-501.

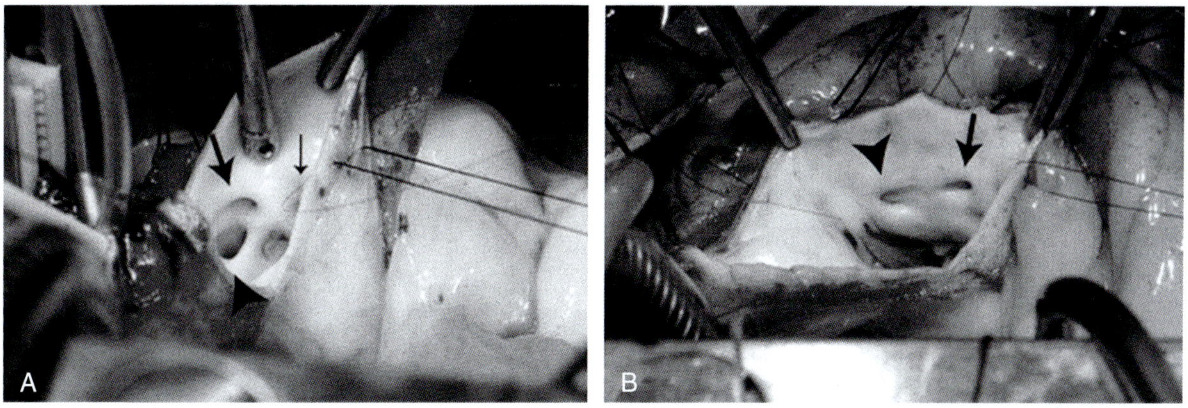

FIGURE 11.22 Anomalous right coronary artery from the left sinus of Valsalva. Surgical findings in patients with AAOCA. (A) A normal round left coronary ostium arising from the left sinus of Valsalva (arrowhead). The right coronary ostium is slitlike (large arrow) and arising from above and to the left of the intercoronary commissure of the aortic valve. The transmural fine stitch (small arrow) marks the location where the anomalous coronary arises from the aorta; the segment between the ostium and the stitch is intramural. (B) A patient that presented with aborted sudden cardiac death. The left coronary ostium (arrowhead) is stenotic with an ostial ridge and arises from the right sinus of Valsalva, above and to the right of the intercoronary commissure. The right coronary artery ostium (arrow) is also abnormal with a smaller ostial ridge. © 2014 Texas Children's Hospital, reprinted with permission; Mery CM, Lawrence SM, Krishnamurthy R, et al. Anomalous aortic origin of a coronary artery: toward a standardized approach. *Semin Thoracic Surg*. 2014;26:110-122.

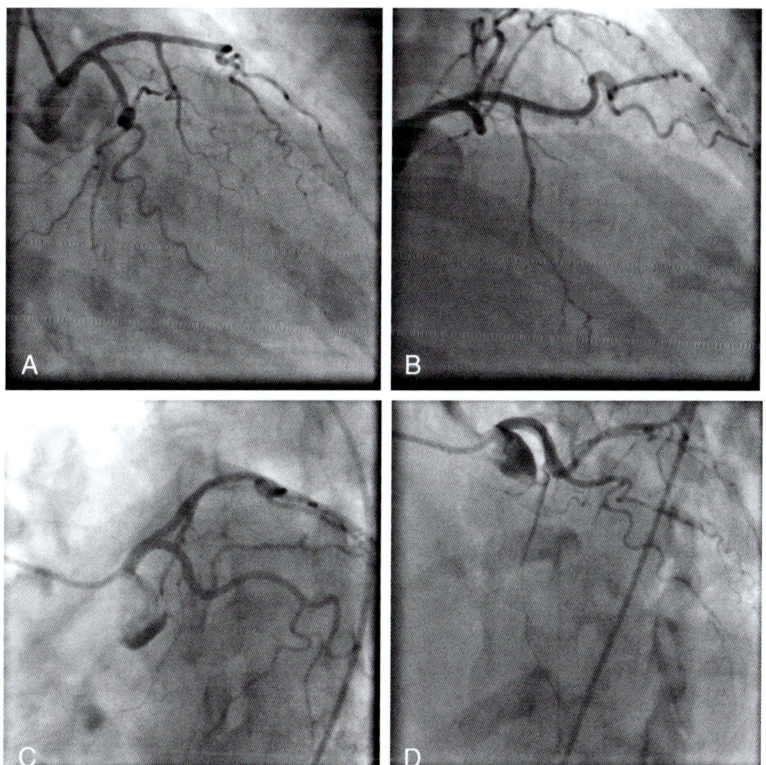

FIGURE 11.23 A-D, Coronary angiography in (A) right anterior oblique (RAO) view, (B) RAO cranial view, (C) left anterior oblique (LAO) caudal, and (D) antero posterior (AP) cranial views. Each view clearly shows the left main coronary trunk, circumflex artery, and the ramus intermedius. Although the RAO view could be inappropriately interpreted as normal coronary anatomy, the correct interpretation is an absent LAD with likely anomalous origin.

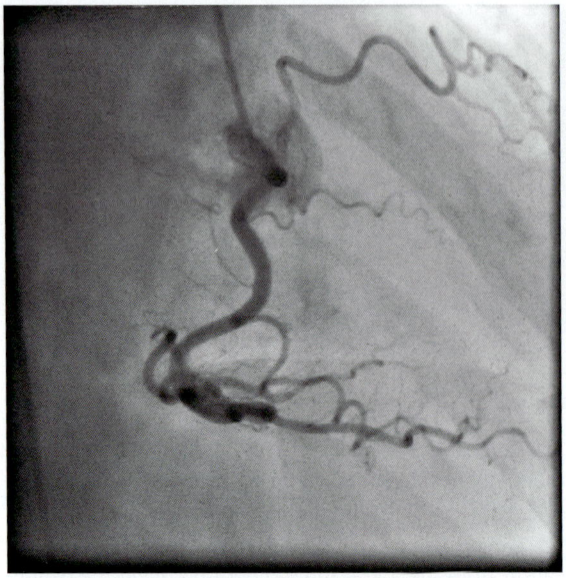

FIGURE 11.24 Right coronary angiography in the case illustrated in **FIGURE 11.21**. The origin of the left anterior descending artery is from the right coronary sinus of Valsalva.

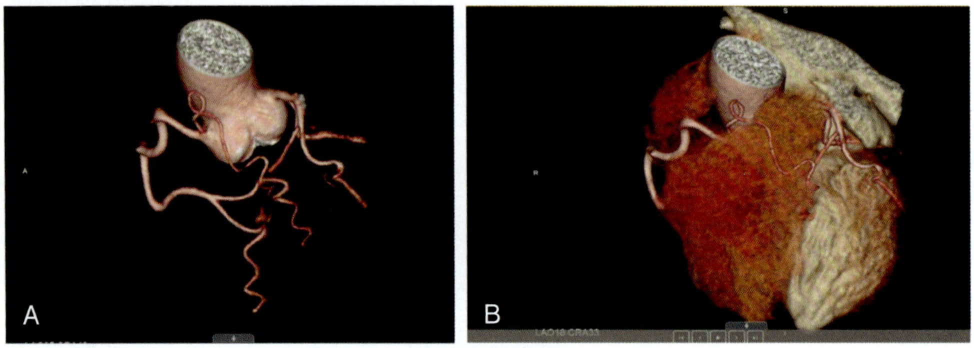

FIGURE 11.25 A and B, CT coronary angiography confirming the anomalous takeoff of the left anterior descending artery from the right sinus of Valsalva, whereas the left circumflex artery and ramus intermedius originate from the correct sinus.

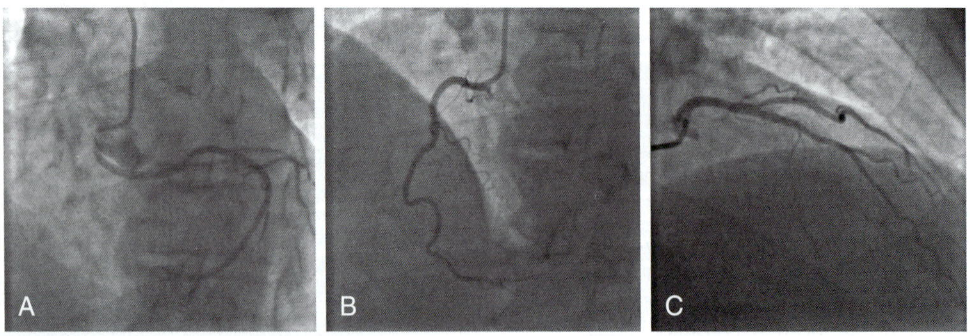

FIGURE 11.26 A relatively common ACAOS is origination of the circumflex artery from the right sinus with either a separate ostium or with a common short trunk. This variant has a retroaortic course (course # 2 in **FIGURE 11.3**) and it is not associated with an increased risk of adverse outcomes. A, Circumflex artery with anomalous origin. B, Right coronary artery with separate ostium from the anomalous left circumflex artery. C, Left anterior descending artery in right anterior oblique cranial view. Note the typical appearance with absence of the circumflex artery branch.

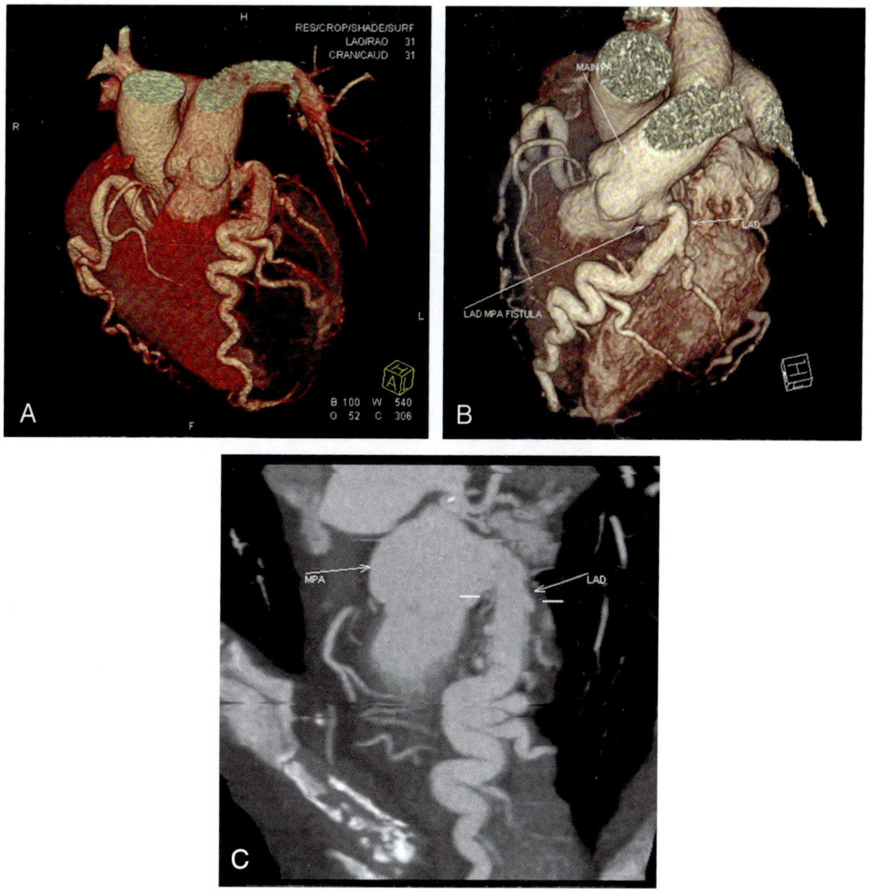

FIGURE 11.27 A-C, Anomalous left coronary artery from the pulmonary artery (ALCAPA). 65-year-old Hispanic woman with a past medical history of uncontrolled hypertension, insulin-dependent diabetes, hyperlipidemia, CAD, TIA. The patient was transferred from an outside hospital, following admission for chest pain radiating to the left side and to her arm. She denied any shortness of breath, fever, or diaphoresis at that time. Further evaluation revealed an anomalous origin of the left coronary artery arising from the pulmonary artery. Surgical repair performed included patch closure of the pulmonary artery to LAD orifice and coronary artery bypass graft with aorta to obtuse marginal 1 and aorta to left anterior descending.

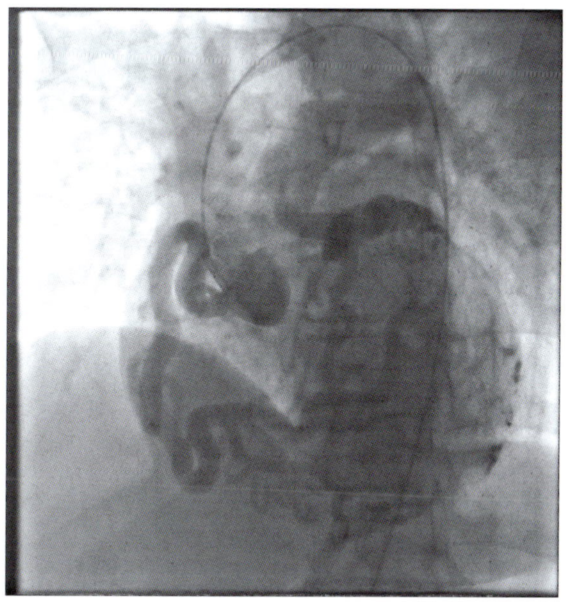

FIGURE 11.28 A 58-year-old woman who presented with a 2-mo history of dyspnea and who was referred for cardiac evaluation. Her past medical history was significant for a "heart murmur" and for mild exertional dyspnea, which, however, worsened over the 2 mo before clinical presentation. An echocardiogram showed moderate-to-severe mitral regurgitation, ejection fraction of 55% with normal left ventricular systolic function, and marked enlargement of the left atrium. Additional complaints included intermittent chest pain at rest with each episode lasting up to 2-3 h. Selective angiography of the right coronary artery revealed an aneurysmatic and tortuous right coronary artery with visualization of the pulmonary artery during contrast injection, thus consistent with a communication between the right coronary artery and the pulmonary artery.

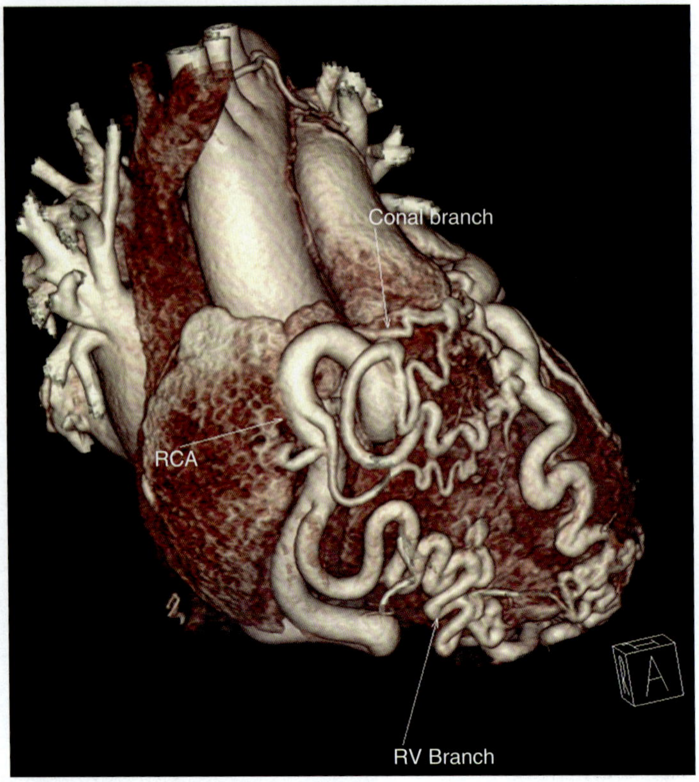

FIGURE 11.29 CT angiography with 3D rendering. The left main artery did not arise from the left sinus of Valsalva and did not communicate directly with the aorta at all. Instead, there was an anomalous connection of the left main coronary artery with the main pulmonary arterial trunk by a small vessel/fistula, which measured approximately 3.5 mm in diameter, and which demonstrated a jet of contrast opacified blood from the left main coronary into the nonopacified main pulmonary artery. The left main coronary artery was aneurysmal, measuring 9.6 mm in diameter, and while patent it bifurcated into the LAD and the left circumflex arteries. Both the LAD and proximal circumflex were also tortuous and ectatic, with the LAD measuring 9.6 mm in short axis diameter in the proximal portion and 10.6 mm in short axis diameter at the midportion. The LAD was also noted to give off/receive numerous large septal perforators, which measured up to 2.9 mm in short axis diameter. The proximal circumflex coronary measured 11 mm in short axis diameter. In addition, the opacification within the left coronary artery and its branches mirrored that of the thoracic aorta and right coronary artery, while the pulmonary arterial system remained relatively unopacified, thus suggesting retrograde filling of the left coronary artery circulation by numerous tortuous collateral vessels arising from prominent RV branches, PDAs, septal perforators, and extensive rich network of mediastinal collateral vessels of uncertain origin.

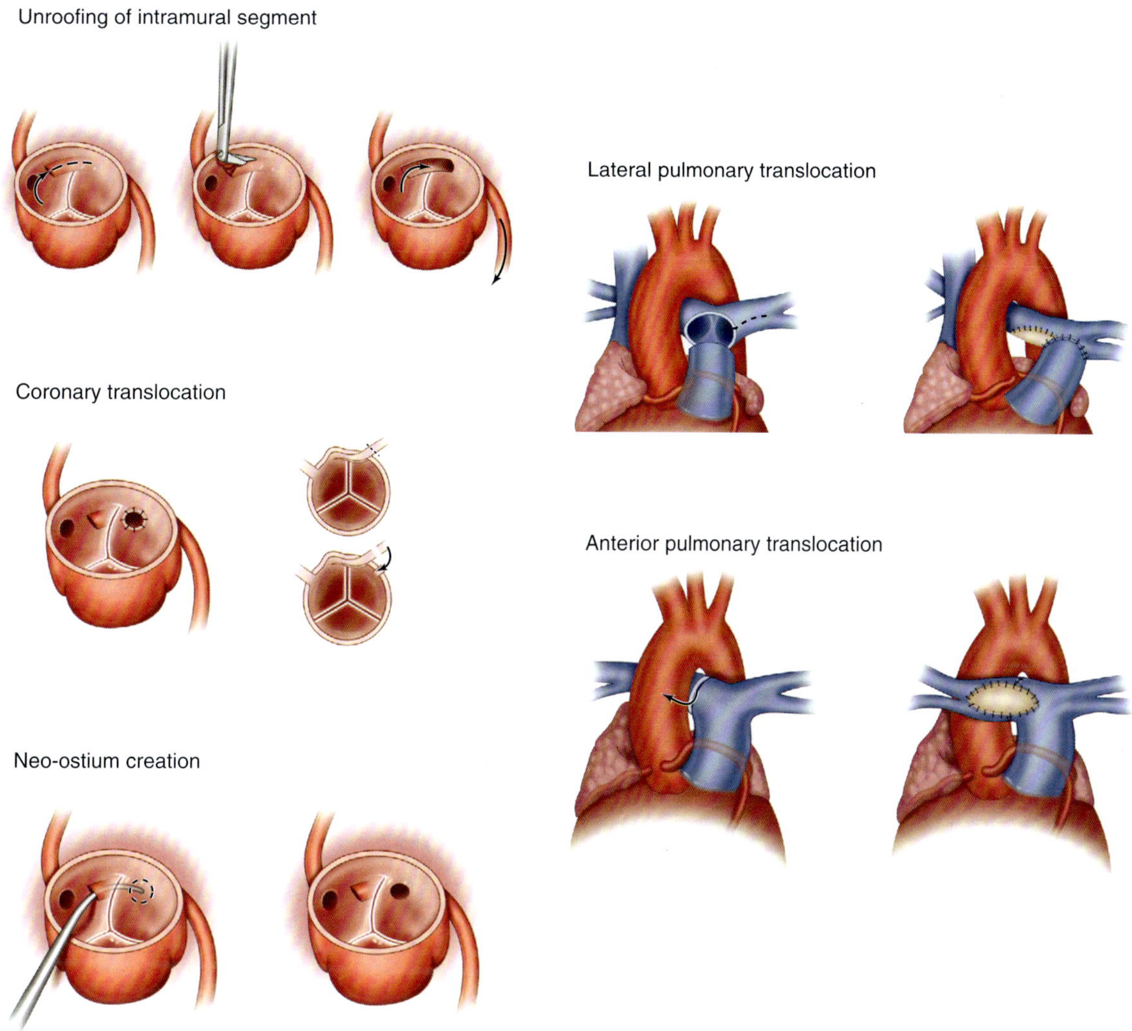

FIGURE 11.30 Surgical techniques currently used for treatment of patients with AAOCA. Adapted from Mery CM, Lawrence SM, Krishnamurthy R, et al. Anomalous aortic origin of a coronary artery: toward a standardized approach. *Semin Thoracic Surg*. 2014;26:110-122.

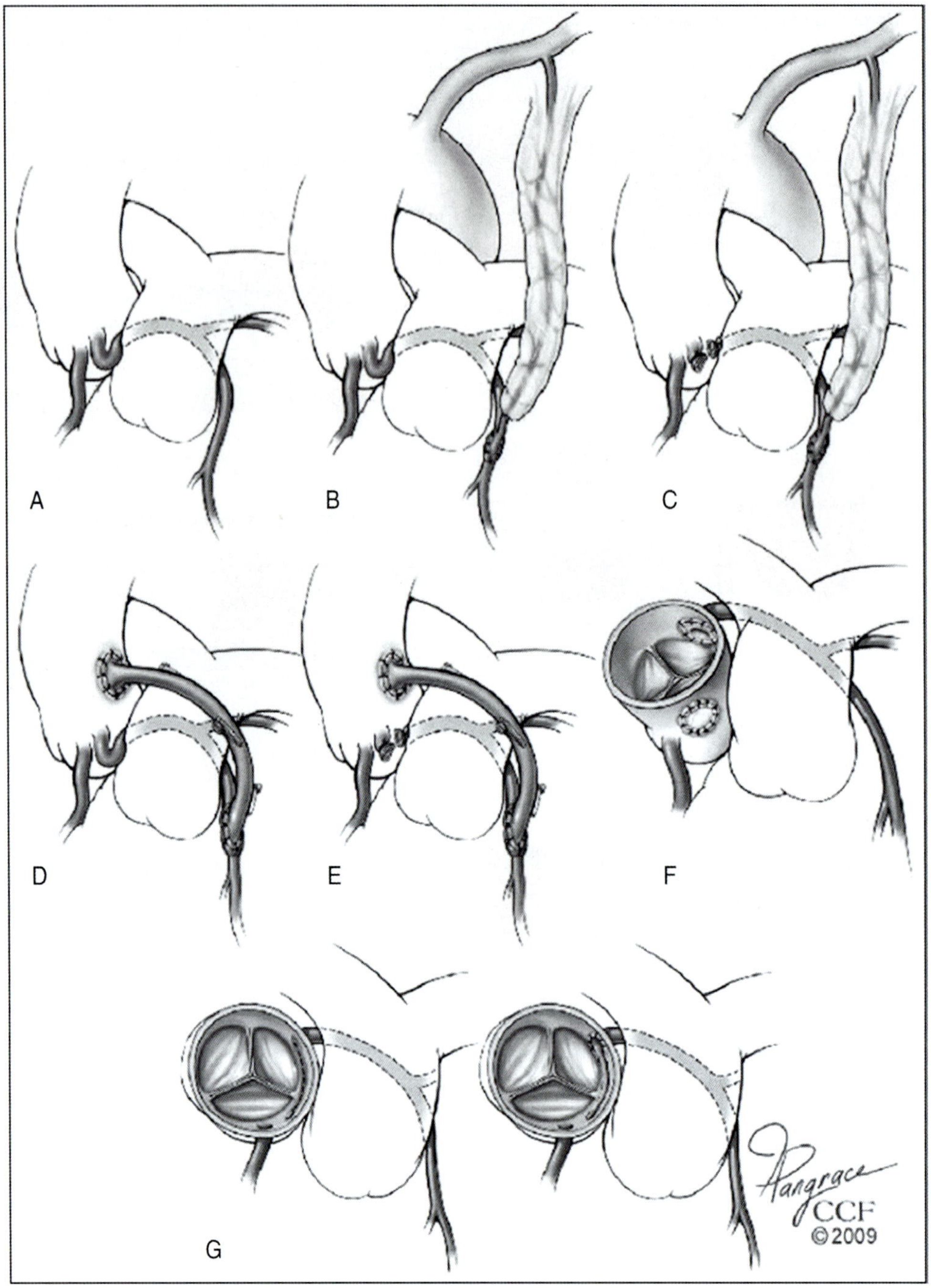

FIGURE 11.31 Additional illustration of a few of the surgical techniques that have been used to correct anomalous coronary arteries; ALCA-R (A) is used for illustrative purposes. These techniques include bypass with an internal thoracic artery (B), bypass with an internal thoracic artery with native vessel ligation (C), bypass with a saphenous vein (D), bypass with a saphenous vein with native vessel ligation (E), reimplantation (F), and coronary unroofing (G). Reproduced with permission from Krasuski RA, Magyar D, Hart S, et al. Long-term outcome and impact of surgery on adults with coronary arteries originating from the opposite coronary cusp. *Circulation*. 2011;123:154-162.

CORONARY FISTULAE

Coronary fistulae are coronary anomalies frequently encountered in the cath lab. They are characterized by abnormal connections between a coronary artery and a systemic vein, the pulmonary artery or a pulmonary vein, a cardiac chamber, and the coronary sinus (**Table 11.3**).[30,33-43] The clinical relevance and management will depend on the amount of blood flow through the fistula, the development of right- or left-sided volume overload, and/or the development of ischemia secondary to a steal phenomenon of blood through the fistulous tract, from a high-pressure system (coronary artery) to a low-resistance system.[30,41,43-46] **FIGURES 11.32-11.38** show examples of coronary fistulae with different hemodynamic significance.

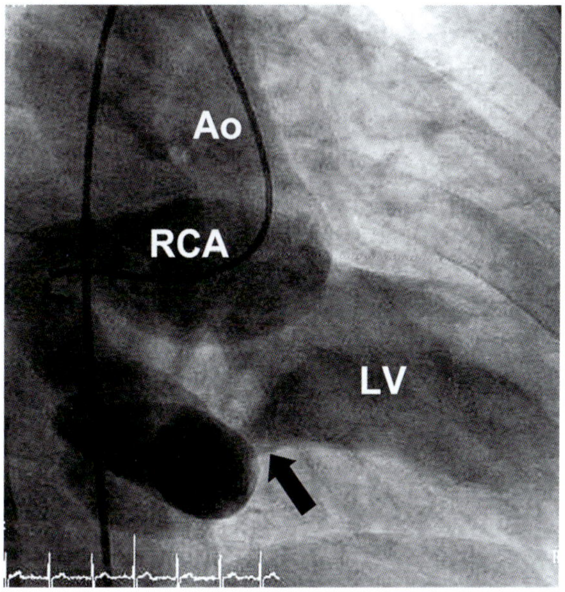

FIGURE 11.32 Selective right coronary angiography showing a huge dilated, tortuous RCA draining into the posterior aspect of the LV through a large fistula (indicated by arrow). Reproduced with permission from Kang SM, Kim JH, Oh J, Shim CY, Choi BW, et al. Giant right coronary aneurysm to left ventricular fistula. *Circ Cardiovasc Imaging*. 2009;2:e15-e16.

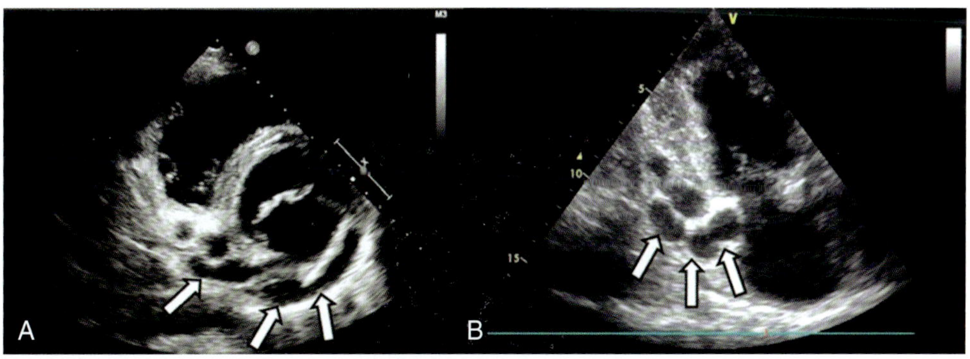

FIGURE 11.33 Giant right coronary artery aneurysm to left ventricular fistula. 58-year-old man admitted with mild dyspnea on exertion and with prior radiographic evidence of cardiac enlargement. Transthoracic echocardiography image of the parasternal short-axis view at the level of the mitral valve (A) shows a complex tubular structure behind the ventricles, which corresponds to the dilated and tortuous right coronary artery (RCA; arrows). The apical 2-chamber view (B) also demonstrates several cross sections of the tortuous RCA (arrows) adjacent to the inferior wall of the left ventricle. Reprinted with permission from Celeng C, Szekely L, Toth A, et al. Multimodality imaging of giant right coronary aneurysm and postsurgical coronary artery inflammation. *Circulation*. 2015;132:e1-e5.

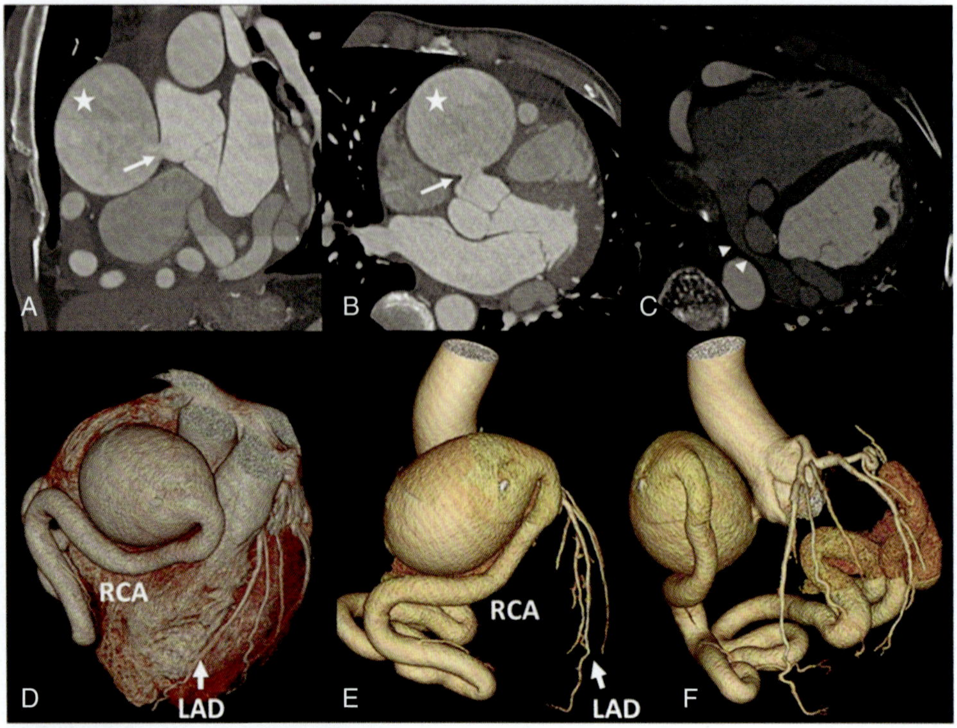

FIGURE 11.34 Maximum-intensity projection images in the coronal (A) and axial (B and C) views obtained from prospective ECG-triggered computed tomography angiography showing dilated ostium (arrows) of the giant aneurysm (asterisk) and its course toward the coronary sinus (arrowheads). Volume-rendered images (D, E, and F) depict the giant right coronary artery (RCA) aneurysm, which originates from the ascending aorta, and its location is anterior to the right atrium, adjacent to the atrioventricular groove. Distal to the aneurysm, the RCA remained enlarged and tortuous. LAD indicates left anterior descending artery. Reproduced with permission from Celeng C, Szekely L, Toth A, et al. Multimodality imaging of giant right coronary aneurysm and postsurgical coronary artery inflammation. *Circulation*. 2015; 132:e1-e5.

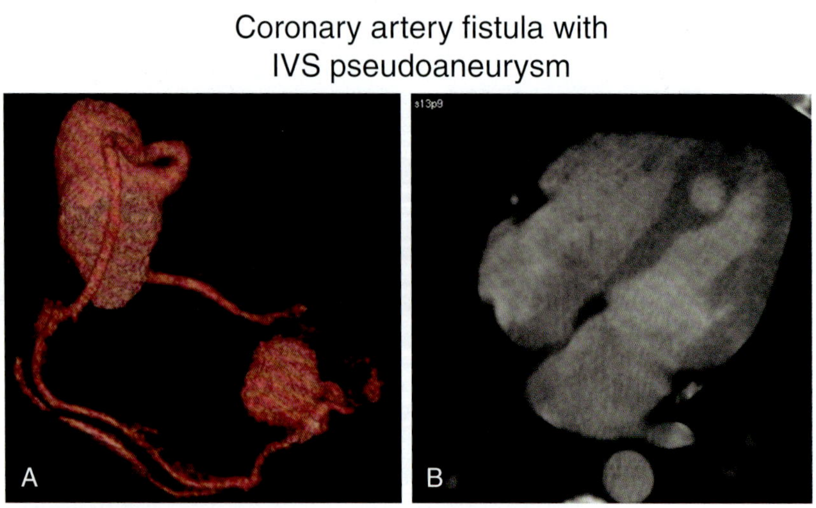

FIGURE 11.35 A 38-year-old man who presented with exertional substernal chest pain. He was evaluated with a nuclear stress test that revealed anterior reversible and septal ischemia. Coronary angiography revealed a right coronary artery to left anterior descending artery fistula. CT angiography confirmed the presence of a right coronary artery to left anterior descending artery fistula through a ventricular septal pseudoaneurysm. IVS, interventricular septum.

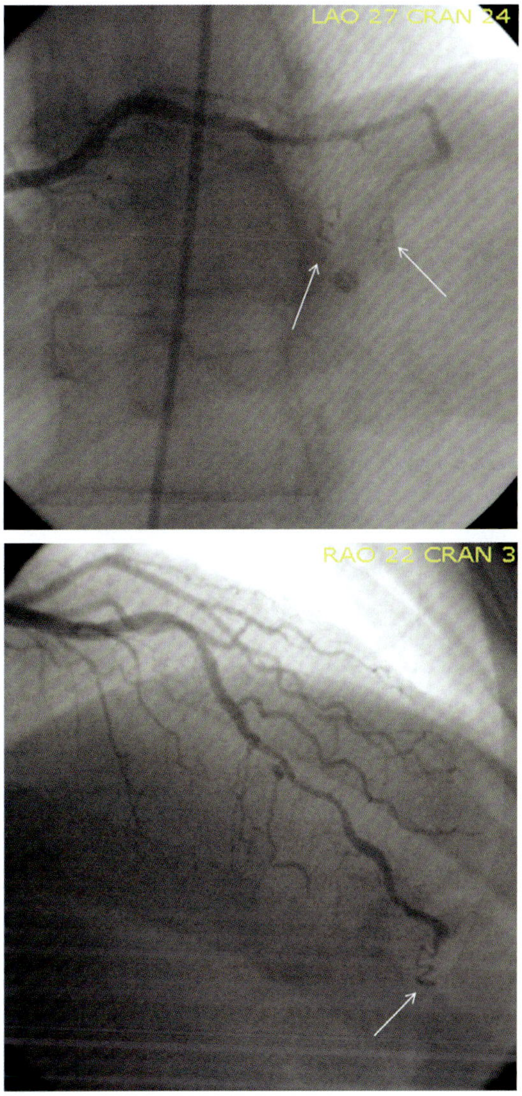

FIGURE 11.36 Coil embolization of the distal left anterior descending artery and of the right coronary artery was performed to exclude the ventricular septal pseudoaneurysm (arrows).

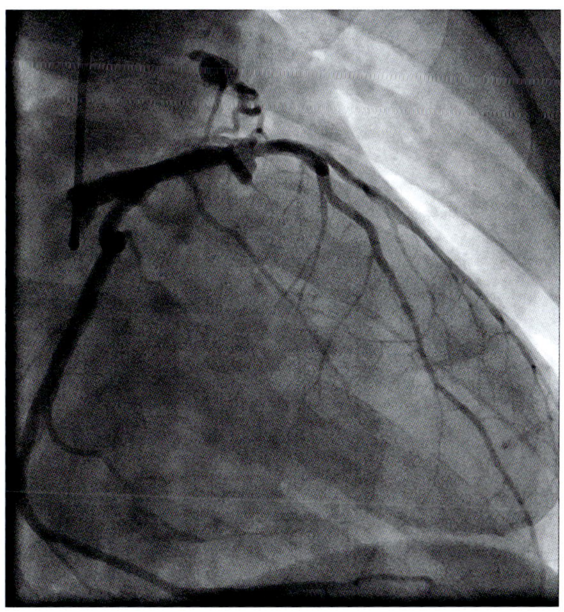

FIGURE 11.37 A 56-year-old man who presented following one episode of diaphoresis and chest discomfort. He was seen by his primary care physician. Electrocardiographic evaluation showed a left bundle branch block. Additional evaluation with a nuclear stress test revealed a fixed septal defect. Therefore he was referred for a diagnostic cardiac catheterization. Coronary angiography revealed an anomalous communication between the left coronary system and the pulmonary artery (PA); a small branch originating in the left main followed by 2 branches originating from the proximal LAD fed an aneurysmatic artery, which drained into the PA.

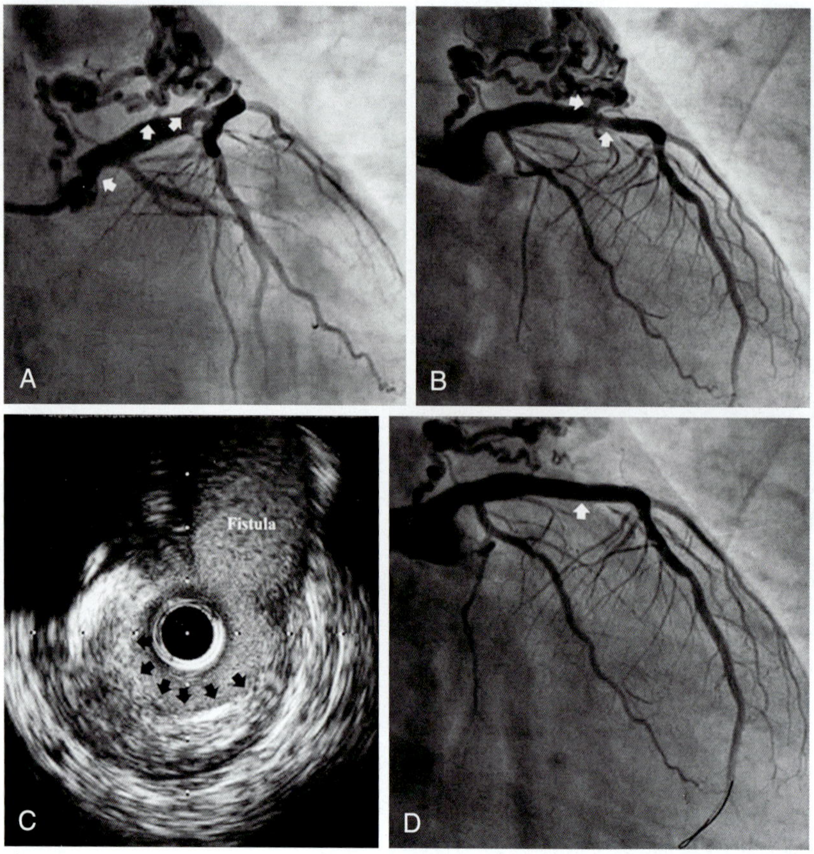

FIGURE 11.38 Covered stent for large coronary arterial fistula and adjacent atherosclerotic plaque with stenosis in a patient with non–ST-segment elevation myocardial infarction. A, Coronary angiography (CAG) of the left coronary artery: 3 coronary arterial fistulae from the left main coronary artery (left white arrow), proximal left anterior descending coronary artery (LAD) (middle white arrow), and mid-LAD (right white arrow) were noted. The largest fistula originated from the mid-LAD. B, CAG of the left coronary artery: the largest coronary fistula (left white arrow) with local haziness (right white haziness) presented at the mid-LAD. C, Intravascular ultrasound study: severe stenosis with extensive atherosclerotic plaque (lower black arrows), and the origins of the coronary fistula originated from here (upper gray shadow). D, Poststented CAG of the left coronary artery: the coronary arterial fistula at the mid-LAD resolved after covered stent deployment (white arrow). Reproduced with permission from Lee WC, Fang HY, Fang CY, et al. Covered stent for large coronary arterial fistula and adjacent atherosclerotic plaque with stenosis in a patient with non–st-segment elevation myocardial infarction. *JACC Cardiovasc Interv*. 2016;9:1512-1513.

REFERENCES

1. Angelini P. Coronary artery anomalies: an entity in search of an identity. *Circulation*. 2007;115(10):1296-1305.
2. Graidis C, Dimitriadis D, Karasavvidis V, et al. Prevalence and characteristics of coronary artery anomalies in an adult population undergoing multidetector-row computed tomography for the evaluation of coronary artery disease. *BMC Cardiovasc Disord*. 2015;15:112.
3. Namgung J, Kim JA. The prevalence of coronary anomalies in a single center of Korea: origination, course, and termination anomalies of aberrant coronary arteries detected by ECG-gated cardiac MDCT. *BMC Cardiovasc Disord*. 2014;14:48.
4. Cheng TO. Prevalence and relevance of coronary artery anomalies. *Cathet Cardiovasc Diagn*. 1997;42(3):276-277.
5. Angelini P. Novel imaging of coronary artery anomalies to assess their prevalence, the causes of clinical symptoms, and the risk of sudden cardiac death. *Circ Cardiovasc Imaging*. 2014;7(4):747-754.
6. Rodriguez-Granillo GA, Rosales MA, Pugliese F, Fernandez-Pereira C, Rodriguez AE. Prevalence and characteristics of major and minor coronary artery anomalies in an adult population assessed by computed tomography coronary angiography. *EuroIntervention*. 2009;4(5):641-647.
7. Erol C, Seker M. Coronary artery anomalies: the prevalence of origination, course, and termination anomalies of coronary arteries detected by 64-detector computed tomography coronary angiography. *J Comput Assist Tomogr*. 2011;35(5):618-624.
8. Park JH, Kwon NH, Kim JH, et al. Prevalence of congenital coronary artery anomalies of Korean men detected by coronary computed tomography. *Korean Circ J*. 2013;43(1):7-12.
9. Safak O, Gursul E, Yesil M, et al. Prevalence of coronary artery anomalies in patients undergoing coronary artery angiography: a review of 16768 patients. A retrospective, single-center study. *Minerva Cardioangiol*. 2015;63(2):113-120.

10. Cademartiri F, Malago R, La Grutta L, et al. Coronary variants and anomalies: methodology of visualisation with 64-slice CT and prevalence in 202 consecutive patients. *Radiol Med.* 2007;112(8):1117-1131.
11. Yorgun H, Hazirolan T, Kaya EB, et al. The prevalence of coronary artery anomalies in patients undergoing multidetector computed tomography for the evaluation of coronary artery disease. *Turk Kardiyol Dernegi Arsivi.* 2010;38(5):341-348.
12. Pillai SB, Khan MM, Diamond A, McKeown PP. The prevalence and types of coronary artery anomalies in Northern Ireland. *Ulster Med J.* 2000;69(1):19-22.
13. Angelini P, Velasco JA, Flamm S. Coronary anomalies: incidence, pathophysiology, and clinical relevance. *Circulation.* 2002;105(20):2449-2454.
14. Davis JA, Cecchin F, Jones TK, Portman MA. Major coronary artery anomalies in a pediatric population: incidence and clinical importance. *J Am Coll Cardiol.* 2001;37(2):593-597.
15. Karabay KO, Yildiz A, Geceer G, Uysal E, Bagirtan B. The incidence of coronary anomalies on routine coronary computed tomography scans. *Cardiovasc J Afr.* 2013;24(9-10):351-354.
16. Ouchi K, Sakuma T, Kawai M, Fukuda K. Incidence and appearances of coronary sinus anomalies in adults on cardiac CT. *Jpn J Radiol.* 2016;34(10):684-690.
17. Krasuski RA, Magyar D, Hart S, et al. Long-term outcome and impact of surgery on adults with coronary arteries originating from the opposite coronary cusp. *Circulation.* 2011;123(2):154-162.
18. Angelini P, Villason S, Chan AV, et al. Normal and anomalous coronary arteries in humans. In: Angelini P, ed. *Coronary Artery Anomalies: A Comprehensive Approach.* Philadelphia: Lippincott Williams & Wilkins; 1999:27-150.
19. Grani C, Benz DC, Schmied C, et al. Prevalence and characteristics of coronary artery anomalies detected by coronary computed tomography angiography in 5 634 consecutive patients in a single centre in Switzerland. *Swiss Med Wkly.* 2016;146:w14294.
20. Basso C, Corrado D, Thiene G. Coronary artery anomalies and sudden death. *Card Electrophysiol Rev.* 2002;6(1-2):107-111.
21. Basso C, Corrado D, Thiene G. Congenital coronary artery anomalies as an important cause of sudden death in the young. *Cardiol Rev.* 2001;9(6):312-317.
22. Cheitlin MD, MacGregor J. Congenital anomalies of coronary arteries: role in the pathogenesis of sudden cardiac death. *Herz.* 2009;34(4):268-279.
23. Gaudio C, Pelliccia F, Evangelista A, et al. Sudden death and physical exercise: timely diagnosis of congenital anomalies of the coronary arteries with the new 320-slide multi-detector computed tomography. *Int Emerg Med.* 2013;8(suppl 1):S35-S39.
24. Basso C, Maron BJ, Corrado D, Thiene G. Clinical profile of congenital coronary artery anomalies with origin from the wrong aortic sinus leading to sudden death in young competitive athletes. *J Am Coll Cardiol.* 2000;35(6):1493-1501.
25. Barriales Villa R, Moris de la Tassa C, Penas Lado M. Sudden death, sports activities and coronary artery anomalies. *Rev Esp Cardiol.* 2002;55(10):1105; author reply 1105-1106.
26. Angelini P. Sudden death and coronary anomalies: the importance of a detailed description. *Tex Heart Inst J.* 2011;38(5):544-546.
27. Angelini P, Uribe C. Anatomic spectrum of left coronary artery anomalies and associated mechanisms of coronary insufficiency. *Cathet Cardiovasc Interv.* July 26, 2018. doi:10.1002/ccd.27656.
28. Angelini P. Coronary artery anomalies–current clinical issues: definitions, classification, incidence, clinical relevance, and treatment guidelines. *Tex Heart Inst J.* 2002;29(4):271-278.
29. Angelini P, Cheong BY, Lenge De Rosen VV, et al. Magnetic resonance imaging-based screening study in a general population of adolescents. *J Am Coll Cardiol.* 2018;71(5):579-580.
30. Angelini P, Monge J. Coronary anomalies. In: Moscucci M, ed. *Grossman & Baim's Cardiac Catheterization Angiography and Intervention.* Philadelphia: Lippincott Williams and Wilkins; 2014:335-353.
31. Grani C, Buechel RR, Kaufmann PA, Kwong RY. Multimodality imaging in individuals with anomalous coronary arteries. *JACC Cardiovasc Imaging.* 2017;10(4):471-481.
32. Mery CM, Lawrence SM, Krishnamurthy R, et al. Anomalous aortic origin of a coronary artery: toward a standardized approach. *Semin Thoracic Surg,* 2014;26:110-122.
33. Kang SM, Kim JH, Oh J, Shim CY, Choi BW. Cardiovascular images. Giant right coronary aneurysm to left ventricular fistula. *Circ Cardiovasc Imaging.* 2009;2(3):e15-e16.
34. Bosher LH Jr, Vasli S, Mc CC, Belter LF. Congenital coronary arteriovenous fistula associated with large patent ductus. *Circulation.* 1959;20(2):254-261.
35. Crawford ES, Turell DJ, Alexander JK. Aorto-inferior vena caval fistula of neoplastic origin. Hemodynamic and coronary blood flow studies. *Circulation.* 1963;27:414-421.
36. DeNofrio D, Barnathan ES, Loh E. Images in cardiovascular medicine. Left anterior descending coronary artery-to-right ventricle fistula. *Circulation.* 1997;96(10):3779.
37. Gensini GG, Palacio A, Buonanno C. Fistula from circumflex coronary artery to superior vena cava. *Circulation.* 1966;33(2):297-301.
38. Gupta V, Truong QA, Okada DR, et al. Images in cardiovascular medicine. Giant left circumflex coronary artery aneurysm with arteriovenous fistula to the coronary sinus. *Circulation.* 2008;118(22):2304-2307.
39. Haller JA Jr, Little JA. Diagnosis and surgical correction of congenital coronary artery-coronary sinus fistula. *Circulation.* 1963;27:939-942.
40. Liberthson RR, Sagar K, Berkoben JP, Weintraub RM, Levine FH. Congenital coronary arteriovenous fistula. Report of 13 patients, review of the literature and delineation of management. *Circulation.* 1979;59(5):849-854.
41. Pascual I, Avanzas P, Hernandez-Vaquero D, et al. Successful percutaneous closure of a well-developed arteriovenous coronary fistula with a giant aneurysm. *Circ Cardiovasc Interv.* 2018;11(7):e006829.
42. Sekarski N, Payot M, Goy JJ. Images in cardiovascular medicine. Giant coronary fistula. *Circulation.* 1998;97(18):1868.
43. Celeng C, Szekely L, Toth A, et al. Multimodality imaging of giant right coronary aneurysm and postsurgical coronary artery inflammation. *Circulation.* 2015;132(1):e1-e5.
44. Lee WC, Sheu JJ, Fang CY. Transcatheter closure of large coronary fistulae via a transradial sheathless approach. *JACC Cardiovasc Interv.* 2016;9(6):e53-e54.
45. Jama A, Barsoum M, Bjarnason H, Holmes DR Jr, Rihal CS. Percutaneous closure of congenital coronary artery fistulae: results and angiographic follow-up. *JACC Cardiovasc Interv.* 2011;4(7):814-821.
46. Armsby LR, Keane JF, Sherwood MC, Forbess JM, Perry SB, Lock JE. Management of coronary artery fistulae. Patient selection and results of transcatheter closure. *J Am Coll Cardiol.* 2002;39(6):1026-1032.

chapter **12**

Pulmonary Angiography

KYUNG J. CHO, MD

INTRODUCTION

The imaging modalities including ventilation-perfusion scan, computed tomography angiography (CTA), and magnetic resonance angiography (MRA) now provide much of the diagnostic information that can be derived from pulmonary angiography with less risk and at lower cost.[1-5] At the same time the number and variety of vascular interventional procedures in the pulmonary vasculature have increased moderately. On balance, the total number of pulmonary angiography performed for the diagnosis of pulmonary embolism (PE) has decreased with the introduction of contrast-enhanced CT, whereas the number of cases for intervention has significantly increased. Pulmonary angiography is generally requested only when pulmonary arterial vascular lesions are suspected or necessary information about the pulmonary arterial vasculature cannot be obtained by CTA or MRA. Pulmonary angiography is performed for the diagnosis of PE, to evaluate the etiology of pulmonary hypertension, to assess the extent and anatomy of the chronic PE before surgical intervention, before pulmonary catheter embolectomy and/or catheter-directed thrombolysis for massive or submissive PE, and for the diagnosis and treatment of pulmonary artery aneurysms and pseudoaneurysms, and arteriovenous malformations. This chapter (atlas) reviews the vascular anatomy as well as the techniques of pulmonary angiography and intervention in the diagnosis and treatment of pulmonary arterial vascular disease.

ANATOMY OF THE PULMONARY ARTERY

The main pulmonary artery arises from the conus of the right ventricle, commencing at the pulmonic valve. It courses 4 to 5 cm posterosuperiorly before dividing into the right and left pulmonary arteries (**FIGURE 12.1**). The right pulmonary artery courses horizontally, passing anterior to the right main stem bronchus and posterior to the ascending aorta and superior vena cava (SVC). The right upper lobe branch arises before reaching the right hilum and divides into the 3 segmental upper lobe arteries (apical, anterior, and posterior segmental). After the takeoff of the upper lobe artery, the pulmonary artery becomes pars interlobaris until the origin of the middle lobe artery (medial and lateral segmental). The artery then divides into 4 basal segmental branches (anterior, medial, lateral, and posterior basal) and superior segmental branch (**FIGURE 12.2**). Left pulmonary artery is a direct posterior continuation of the main pulmonary artery, crossing over the left main stem bronchus and gives rise to 3 segmental branches to the upper lobe and 2 lingular segmental branches (superior and inferior segmental). It then gives rise to 4 lower lobe basal segmental (anterior, medial, lateral, and posterior basal) and superior segmental branch (**FIGURE 12.3**).

Thorough understanding of the segmental anatomy of the lung is important in the performance and interpretation of ventilation and perfusion scan, CTA, and pulmonary angiography for the diagnosis of PE. When performing pulmonary arteriography, oblique views are recommended for optimal visualization of the pulmonary arterial vasculature.

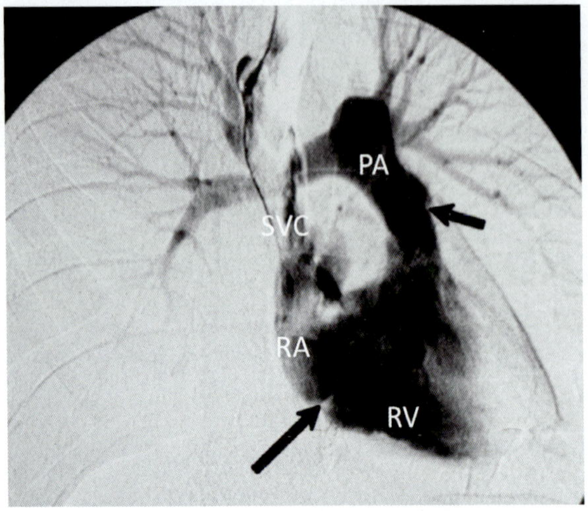

FIGURE 12.1 Intravenous (IV) DSA showing SVC, right atrium (RA), tricuspid valve (longer arrow), right ventricle (RV), pulmonic valve (shorter arrow), pulmonary artery (PA), right and left pulmonary arteries.

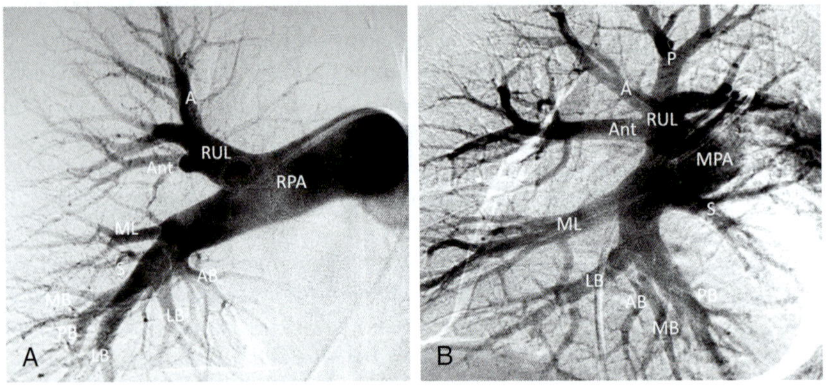

FIGURE 12.2 Right pulmonary arteriogram. A, Right pulmonary DSA (30° RAO). B, Right pulmonary DSA (40° LAO). RPA, right pulmonary artery; RUL, right upper lobe artery; A, apical segmental; P, posterior segmental; Ant, anterior segmental; ML, right middle lobe artery; AB, anterior basal; LB, lateral basal; MB, medial basal; PB, posterior basal, S, superior segmental.

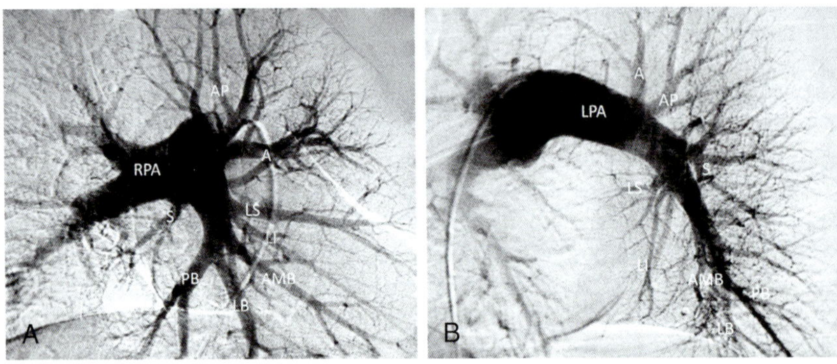

FIGURE 12.3 A, Left pulmonary arteriogram (RAO). B, Left pulmonary arteriogram (LAO). LPA, left pulmonary artery; AP, apical posterior; A, anterior segmental; LS, lingular; LI, lingular inferior; S, superior segmental; PB, posterior basal; LB, lateral basal; AMB, anteromedial basal.

TECHNICAL CONSIDERATIONS

All prior images of the lungs should be reviewed before starting the procedure. Digital subtraction techniques are used in pulmonary angiography.[6] Conventional film-screen imaging techniques are no longer used. Selective and superselective catheterization of the pulmonary artery and the magnification technique are used. Digital subtraction angiography (DSA) is performed using a dilute nonionic contrast medium (240 or 270 mg iodine/mL).

Before the procedure, the operator explains the potential risks and benefits of the procedure and availability of alternative tests to the patient, and obtains a written consent. On the day of the procedure, the patient is allowed to take fluids by mouth, and an intravenous line is placed to hydrate the patient. A mild sedative and an analgesic are given 30 minutes before and during the procedure. During the procedure, electrocardiogram, blood pressure, and oxygen saturation are monitored. Pulmonary angiography can be safely performed as an outpatient procedure. After completion of the procedure, the patient is observed in a radiology recovery room for 2 hours, and ambulation begins. The patient is discharged with an attendant. The attendant is advised to stay with the patient until the following morning and instructed to take certain measures if a complication arises. The patients from the medical intensive care units are usually intubated and attended by the nurse.

Pulmonary Artery Catheterization

Pulmonary angiography is performed using the percutaneous technique. The veins used for pulmonary angiography are the femoral, antecubital or basilic, and internal jugular veins. Of these, the femoral approach is preferable. The puncture site is prepared and draped using the sterile technique and anesthetized with 1% or 2% xylocaine. A small skin incision is made below the inguinal ligament. The common femoral vein is punctured using an 18-gauge double-wall puncture needle, or a 19- or 21-gauge single-wall puncture needle under ultrasound guidance. If ultrasound equipment is not available, the femoral vein is punctured just medial to the femoral artery pulse at the groin crease. When the needle is introduced into the vein, the guide wire is inserted through the needle into the inferior vena cava (IVC), and a diagnostic catheter such as a 5, 6, or 7-Fr pulmonary artery catheter is introduced over the guide wire through a 7 or 8-Fr introducer. The commonly used catheters for pulmonary artery angiography are 7-Fr APC (Cook Medical Inc., Bloomington, IN) and 7-Fr Mont 1 Torcon NB Advantage Catheter (Cook Medical Inc., Bloomington, IN) (**FIGURE 12.4**).

When the catheter is in the right atrium, a right atrial pressure is measured. The pulmonary catheter is passed through the tricuspid valve just above the diaphragm into the right ventricle where it is turned clockwise while advancing it cephalad toward the pulmonary outflow tract (**FIGURE 12.1**). The catheter will likely be passed into the left pulmonary artery, and pulmonary artery pressure is measured. If this maneuver fails, a 0.035-inch Safe-T-J guide wire (Cook Medical Inc., Bloomington, IN) is advanced through the catheter positioned in the right ventricle into the pulmonary artery, and over the wire the catheter is advanced. If the catheter is advanced in the cephalic portion of the right atrium, it may be passed into the left atrium via patent foramen ovale or atrial septal defect, and then into the left pulmonary vein (**FIGURE 12.5**). When the catheter is advanced from the antecubital or jugular vein, the pigtail portion will likely pass through the tricuspid valve and right ventricle into the pulmonary outflow tract. If this maneuver fails, a 0.035-inch Safe-T-J guide wire is advanced through the pulmonary catheter into the pulmonary artery.

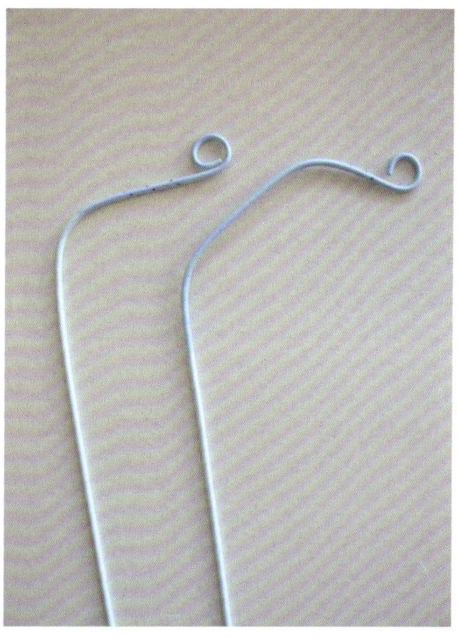

FIGURE 12.4 Two commonly used catheters for pulmonary angiography: 7-Fr APC (left) and 7-Fr MONT 1 (right) (Cook Medical, Bloomington, IN).

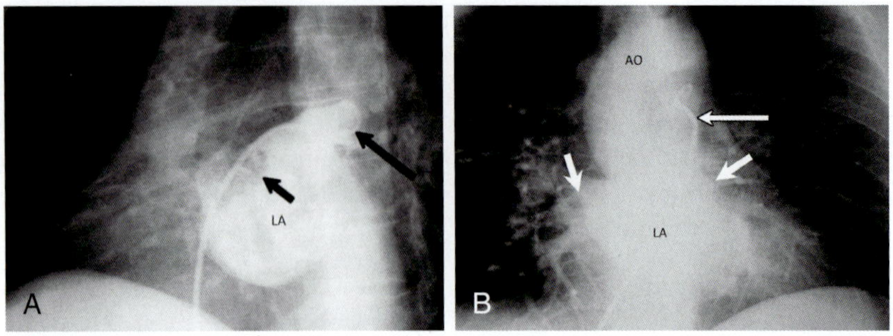

FIGURE 12.5 Inadvertent cannulation of the left pulmonary vein during pulmonary artery catheterization from the right femoral vein. A, The catheter was passed through patent foramen ovale or atrial septal defect into the left atrium, and then into the left pulmonary vein (longer arrow). Contrast medium injection fills the left atrium where flow defect from right pulmonary vein is seen (shorter arrow). B, Pulmonary angiogram (venous phase) shows the catheter in the pulmonary artery (longer arrow), left atrium (LA), pulmonary veins (2 shorter arrows), and the aorta (AO). The pulmonary artery catheter shows a more vertical and superior course than the catheter positioned in the left pulmonary vein of "A."

The presence of a properly placed IVC filter does not necessarily preclude a transfemoral approach. A straight or J-tipped guide wire is passed through the filter and over the wire the catheter is advanced through the filter into the pulmonary artery. A long sheath is placed across the filter to prevent filter dislodgment during pulmonary artery catheterization and intervention.

When congenital anomaly of the IVC or SVC is present, the catheterization of the pulmonary artery can be difficult, and an alternative route should be used. When the guide wire does not pass through the expected course of the IVC or SVC, contrast medium is injected to identify the anomaly such as IVC interruption with azygos continuation (**FIGURE 12.6**). For selective pulmonary artery catheterization, an alternative route such as antecubital or jugular vein access is used. Understanding of the anomalous venous anatomy of the thorax is also important in pulmonary artery catheterization. When both the IVC and SVC is not available owing to its occlusion, percutaneous transhepatic hepatic venous access is used for pulmonary artery catheterization, angiography, and intervention.

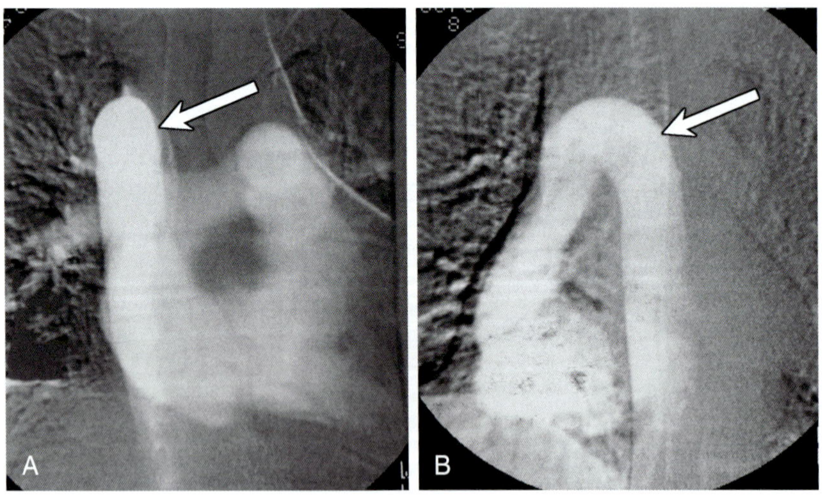

FIGURE 12.6 IVC interruption with azygos continuation in a 52-year-old woman with suspected PE. A, Contrast medium injection in the azygos vein (AP) shows the azygos vein (arrow) opening into the SVC. Right atrium, right ventricle, and pulmonary arteries are visualized. B, Contrast injection in the azygos vein (LAO). The dilated azygos vein (arrow) enters the posterior aspect of SVC.

Injection Factors and Imaging Methods

Pulmonary DSA begins with the injection into the pulmonary artery on the side of perfusion defect on ventilation/perfusion scan or CTA. When the catheter is positioned in the pulmonary artery, 5 cc of contrast medium is injected into the pulmonary artery under fluoroscopic control to estimate the blood flow of the artery being injected. If pulmonary artery pressure is normal, contrast medium should be injected at a rate that approximates as closely as possible the rate of

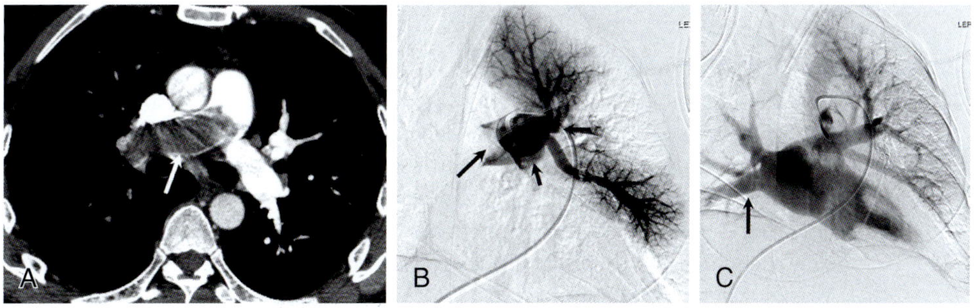

FIGURE 12.7 Massive PE in a patient with severe dyspnea and hypotension. He was treated with systemic tPA infusion and vasopressors. A, CTA showing a large occlusive embolus in right pulmonary artery (arrow). B, Left pulmonary DSA (10 cc/s × 2) showing complete occlusion of right pulmonary artery (arrow) and multiple central embolic occlusion of left pulmonary arteries (shorter arrows) with large perfusion defects. C, The venous phase of the left pulmonary arteriogram showing retrograde filling of the right pulmonary veins (arrow) because of right pulmonary artery occlusion. The patient developed cardiac arrest following pulmonary angiography.

blood flow in the artery being opacified. In general, the injection rate for a normal pulmonary artery is 25 cc per second for 2 seconds for a total contrast volume of 50 cc. In the patient with pulmonary hypertension (pulmonary artery pressure of >50 mmHg) and decreased pulmonary artery blood flow, the injection rate is decreased to 15 cc/s for 2 to 3 seconds for a total volume of 30 to 45 cc. Imaging is acquired with the frame rate of 6 exposures per second using the magnification technique while the patient's breath is held in deep inspiration. The following oblique projections are used: 30° RAO and 40° LAO for right pulmonary arteriography; 40° LAO and 50° RAO for left pulmonary arteriography (**FIGURES 12.2** and **12.3**). Superselective angiography with the magnification technique is used for the evaluation of segmental and subsegmental arteries and pulmonary vascular abnormalities including pulmonary artery aneurysms, pseudoaneurysms, and pulmonary arteriovenous malformations (PAVMs).

DSA has become the standard imaging technique for pulmonary angiography and it has replaced cut film angiography.[6] The technical ability to record radiographic images digitally has allowed image manipulation and various display on monitors. Respiratory motion is a significant problem in pulmonary DSA. Motion between the baseline images (mask image) and the contrast image markedly degrades the digital information obtained. If the patient cannot hold his or her breath in full inspiration, additional mask images (precontrast images) are obtained to choose a suitable mask to reduce motion artifacts. Remasking, pixel shifting, and nonsubtraction image display help correct for misregistration, and thus improve the image quality.

Risks and Contraindications

The major complication of pulmonary angiography was reported in the Prospective Investigation of Pulmonary Embolism Diagnosis (PIOPED), which reported the value of ventilation/perfusion scans in acute PE.[7] The complications include death (0.5%) and major nonfatal complications (1%), renal failure requiring dialysis (0.3%) and hematoma requiring transfusion (0.2%). The risks of pulmonary DSA are generally low and allow its performance for outpatients. There are no absolute contraindications to pulmonary angiography. The risk of complications increases with severe pulmonary hypertension, allergy to iodinated contrast medium, renal insufficiency, left bundle branch block, severe congestive heart failure, or massive PE (**FIGURE 12.7**).

INDICATIONS

Pulmonary angiography is performed for (1) diagnosis of PE, (2) evaluation of chronic PE before operative intervention, (3) specific diagnosis of pulmonary vascular lesions, such as aneurysms, pseudoaneurysms, arteriovenous malformations, anomalous pulmonary venous return, and meandering pulmonary vein, (4) assessment of pulmonary vascular involvement by neoplasm, and (5) evaluation of the cause for hemoptysis.

Pulmonary Embolism

If CT, ventilation-perfusion scan, or ultrasound is equivocal or negative for PE despite high clinical suspicion for PE, pulmonary angiography is requested. The standard technique for pulmonary angiography is used for the diagnosis of PE. Once the femoral vein has been accessed, contrast medium is injected into the iliac vein to confirm patency of the iliac vein and IVC. If thrombosis is present, iliac venography is performed. When the catheter has been passed into the pulmonary artery, pressure is measured. Then a test injection with contrast medium is made under fluoroscopy to estimate pulmonary arterial blood flow. If pulmonary artery pressure is elevated, the injection rate should be decreased to 10 to 15 cc per second for 2 to 3 seconds. If endovascular intervention is contemplated for the treatment of submassive or massive PE, bilateral pulmonary angiography is performed in the anteroposterior projection.

The angiographic findings of acute PE are partially occlusive filling defect with the trailing edge of contrast medium between the clot and vessel wall (**FIGURE 12.8**). When PE causes complete arterial obstruction, it shows concave filling defect at the border of the contrast column (**FIGURE 12.9**). Magnification oblique pulmonary angiography is performed to demonstrate segmental embolism masked by the overlying arteries (**FIGURE 12.10**). Subsegmental and peripheral emboli usually appear as multiple small filling defects at the arterial bifurcation or occlusions. The secondary signs for acute PE include oligemic or avascular regions, local prolonged filling of

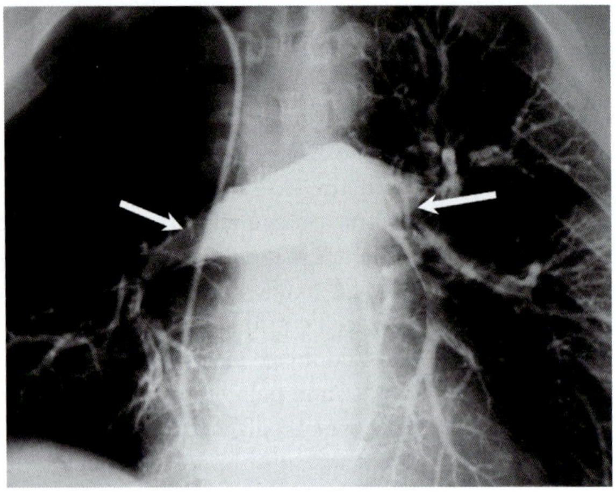

FIGURE 12.8 Bilateral central pulmonary emboli. Pulmonary arteriogram showing bilateral pulmonary emboli extending to the lobar and segmental branches bilaterally (arrows).

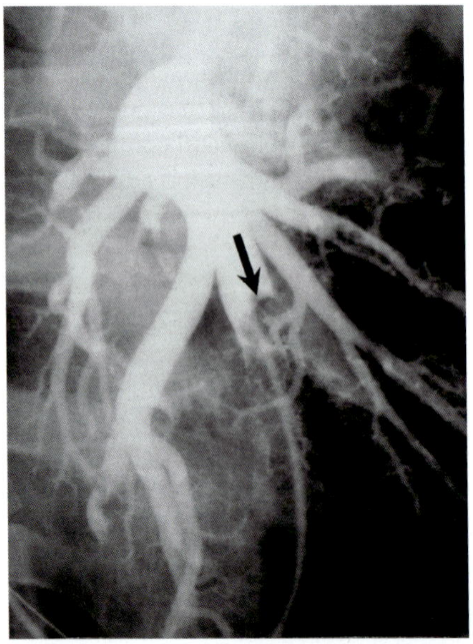

FIGURE 12.9 Acute PE in a 58-year-old woman. Left pulmonary angiogram (RAO) shows occlusion of the left medial basal segmental artery with the concave border of the contrast column (arrow). Small peripheral emboli are present in the inferior lingular and posterior basal segmental branches.

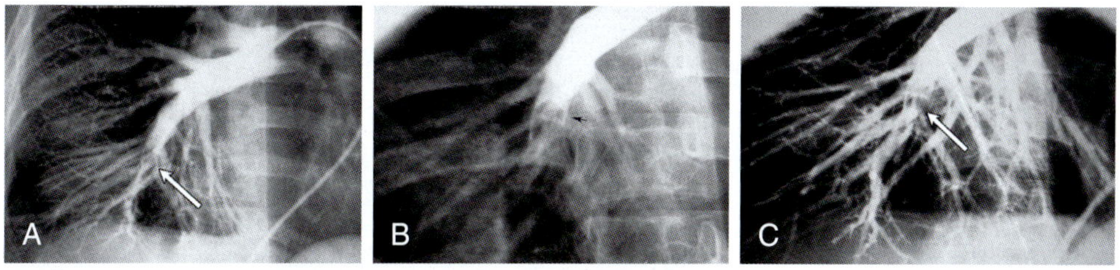

FIGURE 12.10 Segmental PE. A, Right pulmonary arteriogram (RAO) showing possible filling defect in a right lower lobe branch (arrow). B, Selective magnification arteriogram (early arterial phase) showing filling defect with concave border of the contrast column (arrows). C, Late arterial phase also shows the filling defect (arrow).

vessels, and abrupt tapering of the peripheral vessels. These findings alone should be interpreted as PE with caution because the similar findings can be seen in other pulmonary pathologies such as emphysema, pulmonary fibrosis, and even chronic PE. Additional oblique angiograms should be obtained in search of intraluminal filling defect for the diagnosis of PE.

The major problem in the angiographic differential diagnosis of acute PE is chronic PE with complete vessel occlusion, irregular intraluminal filling defects, and arterial wall irregularity. Complete occlusion of the artery caused by chronic PE shows a convex border of the contrast column. Peripheral arterial occlusion of vessel size less than 1 mm in diameter should be interpreted as PE with caution because peripheral arterial occlusion may be seen in primary pulmonary hypertension. Other problems that can mimic PE are pulmonary artery tumors, invasion or compression of the pulmonary artery by bronchogenic carcinoma, mediastinal lymphoma, or sarcoidosis. Contrast-enhanced CT and PET can help differentiate between PE and tumors because the latter usually enhance with contrast medium and positive on PET scan.

The treatment for PE includes supportive measure and prevention of recurrent PE with anticoagulants and caval interruption. Patients with massive PE may present with syncope, systemic arterial hypotension, cardiogenic shock, and cardiac arrest. In patients with submassive PE, right ventricular diameter to left ventricular diameter is usually greater than 0.9 on CT scan.

The percutaneous techniques are used to recanalyze thromboembolic occlusions in patients with life-threatening massive or submissive PE.[8] The goals of this therapy are to rapidly reduce pulmonary arterial pressure, right ventricular strain, and pulmonary vascular resistance and thus to increase arterial perfusion. The techniques include systemic thrombolytic therapy, catheter-directed thrombolysis, thrombofragmentation, and surgical thrombectomy. Because of an increased risk of bleeding from systemic thrombolysis, ultrasound-accelerated catheter-directed thrombolysis is increasingly used. The ultrasound-accelerated thrombolysis using the EkoSonic Endovascular System has been found to be safe and effective and is clinically superior to anticoagulation with survival improvement (FIGURE 12.11).[9-11] The devices that have been used for thrombofragmentation for the treatment of massive PE include the pigtail rotation catheter (Cook Europe, Denmark), the Helix Clot Buster (eV3, Plymouth, MN), AngioJet (Boston Scientific Corp. Natick, MA), and Aspirex catheter (Straub Medical, Wangs, Switzerland).

Chronic Pulmonary Embolism

Most chronic thromboembolic pulmonary hypertension (CTEPH) results from unresolved pulmonary emboli. Embolic volume, location, or repetitive embolic episodes usually lead to incomplete resolution, and the development of pulmonary hypertension. The most common complaints are dyspnea with exertion and fatigue, but in advanced disease, peripheral edema, chest tightness, and syncope may develop owing to low cardiac output.

The diagnostic workup in patients with suspected CTEPH includes pulmonary function tests, transthoracic echocardiogram to screen for pulmonary hypertension, and heart catheterization. The imaging evaluation usually includes chest radiograph, V/Q scan, CTA, MRA, and pulmonary angiography.[12,13]

Pulmonary angiography is generally requested only when necessary information about pulmonary arteries cannot be obtained by CTA or MRA, or when a pulmonary thromboendarterectomy

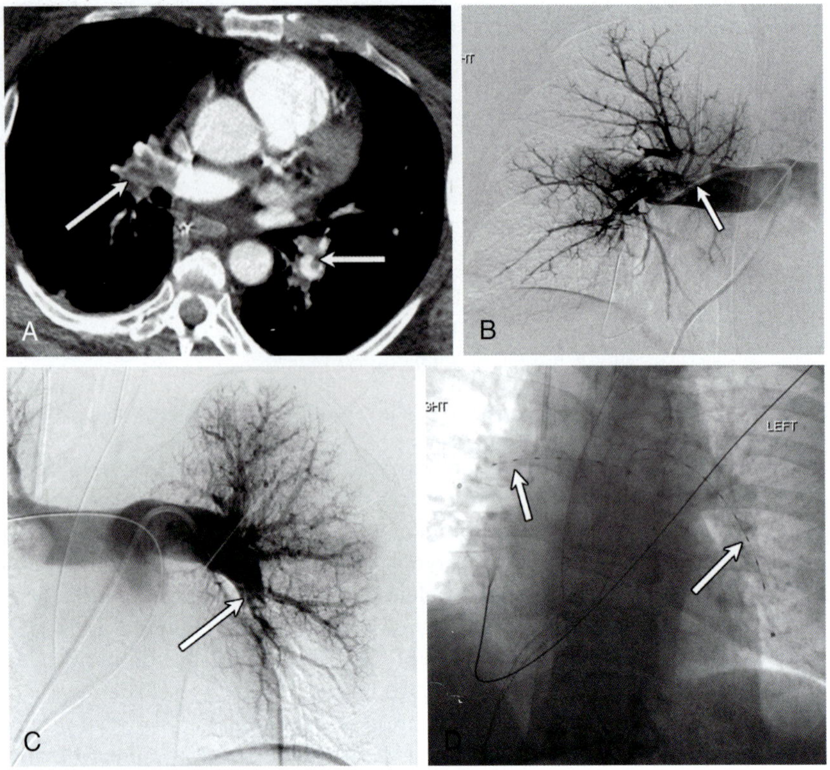

FIGURE 12.11 Massive PE and PEA arrest in a 58-year-old woman. A, CT scan of the chest showing PE of the right main pulmonary and left lobar artery (arrows). B, Right pulmonary DSA showing a large saddle embolus in the right main pulmonary artery with poor lung perfusion (arrow). C, Left pulmonary DSA showing an embolus in the left lower lobe artery (arrow). D, EkoSonic infusion catheters placed in the right and left pulmonary artery (arrows), respectively (EkoSonic Endovascular System, EKOS Corporation, South Bothell, WA). After a bolus infusion of 2 mg tPA in the pulmonary artery, 1 mg tPA/h was infused via each infusion catheter for 14 hours. The patient fully recovered and was discharged on Coumadin.

is contemplated. The technique of pulmonary angiography for CTEPH is similar to that used for the diagnosis of acute PE, but the injection rate must be tailored to the patient with pulmonary hypertension to avoid sudden volume overload to the right heart. A test injection helps assess the speed of blood flow in the artery to be injected. Attention must be paid to the total volume of the injection for the dilated pulmonary arteries. For example, the standard injection rate in the normal pulmonary artery is 25 cc per second for a total volume of 50 cc of nonionic contrast medium at the exposure rate of 6 frames per second. In the patient with CTEPH, the injection rate is reduced to 10 to 15 cc/s for 2 to 3 seconds at the exposure rate of 3 to 4 frames per second.

The primary angiographic abnormality of CTEPH is complete occlusion of the artery, mural irregularity, webs, bands, synechiae, vessel tapering, and focal stenosis (**FIGURES 12.12** and **12.13**).

Treatment of severe CTEPH include anticoagulation, IVC filter placement, repeated balloon angioplasty of the proximal pulmonary artery stenosis, pulmonary thromboembolectomy, and lung transplantation.

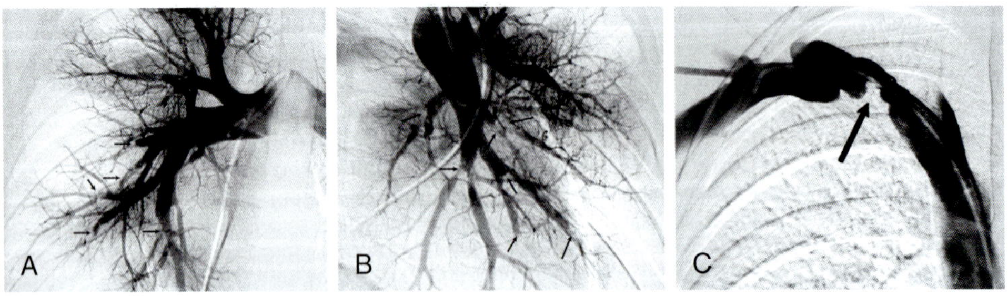

FIGURE 12.12 Chronic recurrent PE in a 17-year-old man with a history of syncopal event while walking. SaO_2 on room air was 80%. CT of the chest showed bilateral pulmonary emboli. A, Right pulmonary DSA (LAO) showing multiple segmental and peripheral arterial stenosis and occlusions (arrows). There are multiple perfusion defects in the middle and lower lobes. B, Left pulmonary DSA (RAO) showing multiple segmental and subsegmental stenosis and occlusions (arrows), and decreased lung perfusion. C, Right subclavian venogram showing partially occlusive thrombosis (arrow), representing the source of PE.

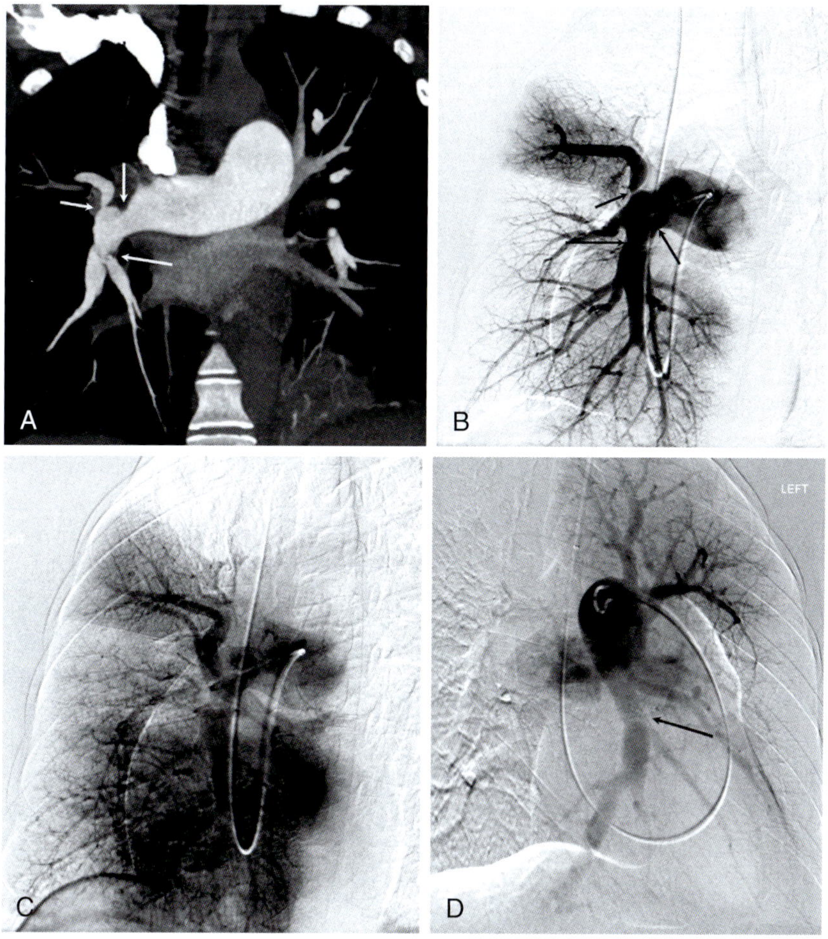

FIGURE 12.13 Chronic thromboembolic pulmonary hypertension (CTEPH) in a 35-year-old woman with a history of multiple DVT and PEs, renal vein thrombosis, heparin-induced thrombocytopenia, and pulmonary hypertension. A, CT (coronal image reconstruction) shows narrowing of the right distal pulmonary artery, the origin of the upper lobe, and descending pulmonary arteries (arrows). B, Right pulmonary arteriogram shows the arterial narrowings (arrows) similar to those of CT. C, The parenchymal phase showing multiple areas of perfusion defect. D, Mild narrowing is seen along the left descending pulmonary artery (arrow). Pulmonary artery pressure = 111/28 mm Hg (mean, 59 mm Hg). The patient underwent a pulmonary thromboendarterectomy.

Primary Pulmonary Hypertension

Primary pulmonary hypertension is a rare disease of unknown etiology characterized by peripheral arterial and capillary stenosis or occlusions. Clinically, the patient presents with shortness of breath or fatigue. The diagnosis is made by excluding diseases such as congenital or acquired pulmonary, cardiac, or collagen vascular disease. Chest radiography is obtained to rule out interstitial or alveolar disease. Echocardiography is performed to document the presence of pulmonary hypertension and evaluate right and left ventricular function. Chest CT is the initial imaging study that can help exclude secondary forms of pulmonary hypertension and lung disease.[14] V/Q scan can rule out PE as the cause of pulmonary hypertension.[15] Right heart catheterization plays an important role in establishing the diagnosis of pulmonary hypertension. Pulmonary venous hypertension can be excluded by demonstration of a normal pulmonary artery wedge pressure.

Pulmonary angiography is generally requested to exclude chronic PE as the cause of pulmonary hypertension. The angiographic technique is similar to that of pulmonary angiography performed for CTEPH. Magnification angiography with selective injection of contrast medium is of value in defining more clearly subtle peripheral arterial abnormalities. The angiographic findings include dilatation of central pulmonary arteries, tortuous segmental and subsegmental arteries, and smooth tapering of the peripheral arteries. The abnormalities are usually bilateral, uniform, and symmetric (**FIGURE 12.14**).

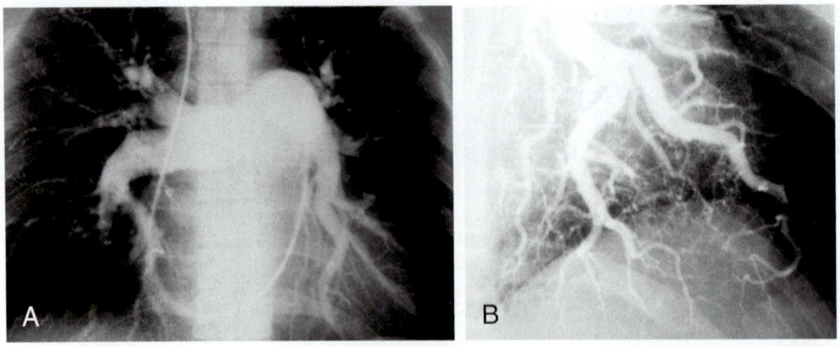

FIGURE 12.14 Primary pulmonary hypertension in a 41-year-old man. A, Pulmonary arteriogram from right antecubital approach showing bilateral central pulmonary artery dilatation and tortuosity with tapering and pruning of the peripheral arteries. B, Magnification left lower lobe pulmonary arteriogram showing tortuous segmental and diminutive peripheral branches with sluggish blood flow and poor capillary filling.

Pulmonary Arteriovenous Malformations

PAVMs are uncommon and represent congenital communication between the pulmonary artery and vein. They are often found as incidental lesions on chest radiograph or computed tomography; however, they may be a source of chest pain, hemoptysis, dyspnea, and paradoxical embolism with stroke or brain abscess. These lesions usually occur in patients with hereditary hemorrhagic telangiectasia (Osler-Weber-Rendu syndrome). The clinical presentations include epistaxis, dyspnea, hemoptysis, polycythemia, gastrointestinal bleeding, superficial telangiectasia, clubbing, cyanosis, and murmur. Pulmonary arteriovenous fistulas and shunting rarely occurs in trauma, malignancy, hepatopulmonary syndrome, and cardiac surgery.

The imaging evaluation of patients suspected of having PAVMS includes chest X-ray, thin-cut CTA or MRA of the chest, radionuclide perfusion scan, and contrast-enhanced echocardiography. MRA is preferable in young patients, pregnant women, and patients with renal failure or a neurologic deficit.

PAVMs present as one of the following types: (1) simple single feeding artery and draining vein, (2) multiple AVMs, (3) complex, large AVM, and (4) capillary malformations. The simple type has a single dilated feeding artery and a draining vein with an intervening aneurysmal sac (**FIGURE 12.15**). PAVMS are often multiple involving both lungs when associated with hereditary hemorrhagic telangiectasia (**FIGURE 12.16**). Complex malformations have multiple subsegmental feeding arteries and a draining vein (**FIGURE 12.17**). The diffuse form of the malformation is rare and characterized by numerous vascular lesions without identifiable feeding arteries and draining veins. Increased vascularity is seen throughout the lesions (**FIGURE 12.18**).

Because of the risk of central nervous system complications, all lesions with the feeding arteries of greater than 3 mm in diameter are treated. Before embolization pulmonary angiography should cover the entire left and right lungs. The study may be focused on the specific area with selective catheterization and contrast injection if prior CTA or MRA has identified and localized the lesion. Transcatheter embolization is the preferred treatment.[16,17] When the malformation and feeding artery have been identified on the angiogram, a 5-Fr catheter with a curved tip is advanced through a 6-Fr or 7-Fr sheath over a 0.035-inch guide wire as selectively as possible into the feeding artery distal to the last normal branch. The feeding artery is then occluded with detachable balloons, coils, or Amplatzer Vascular Plug (AVP) I, II, or IV. The AVP 1V is delivered through a 5-Fr diagnostic catheter with the inner diameter of 0.038 inch. Both coils and AVPs should be 30% to 50% larger than the diameter of the feeding artery being embolized. Postembolization angiogram is obtained to demonstrate complete occlusion of the feeding artery.

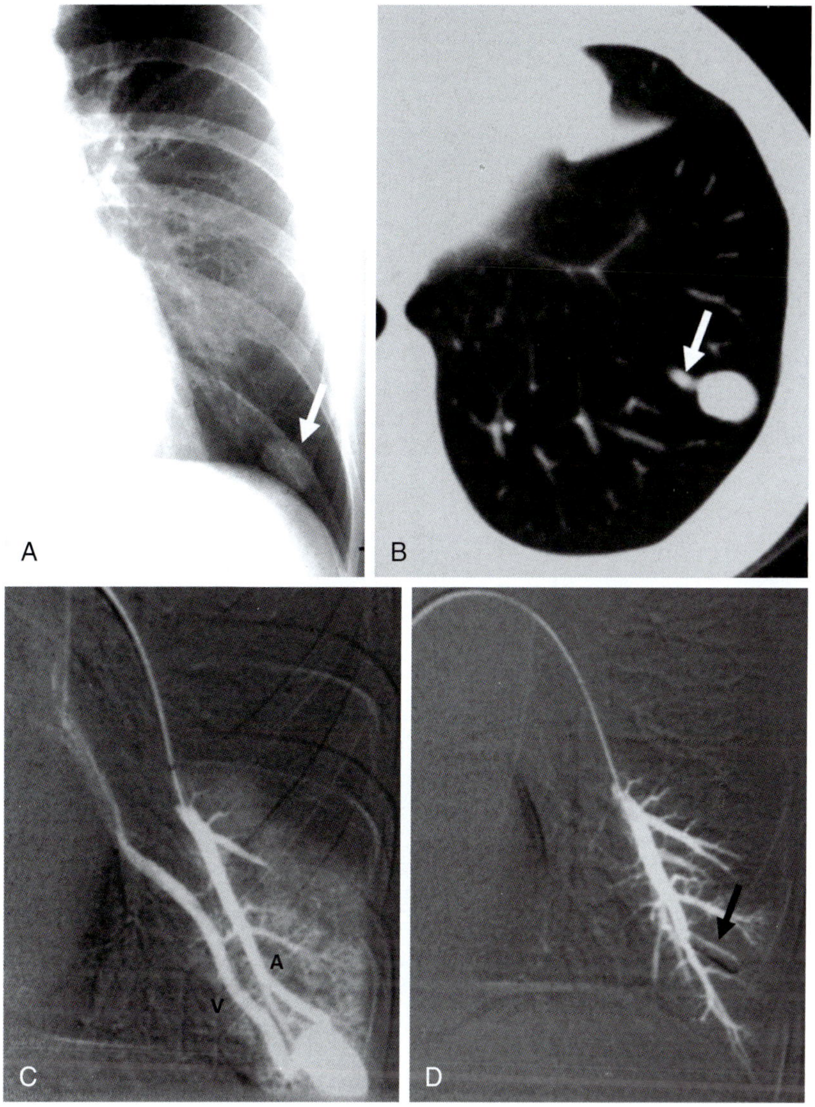

FIGURE 12.15 Pulmonary AVM in a 32-year-old asymptomatic man. A, Chest radiograph showing a left lower lobe nodule (arrow). B, CT scan of the chest showing an aneurysm with a feeding vessel (arrow). C, Selective pulmonary arteriogram showing an aneurysmal sac with the feeding artery (A) and draining vein (V). D, After embolization of the AVM with a detachable balloon (arrow), the feeding artery is completely occluded without filling of the AVM.

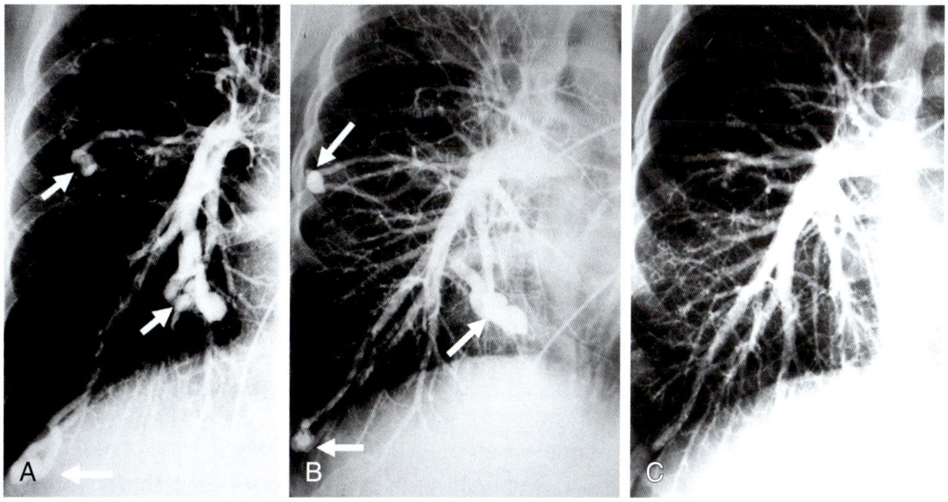

FIGURE 12.16 Pulmonary AVM in a 31-year-old woman with Osler-Weber-Rendu syndrome. A, Right pulmonary angiogram (LAO) showing multiple AVMs in the right lung (arrows). B, Arteriogram (RAO) showing AVMs in the anterior segmental of the upper lobe, the medial basal and lateral basal segmental arteries (arrows). C, After embolization with detachable balloons, all the feeding arteries are occluded. There is no longer filling of the AVMs. Her symptom has abated following the embolization.

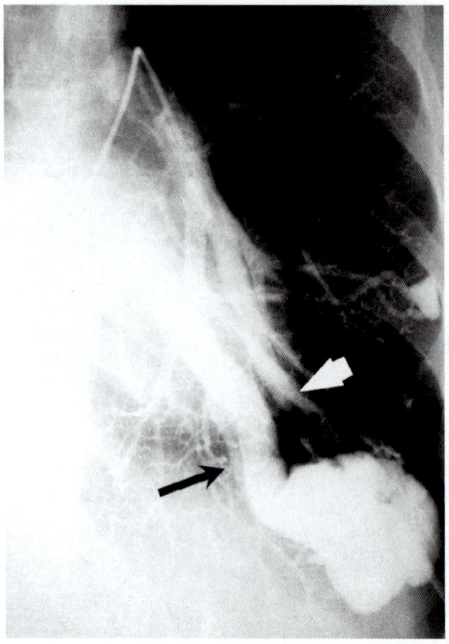

FIGURE 12.17 Left lower lobe complex AVM in a 23-year-old pregnant woman with a history of stroke. Her SaO_2 was 82% on room air. Left pulmonary arteriogram shows a large complex AVM with a dilated feeding artery (shorter arrow) and a dilated draining vein (longer arrow). A smaller AVM is seen in the lingular segment. The AVMs were embolized with detachable balloon and coils (not shown).

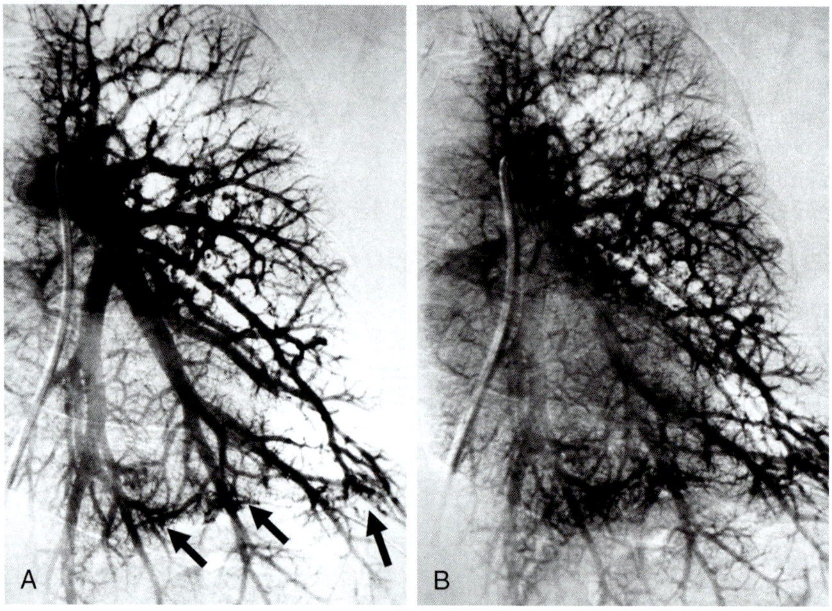

FIGURE 12.18 Pulmonary AVM (capillary type) in a 48-year-old woman with hereditary hemorrhagic telangiectasia. Her SaO_2 was 79% on room air. The shunt volume was estimated to be 35% of the cardiac output on a perfusion lung scan. A, Left pulmonary DSA (RAO) showing multiple capillary malformations (arrows). B, Late arterial phase. Increased vascularity is seen throughout the lesions. She had exertional tolerance and was breathing comfortably. She had undergone evaluation for the possibility of lung transplantation.

Pulmonary Artery Aneurysms and Pseudoaneurysms

Pulmonary artery aneurysms may be found when they rupture, causing massive hemoptysis. They may involve the central, segmental, or peripheral arteries, depending on the etiology. Most aneurysms secondary to pulmonary hypertension or following surgical correction of congenital heart disease occur at the central vessel. Degenerative pulmonary aneurysms can be seen in Marfan syndrome. Rasmussen aneurysms associated with pulmonary tuberculosis usually affect peripheral pulmonary arteries. In Behcet syndrome, pulmonary artery aneurysms may be seen in the central and/or peripheral arteries. The causes of pulmonary artery pseudoaneurysms include (1) injury by Swan-Ganz catheter placement (**FIGURE 12.19**), (2) decelerating injury, (3) penetrating injury, (4) metastatic angiosarcoma, (5) pulmonary artery catheterization, (6) infection (tuberculosis, aspergillomas, and septic emboli), and (7) necrotizing pneumonia (**FIGURE 12.20**).[18,19]

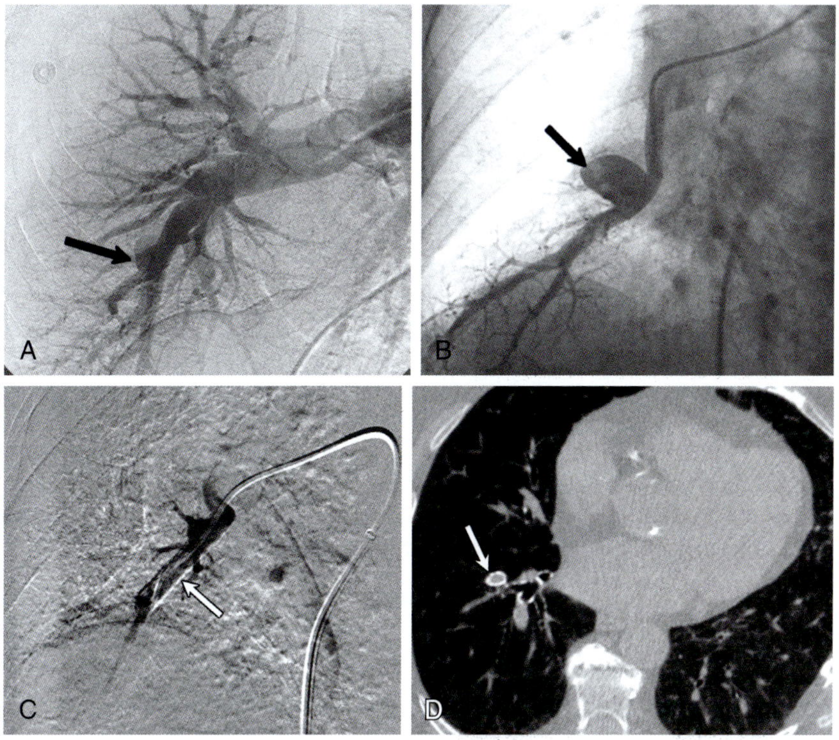

FIGURE 12.19 Right pulmonary artery pseudoaneurysm in a patient who presented with hemoptysis during right heart catheterization. A, Right pulmonary DSA (RAO) showing a 2-cm in diameter pseudoaneurysm of the posterior basal segmental artery (arrow). B, Selective catheterization showing the pseudoaneurysm (arrow). C, After placement of an 6 × 38 mm covered stent (iCAST, Atrium Medical Corp. Hudson, NH) and postdilation to 7 mm, the pseudoaneurysm has been excluded (arrow). D, CT scan showing patent stent (arrow). Hemoptysis has ceased after stent placement.

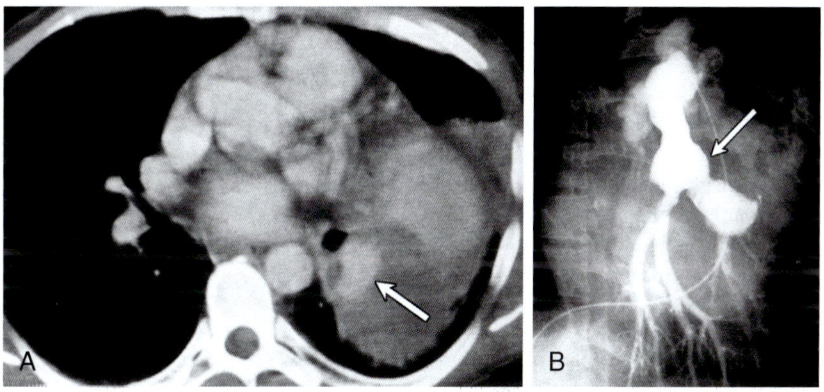

FIGURE 12.20 Mycotic pulmonary artery aneurysms in a 30-year-old man with renal failure and invasive mucormycosis of left lung. A, CT scan of the chest showing a large soft tissue density in the left lower lung with an aneurysm (arrow). B, Left pulmonary arteriogram showing multiple aneurysms of the left pulmonary artery and its branches (arrow). The patient underwent a left-sided pneumonectomy.

Spiral chest CT or MRA can visualize pulmonary artery aneurysms and pseudoaneurysms, and also demonstrate other abnormalities such as lung neoplasm, bronchiectasis, abscess, and acute or chronic inflammatory lung disease. Percutaneous transcatheter therapy is an appealing method for the treatment of pulmonary aneurysms and pseudoaneurysms because it precludes thoracotomy. Most peripheral aneurysms or pseudoaneurysms can be occluded by embolization with coils and AVPs. Medium or large vessel aneurysms are treated with covered stents (iCAST, Advanta V12, Atrium Med. Corp, Hudson, NH).

Pulmonary Artery Stenosis

Pulmonary artery stenosis may involve the main pulmonary artery, the right or left pulmonary artery branches, depending on the underlying disease. If the stenosis is hemodynamically significant, right ventricular and pulmonary artery pressures are elevated. Pulmonary artery stenosis may clinically mimic PE. The causes of pulmonary artery stenosis include (1) congenital with or without other congenital heart disease, (2) surgical procedures used to correct cardiac defects, (3) rubella syndrome, (4) Williams syndrome, (5) central bronchogenic carcinoma, (6) mediastinal lymphoma (**FIGURE 12.21**), (7) pulmonary sarcoidosis, (8) fibrous mediastinitis, (9) vasculitis (Takayasu disease), and (10) chronic PE.[20,21] Rarely systemic-pulmonary artery communication mimics pulmonary artery stenosis or occlusion (**FIGURE 12.22**).

Meandering Pulmonary Vein

Meandering pulmonary vein is a rare congenital venous anomaly in which the pulmonary vein take a tortuous course through the lung before entering the left atrium. Both CTA and MRA of the chest can delineate the meandering course of this anomalous vein.[22] Pulmonary angiography can be definitive in diagnosing the meandering pulmonary vein (**FIGURE 12.23**).

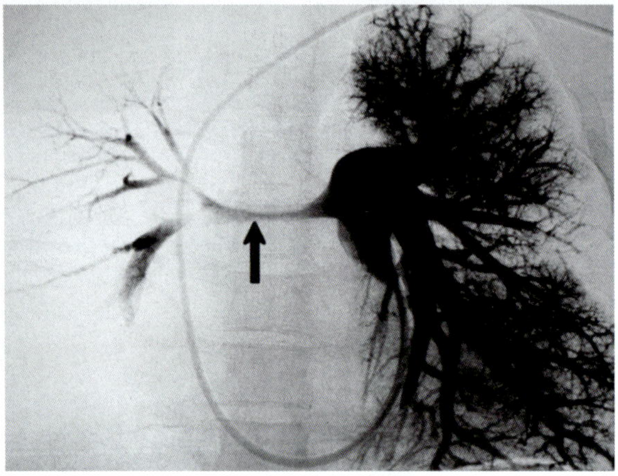

FIGURE 12.21 Pulmonary artery constriction by mediastinal lymphoma in a 32-year-old man with suspected PE. Radionuclide scans showed no perfusion to the right lung. Pulmonary arteriogram from the left antecubital approach showing severe encasement of the right pulmonary artery (arrow) extending to the lobar branches.

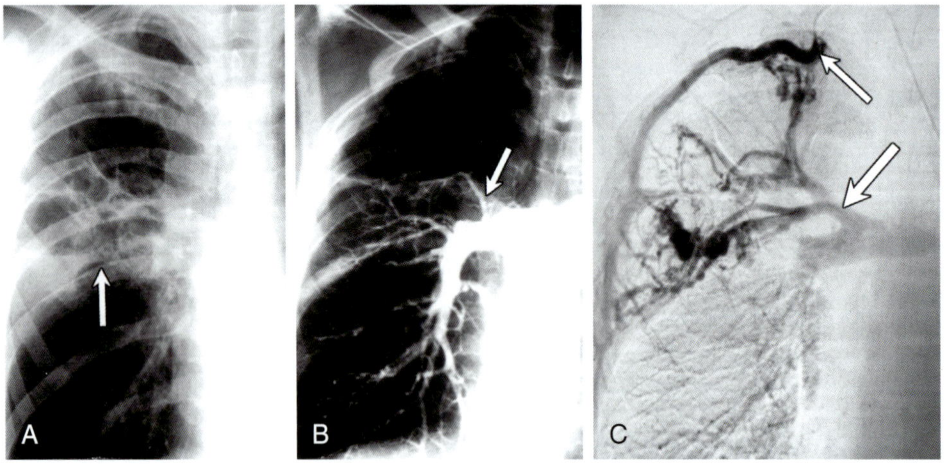

FIGURE 12.22 Pseudoocclusion of right upper pulmonary artery in a 17-year-old asymptomatic man with congenital cystic adenomatoid malformation of right upper lobe. A, Right chest radiograph showing multiple cystic lesions replacing the entire right upper lobe (arrow). B, Right pulmonary arteriogram showing no filling of the upper lobe artery (arrow). C, Right internal mammary arteriogram (shorter arrow). The upper lobe arteries (longer arrow) fill via the transpleural collateral from the lateral thoracic branch of the internal mammary artery.

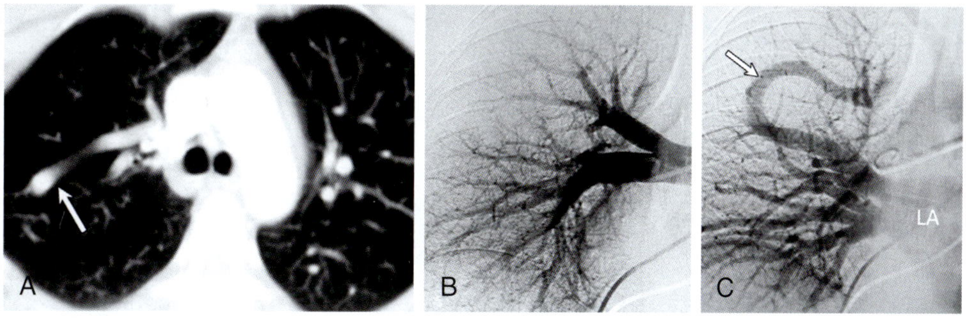

FIGURE 12.23 Meandering right upper lobe pulmonary vein to the left atrium in a 28-year-old woman with a history of respiratory infection and persistent cough. A, Enhanced CT scan of the chest showing a dilated pulmonary vein (arrow) from the right upper lobe. B, Arterial phase of right pulmonary DSA showing a normal right pulmonary arteriogram. C, During the venous phase, the right upper lobe vein shows a meandering course (arrow) before draining into the left atrium (LA).

Partial Anomalous Pulmonary Venous Connection

Partial anomalous pulmonary venous connection (PAPVC) is a rare developmental malformation in which one or more of the pulmonary veins are connected to the right atrium or one of its tributaries such as the innominate vein, SVC or IVC, or coronary sinus. This condition generally involves a part of one lung (segment, lobar, or entire lung). Partial anomalous pulmonary venous return results in a left-to-right shunt but is usually asymptomatic if the shunt involves a pulmonary segment or lobe. The pulmonary veins and anomalous venous return can be visualized following the injection of contrast medium in the pulmonary artery (**FIGURE 12.24**).

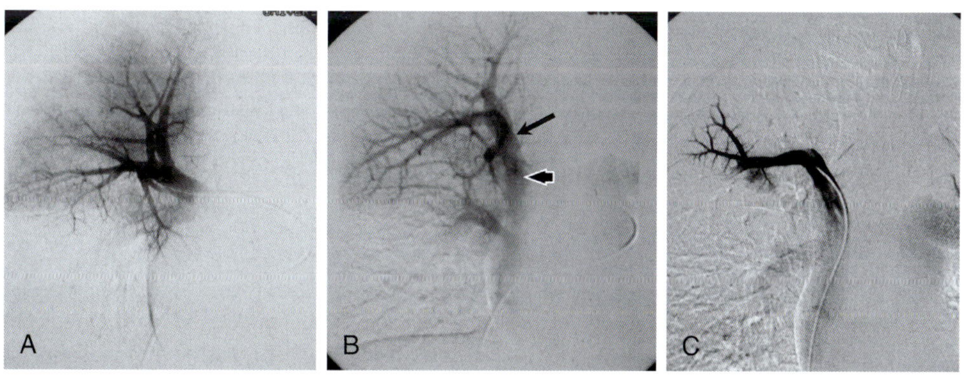

FIGURE 12.24 PAPVC in a patient with suspected PE. A, Right upper pulmonary artery injection showing no evidence of PE. B, During the venous phase, the right upper pulmonary vein (arrow) drains into the SVC (arrowhead). C, After catheterization of the right upper pulmonary vein from the femoral vein, contrast medium injection confirms the anomalous pulmonary venous return to the SVC.

Retrieval of Pulmonary Artery Foreign Body

The pulmonary arterial system is the final destination for fractured and embolized devices placed in the venous system. Foreign bodies that have been found in the pulmonary circulation include catheter fragments, Swan-Ganz catheter, dilator and sheath fragments, guide wire fragments, pacemaker leads or fragments, migrated vena cava filters, migrated intravascular coils, angioplasty balloon fragments, vascular stents, intravascular biopsy devices or fragments, fragments of artificial heart valve, and bullet fragments.

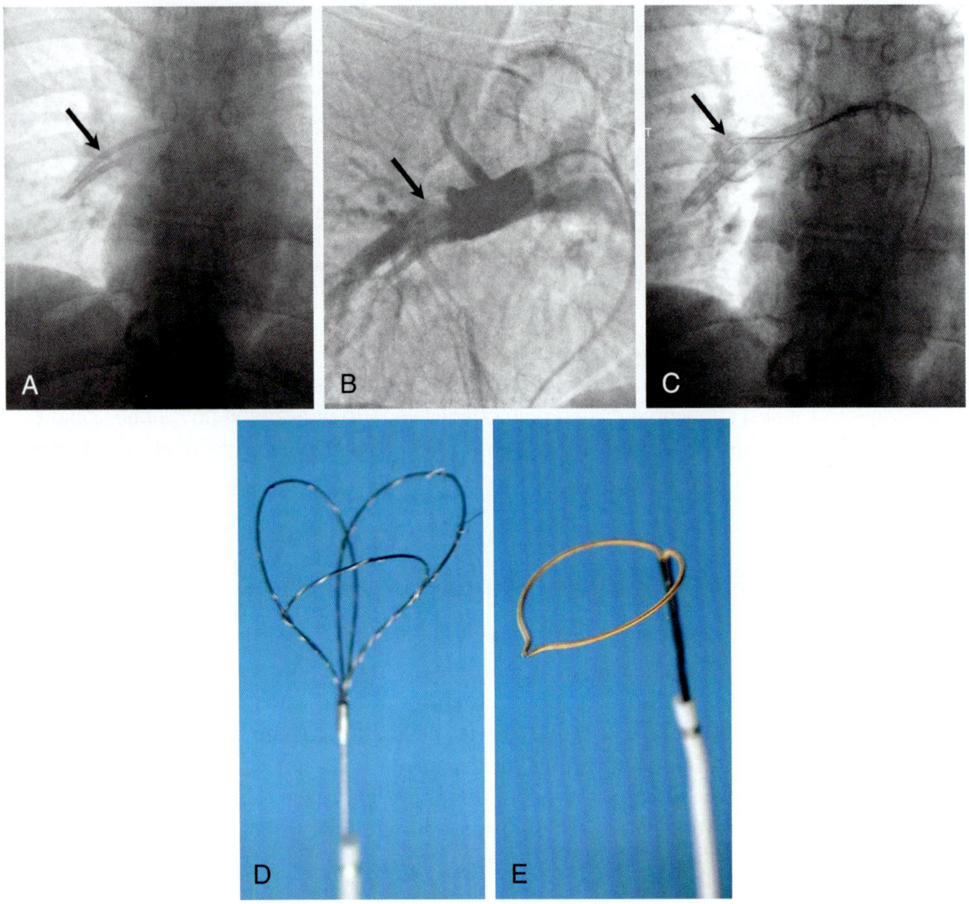

FIGURE 12.25 Retrieval of a retained catheter fragment incidentally found in right pulmonary artery in a 66-year-old woman. She has a history of left chest port for chemotherapy for breast cancer 3 years ago. A, Digital image of the chest showing a catheter fragment in the right pulmonary artery (arrow). B, Right pulmonary DSA (RAO) showing chronic thrombus around the catheter (arrow). C, The catheter fragment was snared by EN Snare (25 mm in diameter) and removed. D and E, Photograph of the EN Snare (MeritMedical, South Jordan, UT) and Amplatz GooseNeck Snare (ev3 Endovascular, Inc., Covidien, Plymouth, MN).

Percutaneous retrieval devices have simplified retrieval of foreign body from the pulmonary artery (**FIGURE 12.25**). The retrieval devices include Amplatz Gooseneck Snare (ev3, Plymouth, MN), EN Snare (MeritMedical, South Jordan, UT), basket and grasping forceps.

The retrieval technique involves (1) percutaneous catheterization of right common femoral vein and insertion of a 12 to 14-Fr sheath (75 cm long), (2) catheterization of the pulmonary artery using the APC catheter, (3) pulmonary angiography (RAO and LAO) to determine the size and orientation of the vessel containing the foreign body, (4) selective catheterization of the affected artery and arteriography, (5) advance the sheath over the guide wire, (6) snare the central end of the foreign body, (7) removal of the foreign body, and (8) completion pulmonary angiography.

REFERENCES

1. Stein PD, Fowler SE, Goodman LR, et al. Contrast enhanced multidetector spiral CT of the chest and lower extremities in suspected acute pulmonary embolism: results of the Prospective Investigation of Pulmonary Embolism Diagnosis II (PIOPED II). *N Engl J Med*. 2006;354:2317-2327.
2. Sostman HD, Stein PD, Gottschalk A, et al. Acute pulmonary embolism: sensitivity and specificity of ventilation-perfusion Scintigraphy in PIOPED II Study. *Radiology*. 2008;246:941-946.
3. Schoepf UJ, Costello P. CT angiography for diagnosis of pulmonary embolism: state of the art. *Radiology*. 2004;230:329-337.

4. Yazdani M, Lau CT, Lempel JK, et al. Historical evolution of imaging techniques for the evaluation of pulmonary embolism. *Radiographics*. 2015;35:1245-1262.
5. Kalb B, Sharma P, Tigges S, et al. MR imaging of pulmonary embolism: diagnostic accuracy of contrast-enhanced 3D MR pulmonary angiography, contrast-enhanced low–flip angle 3D GRE, and non-enhanced free-induction FISP sequences. *Radiology*. 2012;263:271-278.
6. Beek EJV, Bakker AJ, Reekers JA. Pulmonary embolism: interobserver agreement in the interpretation of conventional angiographic and DSA images in patients with nondiagnostic lung scan results. *Radiology*. 1996;198:721-724.
7. Stein PD, Athansoulis C, Alavi A, et al. Complications and validity of pulmonary angiography in acute pulmonary embolism. *Circulation*. 1992;85:462-468.
8. Kuo WT. Endovascular therapy for acute pulmonary embolism. *J Vasc Intervent Radiol*. 2011;23:167-179.
9. Kennedy R, Kenny HH, Dunfee BL. Thrombus resolution and hemodynamic recovery using ultrasound-accelerated thrombolysis in acute pulmonary embolism. *J Vasc Intervent Radiol*. 2013;24:841-848.
10. Kucher N, Boekstegers P, Muller OJ, et al. Randomized, controlled trial of ultrasound-assisted catheter-directed thrombolysis for acute intermediate-risk pulmonary embolism. *Circulation*. 2014;129(4):479-486.
11. Engelberger RP, Kucher N. Ultrasound-assisted thrombolysis for acute pulmonary embolism: a systematic review. *Eur Heart J*. 2014;35(12):758-764.
12. Castañer E, Gallardo X, Ballesteros E. CT diagnosis of chronic pulmonary thromboembolism. *Radiographics*. 2009;29:31-50.
13. Lang MI, Madani M. Update on chronic thromboembolic pulmonary hypertension. *Circulation*. 2014;130:508-518.
14. Mortani Barbosa EJ Jr, Gupta NK, Torigian DA, et al. Current role of imaging in the diagnosis and management of pulmonary hypertension. *AJR (Am J Roentgenol)*. 2012;198:1320-1331.
15. Lisbona R, Kreisman H, Novales-Diaz J, et al. Perfusion lung scanning: differentiation of primary from thromboembolic pulmonary hypertension. *AJR (Am J Roentgenol)*. 1985;144:27-30.
16. Meek ME, Meek JC, Beheshti MV. Management of pulmonary arteriovenous malformations. *Semin Intervent Radiol*. 2011;28(1):24-31.
17. Kucukay F, Ozdemir M, Senol E, Okten S, Ereren M. Large pulmonary arteriovenous malformations: long-term results of embolization with AMPLATZER vascular plugs. *J Vasc Intervent Radiol*. 2014;25:1327-1332.
18. Elsie N, Isabella SS, Jean MS, et al. Pulmonary artery aneurysms and pseudoaneuryms in adults: findings at CT and radiography. *AJR (Am J Roentgenol)*. 2007;188:W126-W134.
19. Laurie AL, James CA, Isaac RF. Multiple mycotic pulmonary artery aneurysms: complication of invasive mucormycosis. *AJR (Am J Roentgenol)*. 1992;158:761-762.
20. Shields JJ, Cho KJ, Geisinger KR. Pulmonary artery constriction by mediastinal lymphoma simulating pulmonary embolism. *AJR Am J Roentgenol*. 1980;135:147-150.
21. Damuth TE, Bower JS, Cho KJ, Dantzker DR. Major pulmonary artery stenosis causing pulmonary hypertension in sarcoidosis. *Chest*. 1980;78:888-891.
22. Tortoriello TA, Vick GW, Chung T, et al. Meandering right pulmonary vein to the left atrium and inferior vena cava: the first case with associated anomalies. *Tex Heart Inst*. 2002;29:319-323.

chapter **13**

Angiography of the Aorta and Peripheral Arteries

HECTOR TAMEZ, MD, THOMAS M. TU, MD, RUBY LO, MD, and
DUANE S. PINTO, MD, MPH

INTRODUCTION

The aorta and peripheral arteries are of significant importance to the interventional cardiologist. The angiographic appearance of a number of clinical entities including aneurysmal disease, dissection, and occlusive disease is important to know. Moreover, knowledge of important complications of vascular access procedures and intervention as well as anatomic variants that may complicate catheter-based procedures is important to recognize. This chapter focuses on the aorta and major branches as well as several disease processes that are relevant to the interventional cardiologist.

ASCENDING AORTA

The aorta can be divided into the ascending, transverse, descending, and abdominal segments (**FIGURE 13.1A**; Video 13.1). The ascending aorta arises after the aortic valve, and its first branches are the coronary arteries. The brachiocephalic artery, also known as innominate artery, arises from the ascending aorta and gives rise to the right subclavian artery and the right carotid artery. Most commonly, the left carotid artery is the next branch arising from the transverse aorta followed by the left subclavian artery. Typically, the vertebral arteries arise as the first branches of the subclavian arteries (**FIGURE 13.1**).

Commonly, the left carotid artery can arise from the innominate artery (**FIGURE 13.2**). This variation is often called a "bovine arch", an inaccurate term. A true bovine arch has a single brachiocephalic origin that gives rise to a right subclavian, a bicarotid vessel that gives rise to the right and left carotid arteries and a left subclavian branch. The next most common aortic variant occurs when the left vertebral artery arises directly from the aorta (**FIGURE 13.3**).

When an aberrant right subclavian artery variant is present, the brachiocephalic trunk is absent. The right common carotid artery, the left common carotid artery, and the left subclavian artery arise from the aorta followed by the right subclavian artery, which arises from the aorta at the proximal descending aorta (**FIGURE 13.3**). Also called the arteria lusoria, it crosses the middle line of the body while traveling to the right arm and usually passes behind the esophagus. If the artery compresses the esophagus, it may produce a condition called dysphagia lusoria. Frequently, it arises from an aortic arch diverticulum at the proximal descending aorta, first described by Kommerell. This anomaly can make catheterization via the right radial approach challenging.

Acute aortic ascending arch dissection may be identified during cardiac catheterization for patients with suspected myocardial infarction or cardiac tamponade (**FIGURE 13.4A**; Video 13.2). The intimal flap is visible as well as a dilated ascending arch with contrast filling both the true and false lumens. Moderate aneurysmal dilation of the ascending aorta is seen with magnetic resonance angiography in **FIGURE 13.4B**. Pseudocoarctation may be present if the aorta is

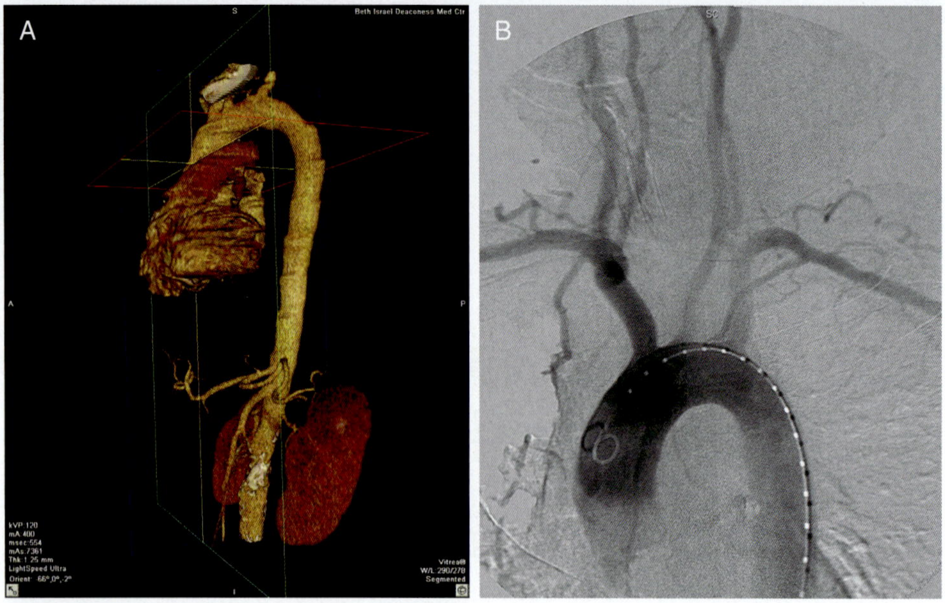

FIGURE 13.1 **A and B**, Aortography and CT angiography with 3D reconstruction illustrating the ascending, transverse, descending, and abdominal segments of the aorta. The first branch is the innominate giving the right subclavian and carotid. Next, is the left carotid and then left subclavian artery, which gives the vertebral artery.

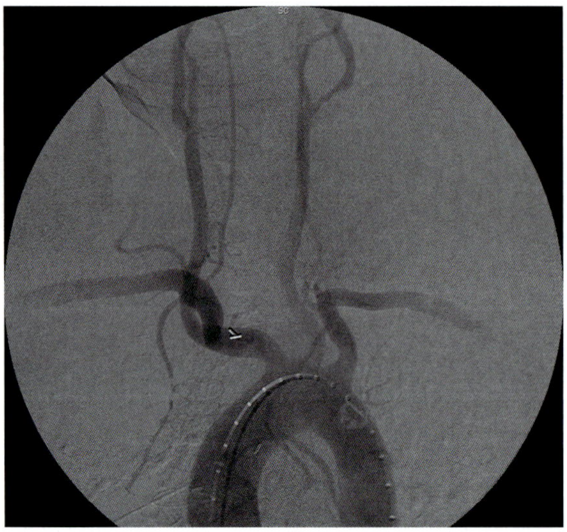

FIGURE 13.2 Left carotid artery originating from the innominate artery.

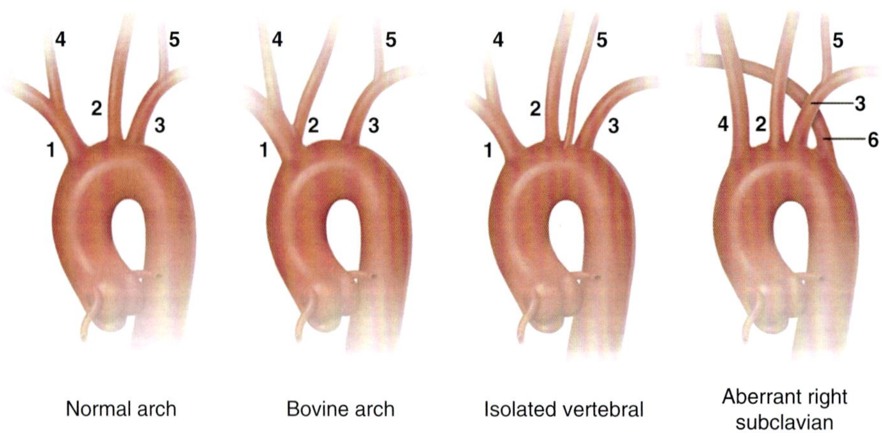

FIGURE 13.3 Aortic variants. 1-Subclavian artery. 2-Left carotid artery. 3-Left subclavian artery. 4 and 5 – Vertibral arteries. 6 - Aberrant right subclavian artery. In the bovine arch, a single brachiocephalic artery gives rise to the right subclavian artery and to a bicarotid vessel. Additional variants include an isolated origin of the left vertebral artery and an aberrant right subclavian artery.

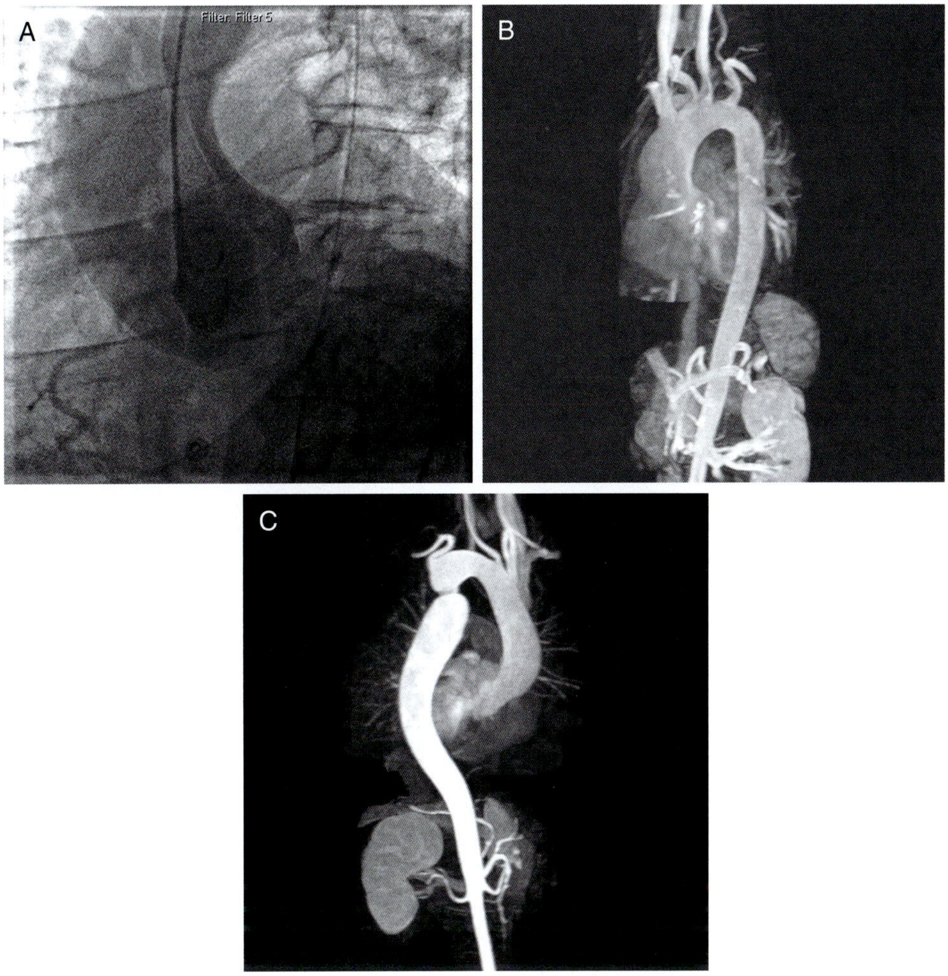

FIGURE 13.4 **A**, Acute aortic ascending arch dissection. The intimal flap is visible as well as a dilated ascending arch with contrast filling both the true and false lumens. **B**, Magnetic resonance angiography showing aneurysmal dilatation of the ascending aorta. **C**, Pseudocoarctation may be present if the aorta is redundant. Note the absence of dilated intercostal vessels suggesting the diagnosis of pseudocoarctation rather than true coarctation.

redundant as in the magnetic resonance angiogram in FIGURE 13.4BC. The absence of dilated intercostal vessels and reduced blood pressure in the lower extremities suggests the diagnosis of pseudocoarctation.

The angiogram in FIGURE 13.5 shows a right aortic arch with true coarctation. This patient has had a bypass graft for this disorder. FIGURE 13.6 shows a graft with numerous stents arising most proximally and then the right carotid artery; the coarcted portion of the aorta appears next, and then the right subclavian originates. The graft attaches to the descending aorta and finally an aberrant left innominate giving rise to the subclavian and left common carotid artery. FIGURE 13.7 demonstrates filling of the graft.

Selective left subclavian angiography reveals the left vertebral artery and left internal mammary artery as well as stenosis before and after repair (FIGURE 13.8A and B). Subclavian stenosis may compromise flow to the left internal mammary artery, which may lead to coronary ischemia if this vessel has been used for coronary artery bypass surgery. The subclavian stenosis in FIGURE 13.9A and Video 13.3 was found in a patient with shock and acute myocardial infarction. FIGURE 13.9B and Video 13.4 show the artery after stent placement with improved flow in the mammary artery.

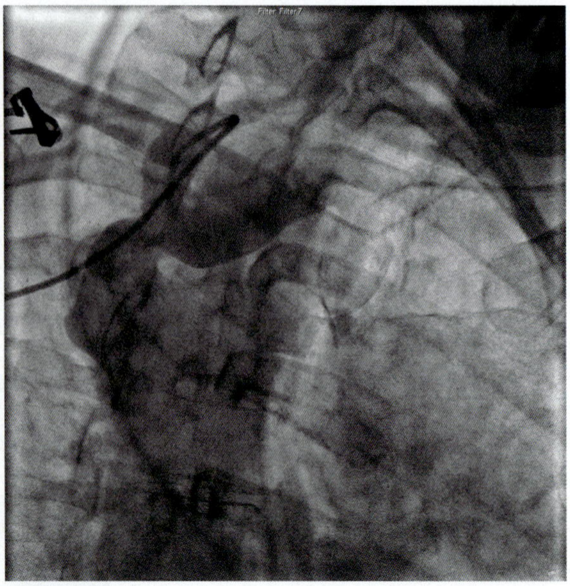

FIGURE 13.5 Aortic arch with true coarctation. The patient had a bypass graft for this disorder.

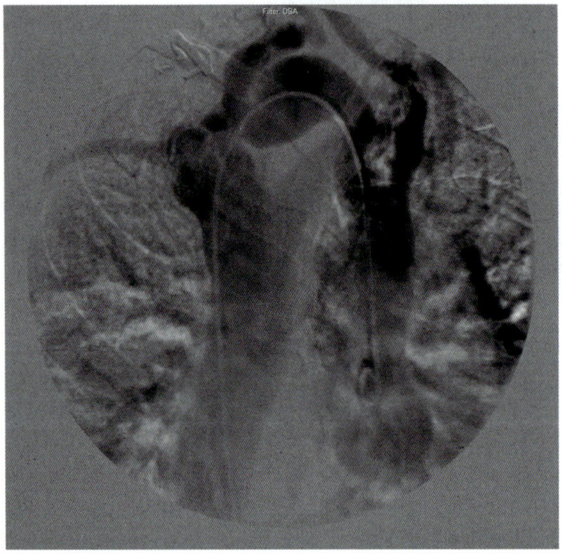

FIGURE 13.6 In sequence from left to right clockwise, bypass graft with numerous stents arising most proximally, right carotid artery, coarcted portion of the aorta, and right subclavian artery. The graft is anastomosed to the descending aorta and an aberrant left innominate gives rise to the subclavian and left common carotid artery.

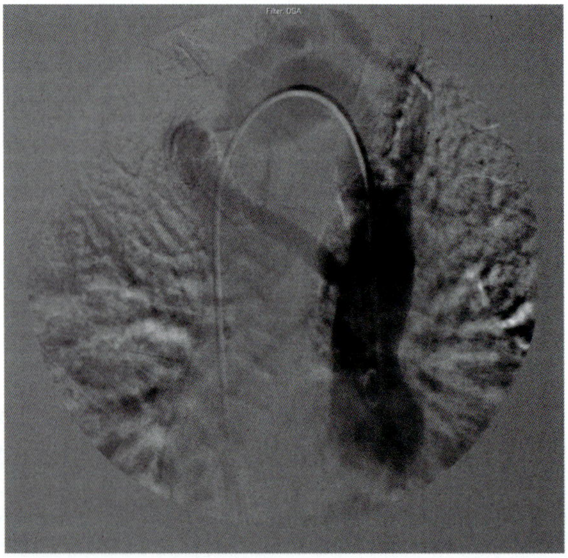

FIGURE 13.7 Filling of the graft shown in **FIGURE 13.6**.

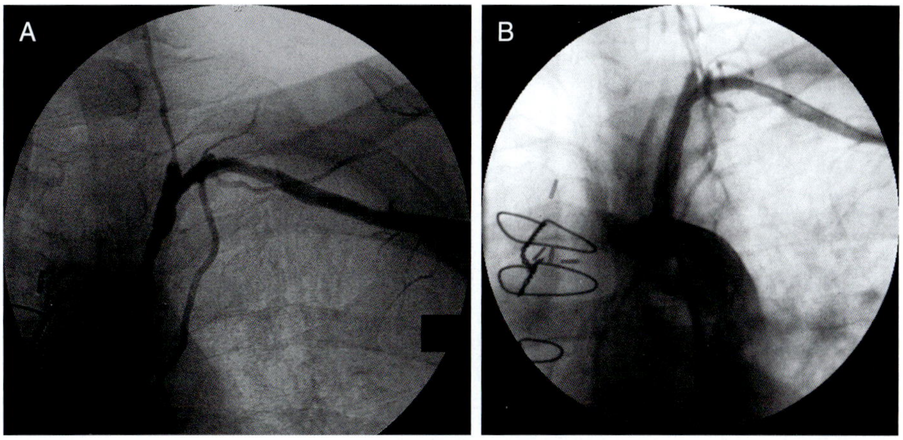

FIGURE 13.8 Selective left subclavian angiography revealing the left vertebral artery and left internal mammary artery as well as stenosis before **(A)** and after **(B)** repair.

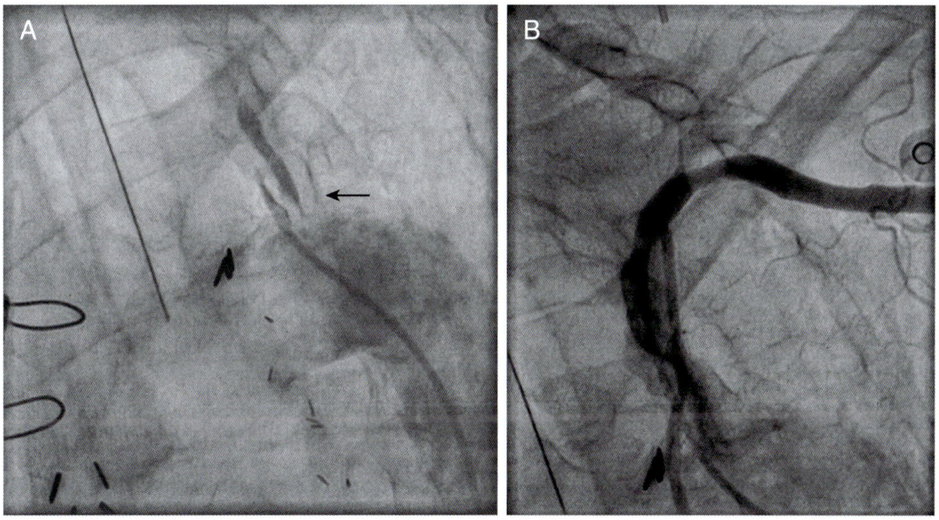

FIGURE 13.9 **A**, The subclavian stenosis shown in this figure was found in a patient with shock and acute myocardial infarction (arrow). **B**, Subclavian artery after stent placement with improved flow in the mammary artery.

THORACIC AORTA

The thoracic aorta can develop aneurysmal disease. Fusiform dilation is common. **FIGURE 13.10** demonstrates dilation due to contained rupture of mycotic aneurysm. This was repaired with an aortic stent graft as shown in **FIGURE 13.11**. The left subclavian artery is partially occluded by the covered stent and fills faintly. **FIGURE 13.12** demonstrates significant thoracic aortic tortuosity on computed tomography (CT) in a patient with severe kyphoscoliosis.

ABDOMINAL AORTA

The abdominal aorta begins at the aortic hiatus of the diaphragm. **FIGURE 13.13A** is a lateral view where the celiac artery takes off as the most superior vessel and courses anteriorly in this view. The superior mesenteric artery also takes off anteriorly and then courses inferiorly. The renal arteries can be seen to take off and course posteriorly. **FIGURE 13.13B** demonstrates these

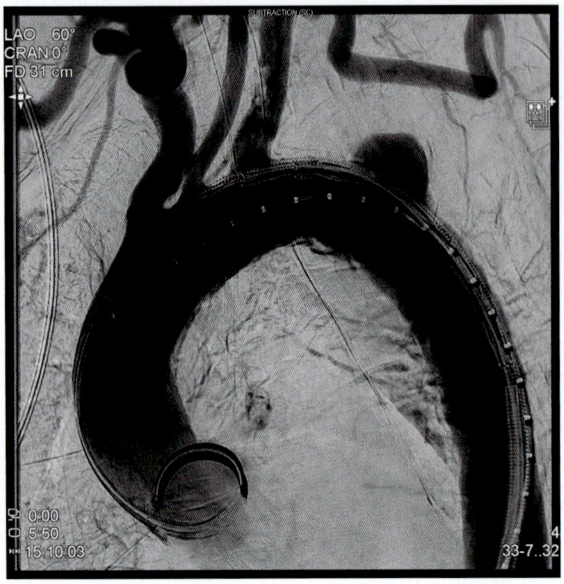

FIGURE 13.10 Dilation of the thoracic aorta due to contained rupture of mycotic aneurysm.

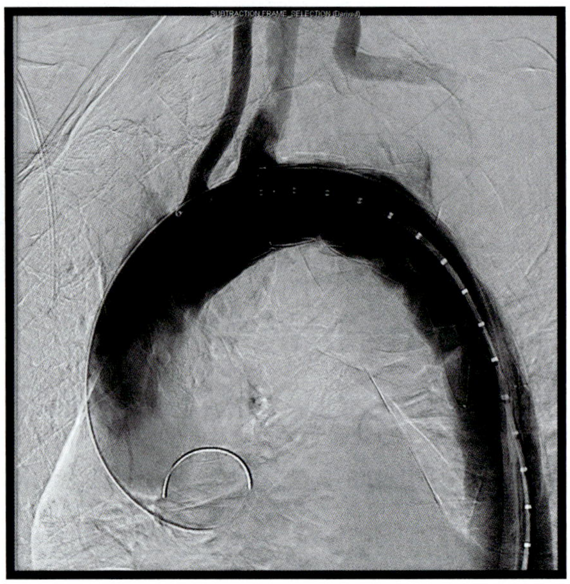

FIGURE 13.11 The ruptured aneurysm shown in **FIGURE 13.10** has been repaired with an aortic stent graft. The left subclavian artery is partially occluded by the covered stent and fills faintly.

same vessels in the anteroposterior projection. Nonselective angiography in the lateral projection demonstrates a stenosis in the celiac artery and occlusion of the superior mesenteric artery (**FIGURE 13.14**).

Selective celiac angiography in the anteroposterior projection shows the artery dividing into the common hepatic and splenic arteries (**FIGURE 13.15A**). The common hepatic artery divides into the proper hepatic and gastroduodenal arteries (**FIGURE 13.15B**). After giving off duodenal branches, the right gastroepiploic artery continues. This artery is sometimes used in coronary artery bypass graft surgery. **FIGURE 13.16** shows a gastroepiploic artery that has been used as a graft to the posterior descending artery (PDA) (Video 13.5).

FIGURE 13.17 is a nonselective angiogram demonstrating normal single bilateral renal arteries. A single renal artery on the right and 2 renal arteries on the left are shown in the angiogram in **FIGURE 13.18. FIGURE 13.19A** shows severe renal artery stenosis that was successfully treated with stenting (**FIGURE 13.19B**) in a patient with uncontrolled hypertension and pulmonary edema. In the same patient, stenosis of the left upper pole renal artery was present (**FIGURE 13.20A**). **FIGURE 13.20B** shows the left upper pole renal artery after stent placement

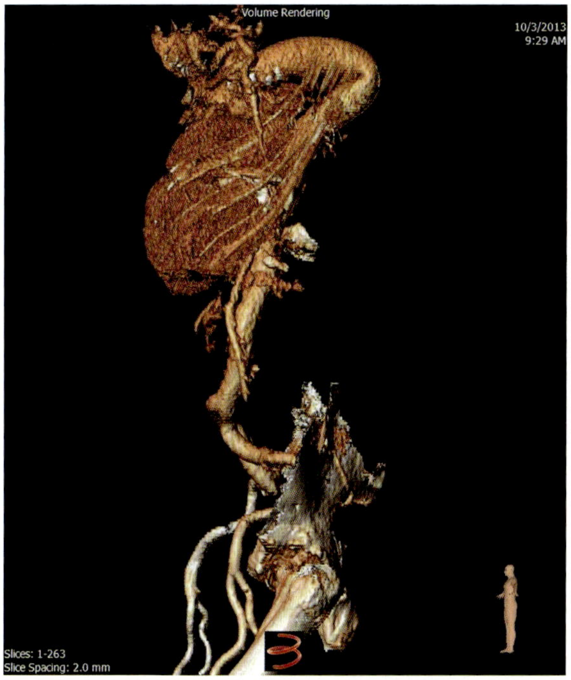

FIGURE 13.12 Significant thoracic aortic tortuosity on CT in a patient with severe kyphoscoliosis.

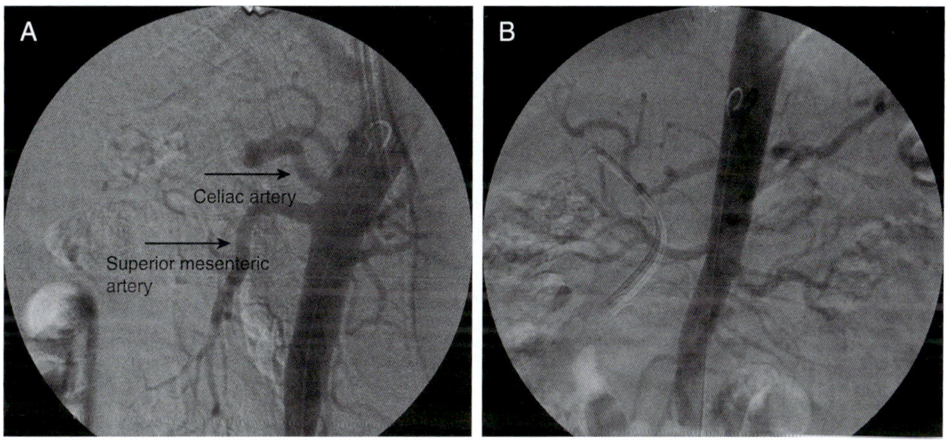

FIGURE 13.13 **A**, Lateral view of the abdominal aorta. The celiac artery takes off as the most superior vessel and courses anteriorly in this view. The superior mesenteric artery also takes off anteriorly then courses inferiorly. The renal arteries can be seen to take off and course posteriorly. **B**, Anteroposterior projection.

with stenosis of the left lower pole that was left untreated. **FIGURE 13.20C** and **Video 13.6** show the celiac artery dividing into the hepatic and splenic arteries. The superior mesenteric and renal arteries are also visualized.

Aortography in **FIGURE 13.21** demonstrates normal aorta and common iliac arteries. There is a superior and inferior pole of the left renal artery. The right renal artery has the characteristic appearance of fibromuscular dysplasia. Selective angiography if this vessel is shown in **FIGURE 13.22**.

DISTAL AORTA

A normal distal aorta is demonstrated in **FIGURE 13.23**. Distal aortography in **FIGURE 13.24** demonstrates filling of the celiac, superior mesenteric, inferior mesenteric, and renal vessels. The proximal portion of an aorto-bifemoral graft can be seen with serrations of the fabric evident in both the right and left limbs. **FIGURE 13.25A** demonstrates occlusion of the left iliac artery with reconstitution of the vessel via collaterals evident in **FIGURE 13.25B**.

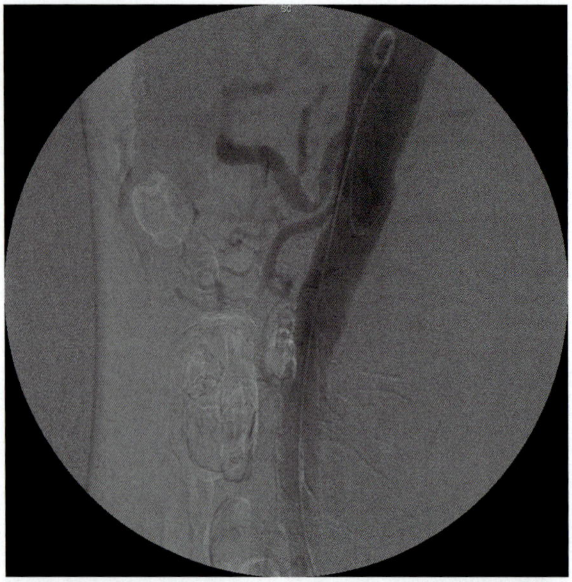

FIGURE 13.14 Nonselective angiography of the abdominal aorta in the lateral projection. There is a stenosis in the celiac artery and occlusion of the superior mesenteric artery.

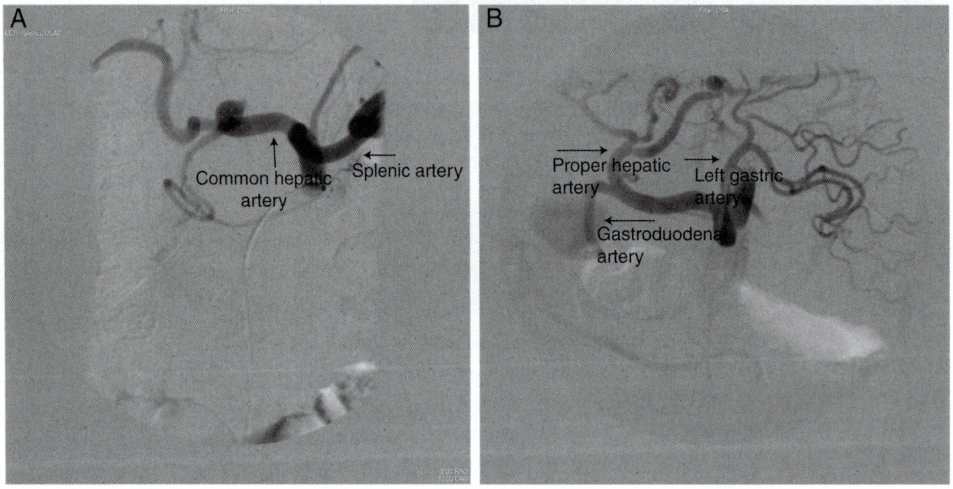

FIGURE 13.15 **A**, Selective celiac angiography in the anteroposterior projection shows the artery dividing into the common hepatic and splenic arteries. **B**, The common hepatic artery divides into the proper hepatic and gastroduodenal arteries. After giving off duodenal branches, the right gastroepiploic artery continues. This artery is sometimes used in coronary artery bypass graft surgery.

Bilateral iliac artery aneurysms are noted in **FIGURE 13.26**. Commonly associated with aortic and popliteal aneurysms, these were not evident in this patient. A saccular abdominal aortic aneurysm (AAA) is demonstrated in **FIGURE 13.27A** before and after repair (**FIGURE 13.27B**).

LOWER EXTREMITY

Popliteal artery aneurysms are shown in **FIGURE 13.28A** and **B**. They are bilateral in 50% to 70% of cases. They can be either true or false aneurysms. The main consequence of this entity is thromboembolism rather than rupture. Of patients with a popliteal artery aneurysm, 40% have an AAA; however, only 10% to 15% of patients with AAA have popliteal artery aneurysms.

The external iliac artery gives off the inferior epigastric artery before the inguinal ligament. The external iliac ends at the inguinal ligament where it becomes the common femoral artery, a commonly used access point for catheter-based procedures (**FIGURE 13.29**). Occasionally, the inferior epigastric artery can become injured during catheterization procedures. **FIGURE 13.30** demonstrates bleeding from a perforation in the inferior epigastric artery with cessation of bleeding after coil placement shown in **FIGURE 13.31A** and **B**.

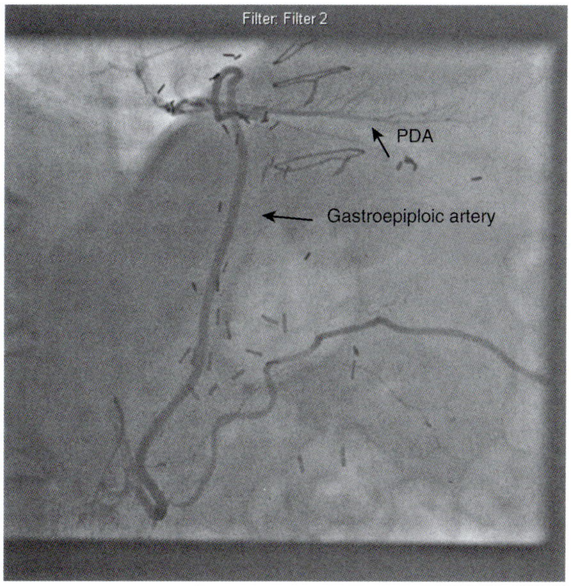

FIGURE 13.16 Gastroepiploic artery that has been used as a graft to the PDA.

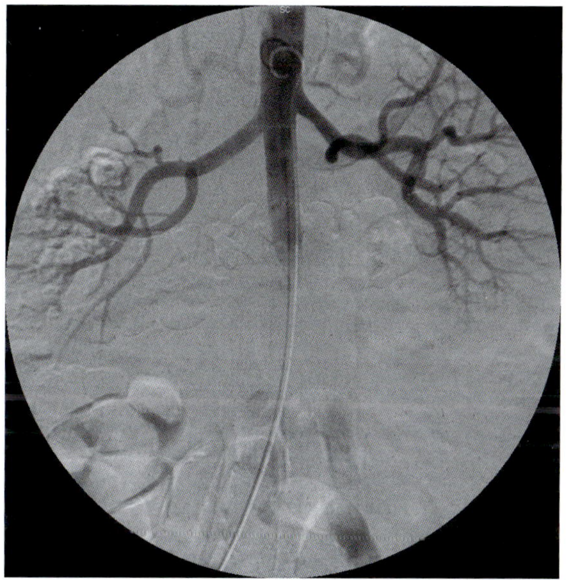

FIGURE 13.17 Nonselective angiography of the abdominal aorta demonstrating normal single bilateral renal arteries.

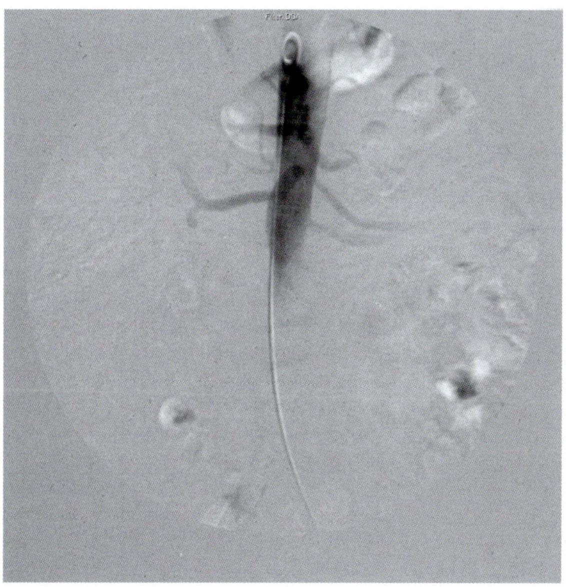

FIGURE 13.18 Nonselective angiography of abdominal aorta demonstrating single renal artery on the right and 2 renal arteries on the left.

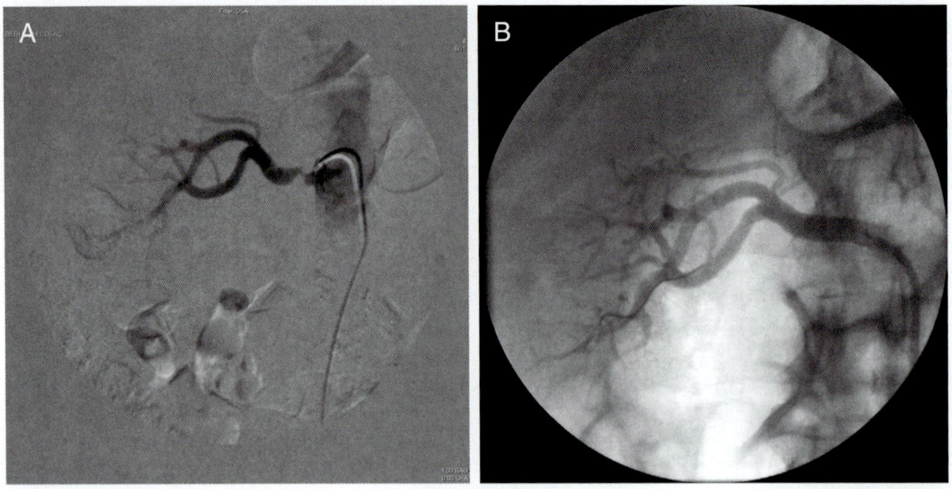

FIGURE 13.19 **A**, Severe renal artery stenosis in a patient with uncontrolled hypertension and pulmonary edema. **B**, The stenosis was successfully treated with stenting.

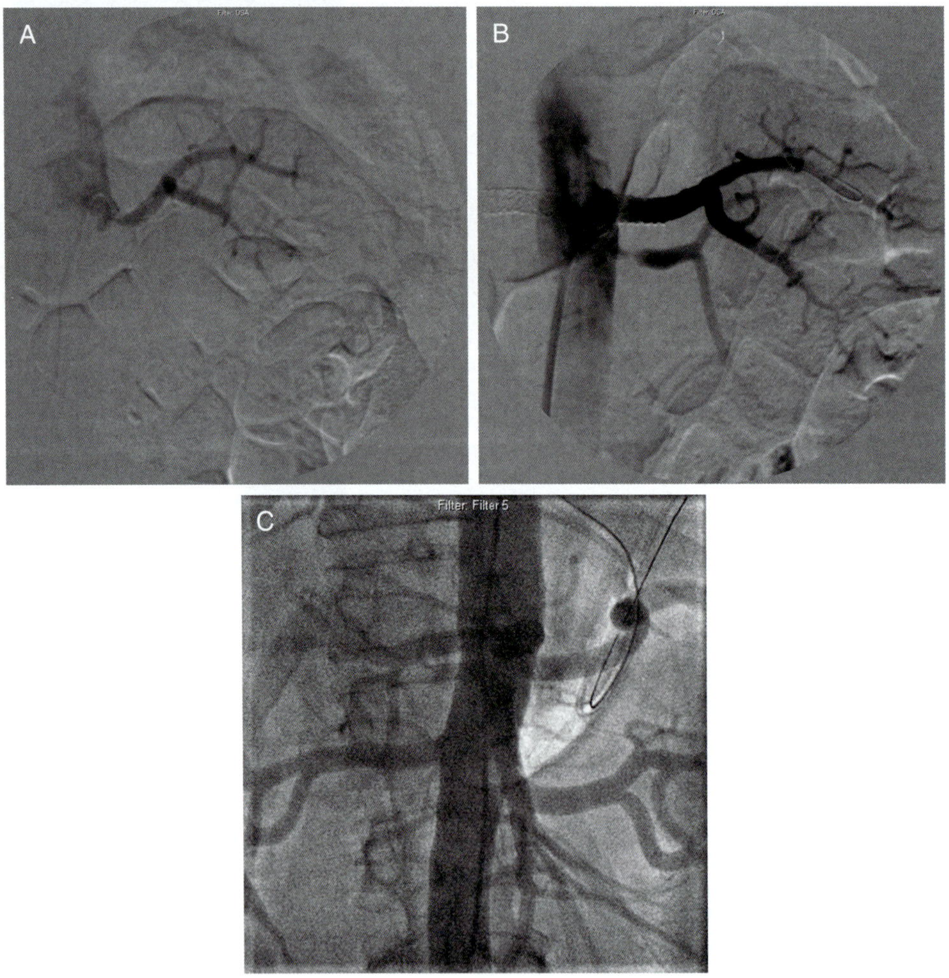

FIGURE 13.20 **A**, Stenosis of the left upper pole renal artery in the same patient shown in **FIGURE 13.19**. **B**, Left upper pole renal artery after stent placement with stenosis of the left lower pole that was left untreated. **C**, Celiac artery dividing into the hepatic and splenic arteries. The superior mesenteric and renal arteries are also visualized.

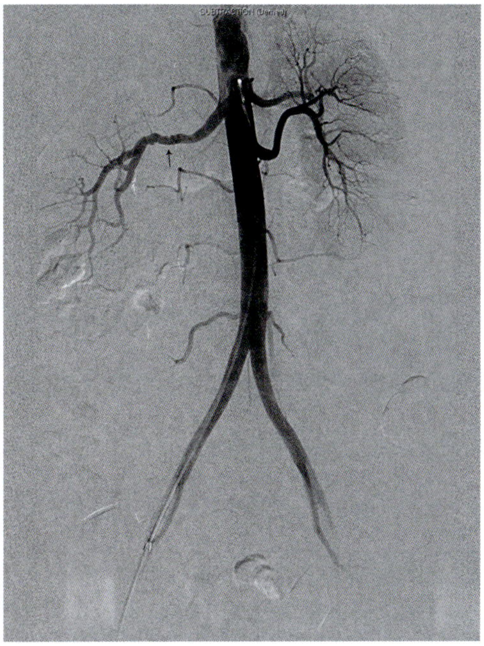

FIGURE 13.21 Normal aorta and common iliac arteries. There is a superior and an inferior pole of the left renal artery. The right renal artery has the characteristic appearance of fibromuscular dysplasia (arrow).

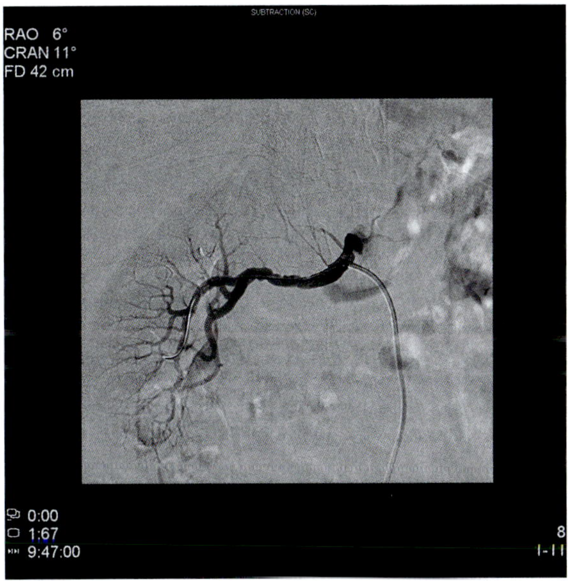

FIGURE 13.22 Selective angiography of the right renal artery shown in **FIGURE 13.21**.

It should be noted that the inferior epigastric artery may have anastomotic connections to the superior epigastric artery, a branch of the internal mammary artery (**FIGURES 13.32** and **13.33**). As such, if the inferior epigastric artery is injured and then successfully occluded proximally, bleeding may still continue if such collateral blood supply is present.

The principal branches of the common femoral artery are the lateral circumflex femoral, profunda femoris, and superficial femoral arteries (**FIGURE 13.33**). Occasionally, the superficial femoral artery or profunda artery may arise in the pelvis. **FIGURE 13.34A** demonstrates access site bleeding from a sheath that had inadvertently been placed in the pelvis. Ultrasound guided access above the superficial femoral artery, but in this case, the superficial femoral artery arose above the inguinal ligament.

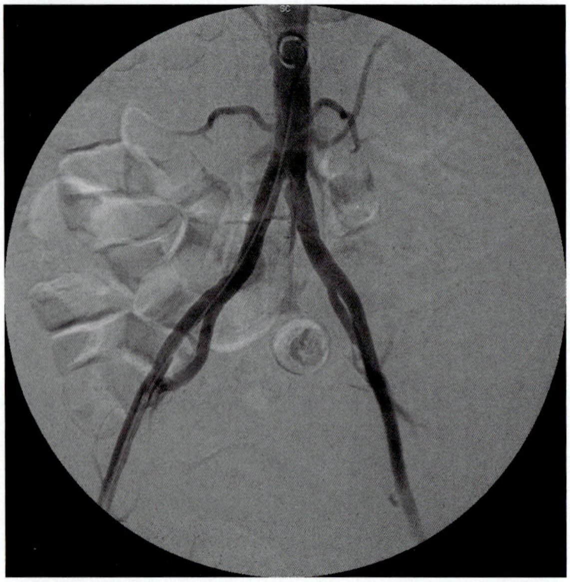

FIGURE 13.23 Normal distal aorta.

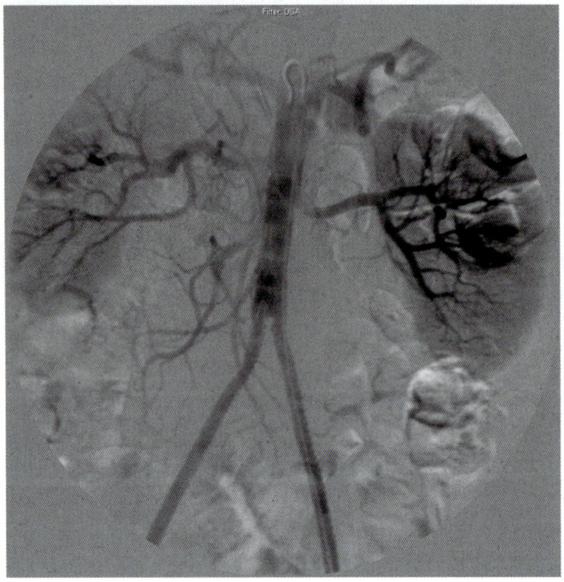

FIGURE 13.24 Distal aortography with filling of the celiac, superior mesenteric, inferior mesenteric, and renal vessels. The proximal portion of an aorto-bifemoral graft can be seen with serrations of the fabric evident in both the right and left limbs.

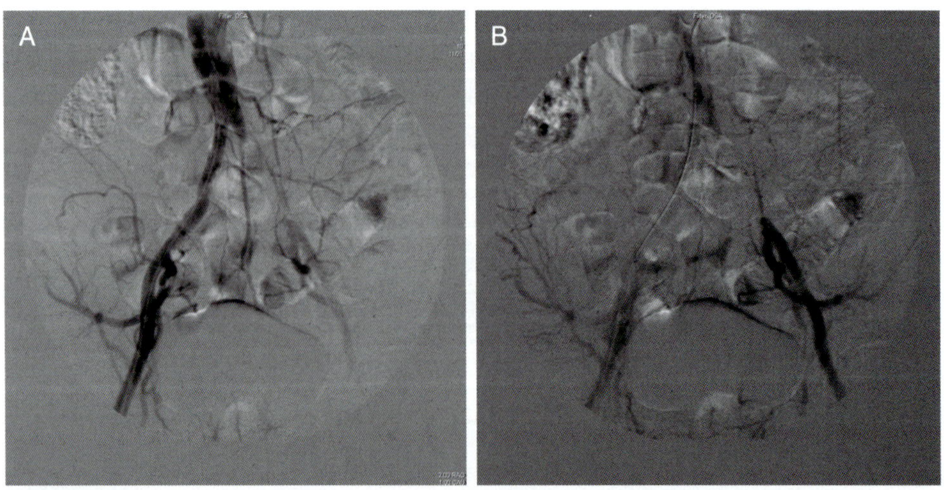

FIGURE 13.25 **A**, Occlusion of the left iliac artery. **B**, Reconstitution of the vessel via collaterals.

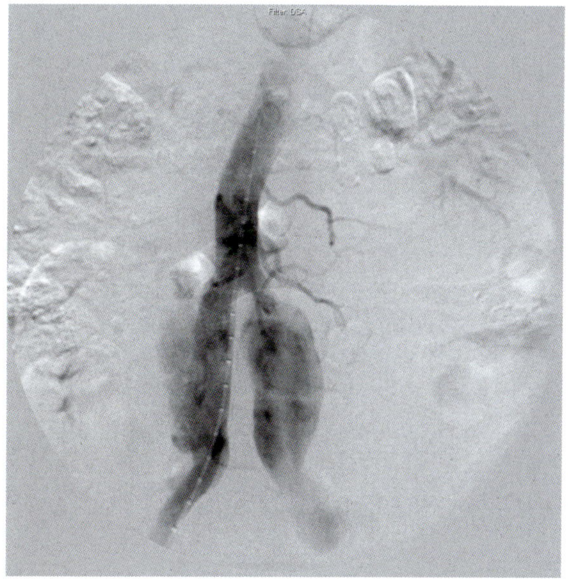

FIGURE 13.26 Bilateral iliac artery aneurysms.

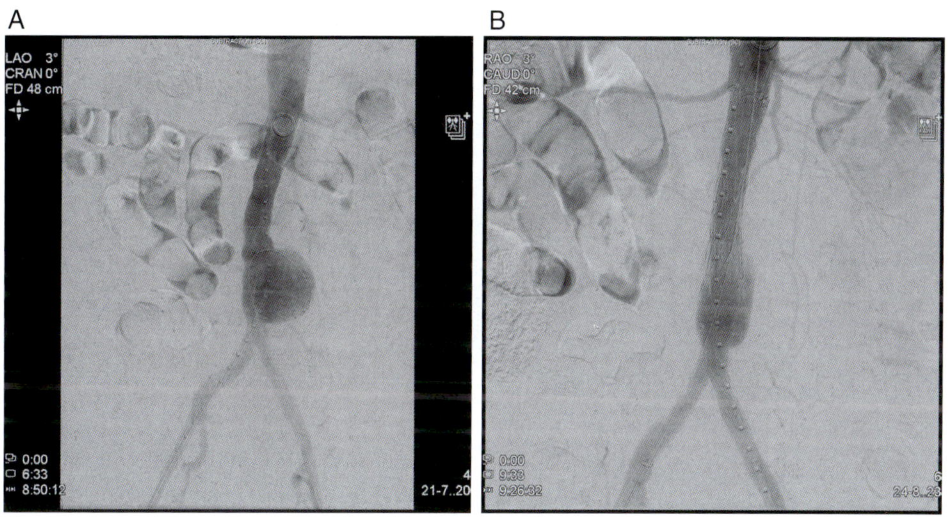

FIGURE 13.27 Saccular AAA **(A)** before and **(B)** after repair.

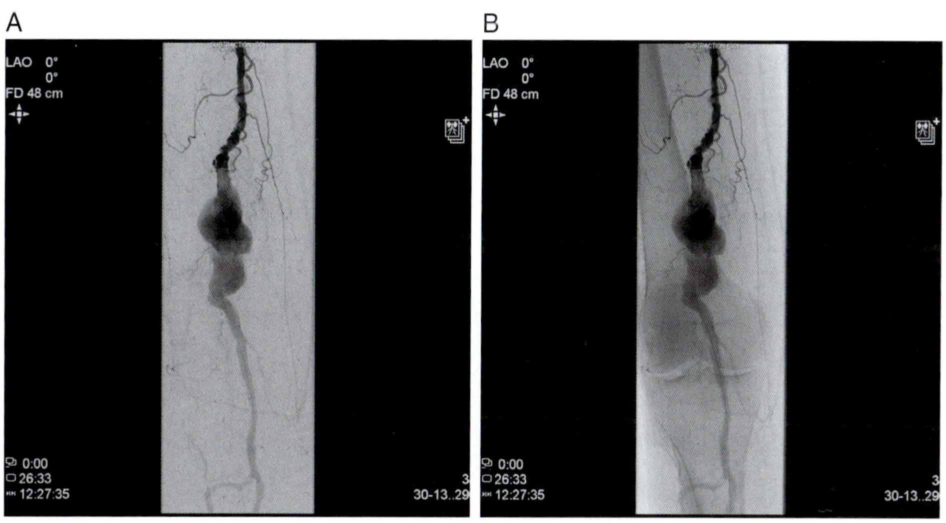

FIGURE 13.28 **A and B**, Popliteal artery aneurysm.

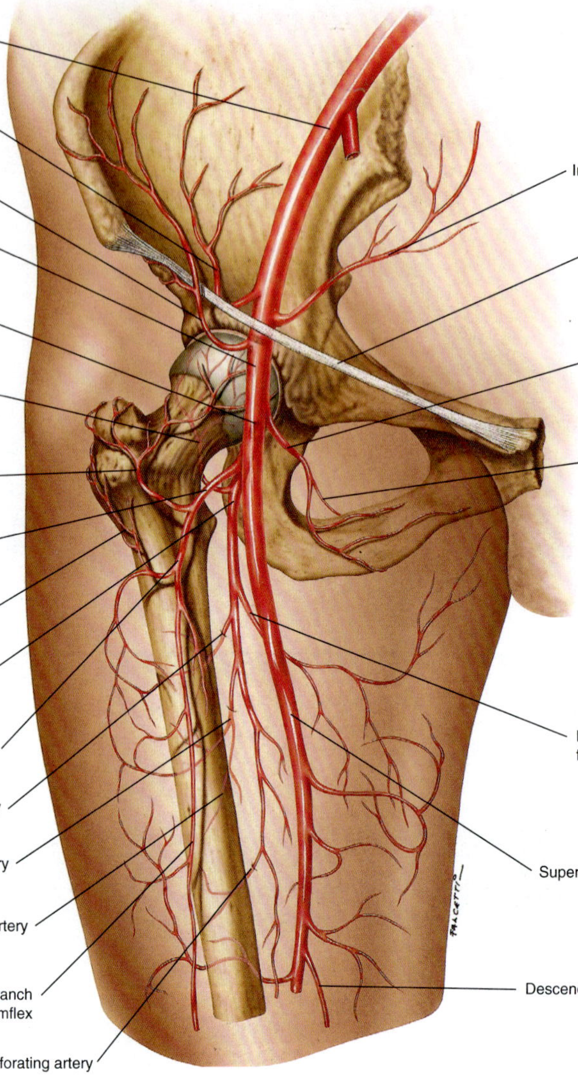

FIGURE 13.29 The external iliac ends at the inguinal ligament where it becomes the common femoral artery, a commonly used access point for catheter-based procedures. Occasionally, the inferior epigastric artery can become injured during catheterization procedures. Reproduced with permission from Uflacker R. *Atlas of Vascular Anatomy*. 2nd ed. Philadelphia, PA: Wolters Kluwer; 2006.

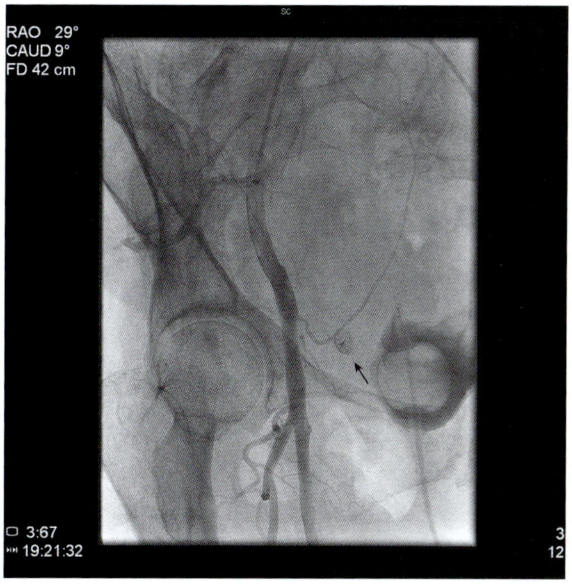

FIGURE 13.30 Bleeding from a perforation in the inferior epigastric artery (arrows).

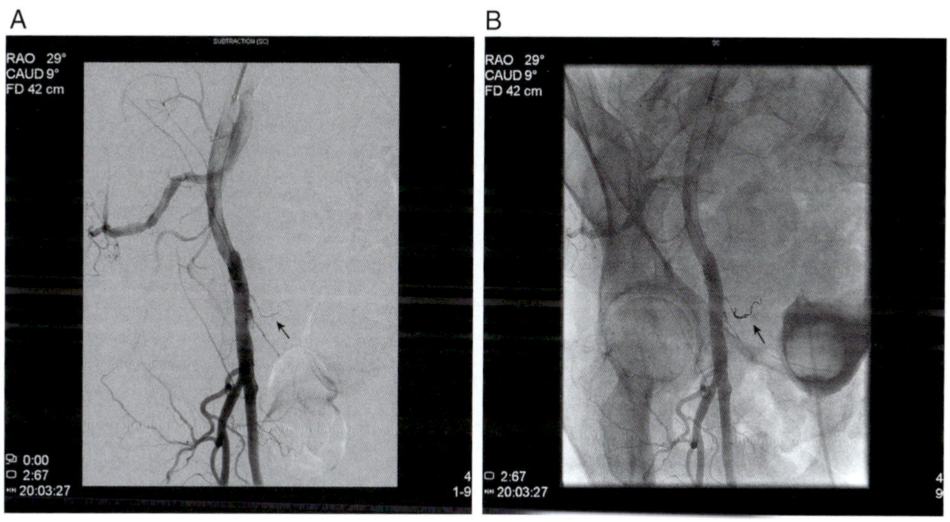

FIGURE 13.31 **A and B**, Cessation of bleeding from the inferior epigastric artery shown in FIGURE 13.30 after coil placement (arrows).

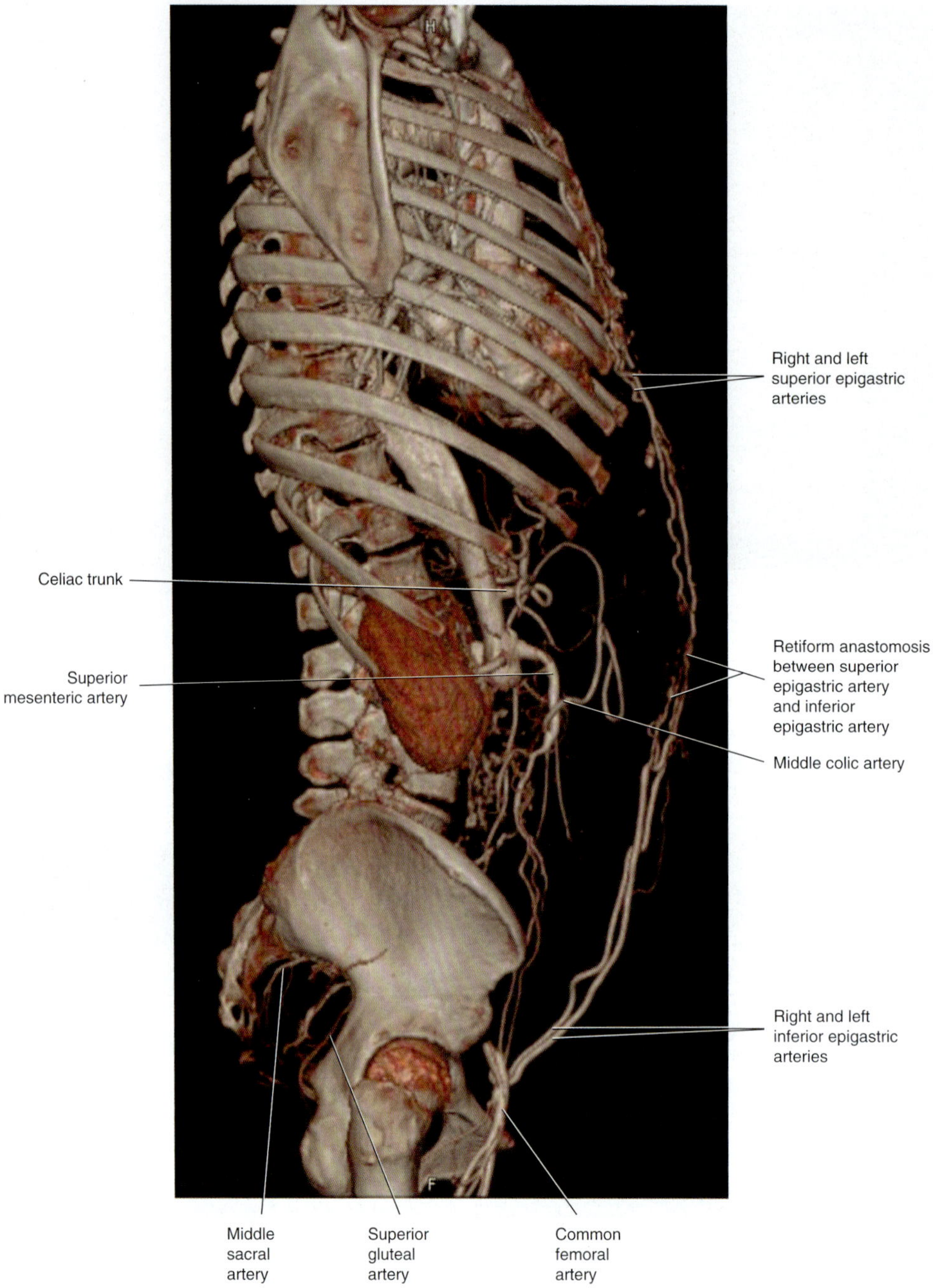

FIGURE 13.32 The inferior epigastric artery may have anastomotic connections to the superior epigastric artery, a branch of the internal mammary artery. As such, if the inferior epigastric artery is injured and then successfully occluded proximally, bleeding may still continue if such collateral blood supply is present. Reproduced with permission from Uflacker R. *Atlas of Vascular Anatomy*. 2nd ed. Philadelphia, PA: Wolters Kluwer; 2006.

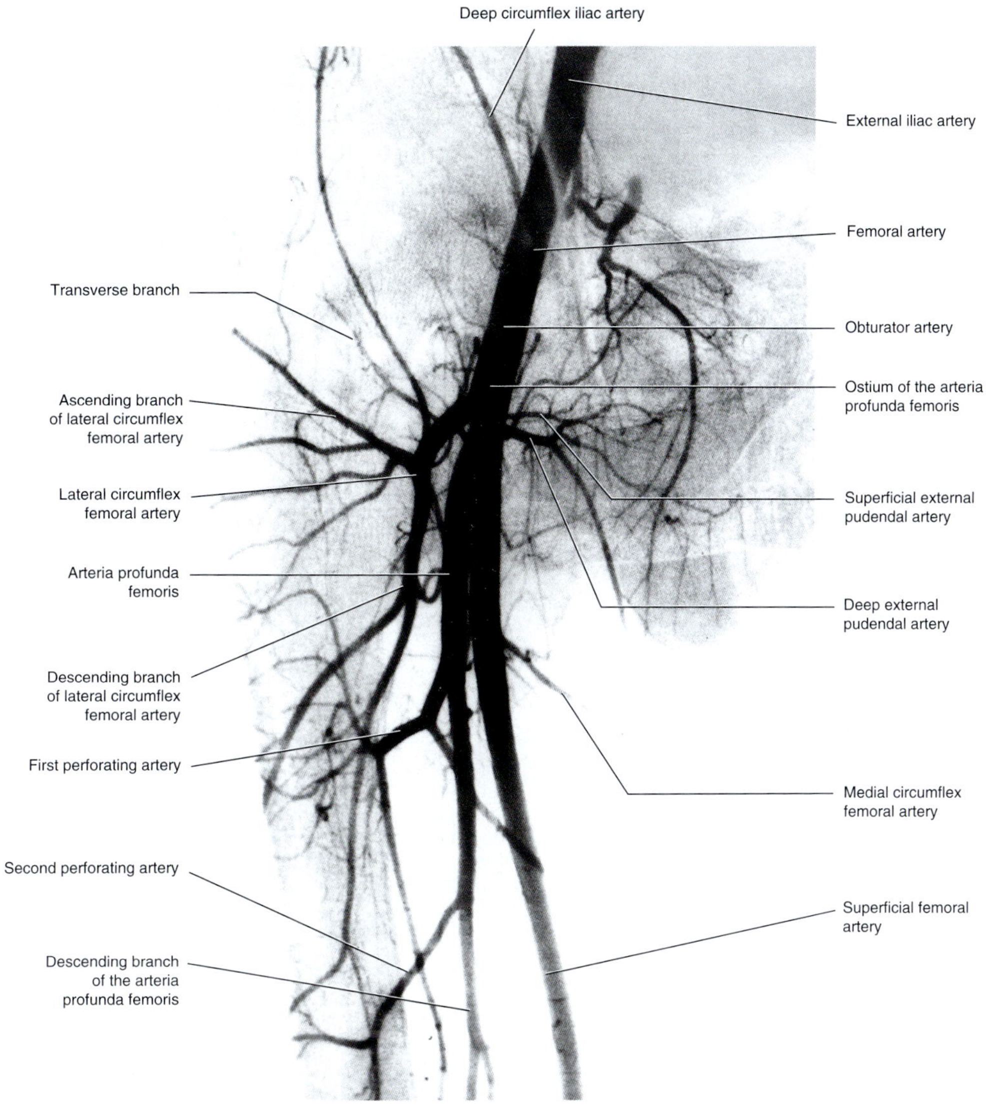

FIGURE 13.33 Principal branches of the common femoral artery. Reproduced with permission from Uflacker R. *Atlas of Vascular Anatomy*. 2nd ed. Philadelphia, PA: Wolters Kluwer; 2006.

FIGURE 13.34B and C show the right and left common femoral arteries as well as proximal portions of the profunda femoris and superficial femoral arteries. Bilateral leg angiography in FIGURE 13.35 demonstrates normal profunda femoris arteries and diffuse disease affecting the proximal and mid portions of the superficial femoral arteries on the right. The left superficial femoral artery has mild luminal irregularities. The distal superficial femoral artery at the adductor hiatus, also known as Hunter canal, has mild disease. The popliteal arteries bilaterally are normal.

Angiography demonstrates perforation (FIGURE 13.36A and B; Video 13.7) of the right superficial femoral artery during transcatheter aortic valve procedure before and after being repaired with covered stent implantation (FIGURE 13.36C; Video 13.8).

The anterior tibial artery is seen on the left with a normal tibioperoneal trunk dividing into the peroneal and posterior tibial arteries. The tibial vessels are not well seen on the right (FIGURE 13.37). FIGURE 13.38A and B show a right popliteal artery with a normal takeoff of the anterior tibial artery followed by the tibioperoneal trunk that divides into the posterior tibial and peroneal arteries. In this variant, the posterior tibial artery arises directly from the popliteal (FIGURE 13.39). A high takeoff of the anterior tibial artery is seen in FIGURE 13.40 with the artery arising in the popliteal fossa.

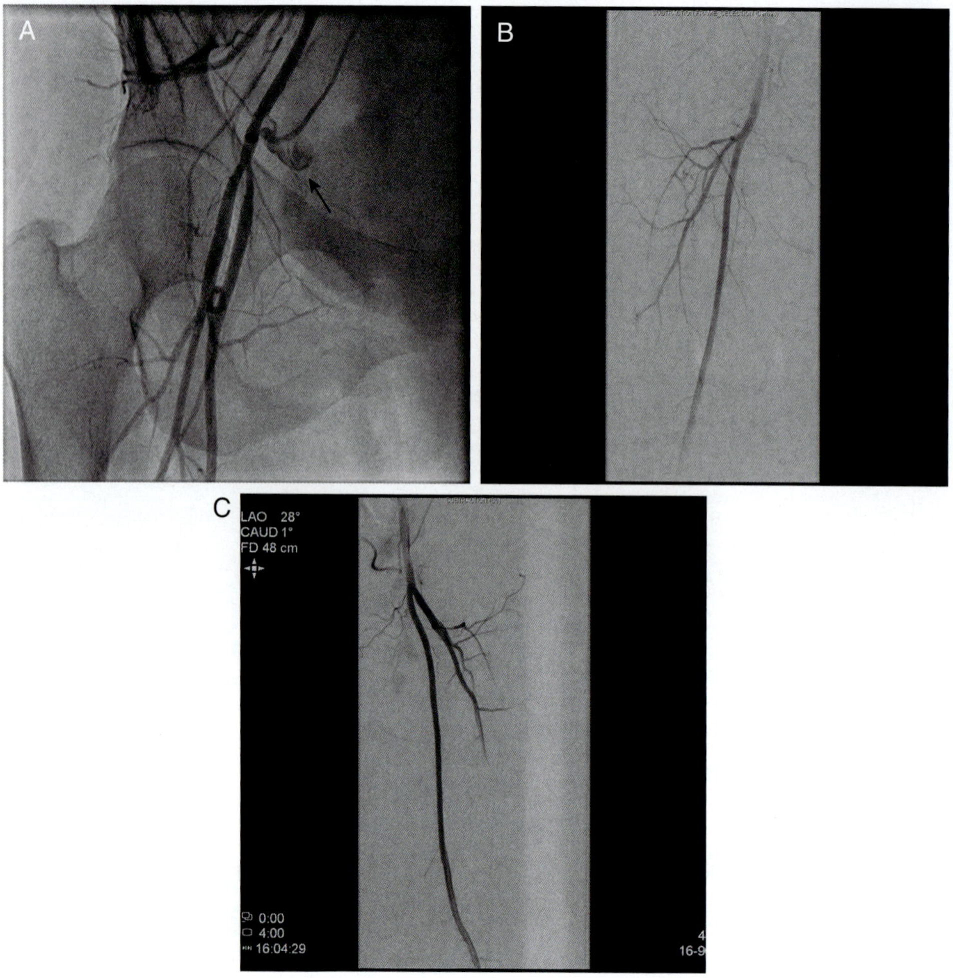

FIGURE 13.34 **A**, Access site bleeding from a sheath that had inadvertently been placed in the pelvis (arrow). Ultrasound guided access above the superficial femoral artery, but in this case, the superficial femoral artery arose above the inguinal ligament. **B and C**, Right and left common femoral arteries as well as proximal portions of the profunda femoris and superficial femoral arteries.

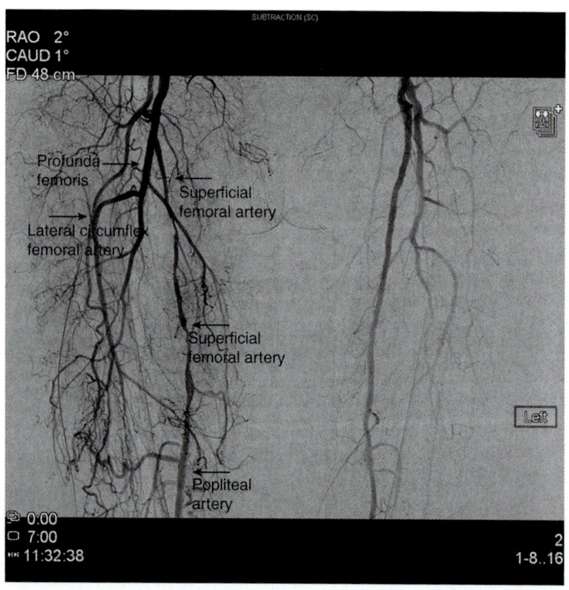

FIGURE 13.35 Bilateral leg angiography demonstrating normal profunda femoris arteries and diffuse disease affecting the proximal and mid portions of the superficial femoral arteries on the right. The left superficial femoral artery has mild luminal irregularities. The distal superficial femoral artery at the adductor hiatus, also known as Hunter canal, has mild disease. The popliteal arteries bilaterally are normal.

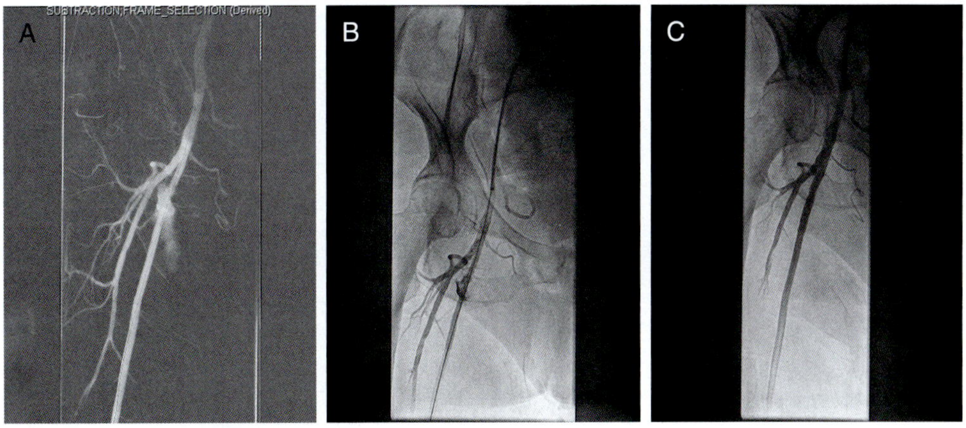

FIGURE 13.36 **A**, Perforation of the right superficial femoral artery during transcatheter aortic valve procedure. **B and C**, Angiography after covered stent implantation.

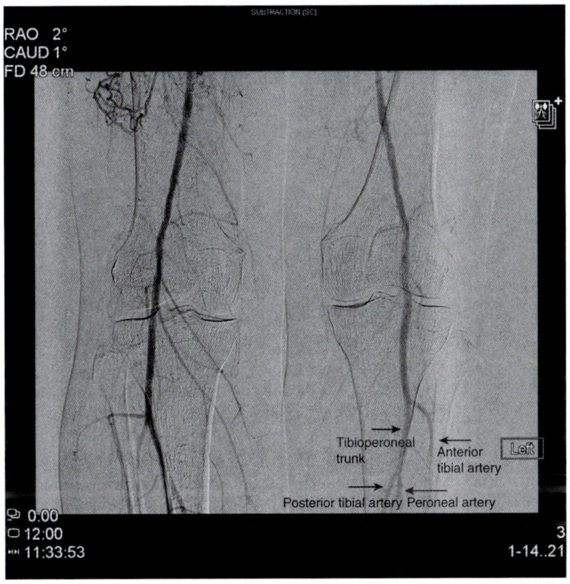

FIGURE 13.37 The anterior tibial artery is seen on the left with a normal tibioperoneal trunk dividing into the peroneal and posterior tibial arteries. The tibial vessels are not well seen on the right.

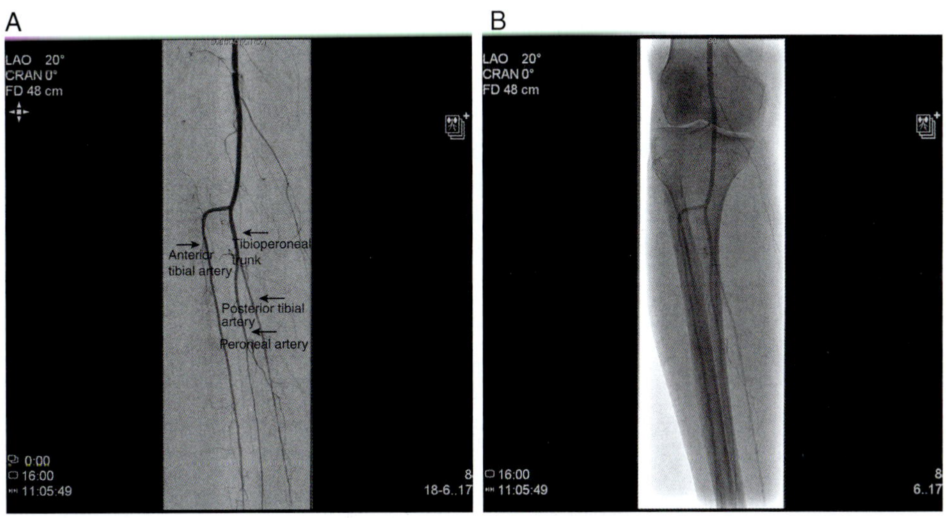

FIGURE 13.38 **A and B**, Right popliteal artery with a normal takeoff of the anterior tibial artery followed by the tibioperoneal trunk that divides into the posterior tibial and peroneal arteries.

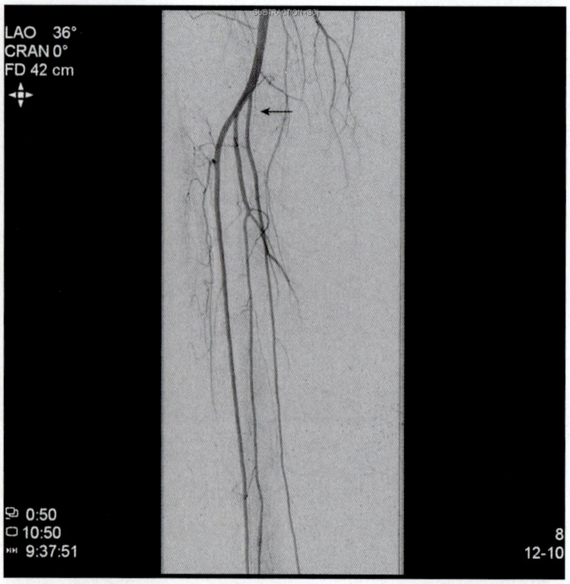

FIGURE 13.39 Posterior tibial artery arising directly from the popliteal artery (arrow).

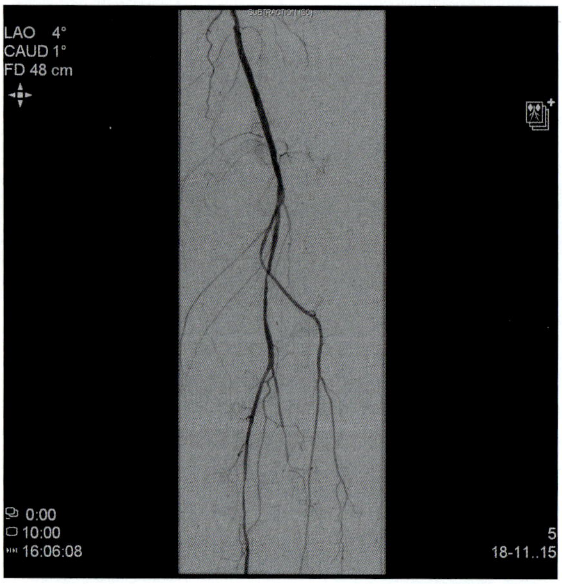

FIGURE 13.40 High takeoff of the anterior tibial artery arising in the popliteal fossa.

The arterial circulation of the foot is shown in **FIGURE 13.41**. The distal tibial vessels are demonstrated in **FIGURES 13.42** and **13.43**. In the anteroposterior view, the dorsalis pedis vessel can be seen as well as the posterior tibial artery. The peroneal artery is seen to terminate at the ankle as is typical. An oblique view of the same vessels is shown.

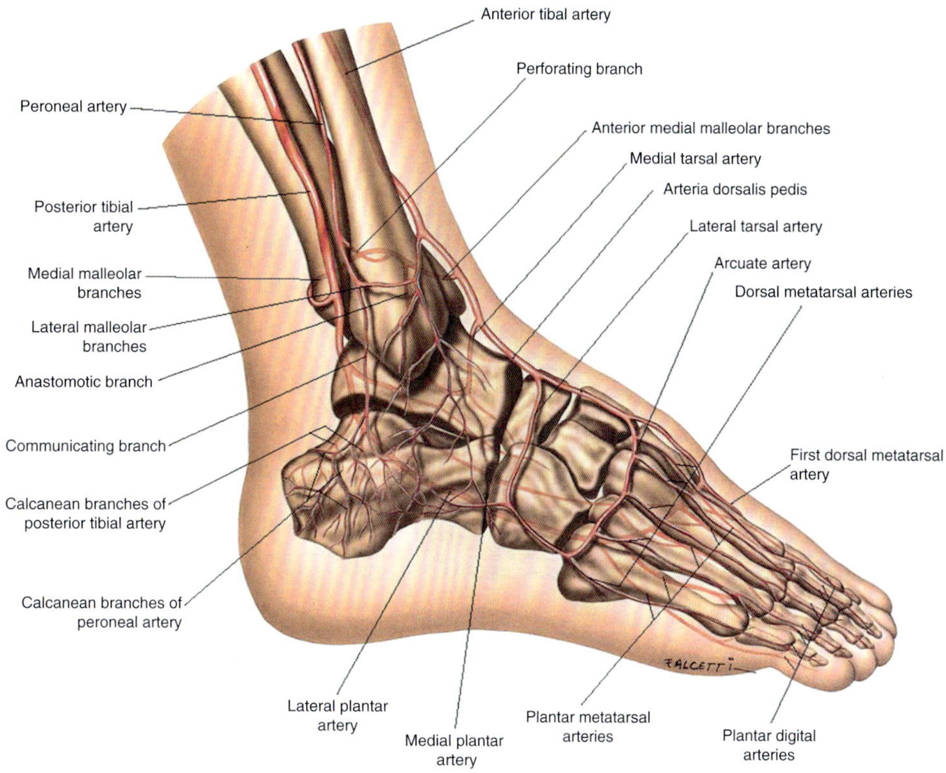

FIGURE 13.41 Arterial circulation of the foot. Reproduced with permission from Uflacker R. *Atlas of Vascular Anatomy*. 2nd ed. Philadelphia, PA: Wolters Kluwer; 2006.

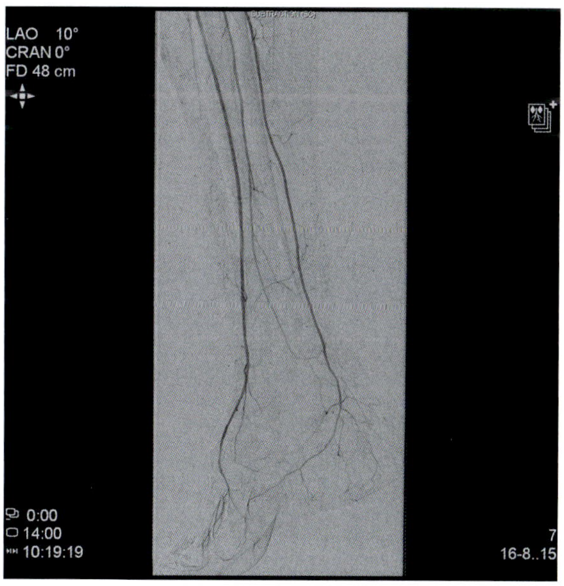

FIGURE 13.42 Distal tibial vessels. In the anteroposterior view, the dorsalis pedis vessel can be seen as well as the posterior tibial artery. The peroneal artery is seen to terminate at the ankle as is typical.

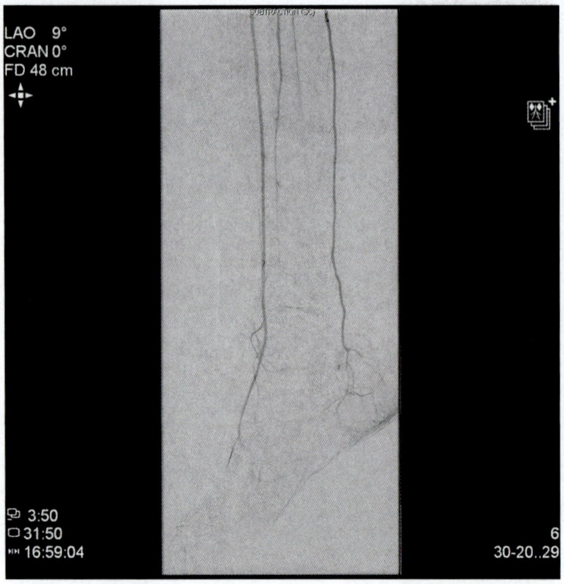

FIGURE 13.43 An oblique view of the distal tibial vessels.

chapter **14**

Myocardial and Coronary Blood Flow and Metabolism

MATHEW LIAKOS, MD, KIRAN V. REDDY, MD, FACC, and ALLEN JEREMIAS, MD, MSC

BASIC PRINCIPLE OF FFR

Epicardial Coronary Artery Versus Microcirculation

FIGURE 14.1 illustrates the importance of the coronary microcirculation in comparison with the epicardial coronary arteries, which represent only a small fraction (about 5%) of the total coronary vasculature. The left panel demonstrates a coronary angiogram of the left coronary system. The epicardial macrocirculation represents the conductance vessels that under normal conditions (in the absence of any critical coronary lesions) offer little resistance to blood flow. The right panel shows an ex vivo angiogram of the human heart submerged in saline to eliminate myocardial tissue shadowing and allowing visualization of the microvasculature that is not seen on typical coronary angiogram.[1]

Regulation of Coronary Blood Flow

The graph depicted in **FIGURE 14.2** demonstrates coronary blood flow at rest and with maximal hyperemia.[2] With maximal hyperemia, the coronary flow can normally increase 3- to 5-folds. As the luminal diameter of the vessel narrows to greater than 50%, the hyperemic flow reserve begins to diminish while resting flow is preserved. As the diameter stenosis further increases, both resting and hyperemic flows are affected, with coronary reserve flow diminishing in greater proportion to resting flow.

Derivation and Experimental Basis for FFR

The theoretical derivation of FFR was first described by Pijls et al in 1993[3] (**FIGURE 14.3**). While direct measurement of coronary blood flow may be ideal to determine the myocardial metabolism, in clinical practice, determination of coronary flow is technically difficult and thus impractical. The basic concept of coronary pressure–based measurements is to induce maximal hyperemia to eliminate the resistance of the microcirculation and thus "isolate" the epicardial vessel. Under those circumstances, based on the illustrated equations, coronary pressure equals coronary blood flow and allows the assessment of coronary stenoses on myocardial metabolism.

As the illustration demonstrates, aortic pressure (Pa) is used as a "reference" pressure. In the absence of coronary artery disease, the pressure within the coronary tree should be equal to the aortic pressure. A coronary stenosis will introduce a resistance in the artery (Rs) and diminish both coronary pressure (Pd) and blood flow (Qs). In the presence of collaterals, total myocardial blood flow (Q) will be the sum of coronary flow through the coronary stenosis (Qs) and collateral blood flow (Qc). The original equations separate FFRcor, which represents a pressure measurement in the coronary artery distal to the stenosis, from FFRmyo which adds collateral

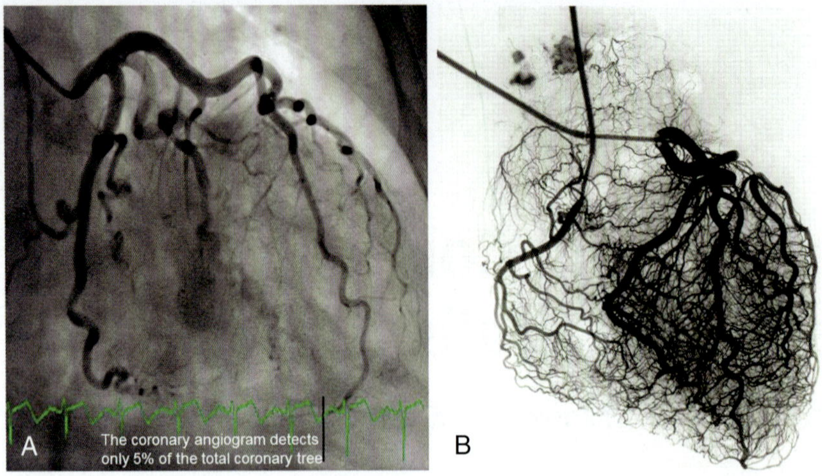

FIGURE 14.1 **A and B**, Epicardial coronary artery versus microcirculation. Reprinted with permission from Fulton WF. Immersion Radiography Of Injected Specimens. *Br J Radiol*. 1963;36:685-688.

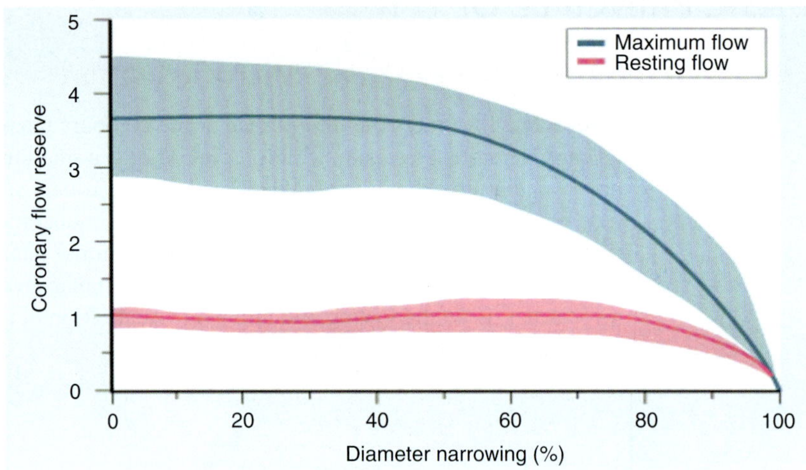

FIGURE 14.2 Regulation of coronary blood flow. Reprinted with permission from Gould KL, Lipscomb K, Hamilton GW. Physiologic basis for assessing critical coronary stenosis. Instantaneous flow response and regional distribution during coronary hyperemia as measure of coronary flow reserve. *Am J Cardiol*. 1974;33:87-94.

Equations for FFR and collateral blood flow. Equation 1, also derived in the appendix, states the fundamental observation that the ratio $(P_a - P_v)$ to $(P_w - P_v)$ is constant under conditions of maximum vasodilation:

$$\frac{P_a - P_v}{P_w - P_v} = 1 + \frac{R_c}{R} = \text{constant} \qquad (1)$$

$$\frac{Q_s^{(2)}}{Q_s^{(1)}} = \frac{P_d^{(2)} - P_w^{(2)}}{P_d^{(1)} - P_w^{(1)}}$$

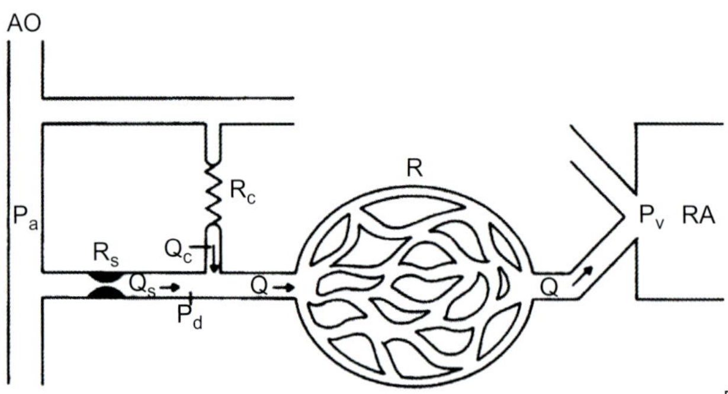

$$\frac{FFR_{cor}^{(2)}}{FFR_{cor}^{(1)}} = \left(1 - \frac{\Delta^{(2)}P}{P_a^{(2)} - P_w^{(2)}}\right) : \left(1 - \frac{\Delta^{(1)}P}{P_a^{(1)} - P_w^{(1)}}\right)$$

$$\frac{Q^{(2)}}{Q^{(1)}} = \frac{P_d^{(2)} - P_v^{(2)}}{P_d^{(1)} - P_v^{(1)}}$$

$$\frac{FFR_{myo}^{(2)}}{FFR_{myo}^{(1)}} = \left(1 - \frac{\Delta^{(2)}P}{P_a^{(2)} - P_v^{(2)}}\right) : \left(1 - \frac{\Delta^{(1)}P}{P_a^{(1)} - P_v^{(1)}}\right)$$

$$\frac{Q_c^{(2)}}{Q_c^{(1)}} = \frac{\Delta^{(2)}P}{\Delta^{(1)}P}$$

FIGURE 14.3 Derivation and experimental basis for FFR. Reprinted with permission from Pijls NH, van Son JA, Kirkeeide RL, De Bruyne B, Gould KL. Experimental basis of determining maximum coronary, myocardial, and collateral blood flow by pressure measurements for assessing functional stenosis severity before and after percutaneous transluminal coronary angioplasty. *Circulation*. 1993;87:1354-1367.

flow and the subsequent rise in distal coronary pressure. For clinical purposes, FFRmyo is now commonly equated to an "FFR" measurement, as it more comprehensively predicts myocardial perfusion pressure and thus the extent of myocardial ischemia.

Finally, the original FFR equation also incorporated right atrial pressure, as it represents a resistance distal to the myocardial capillary system. However, right atrial pressure is typically very low and, for simplicity reasons, can be negated in most clinical FFR measurements.[4]

Core Concept of FFR

The core FFR concept demonstrates the relationship between hyperemic myocardial blood flow and hyperemic coronary perfusion pressure, which are directly related (**FIGURE 14.4**). FFR is thus the theoretical construct of hyperemic coronary blood flow in the presence of a coronary stenosis divided by hyperemic coronary blood flow in the hypothetical case of absence of any coronary artery disease. Under those circumstances, any degree of stenosis or pressure drop will be compared with the normal state and thus the "normal" value for FFR is 1.

FFR is derived by dividing the pressure distal to a coronary stenosis or Pd by the pressure proximal to a stenosis or Pa under maximal hyperemia (for practical purposes aortic pressure is used and measured from the tip of the guiding catheter). As demonstrated in the illustration, a normal FFR is 1 in the absence of any coronary lesions. In the presence of a focal stenosis, there may be a pressure drop distal to the lesion; in this example the proximal or aortic pressure is 100 mm Hg and the distal coronary pressure is 70 mm Hg, yielding an FFR of 0.70. Note that the right atrial or venous pressure is assumed to be ~0 mm Hg and thus not incorporated into the equation.

The importance of inducing myocardial hyperemia has been elegantly demonstrated by Gould et al in a dog model of coronary physiology (**FIGURE 14.5**).[5] The coefficient for pressure loss across a stenotic lesion increases with the degree of stenosis. However, an increase in coronary flow velocity will produce a substantial increase in stenosis resistance and thus will cause an increase in pressure gradient. Depending on the severity of the stenosis, the pressure/flow relationship will result in various steepness of the curve with more significant stenosis producing a steeper curve. In the presence of a moderate stenosis, an increase in coronary flow velocity (which is achieved by inducing coronary hyperemia) will create a significant pressure gradient from 10 mm Hg at baseline to 37 mm Hg with hyperemia and thus "unmask" a significant coronary stenosis.

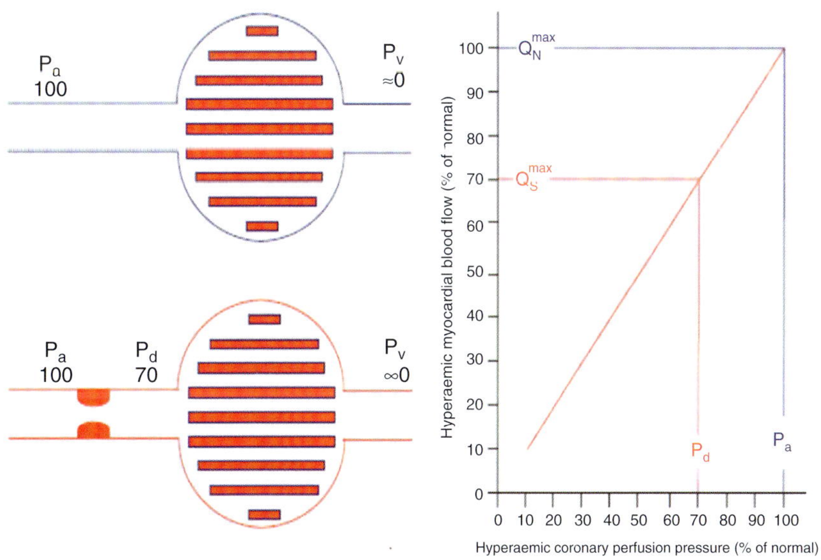

$$FFR_{myo} = \frac{\text{Hyperemic CBF}_{\text{lesion}}}{\text{Hyperemic CBF}_{\text{no lesion}}}$$

FIGURE 14.4 Core concept of FFR. Redrawn from Pijls NH, van Son JA, Kirkeeide RL, De Bruyne B, Gould KL. Experimental basis of determining maximum coronary, myocardial, and collateral blood flow by pressure measurements for assessing functional stenosis severity before and after percutaneous transluminal coronary angioplasty. *Circulation.* 1993;87:1354-1367.

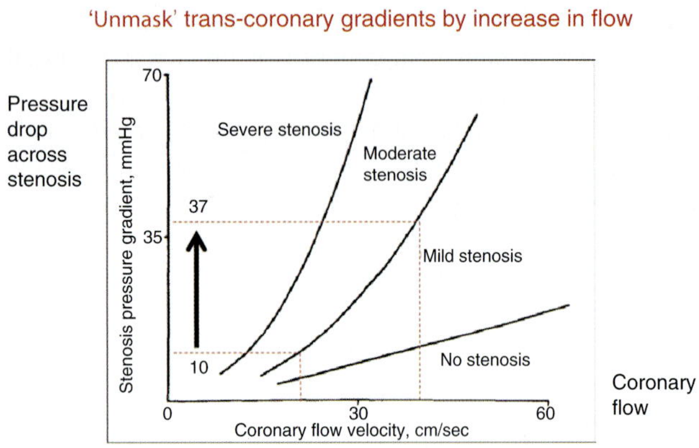

FIGURE 14.5 Pressure/flow relationship. Redrawn from Gould KL. Pressure-flow characteristics of coronary stenoses in unsedated dogs at rest and during coronary vasodilation. *Circ Res*. 1978;43:242-253.

Coronary Pressure Remains Constant Throughout the Coronary Tree

The coronary pressure tree exhibits the hemodynamic principle of sustained pressure through a system in parallel (**FIGURE 14.6**). As resistance increases with lower luminal diameter, flow in the individual branches decreases. However, coronary pressure remains unchanged in the absence of significant coronary artery disease. This constitutes one of the reasons why it is preferable to measure coronary pressure instead of coronary flow.

Myocardial Perfusion Area Factored in by FFR

FFR is affected by both degree of coronary stenosis and myocardial bed supplied by the epicardial coronary vessel. FFR will be higher (and more likely negative) in vessels that do not supply a large myocardial bed (**FIGURE 14.7**). Consequently, a coronary stenosis has to be of higher severity to produce the same degree of FFR reduction when compared with a lesion located in a large coronary artery that serves a large amount of myocardium. This is a very important concept and frequently leads to a "visual versus physiology" mismatch, where coronary lesions appear to be severe by coronary angiography but only have a modest impact on producing myocardial ischemia (**FIGURE 14.8**).[6] Other reasons that result in the same phenomenon are previous myocardial infarction with significant scar formation, microvascular disease, nondominant vessel or coronary branches that supply a small amount of myocardium.

FIGURE 14.7 exhibits that for the same degree of coronary stenosis, the FFR value can be very different based on the amount of viable myocardium that is supplied by the vessel. If half of the myocardial territory is replaced by scar tissue from a prior myocardial infarction, the resulting FFR will be substantially higher (indicating less myocardial ischemia) when compared with a large amount of viable myocardium.

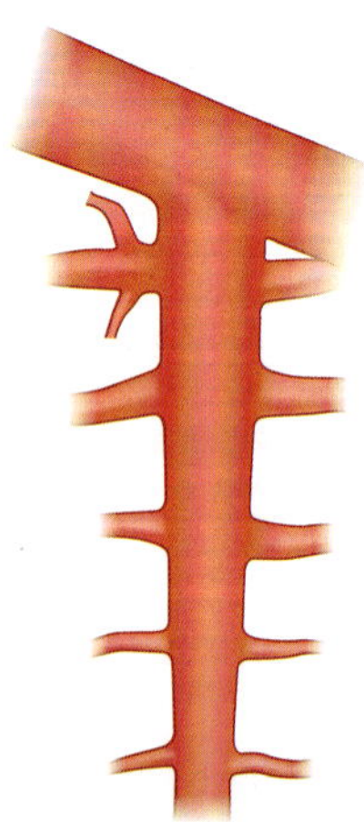

Pressure (mm Hg)	Flow (mL/m)	Resistance (mm Hg/mL/m)	Vessel diameter (mm)
90	200	0.5	4.1
90	150	0.7	3.5
90	100	1.0	3.0
90	75	1.5	2.5
90	50	2.1	2.0
90	25	4.0	1.6

FIGURE 14.6 Coronary pressure remains constant throughout the coronary tree.

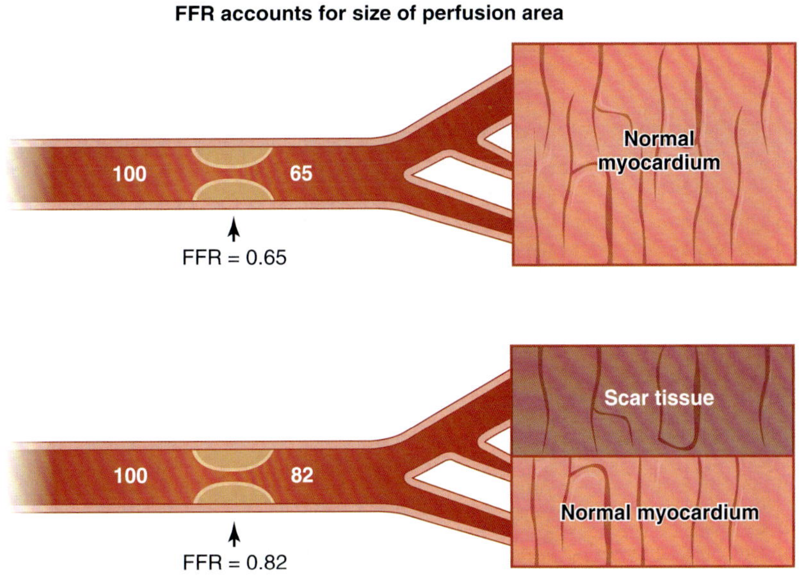

FIGURE 14.7 Myocardial perfusion area factored in by FFR.

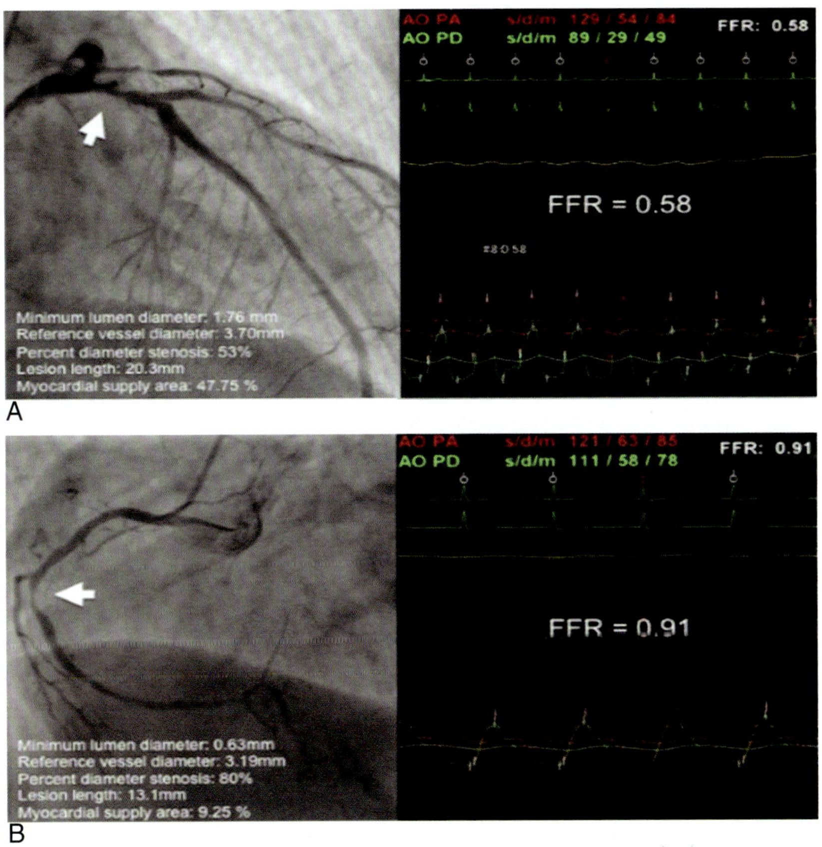

FIGURE 14.8 **A and B**, Myocardial perfusion area factored in by FFR. Reprinted with permission from Shiono Y, Kubo T, Tanaka A, et al. Impact of myocardial supply area on the transstenotic hemodynamics as determined by fractional flow reserve. *Cathet Cardiovasc Interv*. 2014;84:406-413.

Similarly, in the presence of significant collateral flow, the distal perfusion pressure will increase, leading to higher Pd and thus to a higher FFR, despite a similar degree of coronary stenosis (FIGURE 14.9). The fundamental advantage of using FFR, therefore, is the fact that it accurately reflects myocardial perfusion pressure and thus potential for myocardial ischemia, factoring in variables such as size of myocardial territory, viability of myocardium, and collateral blood flow beyond coronary stenosis severity. The impact of myocardial supply area on transstenotic hemodynamics as determined by FFR has been well demonstrated in a recent publication, which showed that coronary lesion severity and myocardial supply area were similarly predictive of FFR (FIGURE 14.10).[6]

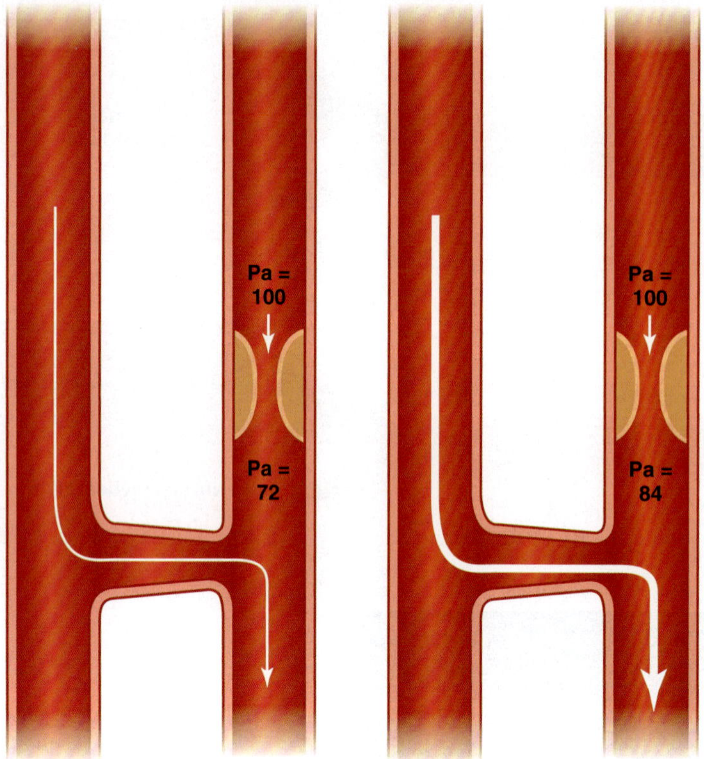

FIGURE 14.9 Myocardial perfusion area factored in by FFR.

FFR as a Continuum of Risk

Although clinical trials have initially used an FFR of ≤0.75 and later ≤0.80 to set the ischemic threshold as a cutoff point for an abnormal or "positive" FFR, it is important to remain cognizant that the risk associated with FFR is a continuum. The lower the FFR value, the more ischemia is present in the myocardial territory that is supplied by the coronary artery and conceptually the greater the risk of an adverse event. Like other biological variables, FFR thus represents a continuum of risk, with lower risk, the closer the FFR gets to the normal range of 1 (**FIGURE 14.11**). Conceptually, patients with very low FFR will have the greatest benefit from revascularization, whereas patients with a normal FFR will have no benefit at all and even potential harm from the

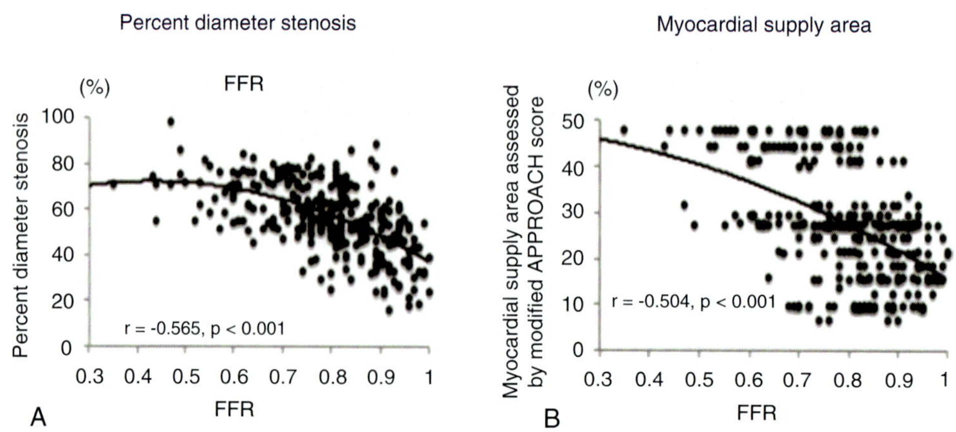

FIGURE 14.10 **A and B**, Myocardial perfusion area factored in by FFR. Reprinted with permission from Shiono Y, Kubo T, Tanaka A, et al. Impact of myocardial supply area on the transstenotic hemodynamics as determined by fractional flow reserve. *Cathet Cardiovasc Interv*. 2014;84:406-413.

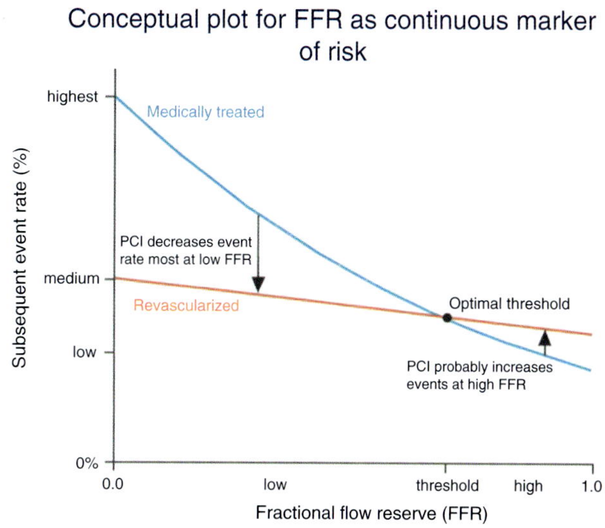

FIGURE 14.11 FFR as a continuum of risk. Reprinted with permission from Johnson NP, Tóth GG, Lai D, et al. Prognostic value of fractional flow reserve: linking physiologic severity to clinical outcomes. *J Am Coll Cardiol.* 2014;64(16):1641-1654. doi:10.1016/j.jacc.2014.07.973.

procedure. Theoretically, there is an optimal threshold at which point coronary revascularization will reduce the risk over medical therapy alone and that will represent the patient population that may benefit most from revascularization therapy. In a retrospective meta-analysis of published data reporting patient outcomes, Johnson et al demonstrated that this optimal threshold for FFR is 0.75 with a gray zone between 0.75 and 0.80 (**FIGURE 14.12**).[7] Similar data have been reported from FAME-2, showing a curvilinear relationship between major adverse cardiovascular events (MACE) and FFR values in the cohort randomized to medical therapy alone (**FIGURE 14.13**).[8] Based on these data, it is recommended to utilize FFR as a marker of overall cardiac risk and not solely as a decision tree for coronary revascularization.

FFR Cutoff Point

Although there is a gray zone between 0.75 and 0.80, an FFR value of <0.80 has been accepted as the cutoff to guide clinical decision-making. A recent observational study by Adjedj et al examined 1459 patients in that gray zone who were treated medically (69%) versus coronary revascularization (31%). MACE was similar between the 2 groups. However, there was a strong trend toward higher mortality or MI (9.4% vs 4.8%, $P = .06$) and overall death (7.5% vs 3.2%, $P = .059$) in the medically treated group[9] (**FIGURE 14.14**).

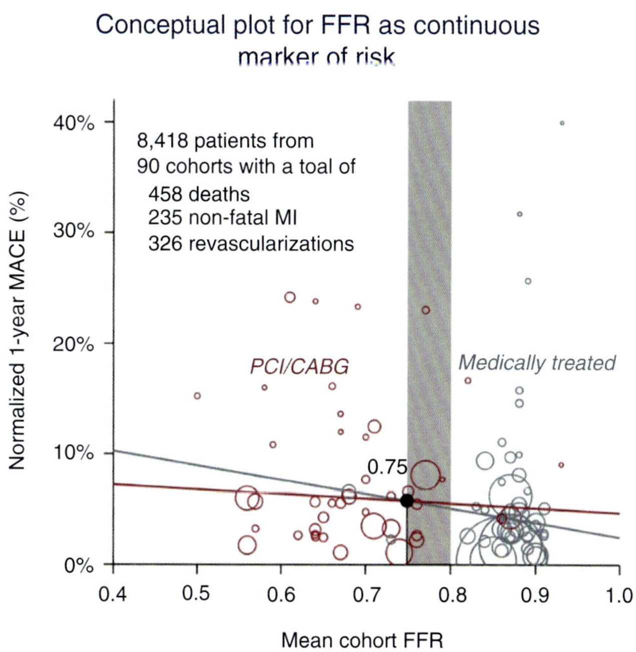

FIGURE 14.12 FFR as a continuum of risk. Reprinted with permission from Johnson NP, Tóth GG, Lai D, et al. Prognostic value of fractional flow reserve: linking physiologic severity to clinical outcomes. *J Am Coll Cardiol.* 2014;64(16):1641-1654. doi:10.1016/j.jacc.2014.07.973.

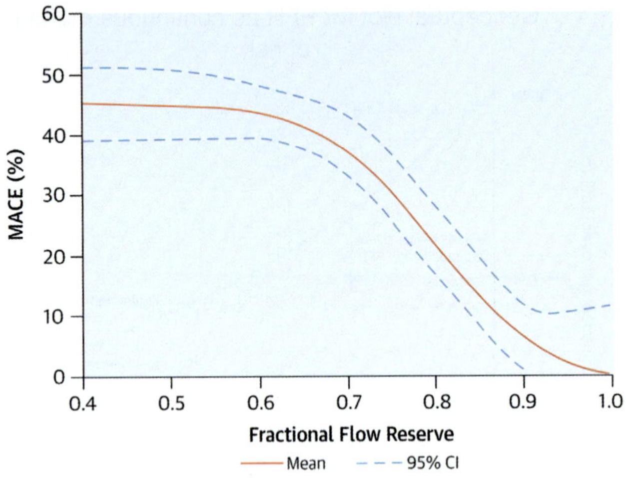

FIGURE 14.13 FFR as a continuum of risk. Reprinted with permission from Barbato E, Toth GG, Johnson NP, et al. A prospective natural history study of coronary atherosclerosis using fractional flow reserve. *J Am Coll Cardiol*. 2016;68(21):2247-2255.

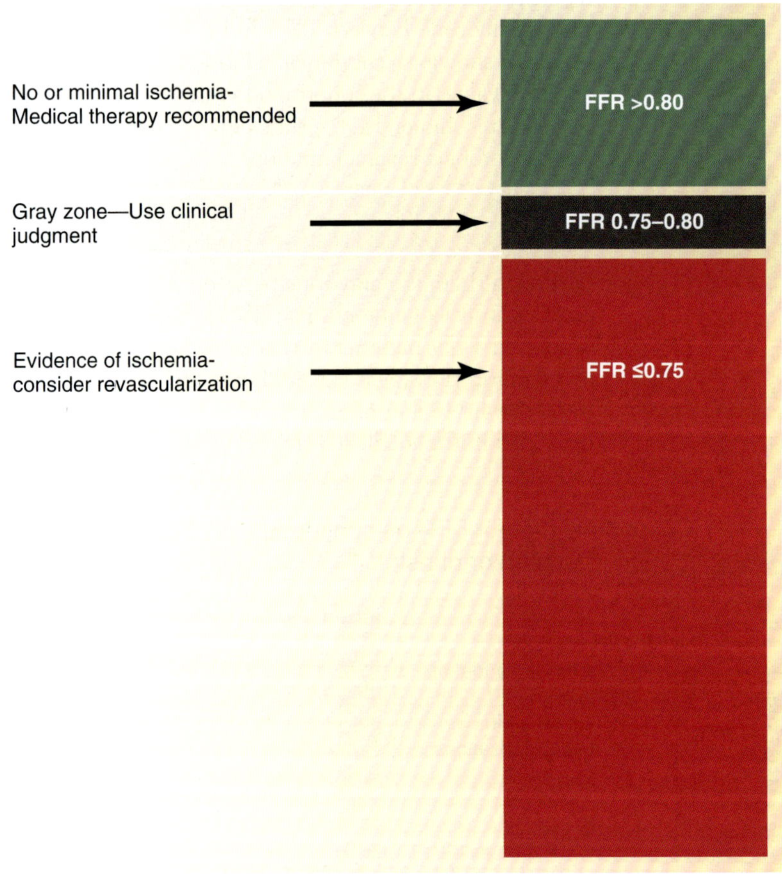

FIGURE 14.14 FFR cutoff point.

FFR TECHNIQUE AND INDUCTION OF HYPEREMIA

Basic FFR Setup

1. Confirm pharmacologic pretreatment with anticoagulation and IC nitroglycerin.
2. "Zero" guide and pressure wire ex vivo to atmosphere on table after flushing with saline (**FIGURE 14.15**).
3. Insert the wire into guide until the pressure sensor and proximal end of opaque wire tip are immediately outside of guide catheter either into aorta or coronary artery (**FIGURE 14.15**, upper right panel). If there is ostial disease, the guide can be pulled slightly back into the aorta, allowing equalization to take place using the aortic pressure.
4. "Equalize" or "Balance" just outside of guide (**FIGURE 14.15**, lower left panel). Confirm that the introducer needle has been removed and guide catheter is flushed free of contrast (**FIGURE 14.15**, lower right panel). The pressure transducer setup should be zeroed at the correct height. The guide catheter pressure should represent aortic pressure. The purpose of this step is to ensure that the pressure from the pressure sensor is equalized to the aortic pressure and thus the starting point is the same for both pressures.
5. Advance wire into the distal coronary artery or at least 2 to 3 cm distal to the lesion (**FIGURE 14.16**). This should be a point at which laminar blood flow is reconstituted distal to the stenosis. Again, confirm that the introducer needle has been removed and guide catheter is flushed free of contrast.
6. Note the resting Pd/Pa and confirm adequate waveforms. It is important to ensure that the aortic pressure is not ventricularized or distorted.
7. **FIGURE 14.17**: Administer hyperemic agent (preferably IV or IC adenosine, see **Table 14.1** and **FIGURE 14.19** for properties and dosing of these medications).
8. Confirm maximal hyperemia—1 to 2 minutes for IV adenosine and 20 seconds for IC adenosine. For IC adenosine, the guide catheter must be well engaged during the injection to ensure adequate delivery of adenosine; it can be slightly disengaged thereafter.
9. Measure the FFR—The length of the recording is generally ~2 minutes with IV adenosine. For IC adenosine, the recording should last about 30 seconds to 1 minute. The baseline, maximal hyperemic phase, and recovery phase should be recorded. The FFR value is measured as the pressure difference at the nadir of the Pd and Pa tracings.
10. Confirm accuracy with pressure pullback (**FIGURE 14.18**) across stenosis and verify that no drift is present with remeasuring Pd/Pa at tip of guide catheter. The 2 pressures should be identical if no drift has occurred.

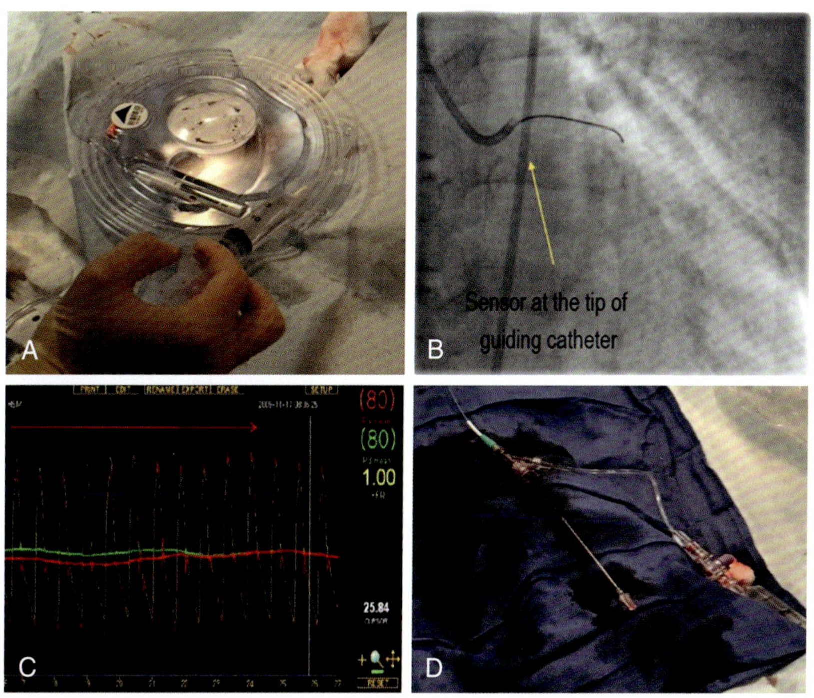

FIGURE 14.15 **A-D**, Basic FFR setup.

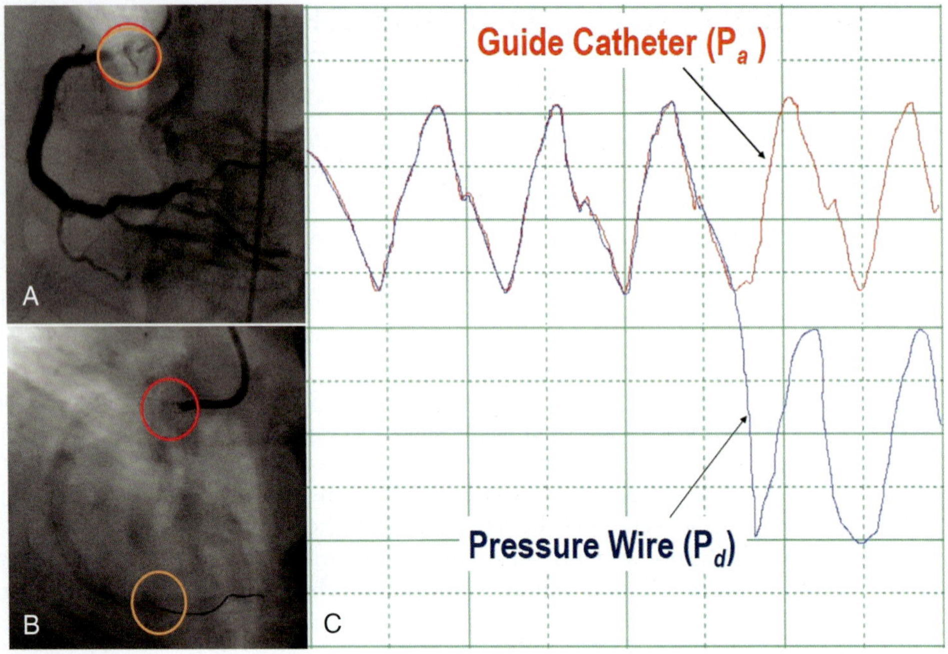

FIGURE 14.16 Basic FFR setup.

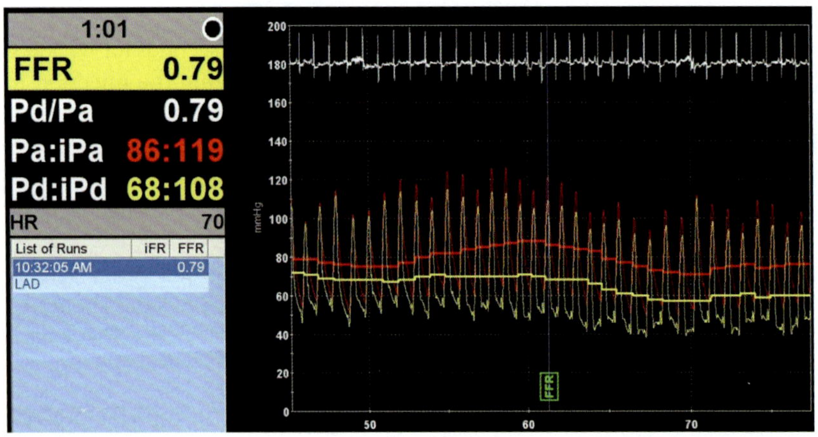

FIGURE 14.17 Basic FFR setup.

Hyperemic Agents

Although intravenous adenosine and intracoronary adenosine are used most often to achieve hyperemia, intracoronary papaverine and nitroprusside and intravenous dobutamine have been used for this purpose. However, they are less popular owing to limiting properties with these medications. Intracoronary papaverine is as effective as adenosine but is associated with QT prolongation and (rarely) torsades de pointes. Additionally, it cannot be used concomitantly with heparin infusions. Dobutamine may cause tachycardia, increasing myocardial oxygen demand; nitroprusside can precipitate undesired hypotension (**Table 14.1**).

Inducing Hyperemia With Adenosine

Adenosine is the most frequently used pharmacologic agent for inducing hyperemia owing to its short half-life and limited side effects (**Table 14.2**). Adenosine can be administered IV or IC. Adenosine IV is administered by nursing through a peripheral IV and should be dosed at 140 μg/kg per minute for 2 to 4 minutes. Adenosine IC should be given in bolus doses of 100μg in the right coronary artery and 200 μg in the left coronary artery (**FIGURE 14 19**).[10] A fluctuating baseline with IC adenosine suggests submaximal hyperemia.

TABLE 14.1

Hyperemic Agents

Drug	Dose	Plateau	Half Life	Side Effect	Pitfall
Adenosine IV	140 mcg/kg/m	<2m		AV block, bronchospasm	Short half life, IV access
Adenosine IC	100mcg in LCA	10s		AV block; pressure damping	No pullback curve; submaximal hyperemia needing increased dosages
Papaverine IC	15mg LCA 10mg RCA	30-60s	2 m	Transient QT prolongation and T-wave abnormalities; very rarely, VT and torsades de pointes	Contraindicated with heparin or heparinized saline due to precipitate formation
Dobutamine IV	10-40mcg/kg/m	1-2 m	3-5 m	Tachycardia, mild increase in blood pressure	
Nitroprusside IC	0.3-0.9 mcg/kg	20 s	1 m	20% decrease in blood pressure	

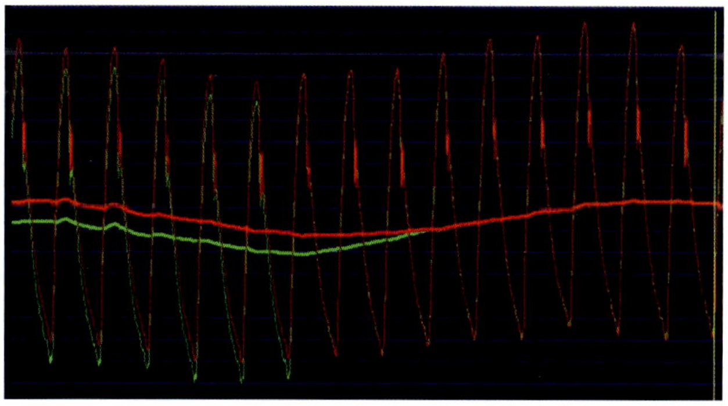

FIGURE 14.18 Basic FFR setup.

Limitations of IV Adenosine as Hyperemic Agent

Although IV and IC adenosine can reliably offer accurate FFR measurements, there is some variability in the hyperemia achieved. Seto et al performed FFR measurements with IV adenosine in 51 patients to examine the variability of hyperemia.[11] FFR was measured for 150 seconds with at least 30 seconds extending past the lowest Pd/Pa measurement. In 28% of the patients, the Pd/Pa ratio changed from greater than 0.80 to lower or vice versa. The valid FFR measurement remains the lowest Pd/Pa observed during the infusion, the so called smart minimum[12] (**FIGURE 14.20**).

TABLE 14.2

Inducing Hyperemia With adenosine

IV Adenosine	
Side effects	
AV block	Rare
Do NOT use in patients with severe (active) asthma/COPD	Bronchospasm
↓BP and ↑HR	Usually 10-20%
Advantages	
Steady state hyperemia	Pullback curve
Measurement of CFR possible	Assessment of microvascular disease
Limitations	
Infusion in femoral vein	Large cubital vein alternative
High-volume infusion pump required	Inadequate infusion leads to suboptimal hyperemia
Setup cumbersome and time consuming	Routine use improves efficiency
Intracoronary Adenosine	
Side effects/Precautions	
AV block	Common; transient
Do NOT use guide with SH	Inadequate drug delivery
Do NOT use guide when pressure damped	Pa underestimated, FFR ↑
Interruption of Pa as short as possible	If too long, peak hyperemia may be missed
Advantages	
Easy administration	No IV setup required No central vein access
Rapid testing	No wait for max. hyperemia
Limitations	
Pull-back curve not possible	Hyperemia too transient
Measurement of CFR not possible	Hyperemia too transient
Dose escalation frequently necessary	Sub-maximal hyperemia at lower doses

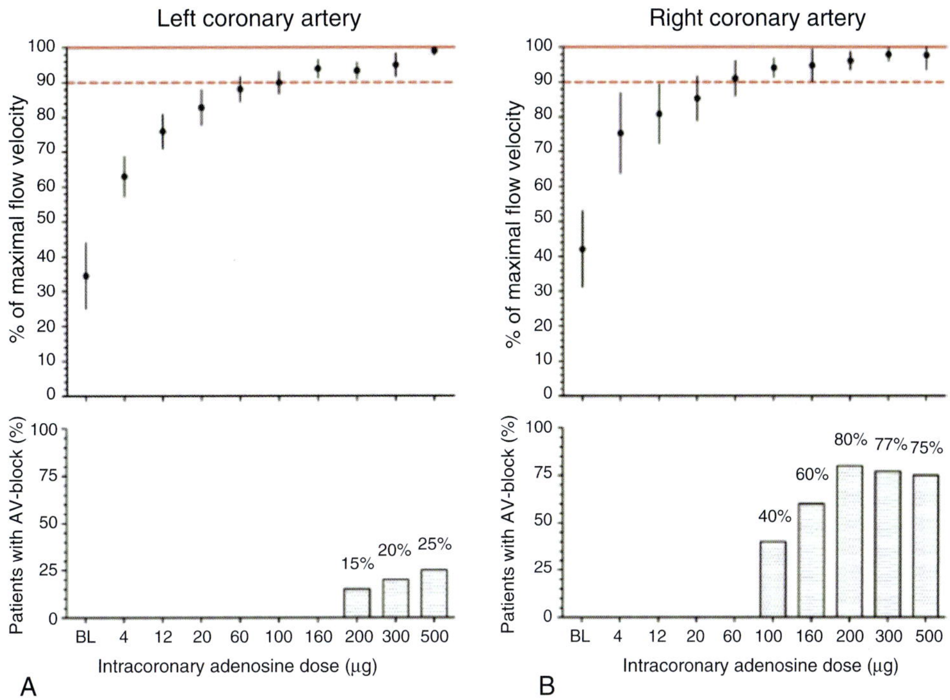

FIGURE 14.19 **A and B**, Inducing hyperemia with adenosine. Reprinted with permission from Adjedj J, Toth GG, Johnson NP, et al. Intracoronary adenosine: dose-response relationship with hyperemia. *JACC Cardiovasc Interv*. 2015;8:1422-1430.

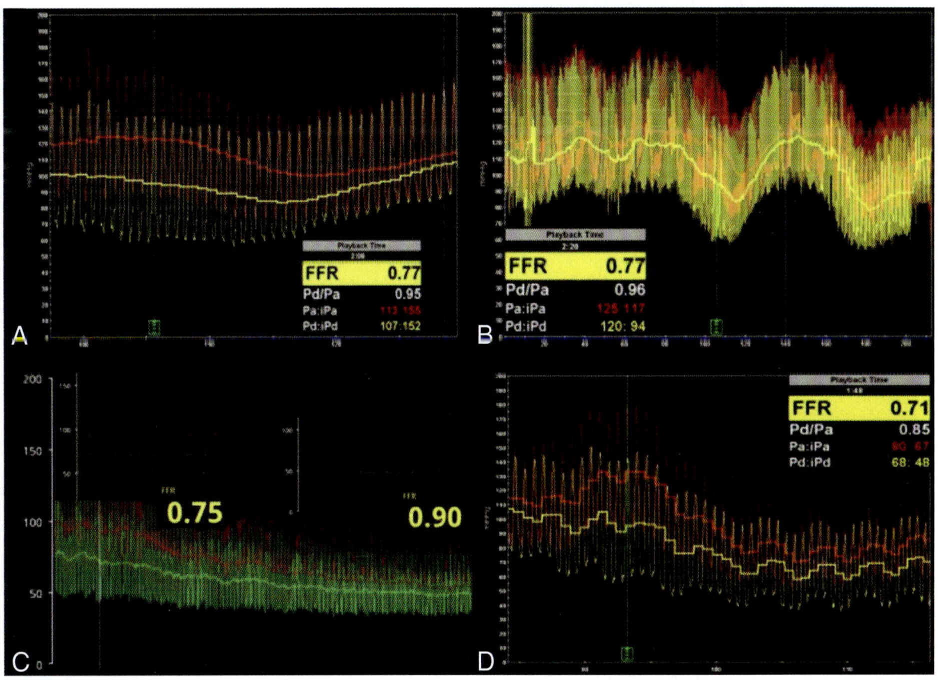

FIGURE 14.20 **A-D**, Limitations of IV adenosine as hyperemic agent. Reprinted with permission from Seto AH, Tehrani DM, Bharmal MI, Kern MJ. Variations of coronary hemodynamic responses to intravenous adenosine infusion: implications for fractional flow reserve measurements. *Cathet Cardiovasc Interv*. 2014;84:416-425.

FFR TECHNOLOGY

Piezoelectric Wires

The most commonly used FFR wires are piezoelectric with a pressure sensor located 30 mm proximal to the wire tip. They are 0.33 mm (0.014″) guidewires with a floppy tip. Piezoelectric wires work on the principle of quartz crystal pressure sensors. When deformed by pressure, they generate an electrical charge that is propagated along 3 electrical wires in the catheter. Some systems offer a wireless system with automatic software connection that reduces the need for peripheral help. The limitations of this technology include electrical pressure drift and suboptimal handling performance of the wire due to the bulky electrical cable inside (**FIGURE 14.21**).

Fiberoptic FFR Technology

Optical sensor wires utilize fiberoptic sensors to detect changes in pressure over a membrane deflector. This technology nearly eliminates signal drift. In addition, the fibers run inside a nitinol or cobalt chromium core, making maneuverability and torqueing close to a typical coronary wire. Similar to the piezoelectric wires, the pressure sensor is 30 to 35 mm proximal to the wire tip (**FIGURES 14.22** and **14.23**).

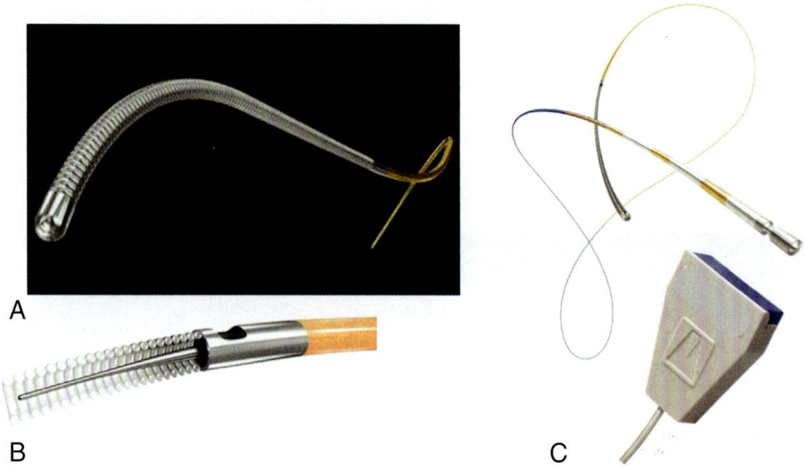

FIGURE 14.21 **A-C**, Piezoelectric wires. Courtesy of Philips Volcano. © 2016 Koninklijke Philips N.V. All rights reserved.

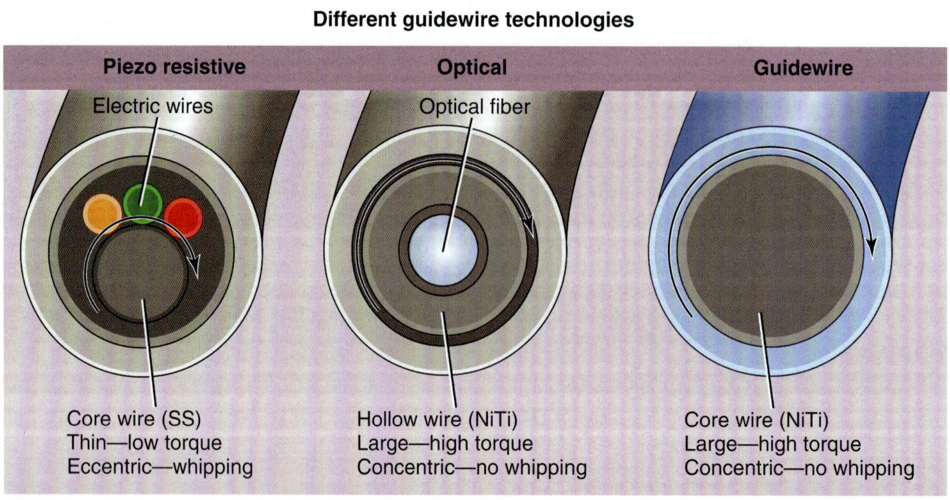

FIGURE 14.22 Fiberoptic FFR technology. Courtesy of Opsen Medical, 750, Boul. du Parc Technologique, Québec, QC Canada G1P 4S3.

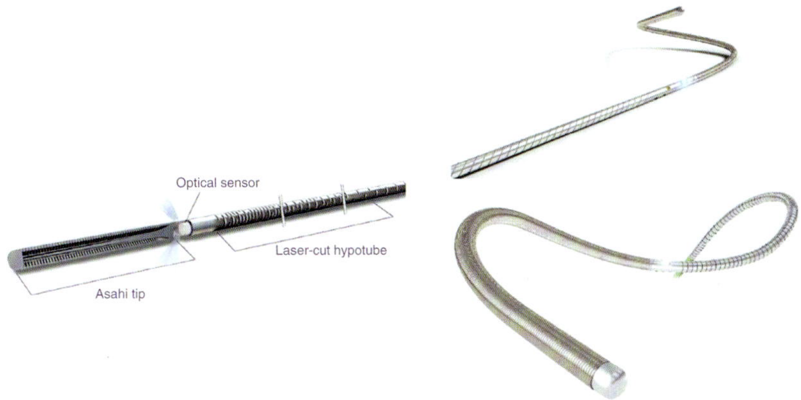

FIGURE 14.23 Fiberoptic FFR technology. Courtesy of Philips Volcano. © 2016 Koninklijke Philips. N.V. All rights reserved.

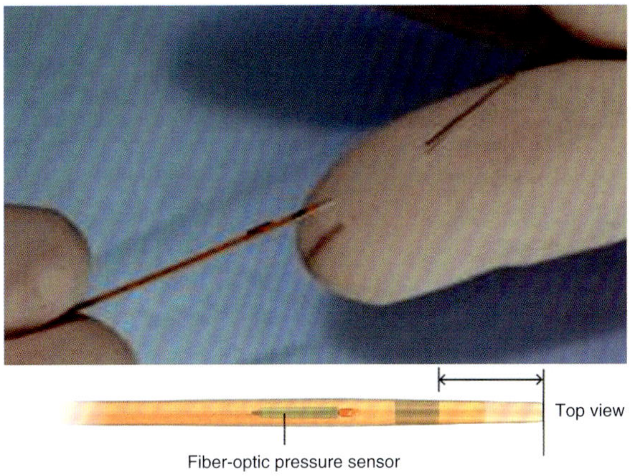

FIGURE 14.24 Rapid exchange fiberoptic microcatheter.

Rapid Exchange Fiberoptic Microcatheter

FIGURE 14.24 depicts a fiberoptic microcatheter that is used as a 0.020 inch monorail over a guide wire of choice. Benefits of the microcatheter include minimal drift due to its fiberoptic technology, evaluation of more complex lesions as the stenosis can be crossed with a regular guide wire, and the ability to do an FFR pullback while the wire remains distal to the lesion.

FFR EVIDENCE

Intermediate Lesions Ideal for FFR Measurement

FFR is ideal for evaluating intermediate grade lesions. **FIGURE 14.25** shows 4 examples of angiograms with intermediate lesions that should be evaluated with FFR to determine their hemodynamic significance, if no adequate noninvasive testing is available.

DEFER Trial

The DEFER trial included 325 patients with a new stenosis >50% of a coronary vessel >2.5 mm in diameter and no evidence of reversible ischemia found on noninvasive testing (**FIGURE 14.26**).[13] Patients were excluded if they had a total occlusion, q wave MI, or unstable angina. Before the angiogram, patients were randomized to deferral of PCI versus performance. FFR was then performed with IV or IC adenosine. Patients with an FFR <0.75 underwent PCI, whereas patients with an FFR >0.75 were randomized to deferral versus performance of PCI. The primary endpoint included all-cause mortality, MI, repeat revascularization as well as freedom from angina and the use of antianginal drugs as secondary endpoints.

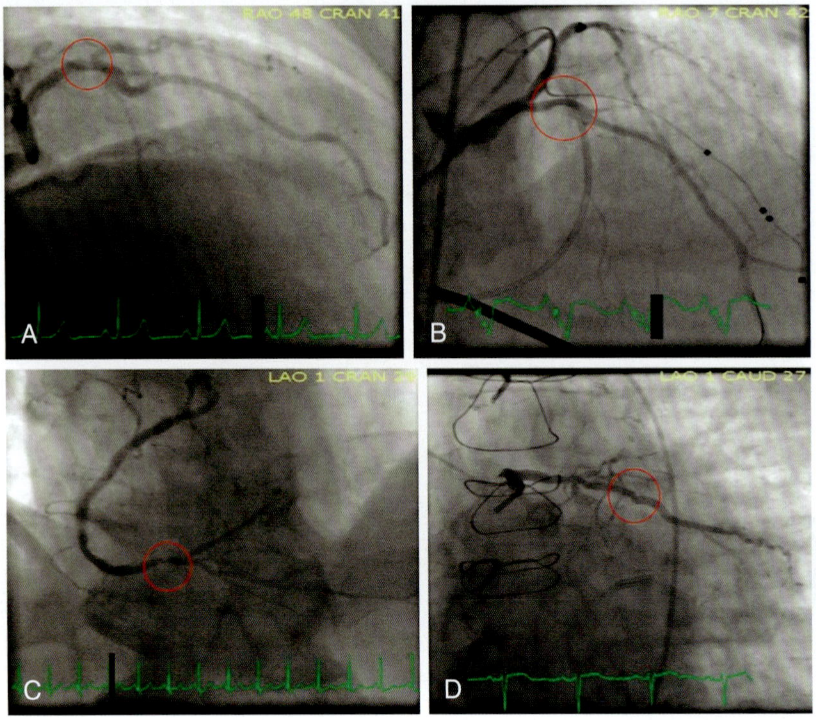

FIGURE 14.25 **A-D**, Intermediate lesions ideal for FFR measurement.

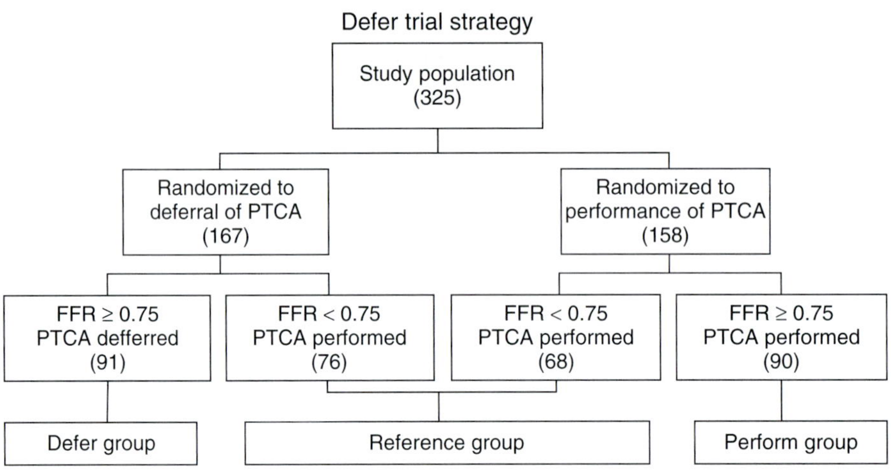

FIGURE 14.26 DEFER trial. Reprinted with permission from Bech GJ, De Bruyne B, Pijls NH, et al. Fractional flow reserve to determine the appropriateness of angioplasty in moderate coronary stenosis: a randomized trial. *Circulation*. 2001;103:2928-2934.

A total of 91 patients were assigned to the deferral group while 90 patients were randomized to PCI. Additionally, 144 patients had an FFR of <0.75 and underwent PCI; these patients were followed as the "reference" group.

At 2 years of follow-up (in 98% of the patient population), the event-free survival was 89% in the deferral group versus 83% in the PCI arm (**FIGURE 14.27**) (P = .27). Event-free survival was 78% in the reference group, which was significantly worse than the deferral group. Use of antianginal and lipid-lowering medications were similar in the 3 groups, but there were significantly more patients free from angina in the deferral group as compared with the PCI group (**FIGURE 14.28**). PCI of lesions that were not hemodynamically limiting did not appear to improve patient outcomes in this trial, supporting the strategy of deferral in patients without documented ischemia on noninvasive testing and an FFR >0.75.[13]

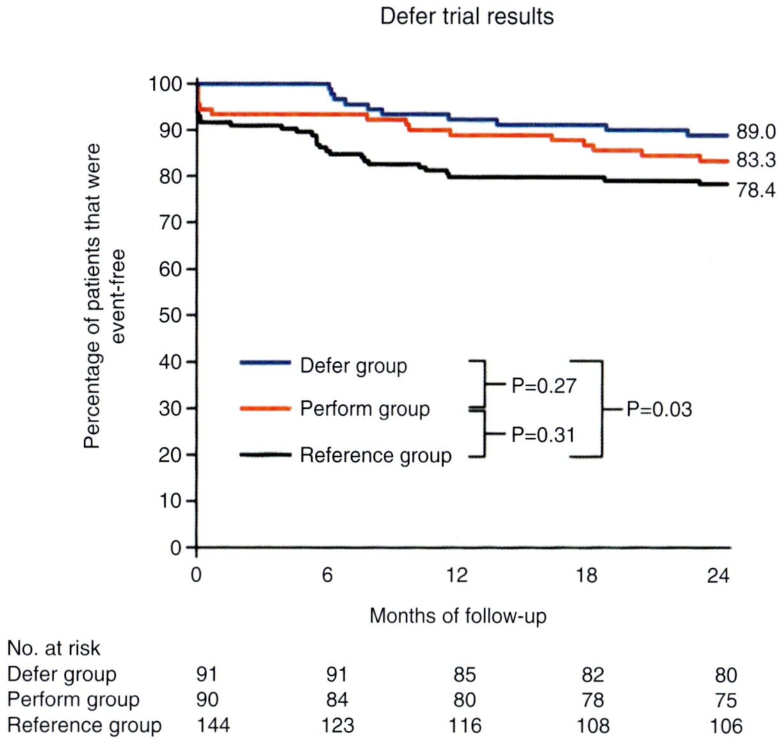

FIGURE 14.27 DEFER trial. Reprinted with permission from Bech GJ, De Bruyne B, Pijls NH, et al. Fractional flow reserve to determine the appropriateness of angioplasty in moderate coronary stenosis: a randomized trial. *Circulation*. 2001;103:2928-2934.

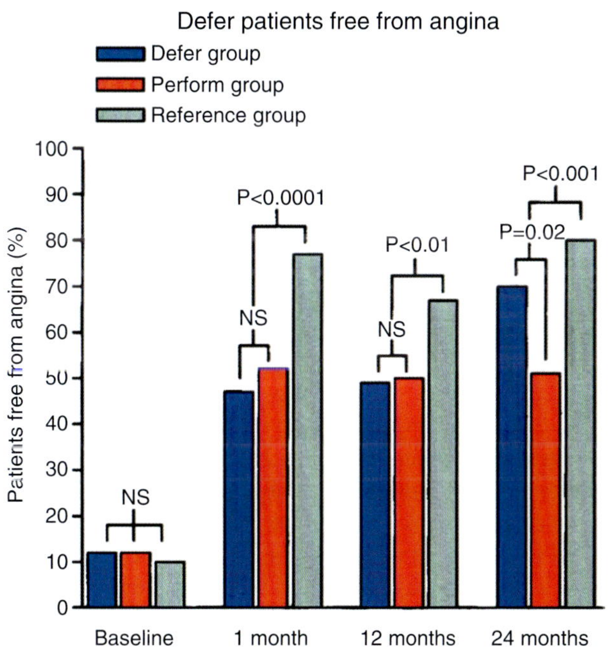

FIGURE 14.28 DEFER trial. Reprinted with permission from Bech GJ, De Bruyne B, Pijls NH, et al. Fractional flow reserve to determine the appropriateness of angioplasty in moderate coronary stenosis: a randomized trial. *Circulation*. 2001;103:2928-2934.

FAME Trial

The FAME trial compared treatment of coronary artery disease based on angiography alone versus physiology-guided PCI by FFR. Patients were eligible for the trial if they had a 50% stenosis in at least 2 major epicardial vessels requiring PCI based on angiographic and clinical criteria (**FIGURE 14.29**). Exclusion criteria included significant left main disease, CABG, cardiogenic shock, prohibitively tortuous or calcified vessels, pregnancy, contraindication to PCI, or life expectancy less than 2 years. Patients were randomized to angiographically guided PCI versus FFR guidance with PCI performed to lesions with an FFR of 0.80 or less. The primary endpoint was rate of major adverse cardiac events (death, MI, or repeat revascularization) at

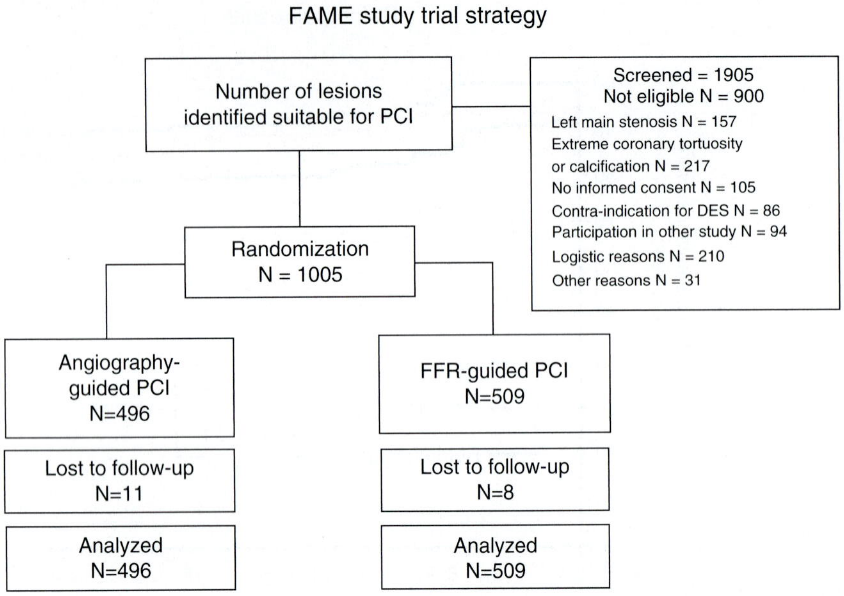

FIGURE 14.29 FAME trial. Adapted from Tonino PA, De Bruyne B, Pijls NH, et al. Fractional flow reserve vs angiography for guiding percutaneous coronary intervention. *N Engl J Med*. 2009;360:213-224.

1 year. Secondary endpoints included procedure time, contrast used, functional class, quality of life score, MACE at 30 days and 6 months, number of antianginal medications used, and cost-effectiveness.

From January 2006 through September 2007, 1005 patients at 20 US and European centers were randomized—496 to angiography-guided PCI and 509 to FFR-guided PCI. 2415 stents were implanted, 96.9% of which were drug-eluting. At least one significant lesion was found in 89.6% of the FFR-guided patients, and overall 63% of the lesions measured were flow limiting. There were significantly more stents placed in the angiography group (2.7 vs 1.9 $P < .001$); while procedure times were similar, more contrast was administered in the angiography group.

Among the 98.1% of patients who completed follow-up, the primary endpoint occurred in 18.3% of the angiography group and 13.2% of the FFR group ($P = .02$). There was a worse, but statistically insignificant, rate of death (3.0 vs 1.8%), MI (8.7% vs 5.7%), repeat revascularization (9.5% vs 6.5%), and angina in the angiography group compared with the FFR group. The authors concluded that the FFR-guided strategy resulted in complete revascularization with fewer stents placed, leading to a significant reduction in 1 and 2 years MACE (**FIGURES 14.30** and **14.31**).[14,15] This strategy was also found to be cost-saving (**FIGURE 14.32**).[16]

FAME II Trial

The FAME II trial set out to determine whether FFR-guided PCI with DES plus optimal medical therapy (OMT) is superior to medical therapy alone in patients with stable coronary artery disease. Patients with stable angina and at least one coronary vessel suitable for PCI were enrolled in the trial (**FIGURE 14.33**). FFR was measured in all patients with adenosine used as the hyperemic agent. Patients with an FFR of 0.80 or less were randomly assigned to PCI plus OMT or to medical therapy alone. Medical therapy included aspirin; a β-1-selective blocker; ACE inhibitor or angiotensin receptor blocker; and a statin with or without ezetimibe to reduce LDL to less than 70. Patients were counseled on smoking cessation and referred to a diabetes specialist if indicated. Those who underwent PCI were given clopidogrel for 12 months. The primary endpoint was a composite of death, nonfatal MI, or hospitalization leading to urgent revascularization. Additional outcomes were the individual components of the primary endpoint, cardiac death, angina class, and nonurgent revascularization. Urgent revascularization was defined as admission to a hospital with persistent or increasing chest pain with or without positive biomarkers or ECG changes with revascularization on that admission.

The trial was stopped early owing to efficacy of PCI in reducing urgent revascularization. By that point, 888 patients had been randomized—447 to the FFR-guided PCI strategy and 441 to medical therapy alone. The primary event rate was 4.3% vs 12.7% ($P < .001$) in the PCI and the medical group, respectively, predominantly owing to an increase in urgent revascularization in the medical therapy group (**FIGURE 14.34**). The rate of all-cause mortality and rate of MI did not differ significantly.[17]

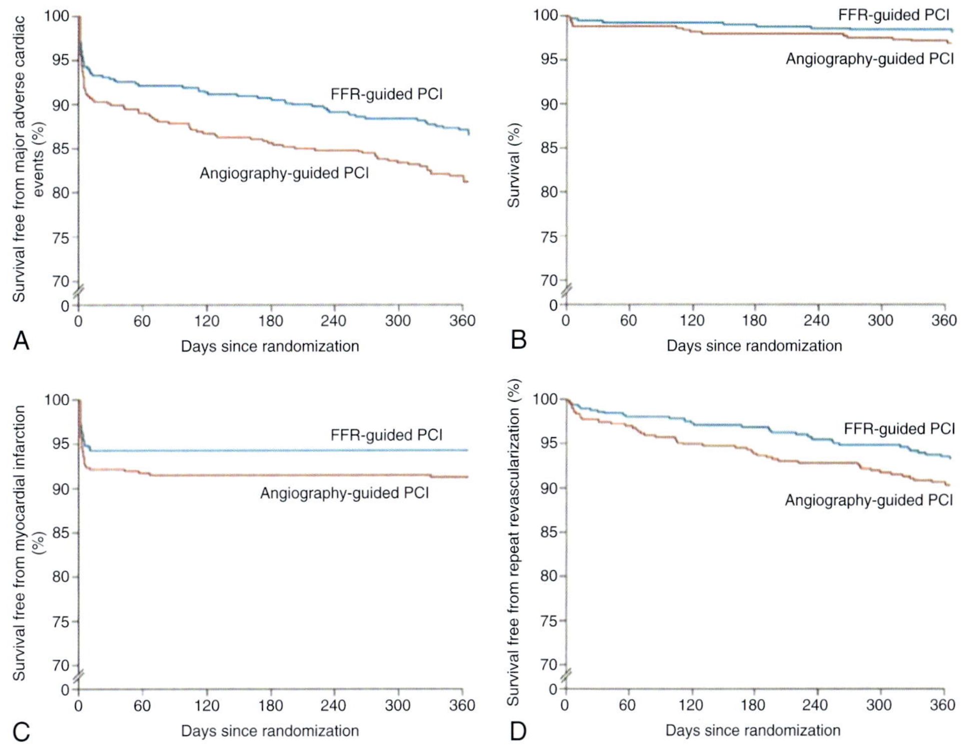

FIGURE 14.30 **A-D**, FAME trial. Reprinted with permission from Tonino PA, De Bruyne B, Pijls NH, et al. Fractional flow reserve vs angiography for guiding percutaneous coronary intervention. *N Engl J Med*. 2009;360:213-224.

FAME: Death and MI at 2 years

	ANGIO-group N=496	FFR-group N=509	P-value
# Indicated lesions per patient	2.7 ± 0.9	2.8 ± 1.0	0.34
DES per patient	2.7 ± 1.2	1.9 ± 1.3	<0.001

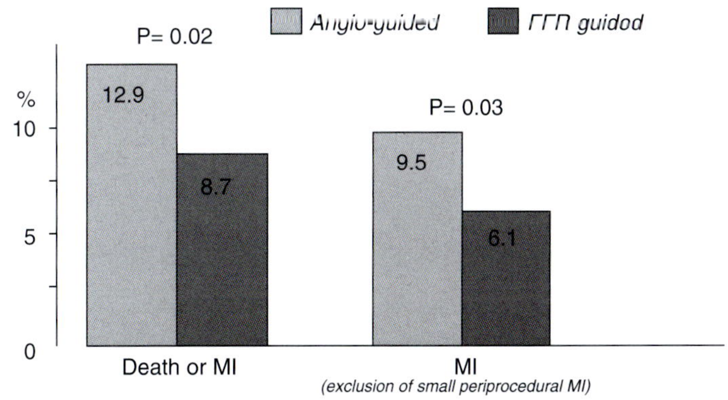

FIGURE 14.31 FAME trial. Data from Tonino PA, De Bruyne B, Pijls NH. Fractional flow reserve vs angiography for guiding percutaneous coronary intervention. *N Eng J Med*. 2009;360:213-224.

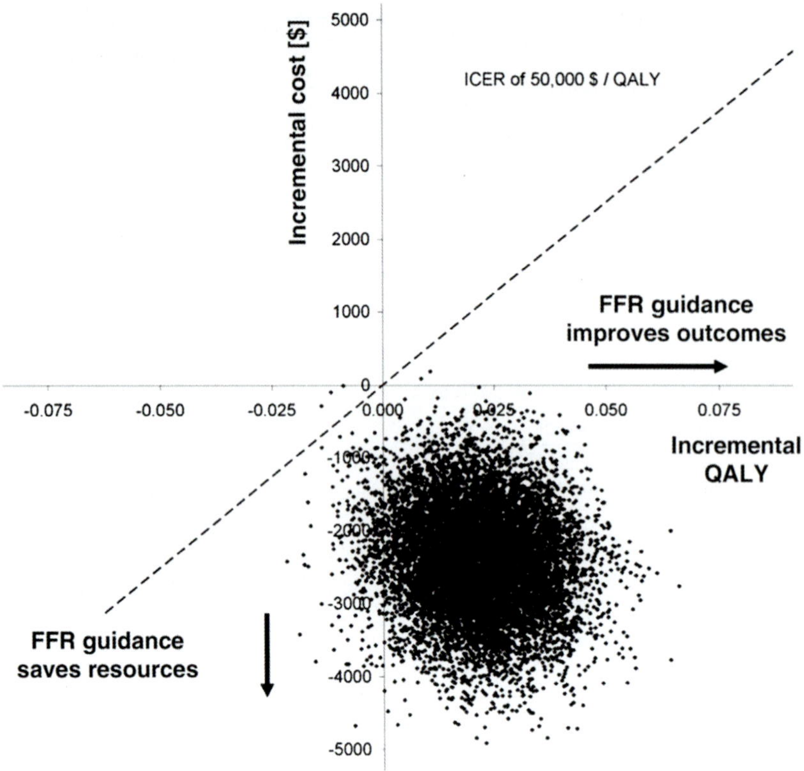

FIGURE 14.32 FAME trial. Reprinted with permission from Fearon WF, Bornschein B, Tonino PA, et al. Economic evaluation of fractional flow reserve-guided percutaneous coronary intervention in patients with multivessel disease. *Circulation*. 2010;122:2545-2550.

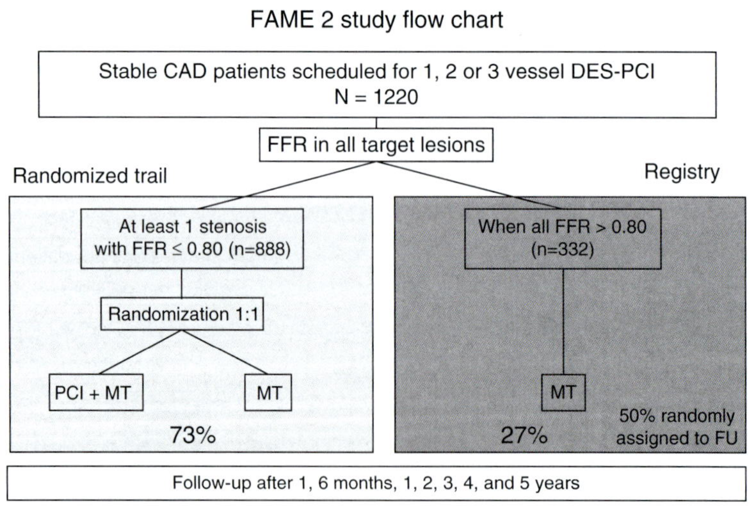

FIGURE 14.33 FAME II trial. Reprinted with permission from De Bruyne B, Pijls NH, Kalesan B, et al. Fractional flow reserve-guided PCI vs medical therapy in stable coronary disease. *N Engl J Med*. 2012;367:991-1001.

R3F Trial

The R3F trial was designed as a prospective cohort study at 20 sites in France. It included 1075 patients with at least 1 angiographically ambiguous lesion (35% to 65%) in a major vessel.[18] Physicians created a revascularization plan based on coronary angiography. The stenosis was then assessed with FFR via intracoronary or intravenous adenosine and the final revascularization strategy was created based on FFR.

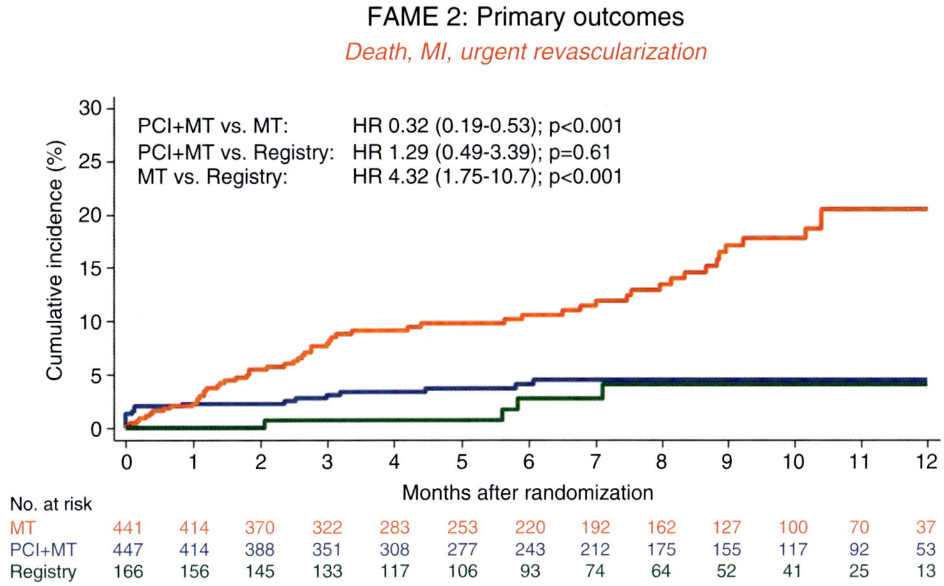

FIGURE 14.34 FAME II trial. Reprinted with permission from De Bruyne B, Pijls NH, Kalesan B, et al. Fractional flow reserve-guided PCI vs medical therapy in stable coronary disease. *N Engl J Med*. 2012;367:991-1001.

A total of 464 (43%) of the patients' strategies were reclassified based on FFR. Among patients with an initial plan for either medical therapy, PCI, or CABG, 33%, 56%, and 51% were reclassified, respectively (**FIGURE 14.35**). Despite the amount of patients reclassified, the percentage or patients prescribed to each strategy remained similar to the percentage before FFR (**FIGURE 14.36**). There was no significant difference in major cardiac events between reclassified versus nonreclassified patients (11.2% vs 11.9%, *P* = .78). The characteristics that made reclassification more likely were percent stenosis, lesion length, and LAD location. This trial demonstrated that a substantial proportion of revascularization plans were changed based on coronary physiology.[18]

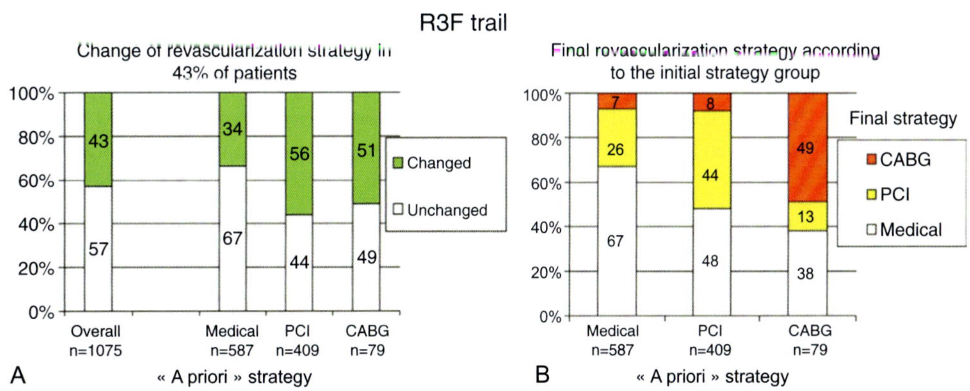

FIGURE 14.35 **A and B**, R3F trial. Reprinted with permission from Van Belle E, Rioufol G, Pouillot C, et al. Outcome impact of coronary revascularization strategy reclassification with fractional flow reserve at time of diagnostic angiography: insights from a large French multicenter fractional flow reserve registry. *Circulation*. 2014;129:173-185.

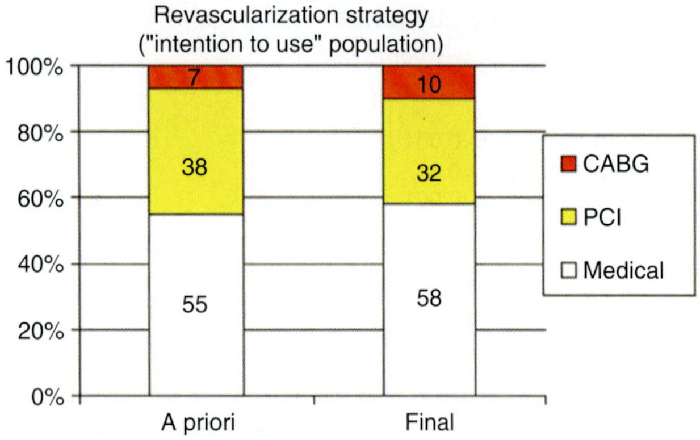

FIGURE 14.36 R3F trial. Reprinted with permission from Van Belle E, Rioufol G, Pouillot C, et al. Outcome impact of coronary revascularization strategy reclassification with fractional flow reserve at time of diagnostic angiography: insights from a large French multicenter fractional flow reserve registry. *Circulation*. 2014;129:173-185.

RIPCORD Study

The RIPCORD trial was an observational cohort including 200 patients with a chest pain history requiring cardiac catheterization. Patients with previous CABG, acute coronary syndrome, severe valvular disease, life-threatening comorbidity, significant renal dysfunction, and angiography within 12 months were excluded. Patients underwent an angiogram and were included if any epicardial vessel >2.25 mm had a stenosis of >30%. The diagnosing physician created a treatment plan based on the angiogram. FFR was performed with intravenous or intracoronary adenosine by a separate cardiologist (**FIGURE 14.37**), and an FFR of <0.80 was considered significant. The initial cardiologist was free to change the treatment plan based on the combined angiographic and FFR data, which occurred in 26%. **FIGURE 14.38** shows a scatter plot representing the FFR measurements in each category of stenosis severity. Even in angiographically severe lesions of >70%, FFR was positive in only 53% of cases. This study reiterates the importance of FFR-guided therapy over angiography alone, as FFR measurements are frequently discordant with visual estimation of epicardial vessel stenosis.[19]

ISIS Trial

The ISIS trial aimed to examine the decision-making processes of interventional cardiologists based on the European Society of Cardiologists recommendation that revascularization should be limited to stenosis causing ischemia and jeopardizing >10% of the left ventricular function (I, evidence A) and the AHA/ACC guidelines to use FFR for patients with stable ischemic heart disease (IIa, evidence A). It was a Web-based study performed among experienced interventional cardiologists who developed treatment plans based on 5 complete angiograms of 12 focal intermediate lesions. Only half of the lesions were functionally significant (FFR <0.80). The FFR and quantitative coronary angiography (QCA) were not revealed to the subjects.

The participants were asked to localize all stenosis, visually estimate the percent stenosis, and determine the significance of each one. If uncertain, QCA, IVUS, OCT, or FFR could be chosen to guide diagnostics. There were 495 participants enrolled in the study, 291 of whom answered all cases. The average stenosis was overestimated by 18% when compared with QCA,

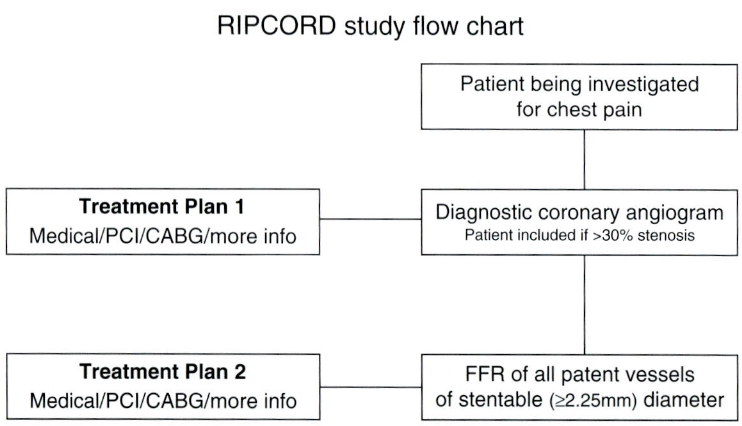

FIGURE 14.37 RIPCORD study. Reprinted with permission from Curzen N, Rana O, Nicholas Z, et al. Does routine pressure wire assessment influence management strategy at coronary angiography for diagnosis of chest pain?: the RIPCORD study. *Circ Cardiovasc Interv*. 2014;7:248-255.

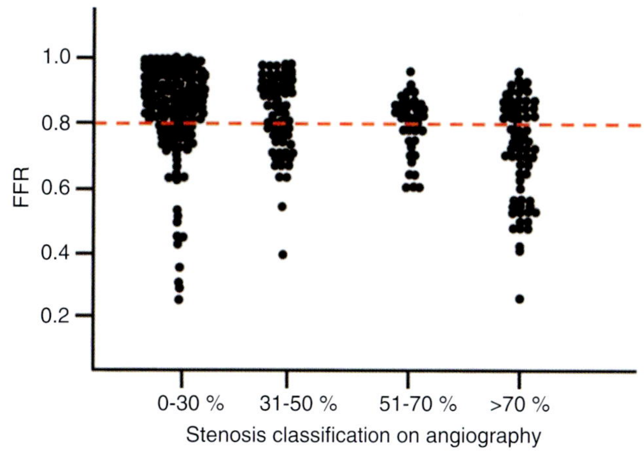

FIGURE 14.38 RIPCORD study. Reprinted with permission from Curzen N, Rana O, Nicholas Z, et al. Does routine pressure wire assessment influence management strategy at coronary angiography for diagnosis of chest pain?: the RIPCORD study. *Circ Cardiovasc Interv*. 2014;7:248-255.

and there were 4421 decisions made regarding stenosis significance. **FIGURE 14.39** shows the individual decision patterns for the 5 cases. Of note, there was significant discrepancy between observers in each of the examined stenoses. Of these, 71% were made on visual estimation alone, ie, without the participants asking for additional diagnostics such as intravascular imaging or FFR. A second modality was requested in 29% of the stenosis with the majority of those being FFR (21% of lesions). **FIGURE 14.40** demonstrates that treatment decisions that were solely based on angiographic assessment correlated with FFR evaluation in only 53% of cases.

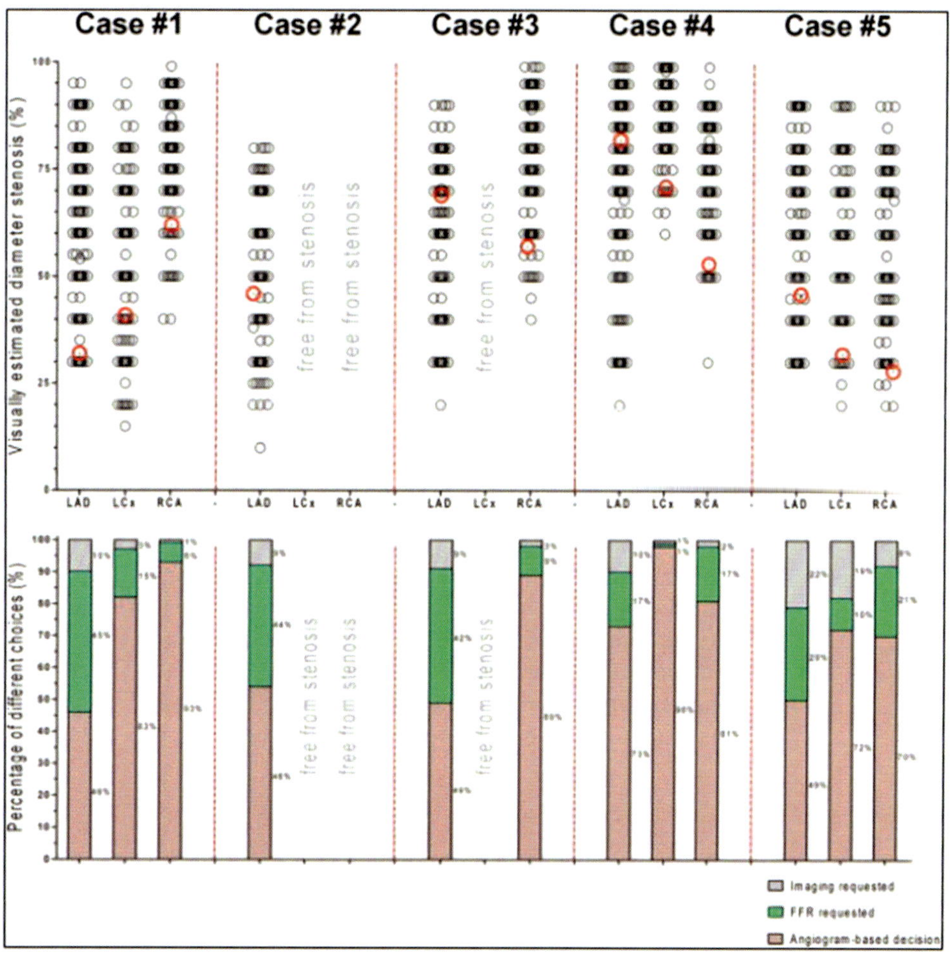

FIGURE 14.39 ISIS trial. Reprinted with permission from Toth GG, Toth B, Johnson NP, et al. Revascularization decisions in patients with stable angina and intermediate lesions: results of the international survey on interventional strategy. *Circ Cardiovasc Interv*. 2014;7:751-759.

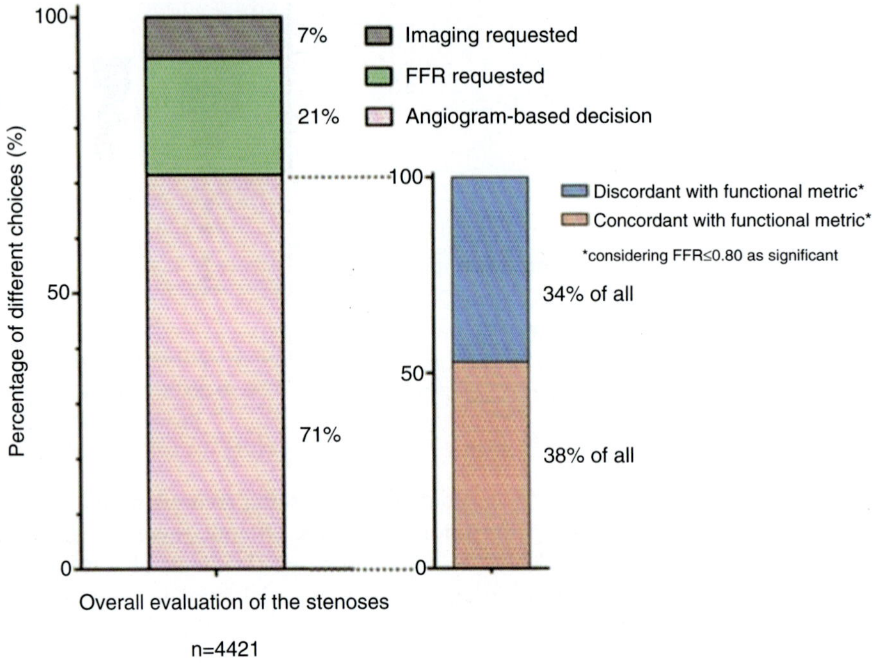

FIGURE 14.40 ISIS trial. Reprinted with permission from Toth GG, Toth B, Johnson NP, et al. Revascularization decisions in patients with stable angina and intermediate lesions: results of the international survey on interventional strategy. *Circ Cardiovasc Interv*. 2014;7:751-759.

This trial sought to determine the adherence of interventional cardiologists with the guidelines for coronary revascularization and the utility of adjunct testing such as FRR and intravascular imaging. The results expose the discrepancy between guideline recommendations and typical clinical practice in which revascularization decisions continue to be primarily based on angiography alone. There was profound interobserver variability of the degree of stenosis and an overestimation when compared with QCA.[20]

HEMODYNAMIC ASSESSMENT OF SPECIFIC CORONARY LESIONS

Tandem Lesions or Serial Epicardial Lesions

Measuring FFR in tandem lesions is challenging, as tandem lesions prevent maximal hyperemia for each individual stenosis and thus "cross-talk" between the separate lesions. A simple FFR distal to both lesions can give adequate information regarding the ischemic burden of the serial lesions in tandem. If the measurement is negative, then none of the lesions are hemodynamically significant. If positive, an FFR pullback during maximal hyperemia can be performed in order to compare the relative pressure drops at each stenotic lesion. In order to maintain distal wire intraluminal presence and second "workhorse" wire can be placed before pullback if necessary. The most obstructive lesion (biggest pressure drop) should be treated first and FFR remeasured to evaluate the residual lesion(s)[21,22] (**FIGURE 14.41**).

Side Branch Evaluation Post-PCI

The approach to treating bifurcation lesions remains challenging as there are higher rates of acute complications as well as an increase in target lesion failure long term. Koo et al followed up patients whose side branch intervention was guided by FFR versus angiography and showed no significant difference in event rates (4.6% vs 3.7%, $P = .7$) with lower rates of side branch interventions in the FFR group.[23] A negative FFR with significant angiographic stenosis can be explained by the small myocardial mass typically supplied by side branches or by an angiographic "Mach" effect induced by the stent strut (**FIGURE 14.42**).

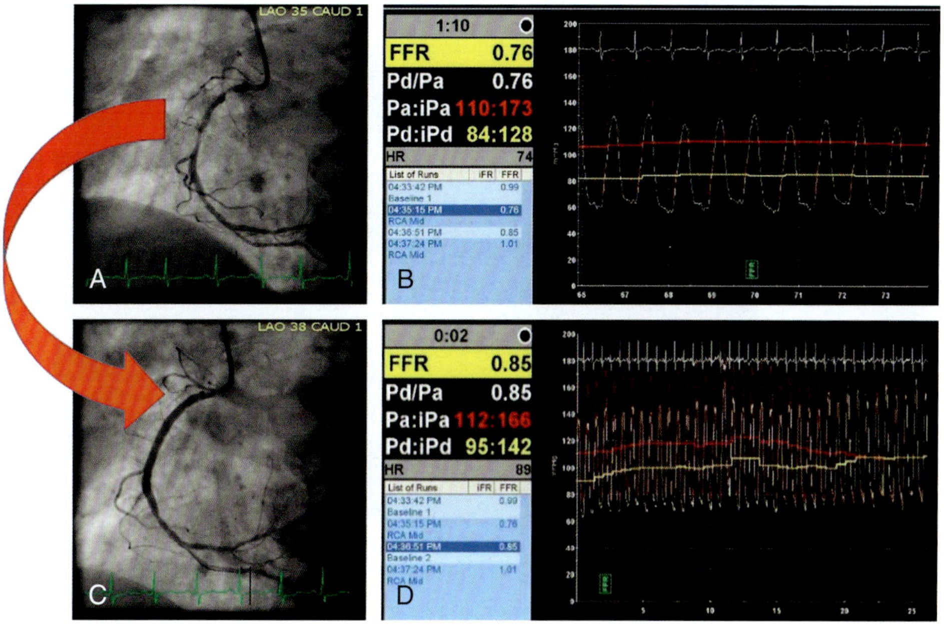

FIGURE 14.41 **A-D**, Tandem lesions or serial epicardial lesions.

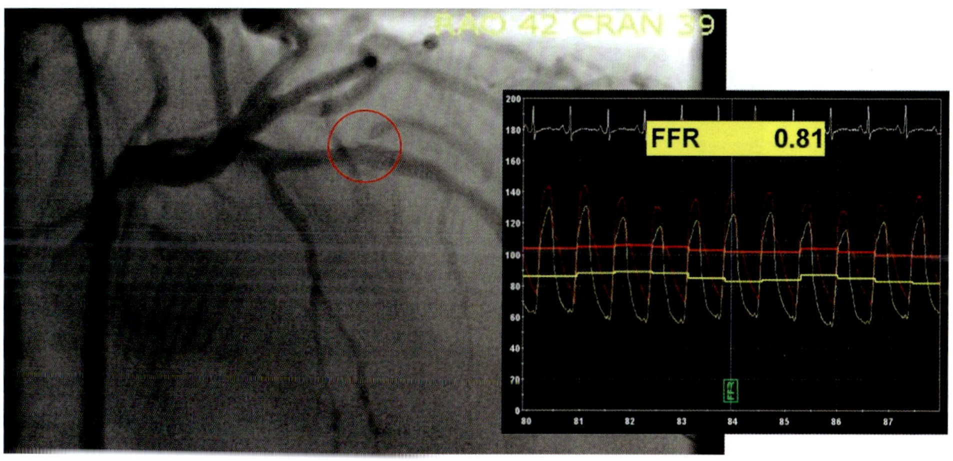

FIGURE 14.42 Side branch evaluation post-PCI.

Collateral Circulation

This figure demonstrates a mild mid-LAD stenosis with a subtotal occlusion of the RCA. Left to right septal collaterals contribute to the right dominant flow. In this case, the FFR is 0.74 because just a mild or moderate lesion on angiography might have a significant hemodynamic effect when the vessel supplies such a large vascular territory (in this case the anterolateral and inferior walls) (FIGURE 14.43).

Branch Vessel Disease

In contrast, when an angiographically significant lesion is present, FFR might be negative if the supplied myocardial mass is small. This occurs frequently in side branches such as diagonal or marginal coronary vessels (FIGURE 14.44).

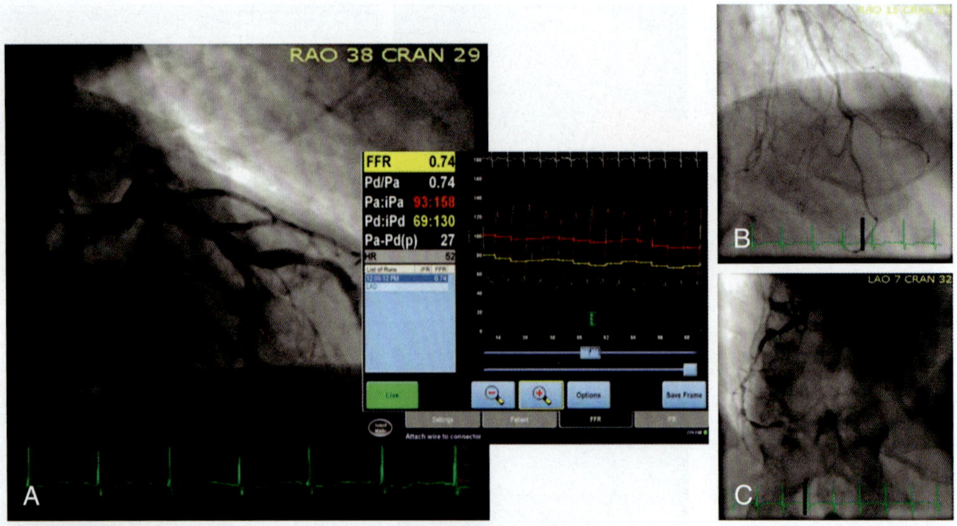

FIGURE 14.43 **A-C**, Collateral circulation.

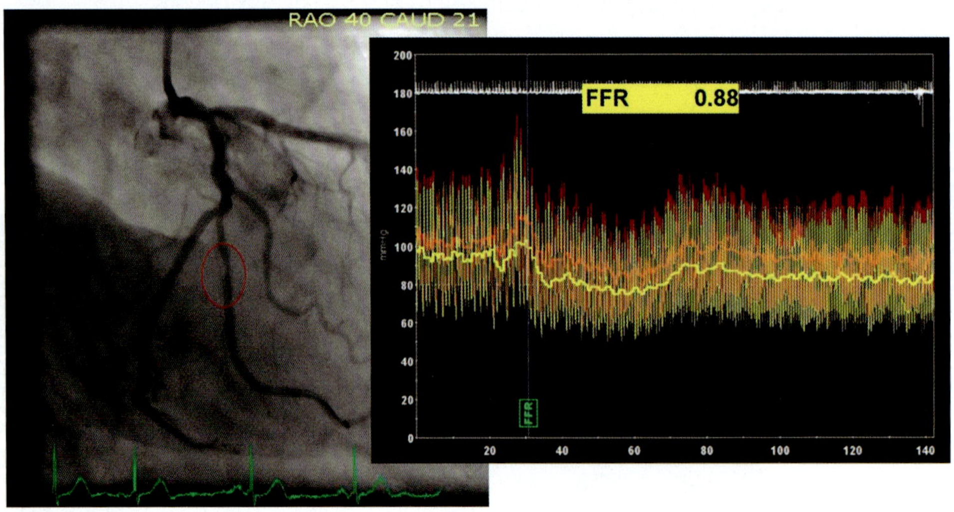

FIGURE 14.44 Branch vessel disease.

Proximal Versus Distal Coronary Stenoses

Despite angiographically similar appearance, proximal vessel disease typically yields lower FFR values than more distal disease. In this example, the proximal LAD stenosis in the upper panel supplies a much larger myocardial territory than the mid-LAD disease in the lower panel and thus the FFR value is substantially lower (**FIGURE 14.45**).

Multivessel CAD

In patients with multivessel disease, FFR can be used to guide the revascularization strategy. Evidence from the FAME trial supports conservative management of lesions that are hemodynamically nonsignificant with an FFR >0.8. This strategy reduced MACE (18.3% vs 13.2, *P* = .02) and was also found to be cost-effective.[14] Using FFR to calculate a "functional SYNTAX" score by including only ischemic lesions led to a reclassification of patients, decreasing the number of high-risk patients, and also proved to be a better predictor of MACE.[24] In this example, a patient with 3-vessel CAD was found to have only single vessel CAD of the LAD after functional assessment with FFR (**FIGURE 14.46**).

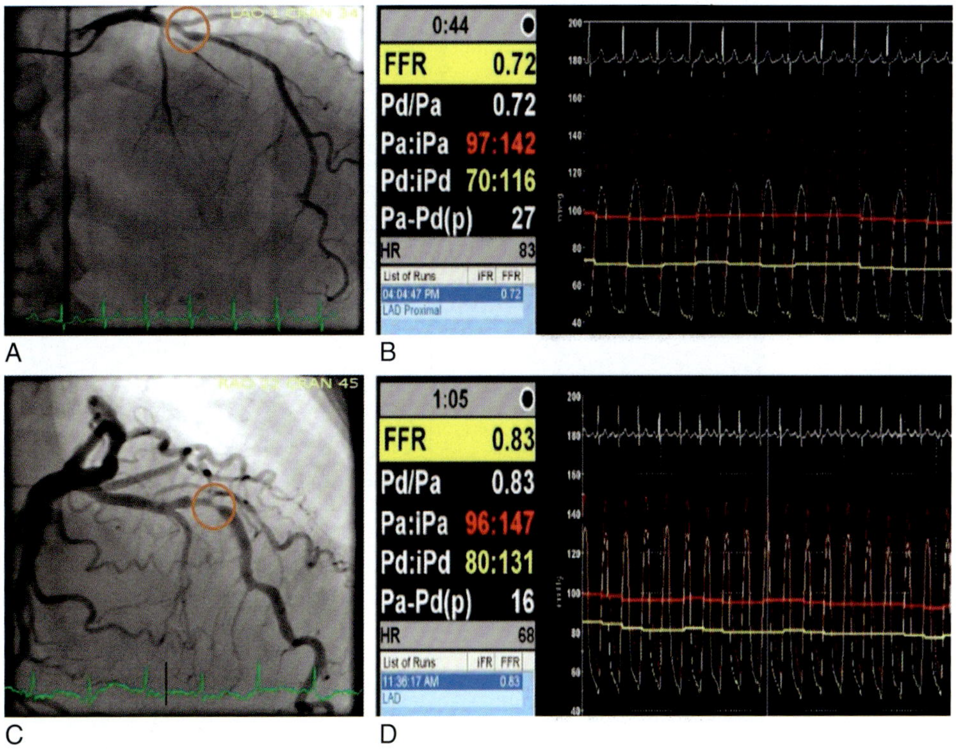

FIGURE 14.45 **A-D**, Proximal vs distal coronary stenoses.

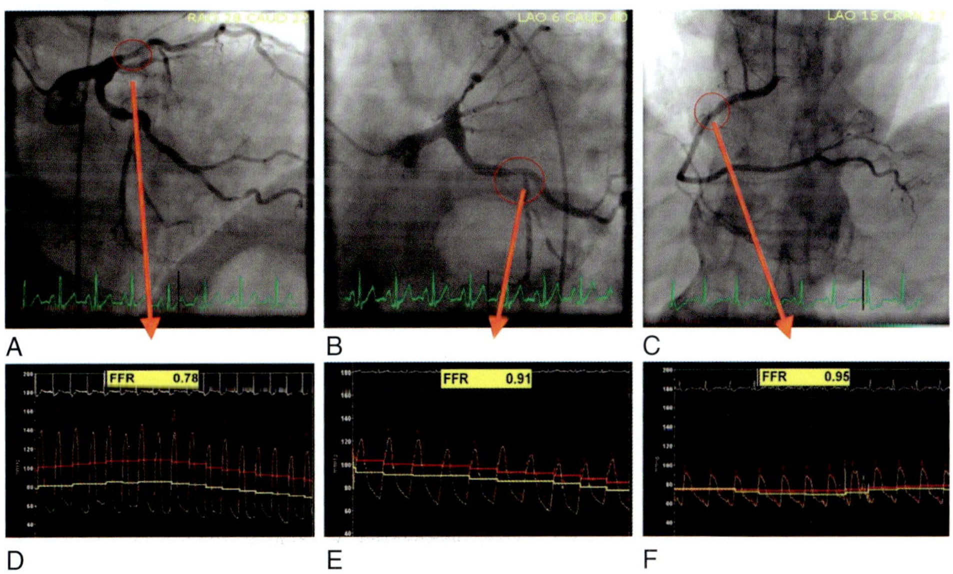

FIGURE 14.46 **A-F**, Multivessel CAD.

Diffuse Atherosclerosis

Diffuse coronary atherosclerosis may lead to significant myocardial ischemia despite the absence of a focal stenosis by angiography. An FFR pullback can help guide therapy and distinguish diffuse disease from multiple focal lesions (**FIGURE 14.47**).

Left Main Disease

Although there are no randomized controlled trials evaluating FFR in the setting of left main disease, a recent meta-analysis demonstrated an FFR cutoff of >0.80 provided reasonable safety for medical management in intermediate left main coronary stenosis.[25] An expert consensus

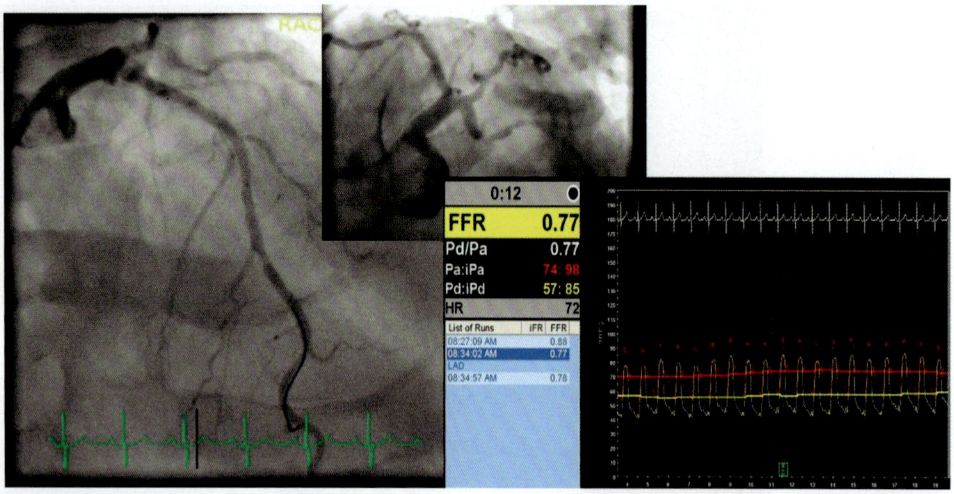

FIGURE 14.47 Diffuse atherosclerosis.

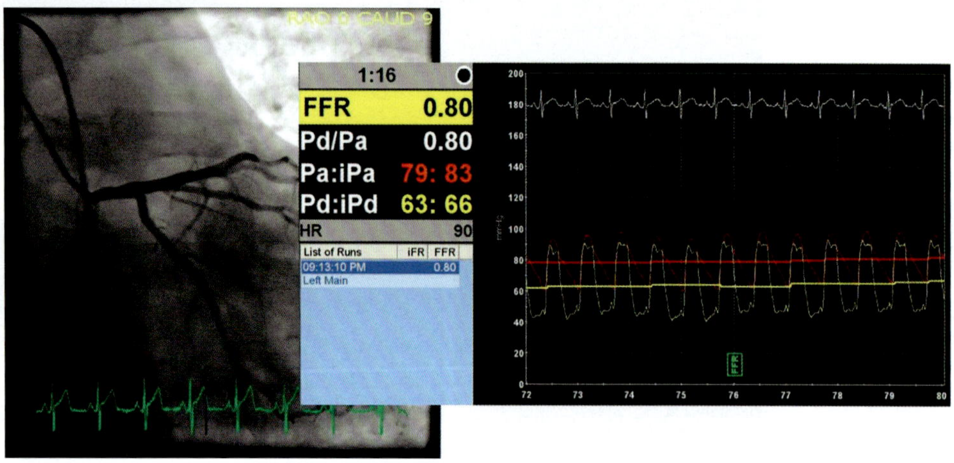

FIGURE 14.48 Left main disease.

suggests a cutoff from 0.75 to 0.80 to guide revascularization decisions.[26] In this example, the left main coronary artery has diffuse atherosclerosis, which is therefore difficult to assess angiographically. FFR was borderline significant at 0.80 (**FIGURE 14.48**).

When ostial left main disease is present, the operator must ensure that the guiding catheter is not engaged too deeply into the vessel to avoid ventricularization of the aortic waveform. Should this occur, removing the guide from the ostium to measure the aortic pressure is critical for an accurate FFR measurement.

Ostial Disease

Similar to ostial left main coronary disease, ostial RCA disease poses a challenge to FFR measurements as catheter ventricularization can occur with deep engagement. This would underestimate the FFR and could cause a false negative reading. In this case example, the guiding catheter is partially removed from the vessel ostium to prevent ventricularization. This should to be done for the equalization of pressures as well as for the actual FFR measurement (**FIGURE 14.49**).

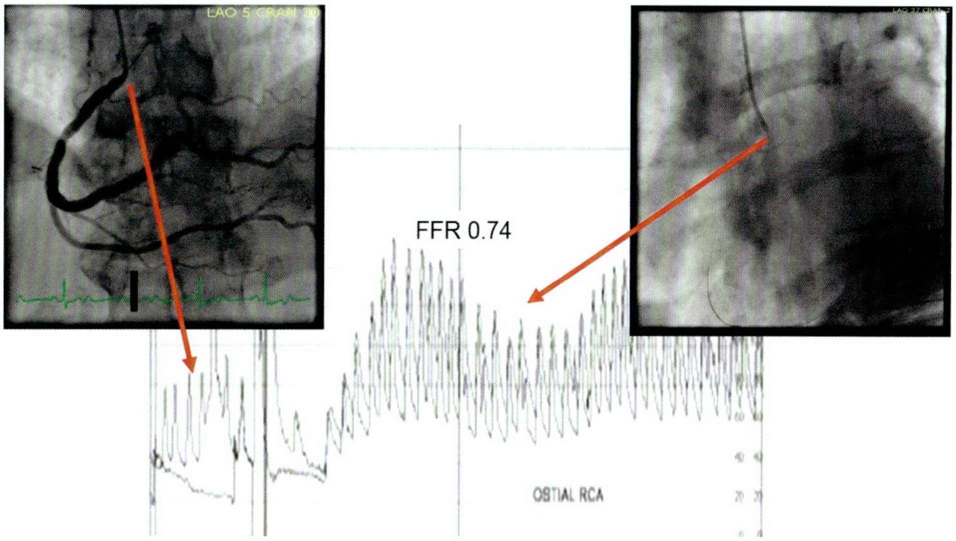

FIGURE 14.49 Ostial disease.

PITFALLS OF FFR MEASUREMENTS

1. **Effect of wire introducer on pressure measurements**

The space surrounding the wire in the introducer may "leak" and decrease the measured aortic pressure. This will underestimate the pressure difference and cause an increase in false-negative results. It is important to remove the introducer before pressure equalization and any FFR measurements (**FIGURE 14.50**).

2. **Aortic waveform distortion**

Distortion of the aortic waveform can occur by contrast residue in the guiding catheter, effectively blunting of the waveform. This can be recognized by a loss of the dicrotic notch and "sinus" waveform pattern. Also, the systolic aortic pressure is frequently lower than the systolic distal coronary pressure. This problem can be easily resolved by flushing the catheter with saline to ensure an adequate aortic waveform (**FIGURE 14.51**).

3. **Catheter ventricularization**

Catheter ventricularization increases with larger catheter size or smaller vessel diameter. It is important to note that catheter ventricularization may occur only at maximal hyperemia as

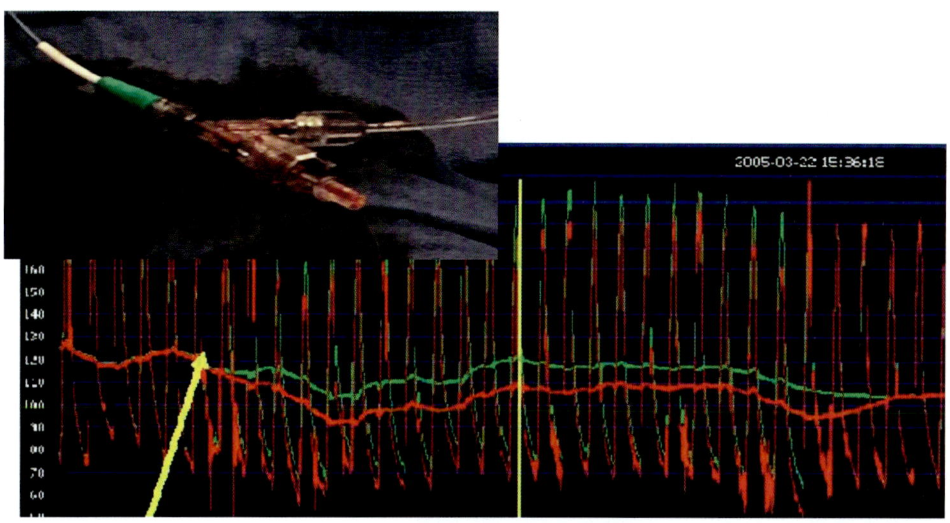

FIGURE 14.50 Effect of wire introducer on pressure measurements.

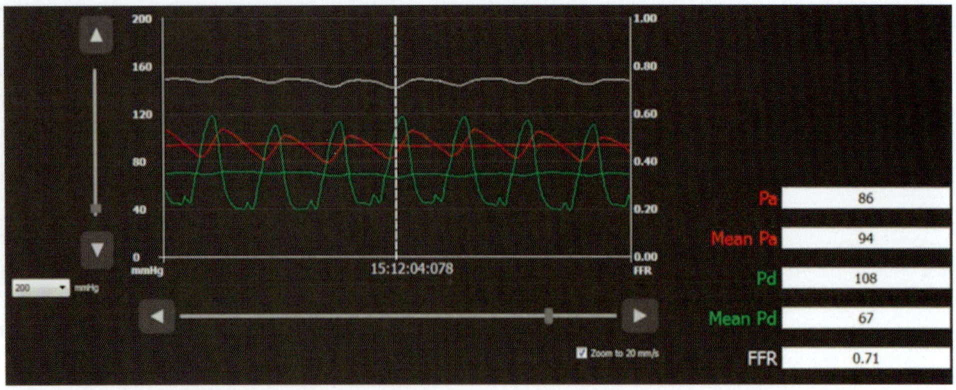

FIGURE 14.51 Aortic waveform distortion.

the increase in coronary flow may "suck in" the guiding catheter into the vessel. Careful evaluation of the waveform is mandatory during FFR measurements. Pressure ventricularization can be corrected by disengaging the catheter from the coronary ostium (**FIGURE 14.52**).

4. **Coronary spasm during FFR measurements**

Coronary vasospasm might occur with the introduction of the FFR wire into the coronary artery. To prevent this, intracoronary nitroglycerin should be administered before all FFR measurements. This is a case example of an ostial LAD spasm that resolved with injection of nitroglycerin. Note that the FFR value increased substantially after the spasm resolved, crossing the threshold from "ischemic" to "nonischemic" (**FIGURE 14.53**).

5. **Signal Drift**

Drift of the pressure sensor is primarily related to changes in the piezoelectric sensor during the measurement and can be minimized by flushing the wire with saline before its use. A large amount of drift could change a decision over the 0.75 to 0.80 "gray zone," and hence a pullback at the completion of the FFR study is critically important to validate the accuracy of the results. The left panel demonstrates signal drift; note that the distal coronary and aortic waveform are identical with the coronary pressure shifted downward. The right panel shows lower distal coronary pressure with significant and adequate distortion of the waveform that is consistent with a significant stenosis (**FIGURE 14.54**).

6. **Whip artifact**

This is an example of a wire artifact that occurs from friction to the pressure transducer. Slight modification of the wire position typically resolves this problem and yields an adequate waveform (**FIGURE 14.55**).

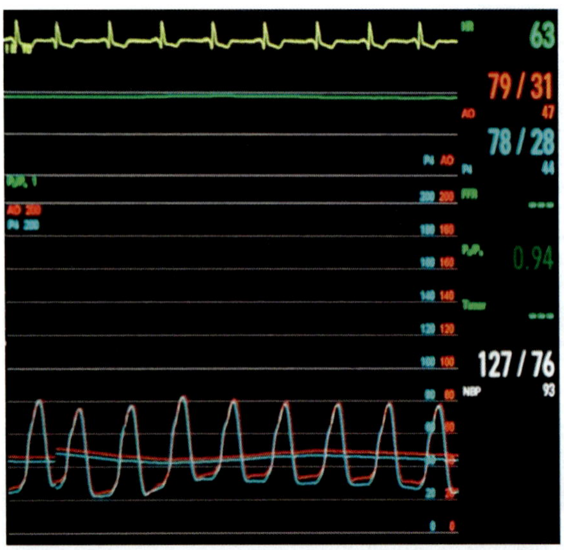

FIGURE 14.52 Catheter ventricularization.

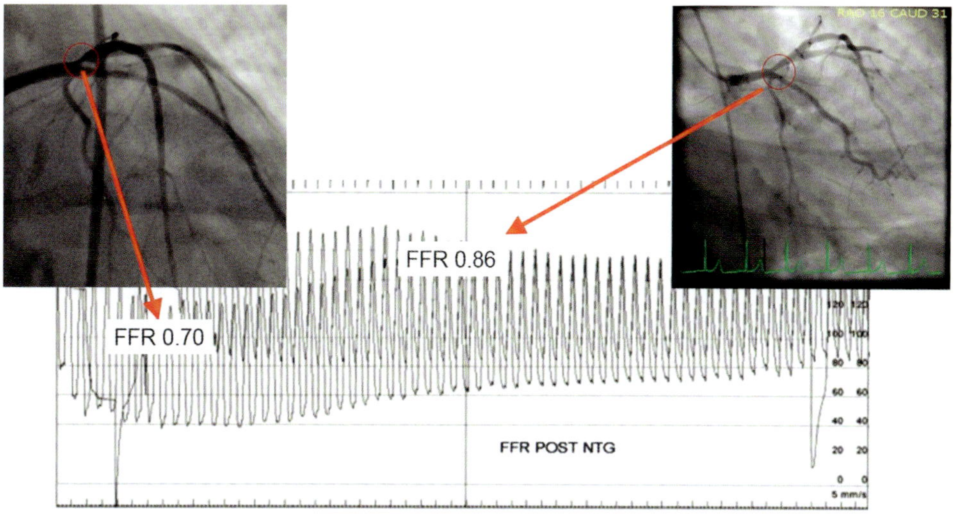

FIGURE 14.53 Coronary spasm during FFR measurements.

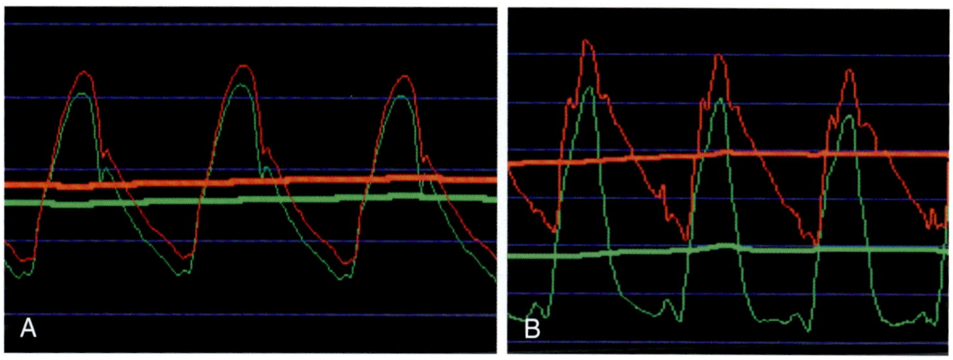

FIGURE 14.54 **A and B**, Signal drift.

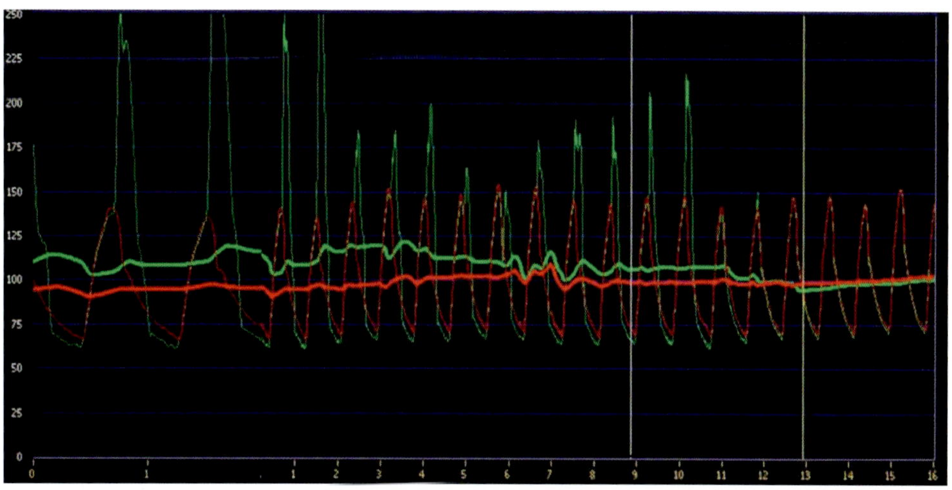

FIGURE 14.55 Whip artifact.

REFERENCES

1. Fulton WF. Immersion radiography of injected specimens. *Br J Radiol*. 1963;36:685-688.
2. Gould KL, Lipscomb K, Hamilton GW. Physiologic basis for assessing critical coronary stenosis. Instantaneous flow response and regional distribution during coronary hyperemia as measure of coronary flow reserve. *Am J Cardiol*. 1974;33:87-94.
3. Pijls NH, van Son JA, Kirkeeide RL, De Bruyne B, Gould KL. Experimental basis of determining maximum coronary, myocardial, and collateral blood flow by pressure measurements for assessing functional stenosis severity before and after percutaneous transluminal coronary angioplasty. *Circulation*. 1993;87:1354-1367.
4. Toth GG, De Bruyne B, Rusinaru D, et al. Impact of right atrial pressure on fractional flow reserve measurements: comparison of fractional flow reserve and myocardial fractional flow reserve in 1,600 coronary stenoses. *JACC Cardiovasc Interv*. 2016;9:453-459.
5. Gould KL. Pressure-flow characteristics of coronary stenoses in unsedated dogs at rest and during coronary vasodilation. *Circ Res*. 1978;43:242-253.
6. Shiono Y, Kubo T, Tanaka A, et al. Impact of myocardial supply area on the transstenotic hemodynamics as determined by fractional flow reserve. *Cathet Cardiovasc Interv*. 2014;84:406-413.
7. Johnson NP, Toth GG, Lai D, et al. Prognostic value of fractional flow reserve: linking physiologic severity to clinical outcomes. *J Am Coll Cardiol*. 2014;64:1641-1654.
8. Barbato E. *Functional Assessment (Invasive) of Coronary Circulation*. Rome, Italy: European Society of Cardiology; 2014.
9. Adjedj J, De Bruyne B, Flore V, et al. Significance of intermediate values of fractional flow reserve in patients with coronary artery disease. *Circulation*. 2016;133:502-508.
10. Adjedj J, Toth GG, Johnson NP, et al. Intracoronary adenosine: dose-response relationship with hyperemia. *JACC Cardiovasc Interv*. 2015;8:1422-1430.
11. Seto AH, Tehrani DM, Bharmal MI, Kern MJ. Variations of coronary hemodynamic responses to intravenous adenosine infusion: implications for fractional flow reserve measurements. *Cathet Cardiovasc Interv*. 2014;84:416-425.
12. Johnson NP, Johnson DT, Kirkeeide RL, et al. Repeatability of fractional flow reserve despite variations in systemic and coronary hemodynamics. *JACC Cardiovasc Interv*. 2015;8:1018-1027.
13. Bech GJ, De Bruyne B, Pijls NH, et al. Fractional flow reserve to determine the appropriateness of angioplasty in moderate coronary stenosis: a randomized trial. *Circulation*. 2001;103:2928-2934.
14. Tonino PA, De Bruyne B, Pijls NH, et al. Fractional flow reserve versus angiography for guiding percutaneous coronary intervention. *N Engl J Med*. 2009;360:213-224.
15. Pijls NH, Fearon WF, Tonino PA, et al. Fractional flow reserve versus angiography for guiding percutaneous coronary intervention in patients with multivessel coronary artery disease: 2-year follow-up of the FAME (Fractional Flow Reserve versus Angiography for Multivessel Evaluation) study. *J Am Coll Cardiol*. 2010;56:177-184.
16. Fearon WF, Bornschein B, Tonino PA, et al. Economic evaluation of fractional flow reserve-guided percutaneous coronary intervention in patients with multivessel disease. *Circulation*. 2010;122:2545-2550.
17. De Bruyne B, Pijls NH, Kalesan B, et al. Fractional flow reserve-guided PCI versus medical therapy in stable coronary disease. *N Engl J Med*. 2012;367:991-1001.
18. Van Belle E, Rioufol G, Pouillot C, et al. Outcome impact of coronary revascularization strategy reclassification with fractional flow reserve at time of diagnostic angiography: insights from a large French multicenter fractional flow reserve registry. *Circulation*. 2014;129:173-185.
19. Curzen N, Rana O, Nicholas Z, et al. Does routine pressure wire assessment influence management strategy at coronary angiography for diagnosis of chest pain?: the RIPCORD study. *Circ Cardiovasc Interv*. 2014;7:248-255.
20. Toth GG, Toth B, Johnson NP, et al. Revascularization decisions in patients with stable angina and intermediate lesions: results of the international survey on interventional strategy. *Circ Cardiovasc Interv*. 2014;7:751-759.
21. Mallidi J, Lotfi A. Fractional flow reserve for the evaluation of tandem and bifurcation lesions, left main, and acute coronary syndromes. In: Price M, Jeremias A, eds. *Intravascular Physiology*. Philadelphia: Elsevier; 2015:472-473.
22. Kern MJ, Kim MJ. Evaluation of myocardial and coronary blood flow and metabolism. In: Moscucci M, ed. *Cardiac Catheterization, Angiography, and Intervention*. Philadelphia: Lippincott Williams & Wilkins; 2014:536-538.
23. Koo BK, Park KW, Kang HJ, et al. Physiological evaluation of the provisional side-branch intervention strategy for bifurcation lesions using fractional flow reserve. *Eur Heart J*. 2008;29:726-732.
24. Nam CW, Mangiacapra F, Entjes R, et al. Functional SYNTAX score for risk assessment in multivessel coronary artery disease. *J Am Coll Cardiol*. 2011;58:1211-1218.
25. Mallidi J, Atreya AR, Cook J, et al. Long-term outcomes following fractional flow reserve-guided treatment of angiographically ambiguous left main coronary artery disease: a meta-analysis of prospective cohort studies. *Cathet Cardiovasc Interv*. 2015;86:12-18.
26. Lotfi A, Jeremias A, Fearon WF, et al. Expert consensus statement on the use of fractional flow reserve, intravascular ultrasound, and optical coherence tomography: a consensus statement of the Society of Cardiovascular Angiography and Interventions. *Cathet Cardiovasc Interv*. 2014;83:509-518.

chapter **15**

Intravascular Imaging

MASAYASU IKUTOMI, MD, PHD, YASUHIRO HONDA, MD, FAHA, FACC
PETER J. FITZGERALD, MD, PHD, FACC, and PAUL G. YOCK, MD

INTRODUCTION

Coronary angiography provides critical information regarding the arterial lumen, and it remains the standard imaging modality to guide coronary and peripheral interventions. For a review of coronary angiography and peripheral angiography, the reader is referred to chapters 10, 11, and 13. In this chapter, we will discuss adjunctive advanced imaging modalities including intravascular ultrasound (IVUS), optical coherence tomography (OCT), and spectroscopy. These modalities can provide a critical insight into the structure of normal and diseased arterial wall, and they can be used to optimize the results of therapeutic interventions.

INTRAVASCULAR ULTRASOUND

Approaches to IVUS Imaging

There are 2 basic approaches to IVUS imaging: solid-state dynamic aperture and mechanical scanning, both generating a 360°, cross-sectional image plane perpendicular to the catheter tip (**FIGURE 15.1**). Solid-state IVUS has an array of multiple piezoelectric transducers that are mounted circumferentially around the distal end of the catheter body. The individual transducer elements are activated sequentially around the device to have an ultrasound beam electronically sweep the circumference of the vessel. Mechanical IVUS uses a single piezoelectric transducer located at the distal end of a drive cable that rotates within a protective outer sheath. Images from each angular position of the transducer are collected by a computerized image array processor, which synthesizes a cross-sectional ultrasound image of the vessel.

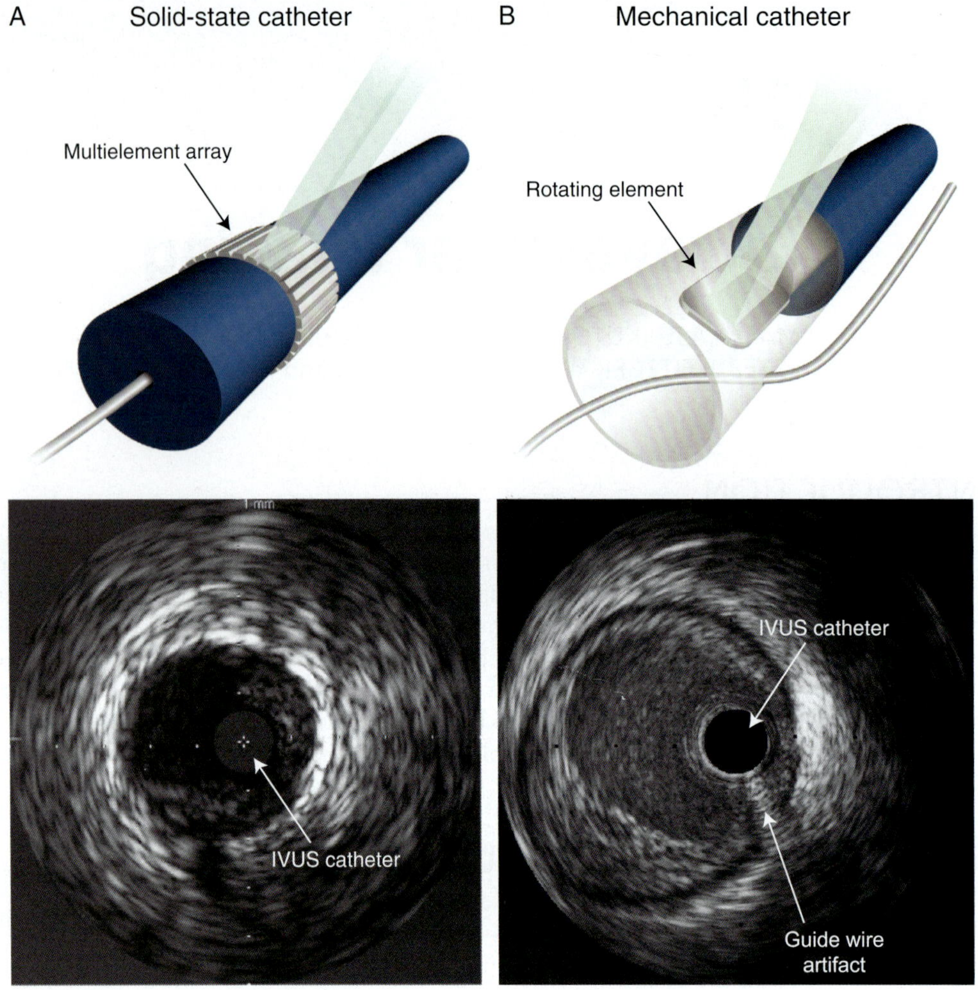

FIGURE 15.1 Basic diagrams of the two imaging catheter designs with representative IVUS images. **A**, The solid-state coronary catheter has 64 transducer elements arranged around the catheter tip and uses a center frequency of 20 MHz. The imaging catheter includes no moving parts and thus is free of nonuniform rotational distortion (NURD). The longer rapid exchange design of the solid-state catheter may track better than the short rail design of mechanical systems in complex coronary anatomy. The distance from the transducer to the catheter tip is shorter than that of mechanical systems, which may also be beneficial in IVUS-guided intervention of chronic total occlusion (CTO) lesions. **B**, The mechanical coronary catheters use a single 40- to 60-MHz transducer, offering advantages in image quality compared with the solid-state systems owing to the higher center frequencies and the larger effective aperture of a transducer element. The catheters are advanced over a guide wire using a short rail section at the catheter tip, located beyond the imaging window segment within which the spinning transducer may be advanced or withdrawn. The fact that the guide wire runs outside the catheter parallel to the imaging segment results in a shadow artifact in the image.

Cross-sectional IVUS

The bright-dark-bright, 3-layered appearance is seen in (**FIGURE 15.2**) with corresponding anatomy as defined. IVUS represents the imaging catheter in the blood vessel lumen. The media has lower ultrasound reflectance owing to less collagen and elastin compared with neighboring layers. Because the intimal layer reflects ultrasound more strongly than the media, there is a spillover in the image, known as "blooming," which results in a slight overestimation of the thickness of the intima and a corresponding underestimation of the medial thickness. The adventitia and periadventitial tissues are similar enough in echoreflectivity that a clear outer adventitial border cannot be defined.

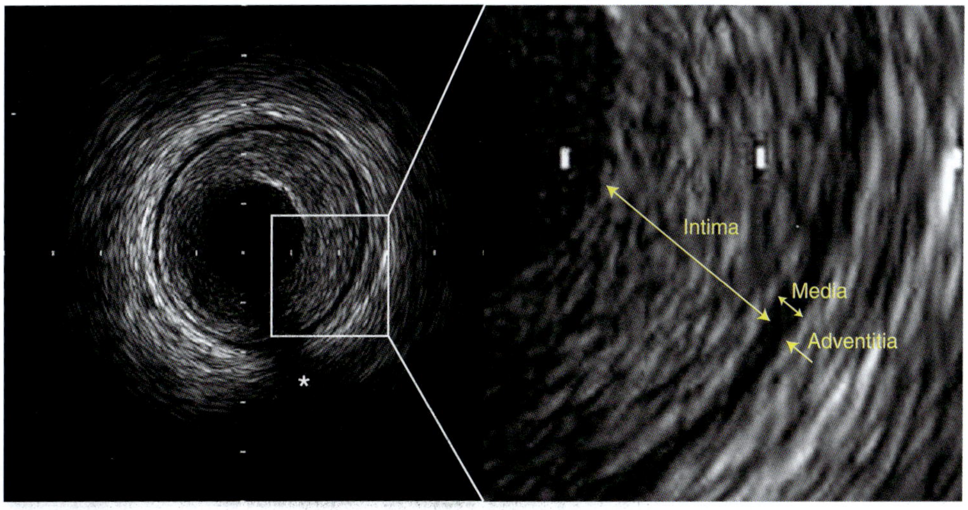

FIGURE 15.2 Typical cross-sectional IVUS image of a diseased coronary artery.

Deviations

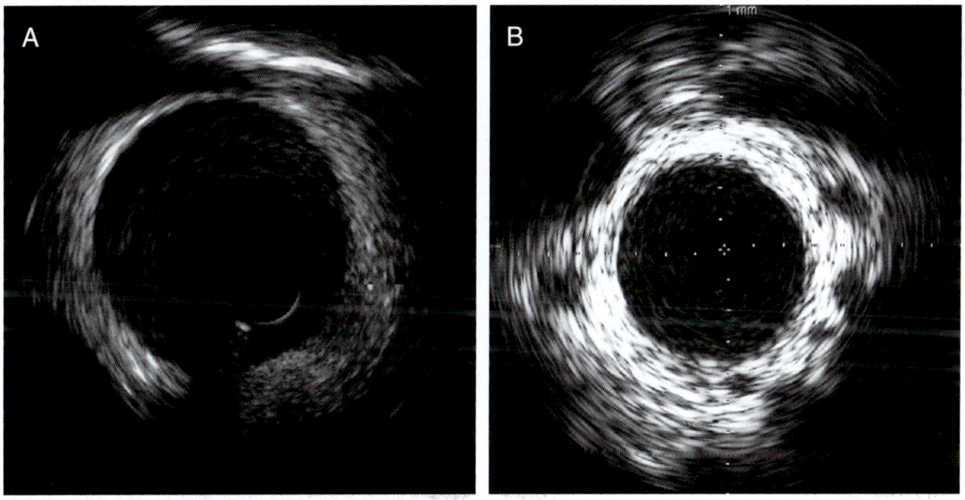

FIGURE 15.3 Deviations from the classic 3-layered appearance. **A**, The classic 3-layered appearance may be undetectable in truly normal coronary arteries of young subjects wherein the intimal thickness is below the effective resolution of IVUS. **B**, Elastic arteries and the transitional zones into muscular arteries, such as the common carotid artery, may also show the media indistinctly, as it contains high amounts of collagen and elastin, causing it to blend with the surrounding layers.

Interpretation of IVUS images relies on the fact that arterial wall structures can be identified as separate layers (FIGURE 15.3). In muscular arteries, such as the coronary tree, the media typically stands out as a thin dark band, as it contains much less echoreflective material (collagen and elastin) than the neighboring intima and adventitia, providing a characteristic 3-layered (bright-dark-bright) appearance on IVUS images. However, several deviations from the classic 3-layered appearance can be encountered in clinical practice.

Image Orienation

Left Anterior Descending Artery (LAD)

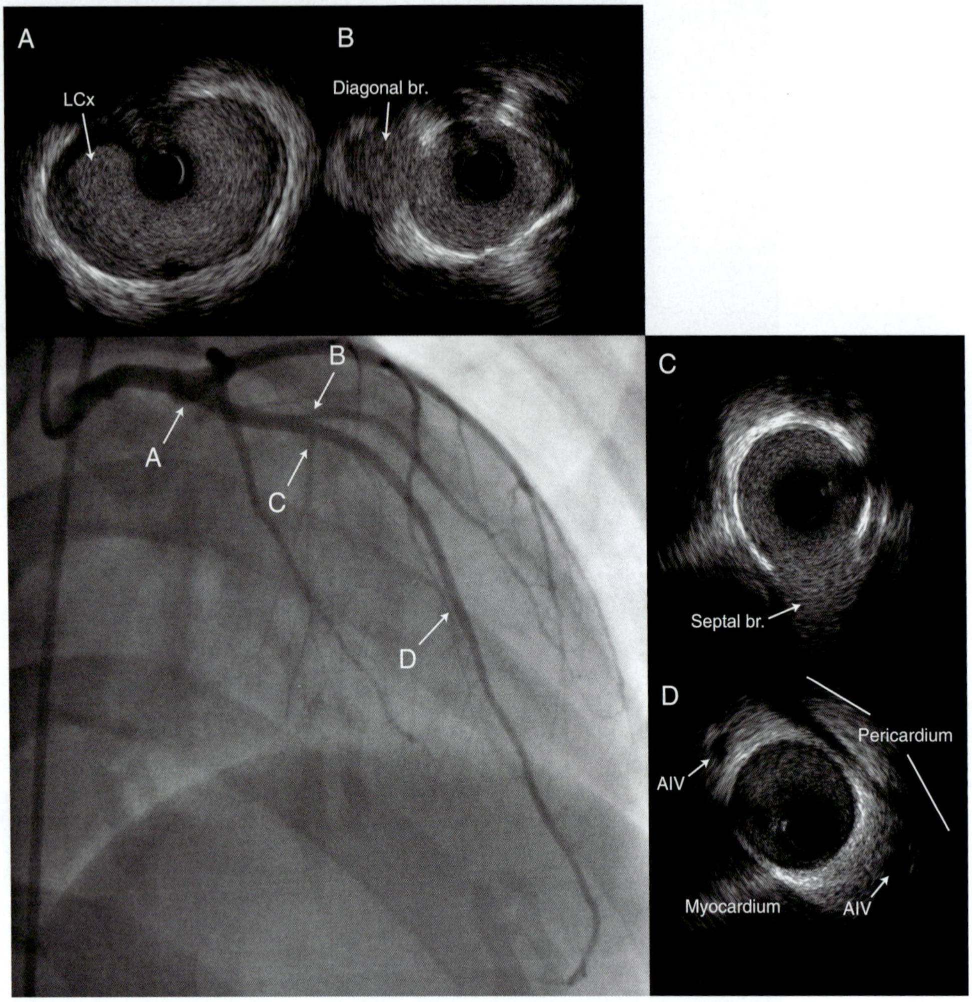

FIGURE 15.4 Image orientation: LAD.

Image orientation within the artery is another important aspect of image interpretation (**FIGURE 15.4**). In general, the IVUS beam penetrates beyond the coronary artery, often providing images of perivascular structures, such as the myocardium, pericardium, and cardiac veins.

These structures have characteristic appearances when viewed from various positions within the arterial tree. Therefore, in combination with the branching patterns of arteries, they can offer useful landmarks. The pericardium appears as a bright and relatively thick layer with varying degrees of "spokelike" reverberations created by the interwoven fibrous strands. The myocardium is often viewed on the side opposite to the pericardium as a variable pattern of homogenous, low-echoic gray-scale signals. The cardiac veins are visualized by IVUS as echolucent luminal structures with no connection to the coronary lumen, often showing compression during the cardiac cycle.

Current IVUS systems display the cross-sectional image as if viewing from a proximal position looking in a distal direction. Therefore, in the left anterior descending artery (LAD), the left circumflex (LCX) artery and the diagonal branches should emerge approximately 90° counterclockwise from the pericardium, whereas septal branches typically emerge on the side opposite to the pericardium (ie, on the myocardium side). The distal LAD is accompanied by 1 or 2 anterior interventricular vein (AIV) branches, which run parallel to the LAD for a variable distance. It is important to recognize that there is no default rotational orientation of the image relative to the anatomy as the image initially appears on the screen—that is, what appears as "up" on the screen depends on where the beam begins its cycle and will be different from case to case. However, it is possible for the operator to rotate the image on the system to a standard view, using the anatomic clues described earlier, to provide the same image orientation for each IVUS examination.

Left Circumflex Artery (LCX)

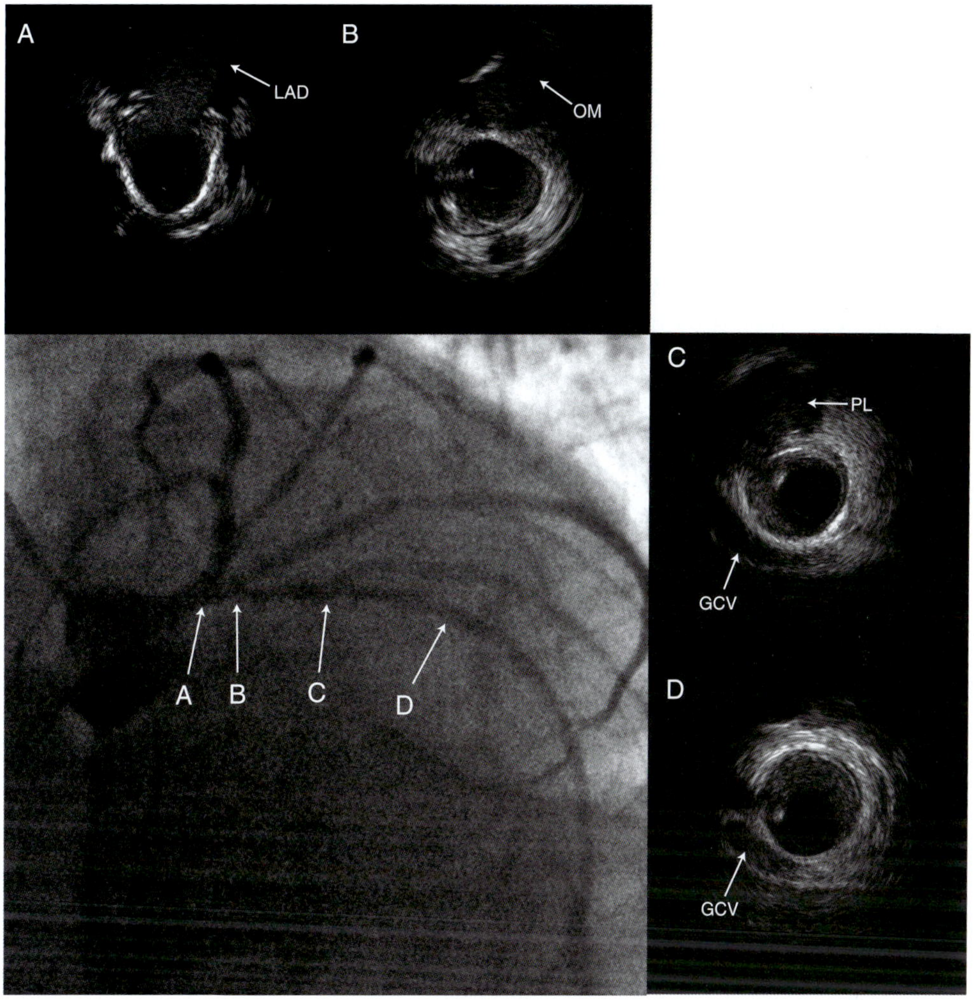

FIGURE 15.5 Image orientation: LCX artery.

In the LCX artery, the great cardiac vein (GCV) runs superior to the LCX in most cases and immediately inferior to the left auricle (FIGURE 15.5). Therefore, viewed from the LCX, the recurrent arterial branches generally emerge in an orientation directed toward the GCV. In contrast, the obtuse marginal (OM) and the posterolateral (PL) branches emerge opposite to the GCV and course inferiorly to cover the lateral myocardial wall.

Left Main Coronary Artery (LMCA)

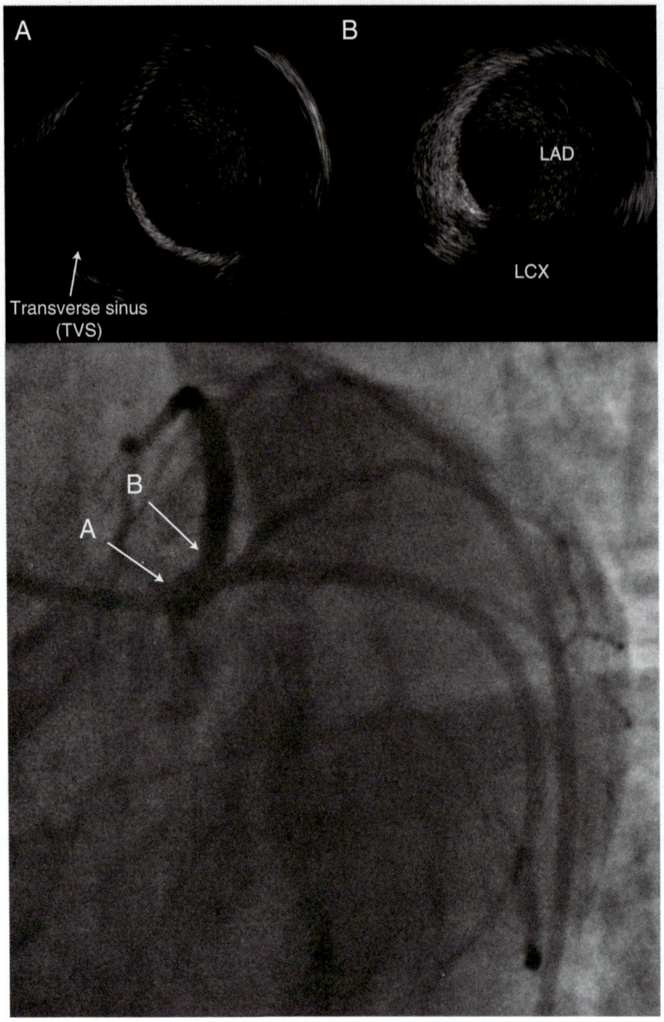

FIGURE 15.6 Image orientation: LMCA.

A clear, echo-free space, called the transverse sinus (TVS), is often observed outside the left main coronary artery (LMCA) (**FIGURE 15.6**). This space is formed by the tenting of pericardium descending from the aorta onto the surface of the heart. Opposite to the plane of imaging, the TVS is appreciated adjacent to the left main lumen, immediately outside the left superior aspect of the aortic root. When imaging near the aorto-ostial junction, the left main lumen enlarges markedly into the aortic root, and often the ultrasound plane captures the inferior aspect of the left coronary cusp.

Right Coronary Artery (RCA)

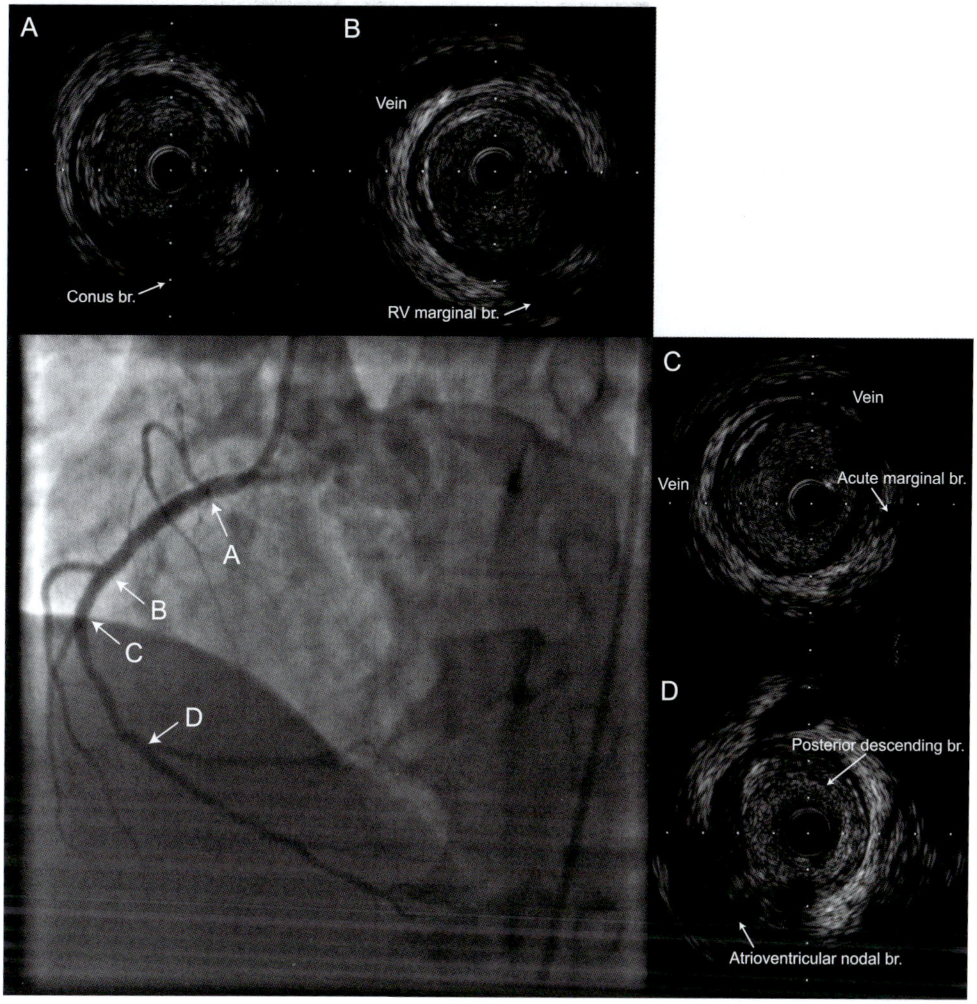

FIGURE 15.7 Image orientation: RCA.

Unlike other epicardial coronary arteries typically accompanied by parallel venous structures, the proximal and mid-right coronary artery (RCA) shows a unique vein appearance—the vein arc crossing around the RCA in a "horseshoe" pattern, often at a position adjacent to the right ventricular (RV) marginal branches (FIGURE 15.7). The RV branches commonly have a geographic relationship with the pericardium similar to the diagonal branches of LAD—roughly 90° counterclockwise from the pericardium. The recurrent atrial branches typically emerge opposite to the RV marginal branches.

Image Artifact

Air Bubbles

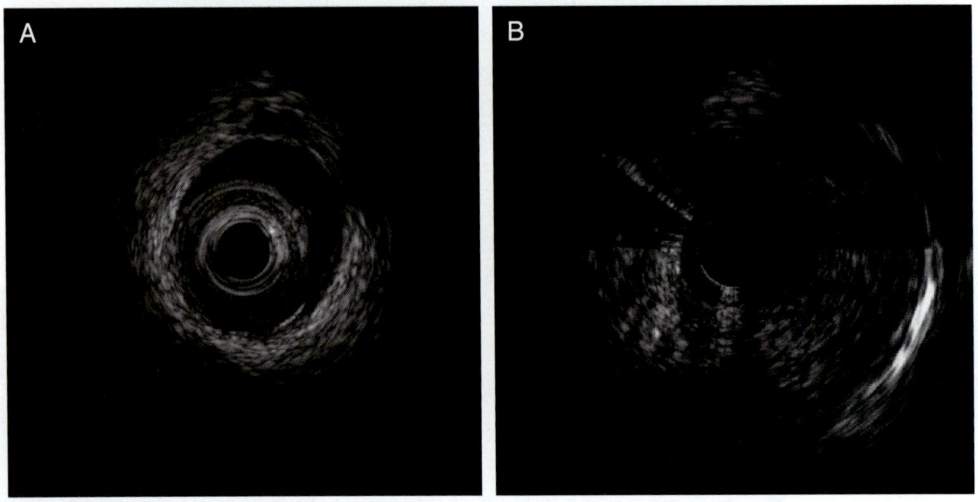

FIGURE 15.8 Image artifact: air bubbles.

Mechanical catheters require flushing with saline to remove air bubbles from inside the catheter (**FIGURE 15.8**). This preparation should be performed before inserting the IVUS catheter to avoid air embolism in the coronary artery. Incomplete flushing can leave microbubbles adjacent to the transducer, resulting in poor image quality. Air bubbles can cause various patterns of noise including concentric rings around the imaging catheter with poor image penetration (**FIGURE 15.8A**) or a deep sector of interference, producing a blind area (**FIGURE 15.8B**).

Blood Stagnation

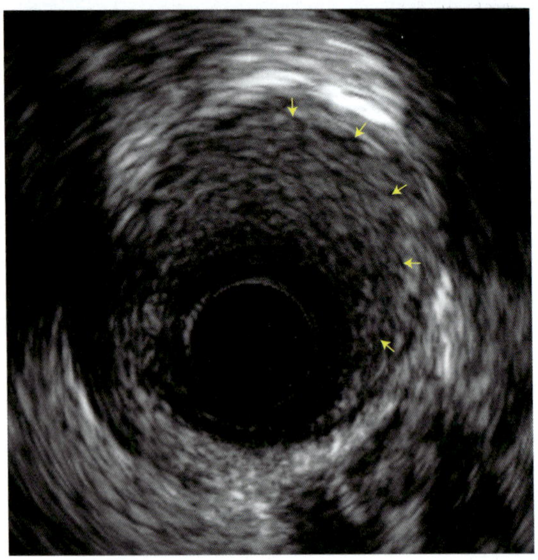

FIGURE 15.9 Image artifact: blood stagnation.

When blood flow is stagnant, red cells aggregate and reflect ultrasound more strongly (**FIGURE 15.9**). This produces an appearance in the lumen that looks white or "foggy" and the lumen-intima boundary (yellow arrows) may be blurred. Injection of contrast or saline may disperse the stagnant flow from the lumen.

Ring-down

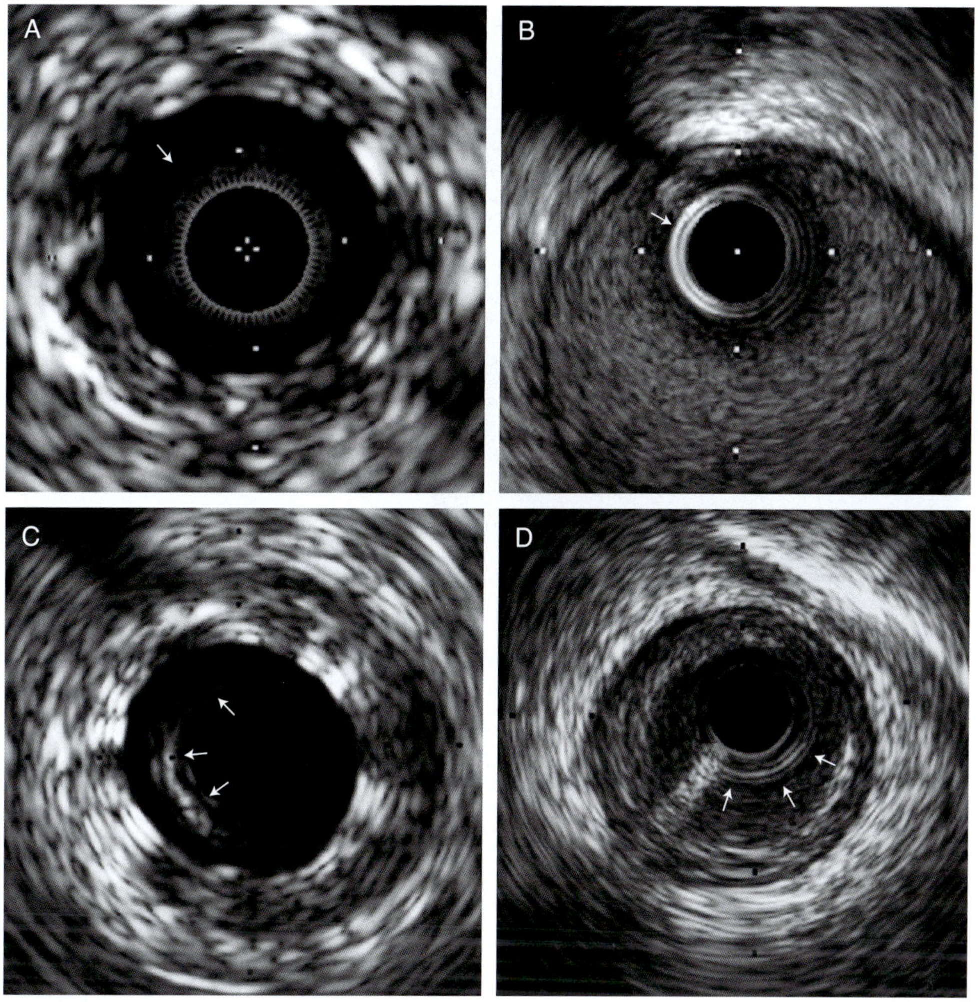

FIGURE 15.10 Image artifact: ring-down.

Ring-down artifact is the most common image artifact with IVUS, which is manifested as multiple bright rings surrounding the catheter (**FIGURE 15.10**). This artifact is more commonly seen with the solid-state systems (**FIGURE 15.10A**) than with mechanical rotational systems (**FIGURE 15.10B**). Solid-state catheters require digital subtraction to mask this artifact before being inserted into the coronary artery. If this is incorrectly performed, digital subtraction can be a potential cause for removal of real information (white arrows in **FIGURE 15.10C**). In mechanical rotating systems, near-field resolution is commonly excellent so that digital subtraction is not required. Ring-down artifact is minimized by the fact that the transducer is offset from the surface of the catheter by design. If a significant ring-down artifact is observed with a mechanical catheter (white arrows in **FIGURE 15.10D**), the likely cause is microbubbles within the protective sheath, requiring repeated saline-flush procedures until the artifact is removed.

Non-Uniform Rotational Distortion (NURD)

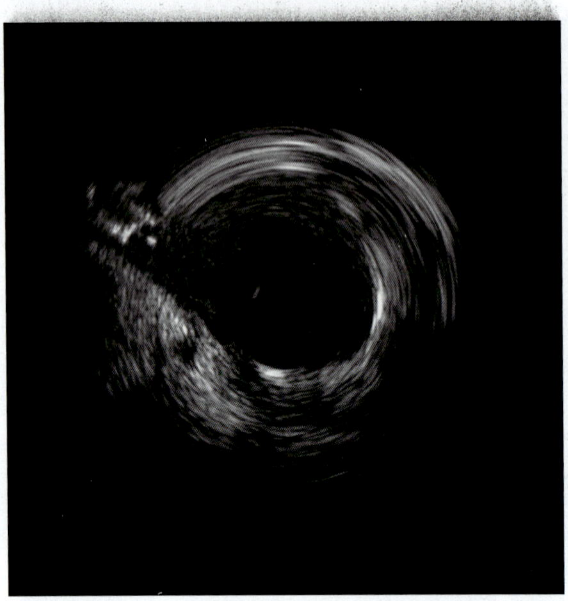

FIGURE 15.11 Image artifact: NURD.

The solid-state catheter includes no moving parts and thus is free of NURD (**FIGURE 15.11**). This artifact can occur with mechanical systems when bending or friction of the drive cable interferes with uniform transducer rotation, causing a wedge-shaped, smeared image to appear in 1 or more segments of the image (between 10 and 6 o'clock in this example).

White Cap

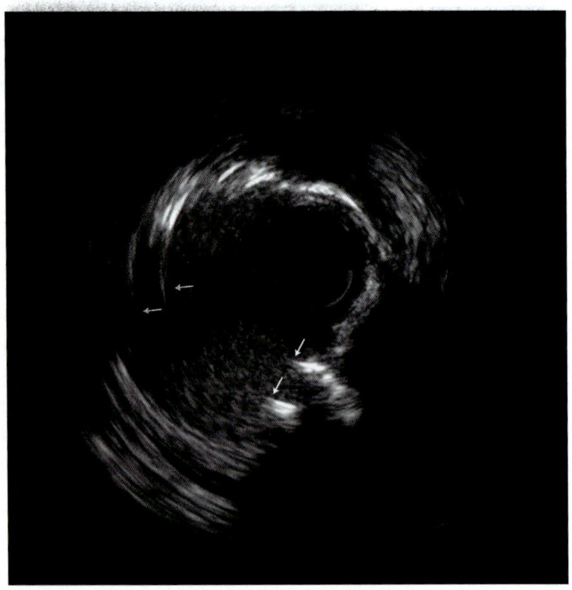

FIGURE 15.12 Image artifact: white cap.

"White cap" artifacts caused by side lobe echoes (arrows) originate at the edges of a strong reflecting surface, such as metal stent struts or calcification (**FIGURE 15.12**). Smearing of the strut image can lead to the mistaken impression that the struts are protruding into the lumen.

Radiofrequency (RF)

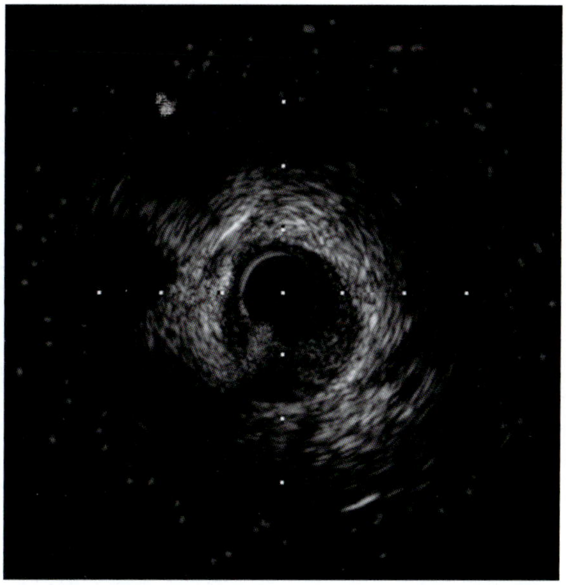

FIGURE 15.13 Image artifact: radiofrequency noise.

Radiofrequency (RF) noise appears as alternating radial spokes or random white dots in the far field (FIGURE 15.13). The interference is usually caused by other electrical equipment in the cardiac catheterization laboratory.

Reverberation

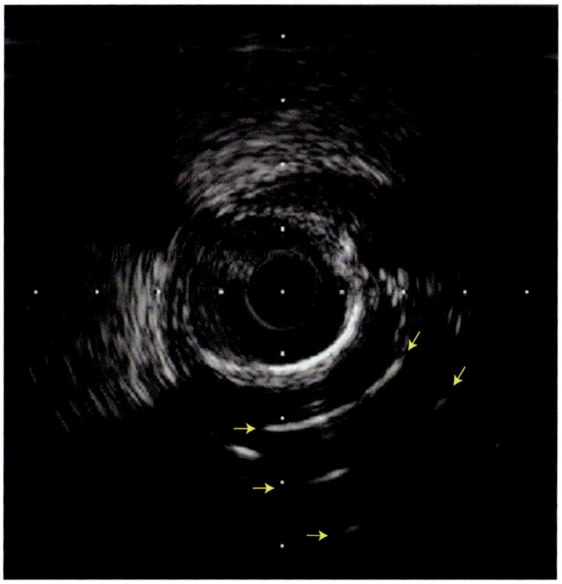

FIGURE 15.14 Image artifact: reverberation.

"Reverberation" refers to an artifact where multiple, radial ghost images are created at regular intervals (yellow arrows) beyond a bright interface such as the leading edge of calcium or a stent strut (FIGURE 15.14). These artifacts are caused by repeated "round trips" of a portion of the ultrasound energy that is reflected back from the bright interface in the vessel and then, in turn, bounces off the transducer and makes another trip (or 2 or 3), which the IVUS scanner presents as ghost images.

Cross-Sectional Ivus Measurements

Non-stented Segments

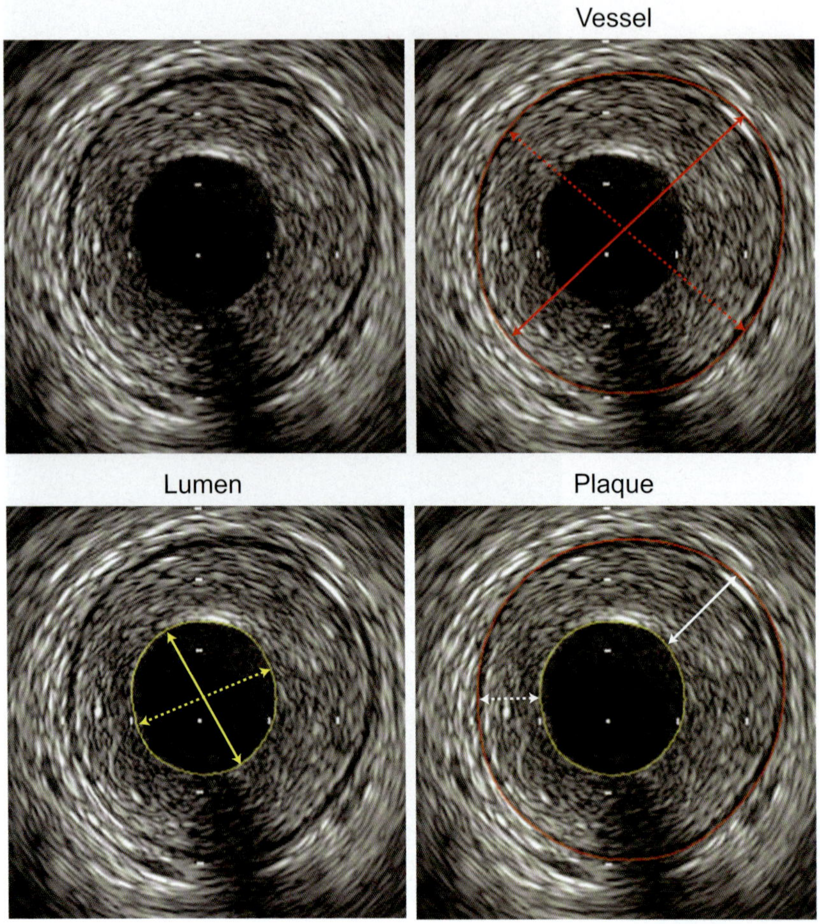

FIGURE 15.15 Cross-sectional IVUS measurements: nonstented segments.

IVUS has an intrinsic distance calibration based on the known speed of ultrasound in tissue. This is implemented in the form of a measurement grid on the image, as calipers and area tracing capability in the system software and as tag information in exported DICOM files. In principle, all ultrasound measurements should be performed at the "leading edge" of boundaries (that is, the edge closest to the transducer) because of the higher accuracy and reproducibility compared with those at the trailing edge.

For cross-sectional analysis, electronic caliper (diameter) and tracing (area) measurements can be performed (**FIGURE 15.15**). For vessel measurement, the interface between the media and the leading edge of adventitia that corresponds to the external elastic membrane (EEM) is used, because the outer border of the adventitial cannot be defined by IVUS. In cross sections with large plaque burden or significant calcification, the circumference of EEM may not be fully identifiable because of ultrasound signal attenuation or acoustic shadowing. Extrapolation from the closest identifiable EEM border is acceptable only if the attenuation or acoustic shadowing involves a relatively small arc (<90°). For lumen measurement, the interface between the lumen and the leading edge of the intima is used. When the blood-tissue interface is obscure on a still image, a review of moving images can help identify the TL border. During the procedure, saline or contrast medium can be injected through the guide catheter to reduce blood speckle. Plaque area (or more accurately, the plaque plus media area) is calculated as the difference between EEM and lumen areas. The ratio of plaque to EEM area is termed the percent plaque area, plaque burden, or cross-sectional narrowing. For EEM and lumen diameter measurements, the maximum (solid arrows) and minimum (dotted arrows) diameters are determined. For plaque, the maximum (solid arrows) and minimum (dotted arrows) thicknesses are measured.

Stented Segments

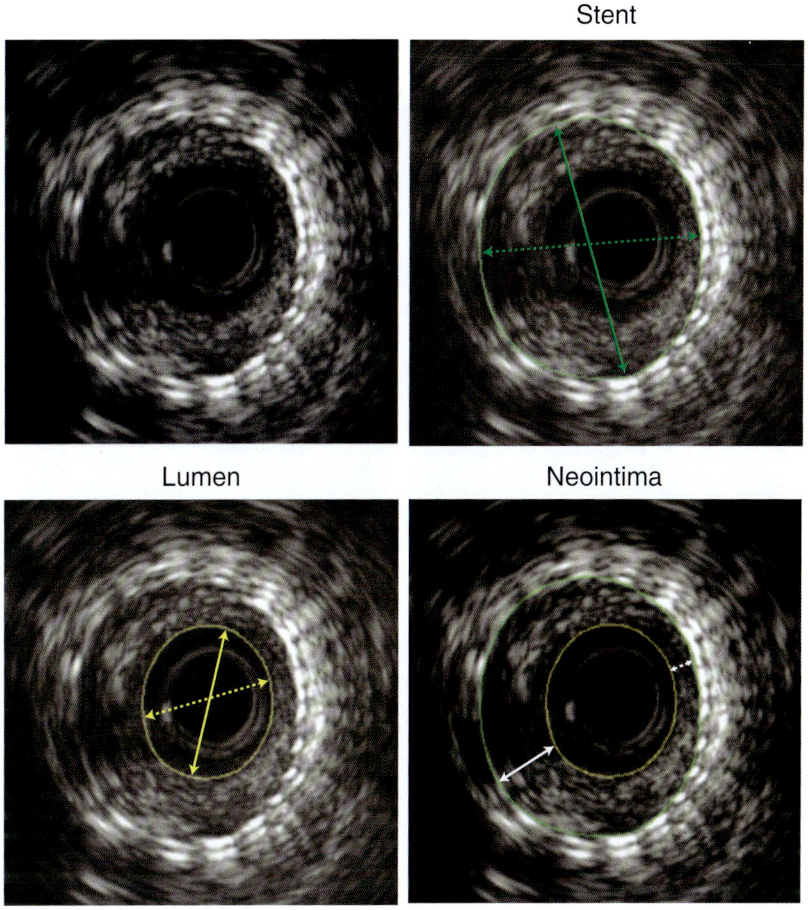

FIGURE 15.16 Cross-sectional IVUS measurements: stented segments.

Metal struts of stents are seen as bright, focal points in a circular-arrayed pattern on the IVUS scan, and stent area is measured by tracing the leading edge of the stent struts (**FIGURE 15.16**). For tissue within the stent (ie, plaque prolapse, in-stent thrombus, or neointimal hyperplasia at follow-up imaging), the area is calculated as the difference between stent area and lumen area. As in the case of nonstented segment analysis, a review of moving images or saline/contrast flush during the procedure can help identify the TL-tissue interface. For diameter measurements, the maximum (solid arrows) and minimum (dotted arrows) stent diameters are determined, and the ratio of maximum to minimum diameter defines a measure of stent symmetry. For neointima, the maximum (solid arrows) and minimum (dotted arrows) thickness are measured.

Arterial Remodeling

Direct Assessment By Serial IVUS

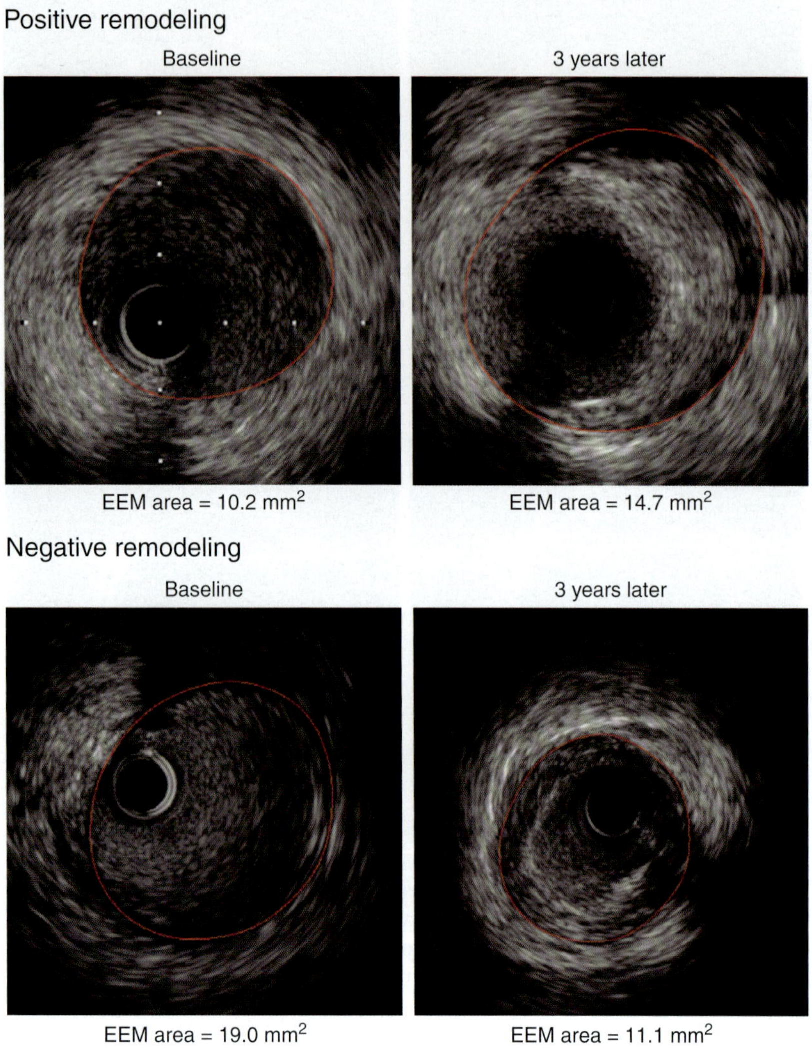

FIGURE 15.17 Arterial remodeling: direct assessment by serial IVUS.

Arterial remodeling refers to a change in vessel caliber (either an increase or decrease) that occurs during the development of atherosclerosis (**FIGURE 15.17**). In serial IVUS studies, evidence of remodeling can be directly derived from serial changes in the EEM area by 2 or more IVUS measurements obtained at different times at the same transducer location. A remodeling index (the ratio of EEM area at the lesion site versus the reference site) as a continuous variable may also be used, in combination with the categorical classifications (positive remodeling = remodeling index >1.0 or 1.05; negative remodeling = remodeling index <1.0 or 0.95).

Indirect Assessment By Single-time Point IVUS

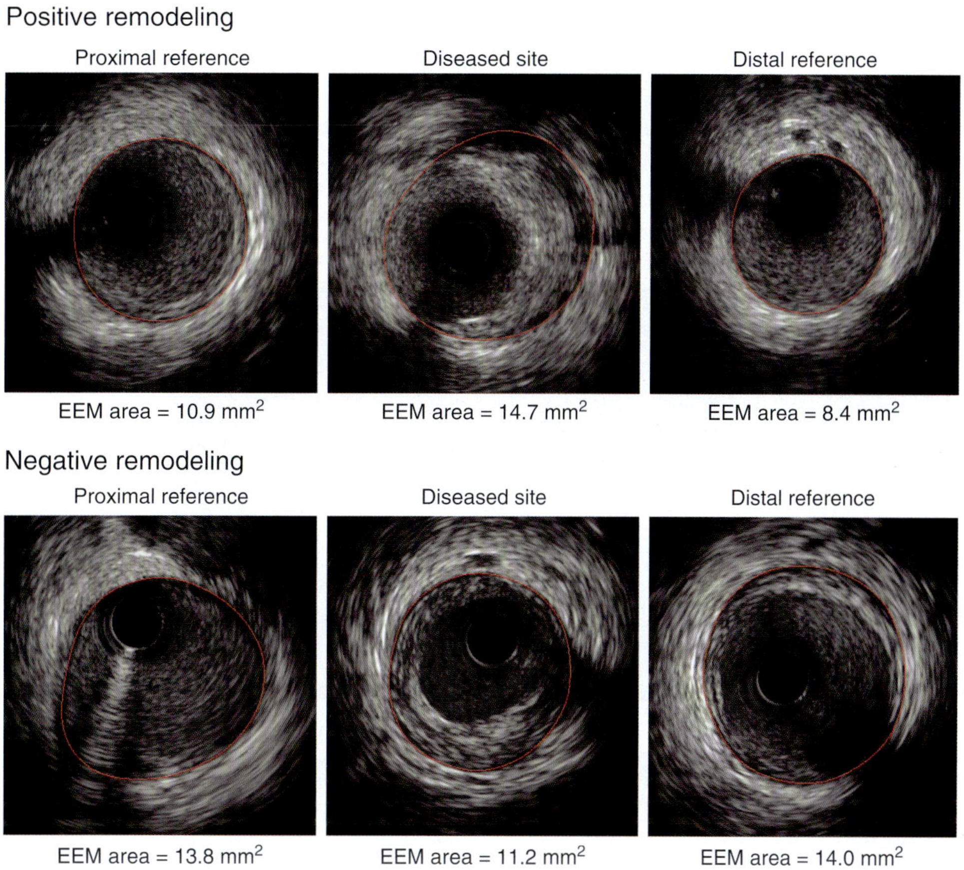

FIGURE 15.18 Arterial remodeling: indirect assessment by single time point IVUS.

In single time point studies, the EEM area measurements at reference sites proximal and/or distal to the segment of interest are used as an indirect surrogate for the original vessel size before the lesion site became diseased (**FIGURE 15.18**). The reference segment is selected as the most normal-looking (largest lumen with smallest plaque burden) cross section within 10 mm from the lesion with no intervening major side branches.

Plaque

Types

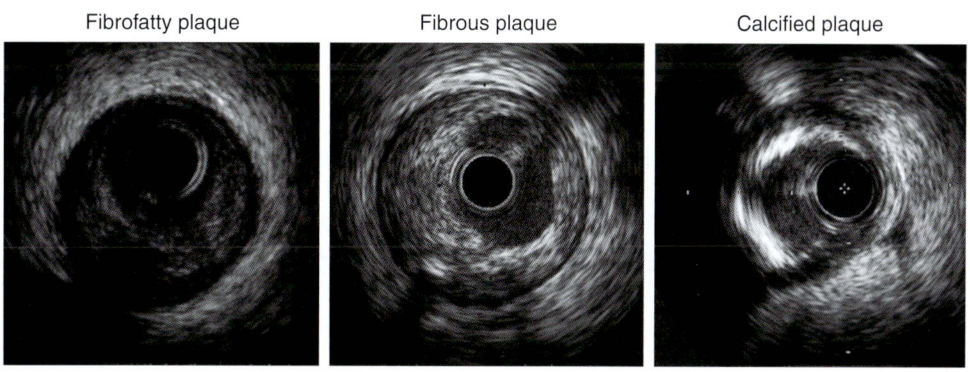

FIGURE 15.19 Plaque types by gray-scale IVUS.

In gray-scale IVUS, atheromatous plaques are classified based on the echogenicity and association with specific acoustic findings, such as signal attenuation, shadowing, and reverberation (FIGURE 15.19). The brightness of the adventitia can be used as a gauge to discriminate between predominantly fatty from fibrous plaque (plaque that appears darker than the adventitia is considered fatty). Regions of calcification are strongly echoreflective and create a dense shadow peripherally from the catheter, known as acoustic shadowing (between 7 and 11 o'clock in the example).

Classifications

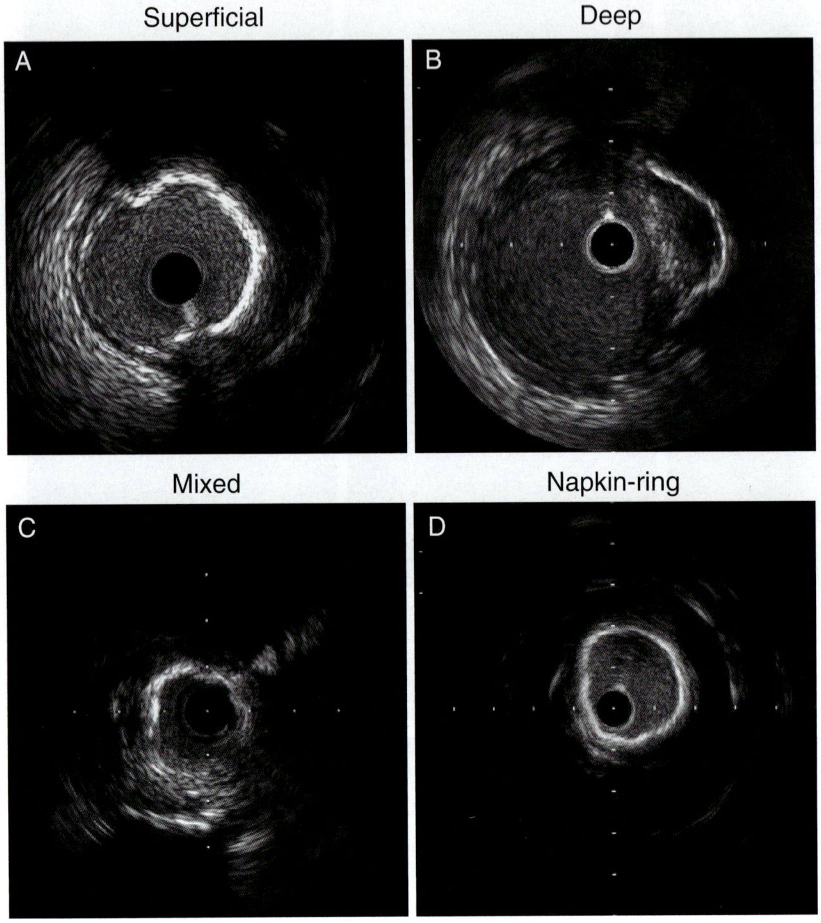

FIGURE 15.20 Classification of calcified plaque **A**, Superficial. **B**, Deep. **C**, Mixed. **D**, Napkin-ring.

Calcium deposits are described qualitatively as superficial (FIGURE 15.20A), deep (FIGURE 15.20B), or mixed (FIGURE 15.20C) according to the leading-edge location of the acoustic shadowing of the deposit. If the edge is within the inner half of the plaque plus media, the deposit is considered superficial. Extensive superficial calcium, particularly circumferential "napkin-ring" calcification (FIGURE 15.20D), may require plaque modification with rotational atherectomy or "scoring" before stent implantation. Conversely, even for lesions with significant calcification on fluoroscopy, IVUS may show that the calcification is distributed in a deep portion of the vessel wall or has a limited arc (less than 180°). In these cases, stand-alone stenting without modifying the calcium deposit usually achieves adequate lumen expansion. The shadowing of the image by calcium precludes determination of the thickness of a calcific deposit as well as visualization of vessel structures behind the calcium. Ultrasound reverberation due to calcium (see FIGURE 15.14) should not be misinterpreted as true vessel structures.

Vulnerable Plaques

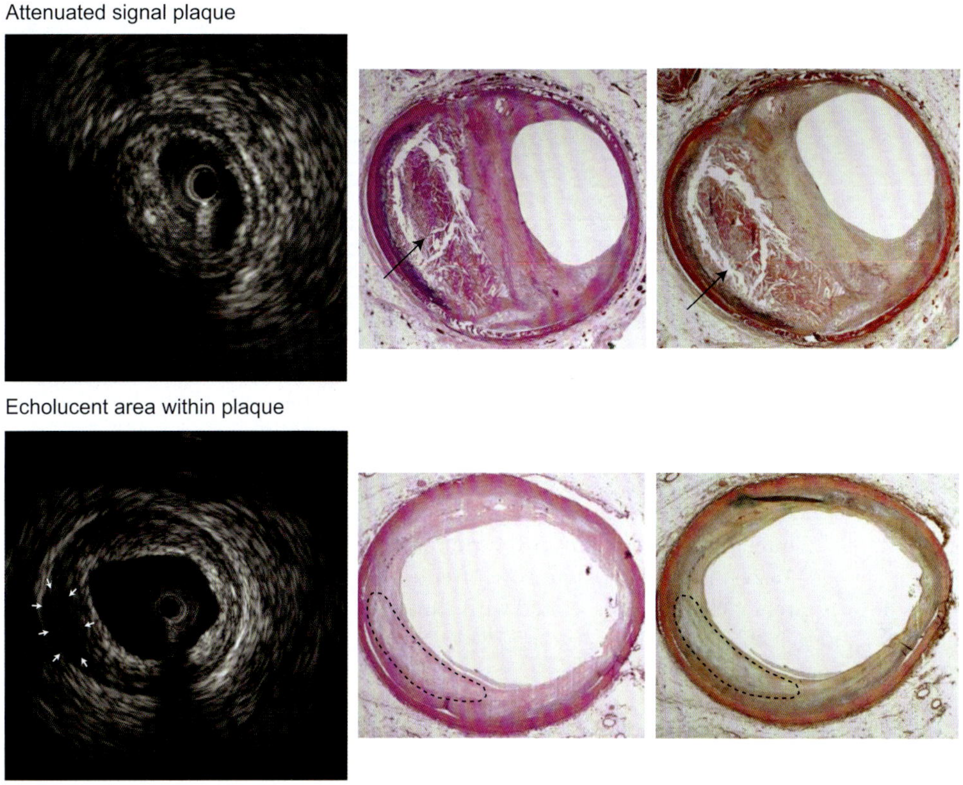

FIGURE 15.21 Vulnerable plaques by gray-scale IVUS. IVUS images (in left) and corresponding histology for vulnerable plaques (histologic staining: hematoxylin and eosin staining in middle; Movat staining in right). **Attenuated signal plaque:** IVUS visualizes large plaque burden with deep ultrasound signal attenuation despite absence of bright calcium (between 6 and 9 o'clock in this example). A corresponding histologic image shows a fibroatheroma containing large necrotic core (black arrows). Attenuation plaque is susceptible to distal emboli during balloon dilatation or stenting. **Echolucent area within plaque:** Lipid deposition appears as an echolucent (hypoechoic) area (white arrows) within the atherosclerotic plaque. A corresponding histologic image shows the lipid pool in this area (black dotted line).

By gray-scale IVUS, morphologic features associated with clinical instability or high risk for cardiovascular events after percutaneous coronary intervention (PCI) include noncalcified plaque with ultrasound attenuation and an echolucent zone within plaque (**FIGURE 15.21**). In particular, echoattenuated plaque (or attenuated signal plaque, defined as the absence of the ultrasound signal behind plaque that is either hypoechoic or isoechoic to the reference adventitia but contains no bright calcium) likely represents either fibroatheroma with a necrotic core or pathologic intimal thickening (PIT) with a lipid pool.

Plaque Rupture

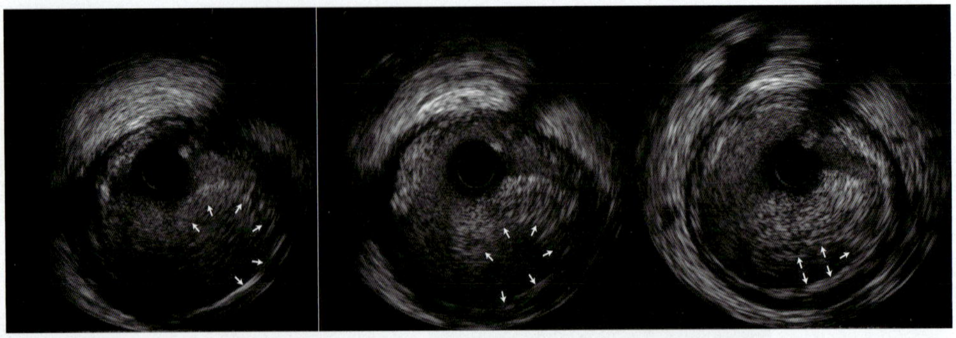

FIGURE 15.22 Serial IVUS images for ruptured plaque. A distinct hole in the plaque (white arrows indicating the border of the hole) is the classic appearance of an ulceration, which may be caused by plaque rupture. It essentially appeared with thrombus.

Plaque rupture is diagnosed when a hypoechoic cavity within the plaque is connected with the lumen and a remnant of the ruptured fibrous cap is observed at the connecting site (**FIGURE 15.22**). Ruptured plaques are often eccentric, less calcified, large in plaque burden, positively remodeled, and associated with thrombus.

Advanced Plaque Characterization

VH-IVUS

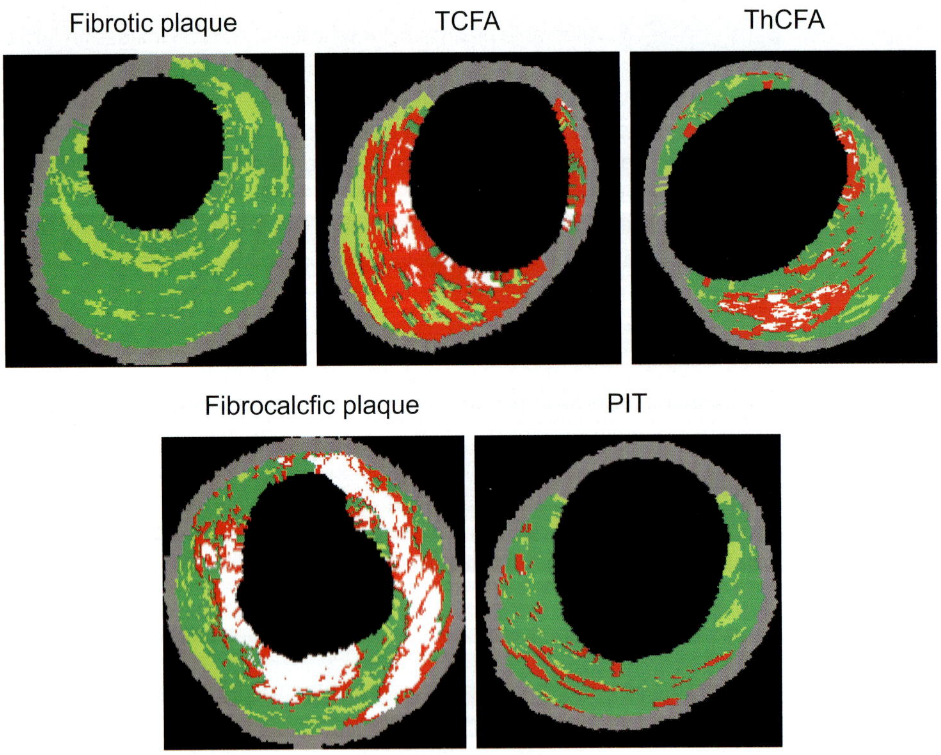

FIGURE 15.23 Advanced plaque characterization: **VH-IVUS**. Types of plaque: dark green (fibrous), light green (fibrofatty), white (calcium), red (necrotic core).

Visual interpretation of conventional gray-scale IVUS images is limited in the precise detection and quantification of specific plaque components, and therefore several advanced signal analysis techniques have been developed. To date, 3 different systems have been commercialized based on computer-assisted analyses of raw RF signals in the reflected ultrasound beam. All systems generate color-mapped images of the vessel wall, with a distinct color for each plaque component category.

The Virtual Histology (VH) IVUS system (Volcano Corp.) (**FIGURE 15.23**) uses spectral RF analyses with a classification tree algorithm developed from ex vivo coronary datasets and groups plaques as 4 types: dark green (fibrous), light green (fibrofatty), white (calcium), and red (necrotic core). VH-IVUS gained significant attention with the PROSPECT trial.[1] In this trial, plaque was classified into 5 phenotypes: fibrotic plaque, thin-cap fibroatheroma (TCFA), thick-cap fibroatheroma (ThCFA), fibrocalcific plaque, and PIT. TCFAs were associated with increased adverse cardiac events (heart rate [HR] = 3.35, $P < .001$). Most importantly, the highest-risk lesions (HR = 11.05, $P < .001$) were a combination of several features, including a greater than 70% plaque burden, low minimal luminal area, and TCFA morphology. One limitation of VH-IVUS is that identification of intraluminal organizing thrombus is currently not possible by RF analysis.

iMap

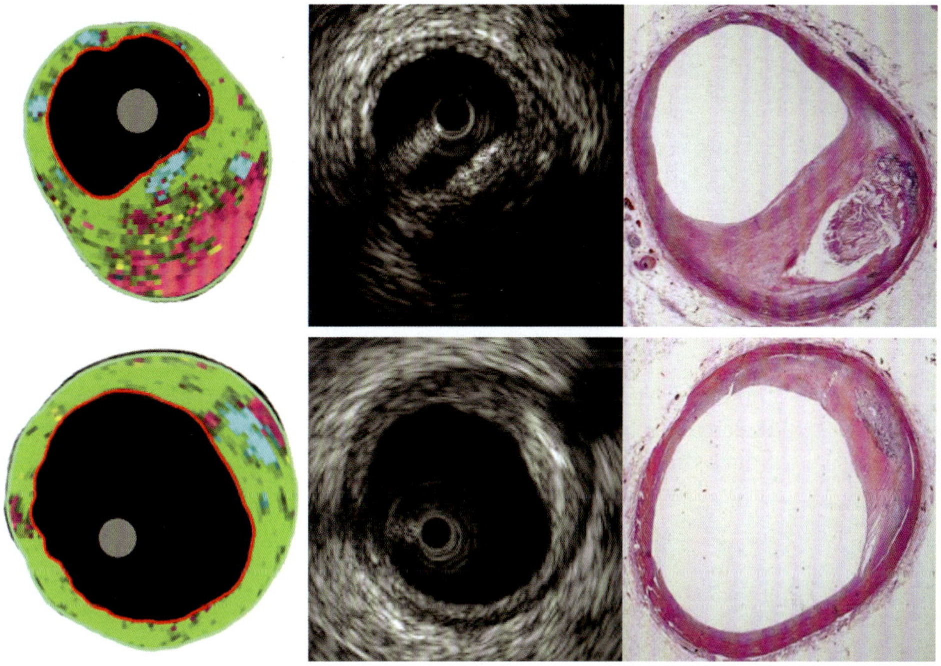

FIGURE 15.24 Advanced plaque characterization: **iMap. Left image:** categories of plaque: fibrous, green; fibrofatty, yellow, calcium, light blue; necrotic core, pink. Two examples for iMap. A corresponding gray-scale IVUS cross section (**middle image**) and hematoxylin and eosin staining (**right image**) are shown. Courtesy of Boston Scientific Co.

In iMap (Boston Scientific), classification of tissue is made based on the degree of similarity between the sample and a reference frequency spectrum (**FIGURE 15.24**). This method enables confidence-level assessment of each plaque component. Tissue is classified into 4 categories: fibrous (green), fibrofatty (yellow), calcium (light blue), and necrotic core (pink).

Integrated Backscatter (IB) IVUS

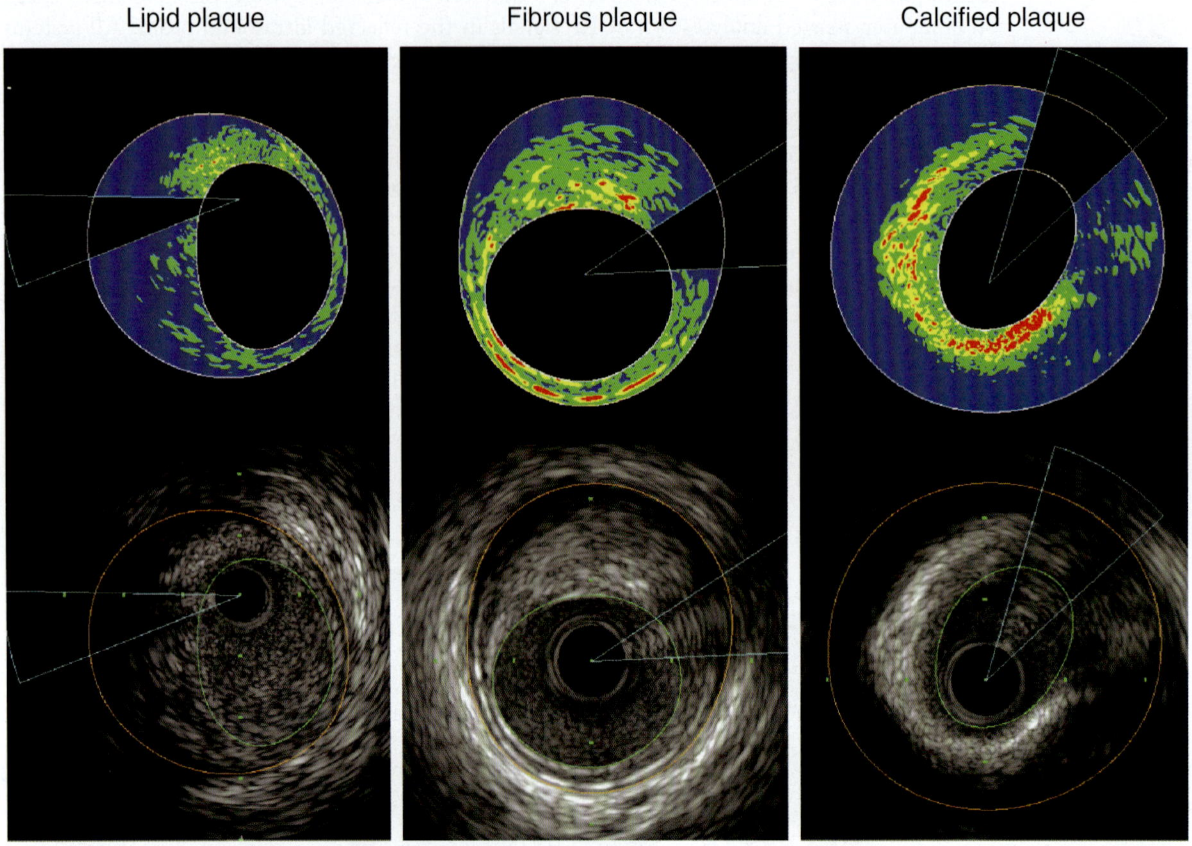

FIGURE 15.25 Advanced plaque characterization: **IB-IVUS**.

Integrated backscatter (IB) IVUS (Terumo Corp.) is another tissue characterization system that directly uses IB values, calculated as the average power of the backscattered ultrasound signal from a sample tissue volume, to differentiate tissue into 4 categories: fibrous (green), dense fibrosis (yellow), lipid pool (blue and purple), and calcification (red) (**FIGURE 15.25**).

Dissection

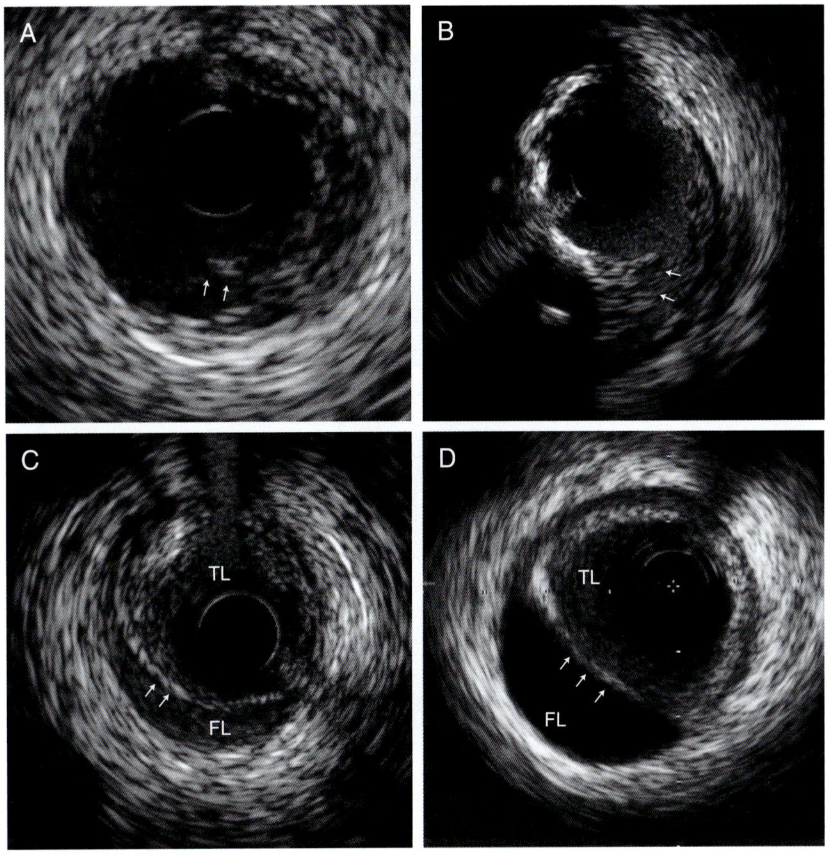

FIGURE 15.26 Four examples of dissection: **A**, Superficial (intima) dissection starting at 6 o'clock and extending counterclockwise (arrows indicating a flap). **B**, Mixed plaque (fibrotic and calcific) with a deeper (medial) dissection at 5 o'clock (arrows). Injection of contrast in this setting may demonstrate free fluid flow behind the flap to better define the extent of the tear. **C**, IVUS image showing a semicircular dissection membrane as an echo-dense flap (arrows) separating a false lumen (FL) from TL. **D**, IVUS showing an echolucent image because of pooled or stagnated contrast medium in the FL (arrows indicating a flap).

Dissection appears as a fissure or separation within the intima or plaque (**FIGURE 15.26**). The severity of a dissection can be characterized according to the depth and extent.

Coronary Artery Spasm

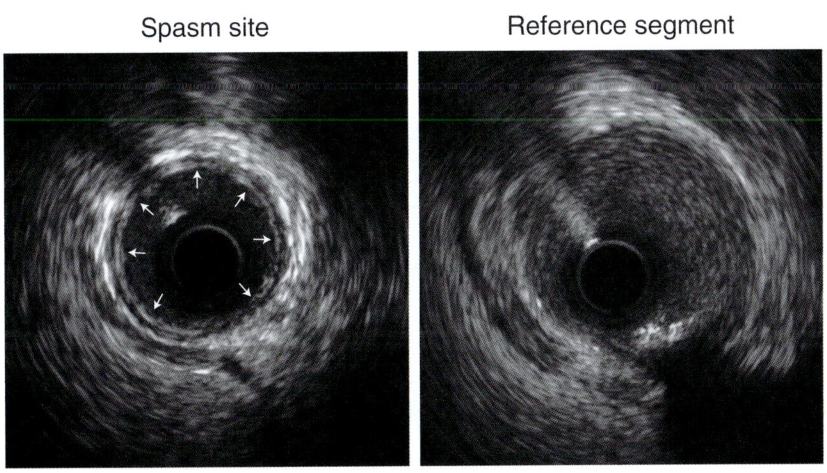

FIGURE 15.27 IVUS images at spasm site and reference segment. Intima is diffusely thickened (arrows) at the spasm site.

Coronary artery spasm has been shown to play an important role in the pathogenesis of not only variant angina but also ischemic heart disease in general, including variant forms of angina pectoris, acute myocardial infarction, and sudden death (**FIGURE 15.27**). Diffuse thickening of intima plus media area is a typical change of coronary spasm in IVUS imaging.

Residual Plaque Burden

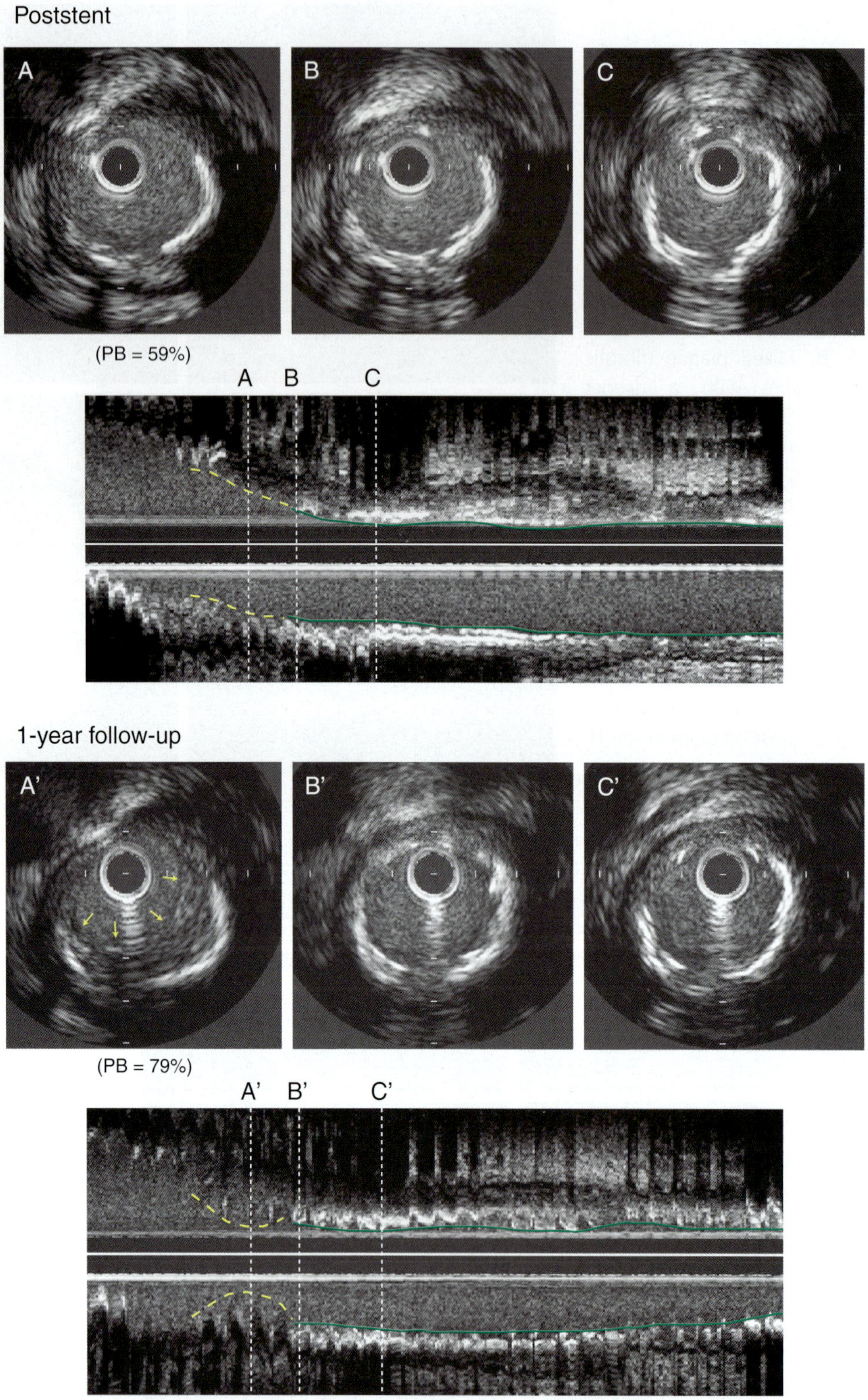

FIGURE 15.28 Residual plaque burden. The IVUS images at baseline (upper) and follow-up (lower) of a patient who developed plaque progression at the proximal reference during 1 year after DES implantation. Minimal neointimal hyperplasia is observed within the stent, whereas obvious plaque progression (yellow arrows in **A′**) is noted in the proximal reference segment where only mild calcified plaque lesion was observed at baseline. The positions in the cross-sectional and longitudinal views at baseline **(A-C)** correspond to the **A′**, **B′**, and **C′** at follow-up. Yellow dotted line tracing lumen and green line tracing stent in longitudinal views. PB, plaque burden.

The ratio of plaque area to total vessel area is termed "plaque burden" (**FIGURE 15.28**). Residual plaque burden after stenting is known as a major and independent influence on the late outcome.[2]

Incomplete Stent Apposition

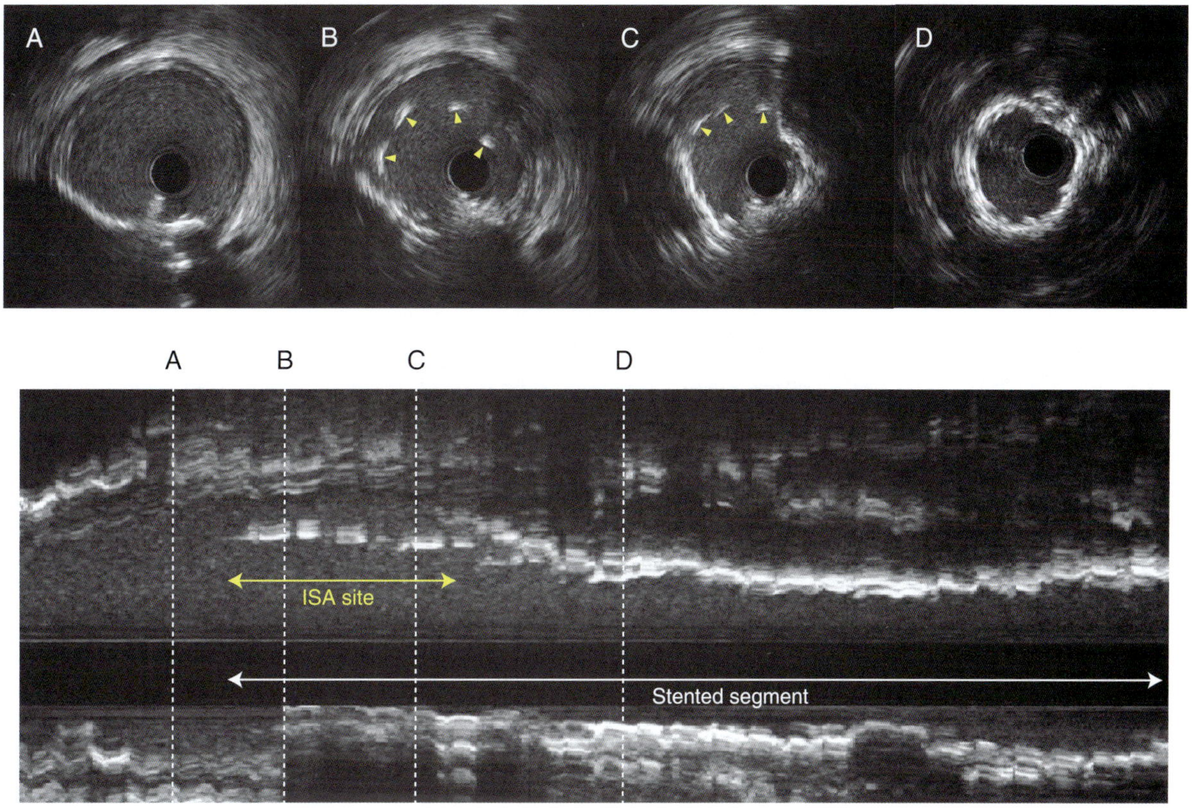

FIGURE 15.29 **A-D**, IVUS images of an ISA case. The malapposed stent struts are shown in the proximal edge of the placed stent both in the cross-sectional IVUS (yellow arrowheads in **B** and **C**) and the longitudinal view.

Incomplete stent apposition (ISA) or stent malapposition occurs when part of the stent structure is not fully in contact with the vessel wall (**FIGURE 15.29**). This is defined by IVUS as 1 or more struts clearly separated from the vessel wall with evidence of blood speckle behind the strut in a segment not associated with any side branches. Isolated ISA observed after deployment usually is not directly linked to adverse clinical events, provided that the lumen is large enough to preserve blood flow. On the other hand, significant ISA possibly increases local flow disturbances, delays healing, and increases the potential risk for stent deformation at subsequent procedures. An early clinical study demonstrated an unexpectedly high percentage of these IVUS-detected stent deployment issues, even after angiographically successful results. These observations led to the concept of the high-pressure stent deployment technique used today.

Classification of ISA (FIGURE 15.30).

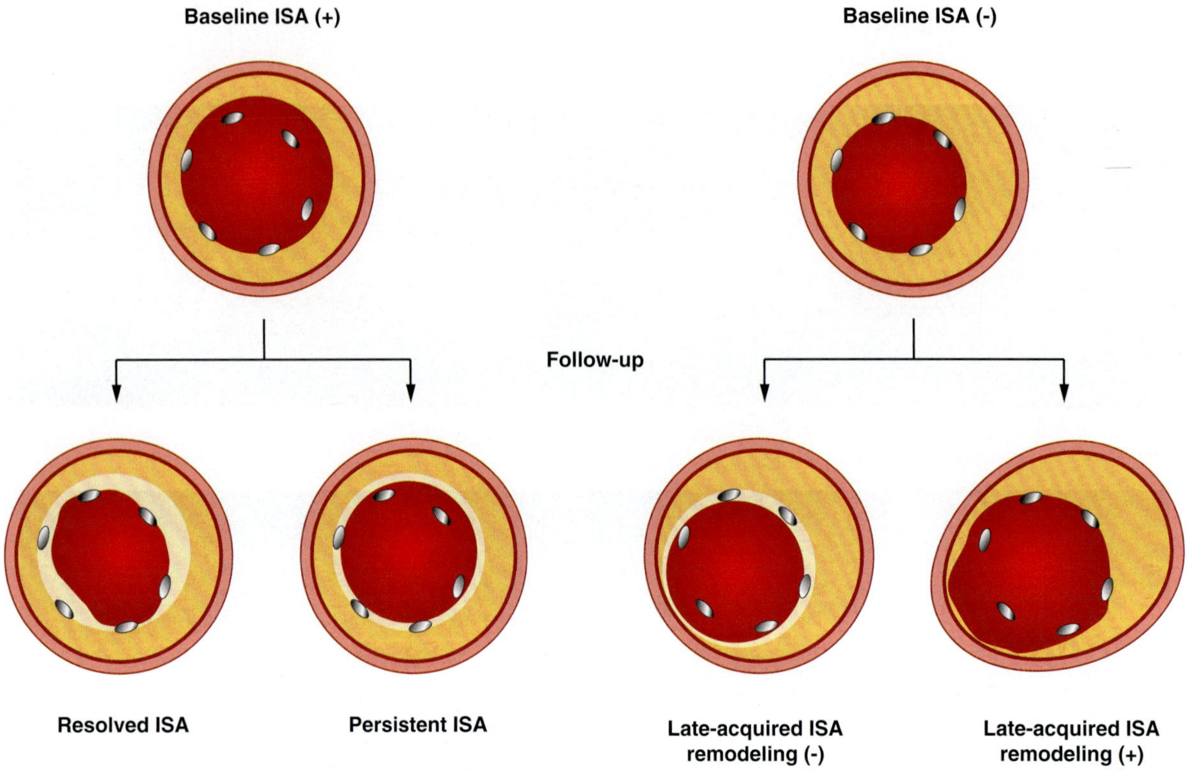

FIGURE 15.30 Classification of ISA.

ISA observed in a baseline study can either be resolved (resolved ISA) or remain (persistent ISA) at follow-up. Late-acquired ISA (LISA) without vessel expansion is typically seen with thrombus-containing baseline lesions, whereas LISA with focal, positive vessel remodeling is more characteristic of segments treated by brachytherapy or drug-eluting stents (DESs).

Incomplete Stent Expansion or Underexpansion

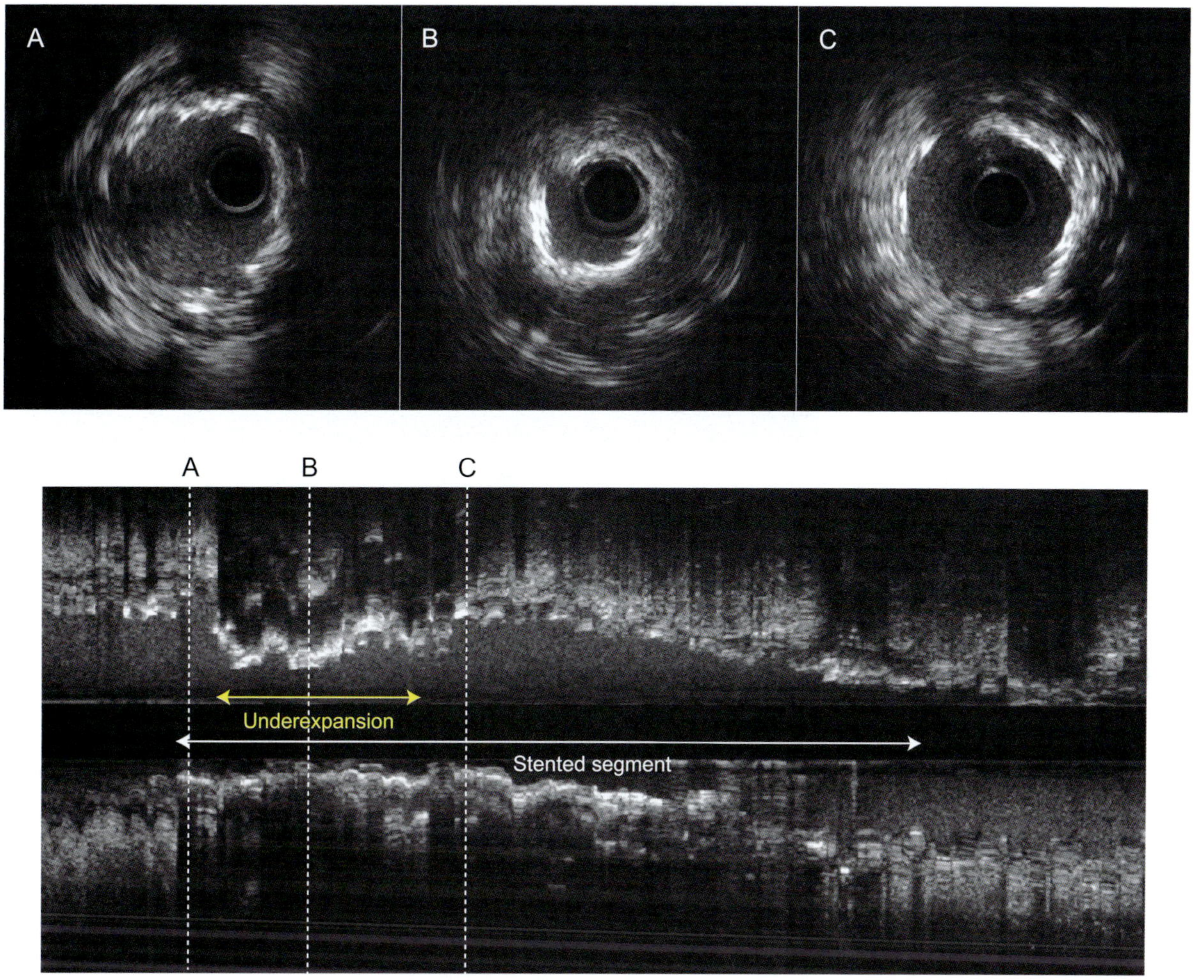

FIGURE 15.31 Incomplete stent expansion or underexpansion. Longitudinal and its corresponding cross-sectional images **(A-C)**. Cross section of **B** shows extensive incomplete expansion (or underexpansion) relative to the proximal and distal segment of the stent. MSA is 2.6 mm^2.

Incomplete stent expansion (or stent underexpansion) is defined as inadequate expansion of a portion of the stent compared with the distal and proximal reference dimensions (**FIGURE 15.31A-C**). This may occur, for example, where dense fibrous or calcified plaque is present. Stent underexpansion represents the most consistent risk factor for both restenosis and thrombosis after stent implantation across clinical IVUS studies. Several investigators have evaluated the predictive value of IVUS-determined minimal stent area (MSA) for in-stent restenosis (ISR) in various types of stents. The optimal diagnostic thresholds of MSA that best predict long-term stent patency were reported to be 5.0 to 5.7 mm^2 for DES and 6.4 to 6.5 mm^2 for bare-metal stent (BMS).[3-6] IVUS-determined MSA remains an independent predictor of restenosis (odds ratio [OR], 0.48-0.77), irrespective of DES type, including sirolimus-, paclitaxel-, zotarolimus-, and everolimus-eluting stents.[5,7]

Instent Thrombus And Tissue Protrusion

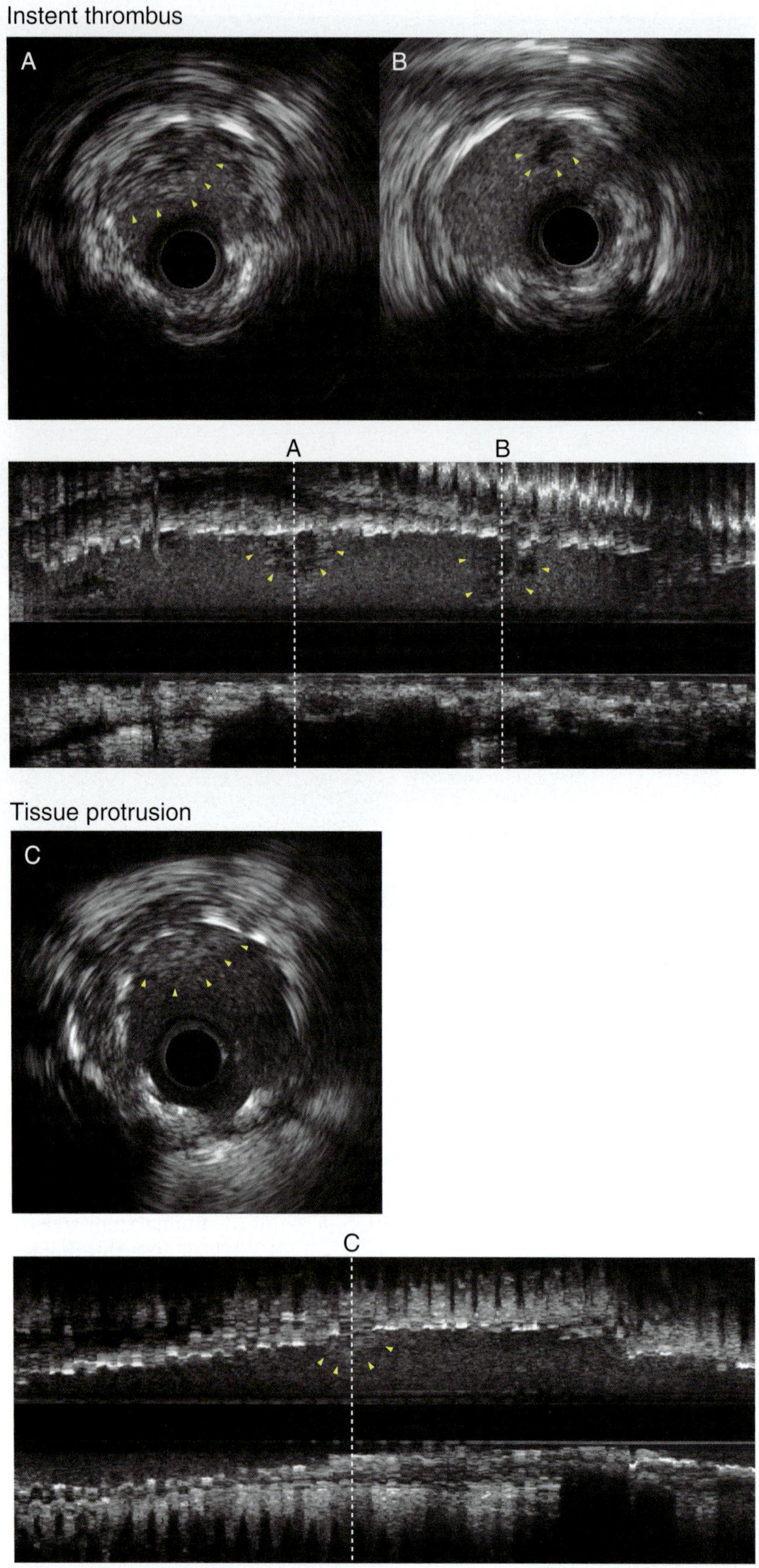

FIGURE 15.32 Instent thrombus and tissue protrusion.

Thrombus is usually recognized as an intraluminal mass (**FIGURE 15.32A** and **B**), often with a layered, lobulated, or pedunculated appearance. Acute thrombus may appear as a relatively echodense mass with speckling or scintillation, while old organized thrombus often has a darker ultrasound appearance. Injection of contrast or saline may disperse the stagnant flow from the lumen, often allowing differentiation of stasis from thrombus.

Tissue protrusions (**FIGURE 15.32C**) are often observed just after placement of stents, and their appearance is essentially similar to that of thrombus.

Hematoma

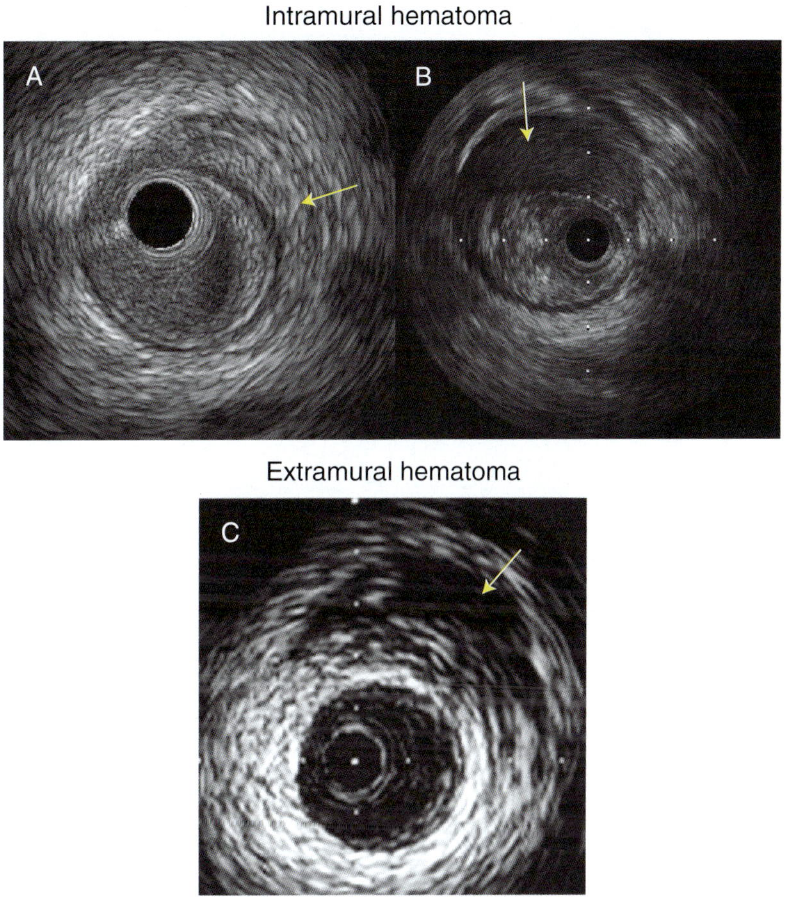

FIGURE 15.33 **Intramural (intravascular) hematoma** is observed typically as a homogenous, hyperechoic, crescent-shaped area **(A)** but may present with a hypoechoic and/or layered appearance when contrast dye or saline is trapped in the FL **(B)**. **Extravascular hematoma (C)** presents as irregularly shaped with an echo-dim pattern owing to the dilution of red blood cell concentration and dissemination throughout an echogenic adventitia.

Intramural (intravascular) hematoma (**FIGURE 15.33A** and **B**) is recognized as an accumulation of blood within the medial space, displacing the internal elastic membrane inward and EEM outward.

Extramural (extravascular) hematoma (**FIGURE 15.33C**) is visualized as an irregularly shaped, echo-dim pattern in the perivascular tissue.

Accordion Artifact

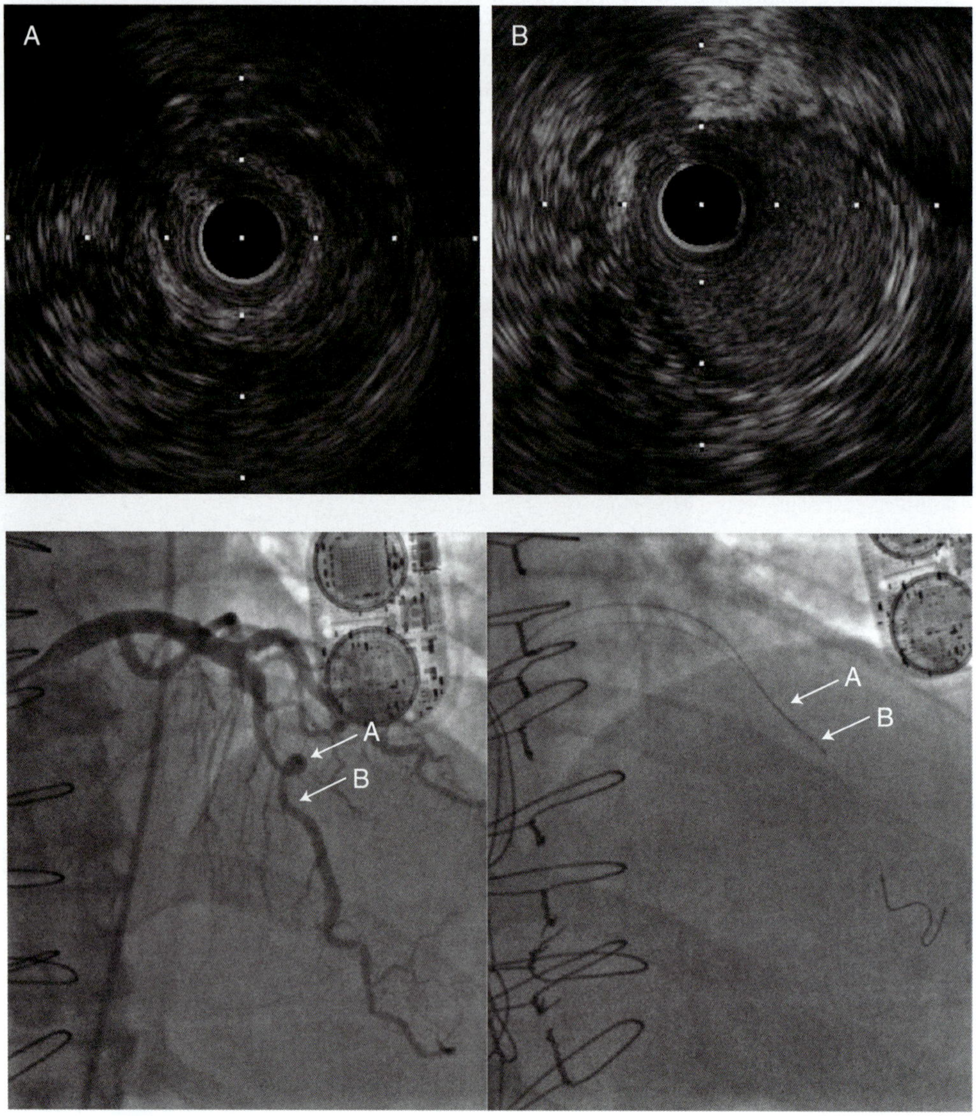

FIGURE 15.34 Accordion artifact. Angiography shows that the guide wire does not conform to the curves in a tortuous artery. Instead, the artery conforms to the straighter guide wire by getting enfolded. The folds in the lumen cause narrowing of the lumen with filling defects. In general, these changes disappear on partial or complete withdrawal of the guide wire, and curvatures in the artery are restored. IVUS cross-sectional image **(A)** shows abrupt change of arterial dimensions with external compression by a heterogeneous or low-echoic structure partially surrounding the artery. **B**, Corresponding to the distal reference of IVUS image.

A "wrinkling" (or "accordion") artifact is caused by an artificial vessel kink associated with intravascular instrumentation (a guide wire or imaging catheter) (**FIGURE 15.34**).

Stent Fracture

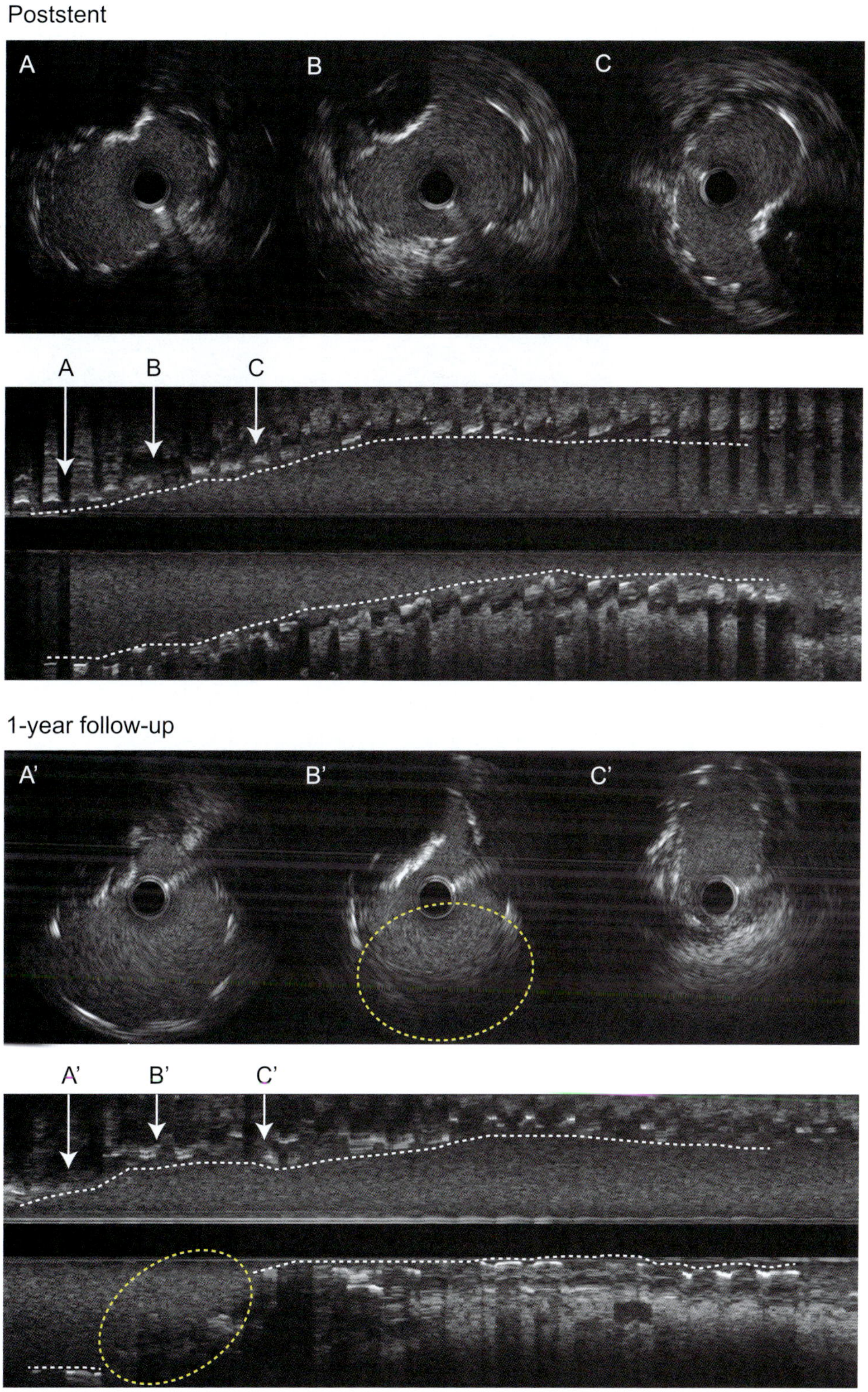

FIGURE 15.35 Stent fracture. Longitudinal view with a schematic diagram of stent struts (white dot lines) and corresponding cross-sectional IVUS images at the poststent (**upper**) and at the 1-year follow-up (**lower**). Although no stent strut collapse is seen at poststent, significant loss of strut discontinuity (yellow dotted circle) is revealed both in the longitudinal and cross-sectional IVUS images at 1-year follow-up.

By IVUS, stent fracture is defined as strut discontinuity and can be categorized based on its morphologic characteristics: (1) strut separation, (2) strut subluxation, or (3) strut intussusceptions (**FIGURE 15.35**).[8] Another proposed classification focuses on potential mechanisms of the strut fracture, categorizing them based on the presence and absence of aneurysm at the fracture site (types I and II, respectively).[9] Stent fracture is reported to be a risk for subsequent ISR or stent thrombosis.

Stent Deformation

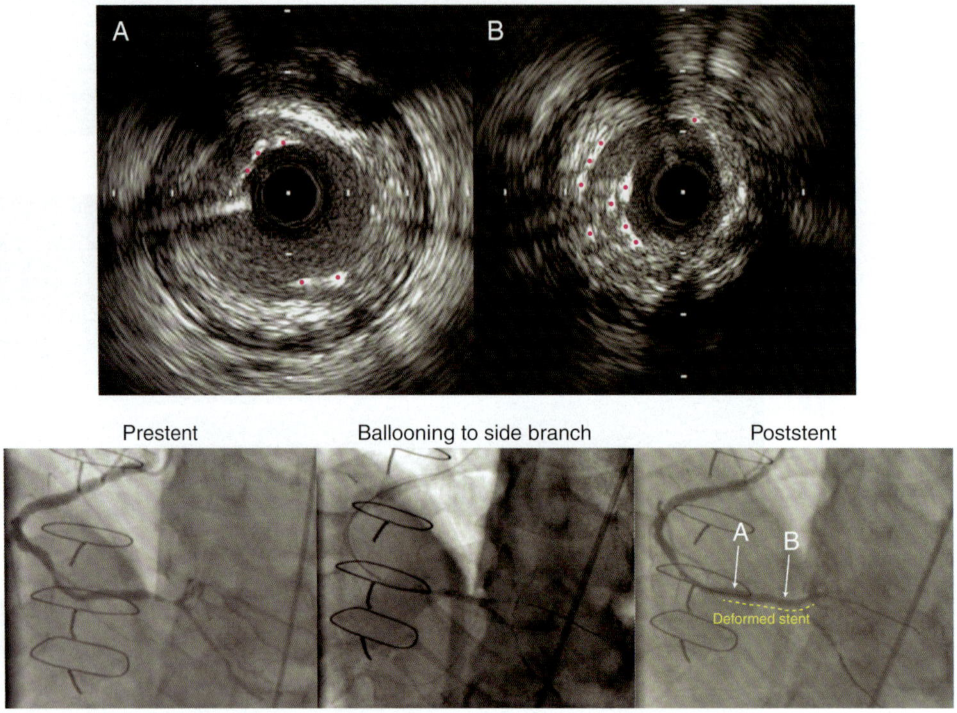

FIGURE 15.36 Example of stent deformation caused by passing and withdrawing a balloon for opening the jailed side branch. Baseline angiogram shows the lesion at the distal RCA involving the crux bifurcation. One stent was placed to cross over the posterior descending artery (PDA) branch. After passing and withdrawing a balloon for opening the jailed PDA branch, stent deformation occurred. Intrastent wrinkling and nonuniform strut distribution **(A)** and multiple strut overlapping and loss of struts in the counter side **(B)** can be visualized by IVUS (pink circles marking the deformed struts in the cross sections).

Stent deformation can be defined as the distortion, shortening, or elongation of a stent caused by mechanical stress following the initial successful stent deployment (**FIGURE 15.36**). It can be induced by guide catheter compression or secondary devices passed into the stent, such as postdilatation balloon, IVUS catheters, filterwire devices, and even by withdrawal of a buddy wire. Intrastent wrinkling and multiple strut layers are found within deformed stents on IVUS, but there is no specific pattern for stent deformation.

Perivascular Microvessels

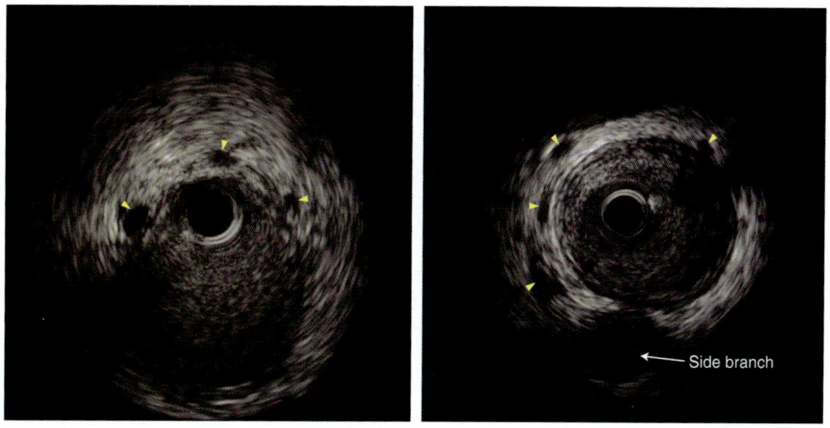

FIGURE 15.37 Perivascular microvessels (or vasa vasorum).

Perivascular microvessels of the coronary artery are a network of blood vessels that supply coronary vessel wall (FIGURE 15.37). IVUS visualized a tubular, low-echoic structure exterior to media, indicating perivascular small vessels (yellow arrowheads).

Myocardial Bridging (MB)

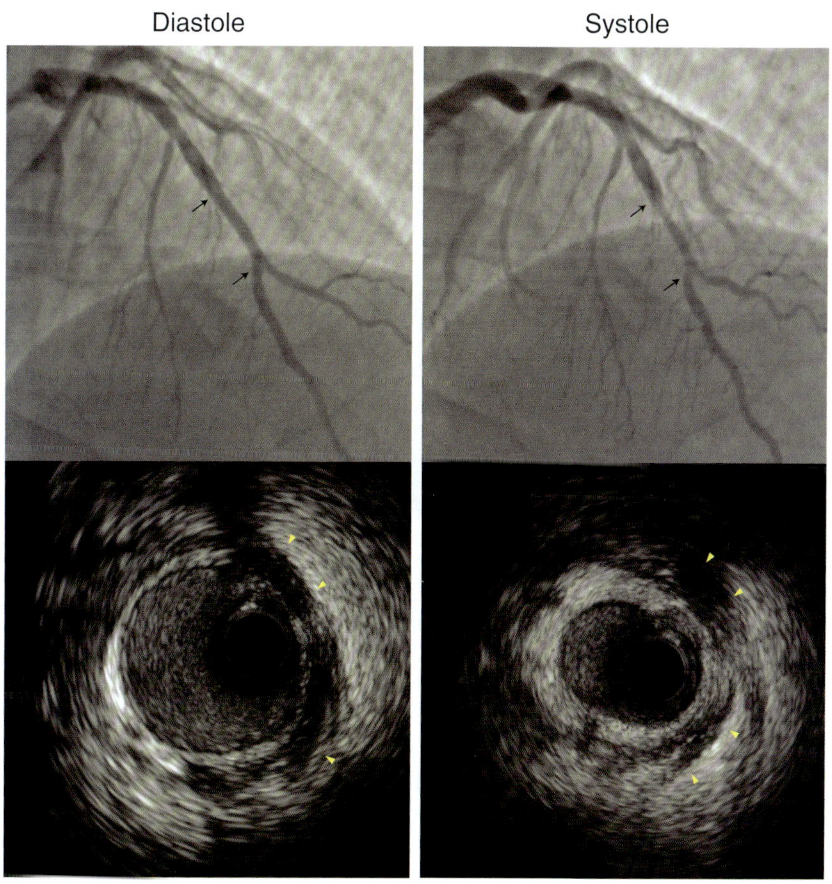

FIGURE 15.38 Myocardial bridging (MB). Angiography showed compression at the middle of the LAD during systole (black arrows indicating the beginning and the end of the MB). Within the MB segment, the IVUS cross-sections visualize systolic arterial compression and the characteristic "halo sign" (yellow arrowheads). The systolic cross-sectional EEM area is 3.6 mm^2, whereas the diastolic is 7.5 mm^2 (52% area stenosis).

Myocardial bridging (MB) is a common congenital coronary anomaly that is located most frequently in the LAD (FIGURE 15.38). Although most patients are presumed to be asymptomatic, MB can cause typical or atypical angina and even myocardial infarction, most likely because of direct compression effects on the MB segment or accelerated atherosclerosis in the segment proximal to the MB. IVUS can detect MB with greater sensitivity than computed tomography or angiography, both by functional assessment (systolic arterial compression) and by a characteristic echolucent band appearance (halo) partially surrounding the artery. The direct assessment of muscle tissue by IVUS regarding length, thickness, and location, in combination with a functional measurement of systolic arterial compression, may provide prognostic information in specific patients and determine the indication and strategy of treatment, especially when unroofing surgery is considered.

Cardiac Allograft Vasculopathy (CAV)

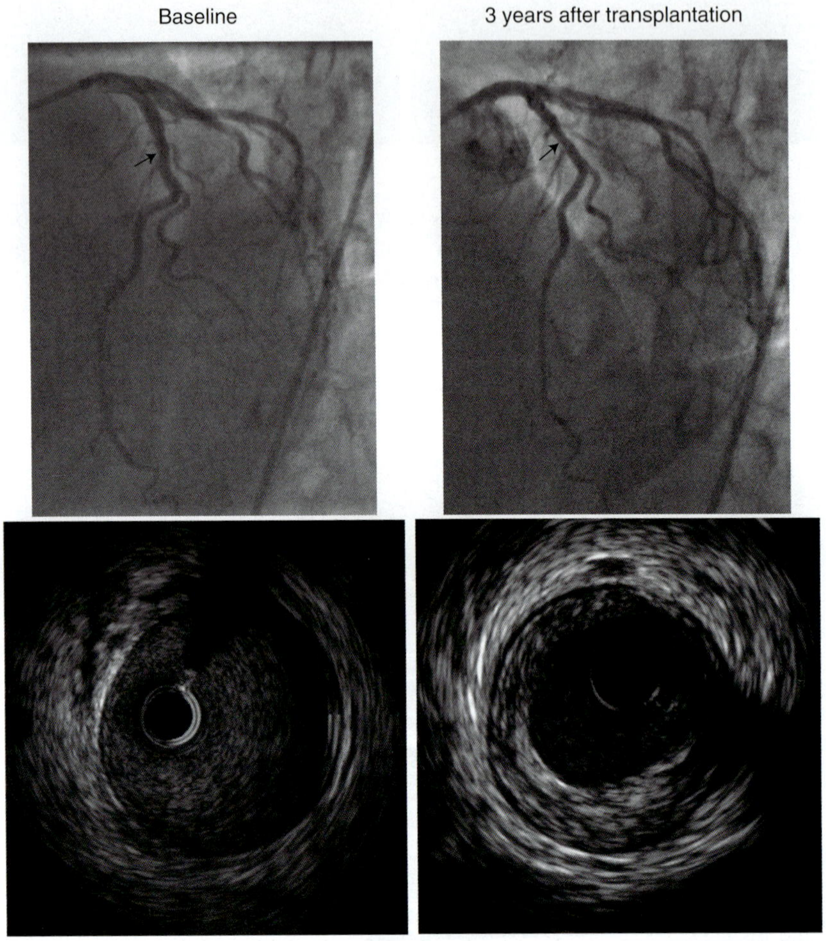

FIGURE 15.39 Example of CAV. Angiography and IVUS cross sections of the LAD at baseline and 3 years after heart transplantation. At baseline, most of the vessel wall appears to be monolayer with no intimal thickening (maximal intimal thickness, 0.27 mm). At 3 years, there is considerable intimal thickening; the maximal intimal thickness of this artery is 1.03 mm, indicating the occurrence of allograft vasculopathy. Angiography is less sensitive for CAV detection than IVUS due to diffuse, longitudinal, and concentric vascular changes. Black arrows indicate the positions of IVUS cross sections.

Cardiac allograft vasculopathy (CAV), a leading cause of long-term mortality after heart transplantation, is the predominant form of chronic rejection (**FIGURE 15.39**). Both immunologic and nonimmunologic factors drive this process, resulting in localized inflammation with persistent vascular injury and endothelial dysfunction. IVUS is the most sensitive tool for the diagnosis of CAV and is considered the gold standard for studies on transplant vasculopathy. IVUS can directly visualize the wall structure, offering a sensitive method to evaluate CAV, which is typically characterized by coronary intimal thickening with pathologic remodeling. Because CAV is frequently diffuse and circumferential, many patients with moderate to severe intimal thickening on IVUS, including those who develop clinical events, do not have significant visible disease on coronary angiography.[10]

Bioresorbable Vascular Scaffold (BRS)

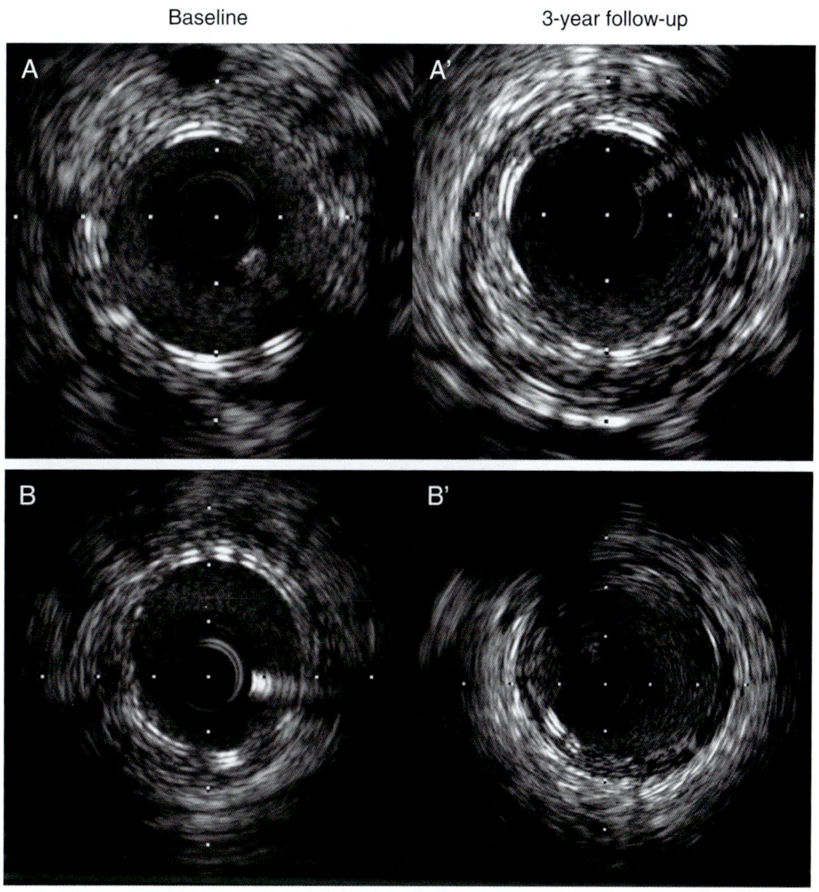

FIGURE 15.40 IVUS image of the Absorb everolimus-eluting BRS (Abbott, Corp.) at baseline **(A and B)** and 3 years after placement **(A′ and B′).** Struts appear as parallel lines without acoustic shadowing because ultrasonic waves pass through the struts with a small reflection from the luminal and abluminal surfaces. At 3-year follow-up, polymeric scaffolds show various patterns of resorption with mild neointimal growth. Most scaffolds are still highly visible even at follow-up in **A′**, whereas only a few scaffolds can be detected in **B′**.

The bioresorbable vascular scaffold (BRS) provides short-term vessel scaffolding of the coronary lesions without permanent implantation (**FIGURE 15.40**).[11] On IVUS, the scaffolds can be seen as double-layered lines (leading and trailing edges of the struts). IVUS can be helpful for optimal BRS sizing and guidance for postdilating, with the goal of avoiding underexpansion or scaffold fracture.

Strut Fracture of BRS

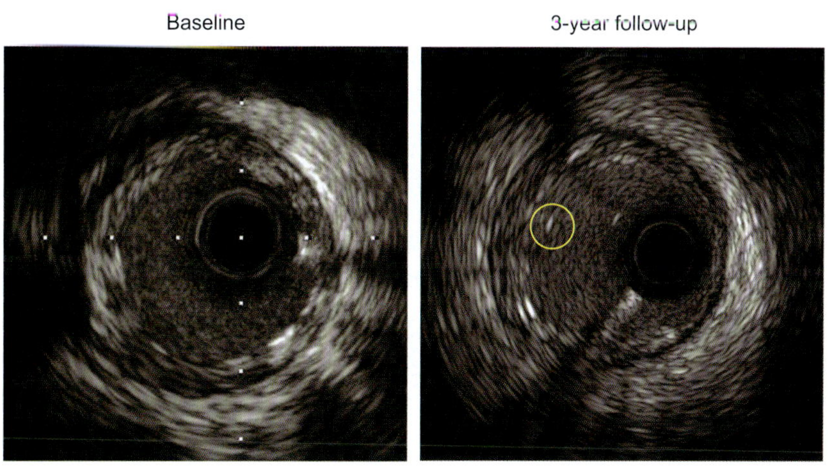

FIGURE 15.41 Strut fracture of BRS.

IVUS cross-sectional images of poststent deployment and 3-year follow-up after BRS implantation (**FIGURE 15.41**). Although IVUS images at poststent deployment show neither strut fracture nor malapposition, IVUS images at 3-year follow-up show that a portion of the scaffold protrudes into the vessel lumen and appeared disorientated (yellow circle), corresponding to strut fracture.

Incomplete Apposition of BRS

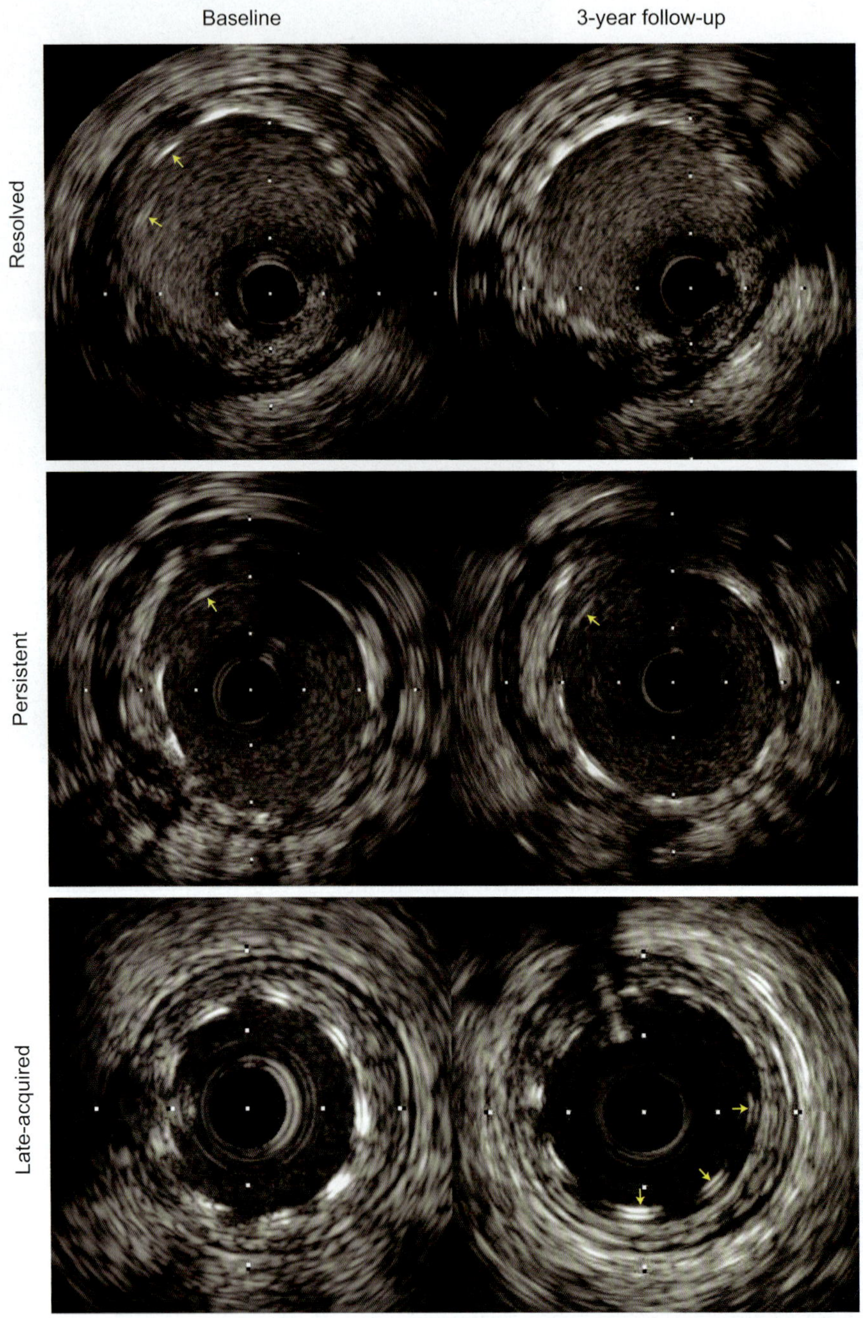

FIGURE 15.42 Three types of incomplete apposition (resolved, persistent, and late-acquired) after BRS implantation. Serial IVUS cross sections at poststent and 3-year follow-up are shown. Yellow arrows indicate malapposed scaffolds.

Incomplete apposition is defined as 1 or more scaffold struts that is separated from the vessel wall and (as with metal stents) is classified as resolved, persistent, or late-acquired (**FIGURE 15.42**). The mechanism of late-acquired malapposition remains unclear; however, it is possible that resorption may be accelerated by secondary inflammation, resulting in vessel and lumen enlargement.

Ivus Guidance For LMCA

In the assessment of LMCA disease, angulations, calcification, or spasm in this location can lead to poor guiding catheter engagement and confounded interpretation of the angiogram (see **FIGURE 15.43**). Several investigators have demonstrated that a high percentage of patients with angiographically normal LMCA are seen to have disease by IVUS. Conversely, another IVUS study demonstrated that fewer than half of the angiographically ambiguous LMCA lesions had significant stenosis.[12]

Cases of LMCA Assesment by IVUS

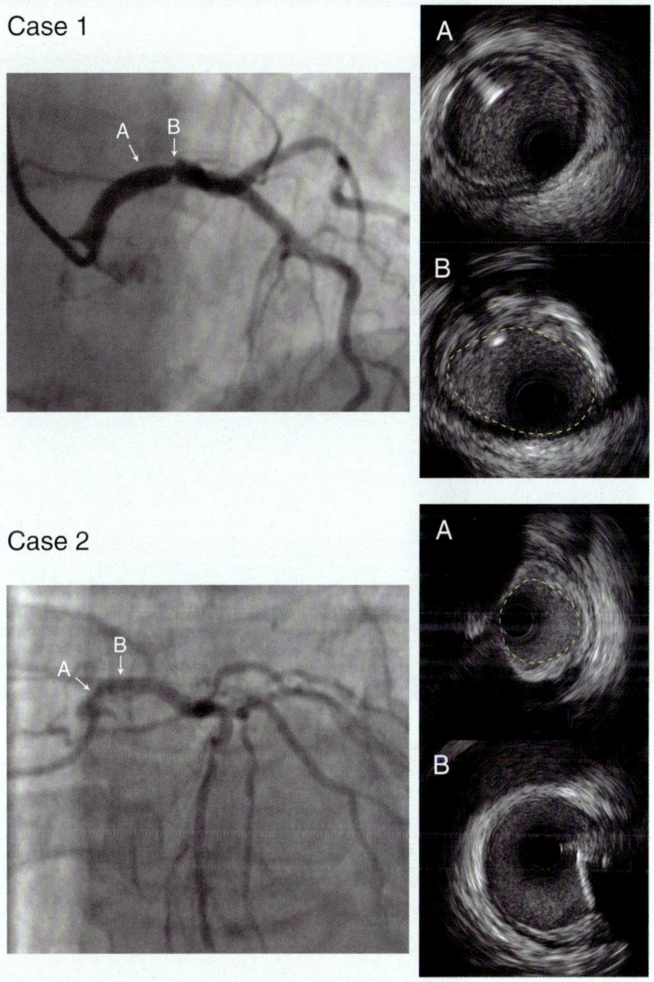

FIGURE 15.43 IVUS guidance for LMCA disease.

In Case 1 (**FIGURE 15.43**), the LMCA appears to have a critical distal stenosis by angiography; however, the fractional flow reserve (FFR) value distal to the LMCA stenosis (=0.88) is not significant. IVUS revealed that a minimum lumen area (MLA) of the distal LMCA is 7.5 mm^2 in compressed shape with plaque accumulation. Because both FFR and IVUS data corroborate that the stenosis of the left main ostium is not significant, revascularization of the LMCA should be deferred.

In Case 2 (**FIGURE 15.43**), only a moderate stenosis can be observed at the ostial LMCA segment by angiography. The IVUS image reveals a significant lumen narrowing (MLA = 3.7 mm^2), with plaque lesion at the corresponding segment. In this case, revascularization is recommended.

Yellow dotted line tracing the lumen at MLA site.

DES Failure

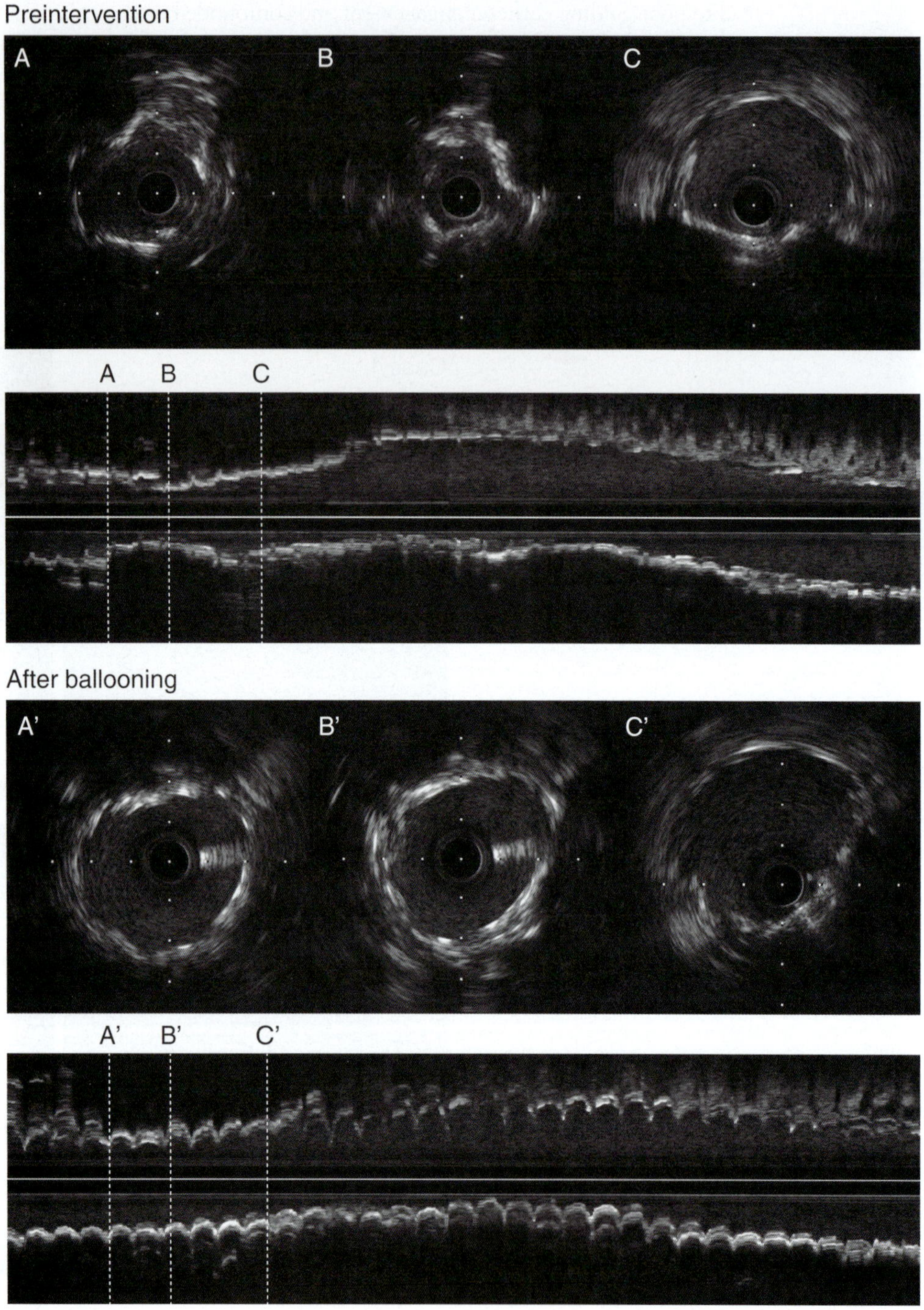

FIGURE 15.44 DES restenosis results primarily from stent underexpansion. Preinteventinal IVUS (upper images) reveals significant stent underexpansion at the proximal segment **(B)** with only a small amount of focal neointima hyperplasia. This type of ISR can often be successfully treated by balloon dilation (lower images) and may not require additional DES implantation within the original restenosed stent.

The most consistent IVUS risk factor for DES restenosis and thrombosis is stent underexpansion, the incidence of which has been reported as 60% to 80% of current DES failures (**FIGURE 15.44**). In the DES era, the relationship between postimplantation MSA and subsequent lumen caliber in the stented segment is more direct than with BMS, as variability of the neointimal proliferation is reduced.

Late-Aquired Incomplete Stent Apposition (LISA)

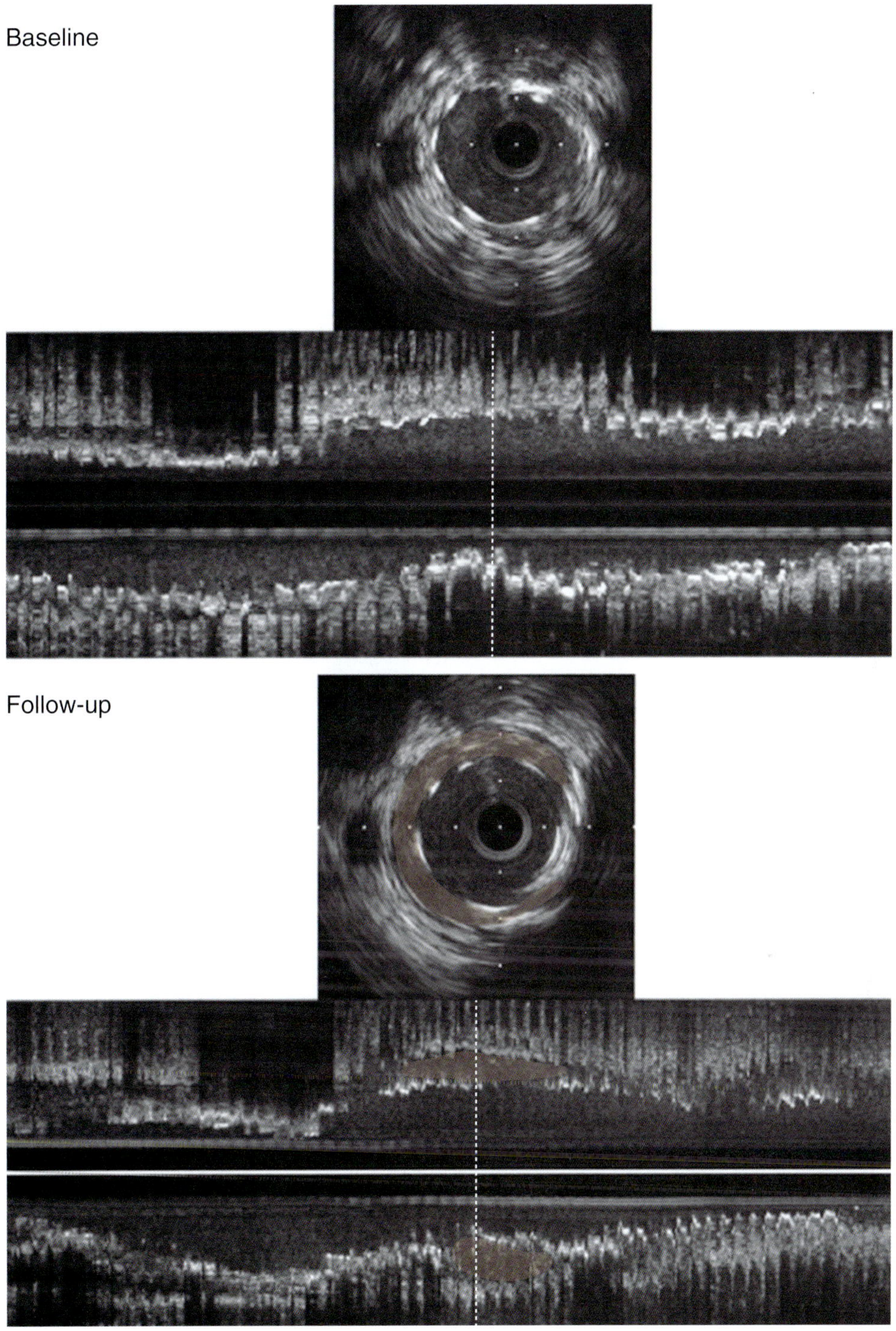

FIGURE 15.45 LISA observed at follow-up (lower images) after implantation of sirolimus-eluting stent, a type of DES. At follow-up, moderate gaps between the stent and the vessel wall are detected (lower images), whereas the stent struts are well apposed to the vessel wall at baseline (upper images).

ISA observed at follow-up could represent either persistent ISA or LISA (FIGURE 15.45). LISA primarily results from structural vessel wall changes that occur during the follow-up period ("biologic ISA"), in contrast to "mechanical ISA" seen with initial stent deployment. The most commonly reported mechanisms for LISA are dissolution of thrombus present at the baseline, and regional positive vessel remodeling that overwhelms plaque area increase.[13] Whereas thrombus dissolution can be seen in patients with any type of stent deployed in thrombus-containing lesions, abnormal positive vessel remodeling is observed more frequently in patients who received a DES or brachytherapy treatment. In cases of remodeling, malapposition is seen primarily with eccentric plaques, and the gaps develop mainly on the disease-free side of the vessel wall.[14] The combination of mechanical injury at stent implantation and biologic injury by DES components may predispose the vessel wall to chronic, pathologic dilatation in the setting of little underlying plaque.[15]

Ivus Guidance For Chronic Total Occlusion (CTO)

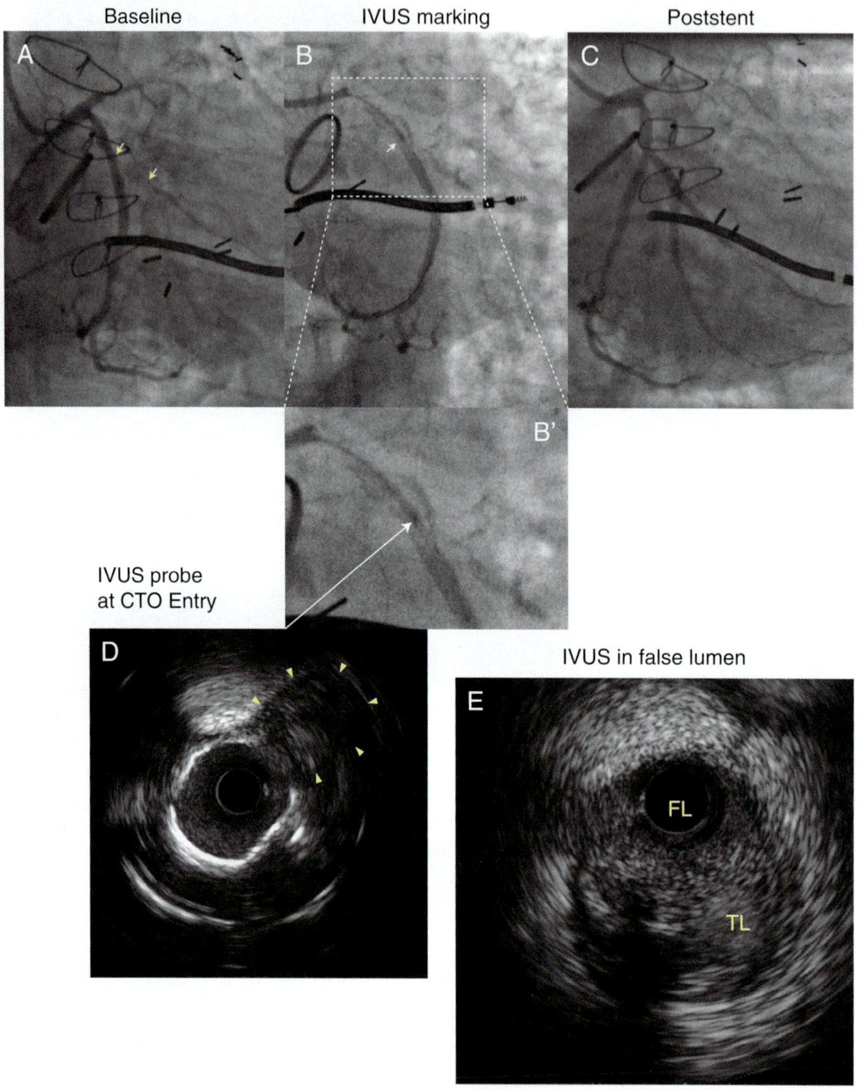

FIGURE 15.46 Example of side branch IVUS for determining the entry point of the CTO and identification of guide wire in FL. Baseline coronary angiography **(A)** shows CTO lesion (yellow arrows indicating the beginning and the end of CTO) in the proximal part of OM branch in LCX with distal vessel filling from collateral arteries. There is no suggestion of entry point of the CTO from the angiography. IVUS pull back from the distal LCX visualizes the proximal entry point of the CTO with simultaneous angiography (white arrow in **B** and **B′** indicating the position of IVUS probe). The IVUS cross section **(D)** shows CTO entry point at 1- to 3-o'clock position (yellow arrowheads). With this landmark from the IVUS image, a stiff guide wire is advanced with microcatheter back up in the direction of proximal entry point, but this wire ends up in FL. The next IVUS **(E)** through this guide wire shows the IVUS probe in FL with compressed TL. Finally, a second tapered stiff wire is successfully advanced into TL with parallel wire technique. Poststent angiogram demonstrates a good result **(C)**.

IVUS is useful in several aspects during intervention on CTO lesions (**FIGURE 15.46**).[16] In lesions with abrupt-type occlusion, the entry point at the CTO ostium is often difficult to identify by angiography. If there is a side branch located near the entrance of CTO, the IVUS catheter can be inserted into the side branch to examine the target for wire penetration. Also, in some cases, the IVUS catheter tracks into the subintimal space, which can provide visualization of the location of the TL. In some cases, it can be challenging to differentiate the TL from the FL. Side branches offer an important clue, as they should communicate with the true but not with the FL. It is important to note that manipulating the IVUS catheter into or along the subintimal space has the potential risk of enlarging this FL.

OPTICAL COHERENCE TOMOGRAPHY

OCT Imaging Systems

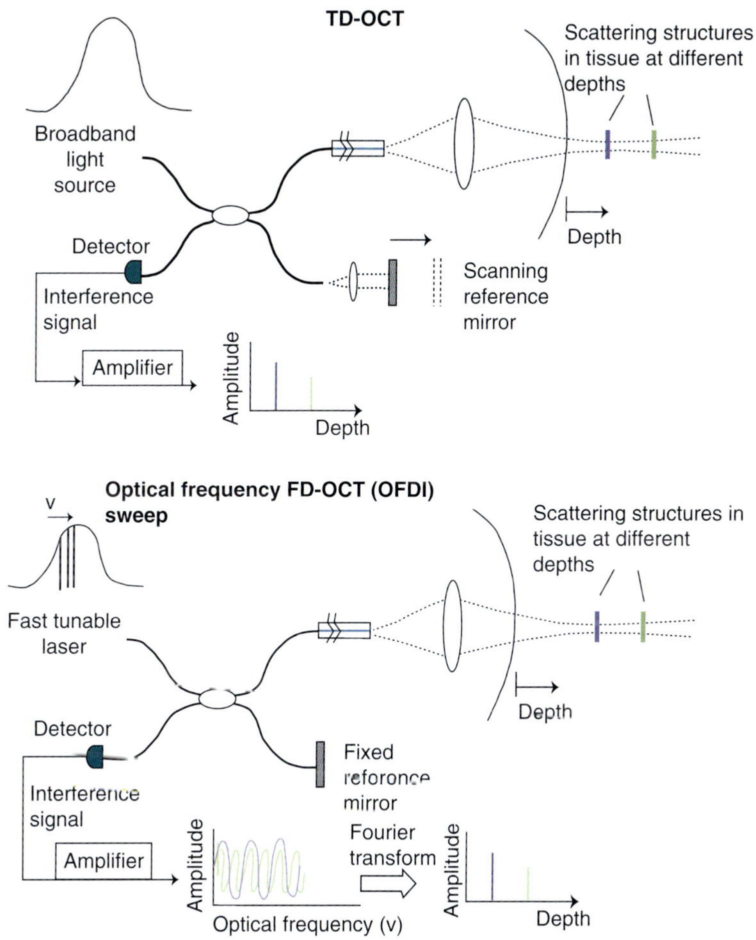

FIGURE 15.47 OCT imaging systems. Reprinted with permission from Bezerra HG, Costa MA, Guagliumi G, Rollins AM, Simon DI. Intracoronary optical coherence tomography: a comprehensive review clinical and research applications. *JACC Cardiovasc Interv*. 2009;2(11):1035-1046.

The ability of OCT to create tomographic cross-sectional images of a vessel is based on optical interference of near-infrared light (**FIGURE 15.47**).[17] Light is emitted and collected back from the tip of a small-diameter optical fiber that rotates rapidly inside a transparent sheath of the catheter. For longitudinal scanning of the vessel, a drive motor unit on the table pulls back the fiber as it rotates within the sheath. In the first-generation systems, called time domain (TD)-OCT, the emitted light is split into a sample beam and a reference beam. When these beams are recombined, positive interference occurs only when the 2 paths are matched—as a result, only the tissue plane that corresponds exactly to the reference arm length is recorded for image reconstruction. In the second-generation frequency domain (FD)-OCT systems, interference is generated using a rapidly swept wavelength source and a stationary reference arm. Each frequency component of the detected interference signal is associated with a discrete depth location within the tissue.

Cross-sectional Format of OCT

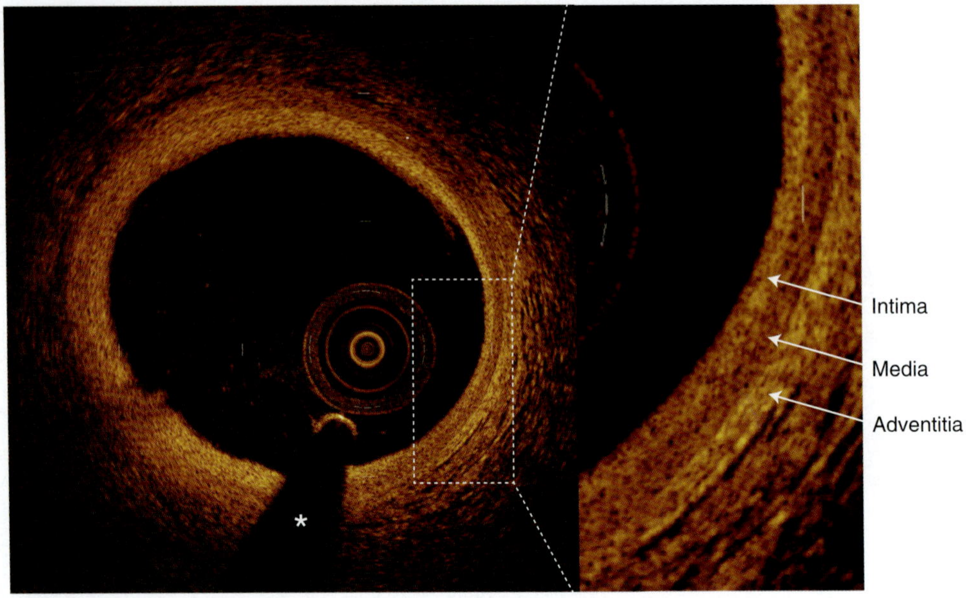

FIGURE 15.48 Cross-sectional format of a typical OCT image. Similar to that seen by IVUS, the normal vessel wall is characterized by a 3-layered architecture on OCT images, comprising a highly backscattering (signal-rich) intima, a media with low backscattering (signal-poor), and a heterogeneous and frequently highly backscattering adventitia. The higher resolution of OCT can often provide superior delineation of each structure with visualization of internal and external elastic membranes as separate thin high-intensity layers. The periadventitial tissues may present an appearance consistent with fat, characterized by large clear structures. A guide wire is seen as a common OCT image artifacts with shadowing (*).

The imaging procedure of intravascular OCT is similar to that of IVUS, except that blood must be displaced by optically transparent liquid (contrast media, low-molecular-weight dextrose, or lactated Ringer solution) while imaging, as red blood cells cause significant scattering of near-infrared light, resulting in very large signal loss. Image acquisition is performed during continuous flushing through the guide catheter typically using a power injector at a flow rate of 3 to 6 mL/s. Because of the very high speed of the pullback, FD-OCT has the ability to scan long segments of artery in few seconds, without need to occlude the vessel, resulting in minimal ischemic electrocardiographic changes and no major arrhythmias during image acquisition.

The greatest advantage of this light-based imaging technology is its significantly higher resolution (10 times or greater) than that of conventional pulse-echo, ultrasound-based approaches (**FIGURE 15.48**).

Common OCT Image Artifacts (FIGURE 15.49)

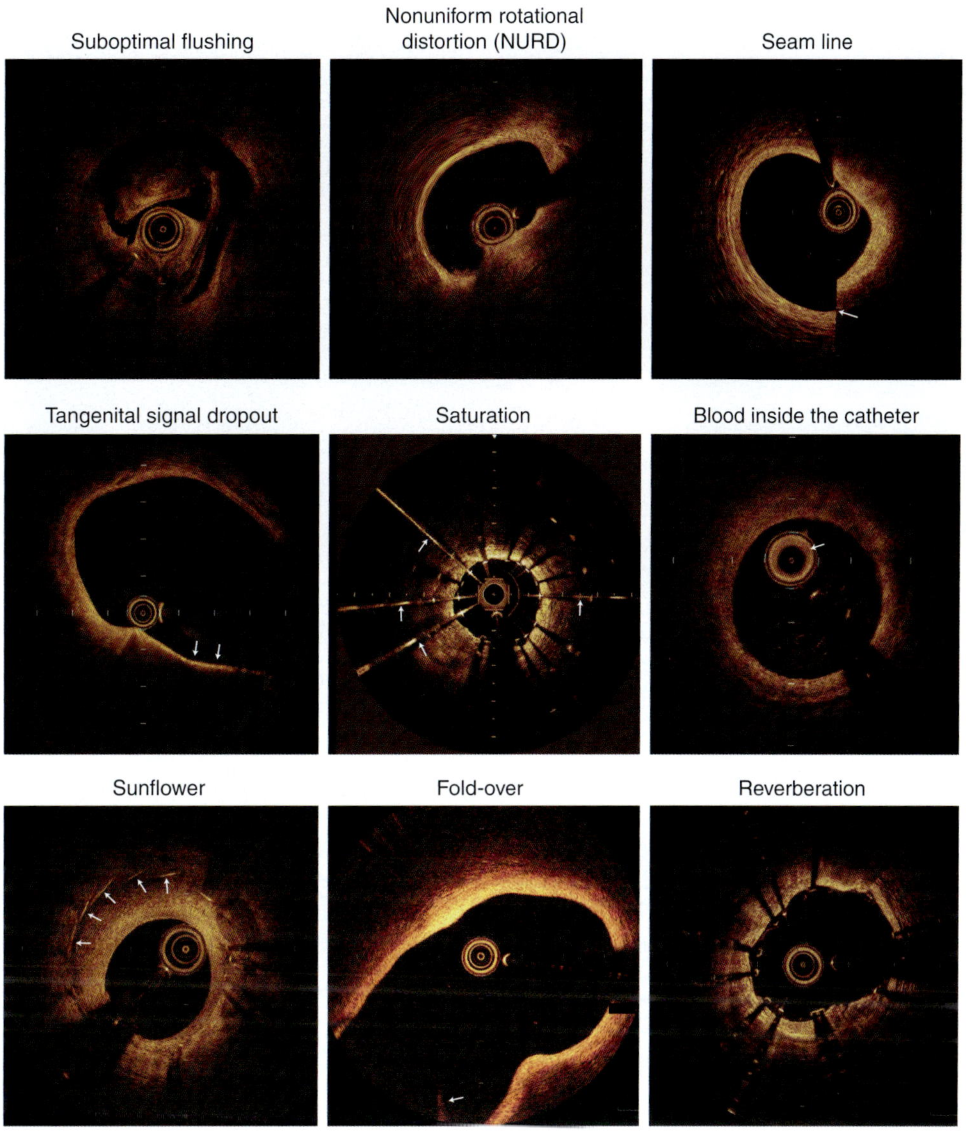

FIGURE 15.49 Common OCT image artifacts. **Suboptimal flushing:** Suboptimal flushing can result in residual blood inside the vessel lumen, leading to deterioration of image quality. **Nonuniform rotational distortion (NURD):** NURD results in a wedge-shaped, smeared appearance in 1 or more segments of the image (7- to 12-o'clock direction). **Seam line or "sew-up" artifact:** Seam line artifact appears as an axial discontinuity (arrow) caused by a catheter motion during the single cross-sectional image acquisition. **Tangential signal dropout:** Tangential signal dropout can occur when the optical beam is directed nearly parallel to the tissue surface, which can resemble OCT appearance of TCFA (arrows). **Saturation artifacts:** Saturation artifacts are linear streaks of high and/or low intensities along the axial direction (arrows). This phenomenon can occur when a strong reflector, such as a guide wire or metal stent strut, backscatters at too high an intensity to be accurately detected by the system. **Blood inside the catheter:** Blood inside the catheter presents as a high-intensity area within the imaging sheath, possibly affecting image quality. **Sunflower or "merry-go-round" artifacts:** Sunflower artifacts appear as smeared stent struts (arrows) facing the OCT probe, which are usually more pronounced when the imaging catheter is off-centered within the artery. **Fold-over:** Fold-over artifact (arrow) is more specifically related to the new generation of FD-OCT devices. It is the consequence of "phase wrapping" or "aliasing" along the Fourier transformation. This can occur when the vessel is larger than the ranging depth (8-9 mm in current systems) and should not be interpreted as real tissue structure. **Reverberation:** Highly reflective objects can also produce a series of ghost reflections, or reverberation, that appear as a replica at a fixed distance from the primary image of an object (6- to 11-o'clock direction).

OCT Assessment of Metal Stent Struts

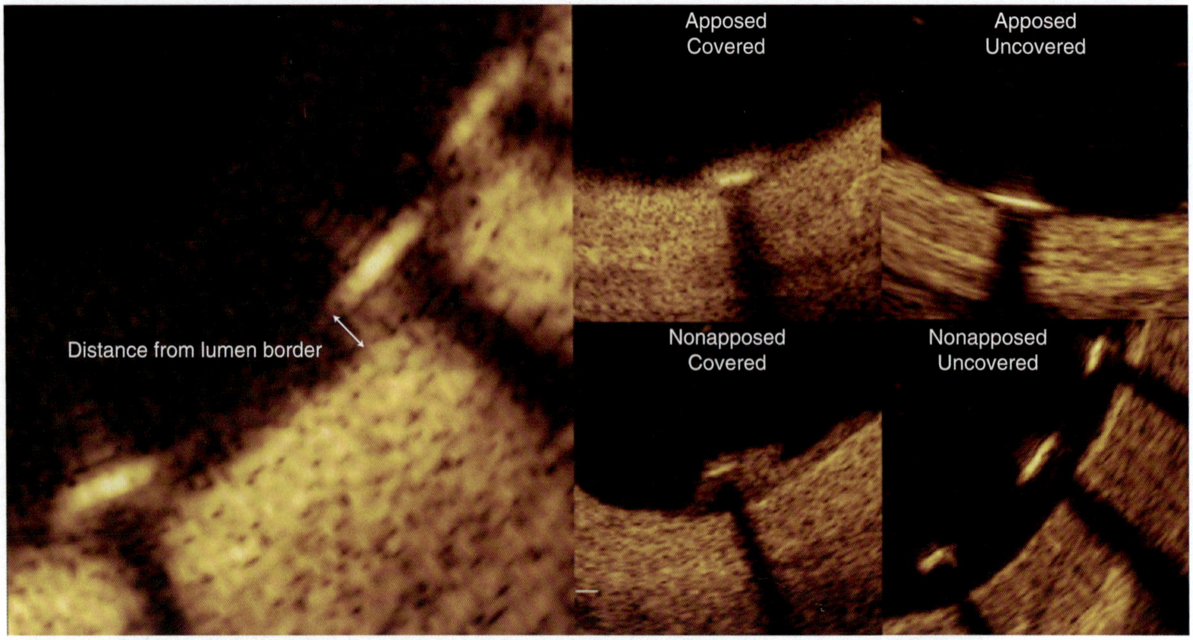

FIGURE 15.50 OCT assessment of metal stent struts.

OCT assessment of metal stent struts in relation to the arterial wall (**FIGURE 15.50**). Strut apposition to the vessel wall is determined by measuring the distance from the stent strut surface to the vessel wall as compared with the nominal strut thickness. Owing to a blooming effect of metal struts, the highest intensity point within the strut image should be used for the measurement. Stent struts at follow-up are classified into 4 categories, based on the apposition and tissue coverage of the struts.

Plaque Types by OCT (FIGURE 15.51)

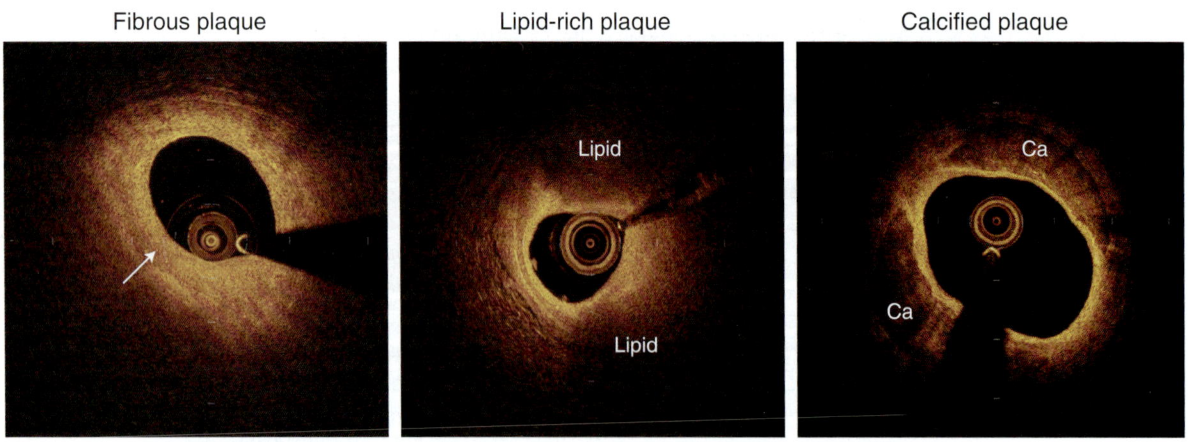

FIGURE 15.51 OCT images for fibrous, lipid-rich, and calcified plaques. In fibrous plaques, the OCT signal is observed to be strong and homogenous (arrow). In contrast, both lipid-rich (Lipid) and calcific (Ca) regions appear as a signal-poor region within the vessel wall. Lipid-rich plaques have diffuse or poorly demarcated borders, whereas the borders of calcific nodules are sharply delineated.

Incomplete Stent Apposition (ISA)

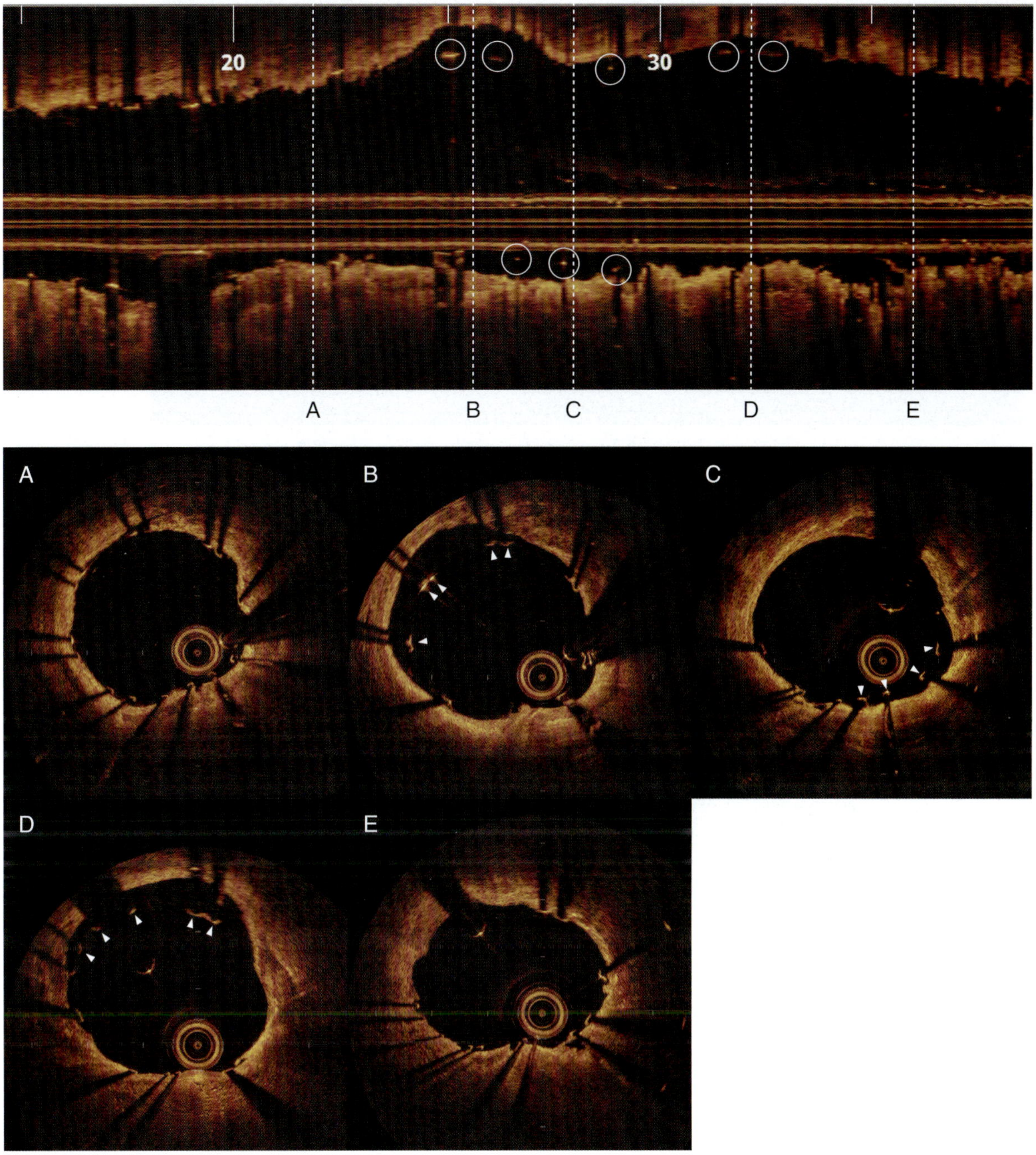

FIGURE 15.52 Longitudinal and the corresponding cross-sectional IVUS images of an ISA case. The cluster of malapposed struts is well visualized (white circles in longitudinal view, white arrowheads in cross sections of **B-D**).

Unlike IVUS, strut apposition is assessed by direct measurement of the distance between the adluminal reflection of the strut and the vessel wall (FIGURE 15.52). ISA is then defined as a strut-vessel distance greater than the nominal strut thickness (including polymer if present).

Tissue Protrusion

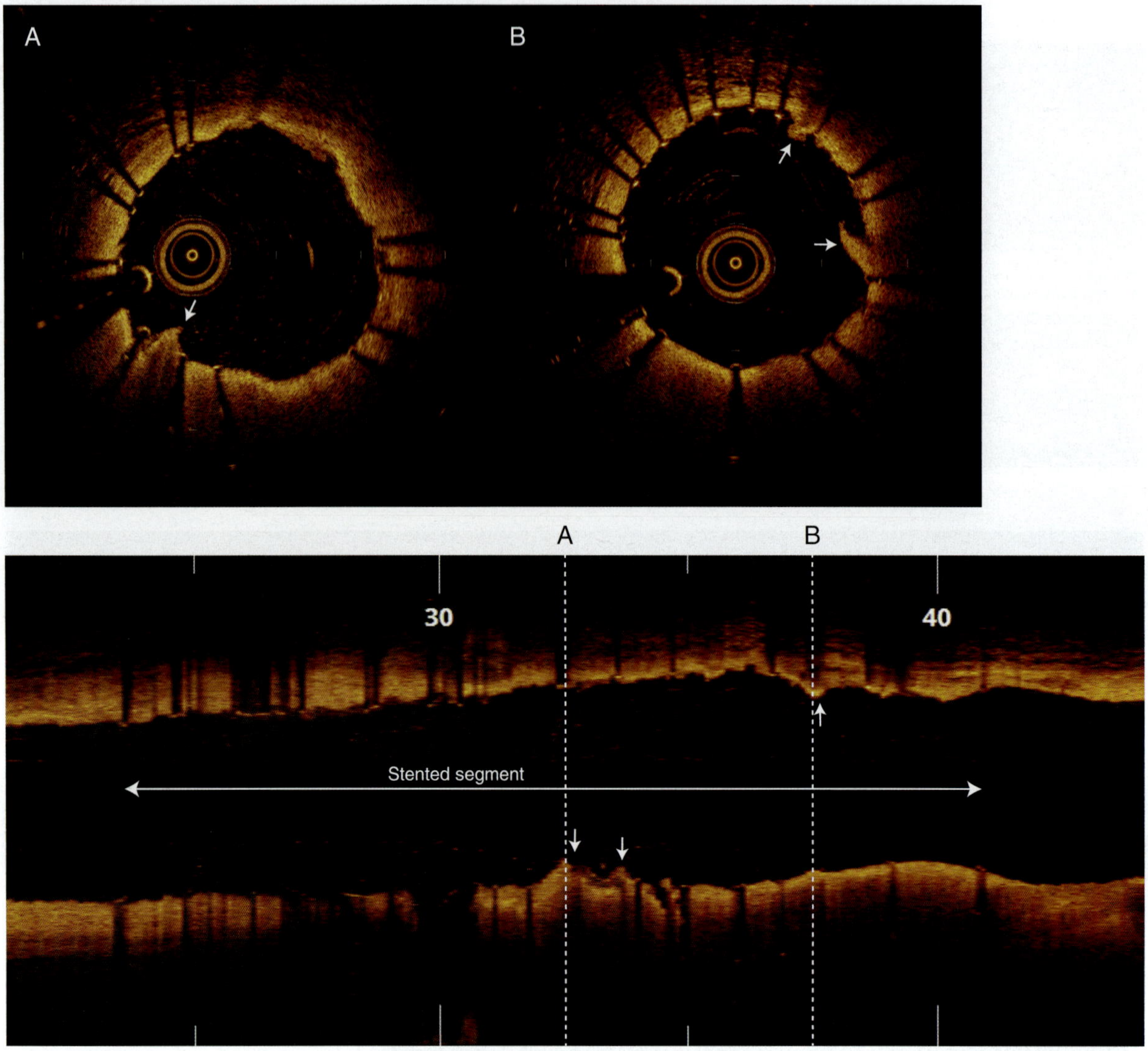

FIGURE 15.53 Longitudinal view and its corresponding cross sections of tissue protrusion. Materials of irregular shape are observed protruding between stent struts (arrows). Struts sometimes appear buried within the disrupted plaque.

Appearances of tissue protrusions are essentially similar between OCT and IVUS (**FIGURE 15.53**). However, the higher resolution, as well as the higher contrast between the lumen and the vessel wall, often allows OCT to visualize those entities in greater detail than IVUS.

Arterial Dissection

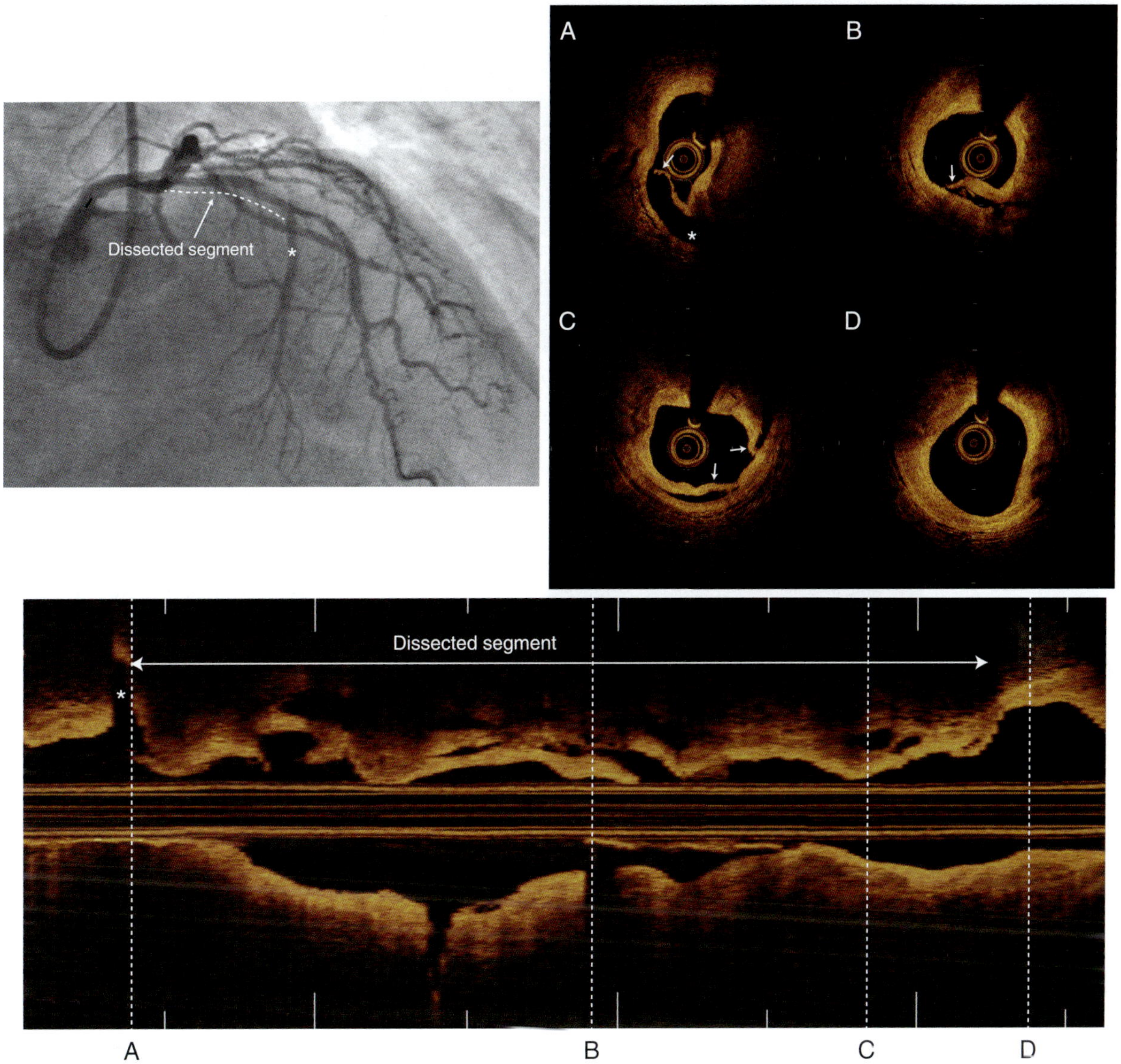

FIGURE 15.54 Angiography and OCT images of arterial dissection. Longitudinal OCT provides the detail about the range of dissection, extending from the beginning of the septal branch (*) to the proximal LAD (the segment is marked by white dotted line in angiography). In the cross-sectional images **(A-D)**, dissection flaps are well visualized (arrows). The dissection flap is also evident on the longitudinal image.

Appearances of arterial dissection are essentially similar between OCT and IVUS (**FIGURE 15.54**).

Thrombus and Ruptured Plaque

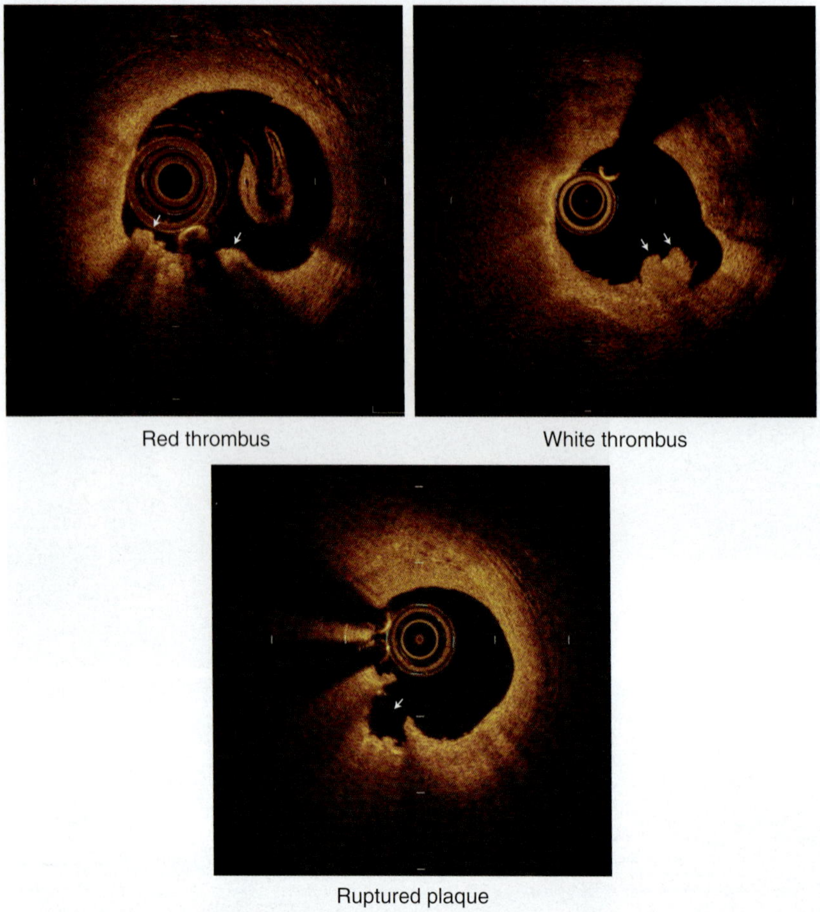

FIGURE 15.55 Thrombus and ruptured plaque. Erythrocyte-rich thrombus (red thrombus) has high backscattering with high signal attenuation (arrows), whereas platelet-rich thrombus (white thrombus) shows a less backscattering and homogeneous appearance with low attenuation (arrows). Ruptured plaque is diagnosed by the presence of fibrous-cap discontinuity and a cavity formation (arrow) in continuity with the lumen. The plaque cavity indicates loss of lipid core due to the rupture. Ruptured plaques usually have an extensive lipid core and a thin fibrous cap and are often associated with thrombus.

Thrombus is recognized as a mass attached to the luminal surface or floating within the lumen (**FIGURE 15.55**).

Cholesterol Crystals

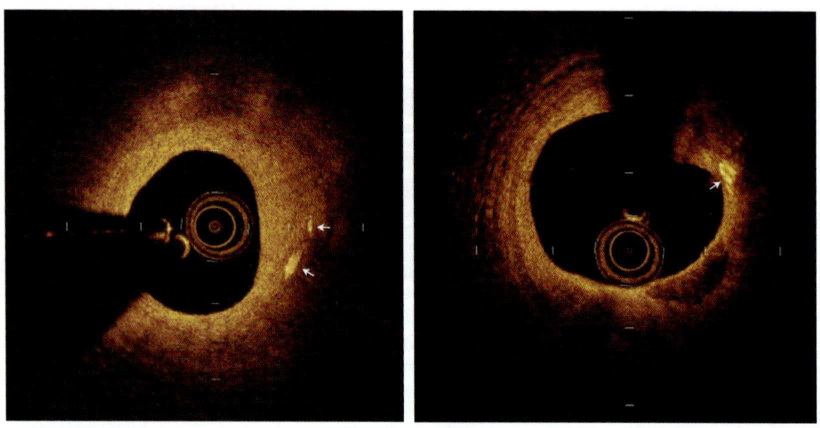

FIGURE 15.56 **Cholesterol crystals** (white arrows) appear as thin, linear regions of high intensity, usually associated with a fibrous cap or necrotic core.

OCT can visualize cholesterol crystals in vivo (**FIGURE 15.56**).[18] Cholesterol crystals, formulated by the high local concentration of cholesterol in foam cells, are reported to trigger a local inflammatory response.[19] Apoptosis of foam cells is induced by intracellular crystals, resulting in further accumulation of macrophages and progression of a lipid-rich necrotic core.[20] These reactions may suggest a potential contribution of cholesterol crystals to plaque instability.

Thin-cap Fibroatheroma (TCFA)

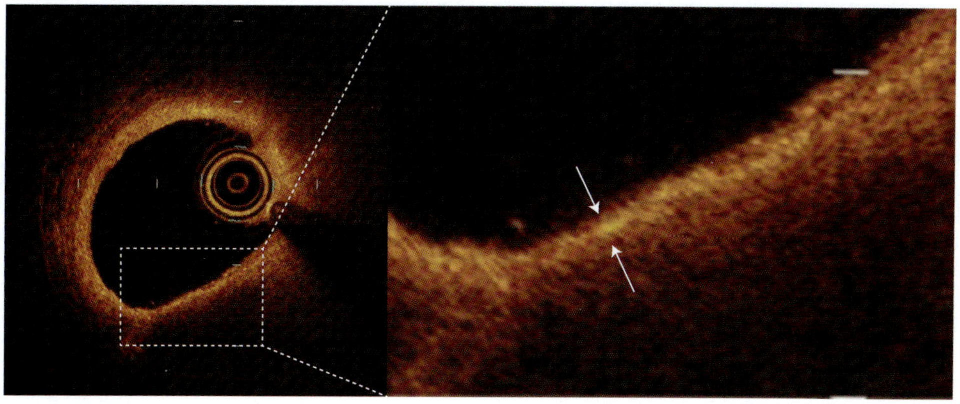

FIGURE 15.57 **TCFA** with a cap thickness of less than 65 μm (arrows).

TCFA is defined as an OCT-delineated lipid or necrotic core with an overlying fibrous cap where the minimum thickness of the fibrous cap is less than a predetermined threshold (FIGURE 15.57). The fibrous cap thickness measured by OCT has been shown to correlate well with that obtained from histologic examination.[21] The most commonly used threshold is 65 μm based on histopathologic studies, although this cutoff may need to be adjusted when applied to in vivo OCT images, accounting for the considerable tissue shrinkage that occurs during histopathologic processing.

Stent Restenotic Tissue

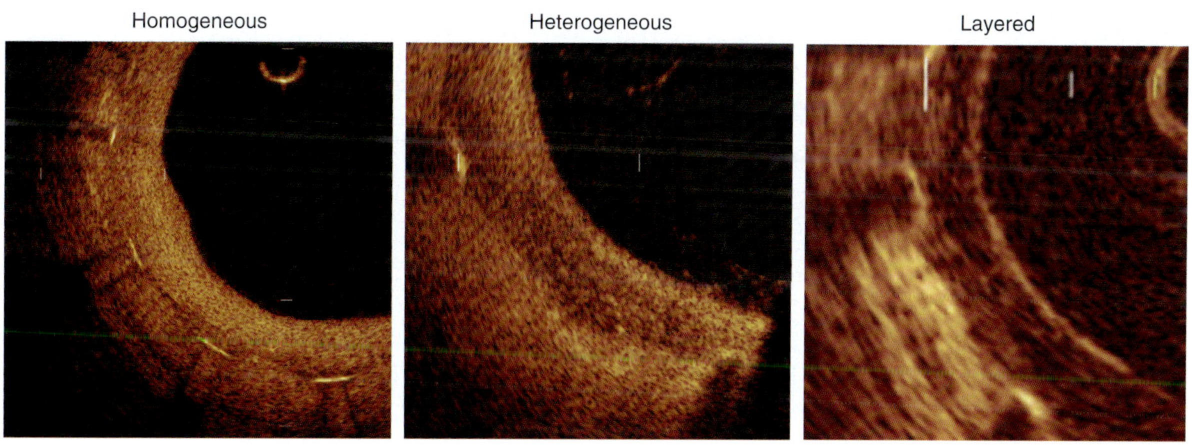

FIGURE 15.58 Chacteristics of stent restenotic tissue. **Homogeneous neointima:** uniform optical properties without focal variation in the backscattering pattern. **Heterogeneous neointima:** changing optical properties and various backscattering patterns. **Layered pattern:** layers with different optical properties (an adluminal high-scattering layer and an abluminal low-scattering layer with stent struts.

Restenotic tissue growth evaluated by OCT can be categorized into 3 main patterns: homogenous, heterogeneous, and layered (FIGURE 15.58).[22]

Calcium Assessment

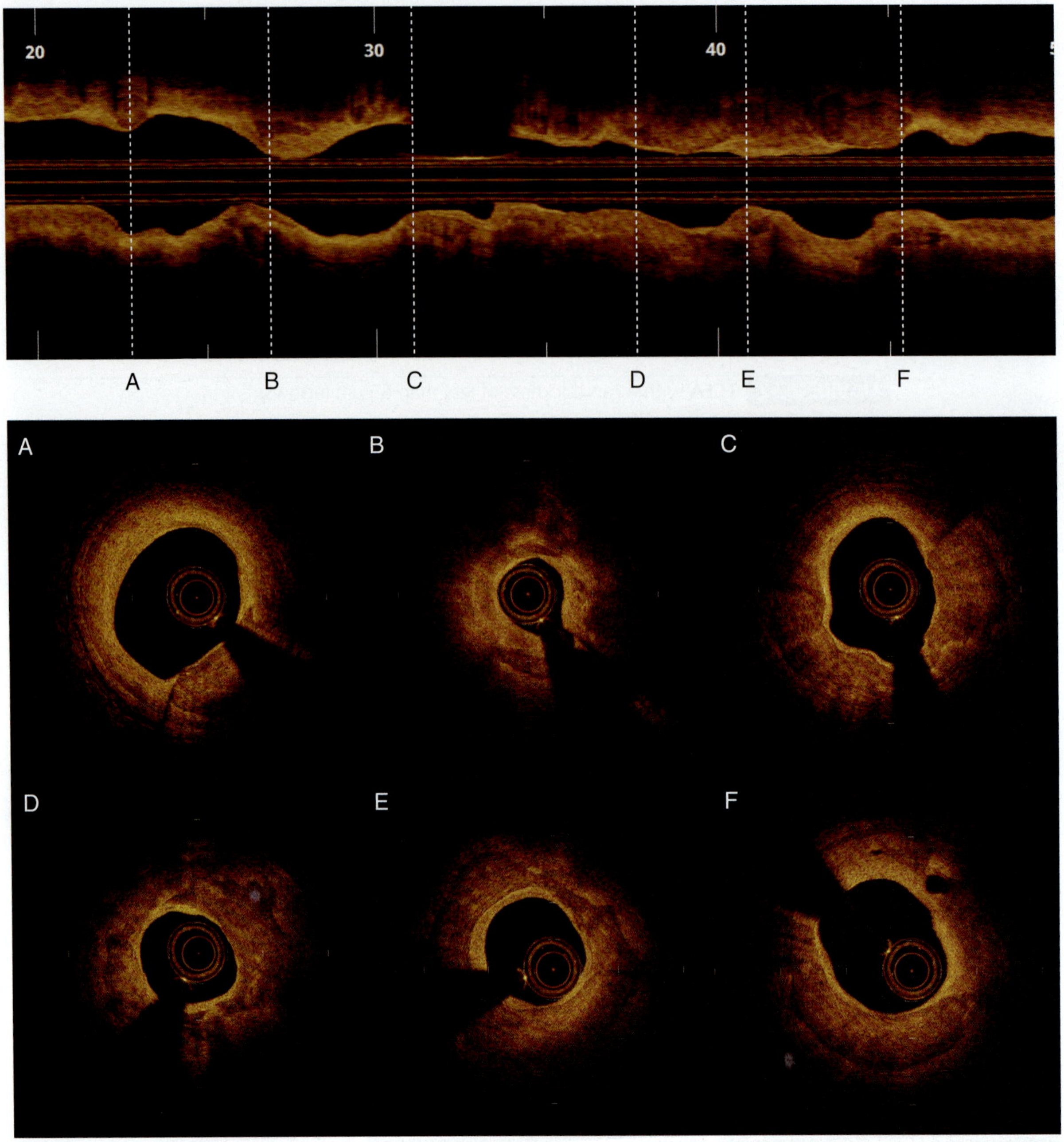

FIGURE 15.59 OCT longitudinal view and its corresponding cross sections **(A-E)** of a heavily calcified segment. These images provide close information on location, distribution, and depth of calcium deposits. The cross sections **(B-E)** show circumferential calcification, which may require plaque modification with rotational atherectomy or cutting balloon dilatation before stent implantation.

Near-infrared light easily penetrates calcium, without any shadowing (different from IVUS) (**FIGURE 15.59**). Therefore, OCT provides a superior imaging tool for calcium detection and quantification, generating information on circumferential extension, thickness, and distance from the luminal surface. Calcified lesions result in signal-poor regions with sharp, well-delineated borders visible in OCT.

OCT Guidance for Severely Calcified Lesion

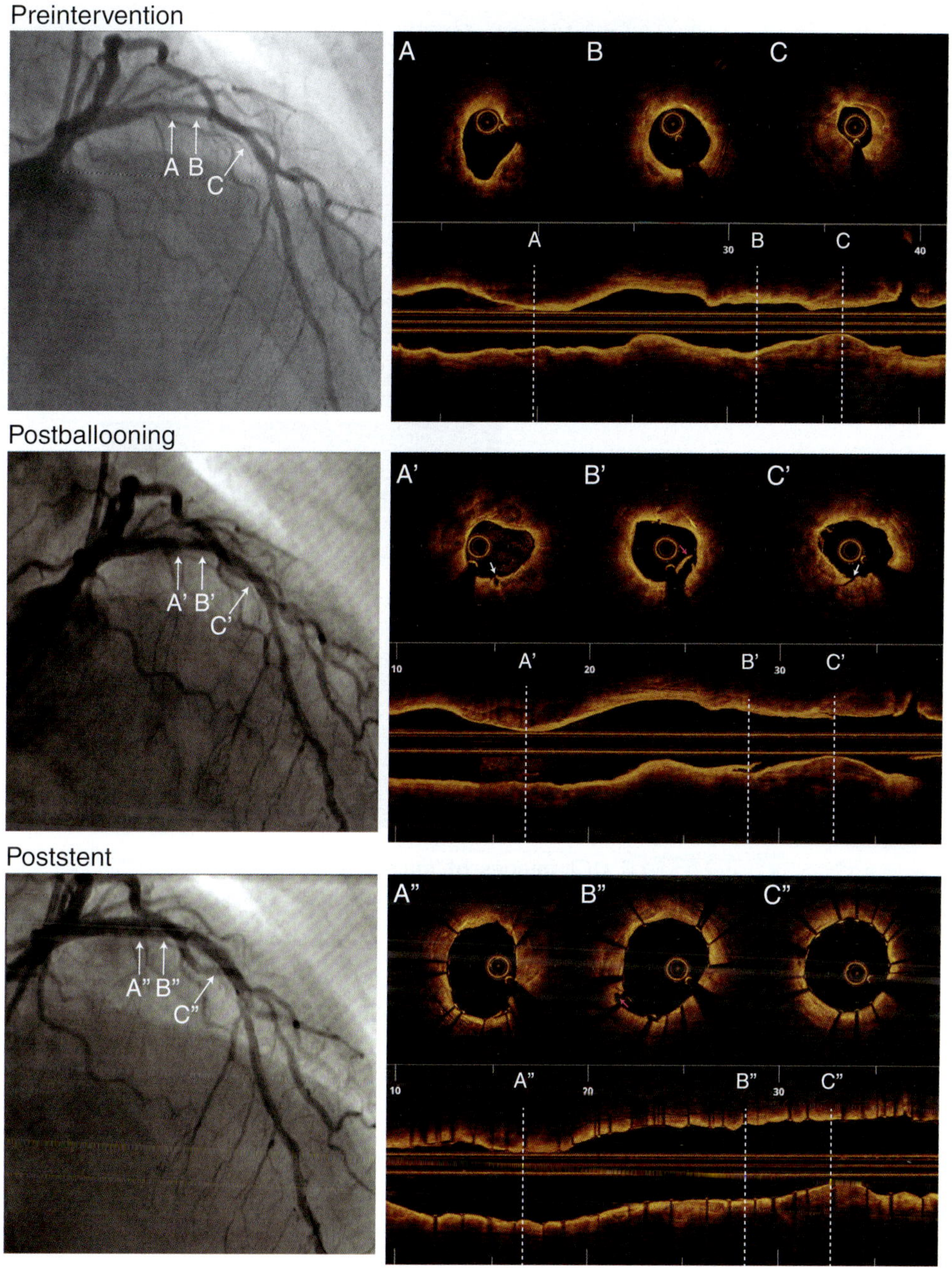

FIGURE 15.60 An example for OCT guidance for severely calcified lesion. Angiography and OCT images at the same position of preintervention (upper), postballooning (middle), and poststent (lower). Pre-intervention OCT shows the distribution of calcification within the lesion in longitudinal view and completely circumferential calcium in the cross-sectional view **(A-C)**. After balloon angioplasty, calcium fracture (white arrows in **A′** and **C′**) and an intimal flap (pink arrow in **B′**) are well visualized. At poststent imaging, the stent is expanded well and the stent sealing of the dissection is observed behind the struts (pink arrow in **B″**).

Heavily calcified lesions in coronary arteries have been known to cause stent underexpansion, which increases the risk of ISR (**FIGURE 15.60**). Plaque modification before stent implantation is considered to be the key for treatment of calcified lesions.[23] OCT offers a unique opportunity to observe plaque modification in the severe calcified lesion. Coronary calcium fracture by PCI is reported to be associated with adequate stent expansion and favorable late outcomes.[24]

Microvessels

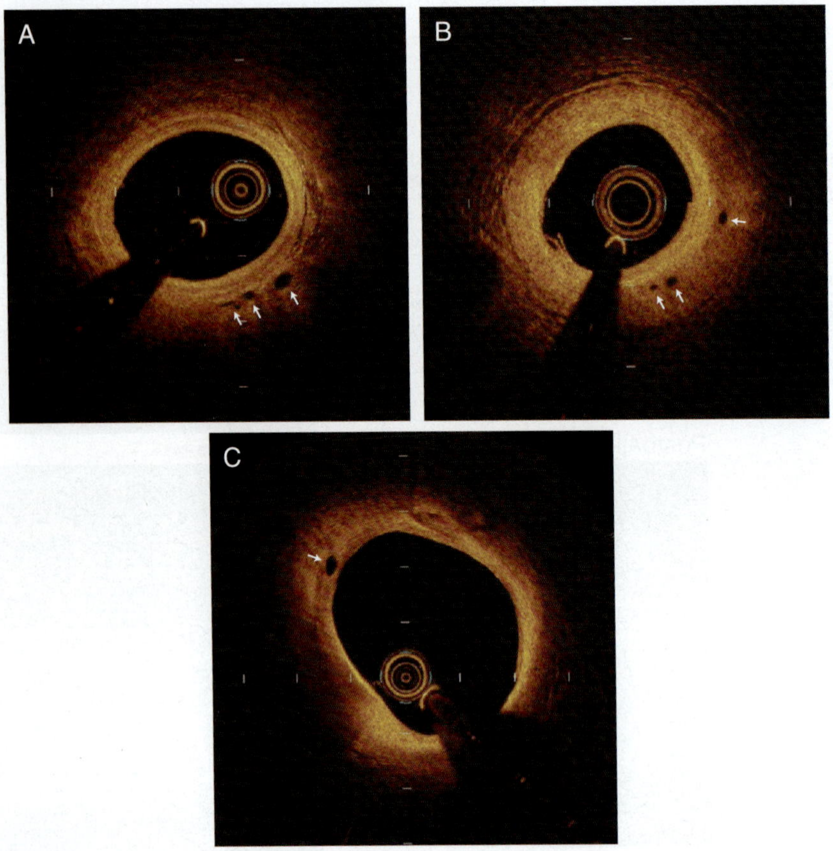

FIGURE 15.61 **OCT images of microvessels** near the adventitia **(A)** and within the lipid-rich plaque **(B** and **C)** can appear as signal-poor voids (arrows) that are sharply delineated.

Intraplaque microvessels (microchannels) are considered to be associated with inflammatory cell infiltration and lipid deposition, leading to plaque progression (**FIGURE 15.61**).[25] While OCT can identify microstructures in atherosclerotic plaques, it is limited by its shallow penetration depth. This makes evaluation of microstructures challenging, particularly when the regions of interest are deep to lipid and calcium deposits.

Peristrut Low-Intensity Area (PLIA)

There are some typical patterns of neointima detected by OCT after stent implantation (**FIGURE 15.62**).

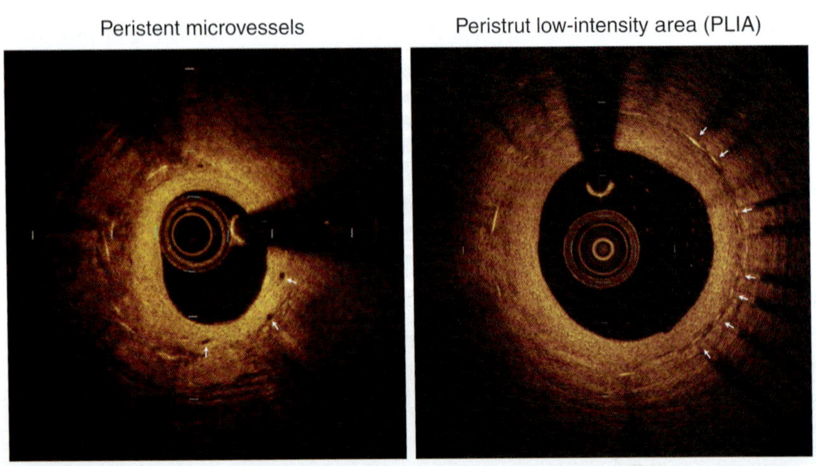

FIGURE 15.62 Neointima with microvessels and PLIA on OCT.

Peristent microvessels are frequently observed in heterogeneous neointima, and this finding is considered to be associated with neointima hyperplasia. Microvessels are imaged as no-signal tubuloluminal structures (arrows) without a connection to the vessel lumen.

The peristrut low-intensity area (PLIA) is defined as a region around stent struts with homogeneous lower intensity (arrows) than the surrounding tissue on OCT images. PLIA is more frequently observed with DES than BMS, and the regions corresponding with the PLIA are distinguishable as hypocellular regions, suggesting the presence of fibrinoid or proteoglycans. Appearance may correlate with delayed arterial healing of the DES.[26]

Macrophage Infiltration

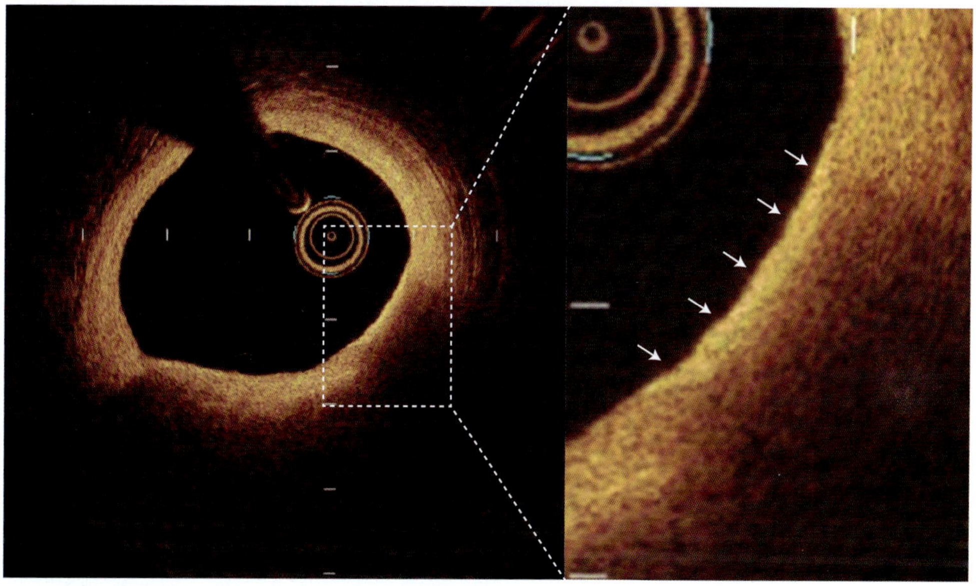

FIGURE 15.63 Macrophage infiltration on OCT.

Macrophage accumulations can be found within the fibrous cap as signal-rich, distinct or confluent punctate regions that exceed the intensity of background speckle noise (arrows) by OCT (**FIGURE 15.63**).[27]

BRS on OCT

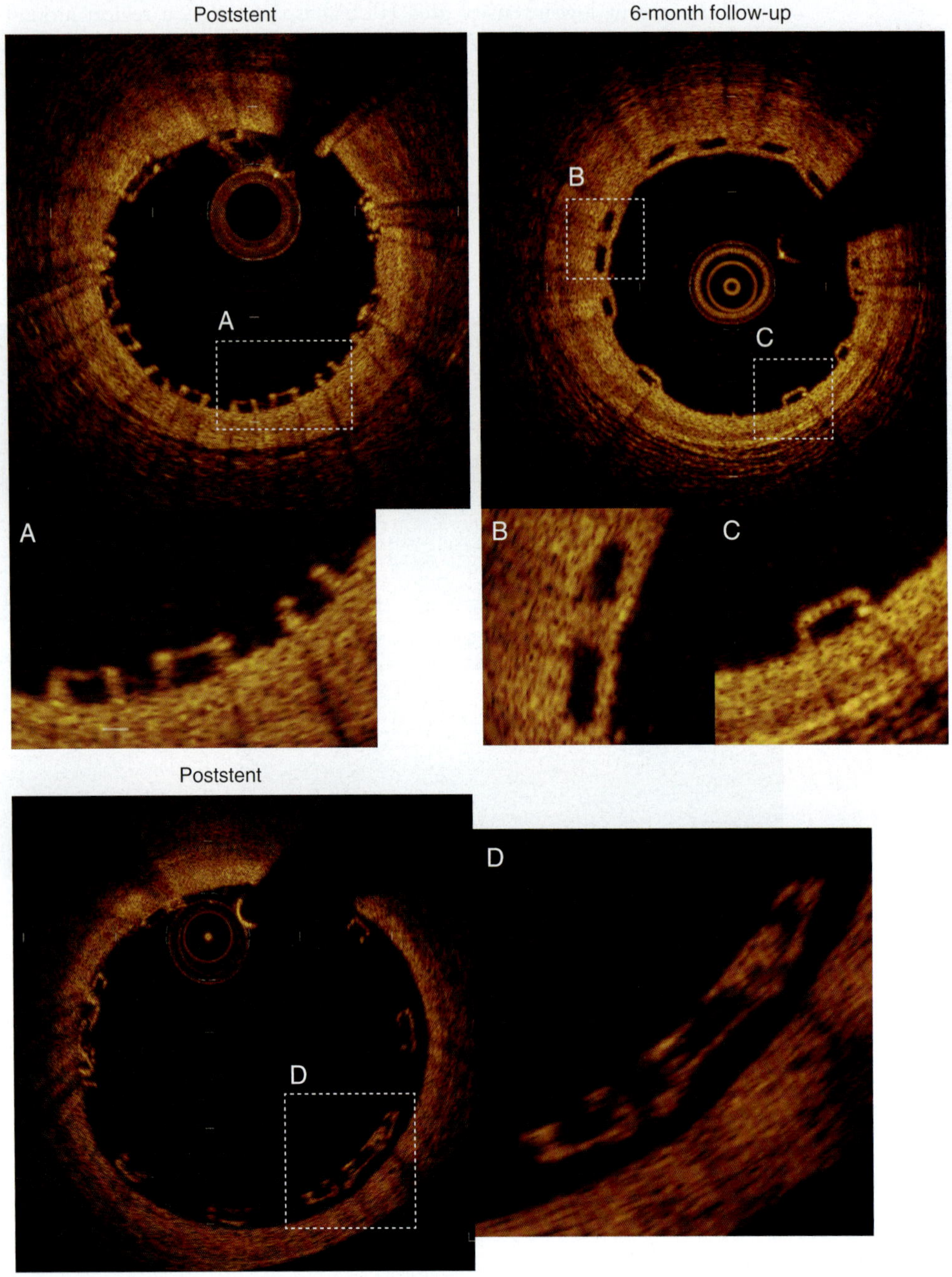

FIGURE 15.64 OCT images of Absorb everolimus-eluting BRS (Abbott, Corp.) at baseline and 6-month follow-up. The scaffold strut is visualized as a box-shaped appearance. Strut apposition to the vessel wall is determined by measuring the distance from the scaffold surface to the vessel wall as compared with the scaffold thickness (well apposed in **A**, malapposed in **D**). At follow-up, OCT images demonstrate one segment with neointima **(B)** or without it **(C)**.

OCT enables full visualization of the box structure of the bioresorbable polymeric strut, permitting accurate assessment of stent expansion and malapposition without shadowing of the underlying pathology (**FIGURE 15.64**). This is possible because a significant amount of the light energy is transmitted through the polymeric struts.[28] As compared with balloon-expandable metallic stents, accurate device sizing with preinterventional imaging is more crucial for BRS, as overdilation of undersized biodegradable stents can damage the polymeric struts.

Spasm on OCT

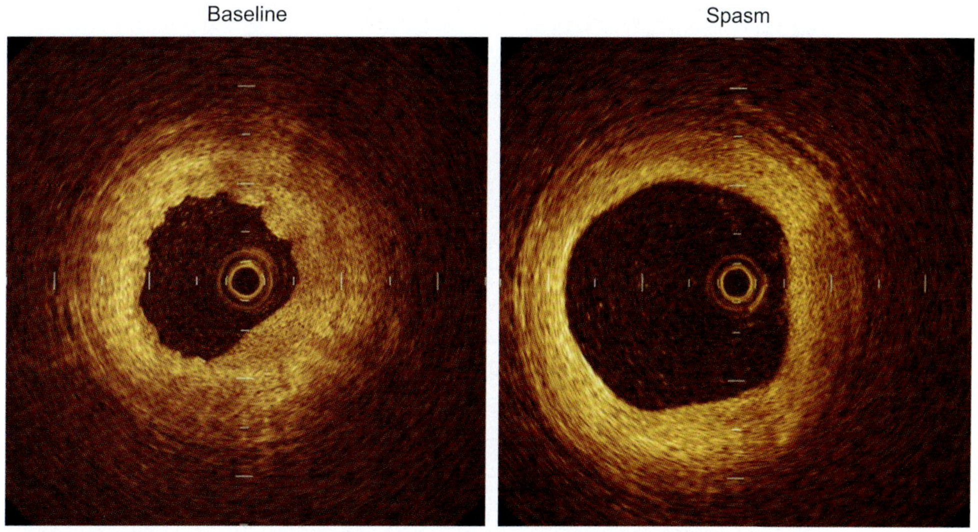

FIGURE 15.65 Coronary spasm on OCT. The lumen is severely narrowed with thickened intima and media. The image shows intimal gathering and protruding humps.

Coronary artery spasm has been shown to play an important role in the pathogenesis of not only variant angina but also ischemic heart disease in general, including other forms of angina pectoris, acute myocardial infarction, and sudden death (FIGURE 15.65).

Bifurcation Treatment and 3D OCT

In bifurcation lesions, 3D OCT imaging can facilitate the visualization of the complex anatomy and the effects of intervention (FIGURE 15.66).[29]

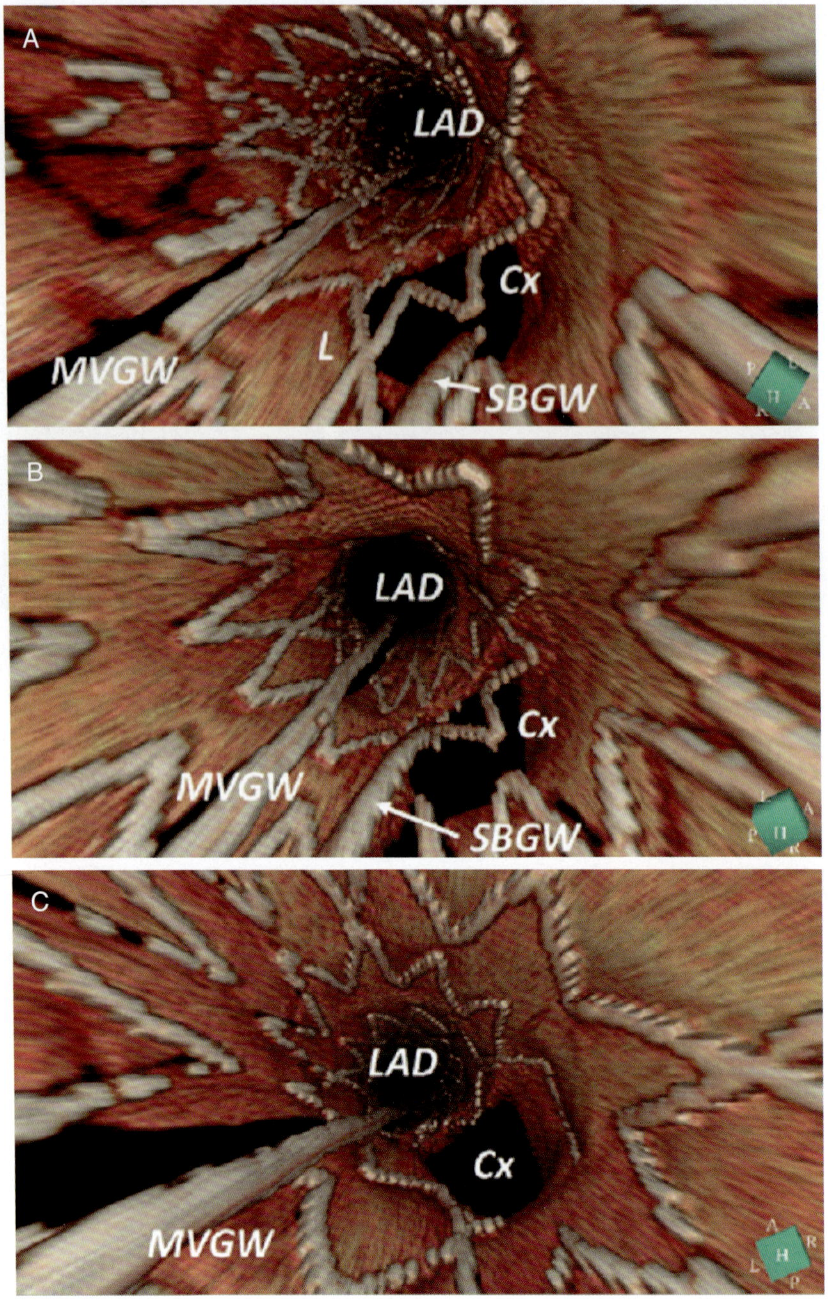

FIGURE 15.66 Representative 3D OCT images during intervention for bifurcation. The recrossing position of the guide wire toward a side branch was changed based on the 3D OCT findings. After the main branch stenting, rewiring passed through the proximal cell in first attempt **(A)**. The recrossing point was changed through the distal cell **(B)** and a kissing balloon inflation was performed, resulting in a wide opening of the side-branch ostium that was free from any metallic structure in front of the side branch **(C)**. L, link; MVGW, main vessel guide wire; SBGW, side branch guide wire. Reprinted from EuroIntervention Vol 10, Takayuki Okamura, Yoshinobu Onuma, Jutaro Yamada, et al. 3D optical coherence tomography: new insights into the process of optimal rewiring of side branches during bifurcational stenting. Pages No. 907-15, Copyright (2017), with permission from Europa Digital & Publishing.

SPECTROSCOPY

Basic Principles of Intravascular Spectroscopy (FIGURE 15.67)

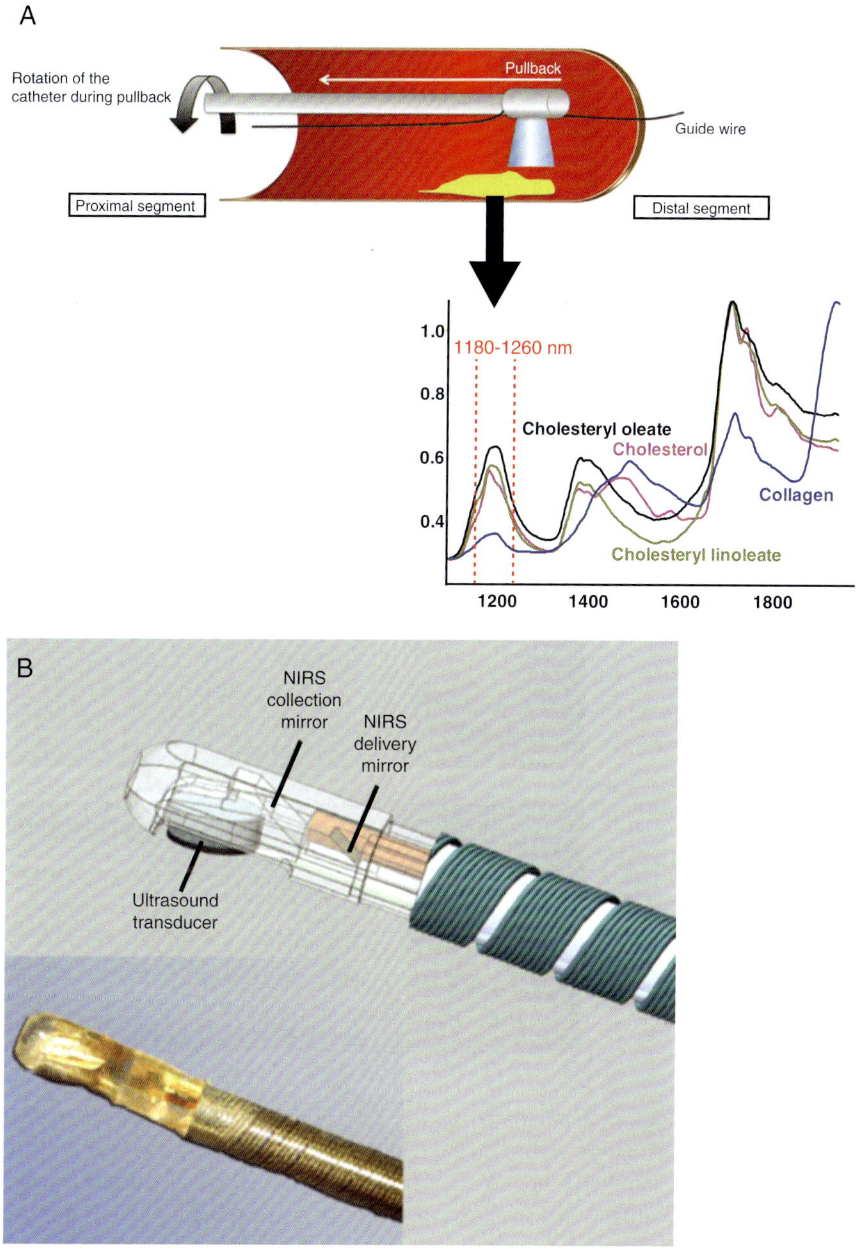

FIGURE 15.67 Basic principles of intravascular spectroscopy. **A**, Spectroscopy displays the chemical composition of plaque substances, based on the analysis of spectra induced by interaction of electromagnetic radiation, or light, with the tissue materials.30 Among the several different optical techniques, the diffuse reflectance NIRS. (near-infrared spectroscopy) system is the frontrunner, showing the ability to identify the lipid component of atherosclerotic plaques in clinical settings. **B**, Image of NIRS-IVUS catheter (The Advanced TVC Imaging System, InfraReDx Inc.). The commercially available coronary spectroscopy system incorporates a dual-modality imaging catheter that provides simultaneous IVUS and NIRS imaging for coregistered acquisition of structural and compositional information. The current system is specifically designed for the detection of lipid-rich plaque. The 40-MHz IVUS transducer is mounted adjacent to the NIRS probe. Image A modified from Bertrand M-J, Lavoie-L'Allier P, Tardif J-C; Near-Infrared Spectroscopy (NIRS). A novel tool for intravascular coronary imaging. In: Kyprianidis KG, Skvaril J, eds. *Developments in Near-Infrared Spectroscopy*. InTech:25-63.

Integrated Display and Quantification of Lipid Burden (FIGURE 15.68)

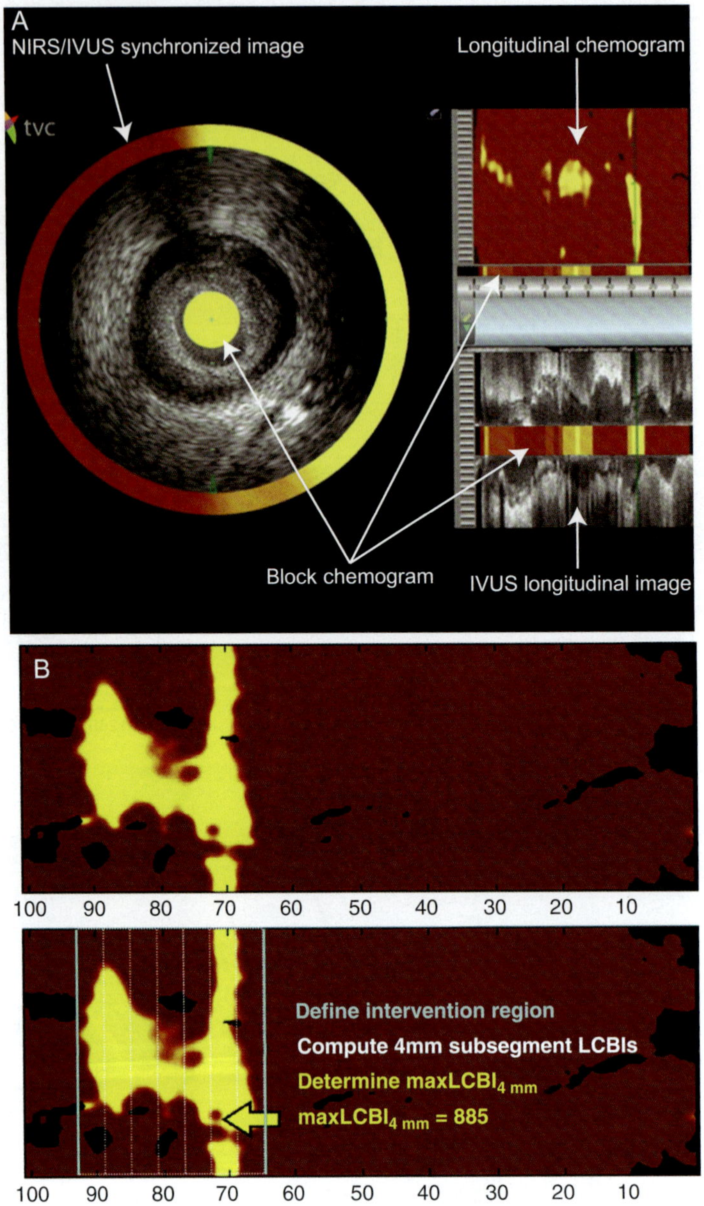

FIGURE 15.68 Integrated display and quantification of lipid burden by NIRS/IVUS. **A**, Example images obtained with a dual-modality IVUS/NIR spectroscopy system (The Advanced TVC Imaging System, InfraReDx Inc.). A color scale from red to yellow indicates increasing algorithm probability of lipid content. The spectroscopy data are displayed in a halo surrounding the cross-sectional IVUS image in a real-time manner (left). In a 2-dimensional map of the vessel called a chemogram (upper right), the x-axis represents millimeters of pullback in the artery and the y-axis represents degrees of rotation. A summary of the results for each 2-mm section of artery is displayed as a block chemogram, which is portrayed in the central catheter artifact of the cross-sectional (left) and longitudinal IVUS images (lower right). **B**, A lipid core burden index (LCBI) is computed as the fraction of valid pixels within the scanned region that exceed a lipid probability of 0.6, multiplied by 1000. Max LCBI4 mm is determined by defining the intervention region, computing LCBI for all 4-mm subsegments within the intervention region and identifying the maximum LCBI subsegment. The presence of a Max LCBI4 mm at the culprit site is associated with a 50% risk of periprocedural myocardial infarction in a substudy of the COLOR (Chemometric Observations of Lipid Core Plaque of Interest in Native Coronary Arteries) registry.[31] **B**, Reprinted with permission from Goldstein JA, Maini B, Dixon SR, et al. Detection of lipid-core plaques by intracoronary near-infrared spectroscopy identifies high risk of periprocedural myocardial infarction. *Circ Cardiovasc Interv*. 2011;4:429-437.

Histological Validation of Spectroscopy

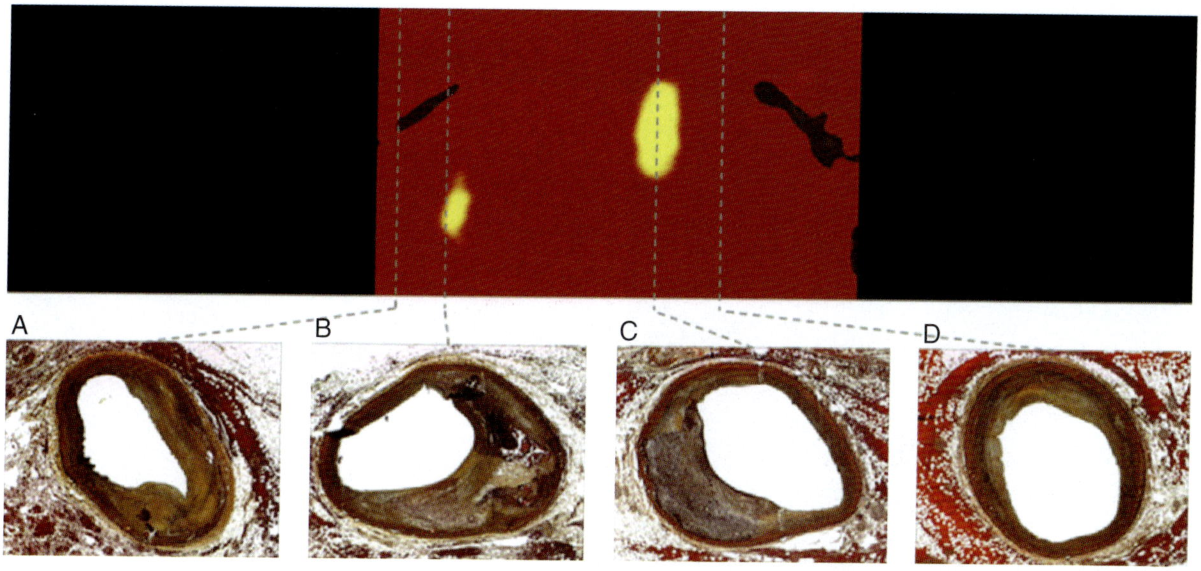

FIGURE 15.69 Correlation between NIRS chemogram and histologic findings. Vessel tissue lacking necrotic lipid core corresponds to "red" in chemogram **(A and D)**, whereas necrotic lipid core plaques correspond to "yellow" **(B and C)**. Movat staining used for histologic evaluation.[32] Reprinted with permission from Kilic ID, Caiazzo G, Fabris E, et al. Near-infrared spectroscopy-intravascular ultrasound: scientific basis and clinical applications. *Eur Heart J Cardiovasc Imaging*. 2015;16(12):1299-1306.

A number of studies have confirmed the ability of spectroscopy to identify the basic chemical components of atherosclerotic plaques in animal models or human arterial samples (**FIGURE 15.69**).

Identification of Fibroatheroma with Calcification

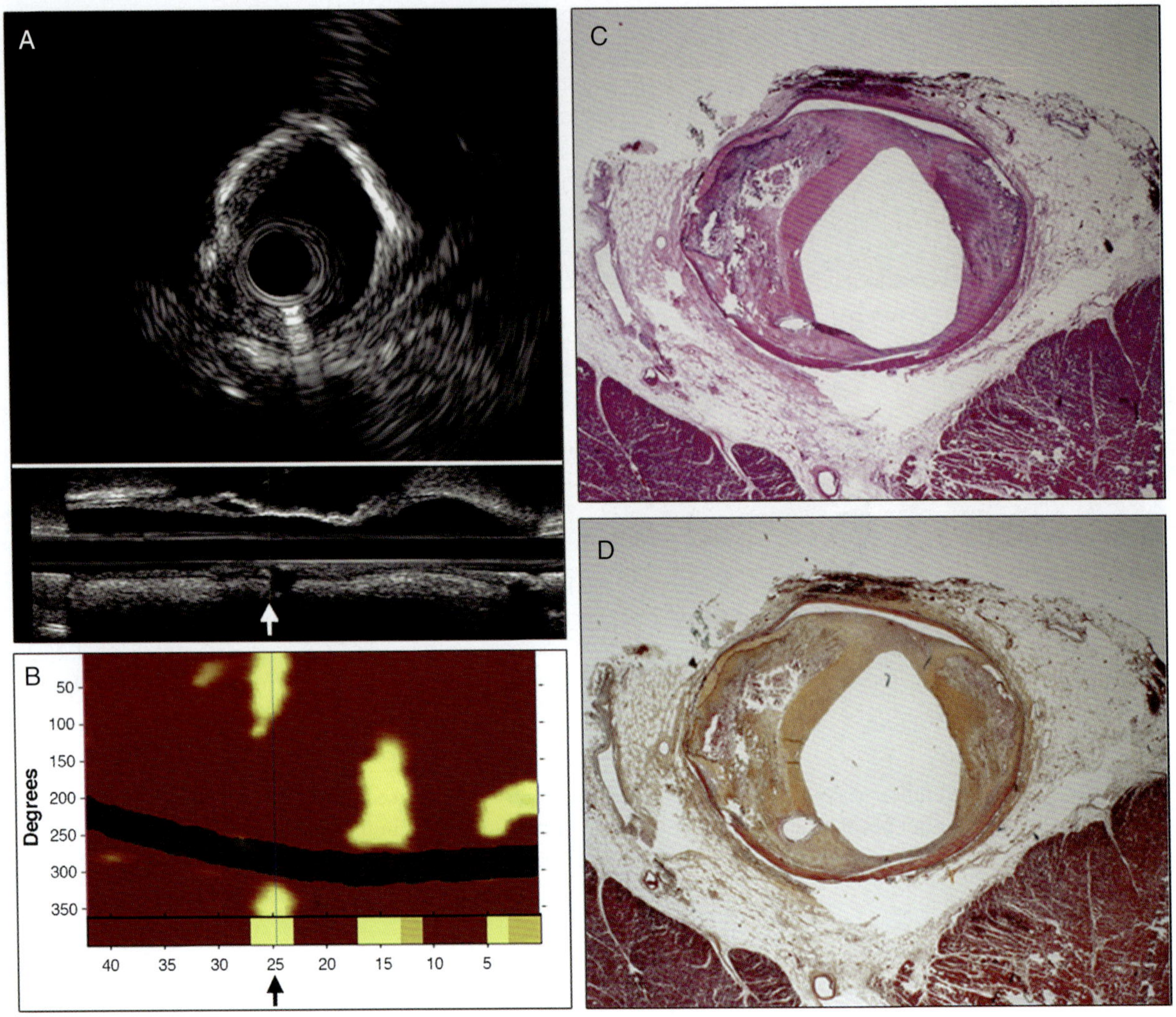

FIGURE 15.70 **A,** Gray-scale IVUS showing extensive superficial calcification. **B,** At the corresponding site (arrow in gray-scale longitudinal view), NIRS chemogram indicates "yellow" lipid-rich plaque. Histopathologic sections demonstrate fibroatheroma with calcified core (hematoxylin-eosin staining in **C**, Movat staining in **D**). Reprinted with permission from Kang SJ, Mintz GS, Pu J, et al. Combined IVUS and NIRS detection of fibroatheromas: histopathological validation in human coronary arteries. *JACC Cardiovasc Imaging*. 2015;8(2):184-194.

A complementary role of IVUS and NIRS to characterize lipid-rich plaque (**FIGURE 15.70**). IVUS is excellent for assessing structures and of calcification, whereas NIRS is well suited to the detection of lipid. NIRS significantly improves the sensitivity for detecting a histologic lipid-rich plaque, especially in calcified lesions.[33]

Implication of NIRS-Detected Lipid-rich Plaque

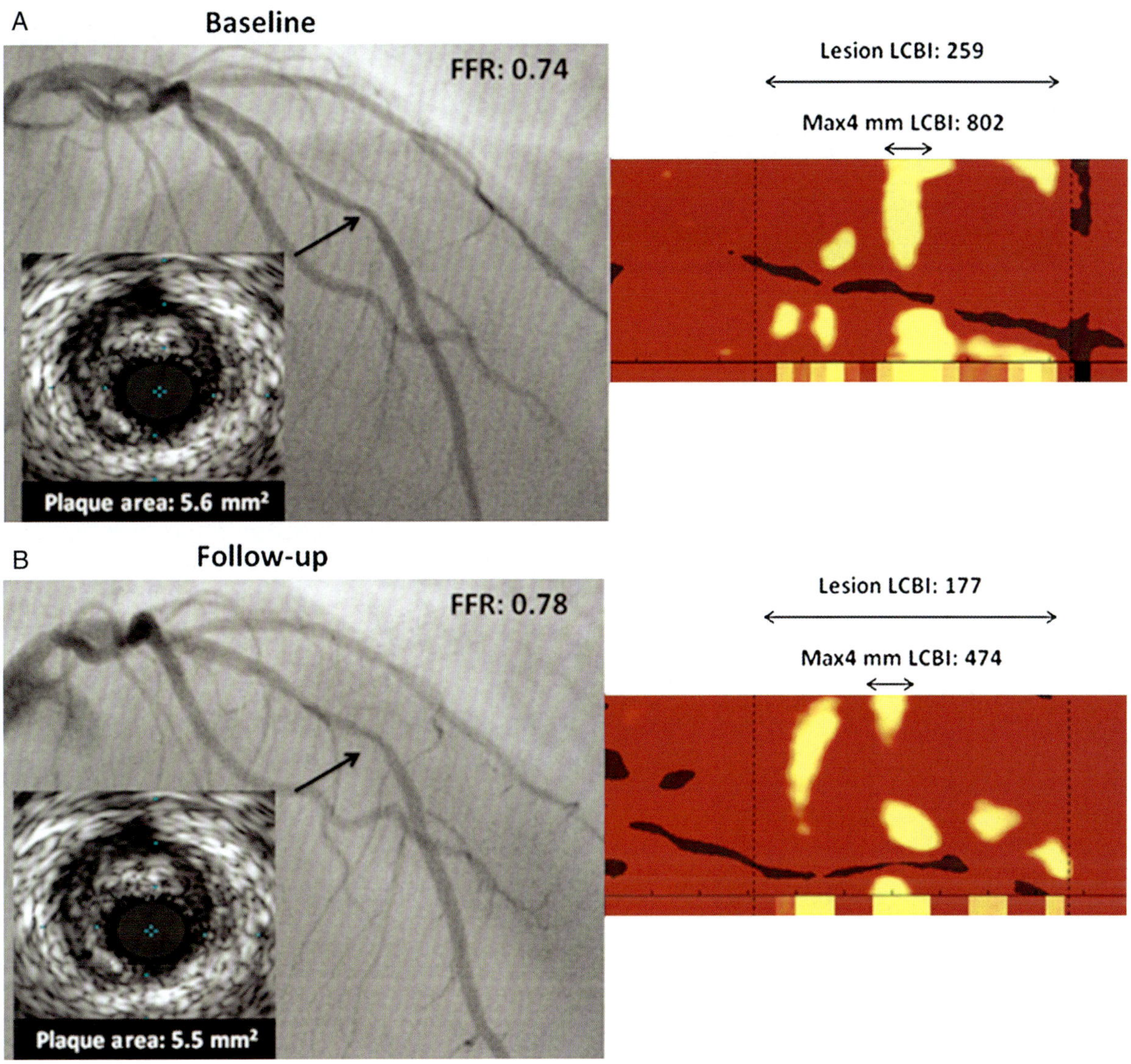

FIGURE 15.71 Image showing an example of angiography, FFR, IVUS, and NIRS at baseline **(A)** and follow-up **(B)** in the trial. Reprinted with permission from Kini AS, Baber U, Kovacic JC, et al. Changes in plaque lipid content after short-term intensive versus standard statin therapy: the YELLOW trial. *J Am Coll Cardiol*. 2013;62(1):21-29.

NIRS/IVUS has been used as a surrogate endpoint to evaluate changes in lipid content in clinical trials (**FIGURE 15.71**). The Reduction in YELlow Plaque by Aggressive Lipid-LOWering Therapy (YELLOW) trial randomized patients with multivessel coronary artery disease who were scheduled to undergo staged PCI.[34] During the initial catheterization, all patients underwent FFR, IVUS, and NIRS of the nontarget lesion, and if the lesion was hemodynamically significant (assessed by FFR) they were randomized to standard care vs high-intensity statin therapy (rosuvastatin 40 mg) for 6 to 8 weeks. Despite the short period of treatment, high-intensity statin therapy significantly reduced the LCBI in patients.

Clinical Practice of Spectroscopy

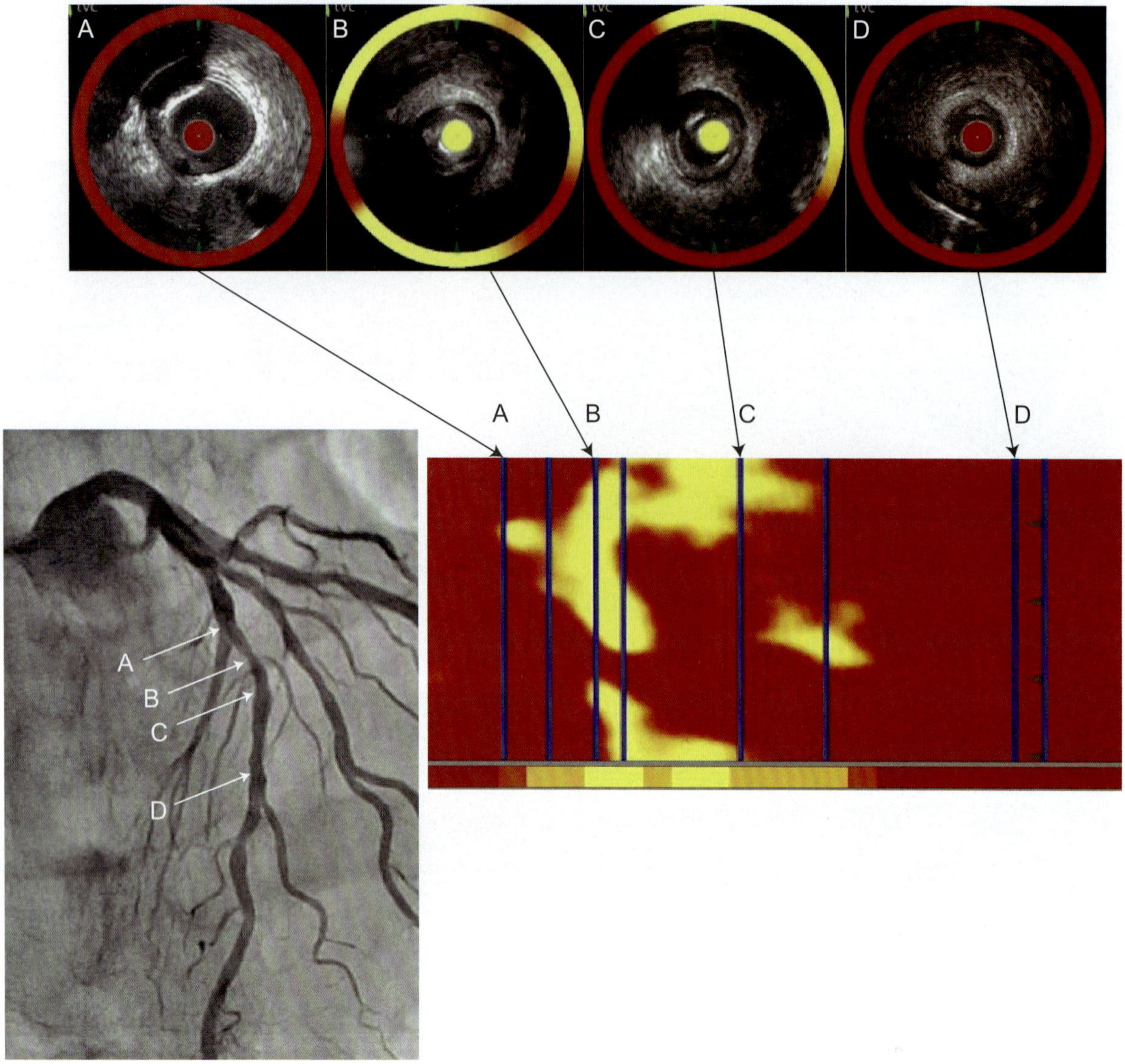

FIGURE 15.72 NIRS-detected vulnerable plaque in FFR-classified gray-zone disease. A case of silent myocardial infarction diagnosed by the troponin elevation without symptom. The LAD appears to have mild stenosis by angiography and the FFR distal to the LAD stenosis was 0.78, indicating a "gray zone" for revascularization. IVUS-NIRS shows a deep lipid pool around the mild stenotic site (from **B** to **C**), as indicated by the longitudinal and cross-sectional yellow chemogram. The LCBI within 70 mm was 187 and the Max LCBI4 mm was 766, suggesting high vulnerability of this lesion.

Aside from the possible utility of NIRS as a diagnostic tool of vulnerable plaque or as a surrogate endpoint of plaque stabilization therapy, peri-interventional NIRS imaging may offer unique guidance for clinical decision-making (**FIGURE 15.72**).

EMERGING TECHNOLOGIES

Hybrid IVUS and OCT

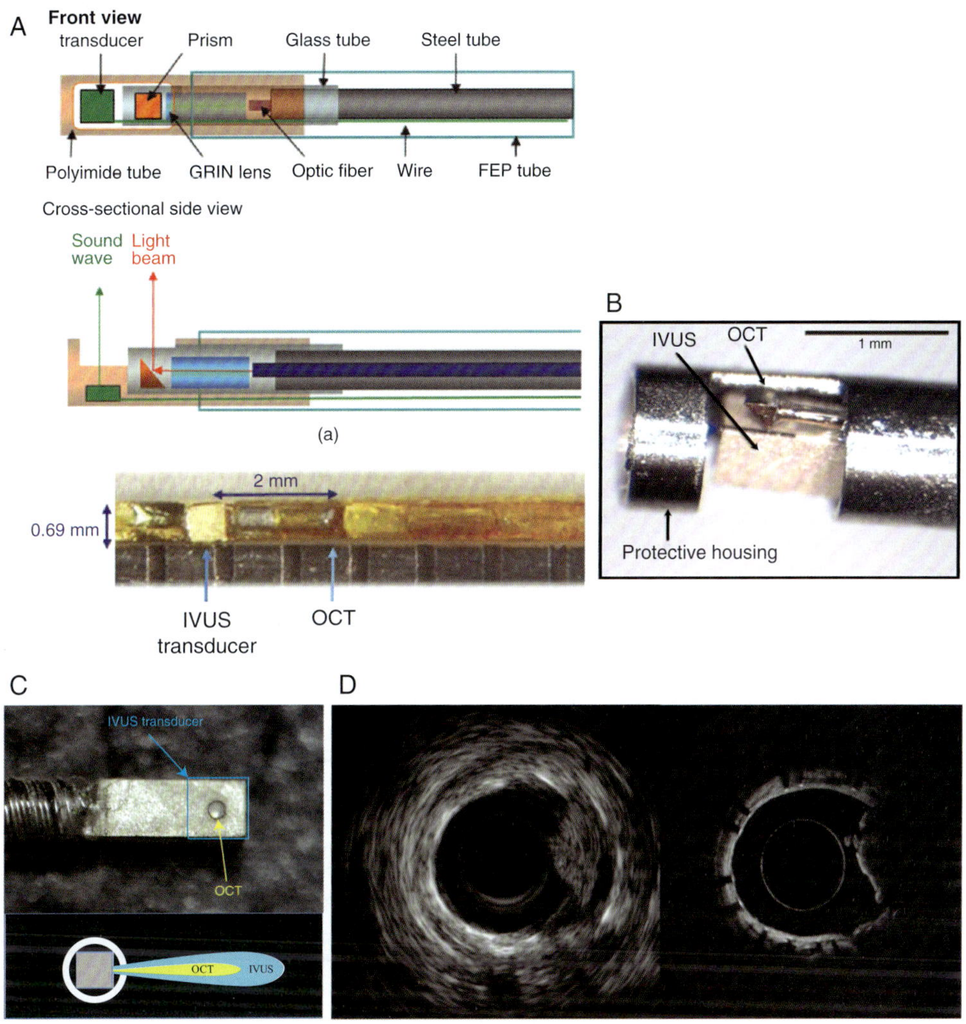

FIGURE 15.73 Hybrid IVUS and OCT. **A**, IVUS and OCT beams were separated from each other by 2 mm along the length of the catheter.[36] **B**, Catheter tip design where the beams for OCT and IVUS are 90° apart, thus potentially subjecting the coregistration of the 2 images to inaccuracy in the event of NURD.[37] **C**, A 3-French rotational custom hybrid IVUS-OCT imaging catheter built using a 40-MHz ultrasound transducer with embedded OCT imaging fiber optics. A collinear alignment of the 2 transducers allows that the IVUS and OCT beams travel in the same direction, providing accurate coregistration of IVUS and OCT images.[35] **D**, A representative coregistered image acquired using the hybrid IVUS-OCT imaging catheter in **C**.[35] OCT image of a coronary vessel showing the implanted struts covered with thin intimal tissue and well-delineated thrombus with high backscattering and signal attenuation at 2 to 4 o'clock. IVUS image of a coronary vessel showing the in-stent thrombus. The neointimal coverage of the stent shown by OCT cannot be resolved using IVUS; on the other hand, IVUS demonstrates vascular remodeling that cannot be seen with OCT owing to lack of penetration.

Combined use of IVUS and OCT can potentially provide synergistic benefits, which may improve the characterization and clinical planning of coronary artery disease (**FIGURE 15.73**). Several probes combining the 2 modalities have been developed and tested in ex vivo and preclinical in vivo settings.[35]

High-definition (HD)-IVUS

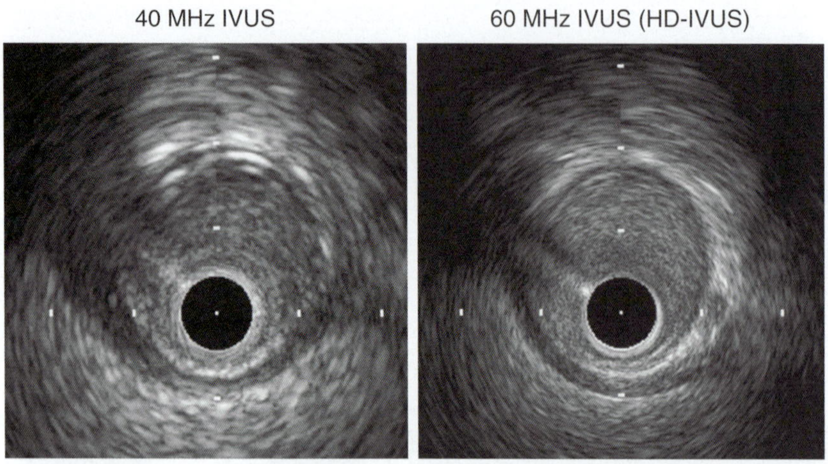

FIGURE 15.74 An example of HD-IVUS system (Terumo, Corp.). Cross-sectional IVUS images of a coronary artery are compared between the conventional 40-MHz IVUS and the 60-MHz HD-IVUS. Resolution is higher at 60 MHz, and differentiation between lumen and vessel wall layers is clearer.

A novel high-definition (HD)-IVUS system based on a 60-MHz mechanical catheter design offers greater resolution than conventional IVUS while still maintaining higher image penetration than OCT (**FIGURE 15.74**).

Hybrid OCT Atherectomy

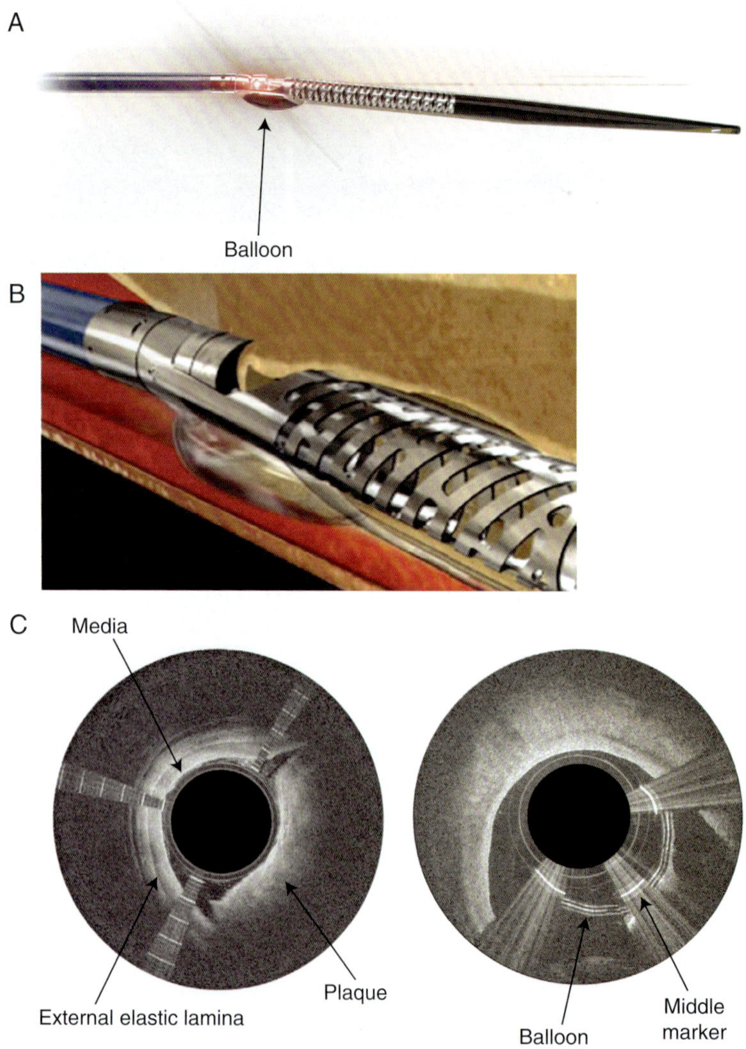

FIGURE 15.75 Images of Pantheris atherectomy device **(A and B)** and OCT image obtained with the Pantheris device **(C)**.

The Pantheris system (Avinger, Corp.) is a novel atherectomy device that uses OCT imaging as an adjunct to fluoroscopy to guide the percutaneous excision of atherosclerotic plaque (**FIGURE 15.75**). With most available devices, atherectomy is performed based on conventional angiography, risking injury to healthy segments of the vessel wall. OCT-guided atherectomy allows selective removal of intimal plaque, preserving the integrity of the medial and adventitial layers.[38]

Co-registration of Angiography and Intravascular Imaging

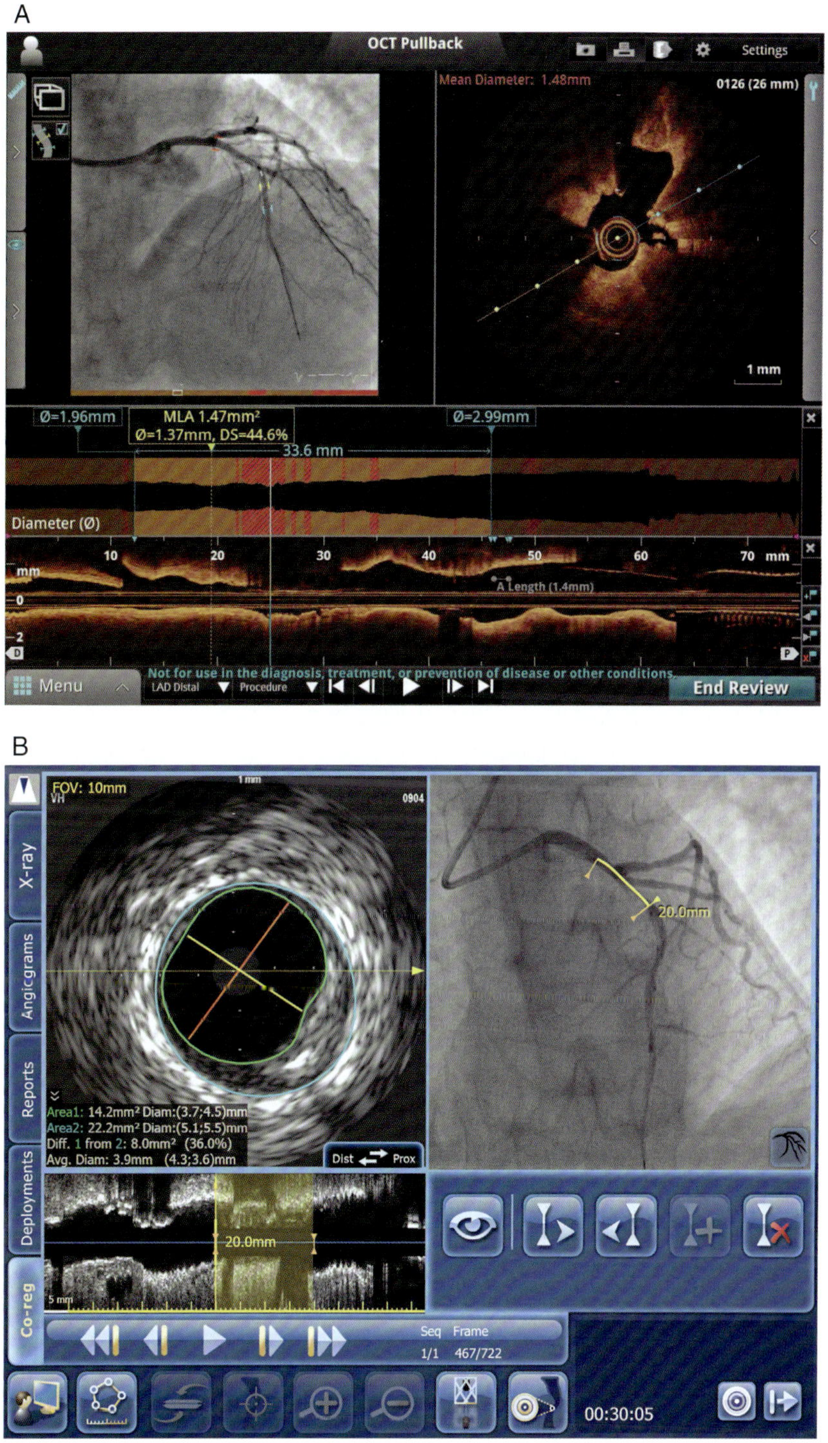

FIGURE 15.76 Coregistration of angiography and intravascular imaging. **A**, OCT coregistration system (the OPTIS integrated system, St. Jude Medical, Corp.). **B**, IVUS coregistration system (SyncVision system, Philips, Corp.).

In a semiautomatic coregistration system, the angiographic image that is recorded during the pullback is projected together with the IVUS or OCT image (**FIGURE 15.76**). The location of the cross-sectional intravascular imaging plane is directly displayed both on the angiogram and in the longitudinal OCT/IVUS view. The integration of structural IVUS or OCT information with the angiographic luminogram allows the operator to understand the location of the detailed intravascular anatomic information relative to the angiographic "roadmap." This enables the operator to take into account the detailed intravascular information in proper positioning of a balloon or stent.

Intracardiac Echocardiography (ICE)

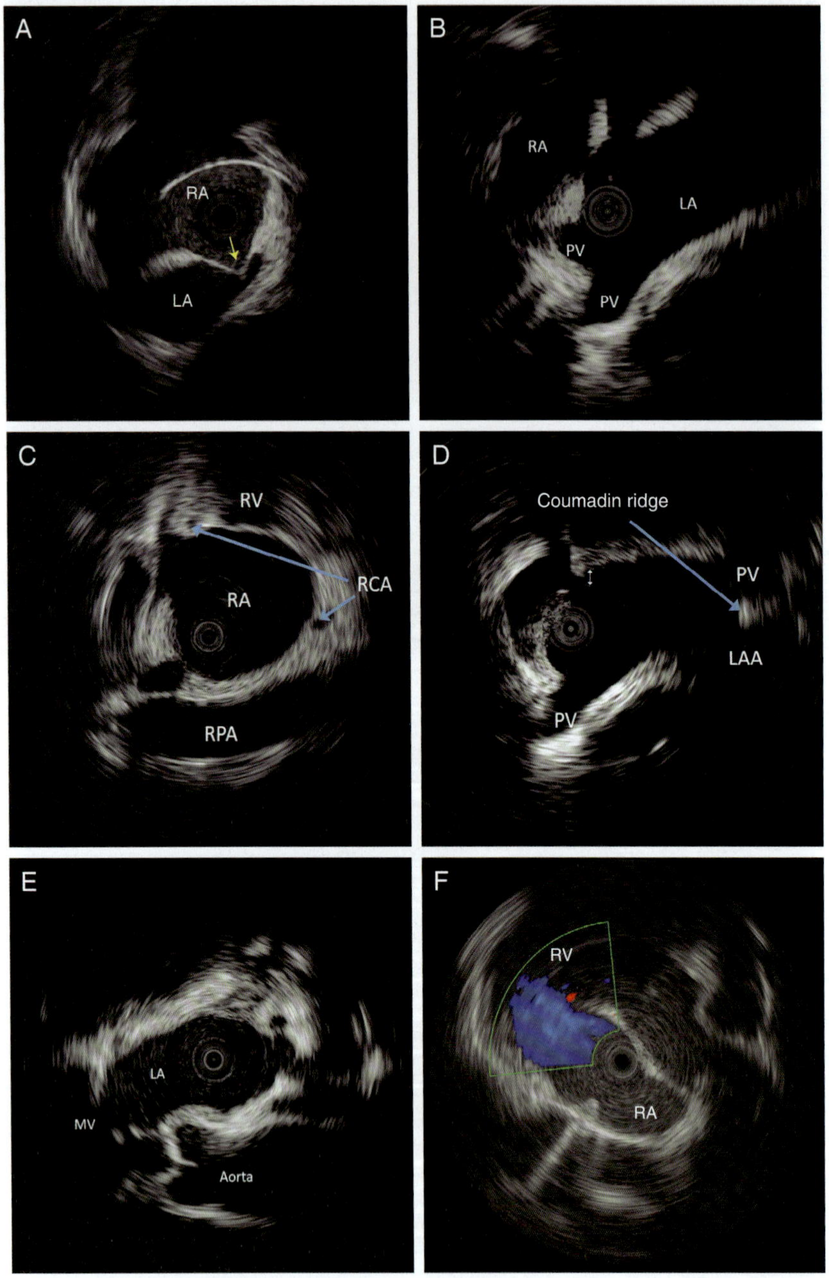

FIGURE 15.77 Intracardiac ecocardiography (ICE). **A**, An ICE image obtained during a transseptal puncture. A thin fossa ovalis is tented from the right atrium (RA) toward the left atrium (LA) by a tip of the transseptal needle (yellow arrow). An EP catheter (a bright arc from 11 o'clock to 2 o'clock) is entering the orifice of the coronary sinus at 2 o'clock. **B**, Anatomy of the pulmonary veins (PVs), the common targets of catheter ablation for atrial fibrillation, and the surrounding structures can be visualized by ICE. **C**, An ICE view from the RA demonstrates the anatomy of the RV, the right pulmonary artery (RPA), and the RCA branches. **D**, The left atrial appendage (LAA) is shown with a connection to the Coumadin ridge, a normal anatomic variant observed in the LA. **E**, The aortic valve and mitral valve (MV) are viewed from the left atrium. **F**, Doppler images of blood flowing away from the RA toward the RV.

Intracardiac echocardiography (ICE) is a catheter-based modality designed to provide real-time ultrasound images of cardiac structures and devices positioned within the heart (**FIGURE 15.77**). Common clinical applications include guidance for electrophysiology (EP) procedures and structural heart interventions, such as transseptal punctures, ablations, closure of septal defects or left atrial appendage, valve repairs, and cardiac biopsy, as an alternative to transesophageal echocardiography (TEE). In general, ICE catheters are larger and use a lower frequency transducer than coronary IVUS catheters to achieve optimal imaging depth and signal penetration for visualization of cardiac anatomy. To date, several different approaches have been commercialized; the most basic design was adapted from mechanical IVUS catheters, but with lower center frequencies. Another approach uses a technology analogous to TEE, providing a sector ultrasound image with color and spectral Doppler capabilities. The most recent approach is similar to mechanical IVUS, but with forward-looking capability and features of Doppler and 3D image reconstruction. Some of those devices have a steerable catheter tip for improved maneuverability within the heart.

ACKNOWLEDGMENTS

Images courtesy of Junya Ako, MD; Brian K. Courtney, MD, MSEE; Yoshiyasu Minami, MD; Hiroyuki Okura, MD; Atsushi Takagi, MD; Shigemitsu Tanaka, MD; Mitsuyasu Terashima, MD; and Atul Verma, MD are gratefully acknowledged.

REFERENCES

1. Stone GW, Maehara A, Lansky AJ, et al. A prospective natural-history study of coronary atherosclerosis. *N Engl J Med.* 2011;364:226-235.
2. Prati F, Di Mario C, Moussa I, et al. In-stent neointimal proliferation correlates with the amount of residual plaque burden outside the stent: an intravascular ultrasound study. *Circulation.* 1999;99:1011-1014.
3. Sonoda S, Morino Y, Ako J, et al. Impact of final stent dimensions on long-term results following sirolimus-eluting stent implantation: serial intravascular ultrasound analysis from the sirius trial. *J Am Coll Cardiol.* 2004;43:1959-1963.
4. Morino Y, Honda Y, Okura H, et al. An optimal diagnostic threshold for minimal stent area to predict target lesion revascularization following stent implantation in native coronary lesions. *Am J Cardiol.* 2001;88:301-303.
5. Doi H, Maehara A, Mintz GS, et al. Impact of post-intervention minimal stent area on 9-month follow-up patency of paclitaxel-eluting stents: an integrated intravascular ultrasound analysis from the TAXUS IV, V, and VI and TAXUS ATLAS Workhorse, Long Lesion, and Direct Stent Trials. *JACC Cardiovasc Interv.* 2009;2:1269-1275.
6. Hong MK, Mintz GS, Lee CW, et al. Intravascular ultrasound predictors of angiographic restenosis after sirolimus-eluting stent implantation. *Eur Heart J.* 2006;27:1305-1310.
7. Song HG, Kang SJ, Ahn JM, et al. Intravascular ultrasound assessment of optimal stent area to prevent in-stent restenosis after zotarolimus-, everolimus-, and sirolimus-eluting stent implantation. *Catheter Cardiovasc Interv.* 2014;83:873-878.
8. Honda Y. Drug-eluting stents. Insights from invasive imaging technologies. *Circ J.* 2009;73:1371-1380.
9. Doi H, Maehara A, Mintz GS, et al. Classification and potential mechanisms of intravascular ultrasound patterns of stent fracture. *Am J Cardiol.* 2009;103:818-823.
10. Tuzcu EM, Kapadia SR, Sachar R, et al. Intravascular ultrasound evidence of angiographically silent progression in coronary atherosclerosis predicts long-term morbidity and mortality after cardiac transplantation. *J Am Coll Cardiol.* 2005;45:1538-1542.
11. Serruys PW, Garcia-Garcia HM, Onuma Y. From metallic cages to transient bioresorbable scaffolds: change in paradigm of coronary revascularization in the upcoming decade? *Eur Heart J.* 2012;33:16-25b.
12. Sano K, Mintz GS, Carlier SG, et al. Assessing intermediate left main coronary lesions using intravascular ultrasound. *Am Heart J.* 2007;154:983-988.
13. Hur SH, Ako J, Honda Y, Sudhir K, Fitzgerald PJ. Late-acquired incomplete stent apposition: morphologic characterization. *Cardiovasc Revasc Med.* 2009;10:236-246.
14. Ako J, Morino Y, Honda Y, et al. Late incomplete stent apposition after sirolimus-eluting stent implantation: a serial intravascular ultrasound analysis. *J Am Coll Cardiol.* 2005;46:1002-1005.
15. Cook S, Ladich E, Nakazawa G, et al. Correlation of intravascular ultrasound findings with histopathological analysis of thrombus aspirates in patients with very late drug-eluting stent thrombosis. *Circulation.* 2009;120:391-399.
16. Rathore S, Terashima M, Suzuki T. Value of intravascular ultrasound in the management of coronary chronic total occlusions. *Catheter Cardiovasc Interv.* 2009;74:873-878.
17. Bezerra HG, Costa MA, Guagliumi G, Rollins AM, Simon DI. Intracoronary optical coherence tomography: a comprehensive review clinical and research applications. *JACC Cardiovasc Interv.* 2009;2:1035-1046.
18. Tearney GJ, Regar E, Akasaka T, et al. Consensus standards for acquisition, measurement, and reporting of intravascular optical coherence tomography studies: a report from the International Working Group for Intravascular Optical Coherence Tomography Standardization and Validation. *J Am Coll Cardiol.* 2012;59:1058-1072.
19. Duewell P, Kono H, Rayner KJ, et al. NLRP3 inflammasomes are required for atherogenesis and activated by cholesterol crystals. *Nature.* 2010;464:1357-1361.
20. Geng YJ, Phillips JE, Mason RP, Casscells SW. Cholesterol crystallization and macrophage apoptosis: implication for atherosclerotic plaque instability and rupture. *Biochem Pharmacol.* 2003;66:1485-1492.
21. Kume T, Akasaka T, Kawamoto T, et al. Measurement of the thickness of the fibrous cap by optical coherence tomography. *Am Heart J.* 2006;152:755.e1-755.e4.
22. Gonzalo N, Serruys PW, Okamura T, et al. Optical coherence tomography patterns of stent restenosis. *Am Heart J.* 2009;158:284-293.
23. Vaquerizo B, Serra A, Miranda F, et al. Aggressive plaque modification with rotational atherectomy and/or cutting balloon before drug-eluting stent implantation for the treatment of calcified coronary lesions. *J Interv Cardiol.* 2010;23:240-248.
24. Kubo T, Shimamura K, Ino Y, et al. Superficial calcium fracture after PCI as assessed by OCT. *JACC Cardiovasc Imaging.* 2015;8:1228-1229.

25. Finn AV, Nakano M, Narula J, Kolodgie FD, Virmani R. Concept of vulnerable/unstable plaque. *Arterioscler Thromb Vasc Biol.* 2010;30:1282-1292.
26. Teramoto T, Ikeno F, Otake H, et al. Intriguing peri-strut low-intensity area detected by optical coherence tomography after coronary stent deployment. *Circ J.* 2010;74:1257-1259.
27. Tearney GJ, Yabushita H, Houser SL, et al. Quantification of macrophage content in atherosclerotic plaques by optical coherence tomography. *Circulation.* 2003;107:113-119.
28. Onuma Y, Serruys PW, Perkins LE, et al. Intracoronary optical coherence tomography and histology at 1 month and 2, 3, and 4 years after implantation of everolimus-eluting bioresorbable vascular scaffolds in a porcine coronary artery model: an attempt to decipher the human optical coherence tomography images in the ABSORB trial. *Circulation.* 2010;122:2288-2300.
29. Okamura T, Onuma Y, Yamada J, et al. 3D optical coherence tomography: new insights into the process of optimal rewiring of side branches during bifurcational stenting. *EuroIntervention.* 2014;10:907-915.
30. Bertrand M-J, Lavoie-L'Allier P, Tardif J-C. A novel tool for intravascular coronary imaging. In: Kyprianidis KG, Skvaril J, eds. *Developments in Near-Infrared Spectroscopy*. InTech:25-63.
31. Goldstein JA, Maini B, Dixon SR, et al. Detection of lipid-core plaques by intracoronary near-infrared spectroscopy identifies high risk of periprocedural myocardial infarction. *Circ Cardiovasc Interv.* 2011;4:429-437.
32. Kilic ID, Caiazzo G, Fabris E, et al. Near-infrared spectroscopy-intravascular ultrasound: scientific basis and clinical applications. *Eur Heart J Cardiovasc Imaging.* 2015;16:1299-1306.
33. Kang SJ, Mintz GS, Pu J, et al. Combined IVUS and NIRS detection of fibroatheromas: histopathological validation in human coronary arteries. *JACC Cardiovasc Imaging.* 2015;8:184-194.
34. Kini AS, Baber U, Kovacic JC, et al. Changes in plaque lipid content after short-term intensive versus standard statin therapy: the YELLOW trial (reduction in yellow plaque by aggressive lipid-lowering therapy). *J Am Coll Cardiol.* 2013;62:21-29.
35. Bourantas CV, Jaffer FA, Gijsen FJ, et al. Hybrid intravascular imaging: recent advances, technical considerations, and current applications in the study of plaque pathophysiology. *Eur Heart J.* 2017;38:400-412.
36. Yin J, Li X, Jing J, et al. Novel combined miniature optical coherence tomography ultrasound probe for in vivo intravascular imaging. *J Biomed Opt.* 2011;16:060505.
37. Li BH, Leung AS, Soong A, et al. Hybrid intravascular ultrasound and optical coherence tomography catheter for imaging of coronary atherosclerosis. *Catheter Cardiovasc Interv.* 2013;81:494-507.
38. Cawich I, Paixao AR, Marmagkiolis K, et al. Immediate and intermediate-term results of optical coherence tomography guided atherectomy in the treatment of peripheral arterial disease: initial results from the VISION trial. *Cardiovasc Revasc Med.* 2016;17:463-467.

chapter **16**

Endomyocardial Biopsy

MAURO MOSCUCCI, MD, MBA

INTRODUCTION

The development of new imaging modalities and particularly of magnetic resonance imaging has provided new tools for the diagnosis of disorders of the myocardium. Despite these advancements, the diagnosis of myocardial diseases continues to be challenging. Endomyocardial biopsy can allow a more precise characterization of the underlying primary myocardial pathology in several diseases, and it remains the gold standard for the assessment of transplant rejection. In this chapter we will review available devices, biopsy techniques and complications, indications for endomyocardial biopsy in the current era, and its utility and findings in specific disease states.

Bioptomes

After the first biopsy performed by Weinberg, Fell, and Lynfield in 1958 through an incision in the left intercostal space at the costochondral junction,[1] Sutton and Sutton in 1960 reported their experience with percutaneous myocardial biopsy performed at the left ventricular apex or at the left costosternal junction. They used a Terry needle, which was made highly flexible by a modified thin wall (**FIGURE 16.1**).[2] Timmis and colleagues in 1965 reported their experience with the use of a modified Silverman needle and Menghini needle (**FIGURE 16.1**).[3] The concept of percutaneous insertion of a heart biopsy needle through the right external or internal jugular vein was introduced by Bulloch[4] in 1965. The technique involved positioning in the right ventricle a 16-gauge, 50-cm-long curved shaft advanced through a large-bore radiopaque catheter. Cutting blades were then advanced through the metal shaft.

In 1962, Sakakibara and Konno introduced the Konno biopsy technique and the Konno bioptome.[5] The device included a 100-cm shaft ending with 2 sharpened cups, connected to a wire (**FIGURES 16.2** and **16.3**). A sliding assembly attached to the proximal end of the catheter activated the wire, and the operation of the wire would open and close the sharpened cups. The operation of the cups allowed "biting" biopsy samples. Caves modified the Konno bioptome for use through the right internal jugular vein. The modification allowed the bioptome to be inserted percutaneously, but the high profile required the use of large no-valve sheaths, which was associated with higher blood losses and the risk of air embolism during insertion and withdrawal of the bioptome. In 1972 Caves introduced the Stanford modification to the Konno bioptome (Stanford or Caves—Schulz bioptome).[6,7] The Stanford bioptome was used until 1995. It was preshaped and had only 1 articulated jaw while the other jaw was fixed. It was developed specifically for right ventricular biopsy using the right internal jugular approach (**FIGURE 16.4**). As of today, there are several disposable and reusable bioptomes, which are available in different lengths and French sizes, with preshaped and straight tips (**FIGURE 16.5**). They can be used from a variety of entry sites including the internal jugular vein, the femoral vein, the subclavian vein, and the transfemoral artery approach for left ventricular biopsy.

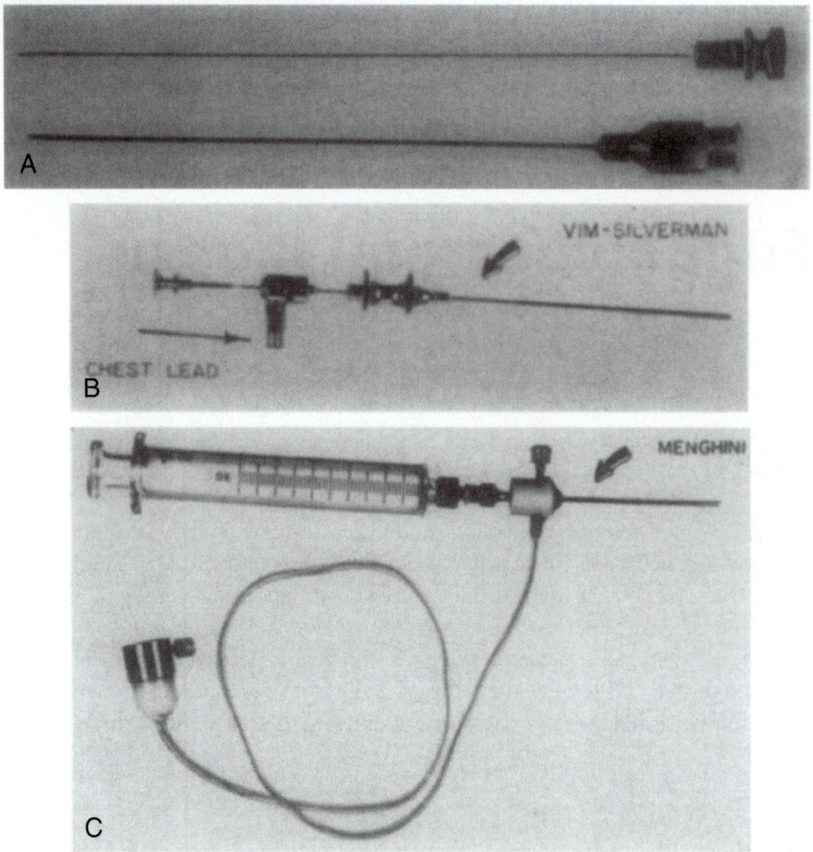

FIGURE 16.1 **A,** Modified Terry biopsy needle used by Sutton and Sutton (1.1 mm inside diameter). **B,** Standard Vim-Silverman needle (14 gauge XI10 mm) fitted with Luer-lock adapter to limit penetration of the cutting piece 1.1 cm beyond the trochar and to serve as an electrode connector for electrocardiographic epicardial sensing. **C,** Menghini biopsy needle (1.6 × 70 mm) and syringe mounted with a special autoclavable platinum ECG electrode extension, which served also to limit penetration of the needle. **A,** Modified with permission from Sutton DC, Sutton GC. Needle biopsy of the human ventricular myocardium: review of 54 consecutive cases. *Am Heart J.* 1960;60:364-370; **B,** Modified with permission from Timmis GC, Gordon S, Baron RH, Brough AJ. Percutaneous myocardial biopsy. *Am Heart J.* 1965;70(4):499-504; **C,** Modified with permission from Timmis GC, Gordon S, Baron RH, Brough AJ. Percutaneous myocardial biopsy. *Am Heart J.* 1965;70(4):499-504.

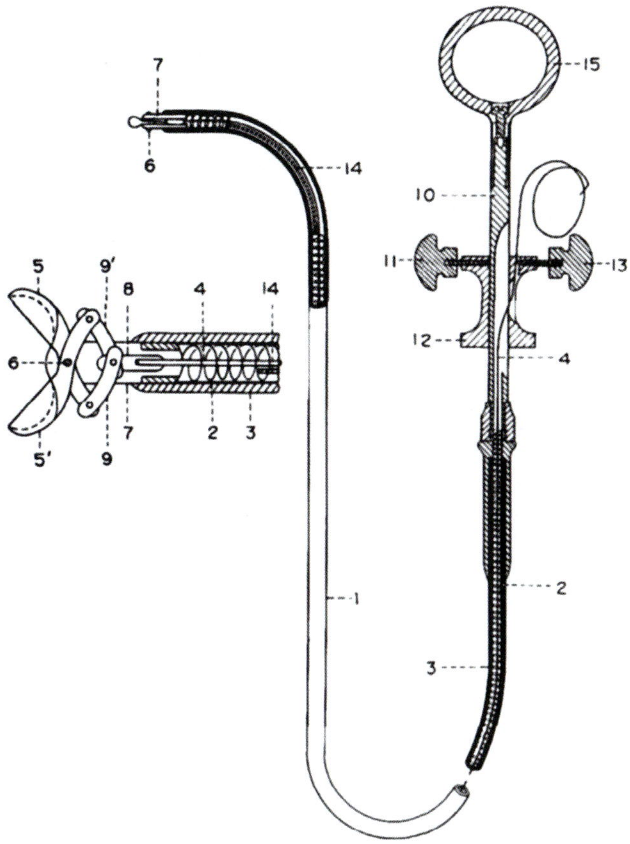

FIGURE 16.2 Instrument for endomyocardial biopsy devised by Konno. Reproduced with permission from Sakakibara S, Konno S. Endomyocardial biopsy. *Jpn Heart J*. 1962;3:537-543.

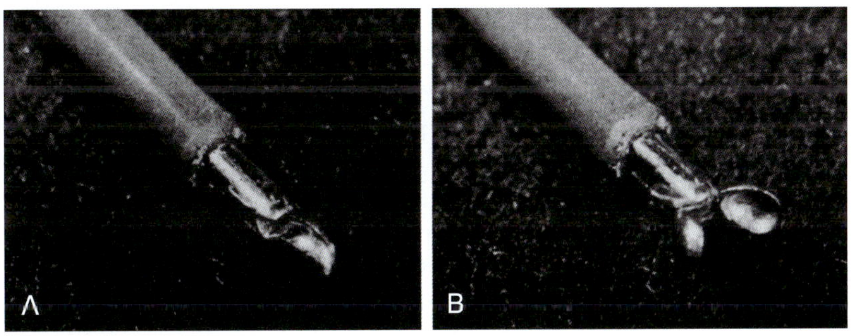

FIGURE 16.3 **A,** Closed top edges of the Konno bioptome. **B,** Opened top edges of the instrument. Reproduced with permission from Sakakibara S, Konno S. Endomyocardial biopsy. *Jpn Heart J*. 1962;3:537-543.

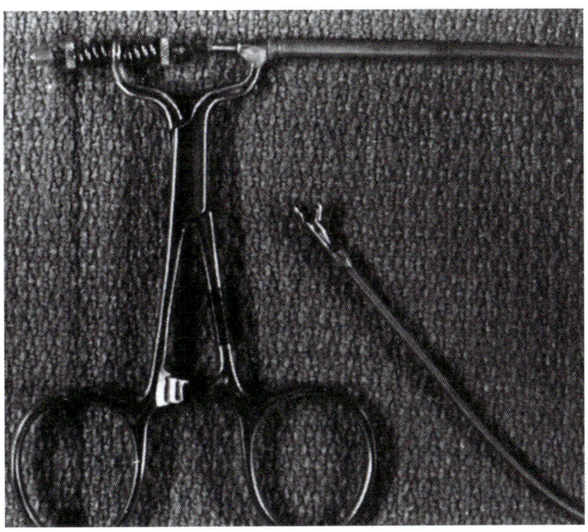

FIGURE 16.4 Stanford (Caves-Schulz) bioptome. The surgical clamp drives a control wire to which it is connected via 2 adjustable nuts, thereby controlling the position of the single mobile jaw at the distal end of the catheter. From Baim DS. *Grossman's Cardiac Catheterization, Angiography, and Intervention*. 7th ed. Philadelphia: Lippincott Williams & Wilkins; 2006.

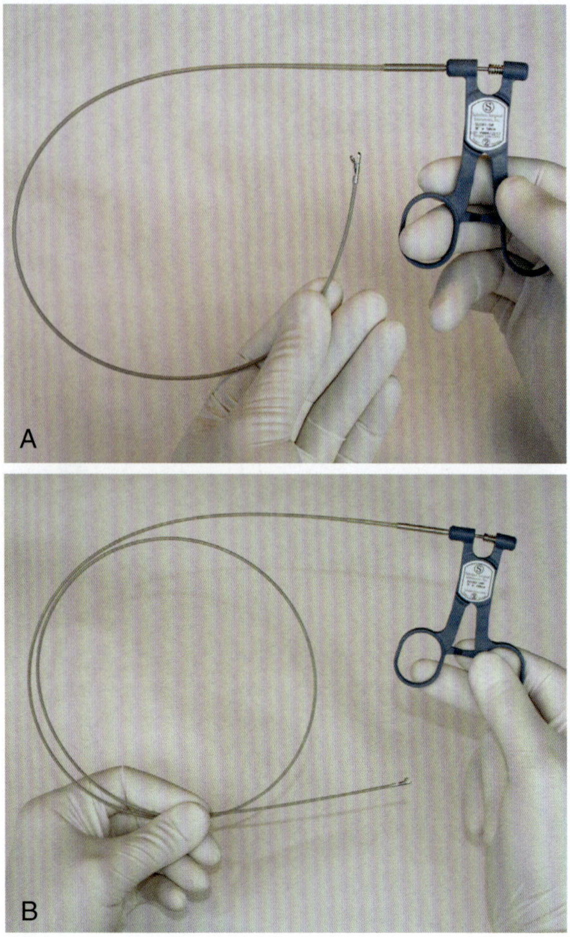

FIGURE 16.5 Single-Use disposable Novatome Bioptome made by Scholten Surgical Instruments, Inc. **A**. 50 cm and **B**. 100 cm lengths. Courtesy of Scholten Surgical Instruments, Inc., Lodi, California.

VASCULAR APPROACH

The right internal jugular approach has been the traditional approach for right ventricular biopsy, with either a preshaped bioptome or a preformed sheath. During the procedures, the patient's electrocardiogram, pulse oximetry, and blood pressure are monitored continuously.

The internal jugular vein is located lateral to the carotid artery, within the triangle formed by the sternal and clavicular head of the sternocleidomastoid muscle and the clavicle (**FIGURE 16.6**). Ultrasound's guidance and the use of micropuncture kits enhance the safety of vascular access (**FIGURES 16.7** and **16.8**). With the preshaped bioptome, the direction of the bioptome tip is concordant with the position of the handle. The preshaped bioptome is inserted with the tip pointing toward the anterior wall of the right atrium. It is advanced across the tricuspid valve and toward the intraventricular septum with a progressive 180° counterclockwise rotation (**FIGURE 16.9**). Other approaches that have been used include the left internal jugular vein with a flexible sheath and the right femoral vein with a preformed sheath or a guiding catheter (**FIGURES 16.10** and **16.11**). Owing to the vascular anatomy, the subclavian vein is not a preferred approach, but it can be used if needed with long sheaths (**FIGURE 16.12**).[8] Left ventricular biopsy can be performed via the femoral artery or radial artery approach using either a preformed sheath or a guiding catheter, and it might have additional diagnostic value in patients with cardiomyopathies and clinically preserved right ventricular function.[9]

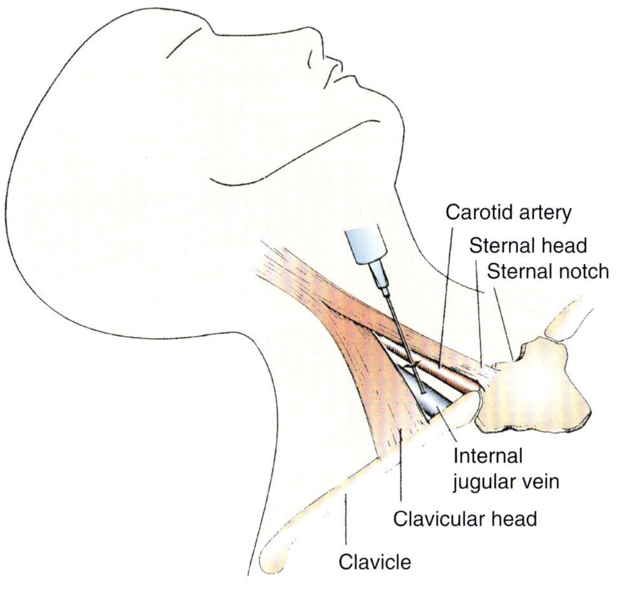

FIGURE 16.6 Regional anatomy for internal jugular puncture. With the patients head rotated to the left, the sternal notch, clavicle, as well as the sternal and clavicular heads of the sternocleidomastoid muscle are identified. A skin nick is made between the 2 heads of this muscle, and 2 fingerbreadths above the top of the clavicle (near the top of the anterior triangle). The needle is inserted at an angle of 30°-40° from vertical, at 20°-30° right of sagittal, aiming the needle away from the more medially located carotid artery. Reproduced with permission from Chaparro SV, Moscucci M. Endomyocardial biopsy. In: Moscucci M, ed. *Grossman & Baim's Cardiac Catheterization Angiography and Intervention*. Philadelphia: Lippincott Williams and Wilkins; 2014.

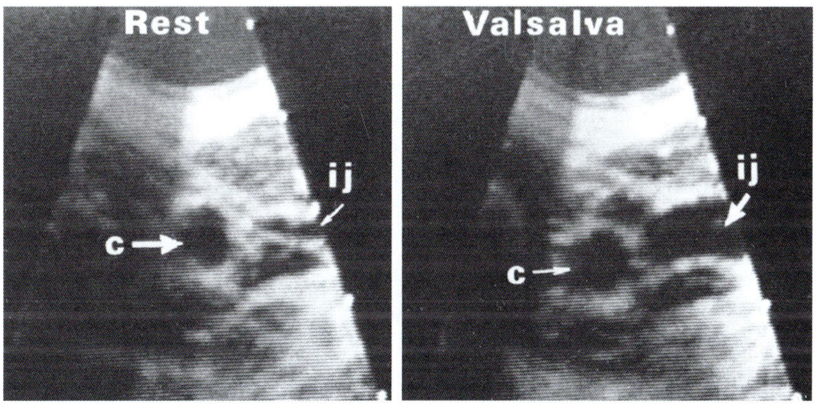

FIGURE 16.7 Ultrasound guidance can facilitate and increase the safety of vascular access. The image on the left side shows the carotid artery (c) and the internal jugular vein (ij) at rest, while the image on the right shows the carotid artery (c) and the distended internal jugular vein (ij) during Valsalva maneuver. Reproduced with permission from Chaparro SV, Moscucci M. Endomyocardial biopsy. In: Moscucci M, ed. *Grossman & Baim's Cardiac Catheterization Angiography and Intervention*. Philadelphia: Lippincott Williams and Wilkins; 2014.

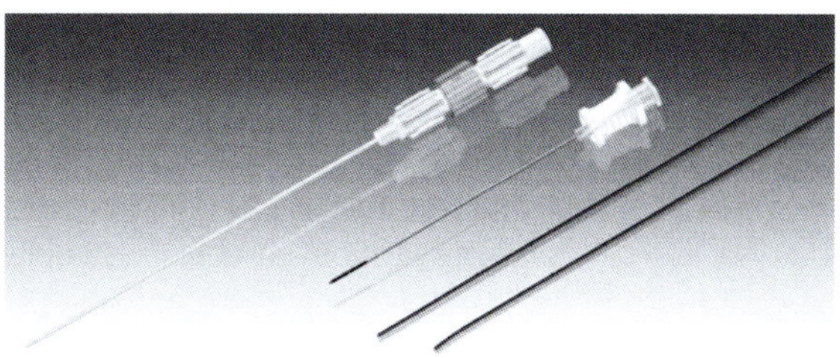

FIGURE 16.8 Micropuncture apparatus: 21-gauge micropuncture needle, 0.018-inch guidewire, 5 Fr guided sheath, and obturator. Glide access® System Photo - © 2018 Terumo Medical Corporation.

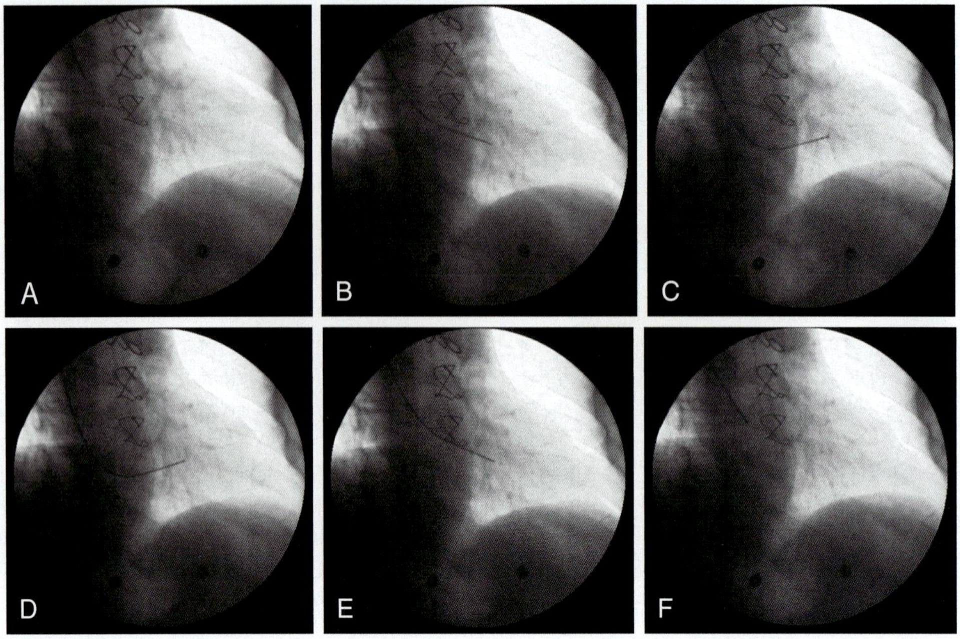

FIGURE 16.9 **A-F,** Cineangiographic frames obtained during right ventricular endomyocardial biopsy using the Stanford bioptome. From left to right, the top rows shows the bioptome against the right atrial wall, against the ventricular septum, withdrawn slightly with jaws open and then against the septum with jaws closed. In the bottom row, the jaws are closed and the bioptome is withdrawn with the sample contained. Reproduced with permission from Chaparro SV, Moscucci M. Endomyocardial biopsy. In: Moscucci M, ed. *Grossman & Baim's Cardiac Catheterization Angiography and Intervention*. Philadelphia: Lippincott Williams and Wilkins; 2014.

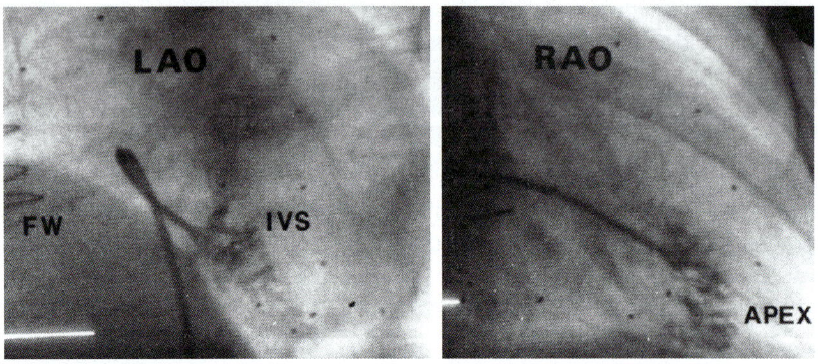

FIGURE 16.10 Right ventricular biopsy from the femoral vein using a double-angulated sheath. Left, in the left anterior oblique projection, contrast injection demonstrates how the terminal sheath curve orients the tip towards the septum (IVS) and away from the free wall (FW). Right, in the right anterior oblique position, contrast injection demonstrates a suitable position about mid-way from the atrial-ventricular groove to the apex. Reproduced with permission from Chaparro SV, Moscucci M. Endomyocardial biopsy. In: Moscucci M, ed. *Grossman & Baim's Cardiac Catheterization Angiography and Intervention*. Philadelphia: Lippincott Williams and Wilkins; 2014.

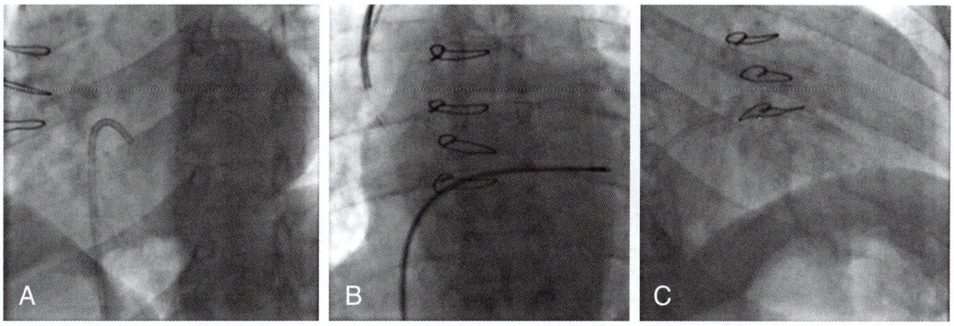

FIGURE 16.11 Endomyocardial biopsy via the femoral vein using a long, curved sheath. **A,** Left anterior oblique (LAO), **(B)** anteroposterior (AP), and **(C)** right anterior oblique (RAO) views of sheath position in the right ventricle. Reproduced with permission from: Naderi N, et al. Endomyocardial Biopsy via the Femoral Vein Using a Long, Curved Sheath. *Transplant Proc.* 2017;49(6):1436-1439.

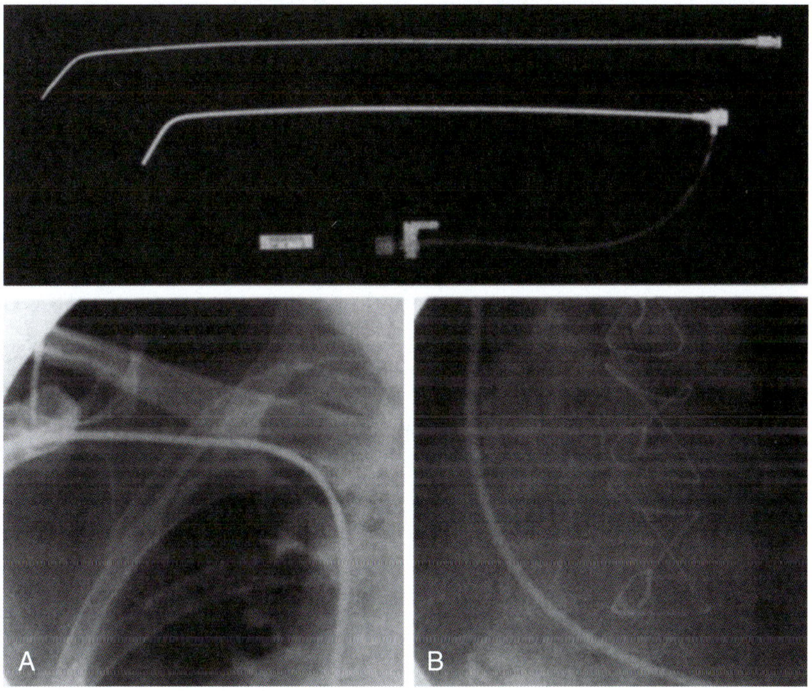

FIGURE 16.12 Top panel. Seven French 35 cm sheath with multipurpose—a curve, side port extension with 3-way stopcock and dilator. Bottom panel: **(A)** sheath course from the right subclavian approach (posterior anterior projection). **B,** sheath positioned in the right ventricle from the right subclavian approach (posterior–anterior projection). Modified with permission from Corley DD, Strickman N. Alternative approaches to right ventricular biopsy. *Cathet Cardiovasc Diagn*. 1994;31:236-239.

ECHOCARDIOGRAPHY-GUIDED BIOPSY

Endomyocardial biopsies are usually performed under fluoroscopic guidance. More recently, echocardiography (transthoracic, intracardiac and transesophageal) has emerged as an additional imaging modality to guide endomyocardial biopsy.[10-16] It is most commonly used as an adjunct to fluoroscopy, particularly during biopsy of intracardiac masses,[17-21] but it has also been used as the only imaging modality (**FIGURES 16.12** and **16.13**).

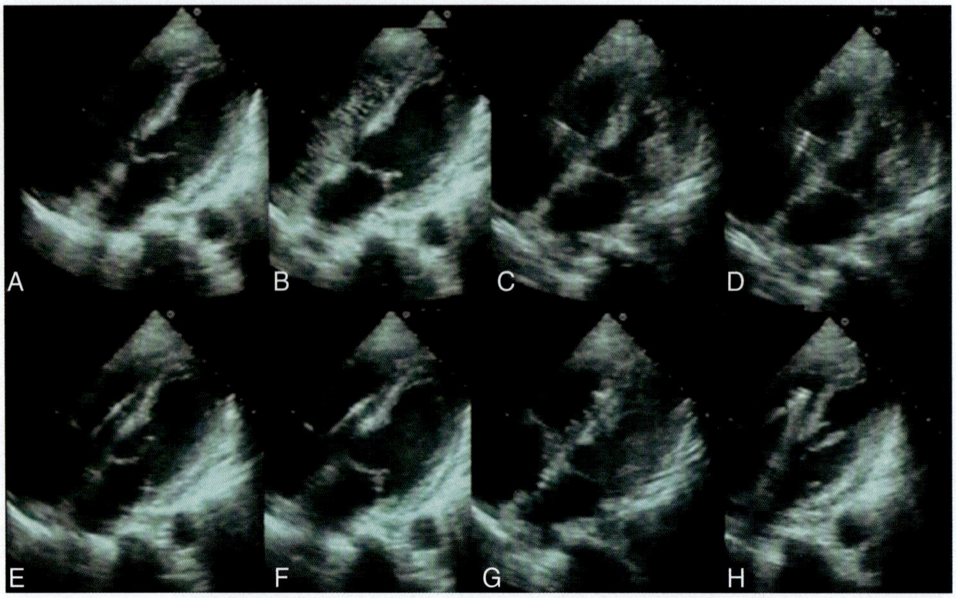

FIGURE 16.13 Sequential images of endomyocardial biopsy guided by 2-dimensional echocardiography. **A,** Apical 4-chamber view. **B,** Contrasted image obtained by saline solution injection. **C,** Bioptome tip on the tricuspid valve. **D,** Bioptome passing across tricuspid valve. **E,** Bioptome advancing against middle of the interventricular septum. **F,** Bioptome withdrawing myocardial fragment. **G,** Bioptome withdrawing myocardial fragment at apex. **H,** Bioptome coming out the right ventricle. © 2011 Fiorelli AI, Junior WM, Groppo Stolf NA. Published in [short citation] under CC BY-NC-SA 3.0 license. Available from http://dx.doi.org/10.5772/22416.

COMPLICATIONS

Several case series have shown that endomyocardial biopsy, in expert hands, is associated with low complication rates (**Tables 16.1-16.3**).[9,22-24] Rare serious complications include cardiac perforation, the development of tricuspid regurgitation due to mechanical damage of the tricuspid valve apparatus (**FIGURE 16.14**), air embolism, and the development of fistulae (**FIGURES 16.15** and **16.16**).

TABLE 16.1

Major Complications of 2505 Retrospective and 543 Prospective EMB Procedures

Major Complications of EMB Procedures	Retrospective, Absolute/%	Prospective, Absolute/%
Pericardial tamponade with pericardiocentesis	2/0.08	0/0
Permanent complete AV block with permanent pacemaker required	1/0.04	0/0
Urgent cardiac surgery	0/0	0/0
Advanced cardiac life support	0/0	0/0
Hemothorax or pneumothorax	0/0	0/0
Death	0/0	0/0

Reproduced with permission from Holzmann M, Nicko A, Kuhl U, et al. Complication rate of right ventricular endomyocardial biopsy via the femoral approach: a retrospective and prospective study analyzing 3048 diagnostic procedures over an 11-year period. *Circulation*. 2008;118:1722-1728.

TABLE 16.2

Minor Complications of 2505 Retrospective and 543 Prospective EMB Procedures

Minor Complications of EMB Procedures	Retrospective, Absolute/%	Prospective, Absolute/%
Small pericardial effusions	.../...	4/0.74
New	.../...	3/0.55
Increase	.../...	1/0.18
Conduction abnormalities	5/0.20	20/3.7
RBBB sustained (>24 h)	.../...	2/0.37
RBBB temporary (<24 h)	.../...	6/1.10
AV block II Mobitz, 2:1 periprocedural (<10 min) requiring 0.5-1 mg atropine	.../...	2/0.37
AV block III periprocedural (<10 min) requiring 0.5-1 mg atropine	.../...	2/0.37
AV block III temporary (<24 h) requiring atropine + temporary pacemaker	5/0.20	8/1.47
Arrhythmias	.../...	6/1.10
Nonsustained ventricular tachycardia (≥10 ventricular complexes)	.../...	0/0
Episode (<12 h) of atrial fibrillation	.../...	5/0.92
Persistent atrial fibrillation with cardioversion	.../...	1/0.18

Reproduced with permission from Holzmann M, Nicko A, Kuhl U, et al. Complication rate of right ventricular endomyocardial biopsy via the femoral approach a retrospective and prospective study analyzing 3048 diagnostic procedures over an 11-year period. *Circulation*. 2008;118:1722-1728.

TABLE 16.3

Complications of LVEMB and RVEMB

	LVEMB (n = 3549), n (%)	RVEMB (n = 3068), n (%)	*P* Value
Major Complication			
Perforation with cardiac tamponade	3 (0.08)	9 (0.29)	0.033
Pericardial effusion without pericardiocentesis	1 (0.028)	5 (0.16)	0.069
Brain embolization with transient cerebral ischemia	8 (0.22)	0	0.007
Pulmonary embolization	0	0	1.0
Permanent AV block	0	0	1.0
Death	0	0	1.0
Overall	12 (0.33)	14 (0.45)	0.116

(continued)

Complications of LVEMB and RVEMB (continued)

	LVEMB (n = 3549), n (%)	RVEMB (n = 3068), n (%)	*P* Value
Minor Complication			
Ventricular or supra-ventricular transient arrhythmias	6 (0.17)	4 (0.13)	0.231
Transient heart block	0	2 (0.06)	0.215
Transient chest pain	7 (0.19)	6 (0.19)	0.218
Intramyocardial hematoma	1 (0.028)	0	0.536
Local Complication			
Vasovagal reaction	47 (1.3)	23 (0.78)	0.007
Local hematoma	16 (0.45)	6 (0.19)	0.035
Femoral arterial venous fistula	1 (0.028)	0	0.536

Reproduced with permission from Chimenti C, Andrea Frustaci A. Contribution and risks of left ventricular endomyocardial biopsy in patients with cardiomyopathies. *Circulation*. 2013;128:1531-1541.

AV, atrioventricular; LVEMB, left ventricular endomyocardial biopsy; RVEMB, right ventricular endomyocardial biopsy.

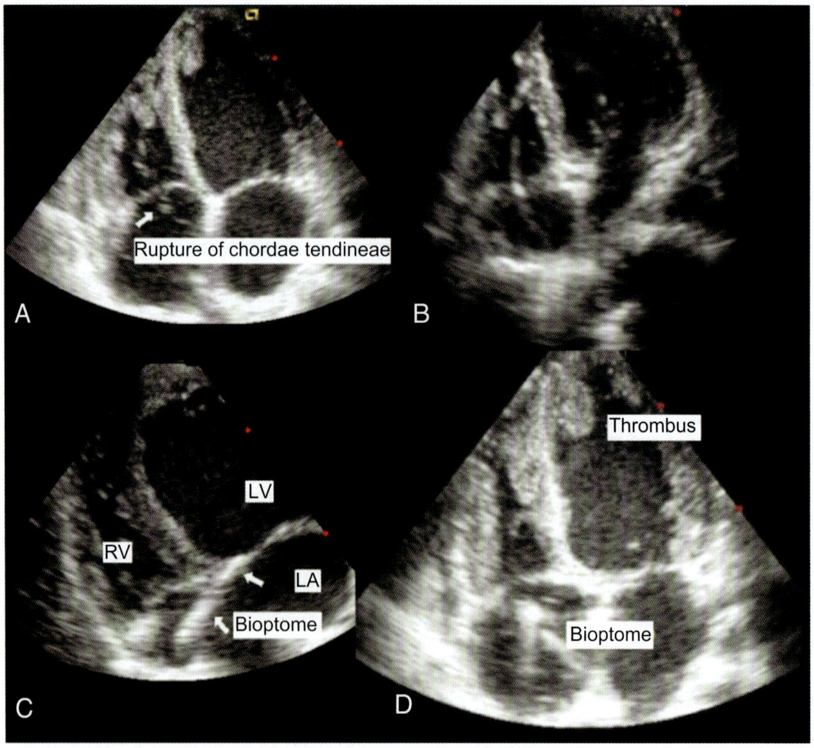

FIGURE 16.14 **A,** Rupture of chordae tendineae due to endomyocardial biopsy. **B,** Bioptome in normal position toward the interventricular septum. **C,** Bioptome inside coronary sinus. **D,** Bioptome in normal position inside right atrium and left intraventricular thrombus finding. © 2011 Fiorelli AI, Junior WM, Groppo Stolf NA. Published in [short citation] under CC BY-NC-SA 3.0 license. Available from http://dx.doi.org/10.5772/22416.

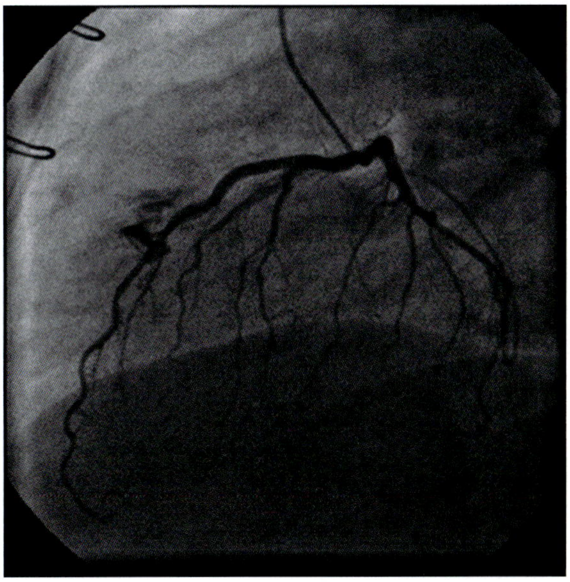

FIGURE 16.15 Fistula between the anterior descending artery and the right ventricle. Reproduced with permission from: Saraiva F, et al. Complications of Endomyocardial Biopsy in Heart Transplant Patients: A Retrospective Study of 2117 Consecutive Procedures. *Transplant Proc*. 2011; 43(5):1908-1912.

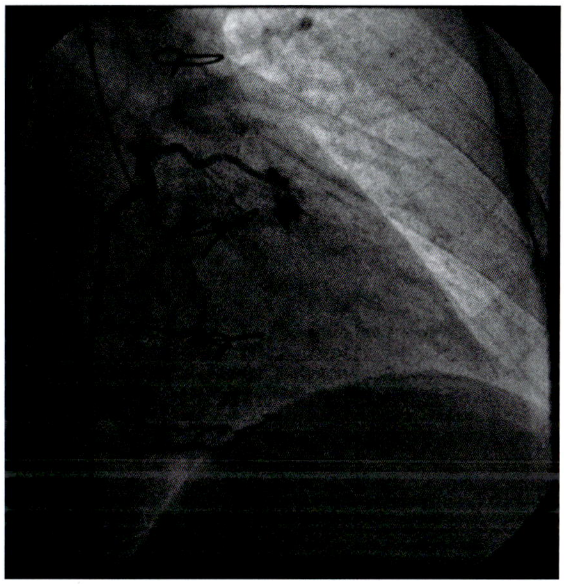

FIGURE 16.16 Fistula originating from the right ventricular branch of the right coronary artery and draining into the right ventricle. Reproduced with permission from: Saraiva F, et al. Complications of Endomyocardial Biopsy in Heart Transplant Patients: A Retrospective Study of 2117 Consecutive Procedures. *Transplant Proc*. 2011;43(5):1908-1912.

ENDOMYOCARDIAL BIOPSY IN THE EVALUATION OF TRANSPLANT REJECTION

Endomyocardial biopsy remains the gold standard in the evaluation and monitoring of heart transplant rejection. **FIGURE 16.17** illustrates biopsy findings according to the International Society for Heart and Lung Transplantation–standardized cardiac biopsy grades, and according to the older classification (**Table 16.4**).

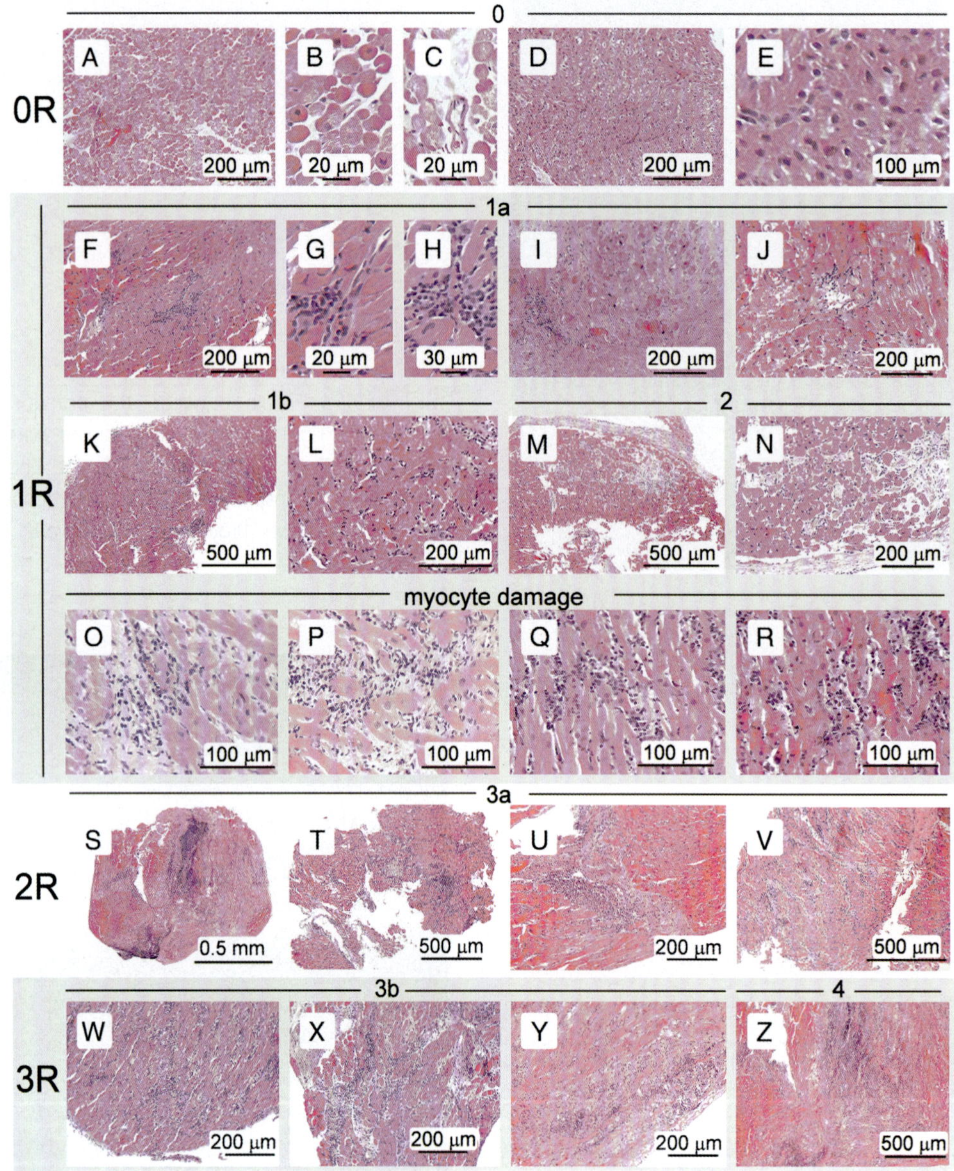

FIGURE 16.17 Cellular rejection in heart transplant biopsies. Vertical axis represents the revised grading scheme, and horizontal axis represents the original grading scheme. **A-C,** Normal, adult. **D and E,** In children, the myocardium appears hypercellular and overall tightly packed. Note the sparse interstitial tissue and many nuclei per cross-section. **F:** Appearance of perivascular **(G)** and interstitial **(H)** infiltrates. **I and J,** Grade 1a is often associated with scars or tissue irregularities (vascular septae). **K and L,** Diffuse infiltration without myocyte damage characterize Grade 1b. Focal **(M)** and diffuse **(N)** infiltration with myocyte damage in Grade 2. **O-R,** Spectrum of myocyte damage with irregular borders of the cardiomyocyte profile and circumferential inflammatory infiltrate. **S-V,** Two or more foci of myocyte damage characterize Grade 3a; note the space-occupying nature of the inflammatory infiltrate and that multiple foci of lower grade-type infiltrates can be present in the same slide. **W-Z,** Grade 3R is characterized by extensive infiltrates with disruption of normal architecture. **W-Y,** Diffuse myocyte damage (Grade 3b), or **(Y)** polymorph-cellular infiltrate, edema, vasculitis, and hemorrhage **(Z)** are associated with extensive myocyte damage in 3R. From Humphrey PA, Dehner LP, Pfeifer JD. *Washington Manual of Surgical Pathology*. Philadelphia, PA: Wolters Kluwer; 2008.

TABLE 16.4

International Society of Lung and Transplant Standardized Cardiac Biopsy Grading

Grade		Histopathological Findings
2004	1990	
0R	0	No rejection
1R	1A	Focal perivascular and or interstitial infiltrate without myocyte damage
	1B	Diffuse infiltrate without necrosis
	2	One focus of infiltrate with associated myocyte damage
2R	3A	Multifocal infiltrate with myocyte damage
3R	3B	Diffuse infiltrate with myocyte damage
	4	Diffuse, polymorphous infiltrate with extensive myocyte damage with edema, hemorrhage or vasculitis

Modified from Stewart S, Winters GL, Fishbein MC, et al. Revision of the 1990 working formulation for the standardization of nomenclature in the diagnosis of heart rejection. *J Heart Lung Transplant*. 2005;24:1710-1720.

ENDOMYOCARDIAL BIOPSY IN THE DIAGNOSIS AND MANAGEMENT OF CARDIOVASCULAR DISEASE

As stated in the introduction, the diagnosis and management of myocardial diseases remain one of the top challenges in cardiovascular medicine. **Table 16.5** and **FIGURES 16.18-16.24** provide examples of clinical scenarios in which endomyocardial biopsy can have a role.[25,26]

TABLE 16.5

The Role of Endomyocardial Biopsy in 14 Clinical Scenarios

Recommendation	Clinical Scenario
I B	New-onset heart failure of 2 wk' duration associated with a normal-sized or dilated left ventricle and hemodynamic compromise
I B	New-onset heart failure of 2 wk' to 3 mo' duration associated with a dilated left ventricle and new ventricular arrhythmias, second- or third-degree heart block, or failure to respond to usual care within 1-2 wk
IIa C	Heart failure of 3 mo' duration associated with a dilated left ventricle and new ventricular arrhythmias, second- or third-degree heart block, or failure to respond to usual care within 1-2 wk
IIa C	Heart failure associated with a DCM of any duration associated with suspected allergic reaction and/or eosinophilia

(continued)

The Role of Endomyocardial Biopsy in 14 Clinical Scenarios (continued)

Recommendation	Clinical Scenario
IIa C	Heart failure associated with suspected anthracycline cardiomyopathy
IIa C	Heart failure associated with unexplained restrictive cardiomyopathy
IIa C	Suspected cardiac tumors
IIa C	Unexplained cardiomyopathy in children
IIb B	New-onset heart failure of 2 wk' to 3 mo' duration associated with a dilated left ventricle, without new ventricular arrhythmias or second- or third-degree heart block, that responds to usual care within 1-2 wk
IIb C	Heart failure of 3 mo' duration associated with a dilated left ventricle, without new ventricular arrhythmias or second- or third-degree heart block, that responds to usual care within 1-2 wk
IIb C	Heart failure associated with unexplained HCM
IIb C	Suspected ARVD/C
IIb C	Unexplained ventricular arrhythmias
III C	Unexplained atrial fibrillation

Modified from Cooper LT, Baughman KL, Feldman AM, et al. The role of endomyocardial biopsy in the management of cardiovascular disease: a scientific statement from the American Heart Association, the American College of Cardiology, and the European Society of Cardiology. Endorsed by the Heart Failure Society of America and the Heart Failure Association of the European Society of Cardiology. *J Am Coll Cardiol*. 2007;50:1914-1931.

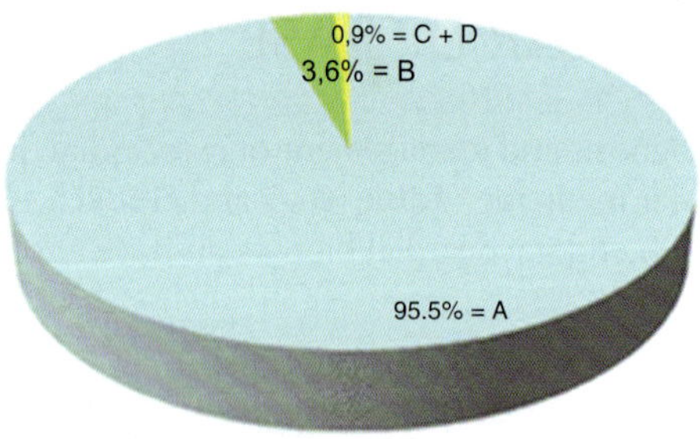

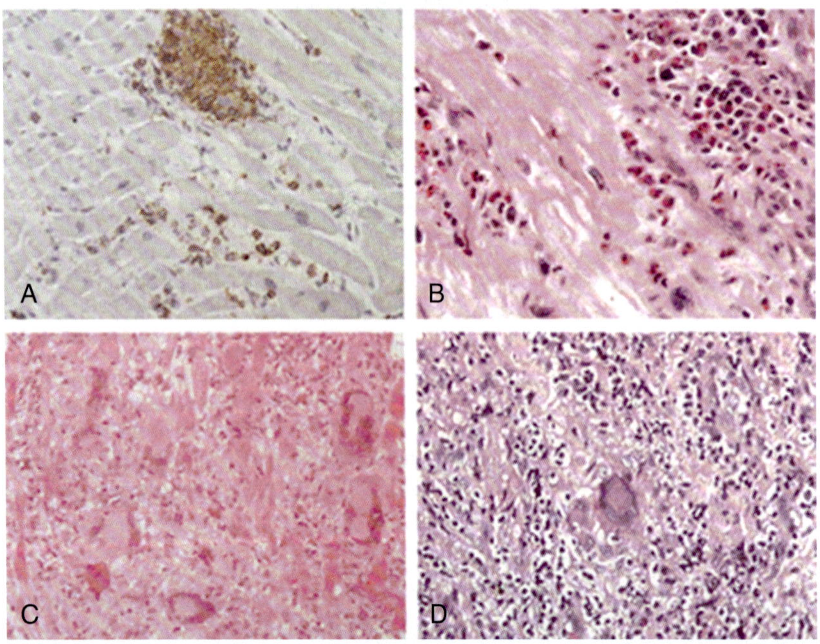

FIGURE 16.18 Myocarditis. Prevalence of different forms of myocarditis in left ventricular endomyocardial biopsy. **A** indicates lymphocytic; **B,** eosinophilic; **C,** giant cell; and **D,** sarcoid. **A,** Immunoperoxidase for CD45RO, ×200. **B,** Hematoxylin and eosin, ×250. **C,** Hematoxylin and eosin, ×200. **D,** Hematoxylin and eosin, ×200. Reproduced with permission from Chimenti C, Andrea Frustaci A. Contribution and risks of left ventricular endomyocardial biopsy in patients with cardiomyopathies. *Circulation*. 2013;128:1531-1541.

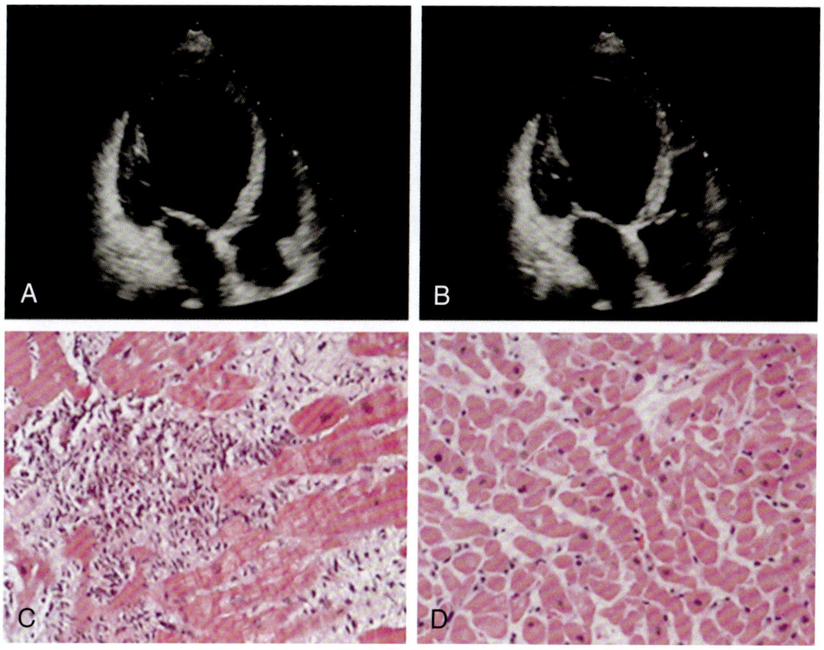

FIGURE 16.19 Active myocarditis in patients with heart failure. Echocardiographic (**A,** diastole; **B,** systole in 4-chamber apical view) and histological (**C,** left ventricle; **D,** right ventricle; hematoxylin and eosin, ×200) comparisons of left ventricular (LV) and right ventricular (RV) involvement in a patient with heart failure. Shown are LV dilation and dysfunction as a result of active myocarditis and a normal RV. Reproduced with permission from Chimenti C, Andrea Frustaci A. Contribution and risks of left ventricular endomyocardial biopsy in patients with cardiomyopathies. *Circulation*. 2013;128:1531-1541.

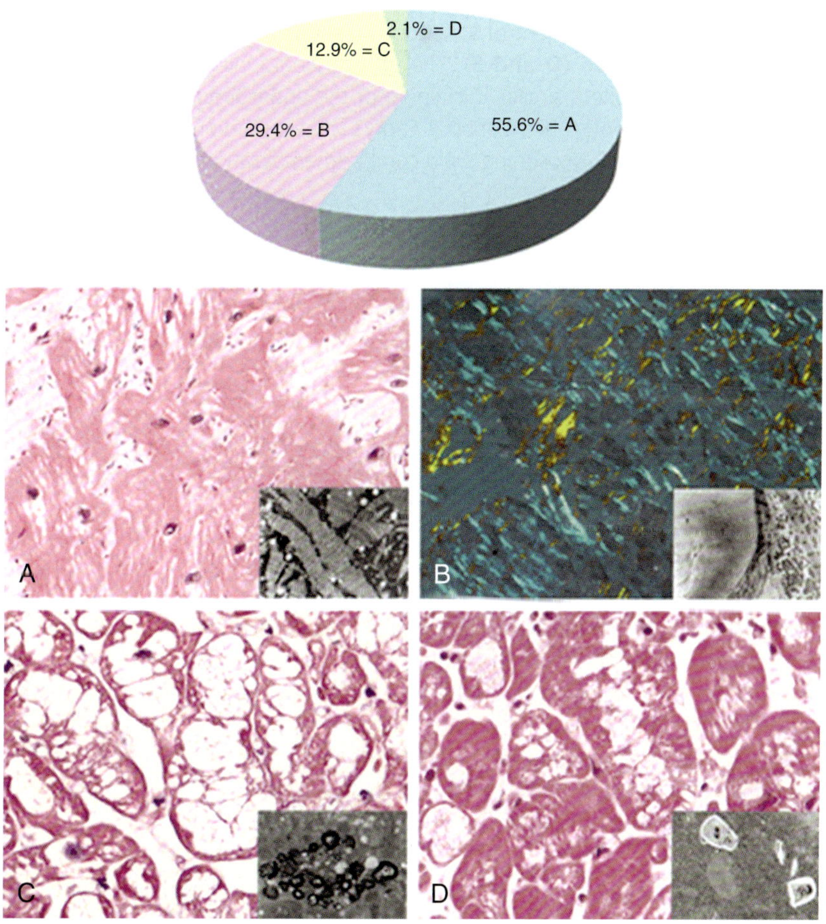

FIGURE 16.20 Prevalence of specific causes of unexplained left ventricular hypertrophy by left ventricular endomyocardial biopsy. **A** indicates hypertrophic cardiomyopathy; **(B)** amyloidosis; **(C)** Fabry disease; and **(D)** glycogenosis. A through **C,** Hematoxylin and eosin, ×200. **B,** Congo red staining, ×100. Insets, Transmission electron microscopy. Reproduced with permission from Chimenti C, Andrea Frustaci A. Contribution and risks of left ventricular endomyocardial biopsy in patients with cardiomyopathies. *Circulation*. 2013;128:1531-1541.

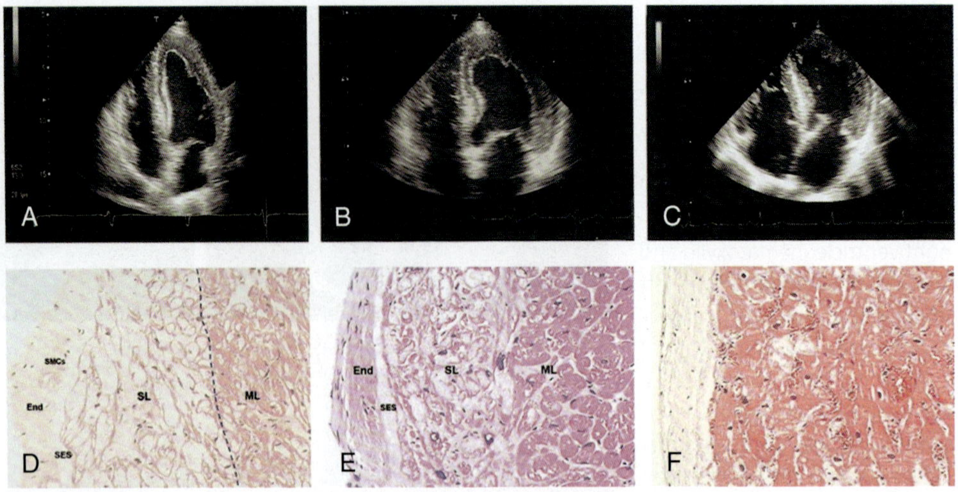

FIGURE 16.21 Fabry disease. Two-dimensional echocardiography in 4-chamber apical view and left ventricular endomyocardial biopsy from 2 patients (Patient #4 and Patient #18 of **Table 16.2**) with Fabry disease cardiomyopathy (A, D and B, E, respectively) and a patient with hypertrophic cardiomyopathy **(C and F)**. Comparison of the 3 echocardiographic frames reveals the presence of a binary appearance of left ventricular endocardial border in the 2 Fabry patients **(A and B)**. This echocardiographic finding reflects the glycosphingolipids compartmentalization involving a thickened endocardium (End) with enlarged and engulfed smooth muscle cells (SMC), a subendocardial empty space (SES), and a prominent involvement of subendocardial myocardial layer (SL), while the middle layer (ML) appears partially spared **(D and E)**. The echocardiographic pattern is absent in hypertrophic cardiomyopathy **(C)**, despite a similar thickening of the endocardium **(F)**. Reproduced with permission from Pieroni M, Chimenti C, De Cobelli F. Fabry's disease cardiomyopathy: echocardiographic detection of endomyocardial glycosphingolipid compartmentalization. *J Am Coll Cardiol*. 2006;47:1663-1671.

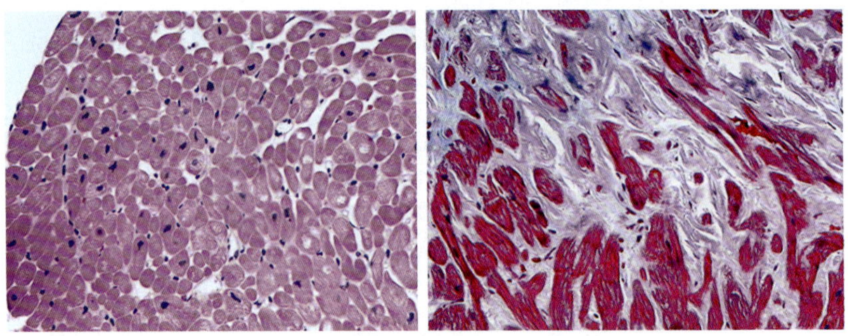

FIGURE 16.22 Cardiac Amyloidosis. Cardiac biopsies (original magnification × 400) showing normal findings (left) and extensive amyloid infiltration (right). In the normal heart, the muscle fibers (stained pink in this slide) are close together with little space between them. In the patient with amyloidosis, the muscle fibers, staining here in red, are disrupted by a large amount of amyloid deposited between them (staining light pink-purple). Courtesy of Dr Paul VanderLaan, Department of Pathology, Brigham and Women's Hospital; Reproduced with permission from Quarta CC, Kruger JL, Falk RH. Cardiac amyloidosis. *Circulation*. 2012;126:e178-e182.

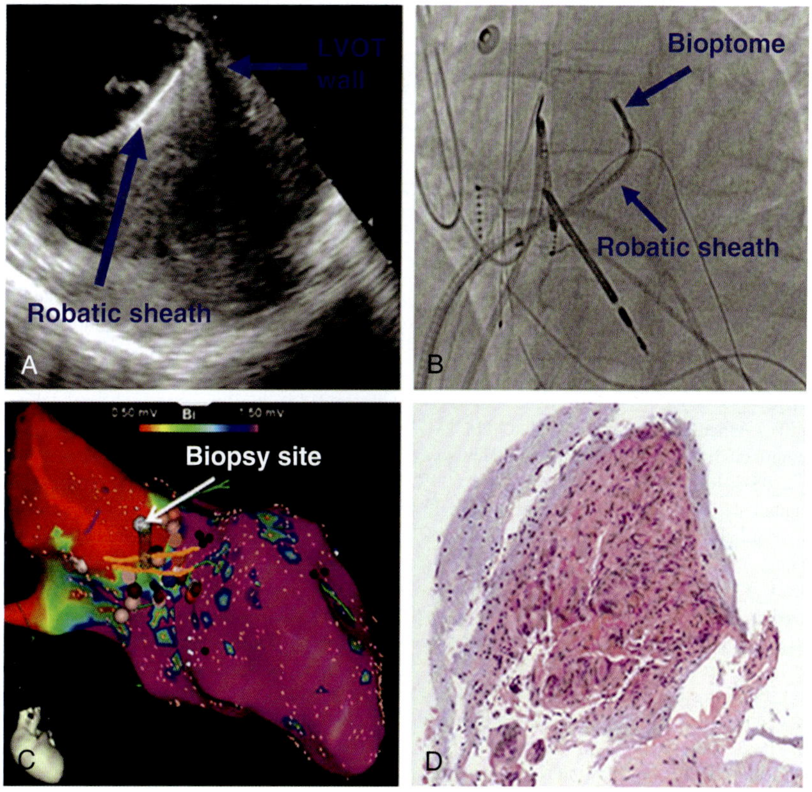

FIGURE 16.23 Sarcoidosis. Robotically Guided Left Ventricular Biopsy to Diagnose Cardiac Sarcoidosis. 44-year-old white woman presented with syncope and dyspnea on exertion. Echocardiographic evaluation was normal, while cardiac MRI showed findings suspicious of infiltrative cardiomyopathy. Standard biopsy, angiography, and CTA were noncontributory. An electrophysiological study showed inducible monomorphic ventricular tachycardia and therefore, a defibrillator was implanted. Two weeks later the patient presented with multiple defibrillator shocks. Therefore, it was decided to obtain a robotically assisted (Sensei Robotic System, Hansen Medical, Mountain View, CA) biopsy using electroanatomic mapping guidance. **A,** Intracardiac echocardiography image monitoring during biopsy of the LVOT showing the bioptome (150 cm) coming out of the robotic sheath; **(B)** fluoroscopy image monitoring during biopsy of the LVOT; **(C)** electroanatomical mapping guidance to the most significant reduction of voltage map in the LVOT; **(D)** H&E staining of the biopsy sample from the LVOT showing a nonnecrotizing granuloma with aggregates of epithelioid histiocytes and giant cells. LVOT indicates left ventricular outflow tract. Adapted with permission from Bhimaraj A, et al. Robotically Guided Left Ventricular Biopsy to Diagnose Cardiac Sarcoidosis: A Multidisciplinary Innovation Leading to First-in-Human Case. *Circ Heart Fail*. 2018;11:e004627.

FIGURE 16.24 Cardiac sarcoidosis, endomyocardial biopsy. **A,** The sarcoid lesion practically replaces the entire biopsy sample. **B,** A different example showing abundant chronic inflammation. From Burke AP, Aubry MC, Maleszewski J, Alexiev B, Tavora F. *Practical Thoracic Pathology*. 1st ed. Philadelphia, PA: Wolters Kluwer; 2016.

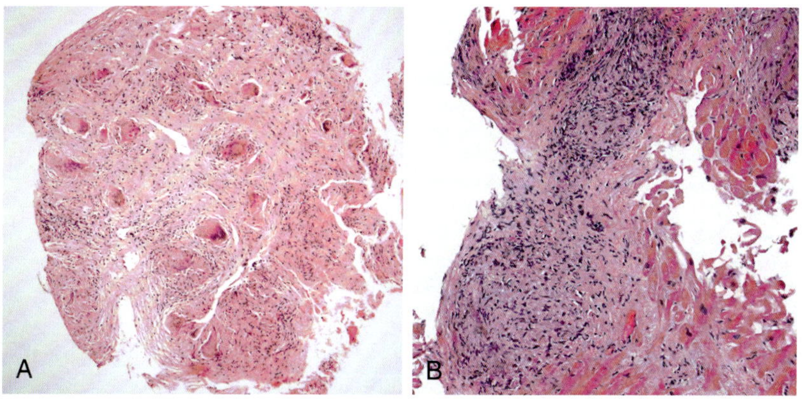

REFERENCES

1. Weinberg M, Fell EH, Lynfield J. Diagnostic biopsy of the pericardium and myocardium. *AMA Arch Surg*. 1958;76(5):825-829.
2. Sutton DC, Sutton GC. Needle biopsy of the human ventricular myocardium: review of 54 consecutive cases. *Am Heart J*. 1960;60:364-370.
3. Timmis GC, Gordon S, Baron RH, Brough AJ. Percutaneous myocardial biopsy. *Am Heart J*. 1965;70(4):499-504.
4. Bulloch RT, Murphy ML, Pearce MB. Intracardiac needle biopsy of the ventricular septum. *Am J Cardiol*. 1965;16:227-233.
5. Sakakibara S, Konno S. Endomyocardial biopsy. *Jpn Heart J*. 1962;3:537-543.
6. Caves PK, Schulz WP, Dong E Jr, Stinson EB, Shumway NE. New instrument for transvenous cardiac biopsy. *Am J Cardiol*. 1974;33(2):264-267.
7. Caves PK, Stinson EB, Graham AF, Billingham ME, Grehl TM, Shumway NE. Percutaneous transvenous endomyocardial biopsy. *JAMA*. 1973;225(3):288-291.
8. Corley DD, Strickman N. Alternative approaches to right ventricular endomyocardial biopsy. *Cathet Cardiovasc Diagn*. 1994;31(3):236-239.
9. Chimenti C, Frustaci A. Contribution and risks of left ventricular endomyocardial biopsy in patients with cardiomyopathies: a retrospective study over a 28-year period. *Circulation*. 2013;128(14):1531-1541.
10. Fiorelli AI, Coelho GB, Santos RH, et al. Successful endomyocardial biopsy guided by transthoracic two-dimensional echocardiography. *Transplant Proc*. 2011;43(1):225-228.
11. Han J, Park Y, Lee H, et al. Complications of 2-D echocardiography guided transfemoral right ventricular endomyocardial biopsy. *J Kor Med Sci*. 2006;21(6):989-994.
12. Kawauchi M, Gundry SR, Boucek MM, de Begona JA, Vigesaa R, Bailey LL. Real-time monitoring of the endomyocardial biopsy site with pediatric transesophageal echocardiography. *J Heart Lung Transplant*. 1992;11(2 pt 1):306-310.
13. Miller LW, Labovitz AJ, McBride LA, Pennington DG, Kanter K. Echocardiography-guided endomyocardial biopsy. A 5-year experience. *Circulation*. 1988;78(5 pt 2):III99-III102.
14. Nelson OL, Robbins CT. Comparison of echocardiography-guided and fluoroscopy-guided endomyocardial biopsy techniques. *Vet Radiol Ultrasound*. 2005;46(2):131-134.
15. Sloan KP, Bruce CJ, Oh JK, Rihal CS. Complications of echocardiography-guided endomyocardial biopsy. *J Am Soc Echocardiogr*. 2009;22(3):324.e1-324.e4.
16. Williams GA, Kaintz RP, Habermehl KK, Nelson JG, Kennedy HL. Clinical experience with two-dimensional echocardiography to guide endomyocardial biopsy. *Clin Cardiol*. 1985;8(3):137-140.
17. Keller DI, Hunziker P, Buser P. Biopsy of right atrial angiosarcoma guided by transesophageal echocardiography. *J Am Soc Echocardiogr*. 2002;15(5):475-477.
18. Burling F, Devlin G, Heald S. Primary cardiac lymphoma diagnosed with transesophageal echocardiography-guided endomyocardial biopsy. *Circulation*. 2000;101(17):E179-E181.
19. Savoia MT, Liguori C, Nahar T, et al. Transesophageal echocardiography-guided transvenous biopsy of a cardiac sarcoma. *J Am Soc Echocardiogr*. 1997;10(7):752-755.
20. Chirillo F, Risica G, Stritoni P. Mobile right atrial mass biopsy guided by biplane transesophageal echocardiography. *Int J Card Imag*. 1995;11(3):201-203.
21. Di Lisi D, Raspante D, Lavanco V, et al. Three-dimensional transesophageal echocardiography in the guide of cardiac mass biopsy: future prospectives. *J Cardiovasc Med*. 2018;19(1):29-30.
22. Deckers JW, Hare JM, Baughman KL. Complications of transvenous right ventricular endomyocardial biopsy in adult patients with cardiomyopathy: a seven-year survey of 546 consecutive diagnostic procedures in a tertiary referral center. *J Am Coll Cardiol*. 1992;19(1):43-47.
23. Saraiva F, Matos V, Goncalves L, Antunes M, Providencia LA. Complications of endomyocardial biopsy in heart transplant patients: a retrospective study of 2117 consecutive procedures. *Transplant Proc*. 2011;43(5):1908-1912.
24. Holzmann M, Nicko A, Kuhl U, et al. Complication rate of right ventricular endomyocardial biopsy via the femoral approach: a retrospective and prospective study analyzing 3048 diagnostic procedures over an 11-year period. *Circulation*. 2008;118(17):1722-1728.
25. Bennett MK, Gilotra NA, Harrington C, et al. Evaluation of the role of endomyocardial biopsy in 851 patients with unexplained heart failure from 2000-2009. *Circ Heart Fail*. 2013;6(4):676-684.
26. Cooper LT, Baughman KL, Feldman AM, et al. The role of endomyocardial biopsy in the management of cardiovascular disease: a scientific statement from the American Heart Association, the American College of Cardiology, and the European Society of Cardiology. Endorsed by the Heart Failure Society of America and the Heart Failure Association of the European Society of Cardiology. *J Am Coll Cardiol*. 2007;50(19):1914-1931.

chapter **17**

Percutaneous Circulatory Support: Intra-Aortic Balloon Counterpulsation, Impella, Tandem Heart, and Extracorporeal Bypass

CARLOS D. DAVILA, MD, MICHELE ESPOSITO, MD, and NAVIN K. KAPUR, MD

INTRODUCTION

The use of percutaneous acute mechanical circulatory support (AMCS) has steadily grown in the last decade. Currently, the main indications for AMCS include (1) high-risk percutaneous coronary and electrophysiological interventions, (2) cardiogenic shock (CS) due to myocardial infarction and myocarditis, (3) postcardiotomy shock, and (4) refractory chronic heart failure as a bridge to durable mechanical support or heart transplantation. Large randomized clinical trials proving benefits of these therapies are scarce. Guidelines and consensus statements addressing proper patient selection, timing of implantation, device choice, and postimplantation protocol are beginning to emerge. Optimization of clinical outcomes in this field requires a critical understanding of the different types of hemodynamic support provided by available devices and their applicability in a particular clinical scenario including best practices to monitor, wean, and optimize each device postimplantation. In this chapter we will review the mechanics of several AMCS devices, specifically discuss the hemodynamic effects of these devices, and review current data available, evaluating their clinical utility.

LVAD AND AMCS

In 2001, the Randomized Evaluation of Mechanical Assistance for the Treatment of Congestive Heart Failure (REMATCH) trial demonstrated that durable, surgically implanted, left ventricular assist devices (LVADs) improved survival in patients with end-stage heart failure compared with medical therapy alone[1]. Moreover, in 2009 continuous flow LVADs (CF-LVADs) showed significantly improved 2-year survival compared with pulsatile LVADS. Since then, the use of permanent CF-LVADs has grown exponentially to more than 2500 implants per year.[3] Consistent with this observation, several recent reports have identified increasing use of AMCS in the setting of CS. A recent analysis of the Nationwide Inpatient Sample from the Healthcare Cost and Utilization Project identified a 1511% increase in the use of AMCS devices and no significant change in intra-aortic balloon pump (IABP) use from 2007 to 2011 compared with

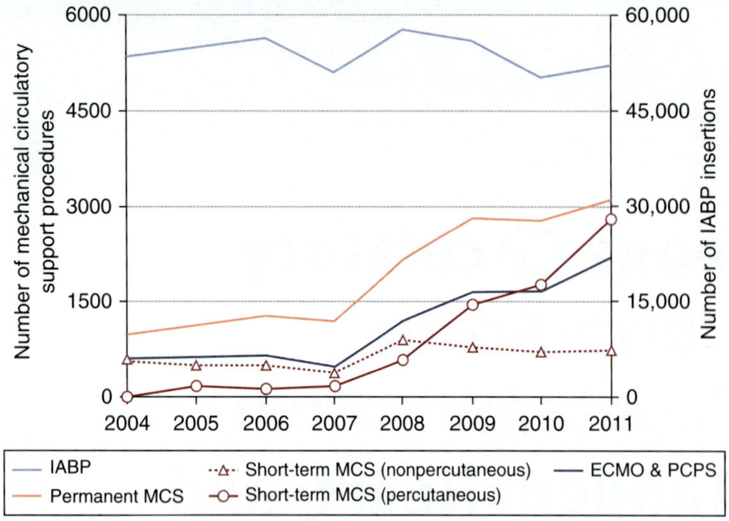

FIGURE 17.1 Trends in the use of percutaneously delivered AMCS devices.[2] PCPS, percutaneous cardiopulmonary support. Reproduced with permission from Stretch R, Sauer CM, Yuh DD, Bonde P. National trends in the utilization of short-term mechanical circulatory support: incidence, outcomes, and cost analysis. *J Am Coll Cardiol.* 2014;64:1407-1415.

2004 to 2007, especially in the setting of high-risk interventions and CS with higher-than-normal-risk profiles for surgically implanted LVADs as a bridge to recovery (BTR) (**FIGURE 17.1**).[2,4] Despite increasing use of AMCS devices, an analysis of the National Cardiovascular Data Registry CathPCI–participating hospitals from 2009 to 2013 identified that the probability of non-IABP AMCS device use for CS was <5% for 1/2 of the hospitals and >20% in less than 1/10th of these hospitals.[4]

Interagency Registry for Mechanically Assisted Circulatory Support (INTERMACS)

See **FIGURE 17.2** for trends.

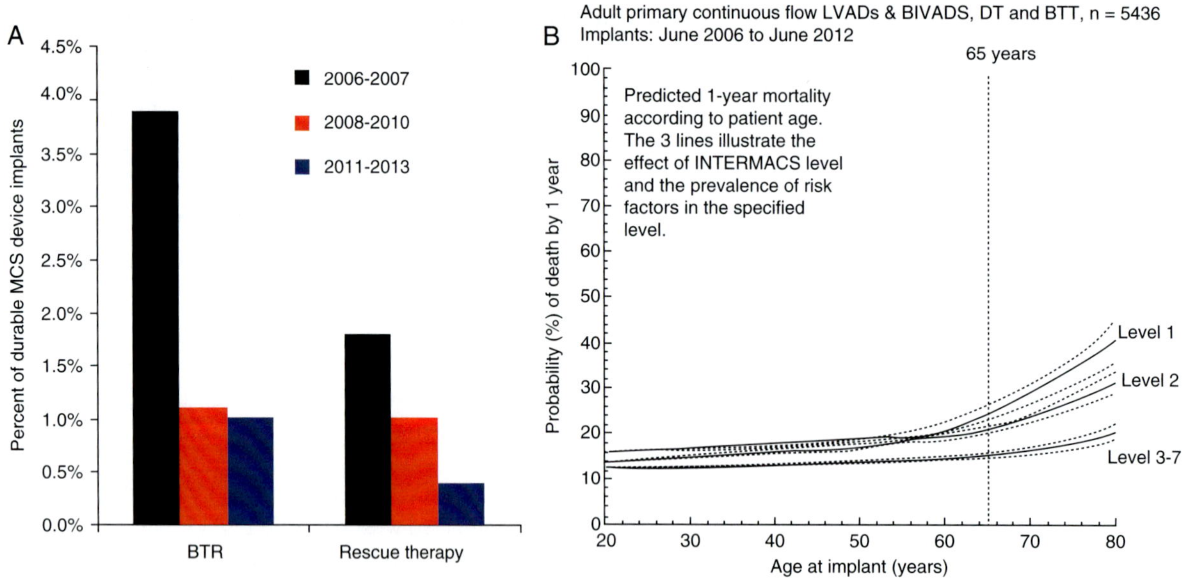

FIGURE 17.2 Trends in the use of surgically implanted durable MCS.[5] **A**, The number of LVADs being implanted as part of a BTR strategy or as a rescue therapy has significantly declined over the past decade. This shift in LVAD use away from unstable, high-risk INTERMACS profiles is partly driven by data showing increased mortality after LVAD implantation for INTERMACS profiles 1 and 2 after the age of 65 years and the increasing availability of AMCS devices, which include short-term, percutaneously inserted devices without the need for cardiac surgery. **B**, The predicted 1 year mortality after LVAD implantation is highest among the sickest patients defined as INTERMACS Levels 1 and 2. Reproduced with permission from Kirklin JK, Naftel DC, Kormos RL, et al. Fifth INTERMACS annual report: risk factor analysis from more than 6000 mechanical circulatory support patients. *J Heart Lung Transplant*. 2013;32:141-156.

AMCS Indications and Complications

See **Tables 17.1** and **17.2**.

TABLE 17.1

Suggested Indications for AMCS[6]

Indication	Comments
Acute myocardial infarction	AMCS devices are commonly used in the setting of cardiogenic shock resulting from a large area of myocardial infarction either during or after PCI or for complications of AMI such as mitral regurgitation, ventricular septal rupture, RVF, or biventricular shock.
High-risk PCI Complex ablation of ventricular tachycardia Structural interventions	Prophylactic use of AMCS during complex coronary interventions involving a large territory of myocardium at risk for ischemia (ie, unprotected left main disease or multivessel disease). AMCS is also used during electrophysiologic procedures (ie, VT ablation) where ventricular support may allow for longer periods of VT during mapping with less hemodynamic compromise. AMCS has more recently been used to support complicated valvular interventions such as high-risk TAVR or mitral therapy.
Refractory heart failure	AMCS devices are commonly used to support advanced heart failure patients with hemodynamic compromise that is refractory to inotropes as part of a BTR, bridge to VAD/OHTx, or bridge to decision pathway. AMCS has also been used to recover patients with reversible causes of cardiomyopathies including myocarditis, peripartum, and stress cardiomyopathy.
Acute allograft failure	Cases of acute cellular or antibody-mediated rejection, organ preservation failure, or prolonged ischemic time.
RVF	Dedicated AMCS devices for RVF are more commonly being used after cardiac transplantation, cardiotomy, and RV myocardial infarction.

TABLE 17.2

Potential Complications Associated with AMCS Devices

Device	Potential Complications
All devices	• Bleeding and vascular injury • Infection • Limb ischemia • Hemolysis • Cerebrovascular accident
IABP	• Subclavian, renal, or mesenteric artery obstruction • Aortic rupture or dissection • Air or atherosclerotic plaque embolism • Balloon rupture
Catheter-mounted axial-flow pumps: Impella device	• Aortic insufficiency • Ventricular arrhythmia
Left atrial-to-femoral artery centrifugal flow pumps: TandemHeart device	• Cannula migration • LA puncture/cardiac tamponade
Venoarterial extracorporeal membrane oxygenation (VA-ECMO)	• LV distension and acute pulmonary edema • Cephalic hypoxemia (North-South syndrome)

THERAPEUTIC OBJECTIVES

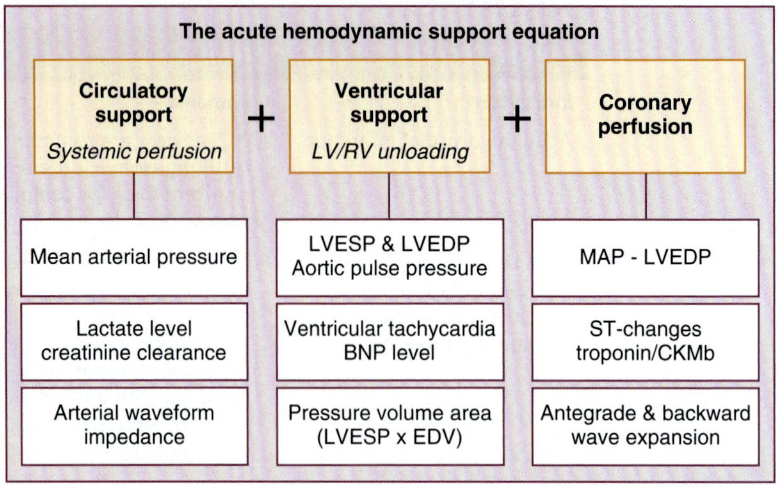

FIGURE 17.3 The acute hemodynamic support equation. BNP, brain natriuretic peptide; EDV, end diastolic volume; MAP, mean arterial pressure.

The main therapeutic objectives of acute percutaneous mechanical support are to provide adequate circulation to vital organs, augment coronary perfusion, improve ventricular unloading, and reduce myocardial oxygen demand (**FIGURE 17.3**). These parameters can be estimated using certain surrogates as shown in **FIGURE 17.3**. Different mechanical circulatory support (MCS) devices are available, and each of them addresses the hemodynamic equation in different degrees. Thus it is of paramount importance to understand the hemodynamics and the initial goal of MCS based on specific clinical scenarios (high-risk percutaneous intervention vs CS). The ideal MCS device would target all elements of the hemodynamic equation and prove to be safe and easy to use in the acute setting.

Mechanical Circulatory Support Systems (MCS)

MCS systems can be classified based on anatomical support provided, mechanism of action, flow pattern, and localization after percutaneous delivery (**FIGURE 17.4A**).

Four primary AMCS device platforms are currently used in clinical practice for left ventricular (LV) hemodynamic support (**FIGURE 17.4B**) and can be broadly categorized as pulsatile and continuous flow systems. These devices include (1) the IABP, (2) centrifugally driven left atrial-to-femoral artery bypass (TandemHeart; TandemLife Inc), (3) centrifugally driven venoarterial extracorporeal membrane oxygenation (VA-ECMO), and (4) micro-axial flow catheters (Impella; Abiomed Inc and Percutaneous Heart Pump [PHP]; St Jude Inc). At present, the PHP device is approved for clinical use in Europe but is under active investigation in the United States.

Right ventricular AMCS (RV-AMCS) device options include VA-ECMO, the TandemHeart centrifugal flow pump (TandemLife, Pittsburgh, PA), and the axial-flow Impella RP catheter (Abiomed Inc, Danvers, MA) (**FIGURE 17.4C**). RV-AMCS devices can be categorized according to their mechanism of action as either RA-PA (right atrium-pulmonary artery) drainage or RA-PA bypass systems. VA-ECMO is a RA-PA drainage system that oxygenates and displaces blood from the RA and/or PA into the arterial circulation. The Impella RP and the TandemHeart RVAD are RA-PA bypass systems that displace blood from the RA into the PA, thereby bypassing the failing RV.

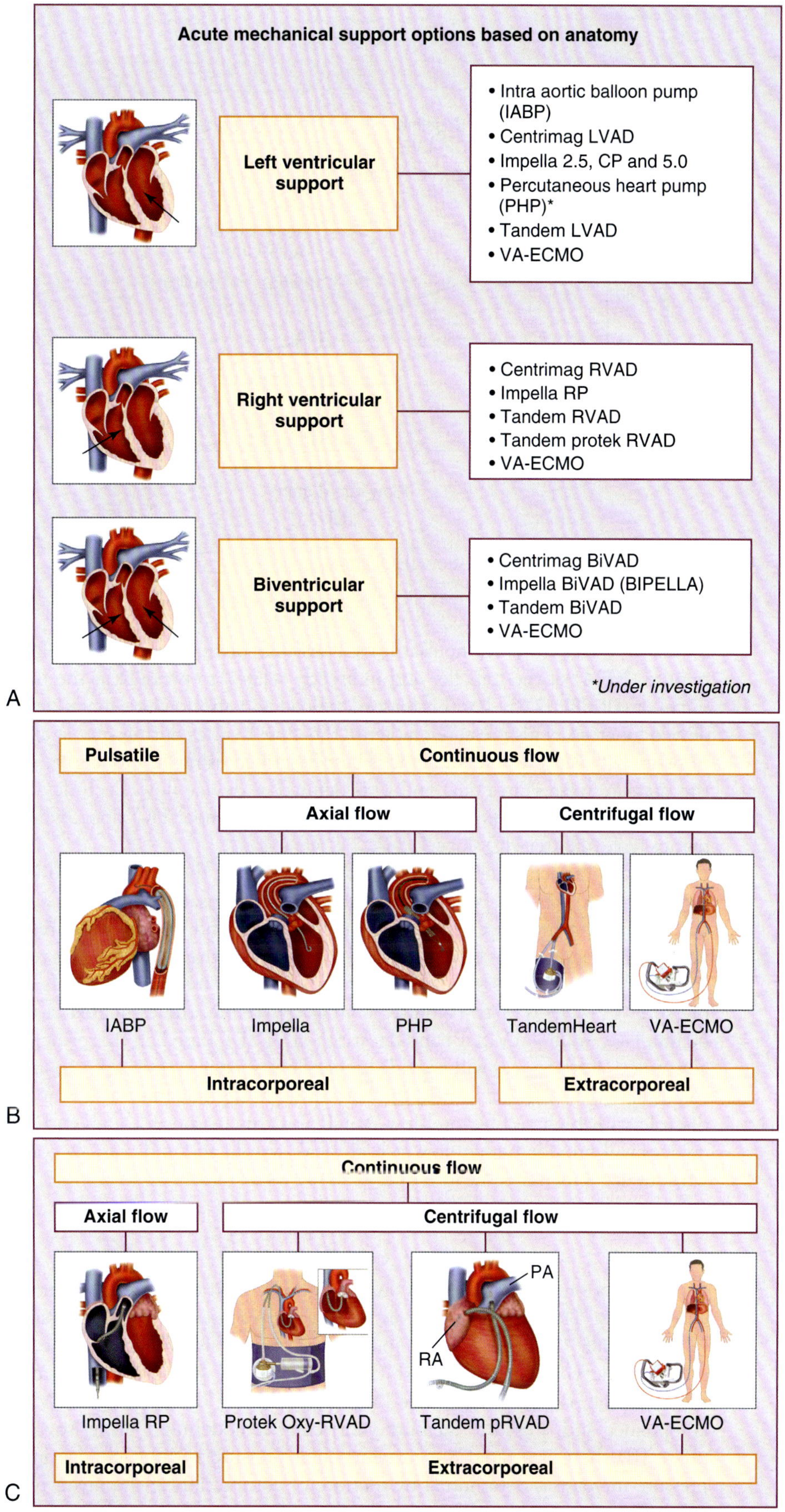

FIGURE 17.4 Options for MCS.

CF-AMCS

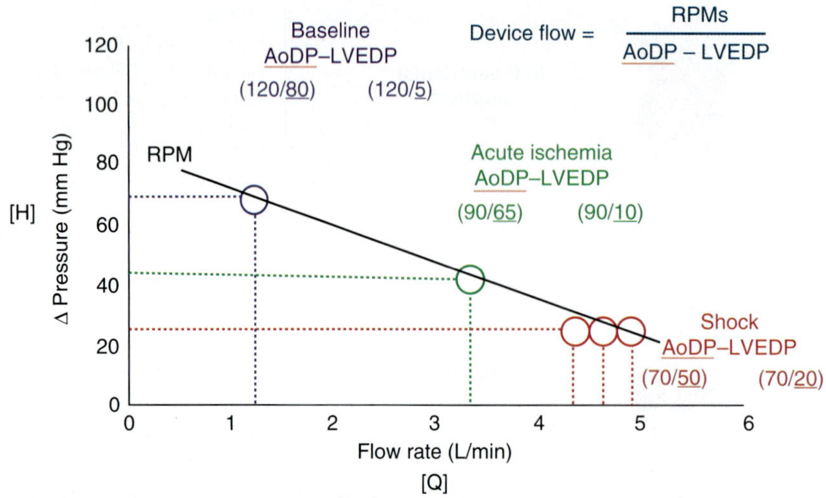

FIGURE 17.5 The pressure-flow (HQ) curve.

Flow through all (nonpulsatile) CF-AMCS devices is directly related to rotations per minute (RPM) of the impeller and indirectly related to pressure at the inlet and outlet of the impeller (**FIGURE 17.5**).[7] For this reason, preload and afterload are major determinants of AMCS device function. This pressure gradient (Pin-Pout) varies during systole and diastole. The relationship between pressure and flow is best described using an HQ curve, where H is defined as the pressure head (Pin-Pout) and Q is defined as device flow. Each device has a specific HQ curve signature. Axial-flow pumps tend to have a steeper HQ slope, whereas centrifugal flow pumps have a flatter HQ slope.[8]

For the TandemHeart, Impella, and PHP devices, the pressure head (H) includes LV pressure and aortic pressure. For patients without decompensated heart failure or aortic valve disease (ie, undergoing high-risk PCI), peak aortic and LV end systolic pressures are matched and at peak systole (ie, AoSP – LVESP = 120 – 120 mm Hg) the estimated H is zero. Throughout diastole, aortic diastolic pressure (AoDP) ranges between 60 and 80 mm Hg and LV end diastolic pressure (LVEDP) is often below 20 mmHg. Therefore, the estimated H ranges between 40 to 60 mm Hg (AoDP – LVEDP) and 0 (AoSP – LVESP). Based on this principle, for a given RPM, continuous flow devices will provide higher flow at peak systole (H = 0) and lower flow in diastole (H = 40 – 60). In contrast, the patient with CS may have a substantially lower H during diastole with high LVEDP and low AoDP. For this reason, for a given RPM, continuous flow devices will provide higher flow at both peak systole and end diastole compared with patients without decompensated heart failure.

PV Loop

LV ejection fraction depends on preloading conditions, afterload, and intrinsic ventricular contractility. These parameters can be visually represented in the pressure-volume loop (PV loop) (**FIGURE 17.6**). Each loop represents a single cardiac cycle, where preload is related to end diastolic volume and pressure **(A)**. End diastolic pressure volume relationship (EDPVR) relates to the passive filling of the LV during diastole; the slope of EDPVR is the reciprocal of compliance and is used to measure ventricular remodeling. During isovolumetric contraction phase **(B)** there is a rapid rise in ventricular pressure without change in volume; the rate of pressure increase is determined by the rate of contraction of the myocytes. The maximal rate of pressure change during this phase is termed dP/dt_{max}. When LV pressure exceeds the aortic

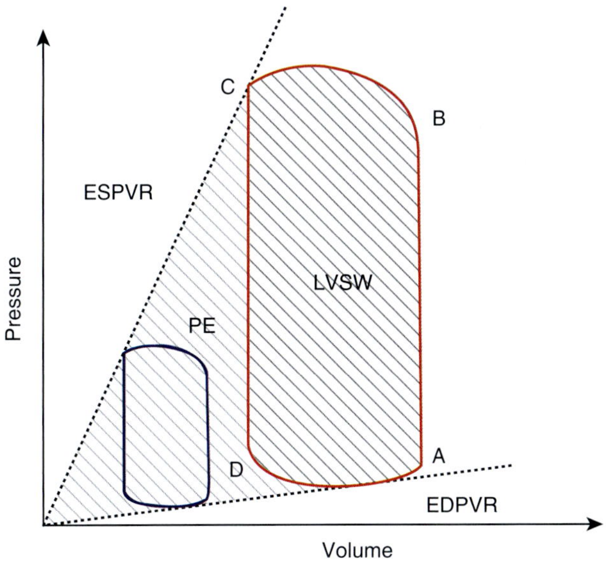

FIGURE 17.6 PV loop and the optimal mechanical support device. Reproduced with permission from Briceno N, Kapur NK, Perera D. Percutaneous mechanical circulatory support: current concepts and future directions. *Heart*. 2016;102(18):1494-1507.

diastolic pressure, the ejection phase begins; during this phase the ventricular volume decreases as the LV pressure reaches peak systolic pressure and then begins to relax **(C)**; the residual LV volume is the end systolic volume. The end systolic pressure volume relationship (ESPVR) is a valuable measure of ventricular systolic function for both clinical and experimental evaluations. Changes in ESPVR represent changes in contractility, whereas the slope measures end-systolic chamber stiffness. Systole is then followed by the isovolumetric relaxation **(D)** before the next cardiac cycle.

It is important to recognize each phase of the cardiac cycle and its graphical representation within the PV loop to understand the different profiles provided by mechanical support devices. The ideal mechanical support device would not only decrease the ventricular volume but also provide enough unloading and pressure relief of the LV while maintaining systemic perfusion (blue PV loop).

Clinical Scenarios

The hemodynamic condition of the LV in different populations is illustrated by the PV loop (FIGURE 17.7). Each clinical syndrome represents a unique set of hemodynamic variables where cardiac function and myocardial oxygen supply or demand is compromised. In acute myocardial infarction (AMI), patients may present with reduced LV contractile function, acute diastolic dysfunction, elevated LV end-diastolic volume (LVEDV) and pressure (LVEDP), and increased LV work, in addition to diminished coronary blood flow.

In CS, LV contractile function is severely reduced with significantly increased LVEDV and LVEDP, markedly reduced stroke volume, but increased myocardial oxygen demand; coronary blood flow may also be impaired by hypotension and elevated wall stress. These PV loops provide hemodynamic characterization only of the LV and do not provide information on right ventricular (RV) function or extra-cardiac problems that may be affected by MCS such as systemic hypoperfusion of the cerebral, visceral, renal, and peripheral arteries.[6]

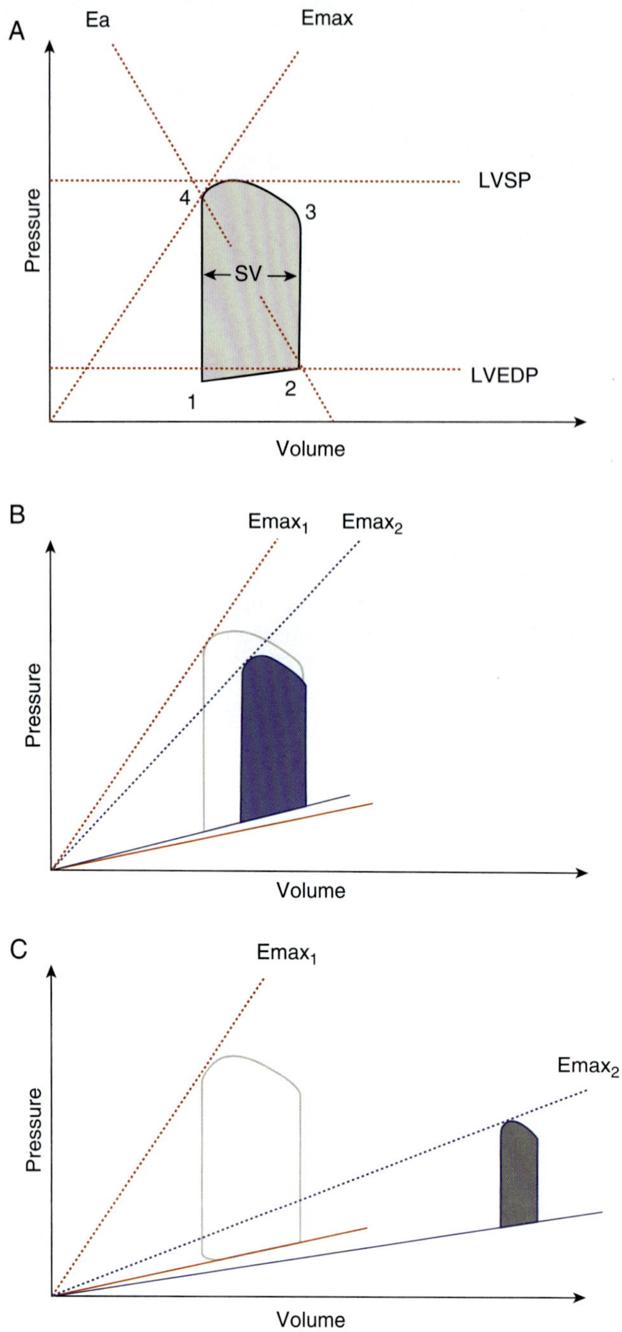

FIGURE 17.7 PV loops in different clinical scenarios. **A**, Steady state. PV loops represent one cardiac cycle in normal conditions. Stroke volume (SV) is represented by the width of PV loop as the volume difference between end-systolic and end-diastolic volumes. The area within the loop represents stroke work. Load-independent LV contractility, also known as Emax, is defined as the maximal slope of ESPV point under various loading conditions, known as the ESPV relationship (ESPVR). Effective arterial elastance (Ea) is a component of LV afterload and is defined as the ratio of end-systolic pressure and stroke volume. Under steady-state conditions, optimal LV pump efficiency occurs when the ratio of EA: E_{max} approaches 1. **B**, AMI. Representative PV loop in AMI (blue loop). LV contractility (E_{max}) is reduced; LV pressure, systolic volume, and LV stroke work may be unchanged or reduced; and LVEDP is increased. **C**, Cardiogenic shock. Representative PV loop in cardiogenic shock (gray loop). Emax is severely reduced; LVEDV and LVEDP are increased; and SV is reduced. Reproduced with permission from Rihal CS, Naidu SS, Givertz MM, et al. 2015 SCAI/ACC/HFSA/STS Clinical Expert Consensus Statement on the Use of Percutaneous Mechanical Circulatory Support Devices in Cardiovascular Care: Endorsed by the American Heart Association, the Cardiological Society of India, and Sociedad Latino Americana de Cardiologia Intervencion; Affirmation of Value by the Canadian Association of Interventional Cardiology-Association Canadienne de Cardiologie d'intervention. *J Am Coll Cardiol*. 2015;65(19):e7-e26.

INTRA-AORTIC BALLOON PUMP (IABP) CONFIGURATION AND FUNCTION

See **FIGURE 17.8.**

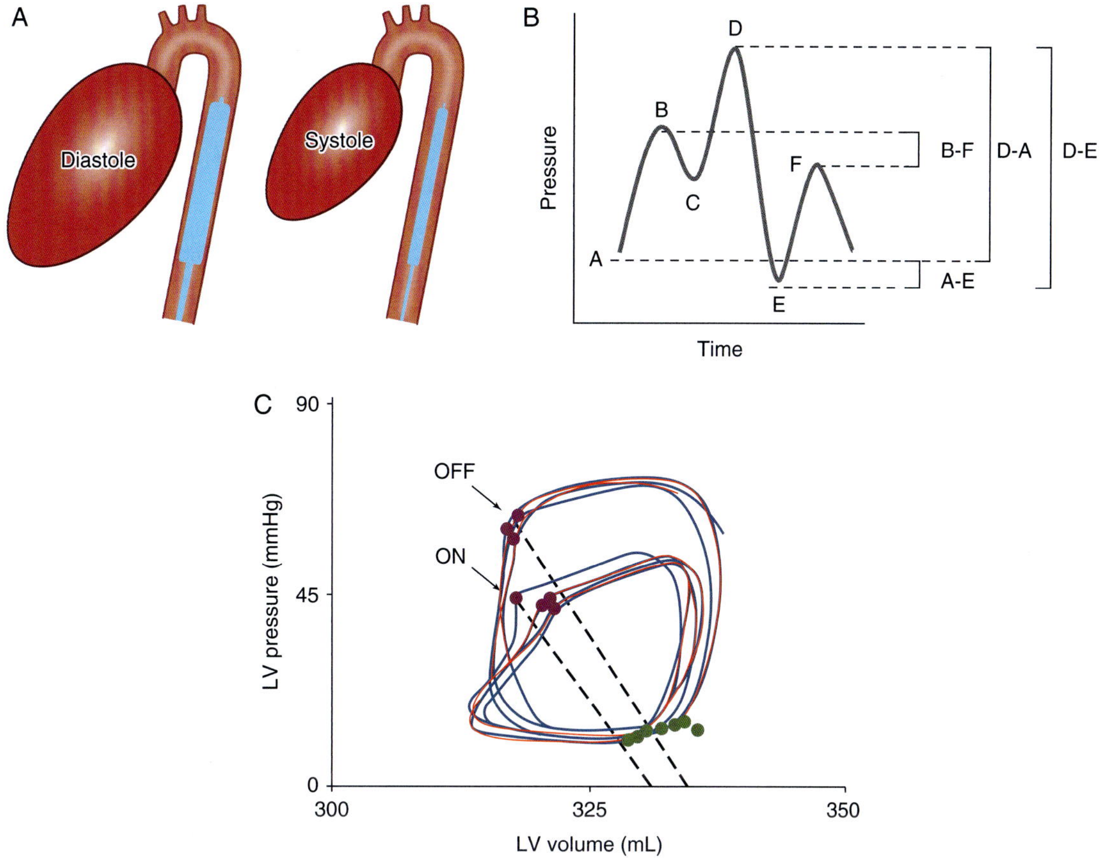

FIGURE 17.8 **A**, Schematic configuration of the IABP . The IABP is the most commonly used form of circulatory support. The IABP has 2 major components: a balloon catheter and a console to control the balloon. The catheter itself is a double-lumen 7.5 to 8.0 French (FR) catheter with a polyethylene balloon attached at its distal end. One lumen is attached to the pump and is used to inflate the balloon with helium. The second lumen is used for guide wire insertion and to transduce aortic pressure. Inflation and deflation is based on electrocardiographic activity or pressure triggers. The balloon inflates with the onset of diastole, which corresponds with repolarization (middle of the T-wave). Following diastole, the balloon rapidly deflates at the onset of LV systole, which is timed to the peak of the R-wave on the surface ECG.[9,10] Thus, poor ECG quality, electrical interference, and cardiac arrhythmias or excessive tachycardia can result in erratic balloon inflation/deflation and inadequate support. **B**, Optimal IABP function is determined by 4 factors: the magnitude of diastolic pressure augmentation, the magnitude of reduced systolic pressure, the magnitude of volume displacement, and the timing of balloon inflation and deflation. This figure shows the arterial pressure tracing analysis for IABP: (A) nonaugmented diastolic pressure, (B) non-augmented systolic pressure, (C) dicrotic notch, (D) augmented diastolic pressure, (E) reduced aortic end-diastolic pressure, (F) augmented reduced systolic pressure. Dotted lines represent: systolic unloading (B-F), diastolic augmentation (D-A), diastolic unloading (A-E), deflation pressure (D-E). **C**, IABPs provide circulatory support by augmenting aortic diastolic pressure, thereby raising mean arterial pressure. Because counterpulsation depends on native ventricular function, severe LV or RV impairment may limit the magnitude of circulatory support achieved with an IABP. IABPs provide limited ventricular unloading because they primarily reduce LV systolic pressure (ie, reduce afterload), which has minimal impact on reducing LV volume. IABPs enhance myocardial perfusion primarily by increasing aortic diastolic pressure and subsequent coronary blood flow.

BCIS-1 AND IABP-SHOCK TRIALS

See **FIGURE 17.9**.

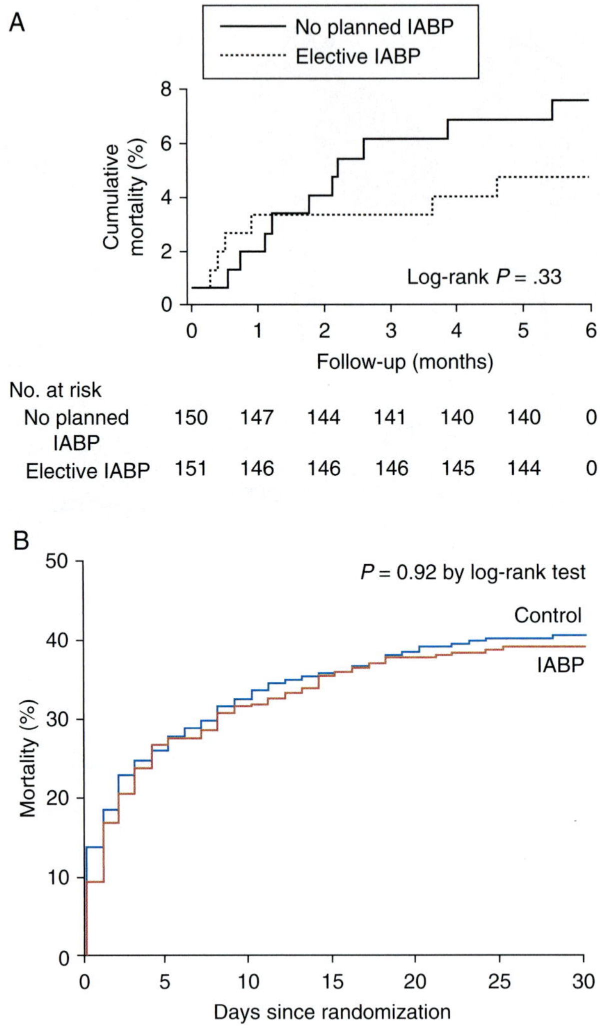

FIGURE 17.9 **A**, The Balloon Pump–Assisted Coronary Intervention Study (BCIS-1), a prospective, open, multicenter RCT, enrolled 301 patients with a LV ejection fraction <30% referred for high-risk PCI as defined by a Jeopardy Score >8/12. Patients were randomized to elective IABP insertion before PCI or no IABP. No difference in the primary endpoint of death, AMI, cerebrovascular event, or further revascularization within 28 days among patients receiving elective or no IABP insertion was observed (15% vs 16%, respectively, $P = .85$). In a subsequent analysis, elective IABP insertion during high-risk PCI was associated with a 34% relative reduction in all-cause mortality at 51 months of follow-up compared with unsupported PCI.[11] **B**, The IABP-SHOCK II trial is the largest contemporary study of IABP therapy in CS. In this study 600 patients with AMI complicated by CS were randomized to IABP or medical therapy. No significant difference in 30-day all-cause mortality was observed between groups. Recent observational studies have supported the observations of IABP-SHOCK II.[12] **A**, Reproduced with permission from Perera D, Stables R, Clayton T, et al. Long-term mortality data from the balloon pump-assisted coronary intervention study (BCIS-1): a randomized, controlled trial of elective balloon counterpulsation during high-risk percutaneous coronary intervention. *Circulation*. 2013;127:207-212. **B**, Reproduced with permission from Thiele H, Zeymer U, Neumann FJ, et al. Intraaortic balloon support for myocardial infarction with cardiogenic shock. *N Engl J Med*. 2012;367:1287-1296.

TANDEMHEART (CARDIACASSIST, INC., PITTSBURG, PA)

See **FIGURE 17.10**.

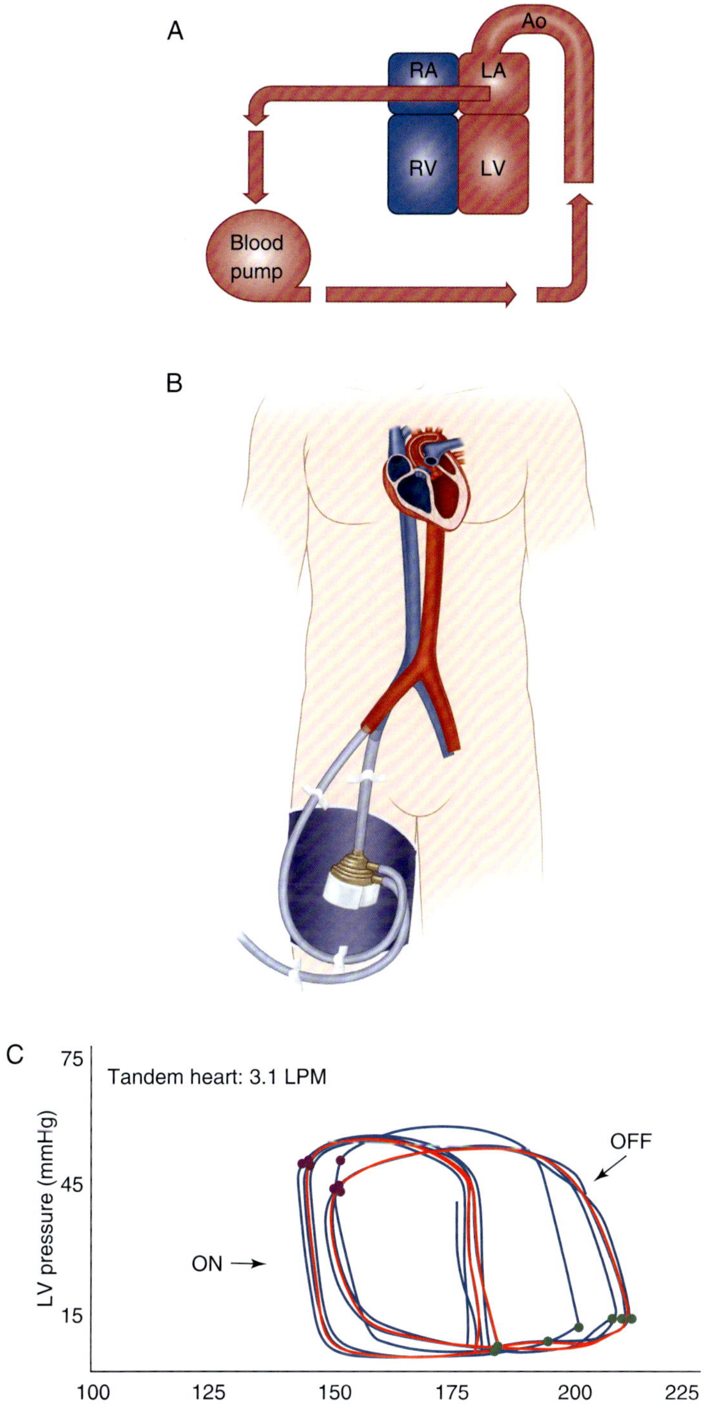

FIGURE 17.10 **A and B,** Schematic configuration of the TandemHeart. After a transseptal puncture, a venous inflow cannula is inserted into the left atrium (LA) and an outflow cannula is placed in the femoral artery (LA-FA bypass) reducing LV preload and augmenting systemic mean arterial pressure. Oxygenated blood is drawn from the LA and returned via an extracorporeal centrifugal pump into the systemic circulation. The flow rate provided by the TandemHeart varies from 3.0 to 5.0 L/min depending on the size of the outflow cannula (15-19F). **C**, PV loop model using the TandemHeart shows a significant decrease in end diastolic volumes. The LA-FA configuration with the TandemHeart works independently of the heart rate or surface ECG tracing and underlying native heart function, making it suitable for CS. However, the delivery of the TandemHeart is limited to specialized center with transseptal puncture; it cannot be placed emergently at the bedside and requires systemic anticoagulation. Also it carries incremental risk for limb ischemia and hemolysis. The TandemHeart device provides circulatory support by increasing aortic systolic, diastolic, and mean arterial pressure. The TandemHeart provides ventricular unloading by reducing both LV pressure and volume. Because the TandemHeart drains the LA, LV preload is reduced and there may be a greater reduction in LV volume than pressure with the TandemHeart device. The TandemHeart device provides myocardial perfusion by increasing aortic diastolic pressure and reducing LV end-diastolic pressure. As a result, the transmyocardial perfusion gradient (coronary diastolic pressure minus LV diastolic pressure) is increased. The TandemHeart can have an oxygenator spliced into the circuit to provide systemic oxygenation and LV unloading.

Clinical Trials

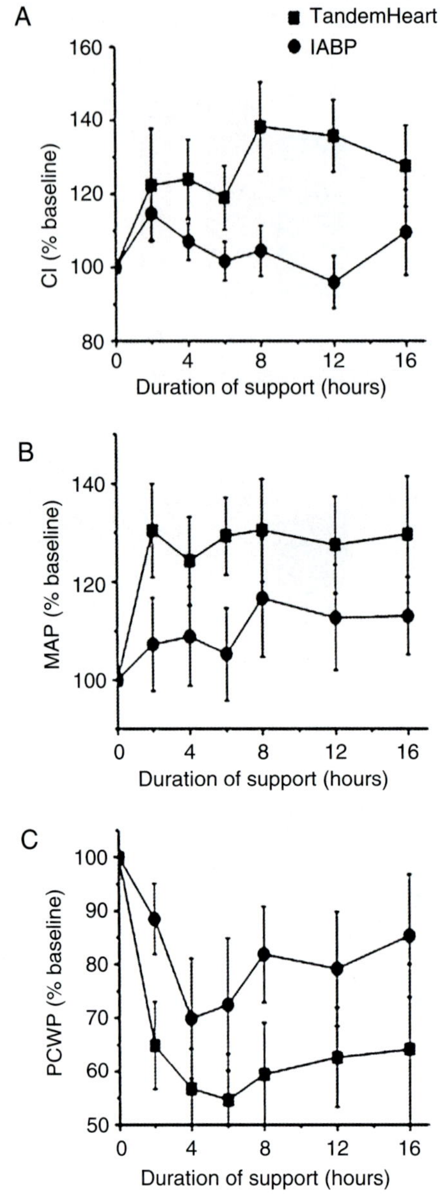

FIGURE 17.11 **A-C**, Change in hemodynamic parameters in TandemHeart and IABP groups. Reproduced with permission from Burkhoff D, Cohen H, Brunckhorst C, O'Neill WW, TandemHeart Investigators Group. A randomized multicenter clinical study to evaluate the safety and efficacy of the TandemHeart percutaneous ventricular assist device vs conventional therapy with intraaortic balloon pumping for treatment of cardiogenic shock. *Am Heart J.* 2006;152:469.e461-469.e468.

The TandemHeart has been examined in clinical trials evaluating the safety and effectiveness of the device in AMI complicated by CS when compared with IABP (**FIGURE 17.11**). In this study, 42 patients presenting within 24 hours of developing CS were treated in an initial roll-in phase (n = 9) or randomized to treatment with IABP (n = 14) or TandemHeart pVAD (n = 19). The mean duration of support was 2.5 days. Compared with IABP, the TandemHeart pVAD achieved significantly greater increases in cardiac index (P = .13) and mean arterial blood pressure (P = .16) and significantly greater decreases in pulmonary capillary wedge pressure (P = .12). Overall 30-day survival and severe adverse events were not significantly different between the 2 groups. Of note, 30 patients (71%) had persistent CS despite having an IABP in place at the time of study enrollment.[13]

IMPELLA AXIAL PUMP CATHETER

See **FIGURE 17.12**.

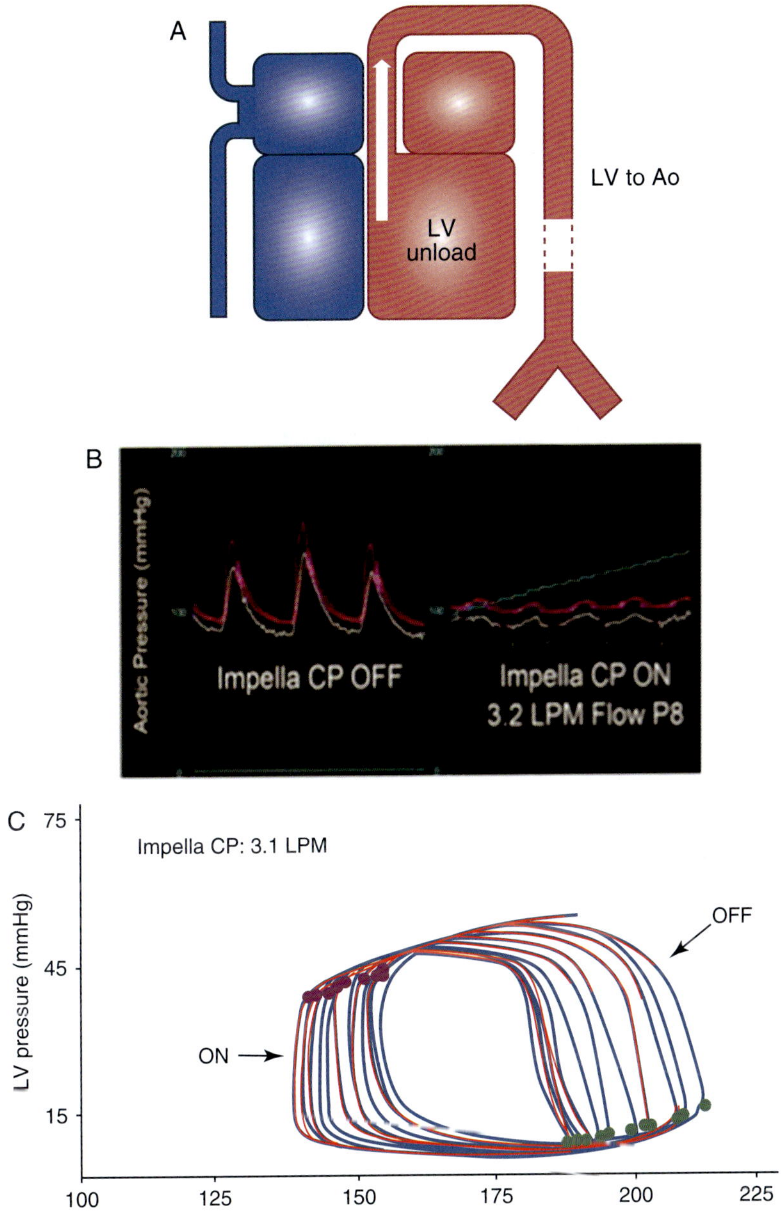

FIGURE 17.12 Impella system (Abiomed, Inc, Danvers, MA). **A**, Schematic representation of the Impella pump catheter. The Impella is an axial flow catheter placed into the LV in retrograde fashion across the aortic valve. The Impella transfers kinetic energy from a circulating impeller to the bloodstream, which results in continuous blood flow from the LV to ascending aorta. The Impella 2.5 LP and CP devices can be deployed without the need for surgery through 13 and 14 FR sheaths, respectively. The Impella 5.0 device requires surgical placement of a vascular graft onto the axillary or femoral artery. It can also be placed during cardiac surgery through an aortotomy into the LV. The Impella devices can achieve mean device flows of 2.5, 3.5, and 5.0 L/min) under optimal hemodynamic conditions. Circulatory support is provided by increasing aortic systolic, diastolic, and mean arterial pressure **(B)**. Because continuous flow pumps do not depend on native LV function, severe LV impairment will augment continuous flow pump efficiency. The Impella device provides ventricular unloading by reducing both LV pressure and volume as shown in the PV loop curve **(C)**. The Impella device provides myocardial perfusion by increasing aortic diastolic pressure and reducing LV end-diastolic pressure. As a result, the transmyocardial perfusion gradient (coronary diastolic pressure minus LV diastolic pressure) is increased.

Safety and Efficacy

The PROTECT II trial randomized 452 patients referred for nonemergent high-risk PCI to insertion of an Impella 2.5 or IABP before PCI (**FIGURE 17.13**).

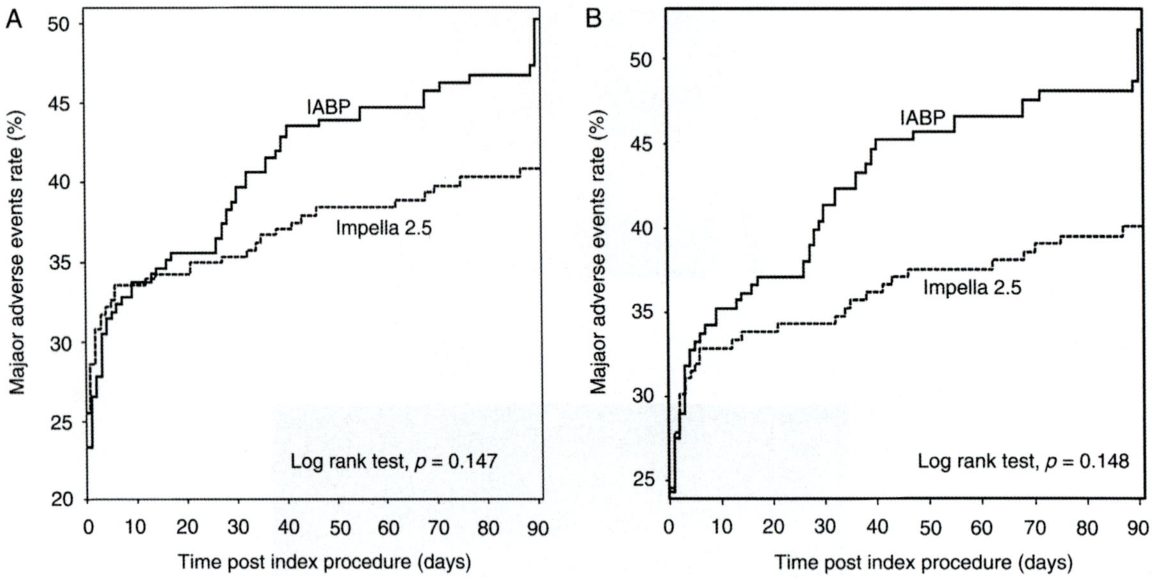

FIGURE 17.13 Safety and efficacy of the Impella axial pump catheter. **A**, High-risk PCI was defined as an LVEF <35% and unprotected left main or last patent coronary conduit or LVEF <30% with 3-vessel coronary disease. The Impella 2.5 demonstrated superior hemodynamic support compared with IABP therapy. No difference in the primary end point (composite rate of intra- or postprocedural major adverse events at discharge or 30-day follow-up) was observed between groups (35% vs 40%, Impella 2.5 vs IABP, *P* = *.227*). At 90 days follow-up a trend toward reduced MAEs was observed in the Impella, not IABP arm (40.6% vs 49.3%, *P* = *.066*) in the intent-to-treat population and (40% vs 51%, *P* = *.02*) **(A)** in the per-protocol population **(B)**.[14] **A**, Reproduced with permission from O'Neill WW, Kleiman NS, Moses J, et al. A prospective, randomized clinical trial of hemodynamic support with Impella 2.5 versus intra-aortic balloon pump in patients undergoing high-risk percutaneous coronary intervention: the PROTECT II study. *Circulation*. 2012;126:1717-1727; **B**, Seyfarth M, Sibbing D, Bauer I, et al. A randomized clinical trial to evaluate the safety and efficacy of a percutaneous left ventricular assist device versus intra-aortic balloon pumping for treatment of cardiogenic shock caused by myocardial infarction. *J Am Coll Cardiol*. 2008;52:1584-1588.

In 2008, the Efficacy Study of LV Assist Device to Treat Patients With Cardiogenic Shock (ISAR-Shock) study randomized 26 patients with CS to IABP or Impella 2.5. The Impella demonstrated a superior increase in cardiac index compared with IABP; however, 30-day mortality was not different between groups.[15]

RIGHT ATRIAL-TO-FEMORAL ARTERY CENTRIFUGAL FLOW PUMPS

VA-ECMO

See **FIGURE 17.14**.

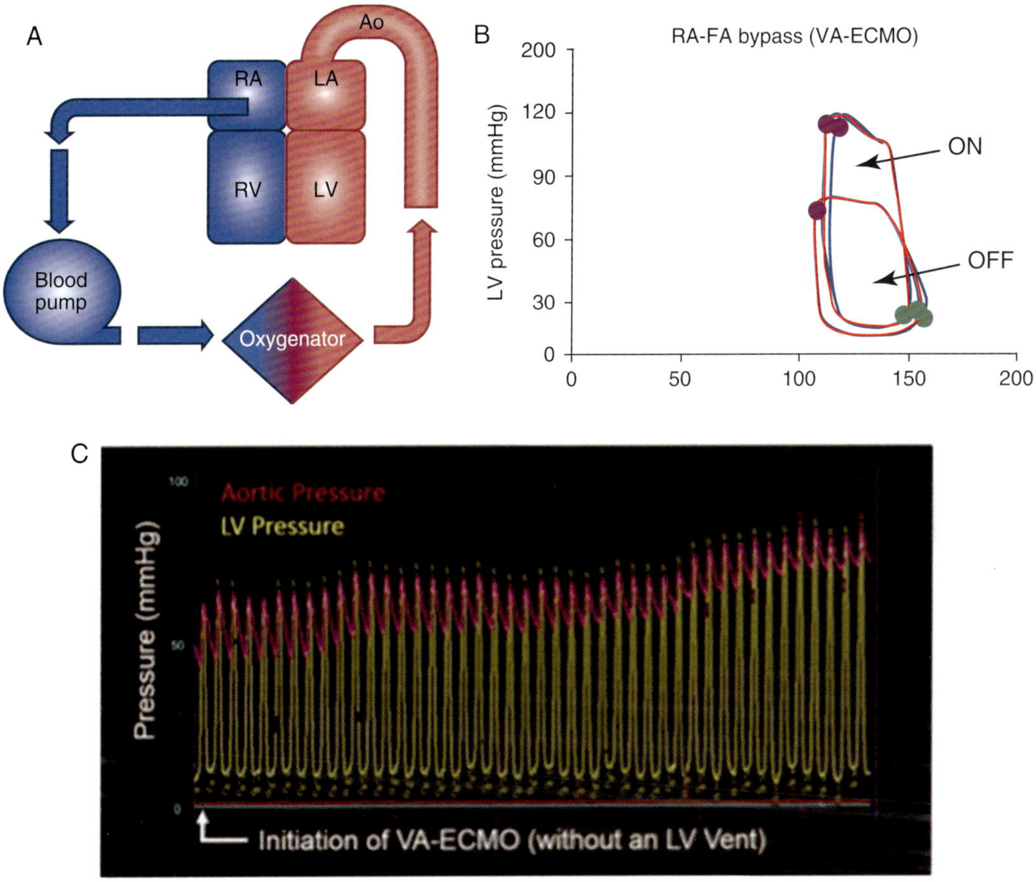

FIGURE 17.14 **A**, Schematic representation of VA-ECMO circuit. VA-ECMO withdraws deoxygenated venous blood into a centrifugal pump, which then delivers blood through an oxygenator and back into the arterial circulation **(B)**. VA-ECMO can be initiated using central (surgical) or peripheral (percutaneous or surgical) access.[16] A percutaneously delivered inflow cannula is often positioned in the superior vena cava and drains the RA using multiple inflow vents. An outflow cannula can be positioned in the femoral or subclavian arteries and commonly ranges in sizes from 15 to 19 FR. VA-ECMO can provide flows ranging between 4 and 8 L/min depending on the type of centrifugal flow pump used. VA-ECMO provides circulatory support by displacing blood volume from the venous to the arterial circulation, which increases aortic systolic, diastolic, and mean arterial pressure. VA-ECMO does not provide ventricular unloading. By pressurizing the arterial circulation, LV afterload is increased. As a result, LV pressure is increased, not decreased. LV volume also may not change significantly with VA-ECMO **(B)**. Depending on native LV function and the presence or absence of aortic valve disease, VA-ECMO can be associated with increased LV diastolic pressures and worsening pulmonary edema. For this reason, VA-ECMO often requires a concomitant system to reduce LV pressure, known as an LV vent, which can include an IABP, Impella, or a LA drainage cannula **(C)**.[8] VA-ECMO may increase myocardial perfusion by increasing aortic diastolic pressure. However, if LV diastolic pressure is also increased, the transmyocardial perfusion gradient may not be greatly augmented with VA-ECMO. In patients with hypoxemia, VA-ECMO plays an important role in increasing systemic oxygenation, which cannot be achieved with Impella or IABP therapy. VA-ECMO with an LV vent is particularly helpful in patients with refractory or recurrent ventricular arrhythmias or systemic hypoxemia. Careful evaluation of cardiac hemodynamics is required when initiating VA-ECMO.[17]

RIGHT VENTRICULAR FAILURE (RVF)

RVF After LVAD Implantation

The development of right ventricular failure (RVF) in patients with an LVAD has a direct effect on morbidity and mortality (**FIGURE 17.15**). Four hundred and eighty four (484) patients enrolled in the HeartMate II left ventricular assist device bridge-to-transplantation clinical trial were analyzed for the incidence of RVF. A total of 98 patients (20%) had some form of RVF defined as patients requiring an RVAD (6%), patients requiring at least 14 days of continuous inotropic support after LVAD implantation (7%), and patients requiring late inotropic support starting after the 14th day (7%). Actuarial survival at 1 year was significantly better for patients without RVF (79%), whereas decreased survival was evident in patients with signs of early RVF.[18] These observations reiterate the need for better selection of patients at high risk for RVF, which can mitigate its occurrence by providing temporary mechanical assistance to the RV simultaneously with LVAD implantation.

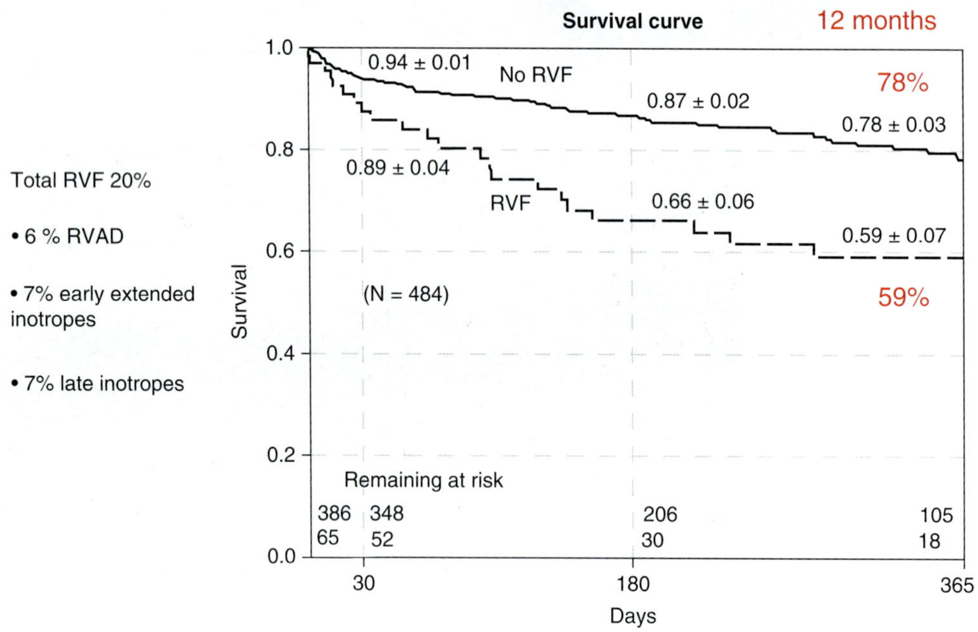

FIGURE 17.15 RVF after LVAD implantation, a major clinical problem. Reproduced with permission from Kormos RL, Teuteberg JJ, Pagani FD, et al. Right ventricular failure in patients with the HeartMate II continuous-flow left ventricular assist device: incidence, risk factors, and effect on outcomes. *J Thorac Cardiovasc Surg*. 2010;139:1316-1324.

RVF After Left Ventricular Support

See FIGURE 17.16.

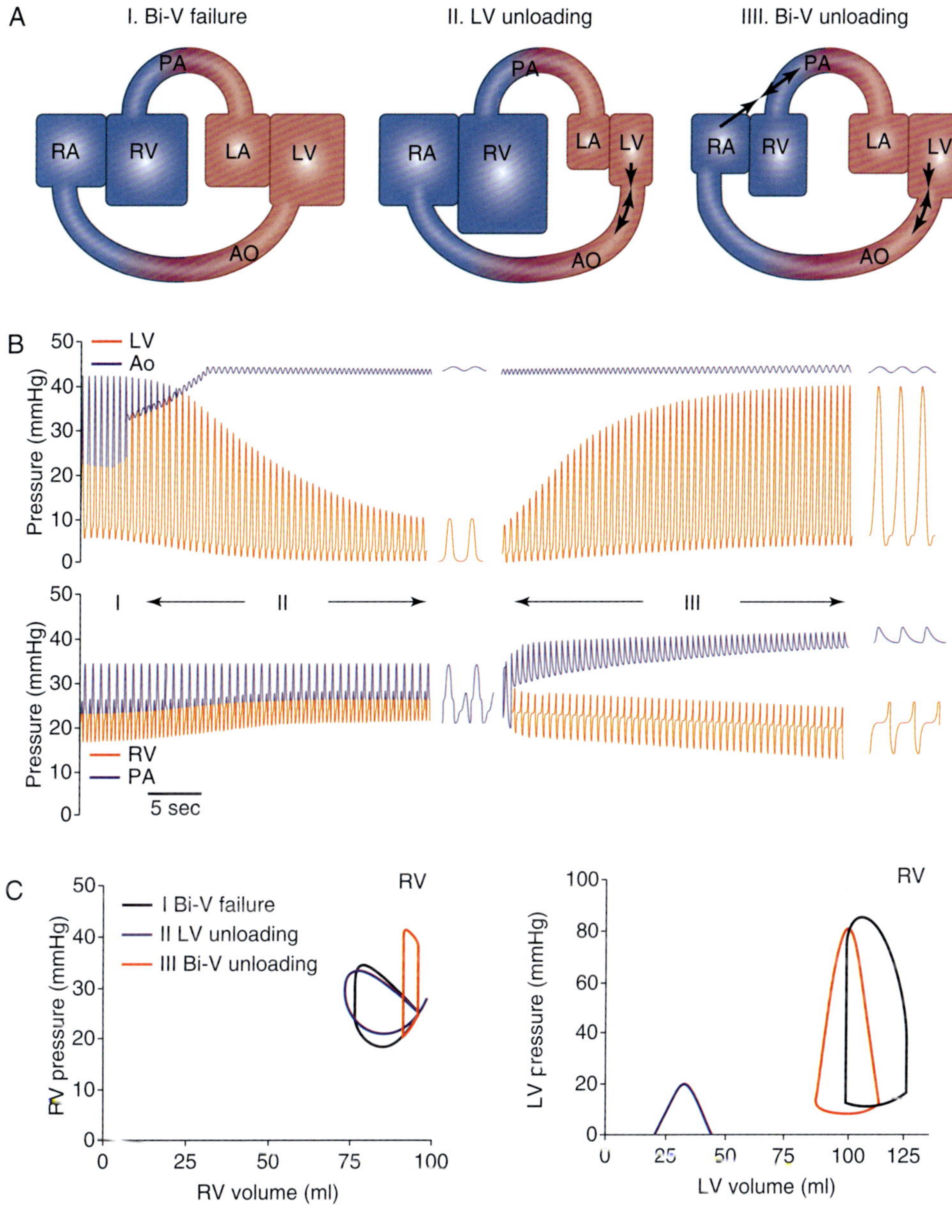

FIGURE 17.16 **A**, Illustration of the LV-RV circuit. **B**, Simulated tracings demonstrate the abrupt development of a gradient between the LV and aorta (Ao) as a marker of concomitant RV failure after activation of a left-sided axial flow catheter (Impella CP or 5.0) (I and II). In case III, activation of an Impella RP bypasses the failing RV and restores LV preload. Impella RP activation decreases RA pressure and increases PA pressure. **C**, Pressure-time and pressure-volume domains. I, Biventricular (BiV) failure is characterized by elevated biventricular filling pressures. II, Activation of a LV pump in BiV failure reduces LV pressure and volume but triggers the abrupt development of an LV-Ao gradient because of insufficient preload generated by the RV. A concomitant increase in RA pressure is observed as the RV is overwhelmed by an increase in venous return from the LV pump. III, Concomitant activation of an RV pump that drives blood from the RA to the PA restores LV preload and unloads the RV. LV pressures increase and the LV-Ao gradient diminishes. PA pressures increase with a loss of PA pulse pressure. RA pressures decrease. Both RV pressure and volume are reduced. **B**, Courtesy of Daniel Burkhoff, MD, PhD.

Pulmonary Artery Pulsatility Index (PAPi) prior and immediately after LVAD

Determining which patients are at highest risk of developing RVF after CF-LVDAs remains a challenge. Previously identified hemodynamic variables that correlate with RVF include elevated RA pressure, elevated RA to pulmonary capillary wedge pressure ratio (RA:PCWP), and reduced RV stroke work index (RVSWI).[19] Moreover, correlates of RV afterload, including pulmonary artery compliance (PAC) and pulmonary artery elastance (PAE), have been explored in patients with pulmonary hypertension due to left heart disease. Recently, the pulmonary artery pulsatility index (PAPi) was also defined as a measure of RVF in AMI.[20]

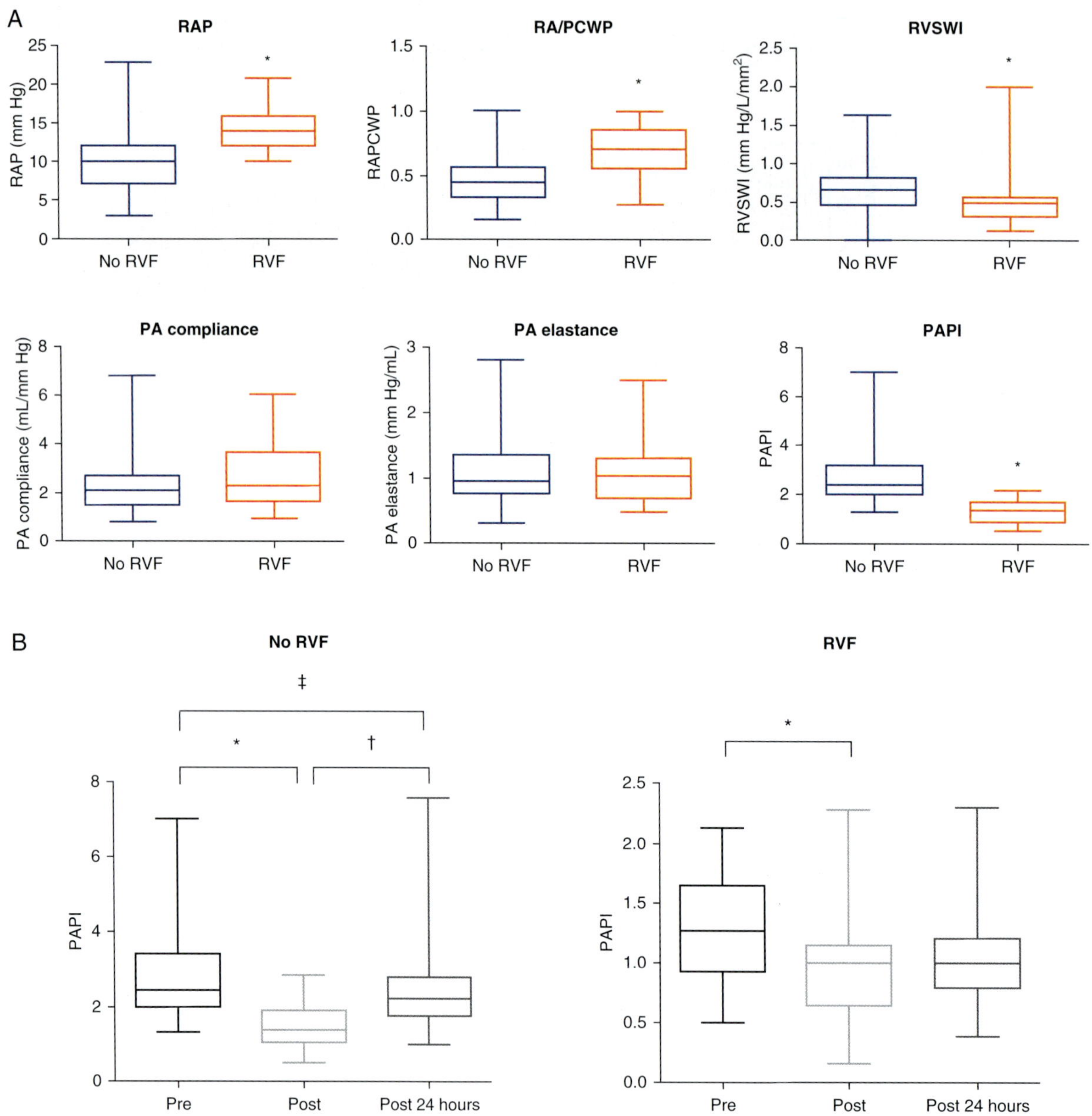

FIGURE 17.17 **A and B**, PAPi before and immediately after LVAD implantation. Reproduced with permission from Morine KJ, Kiernan MS, Pham DT, Paruchuri V, Denofrio D, Kapur NK. Pulmonary Artery Pulsatility Index Is Associated With Right Ventricular Failure After Left Ventricular Assist Device Surgery. *J Card Fail*. 2016;22:110-116.

In a recent study, the preoperative PAPi value was significantly reduced among patients who developed RVF after CF-LVAD implantation (**FIGURE 17.17A**). Furthermore, it was observed that PAPi was significantly reduced in all patients immediately after CF-LVAD surgery and began to recover within 24 hours after surgery in patients who did not develop RVF (**FIGURE 17.17B**). In contrast, patients who developed RVF did not exhibit recovery of PAPi within 24 hours of CF-LVAD implantation.[21] These observations suggest that in addition to serving as a preoperative determinant of risk, monitoring the PAPi value during the postoperative period may be helpful in identifying patients who develop RVF.

Biventricular Failure Support Options

With the recent advent of RV-AMCS devices, mechanical support options for CS due to biventricular failure have evolved beyond surgically implanted biventricular pumps to now include various combinations of percutaneously delivered centrifugal and axial-flow pumps (**FIGURE 17.18**). Biventricular support can be achieved with two TandemHeart devices, which require 4 separate 21 FR cannulas: 2 for LV support and 2 for RV support. Several reports have described the use of an IABP plus TH-RVAD, Impella 2.5 plus TH-RVAD, Impella 5.0 plus TH-RVAD, Impella 5.0 plus Impella RP, and Impella CP plus RP for biventricular support.[22,23]

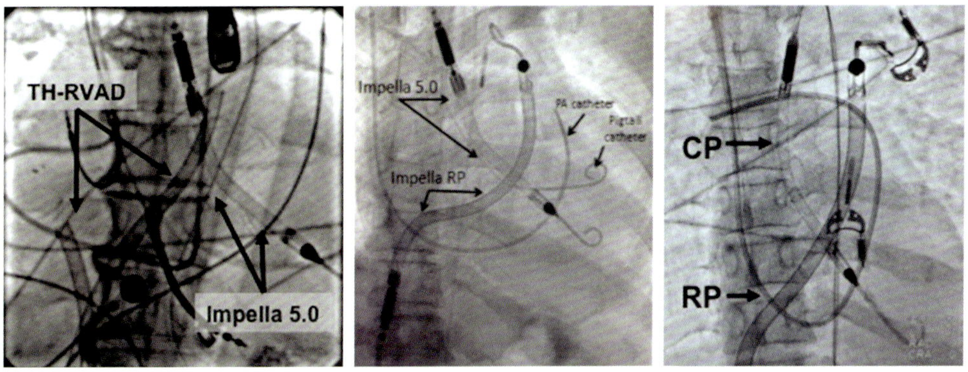

FIGURE 17.18 Acute mechanical support configuration for biventricular failure.

REFERENCES

1. Rose EA, Gelijns AC, Moskowitz AJ, et al. Long-term use of a left ventricular assist device for end-stage heart failure. *N Engl J Med*. 2001;345:1435-1443.
2. Stretch R, Sauer CM, Yuh DD, Bonde P. National trends in the utilization of short-term mechanical circulatory support: incidence, outcomes, and cost analysis. *J Am Coll Cardiol*. 2014;64:1407-1415.
3. Lampropulos JF, Kim N, Wang Y, et al. Trends in left ventricular assist device use and outcomes among Medicare beneficiaries, 2004-2011. *Open Heart*. 2014;1:e000109.
4. Sandhu A, McCoy LA, Negi SI, et al. Use of mechanical circulatory support in patients undergoing percutaneous coronary intervention: insights from the National Cardiovascular Data Registry. *Circulation*. 2015;132:1243-1251.
5. Kirklin JK, Naftel DC, Kormos RL, et al. Fifth INTERMACS annual report: risk factor analysis from more than 6,000 mechanical circulatory support patients. *J Heart Lung Transplant*. 2013;32:141-156.
6. Rihal CS, Naidu SS, Givertz MM, et al. 2015 SCAI/ACC/HFSA/STS clinical expert consensus statement on the use of percutaneous mechanical circulatory support devices in cardiovascular care (Endorsed by the American Heart Association, the Cardiological Society of India, and Sociedad Latino Americana de Cardiologia Intervencion; Affirmation of Value by the Canadian Association of Interventional Cardiology-Association Canadienne de Cardiologie d'intervention). *J Card Fail*. 2015;21:499-518.
7. Moazami N, Fukamachi K, Kobayashi M, et al. Axial and centrifugal continuous-flow rotary pumps: a translation from pump mechanics to clinical practice. *J Heart Lung Transplant*. 2013;32:1-11.
8. Frazier OH, Khalil HA, Benkowski RJ, Cohn WE. Optimization of axial-pump pressure sensitivity for a continuous-flow total artificial heart. *J Heart Lung Transplant*. 2010;29:687-691.
9. Bolotin G, Wolf T, Shachner R, et al. Hemodynamic evaluation of descending aortomyoplasty versus intra-aortic balloon pump performed in normal animals: an acute study. *Eur J Cardiothorac Surg*. 2001;19:174-178.

10. Silva D. Multimarker approach in risk stratification of patients with acute coronary syndromes: towards the ideal stratification. *Rev Port Cardiol.* 2014;33:137-138.
11. Perera D, Stables R, Clayton T, et al. Long-term mortality data from the balloon pump-assisted coronary intervention study (BCIS-1): a randomized, controlled trial of elective balloon counterpulsation during high-risk percutaneous coronary intervention. *Circulation.* 2013;127:207-212.
12. Thiele H, Zeymer U, Neumann FJ, et al. Intraaortic balloon support for myocardial infarction with cardiogenic shock. *N Engl J Med.* 2012;367:1287-1296.
13. Burkhoff D, Cohen H, Brunckhorst C, O'Neill WW, TandemHeart Investigators Group. A randomized multicenter clinical study to evaluate the safety and efficacy of the TandemHeart percutaneous ventricular assist device versus conventional therapy with intraaortic balloon pumping for treatment of cardiogenic shock. *Am Heart J.* 2006;152:469.e461-469.e468.
14. O'Neill WW, Kleiman NS, Moses J, et al. A prospective, randomized clinical trial of hemodynamic support with Impella 2.5 versus intra-aortic balloon pump in patients undergoing high-risk percutaneous coronary intervention: the PROTECT II study. *Circulation.* 2012;126:1717-1727.
15. Seyfarth M, Sibbing D, Bauer I, et al. A randomized clinical trial to evaluate the safety and efficacy of a percutaneous left ventricular assist device versus intra-aortic balloon pumping for treatment of cardiogenic shock caused by myocardial infarction. *J Am Coll Cardiol.* 2008;52:1584-1588.
16. Napp LC, Kuhn C, Hoeper MM, et al. Cannulation strategies for percutaneous extracorporeal membrane oxygenation in adults. *Clin Res Cardiol.* 2016;105:283-296.
17. Aghili N, Kang S, Kapur NK. The fundamentals of extra-corporeal membrane oxygenation. *Minerva Cardioangiol.* 2015;63:75-85.
18. Kormos RL, Teuteberg JJ, Pagani FD, et al. Right ventricular failure in patients with the HeartMate II continuous-flow left ventricular assist device: incidence, risk factors, and effect on outcomes. *J Thorac Cardiovasc Surg.* 2010;139:1316-1324.
19. Kubba S, Davila CD, Forfia PR. Methods for evaluating right ventricular function and ventricular-arterial coupling. *Prog Cardiovasc Dis.* 2016;59:42-51.
20. Korabathina R, Heffernan KS, Paruchuri V, et al. The pulmonary artery pulsatility index identifies severe right ventricular dysfunction in acute inferior myocardial infarction. *Catheter Cardiovasc Interv.* 2012;80:593-600.
21. Morine KJ, Kiernan MS, Pham DT, Paruchuri V, Denofrio D, Kapur NK. Pulmonary artery pulsatility index is associated with right ventricular failure after left ventricular assist device surgery. *J Card Fail.* 2016;22:110-116.
22. Kapur NK, Jumean M, Ghuloom A, et al. First successful use of 2 axial flow catheters for percutaneous biventricular circulatory support as a bridge to a durable left ventricular assist device. *Circ Heart Fail.* 2015;8:1006-1008.
23. Rajagopal V, Steahr G, Wilmer CI, Raval NY. A novel percutaneous mechanical biventricular bridge to recovery in severe cardiac allograft rejection. *J Heart Lung Transplant.* 2010;29:93-95.

chapter **18**

Percutaneous Transluminal Coronary Angioplasty

MAURO MOSCUCCI, MD, MBA

INTRODUCTION

The development and evolution of cardiac catheterization into therapeutic percutaneous coronary intervention (PCI) has been the result of the work of a long list of pioneers and of their forward thinking, persistence, and tolerance to risk taking. In 1964 Dotter and Judkins reported the initial results of dilatation of peripheral vessels' stenosis using tapered, radiopaque, Teflon dilating catheters slipped over a guidewire ("the Dotter effect") (**FIGURES 18.1** and **18.2**).[1] Around the same time, Andreas Gruentzig in Switzerland had been developing the concept of balloon dilatation of vessels' stenosis. His early balloons were made of PVC and connected to a single lumen catheter (**FIGURE 18.3**).[2] After several attempts trying to convince catheter companies to build a double lumen catheter, Gruentzig was finally able to develop a double lumen catheter with the help of Mr Schmidt.[2] The balloon was used in an iliac artery on January 23, 1975 and then it was used on September 16, 1977 to perform the first percutaneous transluminal coronary angioplasty (PTCA).[3,4] As shown in **FIGURES 18.4** and **18.5**, the lesion was in the proximal left anterior descending artery before the bifurcation into a diagonal artery. Two balloon inflations were performed. After the second balloon inflation, the residual pressure gradient across the stenosis resolved. As Gruentzig later stated, "his dreams had come true."[2] The following years were characterized by a tremendous effort focused on the development of new techniques and the introduction of new technology. The introduction of the steerable guide wire and of low-profile balloons (**FIGURE 18.6**) allowed tackling lesions in more distal portions of coronary arteries. New applications of coronary angioplasty beyond stable angina, including the management of patients with acute coronary syndromes and ST segment elevation myocardial infarction, were developed. The introduction in the 1990s of coronary stenting further improved the safety of PCI and long-term outcomes,[5-8] while restenosis was formally "conquered" in 2000 with the introduction of drug-eluting stents. It is unknown whether Gruentzig, at the time of his humble first report, was predicting the revolution that would ensue and the exponential growth in PCI (**FIGURE 18.7**).

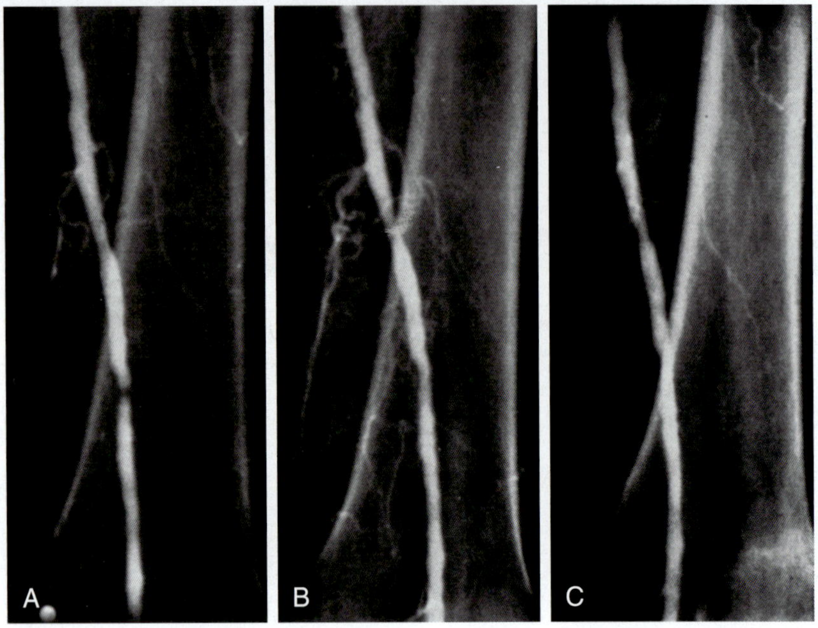

FIGURE 18.1 Transluminal dilatation and segmental narrowing of the left superficial femoral artery. A, Control arteriogram showing threadlike lumen in region of adductor hiatus. B, Immediately after dilation with catheter of 3.3 mm OD. C. Three weeks after transluminal dilatation, Lumen remains open. Clinical and plethysmographic studies indicate continuing patency over 6 mo later. Reproduced with permission from Dotter CT, Judkins MP. Transluminal treatment of arteriosclerotic obstruction. description of a new technic and a preliminary report of its application. *Circulation*. 1964;30:654-670.

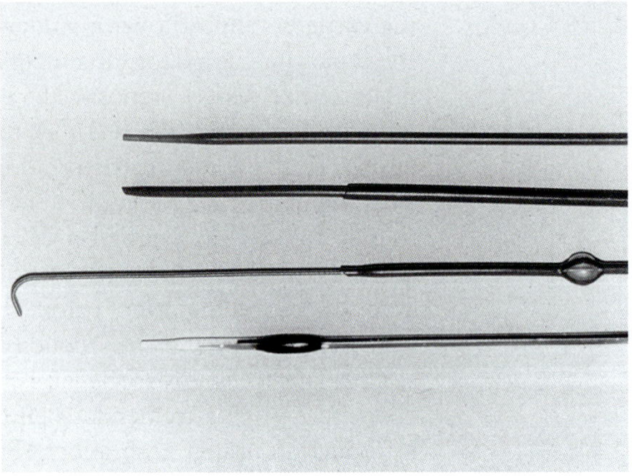

FIGURE 18.2 Top to bottom, single, tapered Dotter catheter; coaxial Dotter catheter system; slotted expanding Porstmann catheter; and early coaxial Gruentzig design. Reproduced with permission from King SB III. Angioplasty from bench to bedside to bench. *Circulation*. 1996;93(9):1621-1629.

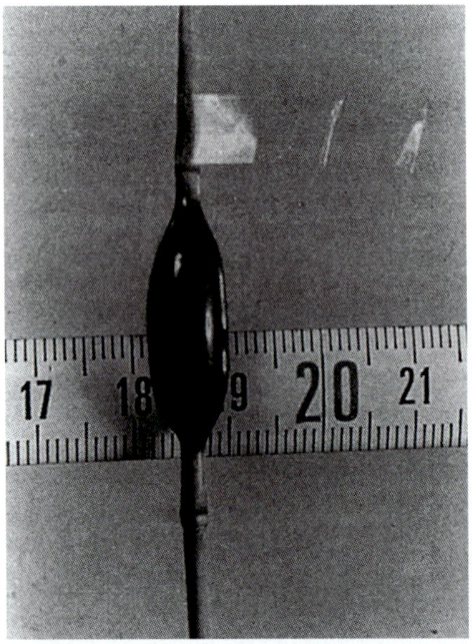

FIGURE 18.3 Early PVC balloon tied to a single-lumen catheter. The first angioplasty balloons were fabricated from flexible polyvinyl chloride (PVC). They were relatively thick walled and designed for low pressure, compared with today's high-pressure balloons. Reproduced with permission from King SB III. Angioplasty from bench to bedside to bench. *Circulation*. 1996;93(9):1621-1629.

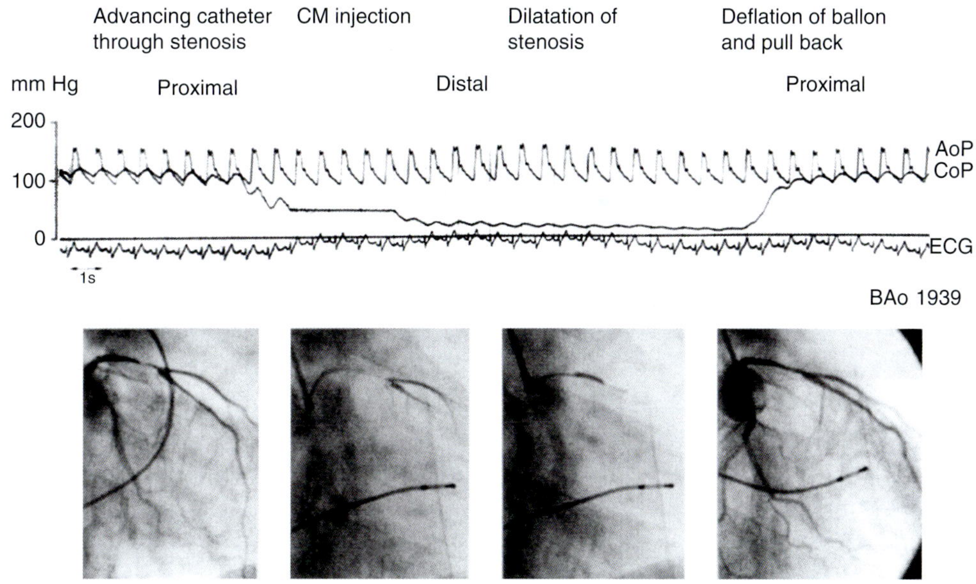

FIGURE 18.4 Angiogram and hemodynamic measurements from the first PTCA performed by Andreas Gruentzig in 1977. Reprinted from EuroIntervention Vol 13. Meier B. His master's art, Andreas Gruntzig's approach to performing and teaching coronary angioplasty. Pages No. 15-27, Copyright (2017), with permission from Europa Digital & Publishing.

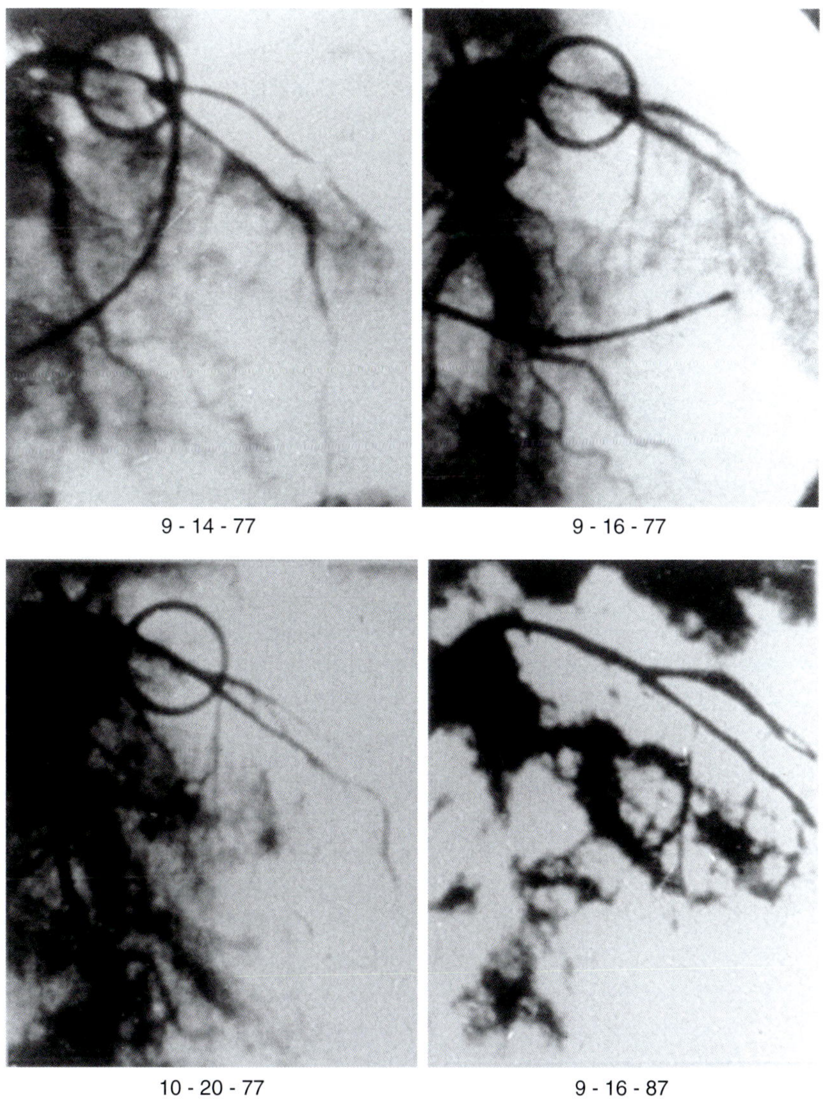

FIGURE 18.5 Angiograms of the first patient to undergo successful angioplasty and follow-up 1 month restudy. Top, The diagnostic angiogram (September 14, 1977) and appearance at the time of angioplasty (September 16, 1977). Bottom, The 1-month restudy (October 20, 1977) and the 10-year repeat study (September 16, 1987). Reproduced with permission from King SB III. Angioplasty from bench to bedside to bench. *Circulation*. 1996;93(9):1621-1629.

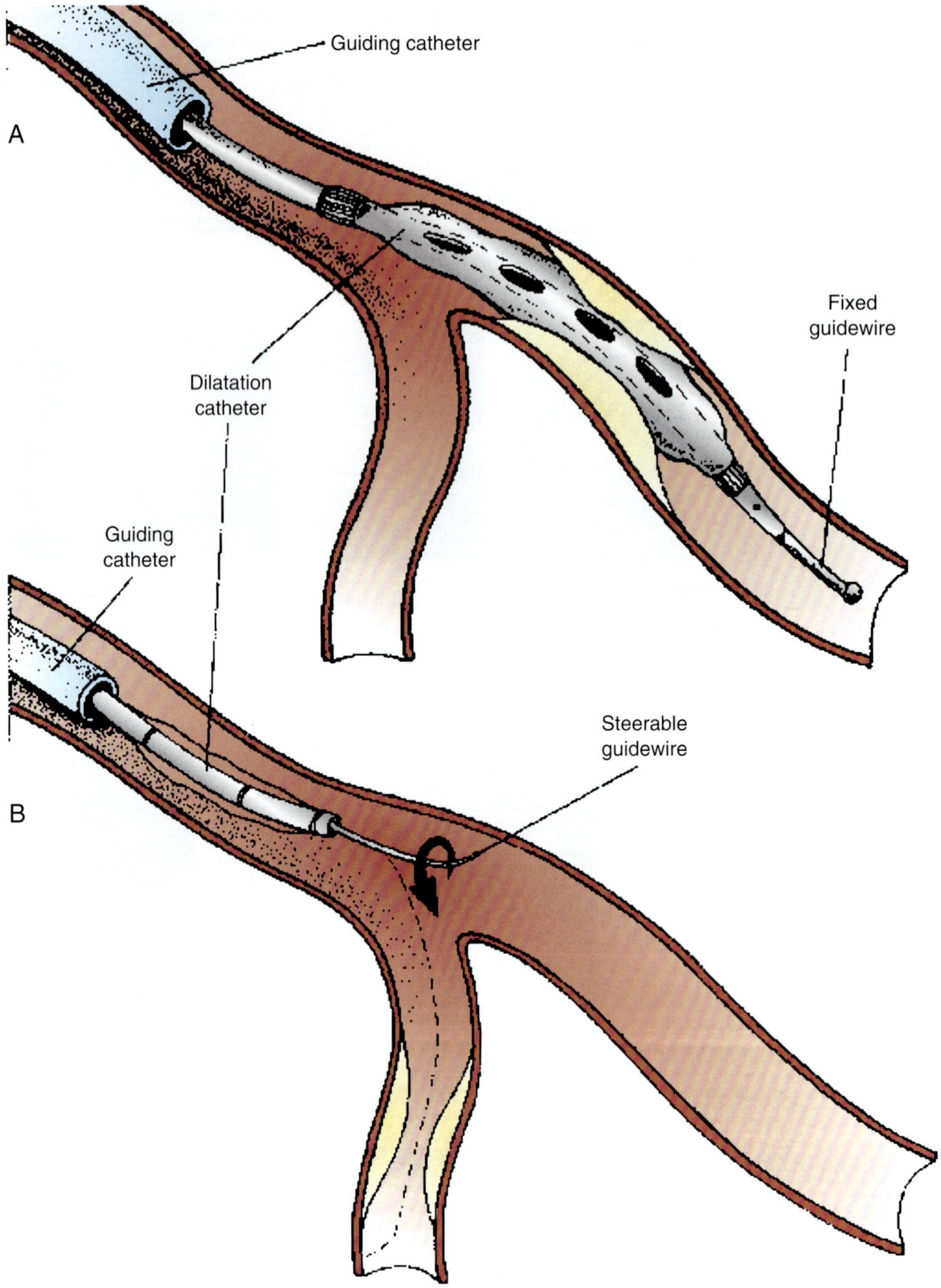

FIGURE 18.6 Components of the coronary angioplasty system. The original Gruentzig fixed guidewire balloon (A) is compared with the steerable guide wire system (B). Although both are advanced through a guide catheter positioned in the coronary ostium, neither the wire shape nor its orientation could be changed once the original Gruentzig catheter was introduced, whereas the steerable design allows the guidewire to be advanced, withdrawn, and reshaped, and steered independently of the balloon catheter to select the desired vessel. Once in place in the distal vessel beyond the target lesion, the guidewire serves as a rail over which the angioplasty balloon or other device can be advanced. Reproduced with permission from Moscucci M, eds. *Grossman & Baim's Cardiac Catheterization, Angiography, and Intervention*. 8th ed. Philadelphia: Lippincott Williams and Wilkins; 2014.

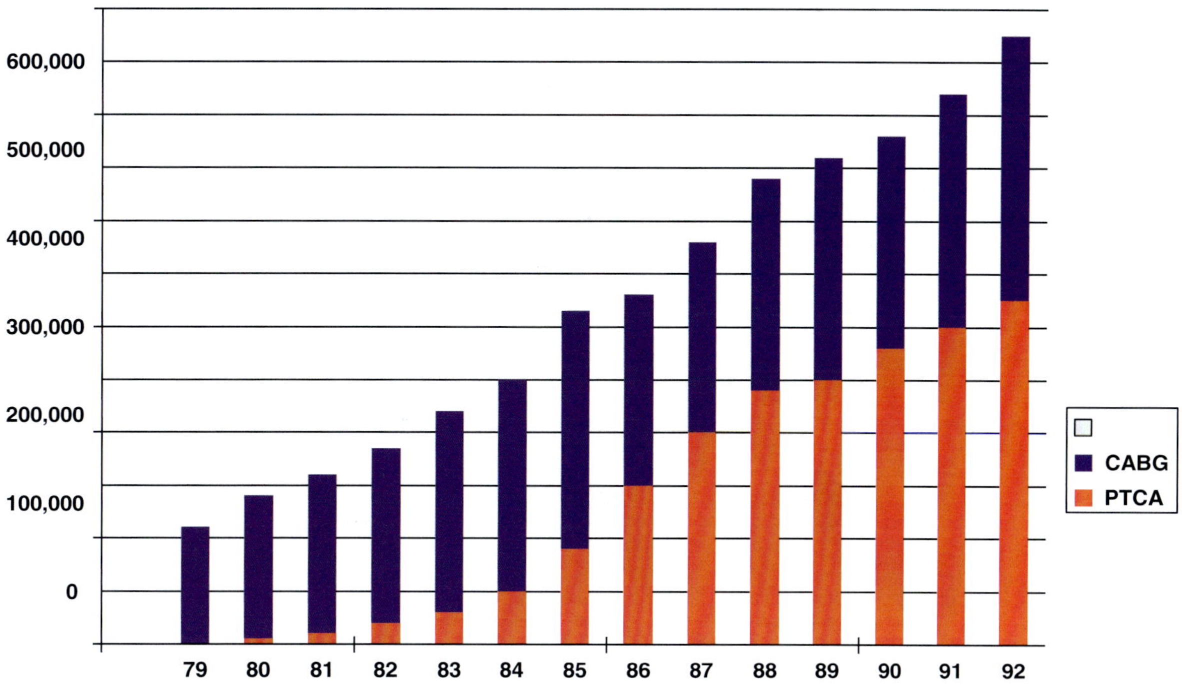

FIGURE 18.7 Coronary revascularization (PTCA and CABG) in the United States, 1979 to 1992.

The mechanism of balloon angioplasty is based on a controlled balloon injury to the arterial wall leading to plaque disruption and enhancement of blood flow (FIGURES 18.8 and 18.9). Ultrasound imaging has shown that the improvement in lumen diameter following PTCA is due to a combination of vessel stretch and local dissection[9] (FIGURE 18.9). The major limitations of balloon angioplasty include abrupt closure secondary to an uncontrolled dissection and the development of restenosis. Elastic recoil, chronic restrictive remodeling, and intimal hyperplasia can lead to progressive renarrowing of the vessel following PTCA (FIGURES 18.8-18.10). By providing a scaffolding system to the artery, coronary stenting has addressed most of the intrinsic limitations of PTCA. Our readers are referred to Chapter 20 for a review of coronary stenting. In this chapter, we will review basic concepts of PTCA, as well as some of the pivotal clinical trials evaluating the role of PTCA in the management of patients with coronary artery disease.

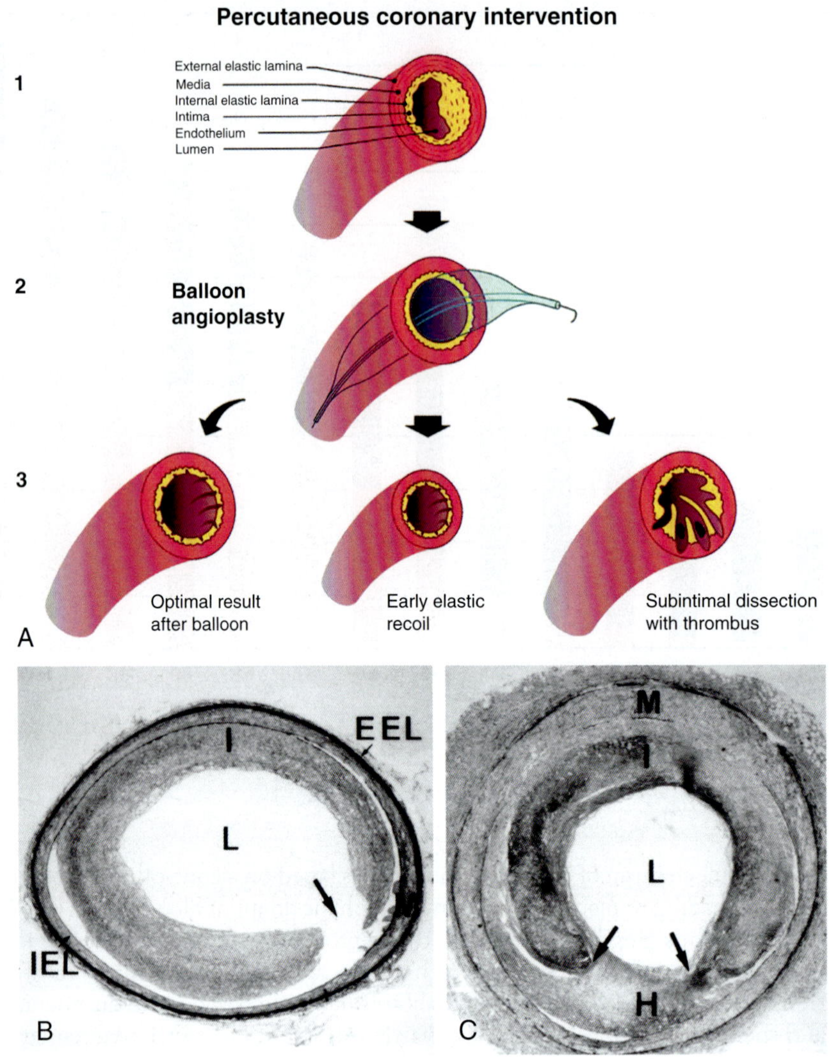

FIGURE 18.8 A, Mechanisms of PTCA and restenosis. Balloon dilatation leads to local injury, a "controlled dissection" and stretching of the arterial wall. The development of restenosis is due to a combination of factors including elastic recoil, geometric remodeling (shrinking of the vessel), and intimal hyperplasia (tissue growth). B and C, Experimental balloon angioplasty of an iliac artery in the hypercholesterolemic rabbit model. B, Immediately after balloon angioplasty, rupture (arrow) of the atherosclerotic lesion is seen. C, Twenty-eight days after balloon angioplasty, the site of plaque rupture is "grouted in" by neointimal hyperplasia (H), maximal at the site of plaque rupture (elastic tissue stain). EEL, external elastic lamina; I, intima; IEL, internal elastic lamina; L, lumen; M, media. A, Reproduced with permission from Windecker S, Meier B. Intervention in coronary artery disease. *Heart*. 2000;83(4):481-90 B and C, Reproduced with permission from Topol EJ, Califf RM, Prystowsky EN, et al. *Textbook of Cardiovascular Medicine*. 3rd ed. Philadelphia: Lippincott Williams & Wilkins; 2006.

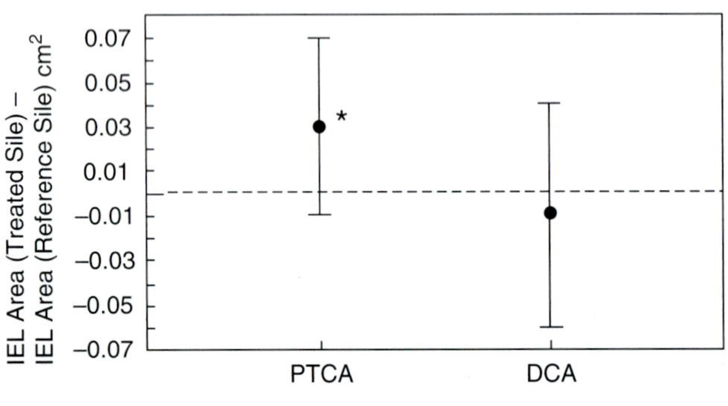

FIGURE 18.9 Vessel stretch, defined as internal elastic lamina (IEL) at treated site minus that of reference site and presented as mean value + SD. $P = .01$ for values different from 0 in the PTCA group. DCA, directional coronary atherectomy. Reproduced with permission from Tenaglia AN, Buller CE, Kisslo KB, Stack RS, Davidson CJ. Mechanisms of balloon angioplasty and directional coronary atherectomy as assessed by intracoronary ultrasound. *J Am Coll Cardiol*. 1992;20(3):685-691.

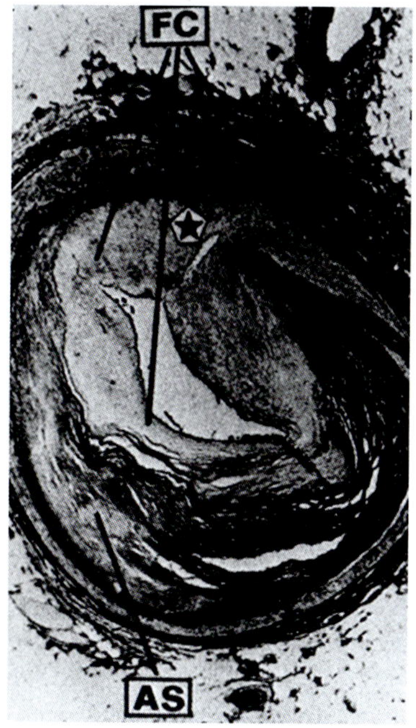

FIGURE 18.10 Mechanisms of restenosis: Cross section of a restenotic lesion in the left anterior descending artery 5 months after initial coronary angioplasty shows the original atherosclerotic plaque (AS), the crack in the medial layer induced by the original procedure (star), and the proliferation of fibrocellular tissues (FC) that constitutes the restenotic lesion. In stent restenosis, the mechanism is purely such proliferation, whereas in nonstent interventions such as balloon angioplasty there is frequently an additional component owing to shrinkage of the overall vessel diameter (unfavorable remodeling) at the treatment site. From Serruys PW, Reiber JHC, Wijns W, et al. Assessment of percutaneous transluminal coronary angioplasty by quantitative coronary angiography: diameter vs videodensitometric area measurements. *Am J Cardiol*. 1984;54:482.

GUIDE CATHETERS

Adequate guide catheter support is a critical component of successful PCIs. The guiding catheter design has evolved with a progressive reduction in outer diameter, an increase in inner lumen without a reduction in catheter stiffness and support, and by the development of atraumatic tips (**FIGURE 18.11**). Critical characteristics of guide catheters include ease of handling, backup support, ability to advance devices through the inner lumen, and atraumatic engagement (**Table 18.1**). In addition, multiple shapes have become available to allow intubation of coronary arteries with different anatomy and takeoff via the transfemoral, transradial, or brachial approach (**FIGURES 18.12-18.23**). An overview of catheters available for transradial approach is provided in Chapter 4. Different shapes are characterized by a primary curve, which is located at the level of the tip of the catheter, and by secondary and occasionally tertiary curves (**FIGURE 18.24**).

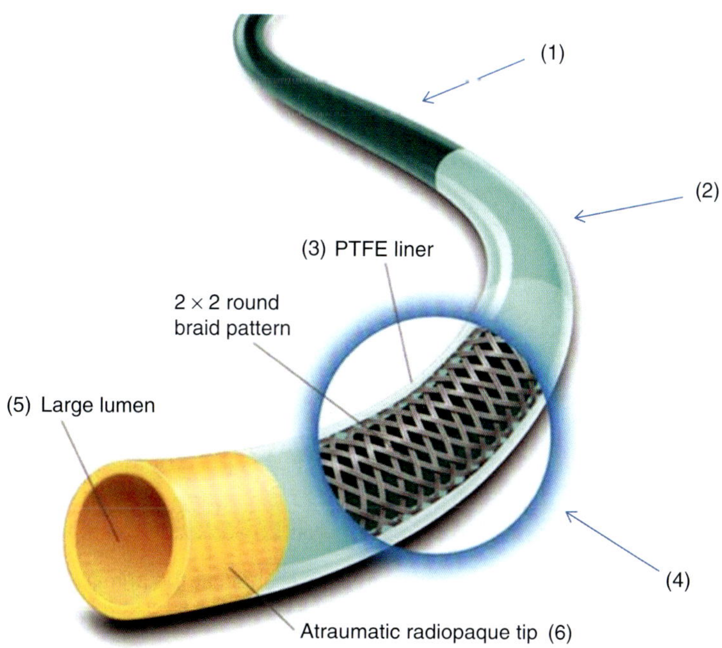

FIGURE 18.11 Layers and sections of a guide catheter. Stiff portion of the body (1); variable softer primary curve (2); lubricious coating (3); wire braiding (4); large lumen (5); atraumatic tip (6). Image provided courtesy of Boston Scientific. ©2018 Boston Scientific Corporation or its affiliates. All rights reserved.

TABLE 18.1

Guide Catheter Characteristics

Handling
• Torque characteristics and tip steerability • Shaft and tip visibility for accurate guide positioning • Kink resistance
Backup Support
• Braiding and polymer technology to ensure curve retention once the catheter has been inserted in the body • Flexibility of the distal curve to allow further manipulation of the catheter and deep engagement for additional support when needed
Device Passage
• Smooth PTFE inner liner combined with large lumens to facilitate advancement of devices
Atraumatic TIP
• Soft distal tip material for gentle engagement of the guide and minimization of the risk of dissection of the origin of engaged coronary artery. • Adequate radio-opacity for visualization of the guide catheter tip

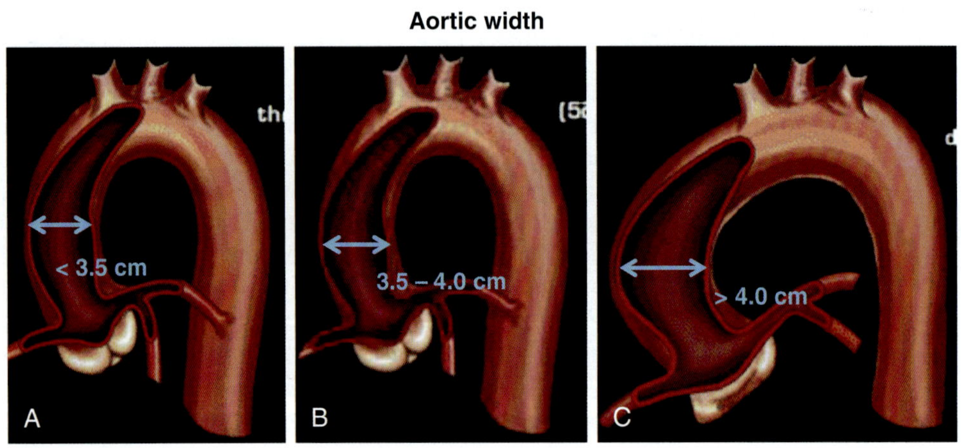

FIGURE 18.12 Aortic width. A, Narrow. B, Normal. C, Dilated. Used with permission by Medtronic ©2018.

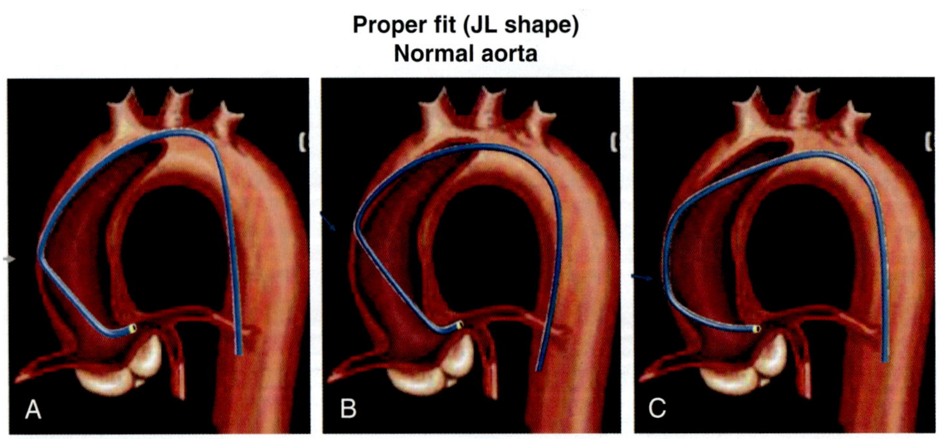

FIGURE 18.13 Guide catheter fit with normal aorta. Proper fit is a 45° angle at the primary curve, and buttressing against the contralateral wall. A, Just right. B, Too long. C, Too short. Used with permission by Medtronic ©2018.

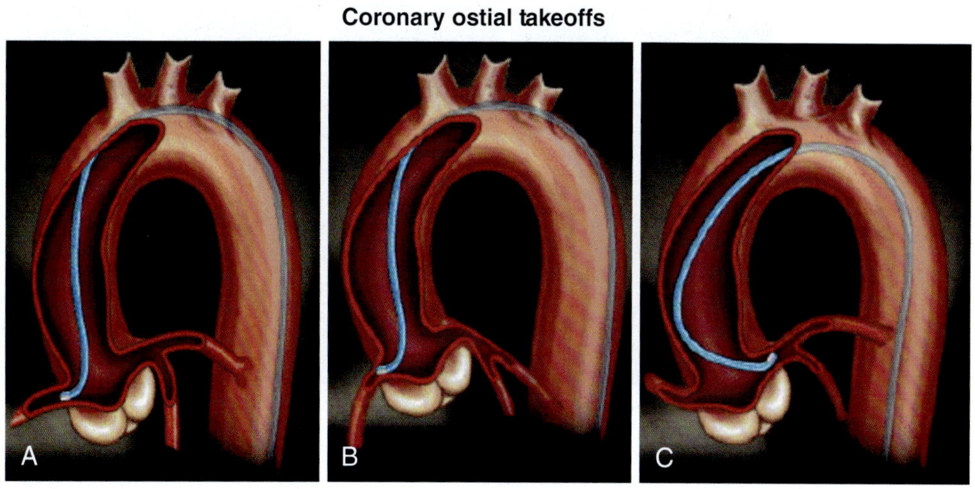

FIGURE 18.14 Right and left coronary artery takeoff variants. A, Horizontal. B, Inferior. C, Superior. Used with permission by Medtronic ©2018.

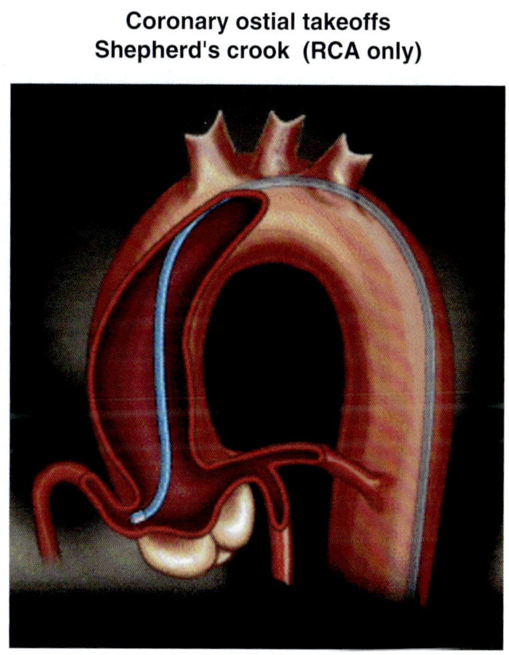

FIGURE 18.15 Shepherd's crook takeoff, right coronary artery (RCA). Used with permission by Medtronic ©2018.

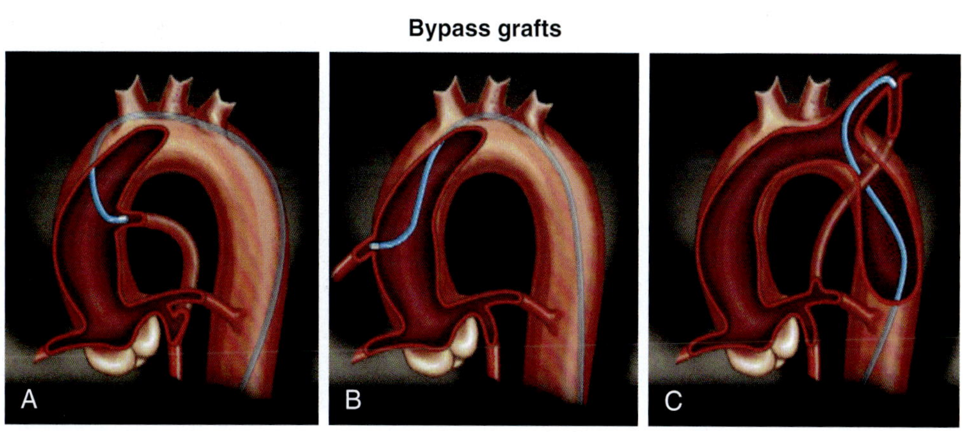

FIGURE 18.16 Grafts anastomosis. Grafts are anastomosed to the anterior wall of the ascending aorta with the exception of the LIMA. A, Left coronary bypass (LCB). B, Right coronary bypass (RCB). C, Left coronary bypass (LCB). Used with permission by Medtronic ©2018.

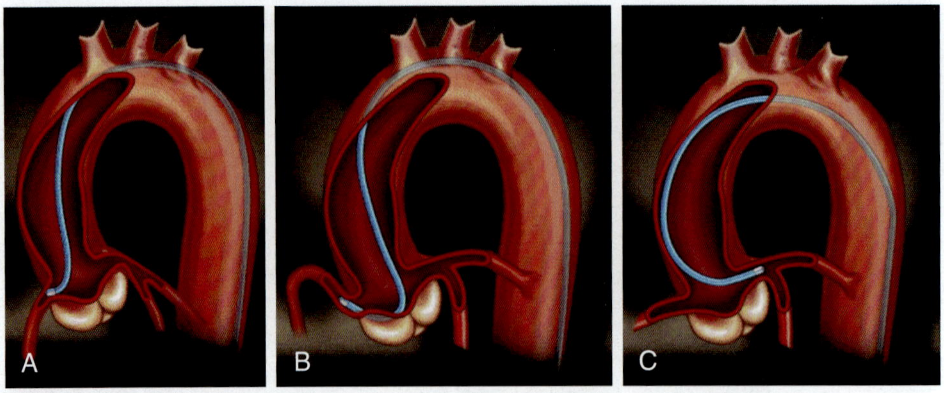

FIGURE 18.17 Examples of guide selection for right coronary inferior takeoff, right coronary shepherd's crook takeoff, and left coronary artery horizontal takeoff. A, JR4. Simple coaxial alignment, without support. B, Hockey stick. Coaxial alignment, with extra support from sinus of Valsalva. C, EBU. Coaxial alignment, with power support from opposite wall of aorta. Used with permission by Medtronic ©2018.

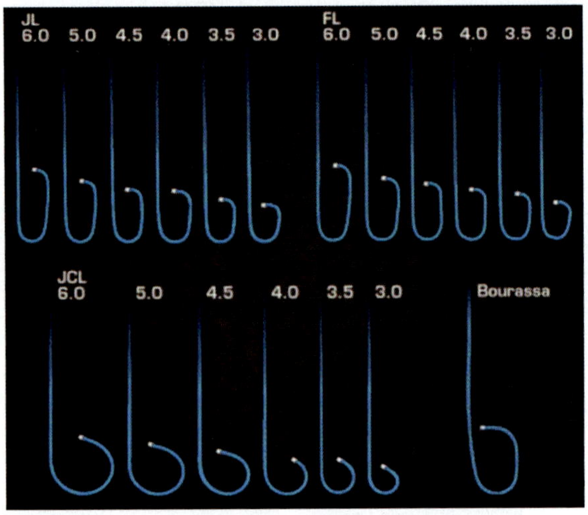

FIGURE 18.18 Left coronary curves. Used with permission by Medtronic ©2018.

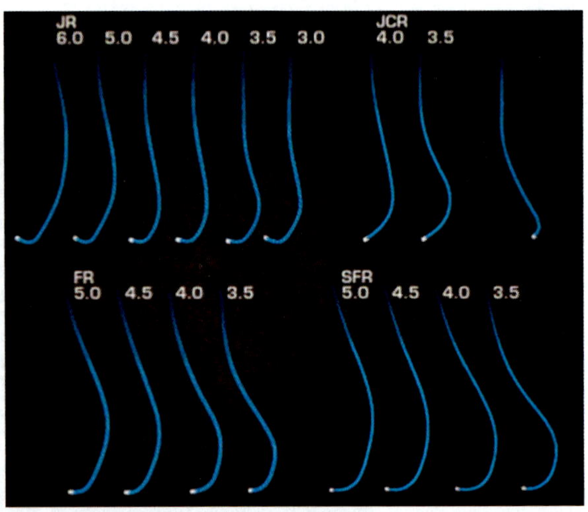

FIGURE 18.19 Right coronary curves. Used with permission by Medtronic ©2018.

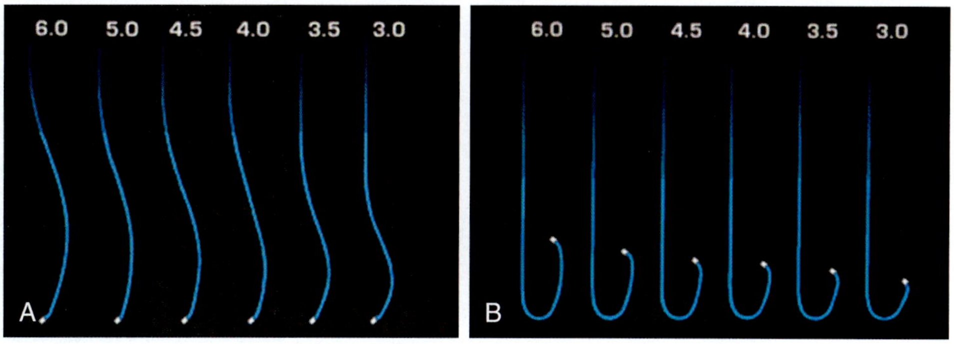

FIGURE 18.20 Short right and left coronary curves. A, Short right curves. B, Short left curves. Used with permission by Medtronic ©2018.

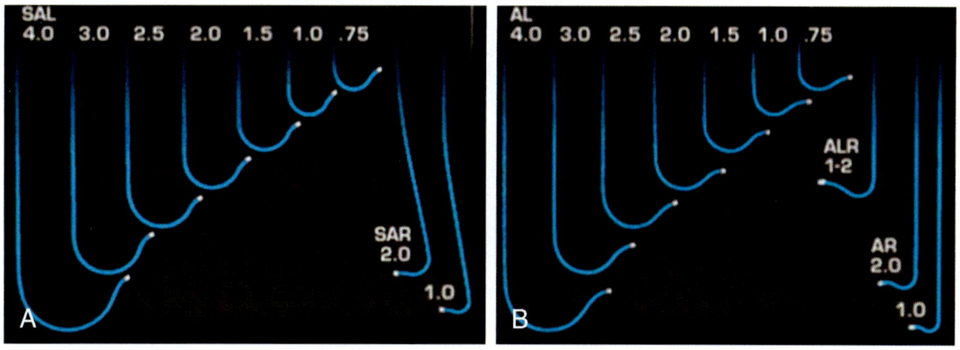

FIGURE 18.21 Short and regular Amplatz curves. A. Short Amplatz curves. B. Amplatz coronary curves. Used with permission by Medtronic ©2018.

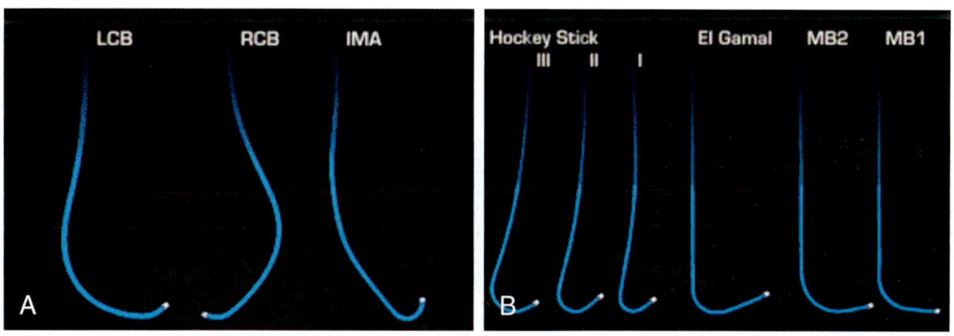

FIGURE 18.22 A, Bypass graft and (B) multipurpose curves. Used with permission by Medtronic ©2018.

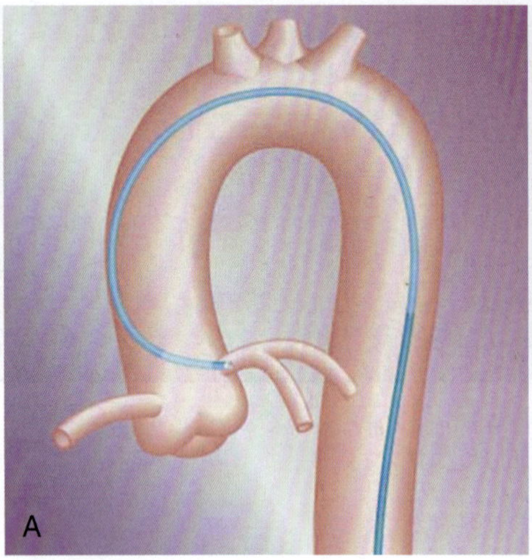

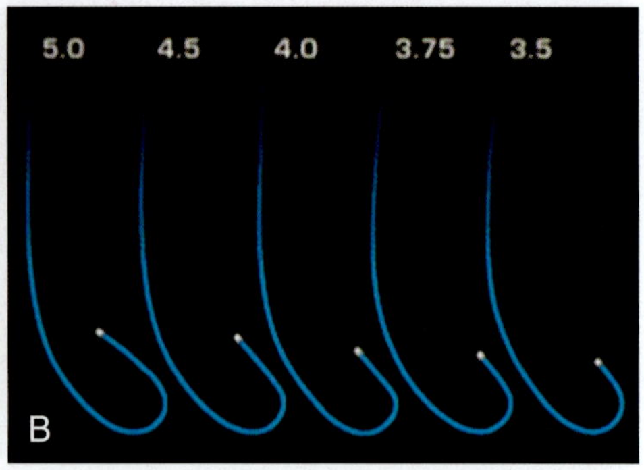

C

Judkins Left Cathetre Used	EBU Curve Used
JL 3.5	EBU 3.5
JL 4.0	EBU 3.75 will engage 2-3 mm into the ostium EBU 4.0 will engage 3-5 mm into the ostium
JL 4.5	EBU 4.5
JL 5.0	EBU 4.5

FIGURE 18.23 A-C, EBU curve. The secondary curve braces against the contralateral wall for EBU. Used with permission by Medtronic ©2018.

Coaxial alignment of the guide catheter with the ostium of the coronary artery is critical to minimize the risk of guide catheter–induced proximal dissection and to optimize guide catheter support and advancement of devices (**FIGURES 18.25** and **18.26**). Guide catheters can be divided into 2 broad categories: passive support and active support. Passive support relies on the property of the catheter shaft and tip to maintain position within the ostium of the coronary artery. They are rarely deep seated and they require minimal manipulation. Active support relies on manipulation of the guide catheter, deep seating when needed through rotation of the catheter and it uses the aortic root with different guide catheter curves to provide backup support. **Table 18.2** lists factors to be considered in the selection of guide catheters.

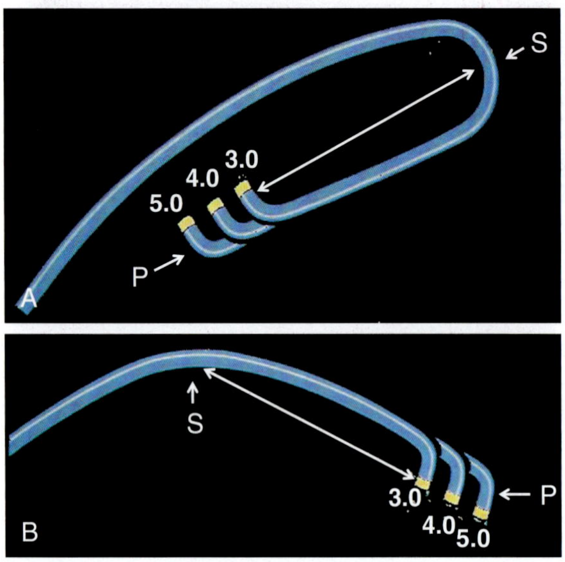

FIGURE 18.24 A, Primary and (B) secondary curves of Judkins left and right guide catheters. P, primary curve; S, secondary curve; curve length, P-S distance (cm).

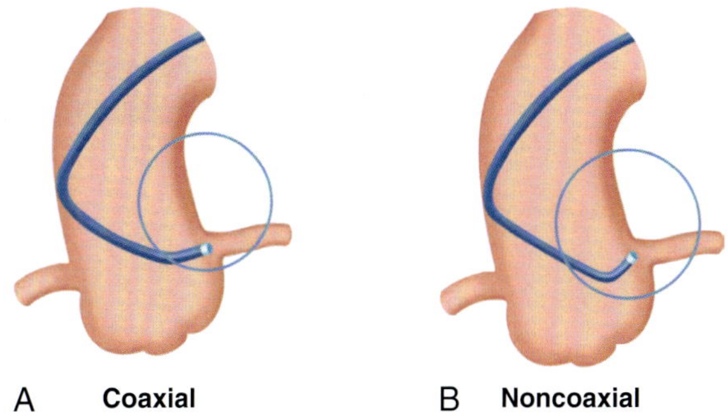

FIGURE 18.25 A, Coaxial and (B) noncoaxial guide catheter position.

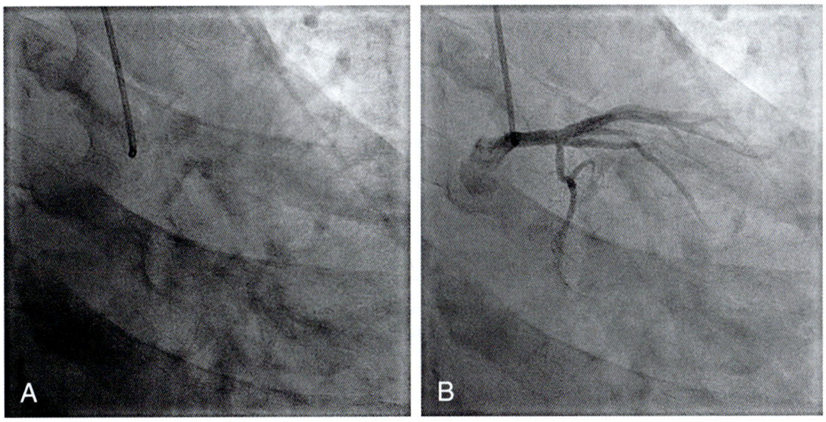

FIGURE 18.26 A and B, Example of noncoaxial engagement of the left main coronary artery.

TABLE 18.2

Factors to Be Considered in Guide Catheter Selection

Access site	Transfemoral, radial, brachial
French size	Bifurcation lesions, planned kissing balloon inflation etc.
Coronary anatomy	Extreme tortuosity, takeoff
Aortic width	Normal, small, large
Native Coronary vs. CABG/IMA	
Location and severity of lesion	Distal lesion, bifurcation, calcification
Type of support	Active vs. Passive

GUIDE WIRES

The introduction of the steerable guide wire in the early 1980s has allowed the expansion of PTCA to the management of stenosis in distal coronary arteries and side branches (**FIGURE 18.6**). **Tables 18.3** and **18.4** illustrate general characteristics of guide wires. Guide wires can be divided into 2 major categories: "work horse guide wires," generally used in the average PCI, and "specialty guide wires," used with more complex coronary anatomy as well as conditions including chronic total occlusion (CTO) (**FIGURES 18.27-18.31**).

TABLE 18.3

Guide Wire Characteristics

Trackability	Ability of the guidewire to be advanced through a vessel around curves and tortuosity. In general, floppy wires can be advanced though tortuosity better than stiff wires. Tractability depends on tip's design and the core wire's material.
Torqueability	Ability of transmitting rotational force from the proximal end of the guidewire to the distal tip. High torqueability allows proper control of the distal tip.
Flexibility	Ability of the guidewire to bend along its long axis while maintaining torque and trackability. It depends on the characteristics of the material of the core wire. Nitinol is very flexible while steel is stiff.
Crossability	Ability to cross a lesion.
Supportability	Ability of a guidewire to support advancement of devices over it. Floppy wires provide good trackability and flexibility, but less support when compared to extra support guide wires.
Tip load	The measurement of tip stiffness, and it is the force needed to bend a wire when exerted on the tip, at a point 1 cm from the tip. As the tip load increases, the penetration force of the guidewire and the risk of perforation increase in parallel.

Data from Fornell D. Understanding the design and function of guidewire technology. Diagnostic and Interventional Cardiology website. https://www.dicardiology.com/article/understanding-design-and-function-guidewire-technology. October 2016. Accessed September 24, 2018.

TABLE 18.4

Guidewire Components

Core	Guidewires have an inner core which tapers at the tip, or it stops before the tip. The inner core is made either of nitinol or stainless steel. Nitinol provides good flexibility and torqueability, it is less prone to bending, but in general it provides less support when compared with stainless steel. Stainless steel provides good support, pushability and torqueability, but it is less flexible when compared with nitinol.
Tip	The core wire either tapers down to the tip of the wire for added support, or stops short of the tip. A shaping ribbon at the tip makes the tip more flexible, and it helps in enhancing torqueability.
Shaping ribbon/tip coils	The inner core of the guidewire is tapered all the way to the tip or it stops right before the tip. A shaping ribbon enhances the flexibility and atraumatic characteristics of the tip. Importantly, the shaping ribbon is critical for retention of the shape of the tip with nitinol guidewires. Wire tactile feedback, torqueability and crossability depend in part on the characteristics of the shaping ribbon.
Coatings	Wires are usually coated with hydrophobic or hydrophilic polymers. Silicone is the most common hydrophobic coating. It repels water to reduce friction, increase trackability, and it offers good tactile feedback. Hydrophilic coatings trap a thin film of water on the surface of the guidewire. The film of water prevents direct contact between the guidewire, the vasculature and the catheters advanced over the guidewire. It makes the wires more slippery, thus reducing friction and increasing trackability. However, hydrophilic wires provide less tactile feedback and are more prone to lead to dissection and perforation.

Data from Fornell D. Understanding the design and function of guidewire technology. Diagnostic and Interventional Cardiology website. https://www.dicardiology.com/article/understanding-design-and-function-guidewire-technology. October 2016. Accessed September 24, 2018.

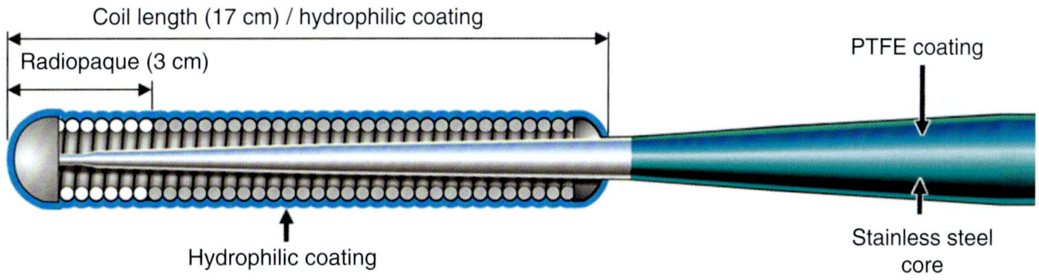

FIGURE 18.27 Work Horse guidewire: Marvel Guidewire: **Compound-Taper Stainless Steel Core**—The unique design of MARVEL's stainless steel core provides 1:1 torque response, outstanding trackability and pushability, and enhanced rail support for increased device deliverability support. **Core-To-Tip Design**—This feature provides an atraumatic tip while promoting torqueability and durability. **Hydrophilic Coating**—The coating over the entire length of the spring coil promotes crossability, trackability, and device deliverability. Image provided courtesy of Boston Scientific. ©2018 Boston Scientific Corporation or its affiliates. All rights reserved.

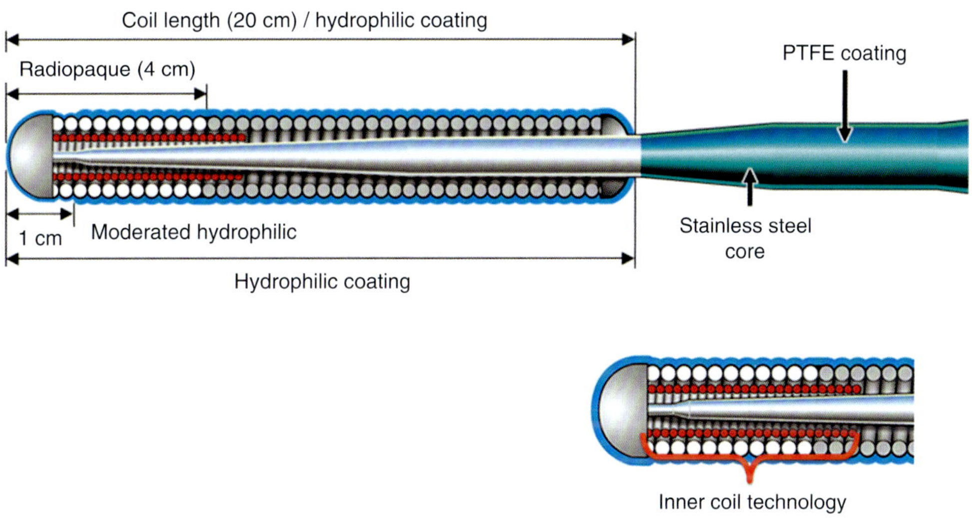

FIGURE 18.28 Work Horse guidewire: Samurai Guidewire. **Inner Coil Technology (ICT)**—A stainless steel inner coil is affixed directly to the distal portion of the stainless steel core and enhances the shape retention and durability of the distal tip, reduces whipping, and provides exceptional torqueability. **Moderated Hydrophilic Coating**—The reduced coating on the distal 1 cm improves tactile feel, while the hydrophilic coating over the rest of the spring coil promotes exceptional trackability and device deliverability. **Compound-Taper Stainless Steel Core**—The unique design of SAMURAI's stainless steel core provides 1:1 torque response, outstanding trackability, torqueability, and moderate rail support for device delivery. Image provided courtesy of Boston Scientific. ©2018 Boston Scientific Corporation or its affiliates. All rights reserved.

Frontline Guidewires / Coil

Rinato / PROWATER

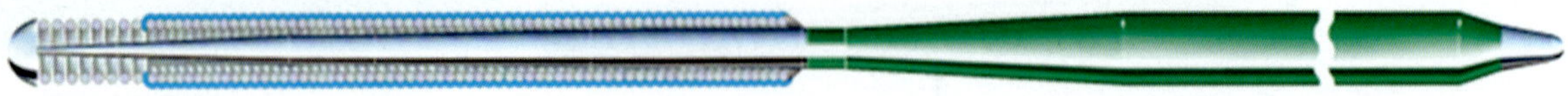

- Tip load ....0.8 g
- Tip radiopacity ....3 cm
- SLIP-COAT® coating over the spring coil*

First choice guidewire with floppy tip and moderate core wire support. Excellent maneuverability and good support for device delivery.
*Silicone coating up to 30mm from the tip for safer procedures.

Route / PROWATERflex

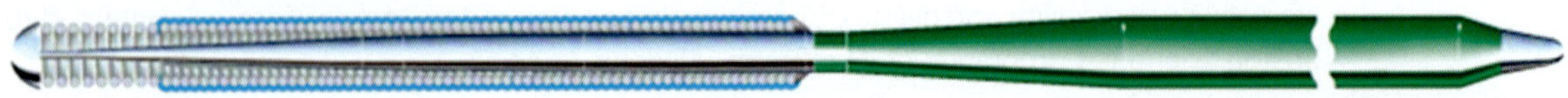

- Tip load ....0.8 g
- Tip radiopacity ....3 cm
- SLIP-COAT® coating over the spring coil*

First choice guidewire featuring a soft tip with good shaping memory and excellent guidewire trackability. Sufficient support for delivery of most interventional devices.
*Silicone coating up to 30mm from the tip for safer procedures.

Soft

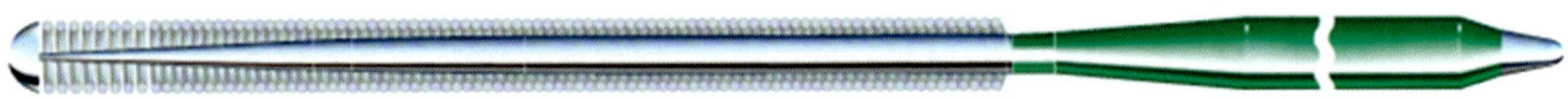

- Tip load ....0.7 g
- Tip radiopacity ....3 cm
- Silicone coating over the spring coil

Basic frontline guidewire with floppy tip and non hydrophilic coating to ensure optimal tactile feedback.

Light

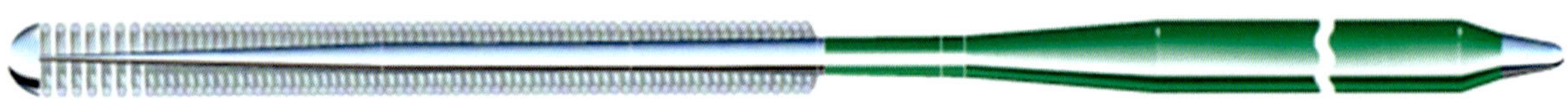

- Tip load ....0.5 g
- Tip radiopacity ....3 cm
- Silicone coating over the spring coil

Basic frontline guidewire with a flexible core and good torqueability for distal side branch selection.

FIGURE 18.29 Examples of "frontline-guidewires." Courtesy of Asahi Intecc Co., Ltd.

Chronic Occlusion Guidewires

Conquest / CONFIANZA

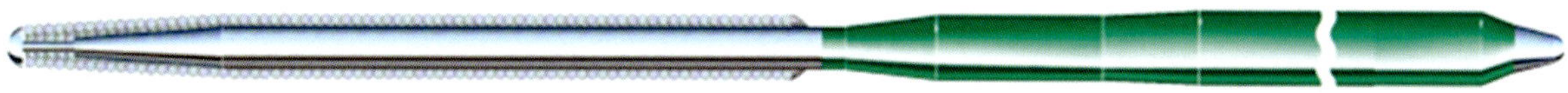

- Tip load ....9.0 g
- Tip radiopacity ....20 cm
- Tip outer diameter ....0.23 mm (0.009 inch)
- Silicone coating over the spring coil

Silicone coated and tapered to 0.23mm (0.009inch) at the tip. The 9g stiff, tapered tip helps to penetrate highly stenosed lesions.

Conquest Pro / CONFIANZA PRO

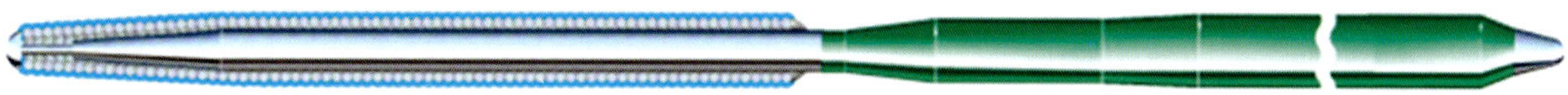

- Tip load ....9.0 g
- Tip radiopacity ....20 cm
- Tip outer diameter ....0.23 mm (0.009 inch)
- SLIP-COAT® coating over the spring coil, excluding the tip

Similar structure and tip stiffness as Conquest with SLIP-COAT® coating for lubricity. The distal tip is not coated to allow it to catch on the entry point of the lesions.

Conquest Pro 12 / CONFIANZA PRO 12

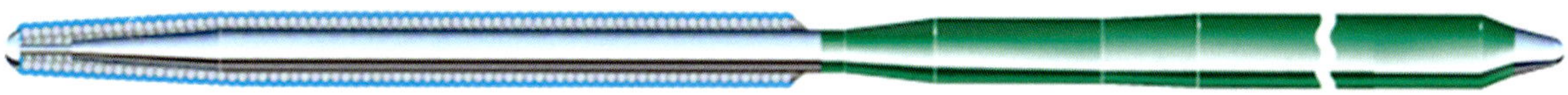

- Tip load ....12.0 g
- Tip radiopacity ....20 cm
- Tip outer diameter ....0.23 mm (0.009 inch)
- SLIP-COAT® coating over the spring coil, excluding the tip

A tapered tip with 12g tip load. For penetration of calcification and proximal or distal thick, fibrous caps.

Conquest Pro 8-20 / CONFIANZA PRO 8-20

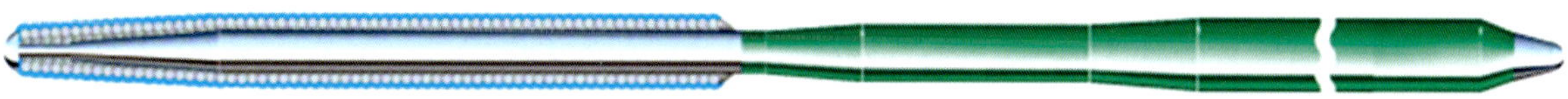

- Tip load ....20.0 g
- Tip radiopacity ....17 cm
- Tip outer diameter ....0.20 mm (0.008 inch)
- SLIP-COAT® coating over the spring coil, excluding the tip

Designed for crossing complex lesions with heavy calcifications and tough fibrous tissues. The wire has a tip load of 20g and is tapered to 0.20mm (0.008inch). It is the finest and stiffest guidewire in the current Asahi series.

FIGURE 18.30 Specialty, chronic occlusion guidewires. Courtesy of Asahi Intecc Co., Ltd.

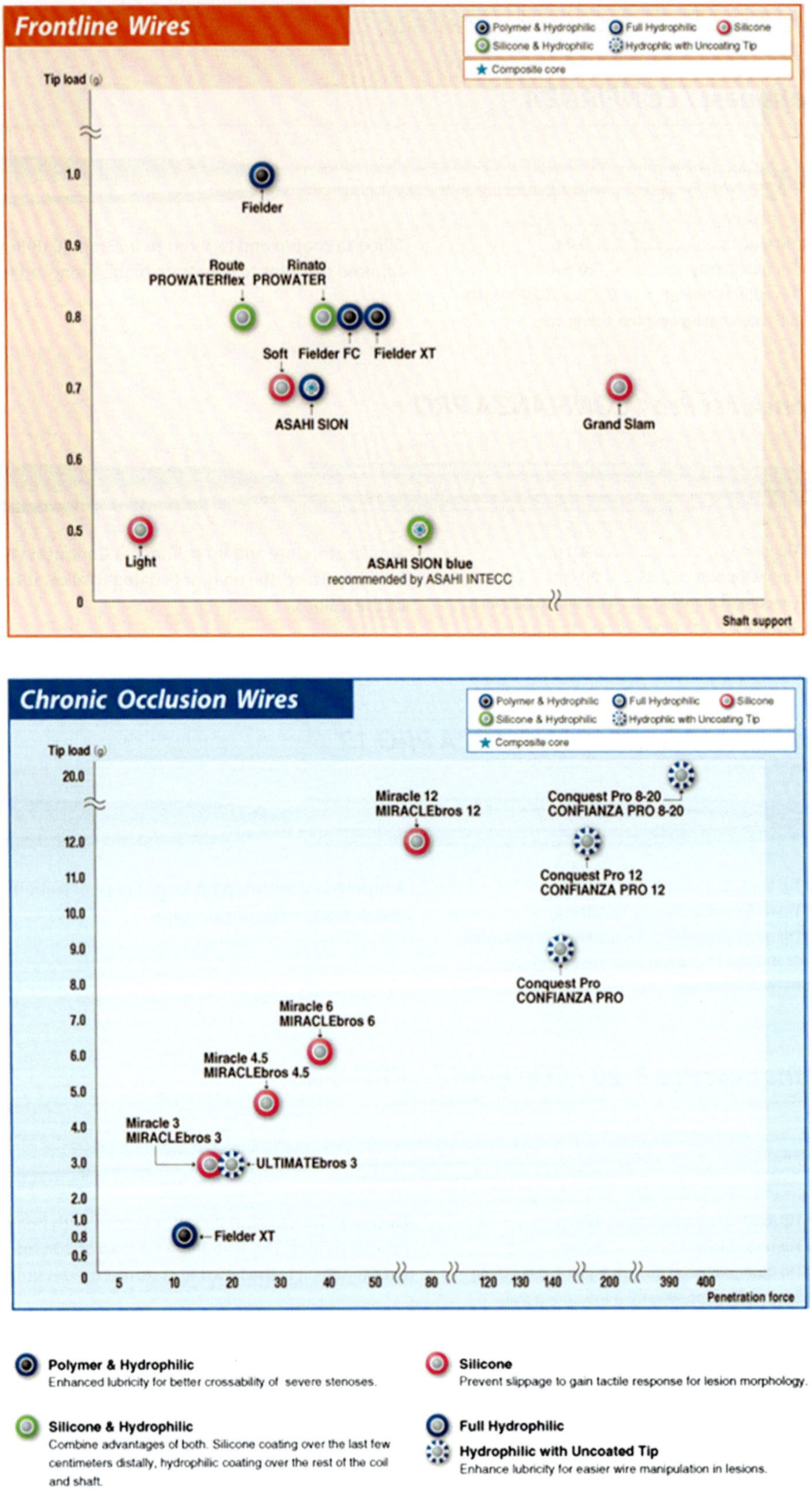

FIGURE 18.31 "Frontline" and "specialty guidewires" (chronic occlusion wires). Mechanical characteristics of frontline and chronic occlusion guide wires. The top panel shows the level of shaft support and tip load for guidewires used as "frontline" wires. The bottom panel shows penetration force and tip load of guide wires commonly used for CTO. As expected, the tip load of chronic occlusion wires is several folds the tip load of frontline or "work horse" guide wires. Courtesy of Asahi Intecc Co., Ltd.

PTCA BALLOONS

The original balloons used in the 1970s were fixed wire balloons made of PVC (**FIGURE 18.3**). They had a high profile, and they were suitable for the management of only proximal coronary artery lesions. Since then, major breakthroughs have included the development of the steerable guide wire and the evolution of balloon technology (**FIGURES 18.32-18.34**). Balloon characteristics include the balloon material, tractability, crossability, dilation properties, and balloon rewrap (**Table 18.5**). Balloon rewrap depends on the type of balloon material. Different manufacturers use different materials including polyethylene terephthalate (PET), polyethylene (PE), polyolefin copolymer (POC), and Pebax (polyether block amide). As shown in **FIGURE 18.34**, in addition to having different rewrap characteristic, these materials have different compliance.

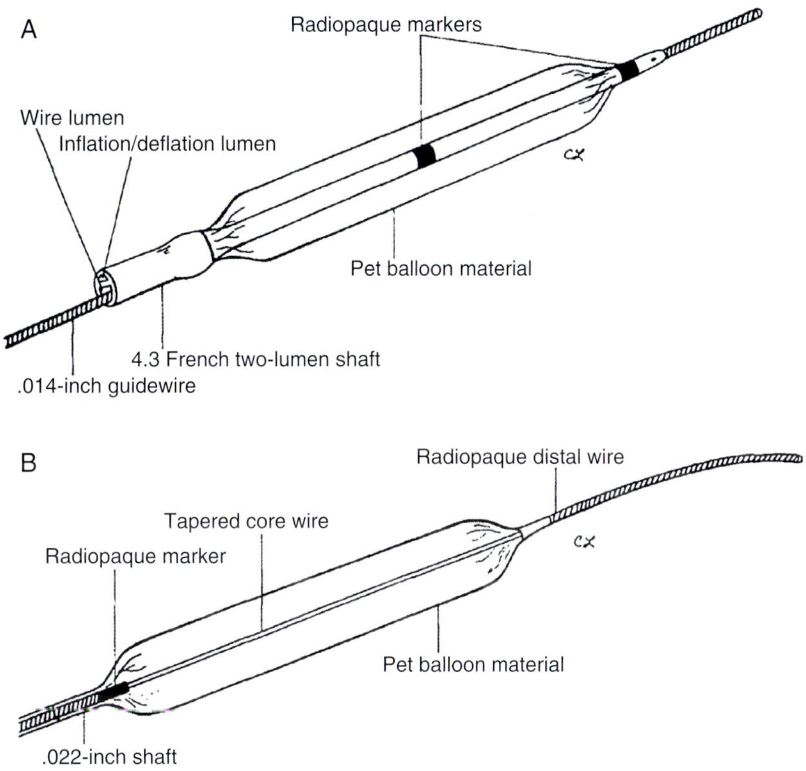

FIGURE 18.32 **A**, Schematic illustration of a typical balloon-over-a-wire system (eg, USCI profile plus) showing eccentric inflation and wire ports, balloon, and radiopaque markers. **B**, Schematic illustration of a typical balloon-on-a-wire system (eg, USCI micro probe) showing 0.22 in shaft, balloon, and radiopaque distal tip wire (in this case 2 cm Flex@ tip). PET, polyethylene terephthalate. Reproduced with permission from Avedissian MG, Killeavy ES, Garcia JM, Dear WE. Percutaneous transluminal coronary angioplasty: a review of current balloon dilatation systems. *Cathet Cardiovasc Diagn*. 1989;18:263-275.

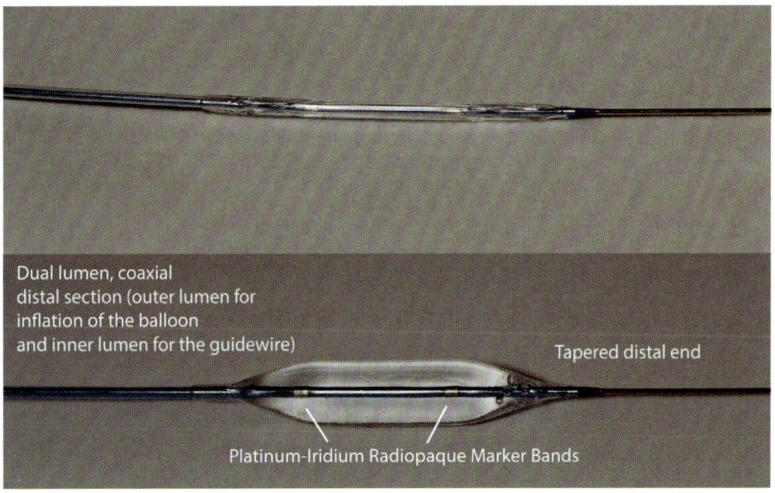

FIGURE 18.33 Modern PTCA balloon. 5.0 mm x 12 mm NC Quantum Apex Monorail Balloon.

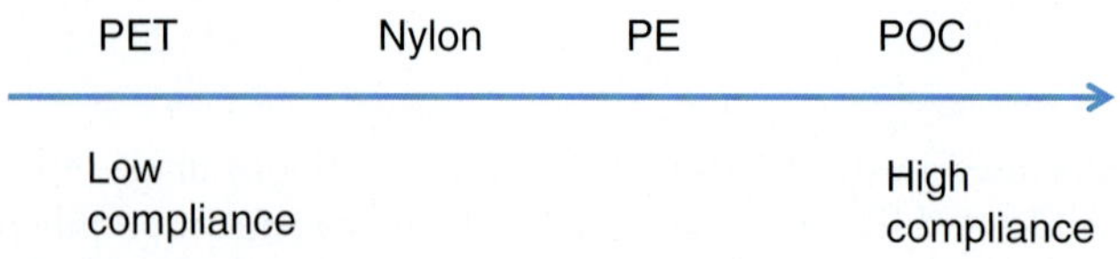

FIGURE 18.34 Balloon material and corresponding compliance. Cross-linked polyethylene (PE) and polyethylene terephthalate (PET) were introduced in the early 1980s, and replaced PVC. Nylon balloons were introduced in the late 1980s, and polyurethane balloons in the early 1990s. Nylon is relatively strong and it can be used in relatively thin designs. Most high-pressure balloons are made from either PET or nylon. Compared with PET balloons, nylon high-pressure balloons require a thicker wall for a given burst pressure. Thus, nylon balloons tend to have a higher profile when compared with PET balloons, but are more easily refolded when deflated.

TABLE 18.5

Balloon Characteristics

Balloon profile	Maximum diameter of the balloon when mounted on a catheter in its deflated and wrapped condition.
Balloon diameter	Nominal inflated balloon diameter measured at a specified pressure.
Balloon length	Length of the straight body section of the balloon.
Nominal pressure	Pressure at nominal balloon diameter.
Burst pressure	Average pressure required to rupture a balloon; usually measured at body temperature.
Rated burst pressure	Maximum statistically guaranteed pressure to which a balloon can be inflated without failing. For PTCA and PTA catheters, this is normally at a 95% confidence/99.9% guaranteed level.
Balloon compliance	Change in balloon diameter as a function of inflation pressure.
Balloon material	The balloon material determines compliance characteristics, burst pressure, rewrap characteristics, and balloon profile. For example, nylon high-pressure balloons require a thicker wall than PET balloons for a given burst pressure. However, they rewrap better than PET balloons.
Balloon rewrap	Ability of the balloon to rewrap after deflation.
Trackability	Ability of the balloon to be advanced through a vessel, particularly around curves and tortuosity.
Crossability	Ability of the balloon to cross the lesion

NEW TECHNOLOGY

The innovation that has occurred in guide catheter, guide wire, and balloon technology has been paralleled by a major expansion of PTCA, by the introduction of new devices and new applications, and by the development of the new term of percutaneous coronary intervention. New devices have included cutting balloons (**FIGURES 18.35-18.37**), atherectomy catheters (Chapter 19), coronary stents (Chapter 20), specialty guidewires (**FIGURES 18.30** and **18.31**), and distal protection devices. New applications encompass CTO[10-14] (**FIGURES 18.38-18.42**), multivessel disease, calcified lesions, thrombotic lesions, left main disease, vein graft disease, and acute coronary syndromes.

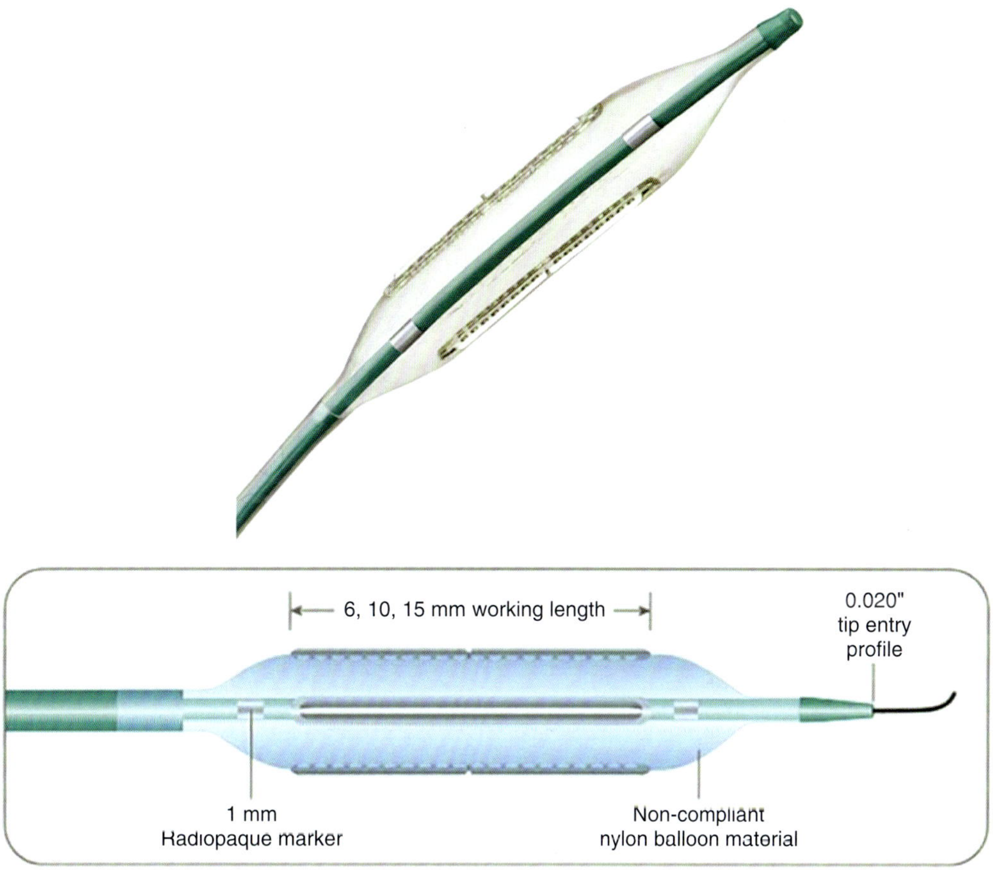

FIGURE 18.35 FLEXTOME Cutting Balloon. The Flextome Cutting Balloon Device is indicated for dilatation of stenoses in coronary arteries for the purpose of improving myocardial perfusion in those circumstances where a high pressure balloon resistant lesion is encountered. Image provided courtesy of Boston Scientific. ©2018 Boston Scientific Corporation or its affiliates. All rights reserved.

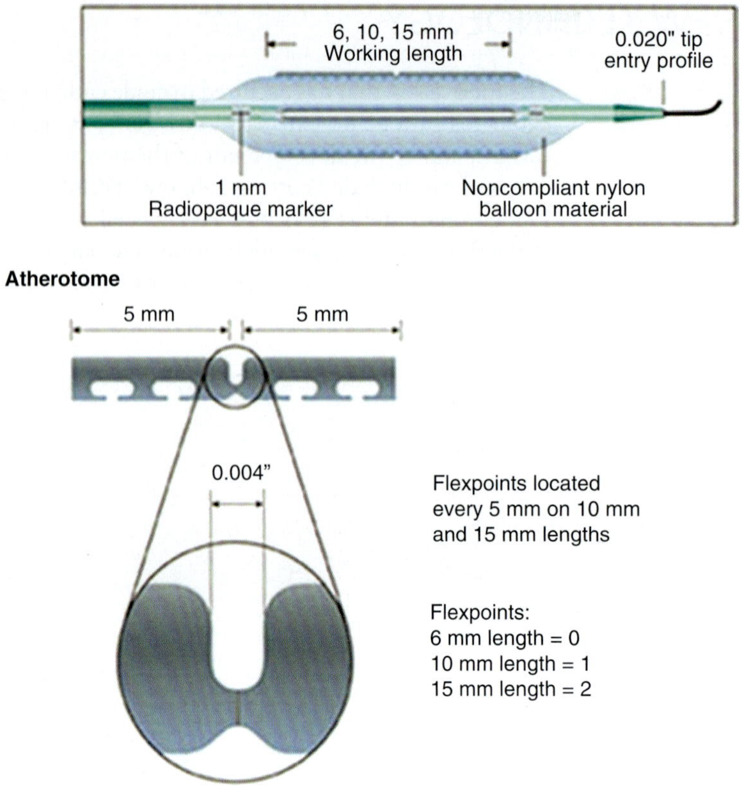

FIGURE 18.36 Atherotomes and flexion points on cutting balloon. Image provided courtesy of Boston Scientific. ©2018 Boston Scientific Corporation or its affiliates. All rights reserved.

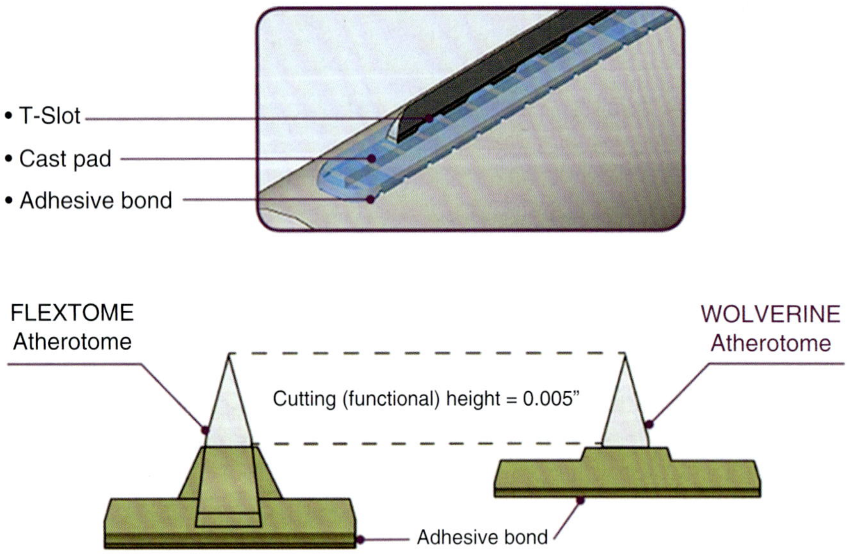

FIGURE 18.37 Comparison of the FLEXTOME and WOLVERINE atherotomes. The WOLVERINE cutting balloon has a smaller profile achieved through the reduction in the T-Slot height, thus resulting in improved crossability and deliverability. Image provided courtesy of Boston Scientific. ©2018 Boston Scientific Corporation or its affiliates. All rights reserved.

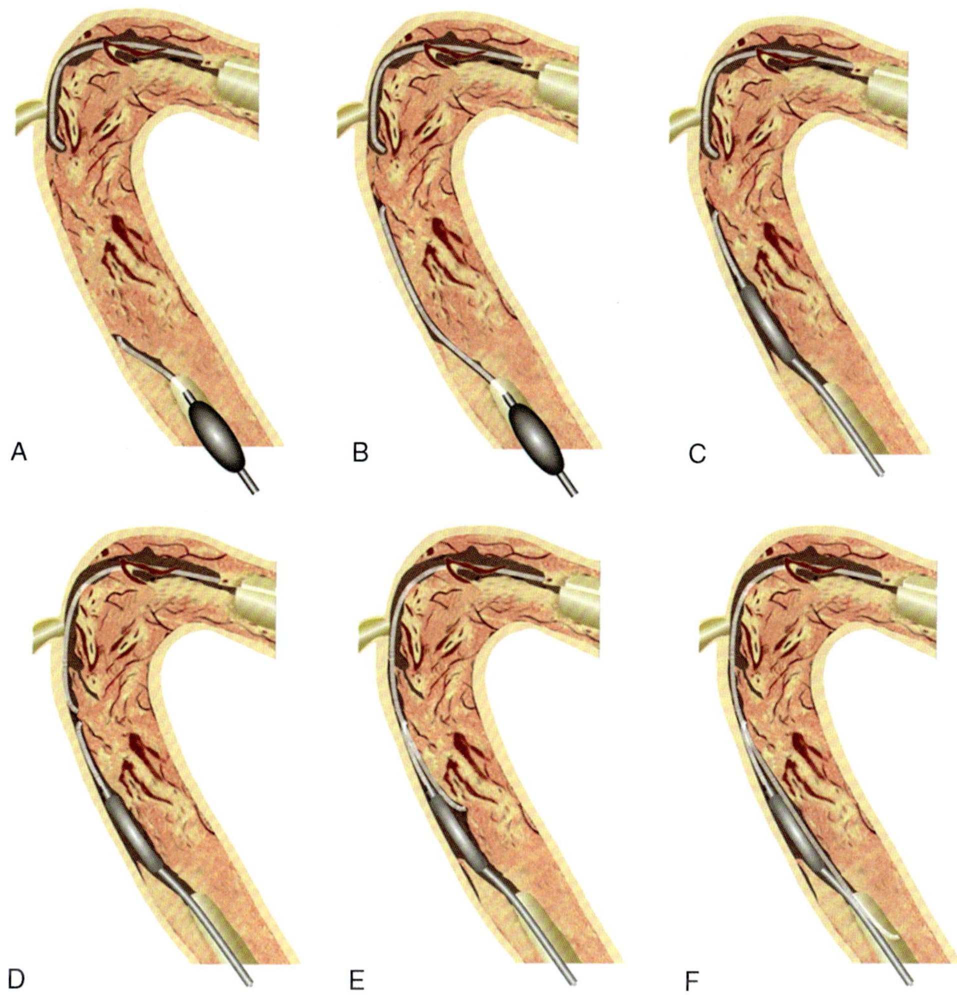

FIGURE 18.38 Controlled antegrade and retrograde subintimal tracking (CART) technique for CTO. A, A wire is advanced antegradely from the proximal true lumen into the CTO, then into the subintimal space at the CTO site. A retrograde wire with an over-the-wire balloon is advanced retrogradely from the distal true lumen into the CTO. B, The retrograde wire is further advanced into the subintimal space at the CTO site. C, Balloon dilatation of the subintimal space and also on the course from this subintimal space to the distal end of the CTO. D and E, The deflated balloon is left in place and the antegrade wire is further advanced in the subintimal space, targeting the deflated balloon. F, The antegrade wire is advanced through the channel done by the retrograde wire into the distal true lumen. Reproduced with permission from Surmely JF, Tsuchikane E, Katoh O, et al. New concept for CTO recanalization using controlled antegrade and retrograde subintimal tracking: the CART technique. *J Invasive Cardiol*. 2006;18(7):334-338.

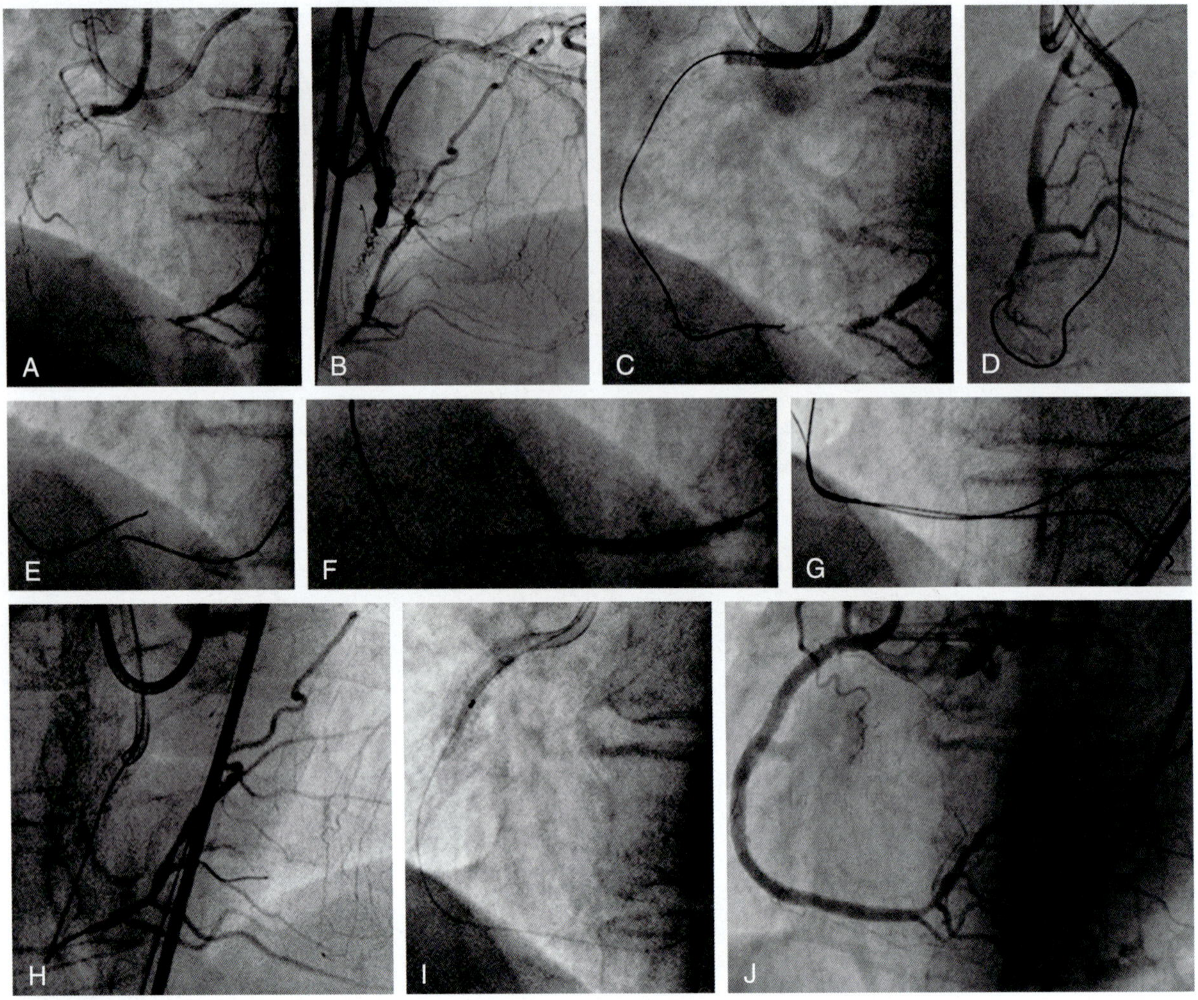

FIGURE 18.39 A-J, Angiographic example of the CART technique. First, a wire is advanced antegradely from the proximal true lumen into the CTO, then into the subintimal space at the CTO site. Experienced operators can recognize the wire entering into the subintimal space by a decreased resistance of the wire tip or wire movement. Next, another wire is advanced through the intercoronary collateral using a microcatheter in order to protect the channel from injury, as well as to achieve better wire maneuverability. This wire is placed at the distal end of the CTO, then it penetrates retrogradely from the distal true lumen into the CTO, and finally into the subintimal space at the CTO site. After advancing a small balloon (1.5-2.0 mm) over the retrograde wire into the subintima, the balloon should be inflated in the subintima as well as on the course from this subintimal space to the distal end of the CTO. In order to keep this subintimal space open, the deflated balloon should be left in place. As a consequence, the 2 dissections created by the antegrade wire and the retrograde balloon lie in the subintima at the CTO site, which allows them to be easily connected. Thereafter, the antegrade wire is advanced further along the deflated retrograde balloon that lies from the subintimal space to the distal true lumen. This technique allows limited subintimal tracking only in the portion of the CTO lesion and avoids the difficulty of reentering the distal true lumen. After successful recanalization, dilatation and stent implantation are performed. Adapted with permission from Surmely JF, Tsuchikane E, Katoh O, et al. New concept for CTO recanalization using controlled antegrade and retrograde subintimal tracking: the CART technique. *J Invasive Cardiol*. 2006;18(7):334-338.

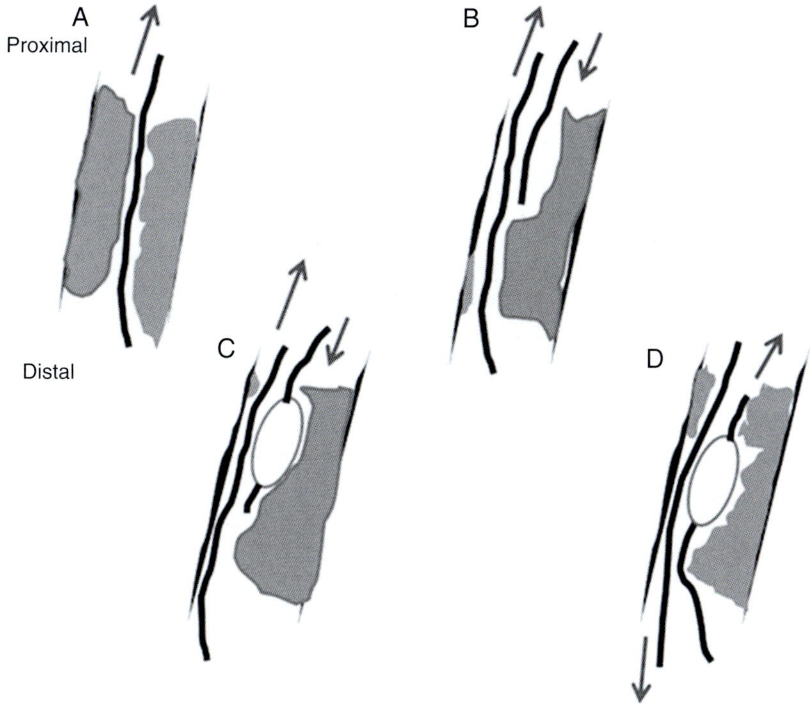

FIGURE 18.40 Approaches to retrograde CTO crossing techniques. A, Retrograde wiring, (B) kissing wire technique, (C) Reverse CART technique, (D) CART technique. Reproduced with permission from Muramatsu T, Tsukahara R, Ito Y, et al. Changing strategies of the retrograde approach for chronic total occlusion during the past 7 years. *Catheter Cardiovasc Interv*. 2012;81(4):E178-E185. doi:10.1002/CCD.24447.

1. CART technique: the basic concept of the CART technique is to create a subintimal dissection limited to the site of the CTO. First a wire is advanced antegrade from the proximal true lumen into the CTO, then into the subintimal space of the CTO. Next a retrograde wire is advanced from the distal true lumen into the CTO and into the subintimal space of the CTO. A balloon is advanced over the retrograde wire and inflated from the subintimal space to the distal end of the CTO. The two subintimal dissections tend to expand toward each other and to connect. Then the antegrade wire is advanced targeting the deflated balloon.
2. The bilateral kissing wire technique combines the simultaneous use of antegrade and retrograde approach. It is similar to a parallel-wire technique.

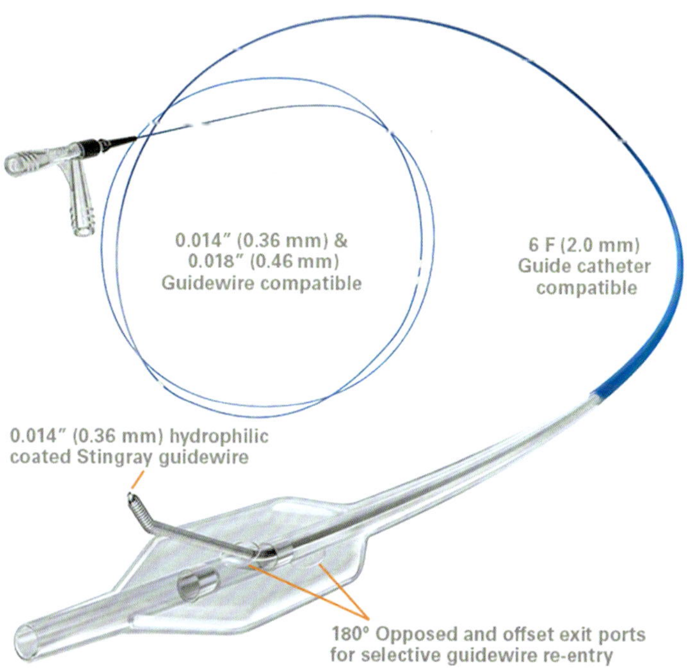

FIGURE 18.41 STINGRAY LP reentry device for CTO. Designed for reliability, safety, and predictability, the STINGRAY LP allows the operator to target and reenter the true lumen from a subintimal position. The self-orienting, flat balloon allows positioning of the exit port toward the true lumen, and the 180° opposed and offsetting exit ports enable selective guidewire reentry. Two radiopaque marker bands facilitate accurate placement and positioning. The hydrophilic coating on the balloon shaft ensures smooth device delivery. Image provided courtesy of Boston Scientific. ©2018 Boston Scientific Corporation or its affiliates. All rights reserved.

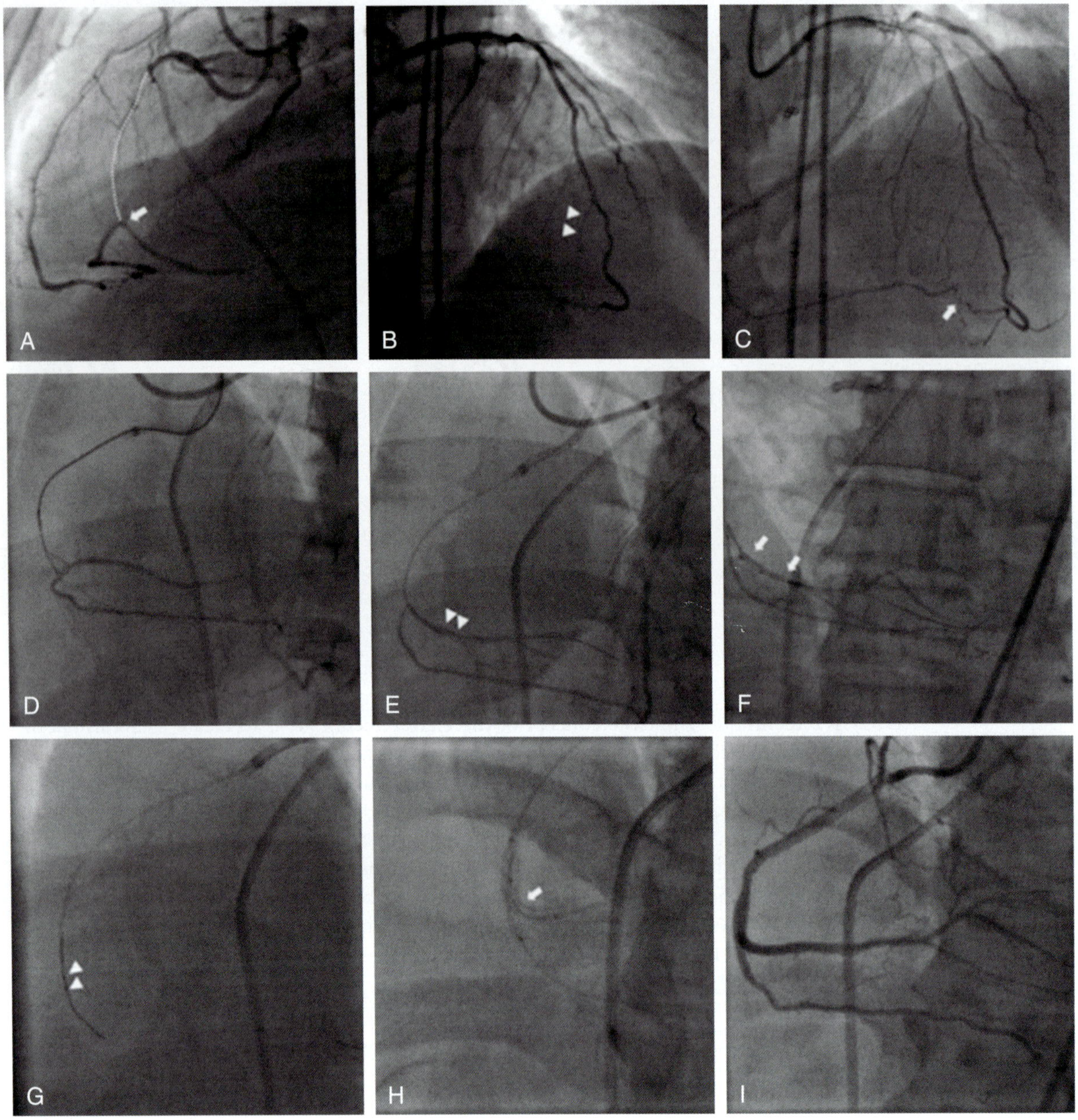

FIGURE 18.42 Successful recanalization of a right coronary artery CTO with bifurcation at the distal cap. A, Diagnostic angiography showing a mid-RCA-CTO with ambiguous proximal cap and a bifurcation at the distal cap (arrow). B-C, Failed retrograde crossing attempts via septal (arrowheads, B) and epicardial (arrow, C) collaterals. D, Antegrade crossing with a knuckled Fielder XT guidewire. E, Reentry into the right posterolateral vessel using the Stingray balloon (arrowheads) and the double-blind stick and swap technique. F, Confirmation of distal true lumen guidewire position using intravascular ultrasound (arrows). G, Successful reentry into the right posterior descending artery using the Stingray system (arrowheads) and the stick and swap technique. H, Kissing balloon inflation (arrow) after stenting of the right posterolateral and right posterior descending artery. I, Final angiography showed TIMI 3 flow in both distal branches Reproduced with permission from Tajti P, Doshi D, Karmpaliotis D, Brilakis ES, et al. The "double stingray technique" for recanalizing chronic total occlusions with bifurcation at the distal cap. *Catheter Cardiovasc Interv*. 2018;91(6):1079-1083.

ROLE OF PTCA IN THE MANAGEMENT OF CORONARY ARTERY DISEASE

In his letter to *Lancet* reporting the first 5 PTCA cases in 1978, Gruentzig concluded, "This technique, if it proves successful in long-term follow-up studies, may widen the indication for coronary angiography and provide another treatment for patient with angina pectoris".[3] Fifteen years later, the results of the first study, the ACME trial (A Comparison of Angioplasty with Medical Therapy in the Treatment of Single-Vessel Coronary Artery Disease) were reported in the *New England Journal Of Medicine*[15] (**FIGURE 18.43**). In the ACME trial, patients at 8 VA hospitals were randomized to PTCA or to medical therapy. When compared with medical therapy, PTCA improved symptoms but did not reduce cardiac events and it was more costly. Following the ACME trial, there have been several studies comparing PTCA with medical therapy[16,17]

ACME Trial 6 months Outcome

	PTCA n=105	Med. n=107	p
Death	0	1	1.0
Infarction	5	3	0.5
CABG	7	0	<0.01
PTCA	116	12	
Asymptomatic	64%	46%	<0.01
ET duration	2.1 min	0.5 min	<0.0001

PTCA versus medical therapy
- Improved symptoms
- No reduction in cardiac events
- Higher cost

8 VA Hospitals
9,573 patients screened
212 patients enrolled

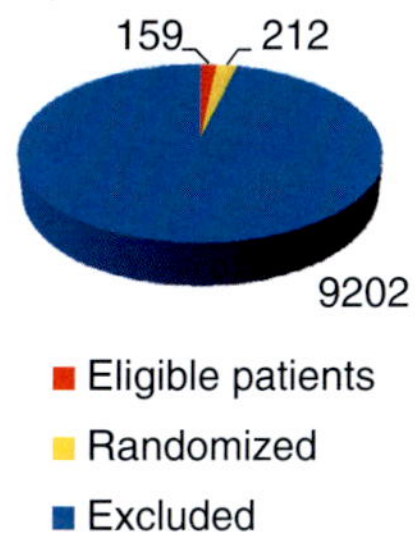

FIGURE 18.43 Angioplasty Compared to Medicine VA Trial (ACME). In the ACME trial, patients at 8 VA hospitals were randomized to PTCA or to medical therapy. When compared with medical therapy, PTCA improved symptoms but did not reduce cardiac events and it was more costly.[15]

(**FIGURES 18.44-18.49**). Although the evidence supports that PTCA, in stable patients with stable coronary artery disease, can improve symptoms[15] (**FIGURES 18.43**, **18.45**, and **18.49**), whether PTCA (and PCI, see Chapter 20) can reduce future adverse cardiovascular events remains the topic of a major debate. It should be noted that early clinical trials have been limited by relatively small sample size, the use of old technology, the inclusion as an endpoint of peri-procedure non-q wave MI, and by the fact that medical therapy was not maximized in the PTCA group. For example, in the AVERT trial randomizing patient to PTCA plus usual care versus aggressive lipid-lowering therapy, the LDL average value in the PTCA group was 119 mg/dL when compared with an LDL value of 77 mg/dL in the group of patients randomized to aggressive medical therapy (**FIGURE 18.48**). By today standards, the medical management of PTCA patients could be considered suboptimal. That said, as discussed earlier, pooled analysis of randomized clinical trials of PTCA versus medical therapy have shown that PTCA can result in improved relief from angina (**FIGURE 18.49**). In contrast, data from clinical trials in acute coronary syndromes fully support the value of PTCA/PCI in improving outcomes[18-23] (**FIGURES 18.50-18.57**). Thus, PCI remains the standard of care for patients presenting with unstable angina, non-ST segment elevation myocardial infarction, and ST segment elevation myocardial infarction.[24-26]

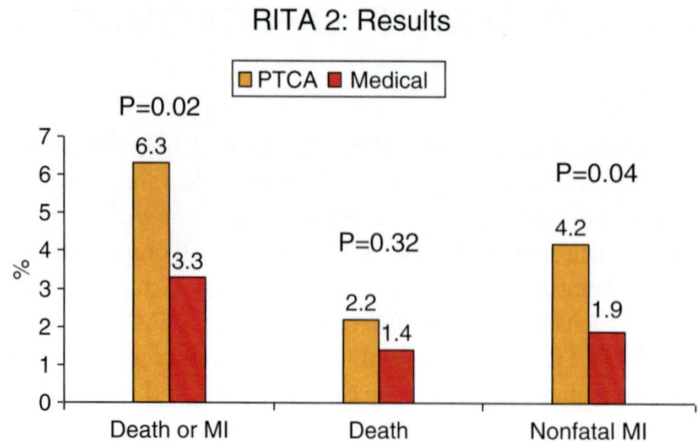

FIGURE 18.44 RITA-2 trial. Coronary angioplasty versus medical therapy for angina: the second Randomized Intervention Treatment of Angina (RITA-2). RITA-2 was a randomized trial comparing the long-term effects of PTCA and conservative (medical) care in patients with coronary artery disease considered suitable for either treatment option. 504 patients were randomized to PTCA and 514 patients were randomized to medical treatment with antianginal drugs. The primary endpoint was the combined frequency of death from all causes and definite nonfatal myocardial infarction. Of note, in the medical group 118 patients (23.0%) underwent a revascularization during follow-up, because of worsening symptoms.[17] Data from Coronary angioplasty versus medical therapy for angina: the second Randomised Intervention Treatment of Angina (RITA-2) trial. RITA-2 trial participants. *Lancet*. 1997;350(9076):461-468.

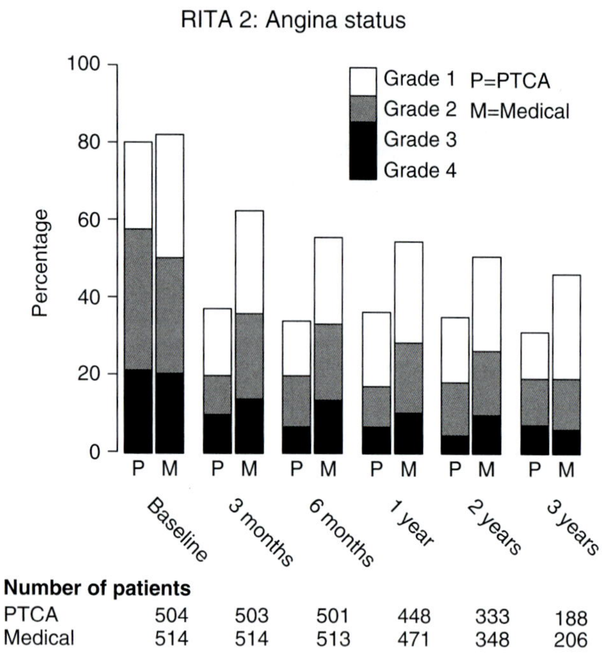

FIGURE 18.45 Angina status in the RITA 2 trial. Reprinted with permission from Coronary angioplasty vs medical therapy for angina: the second Randomised Intervention Treatment of Angina (RITA-2) trial. RITA-2 trial participants. *Lancet*. 1997;350(9076):461-468.

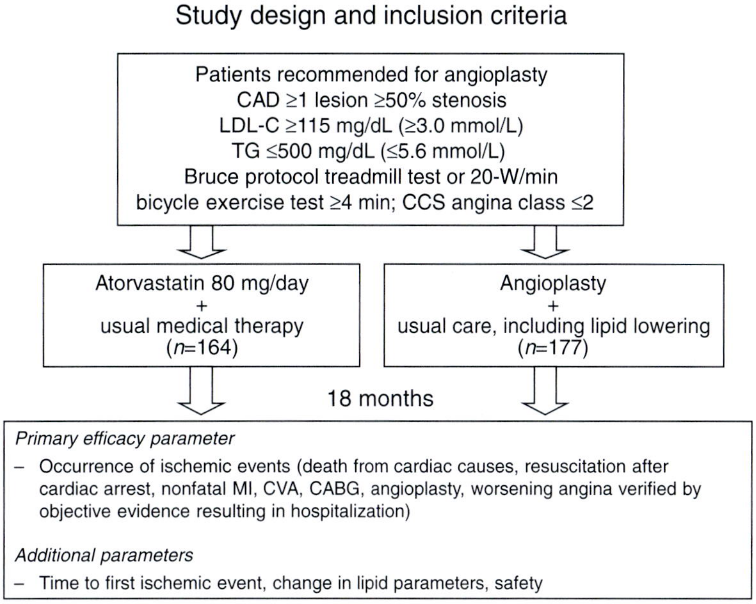

FIGURE 18.46 AVERT trial. The Atorvastatin versus Revascularization Treatment (AVERT) trial compared the efficacy of aggressive lipid-lowering therapy versus PTCA in low-risk, stable patients with coronary artery disease.[16] Data from Pitt B, Waters D, Brown WV, et al. Aggressive lipid-lowering therapy compared with angioplasty in stable coronary artery disease. Atorvastatin versus Revascularization Treatment Investigators. *N Engl J Med*. 1999;341(2):70-76.

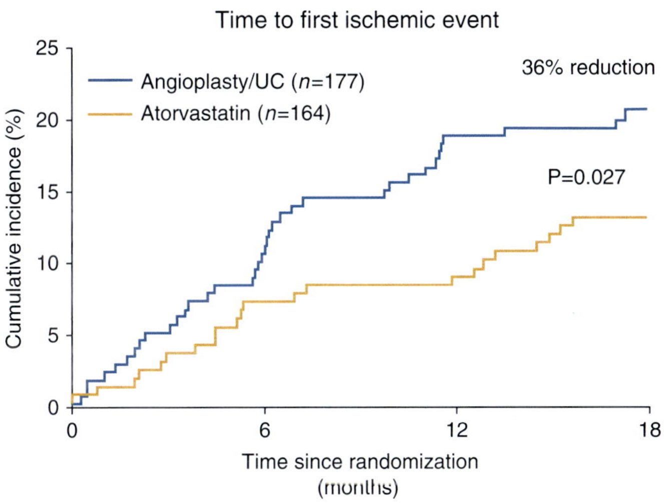

FIGURE 18.47 AVERT trial study results. Reprinted with permission from Pitt B, Waters D, Brown WV, et al. Aggressive lipid-lowering therapy compared with angioplasty in stable coronary artery disease. Atorvastatin versus Revascularization Treatment Investigators. *N Engl J Med*. 1999;341(2):70-76.

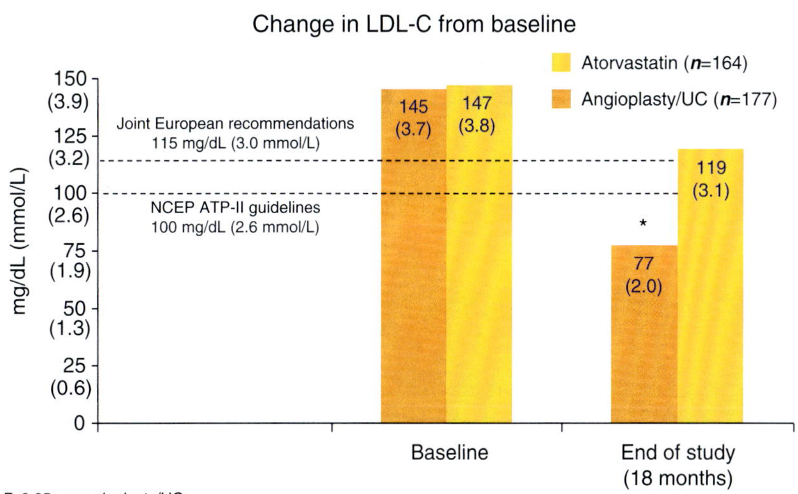

* *P*<0.05 *vs* angioplasty/UC
At randomization, 26% and 19% of patients were taking lipid-lowering medication in the atorvastatin 80 mg/day and angioplasty/UC arms, respectively. 73% of the angioplasty/UC patients were on lipid-lowering therapy at some time during the study.

FIGURE 18.48 Change in LDL-cholesterol in the AVERT trial. Adapted from Pitt B, Waters D, Brown WV, et al. Aggressive lipid-lowering therapy compared with angioplasty in stable coronary artery disease. Atorvastatin versus Revascularization Treatment Investigators. *N Engl J Med*. 1999; 341(2):70-76.

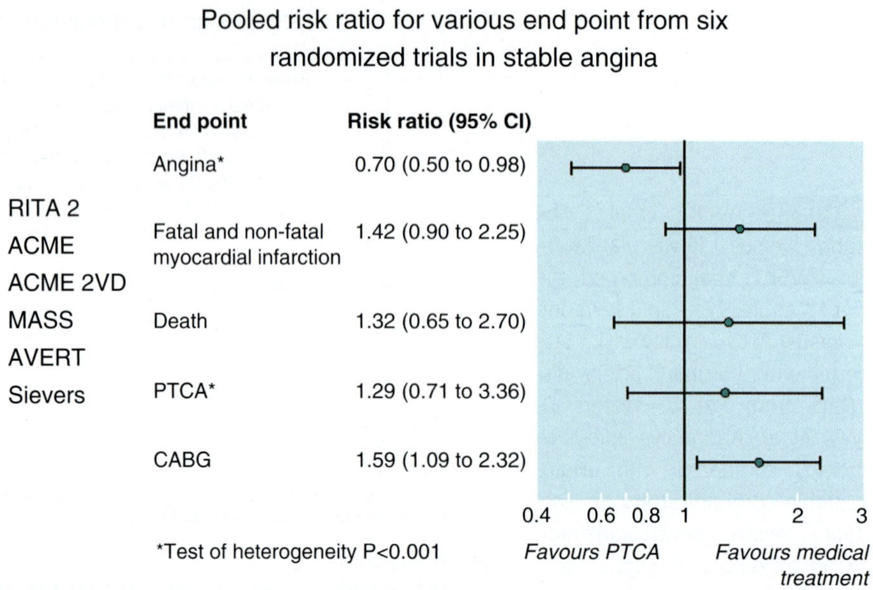

FIGURE 18.49 Pooled risk ratio for various endpoints from 6 randomized trials in stable angina. Reprinted with permission from Bucher HC, Hengstler P, Schindler C, Guyatt GH. Percutaneous transluminal coronary angioplasty vs medical treatment for non-acute coronary heart disease: meta-analysis of randomised controlled trials. *BMJ*. 2000;321(7253):73-77.

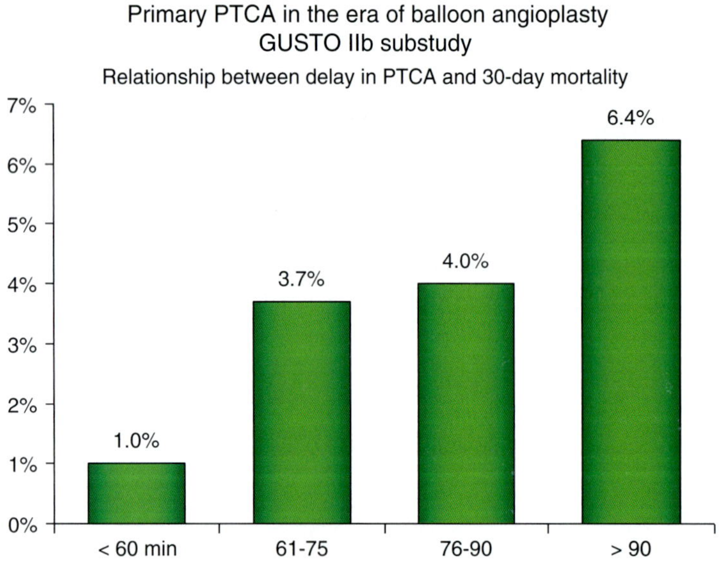

FIGURE 18.50 Gusto II-b substudy. The GUSTO II-b substudy evaluated the role of primary PTCA in the management of patients with STEMI. In addition to showing the benefit of balloon angioplasty when compared with thrombolytic therapy, the GUSTO II-b was the first study to show the important relationship between door to balloon time and mortality in STEMI.

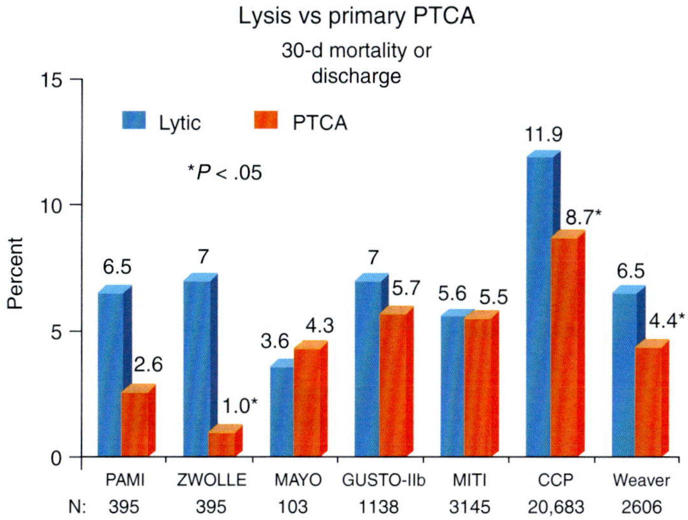

FIGURE 18.51 Thirty-day mortality in clinical trials and a large registry analysis comparing PTCA with thrombolysis in the management of STEMI. Reprinted with permission from Herrmann HC. Triple therapy for acute myocardial infarction: combining fibrinolysis, platelet IIb/IIIa inhibition, and percutaneous coronary intervention. *Am J Cardiol*. 2000;85(8A):10C-16C.

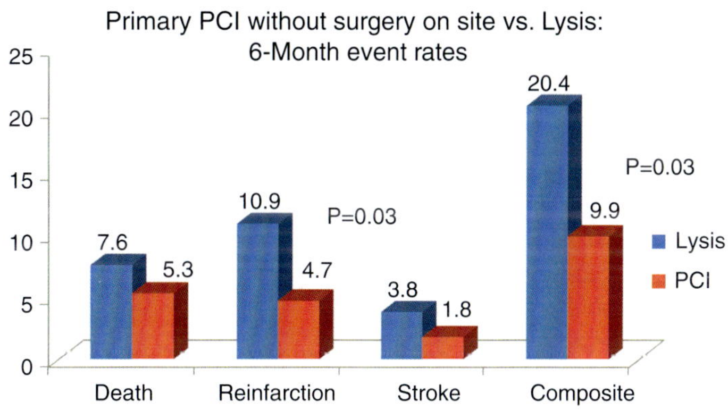

FIGURE 18.52 C-PORT clinical trial. The C-PORT study evaluated the role of PCI in the management of STEMI in hospital without surgical backup on-site. The benefit of PCI observed in the C-PORT trial has led to the introduction of primary PCI in centers without surgical backup on-site.[23] Data from Aversano T, Aversano LT, Passamani E, et al. Thrombolytic therapy vs primary percutaneous coronary intervention for myocardial infarction in patients presenting to hospitals without on-site cardiac surgery: a randomized controlled trial. *JAMA*. 2002;287(15):1943-1951.

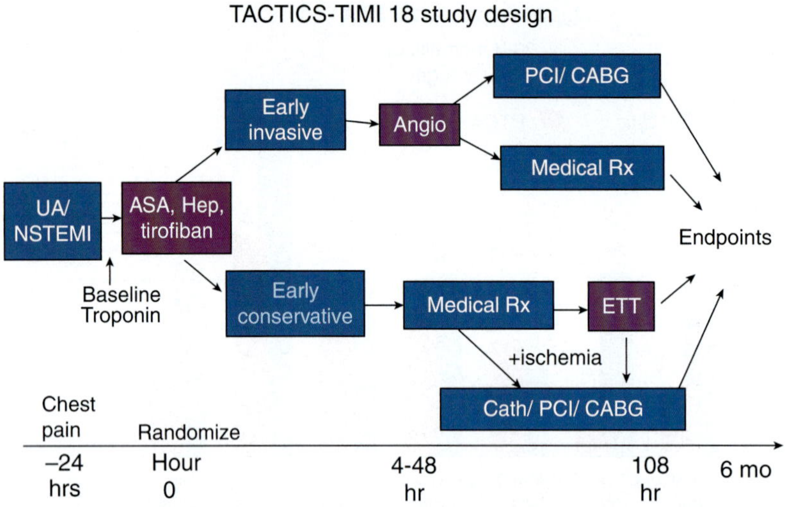

FIGURE 18.53 TACTICS-TIMI 18 study design. The TACTICS-TIMI 18 study compared an early invasive approach with a conservative approach in patients admitted with acute coronary syndromes. Reprinted with permission from Cannon CP, Weintraub WS, Demopoulos LA, Robertson DH, Gormley GJ, Braunwald E. Invasive vs conservative strategies in unstable angina and non-Q-wave myocardial infarction following treatment with tirofiban: rationale and study design of the international TACTICS-TIMI 18 Trial. Treat Angina with Aggrastat and determine Cost of Therapy with an Invasive or Conservative Strategy. Thrombolysis in Myocardial Infarction. *Am J Cardiol*. 1998;82(6):731-736.

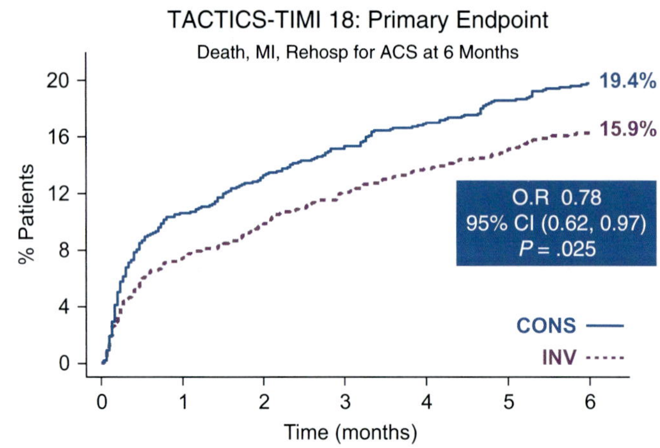

FIGURE 18.54 TACTICS-TIMI 18 primary endpoint. There was a clear benefit from an early invasive approach when compared with a conservative approach. Reprinted with permission from Cannon CP, Weintraub WS, Demopoulos LA, et al. Comparison of early invasive and conservative strategies in patients with unstable coronary syndromes treated with the glycoprotein IIb/IIIa inhibitor tirofiban. *N Engl J Med*. 2001;344(25):1879-1887.

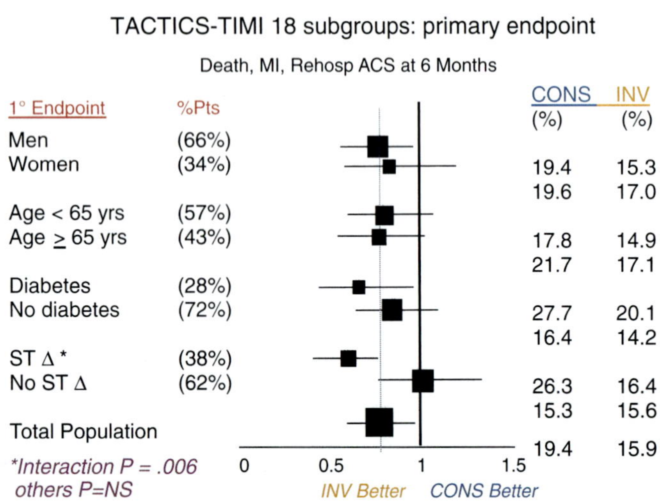

FIGURE 18.55 Subgroups analysis of the TACTICS-TIMI 18 clinical trial. Reprinted with permission from Cannon CP, Weintraub WS, Demopoulos LA, et al. Comparison of early invasive and conservative strategies in patients with unstable coronary syndromes treated with the glycoprotein IIb/IIIa inhibitor tirofiban. *N Engl J Med*. 2001;344(25):1879-1887.

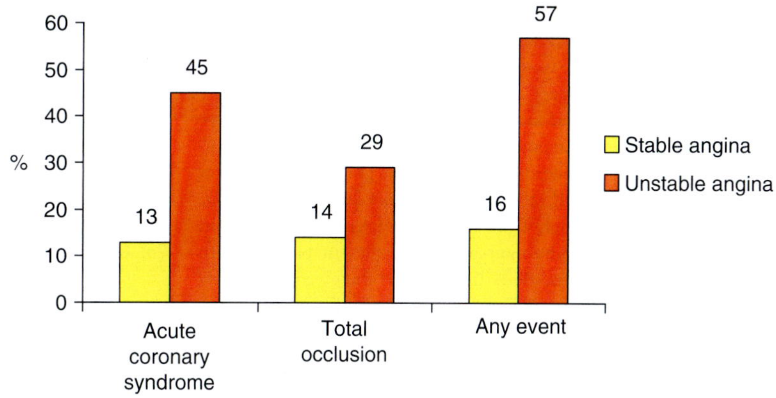

FIGURE 18.56 Waiting time for PTCA and adverse events stratified by unstable and stable angina.[26] Data from Chester M, Chen L, Kaski JC. Identification of patients at high risk for adverse coronary events while awaiting routine coronary angioplasty. *Br Heart J*. 1995;73(3):216-222.

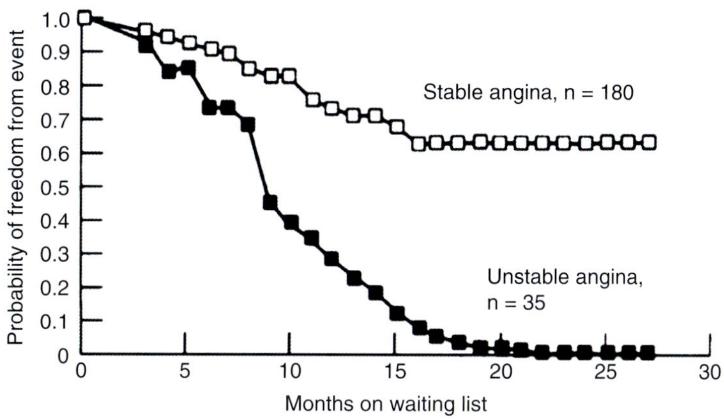

FIGURE 18.57 Waiting time for PTCA. Probability of freedom from events and waiting time in patients with stable angina and unstable angina. Reprinted with permission from Chester M, Chen L, Kaski JC. Identification of patients at high risk for adverse coronary events while awaiting routine coronary angioplasty. *Br Heart J*. 1995;73(3):216-222.

REFERENCES

1. Dotter CT, Judkins MP. Transluminal treatment of arteriosclerotic obstruction. Description of a new technic and a preliminary report of its application. *Circulation*. 1964;30:654-670.
2. King SB III. Angioplasty from bench to bedside to bench. *Circulation*. 1996;93(9):1621-1629.
3. Gruntzig A. Transluminal dilatation of coronary-artery stenosis. *Lancet*. 1978;1(8058):263.
4. Gruntzig AR, Senning A, Siegenthaler WE. Nonoperative dilatation of coronary-artery stenosis: percutaneous transluminal coronary angioplasty. *N Engl J Med*. 1979;301(2):61-68.
5. Roubin GS, King SB III, Douglas JS Jr, Lembo NJ, Robinson KA. Intracoronary stenting during percutaneous transluminal coronary angioplasty. *Circulation*. 1990;81(3 suppl):IV92-100.
6. George BS, Voorhees WD III, Roubin GS, et al. Multicenter investigation of coronary stenting to treat acute or threatened closure after percutaneous transluminal coronary angioplasty: clinical and angiographic outcomes. *J Am Coll Cardiol*. 1993;22(1):135-143.
7. Emanuelsson H, van der Giessen WJ, Serruys PW. Benestent II: back to the future. *J Intervent Cardiol*. 1994;7(6):587-592.
8. Serruys PW, de Jaegere P, Kiemeneij F, et al. A comparison of balloon-expandable-stent implantation with balloon angioplasty in patients with coronary artery disease. Benestent Study Group. *N Engl J Med*. 1994;331(8):489-495.
9. Tenaglia AN, Buller CE, Kisslo KB, Stack RS, Davidson CJ. Mechanisms of balloon angioplasty and directional coronary atherectomy as assessed by intracoronary ultrasound. *J Am Coll Cardiol*. 1992;20(3):685-691.
10. Saito S. Different strategies of retrograde approach in coronary angioplasty for chronic total occlusion. *Cathet Cardiovasc Interv*. 2008;71(1):8-19.
11. Muramatsu T, Tsukahara R, Ito Y. "Rendezvous in coronary" technique with the retrograde approach for chronic total occlusion. *J Invasive Cardiol*. 2010;22(9):E179-E182.
12. Muramatsu T, Tsukahara R, Ito Y, et al. Changing strategies of the retrograde approach for chronic total occlusion during the past 7 years. *Cathet Cardiovasc Interv*. 2013;81(4):E178-E185.
13. Vo M, Brilakis ES. Faster, easier, safer: "guideliner reverse CART" for retrograde chronic total occlusion interventions. *Cathet Cardiovasc Interv*. 2014;83(6):933-935.
14. Vetrovec GW. Chronic total occlusion PCI: is this the ultimate test of the importance of complete revascularization? *JACC Cardiovasc Interv*. 2016;9(6):539-540.
15. Parisi AF, Folland ED, Hartigan P. A comparison of angioplasty with medical therapy in the treatment of single-vessel coronary artery disease. Veterans Affairs ACME Investigators. *N Engl J Med*. 1992;326(1):10-16.
16. Pitt B, Waters D, Brown WV, et al. Aggressive lipid-lowering therapy compared with angioplasty in stable coronary artery disease. Atorvastatin versus Revascularization Treatment Investigators. *N Engl J Med*. 1999;341(2):70-76.
17. Coronary angioplasty versus medical therapy for angina: the second Randomised Intervention Treatment of Angina (RITA-2) trial. RITA-2 trial participants. *Lancet*. 1997;350(9076):461-468.

18. WW OO, de Boer MJ, Gibbons RJ, et al. Lessons from the pooled outcome of the PAMI, ZWOLLE and Mayo clinic randomized trials of primary angioplasty versus thrombolytic therapy of acute myocardial infarction. *J Invasive Cardiol.* 1998;10(suppl A):4A-10A.
19. Kugelmass AD, Sadanandan S, Lakkis N, et al. Early invasive strategy improves outcomes in patients with acute coronary syndrome with previous coronary artery bypass graft surgery: a report from TACTICS-TIMI 18. *Crit Pathw Cardiol.* 2006;5(3):167-172.
20. Cannon CP, Weintraub WS, Demopoulos LA, et al. Comparison of early invasive and conservative strategies in patients with unstable coronary syndromes treated with the glycoprotein IIb/IIIa inhibitor tirofiban. *N Engl J Med.* 2001;344(25):1879-1887.
21. Herrmann HC. Triple therapy for acute myocardial infarction: combining fibrinolysis, platelet IIb/IIIa inhibition, and percutaneous coronary intervention. *Am J Cardiol.* 2000;85(8A): 10C-16C.
22. Stone GW, Grines CL, Browne KF, et al. Predictors of in-hospital and 6-month outcome after acute myocardial infarction in the reperfusion era: the Primary Angioplasty in Myocardial Infarction (PAMI) trail. *J Am Coll Cardiol.* 1995;25(2):370-377.
23. Aversano T, Aversano LT, Passamani E, et al. Thrombolytic therapy vs primary percutaneous coronary intervention for myocardial infarction in patients presenting to hospitals without on-site cardiac surgery: a randomized controlled trial. *JAMA.* 2002;287(15):1943-1951.
24. Bucher HC, Hengstler P, Schindler C, Guyatt GH. Percutaneous transluminal coronary angioplasty versus medical treatment for non-acute coronary heart disease: meta-analysis of randomised controlled trials. *BMJ.* 2000;321(7253):73-77.
25. Cannon CP, Weintraub WS, Demopoulos LA, Robertson DH, Gormley GJ, Braunwald E. Invasive versus conservative strategies in unstable angina and non-Q-wave myocardial infarction following treatment with tirofiban: rationale and study design of the international TACTICS-TIMI 18 Trial. Treat Angina with Aggrastat and determine Cost of Therapy with an Invasive or Conservative Strategy. Thrombolysis in Myocardial Infarction. *Am J Cardiol.* 1998;82(6):731-736.
26. Chester M, Chen L, Kaski JC. Identification of patients at high risk for adverse coronary events while awaiting routine coronary angioplasty. *Br Heart J.* 1995;73(3):216-222.

chapter **19**

Atherectomy, Thrombectomy, and Distal Protection Devices

KARIM M. AL-AZIZI, MD and AARON KUGELMASS, MD

ATHERECTOMY, THROMBECTOMY, AND DISTAL PROTECTION DEVICES

Coronary artery disease is traditionally treated using balloon angioplasty and stenting. However, as the complexity of the disease increases, additional equipment may be needed to ensure success and minimize complications. This may include lesion modification, thrombus removal, or trapping lesion debris produced during the intervention to prevent distal embolization (**FIGURE 19.1**).

Atherectomy

Atherectomy has been a growing technique and is used primarily for lesion modification and debulking to improve stent delivery and expansion. The following section outlines the different atherectomy devices and techniques available with cases (**FIGURES 19.2-19.11**).

Thrombectomy

Myocardial infarction is most often the result of plaque rupture and subsequent intracoronary thrombus formation. Attempting percutaneous coronary intervention (PCI) on vessels with large thrombi has been associated with embolization, no-reflow phenomenon, and abrupt vessel closure. The following section outlines available thrombectomy techniques (**FIGURES 19.12-19.15**).

Embolic Protection

During coronary interventions, fragments of plaque or thrombus may embolize into the distal circulation resulting in no reflow and increased periprocedural myocardial injury. The following section outlines the use of embolic protection devices during PCI (**FIGURES 19.16** and **19.17**).

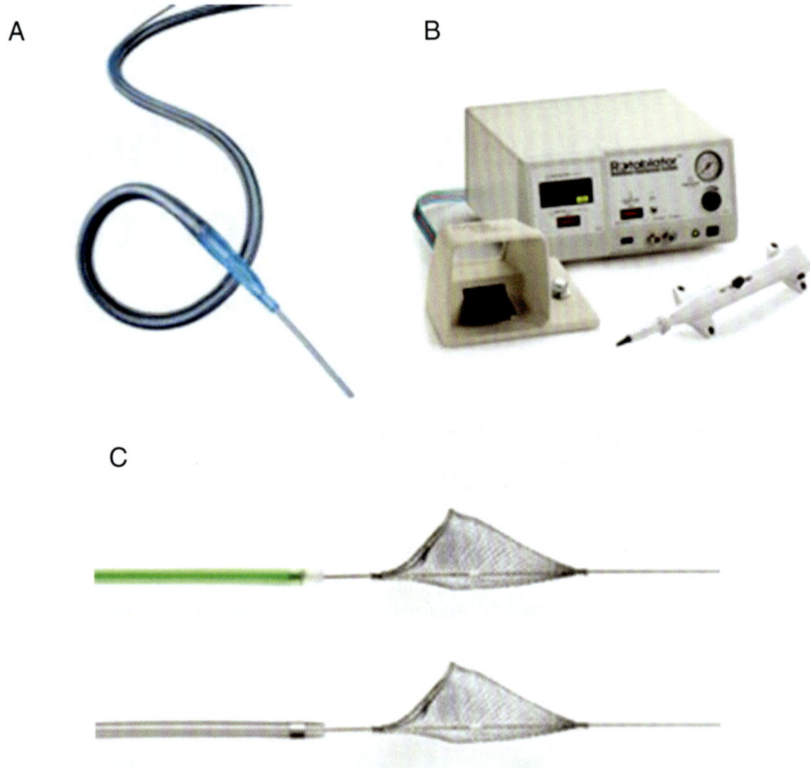

FIGURE 19.1 Atherectomy, thrombectomy, and distal protection devices. The figure illustrates the equipment that may be used in treating complex coronary artery disease. **A**, Medtronic Export AP aspiration thrombectomy catheter is seen in the left panel. **B**, Boston Scientific Rotablator System is seen in the right panel. **C**, A SpiderFX filter is seen in the bottom panel. **A and C**, Used with permission by Medtronic ©2018; **B**, Image provided courtesy of Boston Scientific. ©2018 Boston Scientific Corporation or its affiliates. All rights reserved.

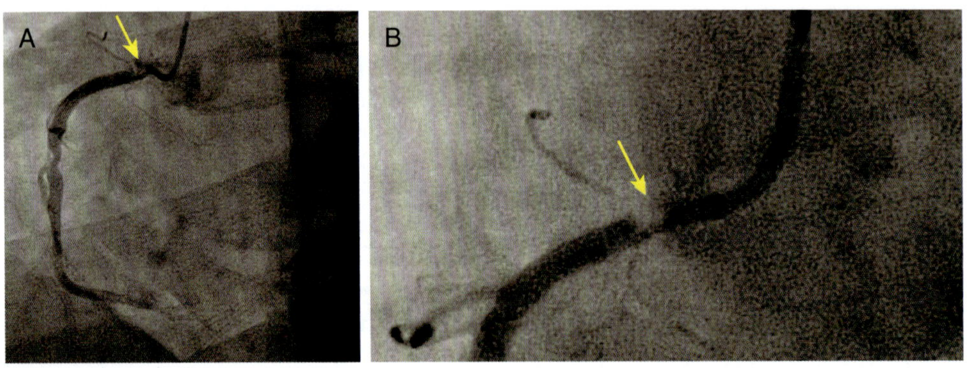

FIGURE 19.2 **A and B**, Calcified coronary lesions. This figure illustrates significant coronary calcification (arrow) that can be encountered during cardiac catheterization and PCI. Atherectomy can modify the arterial wall compliance in heavily calcified vessels. This is accomplished both by plaque removal and micro fracturing of the vessel calcification. The net result is improved stent delivery and expansion.[1]

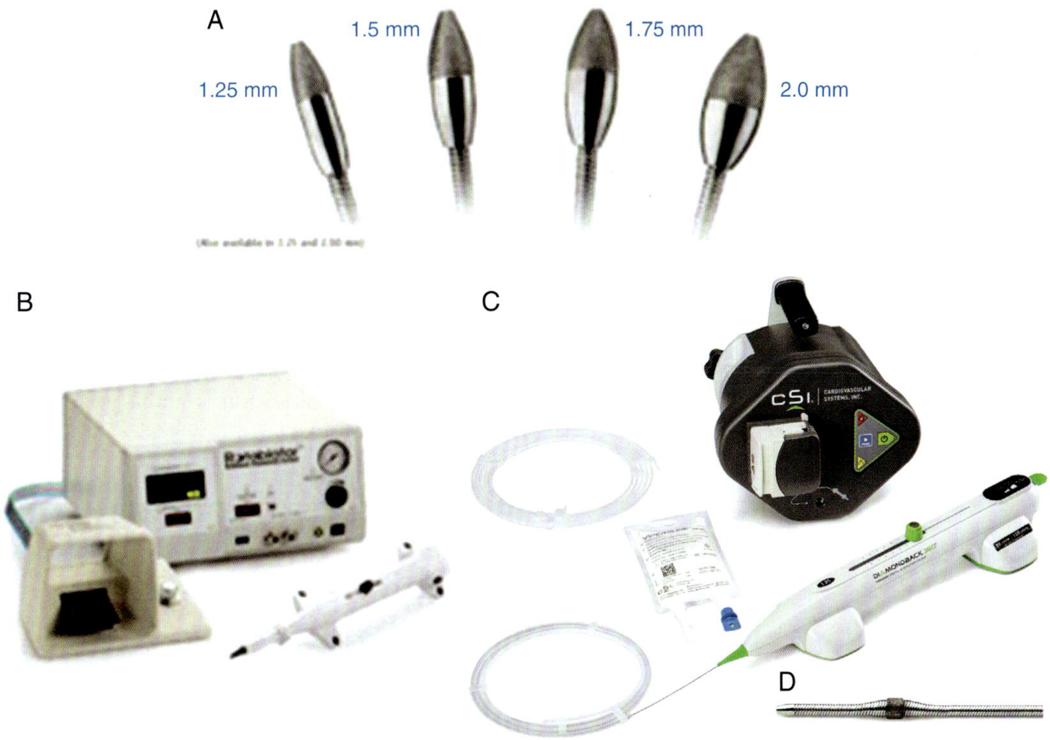

FIGURE 19.3 Types of atherectomy devices and device characteristics. Atherectomy is indicated to facilitate stent delivery and improve stent expansion in patients with coronary artery disease who are acceptable candidates for coronary stenting owing to de novo, severely calcified coronary lesions. There are currently 2 types of atherectomy devices used in coronary interventions. **A and B**, The Boston Scientific Rotablator, which functions as rotational atherectomy. **C and D**, The Cardiovascular Systems, INC (CSI) Diamondback 360 is another device, which is a coronary orbital atherectomy system (seen in the bottom panel). These systems have a different atherotome shapes and drive systems. The Boston Scientific RotaLink catheter consists of an elliptical, nickel-coated burr, with a distal surface embedded with 20 μm diamond chips, protruding 5 μm from the surface. The CSI Diamondback device consists of a diamond-coated 1.25 mm crown, mounted on an asymmetric platform. **A and B**. Image provided courtesy of Boston Scientific. ©2018 Boston Scientific Corporation or its affiliates. All rights reserved; **C and D**. ©2018 Cardiovascular Systems, Inc. CSI®, Diamondback 360®, GlideAssist®, ViperWire Advance® and ViperSlide® are registered trademarks of Cardiovascular Systems, Inc., and used with permission.

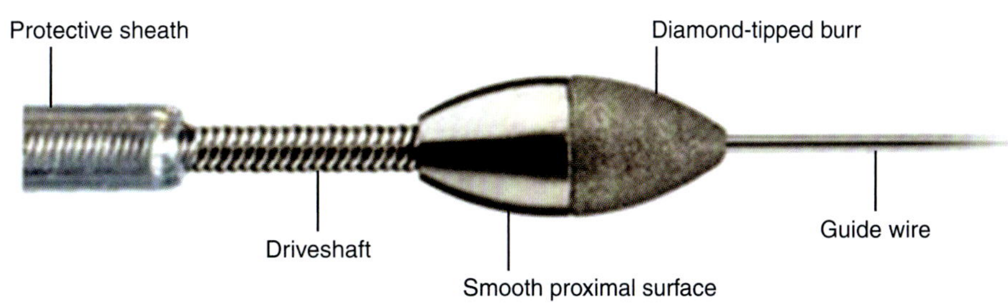

FIGURE 19.4 Rotational atherectomy. Rotablator system burr mounted on a drive shaft and sheath. The burr size is usually selected based on a vessel to burr ratio of approximately 0.7, as demonstrated in the CARAT study (Coronary Angioplasty and Rotablator Atherectomy Trial).[2] In that study, there were higher rates of acute complications if higher burr to artery ratios were used, with no clear benefit or change in target vessel revascularization.

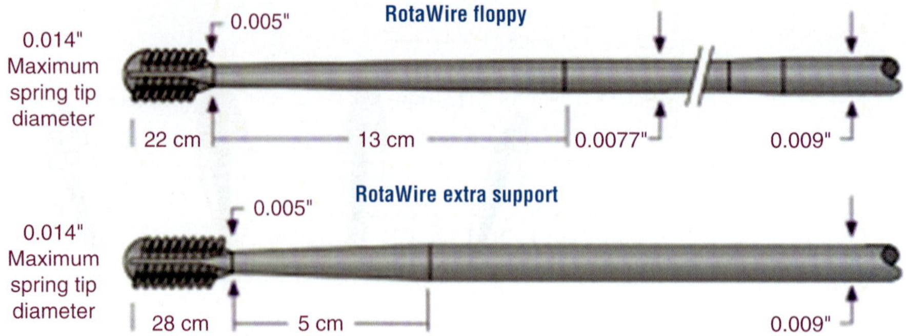

FIGURE 19.5 Rotational atherectomy. The RotaWires are designed specifically for the use with the rotational atherectomy system. They are made of a 0.009" stainless steel core with tapered distal ends for varying degrees of burr support. A 0.014" distal platinum coil prevents the burr from traveling beyond the tip of the wire. Image provided courtesy of Boston Scientific. ©2018 Boston Scientific Corporation or its affiliates. All rights reserved.

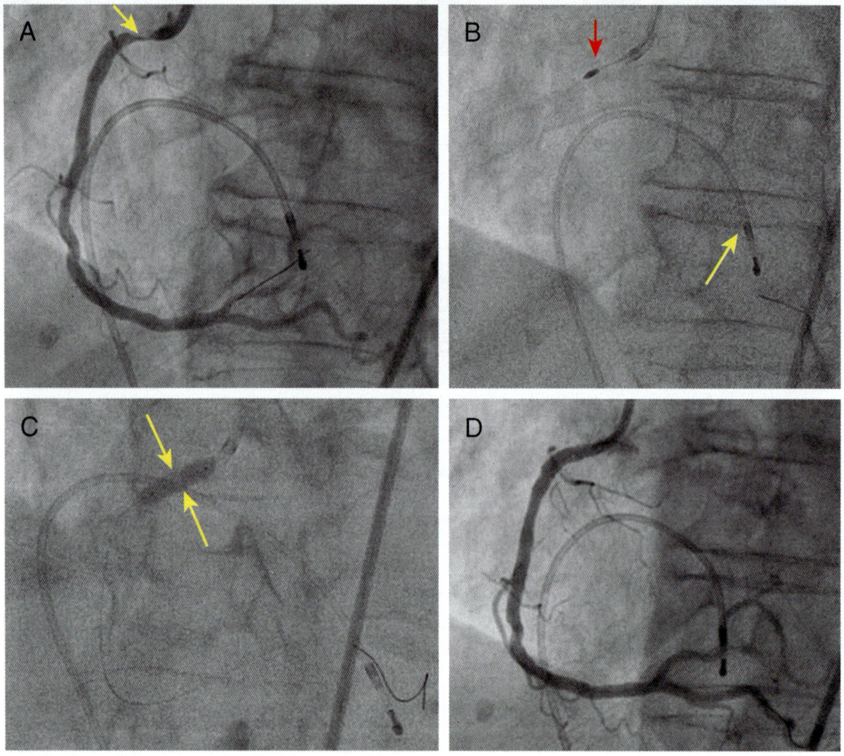

FIGURE 19.6 **A**, Rotational atherectomy in ostial right coronary artery (RCA) lesions. Rotational atherectomy is used to treat heavily calcified lesions, provided the vessel is of adequate size and without significant tortuosity. At times, calcified lesions may be ostial. Depending on the degree of stenosis, size of index vessel and location and intensity of the calcification, different burr sizes may be selected to prepare and treat the lesion. The figure shows a heavily calcified ostial and proximal RCA lesion (arrow). On engaging the artery for angiography, there was significant pressure dampening. **B**, Rotational atherectomy of ostial RCA stenosis. The decision was made to proceed with rotational atherectomy to treat the heavily calcified lesion shown in **Figure 19.6A**. Utilizing a 7 FR Judkins Right 4.0 guiding catheter, the lesion was wired with a BMW (Balance middle weight) guide wire, which was then exchanged for a RotaWire in the distal vessel. A 1.7 mm burr (red arrow) was used to treat the lesion. A venous temporary pacer wire (yellow arrow) was inserted. In many cases, rotational atherectomy of the RCA may be complicated by significant bradycardia and heart block. During this case, the patient developed transient heart block requiring temporary pacing. **C**, Stent deployment postatherectomy. Following atherectomy, the vessel underwent angioplasty and stenting with a 4.0 × 15 mm drug-eluting stent, with no evidence of "waist" in the stent balloon (yellow arrows), at the lesion. **D**, Final result after atherectomy and stenting.

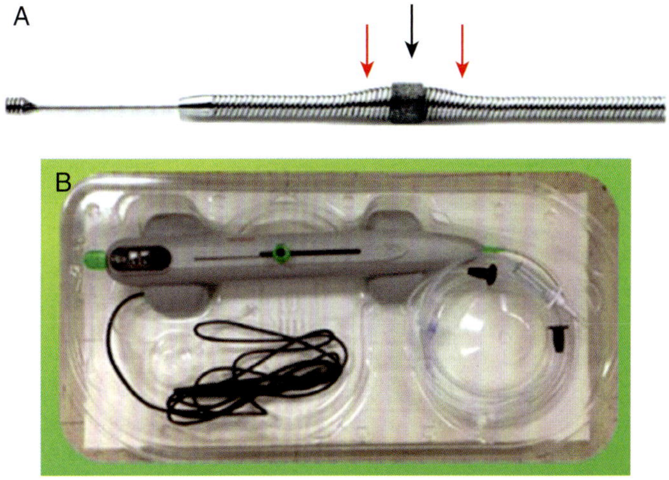

FIGURE 19.7 **A and B**, The orbital atherectomy system. The diamondback 360 Coronary system is an atherectomy system that treats the vessel in an orbital fashion. It is an over-the-wire system, which uses a 0.012″ core guide wire with a 0.014″ spring tip; the ViperWire. The device has a bullet tip bushing followed by a long tip designed to reduce wire bias. The crown (black arrow) is in between a crown-lead-in and crown-lead-out segments (red arrows), which helps the crown track in and out of lesions smoothly. The device operates based on the idea of differential sanding, acting on calcified segments of the artery and not the healthier segments. The system is lubricated with a continuous flow of the ViperSlide solution (emulsion composed of soybean oil, egg yolk phospholipids, glycerin, and water for injection) through the catheter tip. The device exerts its force in a centrifugal manner. The faster the crown orbits the vessel circumferentially, the larger the force it exerts against the vessel wall. The faster speed is typically used to treat larger vessels. ©2018 Cardiovascular Systems, Inc. CSI®, Diamondback 360®, GlideAssist®, ViperWire Advance® and ViperSlide® are registered trademarks of Cardiovascular Systems, Inc., and used with permission.

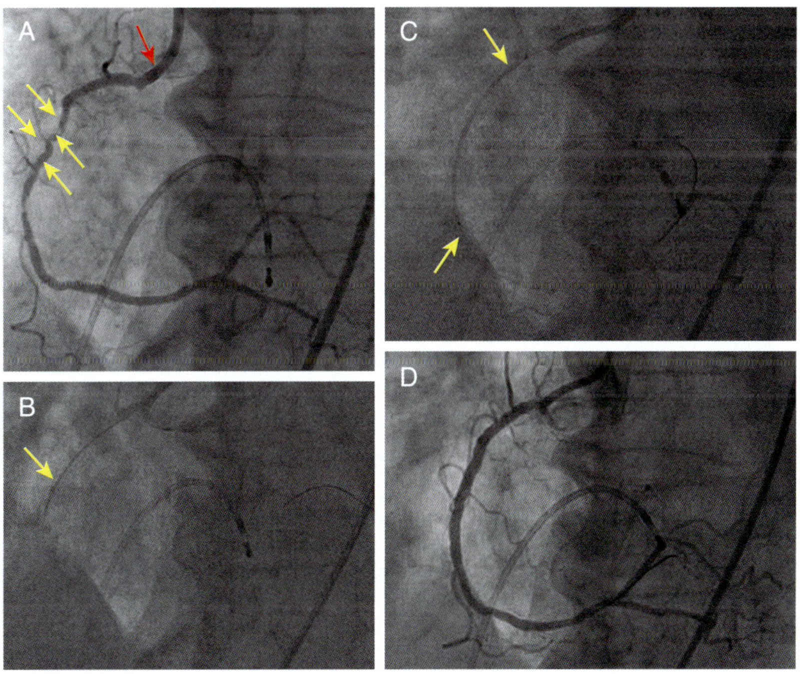

FIGURE 19.8 **A**, Orbital atherectomy of RCA stenosis. This figure demonstrates a long, heavily calcified lesion in the proximal to mid-RCA (yellow arrows). Using a 7 FR Judkins Right 4.0 guiding catheter (red arrow), the lesion was crossed with a regular guide wire. The guide wire was then exchanged for a ViperWire. A temporary pacer wire was inserted in the right ventricle. Treating long lesions requires short, multiple runs. Unlike rotational atherectomy, with orbital atherectomy the vessel is treated bidirectionally as the crown traverses the lesion. **B**, The crown and the artery. In this figure, the crown (yellow arrow) was advanced in the vessel, and atherectomy was initiated to treat the diseased segment. **C**, Stenting after orbital atherectomy. Following atherectomy, a 38 mm long, drug-eluting stent (yellow arrows) was passed into the artery without difficulty. **D**, Final results poststenting. Final angiographic result after angioplasty and stenting with a 3.0 mm × 38 mm drug-eluting stent.

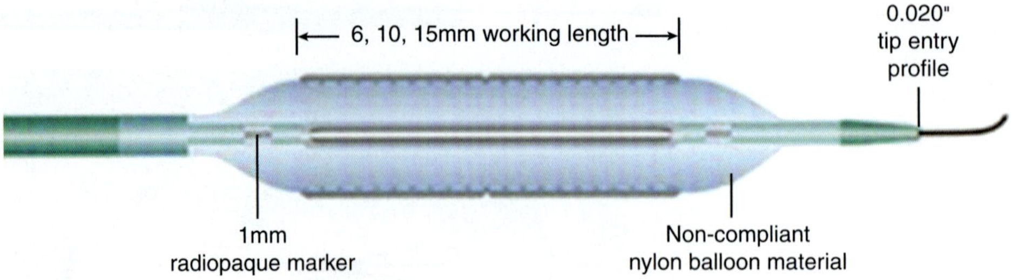

FIGURE 19.9 Cutting balloon angioplasty. Other forms of plaque modification include the cutting balloons. They consist of a noncompliant rigid balloon with multiple long microtomes mounted on it. The microtomes are designed to provide longitudinal incisions in the lesion during inflation of the balloon, thereby causing lesion modification. The Boston Scientific Flextome is seen in this figure. Image provided courtesy of Boston Scientific. ©2018 Boston Scientific Corporation or its affiliates. All rights reserved.

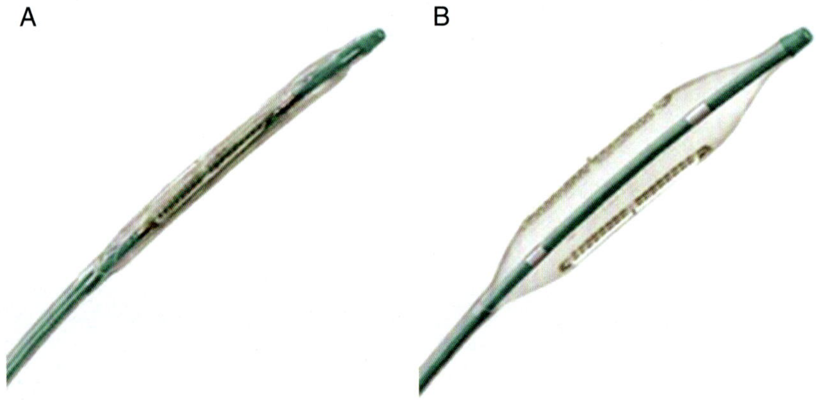

FIGURE 19.10 **A and B**, Cutting balloon angioplasty. With conventional balloon angioplasty, stretching of the vessel occurs with plaque fracture and dissection. This process can also lead to uncontrolled dissections and is associated with significant recoil. In theory, with cutting balloons, similar but more effective plaque modification is achieved at lower balloon pressure, hence reducing the barotrauma and dissection. This was demonstrated in the REDUCE (Restenosis Reduction by Cutting Balloon Evaluation) study,[3] which compared cutting balloon angioplasty with conventional angioplasty and showed better plaque reduction with lower maximal balloon expansion pressures. Despite hypothetical therapeutic benefits, several studies have failed to show reduction in restenosis as compared with conventional balloon angioplasty.[4] Image provided courtesy of Boston Scientific. ©2018 Boston Scientific Corporation or its affiliates. All rights reserved.

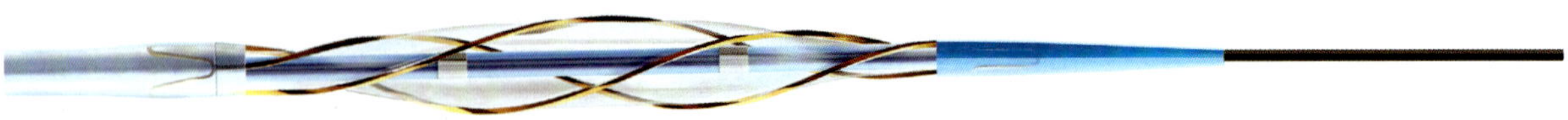

FIGURE 19.11 Scoring balloon angioplasty. The AngioSculpt Scoring Balloon Catheter (AngioScore, Inc Alameda, California) uses a semicompliant balloon, with nitinol scoring element wrapped around it. In a small, nonrandomized trial, predilatation with AngioSculpt resulted in greater stent expansion by ultrasound criteria as compared with direct stenting or predilatation with a standard semi-compliant balloon.[5] Of note, no randomized studies for coronary intervention have been performed with this device. Reproduced with the permission of Koninklijke Philips N.V. and its subsidiary, The Spectranetics Corporation. All rights reserved.

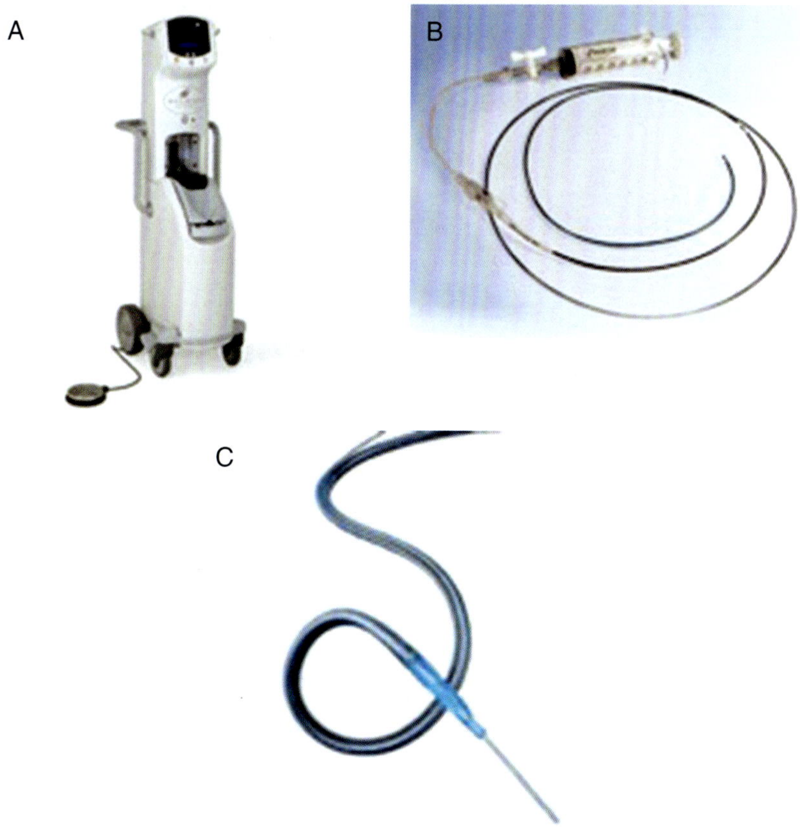

FIGURE 19.12 **A-C**, Aspiration thrombectomy. The TAPAS (Thrombus Aspiration during Percutaneous coronary intervention in Acute myocardial infarction Study)[6] and EXPIRA (Thrombectomy with Export Catheter in Infarct-Related Artery During Primary Percutaneous Coronary Intervention) trials[7] compared aspiration thrombectomy with no aspiration and showed a significant benefit and improved outcomes with aspiration. However, subsequent larger clinical trials have not demonstrated a clinical benefit with routine thrombectomy.[8] This figure illustrates available devices that may be used to remove thrombus from coronary arteries and vein grafts. From left to right: Angiojet, Pronto Catheter, and Export aspiration catheter. **A**, Image provided courtesy of Boston Scientific. ©2018 Boston Scientific Corporation or its affiliates. All rights reserved; **B**, Image courtesy of Teleflex Incorporated. © 2018 Teleflex Incorporated. All rights reserved; **C**, Used with permission by Medtronic ©2018.

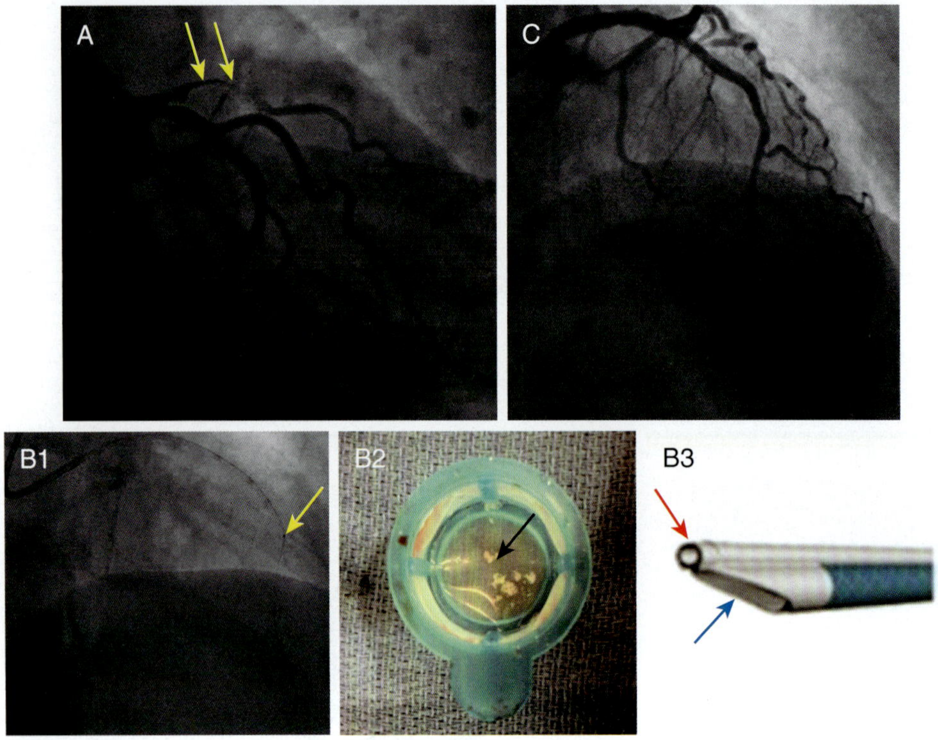

FIGURE 19.13 **A**, Manual aspiration thrombectomy in STEMI (ST segment elevation myocardial infarction) patients. Initial angiogram of a 55-year-old gentleman presenting with anterior ST elevation myocardial infarction. There is significant thrombus at the site of the lesion (yellow arrows). **B1 and 2**, Manual aspiration thrombectomy with the Export AP catheter. This figure illustrates the use of the Medtronic Export AP catheter (yellow arrow). The lower left panel shows white thrombus (black arrow) aspirated with the catheter (black arrow). **B3**, The Export AP catheter (right lower panel) consists of 2 lumens, a smaller lumen for the coronary guide wire (red arrow) and a larger lumen for aspiration (blue arrow). **C**, Final angiography. The figure illustrates the final result following manual aspiration thrombectomy, balloon angioplasty, and stenting. **B3**, Used with permission by Medtronic ©2018.

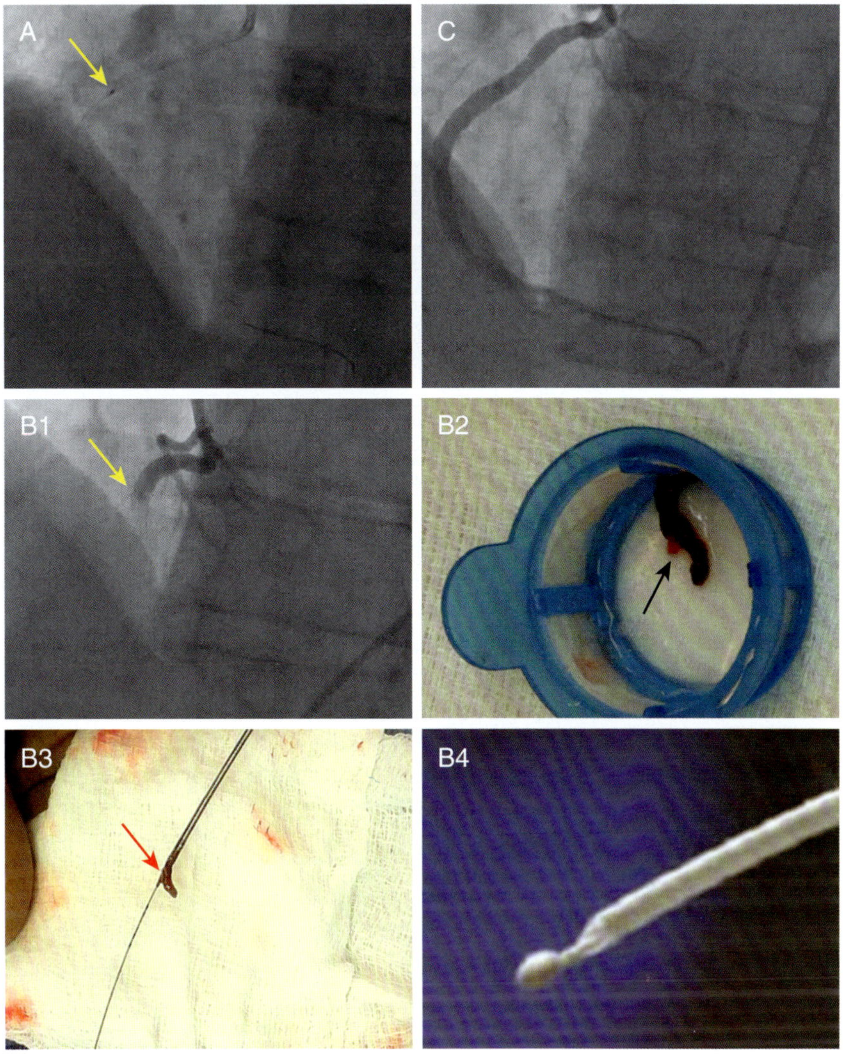

FIGURE 19.14 **A**, Pronto Export device for aspiration. RCA angiography in a 69-year-old male presenting with an inferior ST elevation myocardial infarction. The angiographic appearance is highly suggestive of a large amount of thrombus in the proximal RCA (yellow arrow). **B**, Pronto Export device for aspiration. The Pronto aspiration catheter (yellow arrow) is seen in the RCA **(1)**. A significant amount of red thrombus was aspirated **(2)**. Residual thrombus was identified on the catheter tip when the catheter was removed from the body (red arrow, **3**). The presence of residual thrombus on the catheter tip increases the risk of stroke after aspiration, as demonstrated in the TOTAL (The Trial of Routine Aspiration Thrombectomy with PCI versus PCI Alone in Patients with STEMI) trial.[8] Thus, it is important to maintain negative suction and let the Tuohy valve to back bleed during device retrieval. The Pronto catheter is a dual lumen catheter, with a smaller lumen for the coronary guiding wire and a larger lumen for aspiration **(4)**. **C**, Final angiographic result. Final angiographic result following aspiration thrombectomy, balloon angioplasty, and stenting with a 4.0 × 18 mm bare metal stent.

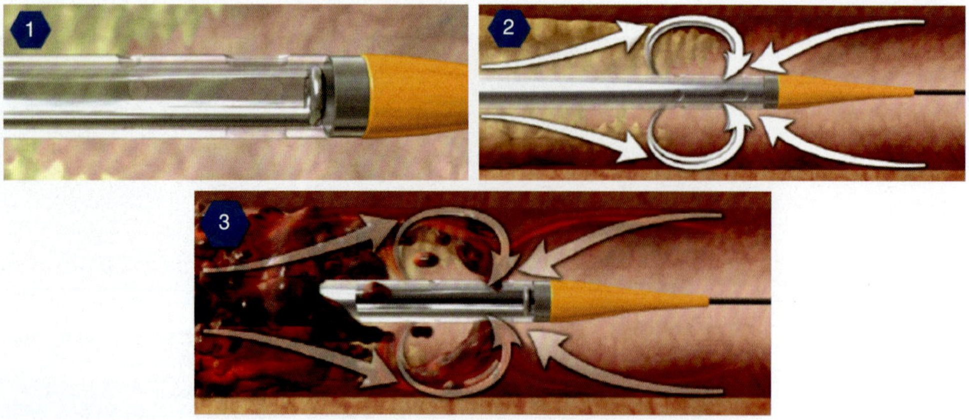

FIGURE 19.15 Angiojet. The AngioJet® (Boston Scientific) **(1)** system operates on the basis of the Bernoulli/Venturi **(2)** effect. On device activation, saline jets travel backward at high speed to create a negative pressure zone (less than -600 mm Hg) causing a powerful vacuum effect. Cross-Stream windows optimize the fluid flow for more effective thrombus removal. Thrombus is drawn into the catheter where it is fragmented by the jets **(3)** and evacuated from the body. In the VEGAS-2 (the Vein Graft AngioJet Study),[9] safety and efficacy of the AngioJet device was compared with intracoronary urokinase with benefit with AngioJet. In the JETSTENT (AngioJet Rheolytic Thrombectomy Before Direct Infarct Artery Stenting in Patients Undergoing Primary PCI for Acute Myocardial Infarction) trial,[10] when compared with usual care, the use of AngioJet in patients with STEMI was associated with better ST elevation resolution, lower mace rate at 6 months, and improved 1-year survival. Conversely, in the AIMI (AngioJet Rheolytic Thrombectomy In Patients Undergoing Primary Angioplasty for Acute Myocardial Infarction) study,[11] there was no benefit in reducing final infarct size, which was higher in the AngioJet group. Image provided courtesy of Boston Scientific. ©2018 Boston Scientific Corporation or its affiliates. All rights reserved.

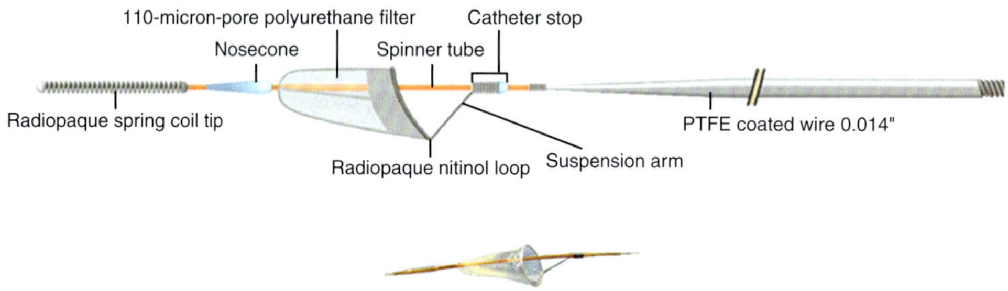

FIGURE 19.16 Embolic protection devices. Current ACC/AHA/SCAI (American College of Cardiology, American Heart Association, Society for Cardiovascular Angiography and Interventions) and ESC (Eurpoean Society of Cardiology) guidelines provide a class I recommendation for embolic protection devices' (EPD) use in saphenous vein graft (SVG) interventions based on the results of the SAFER (Saphenous vein graft Angioplasty Free of Emboli Randomized)[12] and FIRE[13] (FilterWireEX During Transluminal Intervention of Saphenous Vein Grafts) trials. Several devices have been approved for use during SVG interventions. Owing to a lack of proven benefit in native coronary interventions, they are not recommended in coronaries with high thrombus burden. The Boston Scientific FilterWire is illustrated in the figure. Image provided courtesy of Boston Scientific. ©2018 Boston Scientific Corporation or its affiliates. All rights reserved.

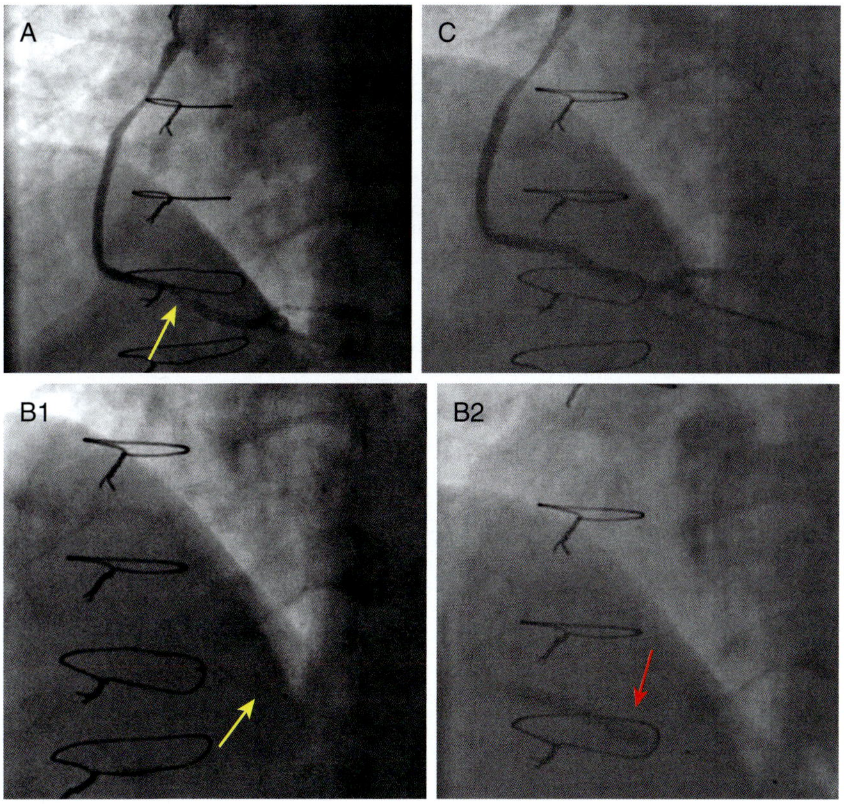

FIGURE 19.17 **A**, Distal filtration embolic protection devices. The 2 most commonly used distal embolic protection devices are the FilterWire and the SpiderFX device. The FilterWire system is a fixed wire device, with the filter net mounted on a wire. The filter is collapsed into a low-profile sheath, and it is advanced across the lesion. Sheath removal allows the filter net to expand and to approximate the vessel. As for the SpiderFX, the vessel is wired using a coronary guide wire of the operator's choice. The SpiderFX filter is inserted over the guide wire, which is then removed to deploy the filter distal to the SVG lesion and proximal to the graft anastomosis. The angiogram shows a significant lesion in the distal segment of the SVG to the RCA (yellow arrow). The vein graft was engaged with a right coronary bypass graft catheter and was wired with a coronary guide wire. Subsequently the SpiderFX device was inserted and deployed. **B1 and 2**, A SpiderFX device has been deployed distal to the lesion (yellow arrow). Following deployment of the SpiderFX device, balloon angioplasty and stenting are performed over the SpiderFX wire (Red arrow). **C**, Final angiographic result.

REFERENCES

1. Moscucci M. *Grossman & Baim's Cardiac Catheterization, Angiography, and Intervention*. 8th ed. 2013;696-670.
2. Safian RD, Feldman T, Muller DW, et al. Coronary angioplasty and Rotablator atherectomy trial (CARAT): immediate and late results of a prospective multicenter randomized trial. *Catheter Cardiovasc Interv*. 2001;53(2):213-220.
3. Bittl JA, Chew DP, Topol EJ, Kong DF, Califf RM. Meta-analysis of randomized trials of percutaneous transluminal coronary angioplasty versus atherectomy, cutting balloon atherectomy, or laser angioplasty. *J Am Coll Cardiol*. 2004;43:936-942.
4. Mauri L, Bonan R, Weiner BH, et al. Cutting balloon angioplasty for the prevention of restenosis: results of the cutting balloon global randomized trial. *Am J Cardiol*. 2002;90:1079-1083.
5. de Ribamar Costa J Jr, Mintz GS, Carlier SG, et al. Nonrandomized comparison of coronary stenting under intravascular ultrasound guidance of direct stenting without predilation versus conventional predilation with a semi-compliant balloon versus predilation with a new scoring balloon. *Am J Cardiol*. 2007;100:812-817.
6. Svilaas T, Vlaar PJ, van der Horst IC, et al. Thrombus aspiration during primary percutaneous coronary intervention. *N Engl J Med*. 2008;358:557-567.
7. Sardella G, Mancone M, Canali E, et al. Impact of thrombectomy with export catheter in infarct-related artery during primary percutaneous coronary intervention (EXPIRA trial) on cardiac death. *Am J Cardiol*. 2010;106:624-629.

8. Džavík V, for the TOTAL Investigators. Randomized trial of primary PCI with or without routine manual thrombectomy. *N Engl J Med.* 2015;372:1389-1398.
9. Kuntz RE, Baim DS, Cohen DJ, et al. A trial comparing rheolytic thrombectomy with intracoronary urokinase for coronary and vein graft thrombus (the Vein Graft AngioJet Study [VeGAS 2]). *Am J Cardiol.* 2002;89(3):326-330.
10. Migliorini A, Stabile A, Rodriguez AE, et al. Comparison of Angio-Jet rheolytic thrombectomy before direct infarct artery stenting with direct stenting alone in patients with acute myocardial infarction. The JETSTENT trial. *J Am Coll Cardiol.* 2010;56:1298-1306.
11. Ali A, Cox D, Dib N, et al. Rheolytic thrombectomy with percutaneous coronary intervention for infarct size reduction in acute myocardial infarction: 30-day results from a multicenter randomized study. *J Am Coll Cardiol.* 2006;48:244-252.
12. Baim DS, Wahr D, George B, et al. Randomized trial of a distal embolic protection device during percutaneous intervention of saphenous vein aorto-coronary bypass grafts. *Circulation.* 2002;105:1285-1290.
13. Halkin A, Masud AZ, Rogers C, et al. Six-month outcomes after percutaneous intervention for lesions in aortocoronary saphenous vein grafts using distal protection devices: results from the FIRE trial. *Am Heart J.* 2006;151:915.e911-915.e917.

chapter **20**

Coronary Stenting

MAURO MOSCUCCI, MD, MBA

INTRODUCTION

Since the first coronary angiography performed by Marvin Stones in 1958, the history of interventional cardiology has been characterized by the work of many pioneers and critical milestones (**FIGURE 20.1**). In this chapter, we will provide a visual overview of the evolution of coronary stenting.

As stated in Chapter 18, the improvement in lumen diameter following balloon angioplasty is secondary to local dissection and vessel stretch. Unfortunately, major limitations of balloon angioplasty beyond heavy calcification and other lesion characteristics include the development of abrupt closure due to uncontrolled dissection and the development of restenosis secondary to a combination of elastic recoil, intimal hyperplasia, and vascular remodeling (**Table 20.1**; **FIGURES 20.2** and **20.3**). By providing a scaffolding system to the artery, coronary stents reduce the risk of abrupt closure secondary to local dissection, they overcome elastic recoil, and they can optimize final lumen diameter and reduce the risk of restenosis. Thus, the introduction of coronary stenting has created a true revolution in interventional cardiology. The objective of this chapter is to provide an historical, chronological, and visual overview of coronary stenting (**FIGURES 20.4-20.51**).

- ☐ 1958 - Introduction of the diagnostic coronary angiogram.
- ☐ 1967 - First coronary artery bypass graft (CABG) surgery.
- ☐ 1977 - Introduction of percutaneous transluminal coronary angioplasty (PTCA) using balloon catheters.
- ☐ 1986 - Introduction of coronary atherectomy devices.
- ☐ 1993 - Introduction of stainless steel coronary stents.
- ☐ 2002 - Introduction of drug-eluting stents.

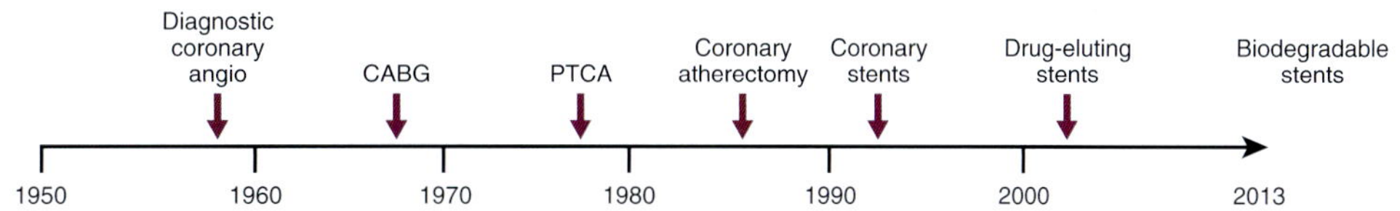

FIGURE 20.1 Milestones in coronary care.

LIMITATIONS OF PERCUTANEOUS TRANSLUMINAL CORONARY ANGIOPLASTY (PTCA)

See **Table 20.1**.

TABLE 20.1

Limitations of Conventional PTCA

- Abrupt closure
- Restenosis
- Calcified lesions
- Bifurcation lesions
- Osteal lesions
- Thrombus
- Vein grafts

DEFINITIONS OF RESTENOSIS

Restenosis can be defined according to angiographic findings at follow-up angiography (angiographic restenosis) and clinically driven revascularization of the target site. Importantly, studies have shown that restenosis rates and target vessel revascularization rates tend to be higher when angiographic follow-up is performed on a routine base. Thus, the concept of "clinical restenosis," defined as clinically driven target lesion and target vessel revascularization, has been developed as a clinically meaningful surrogate of angiographic restenosis (**Table 20.2**).

TABLE 20.2

Angiographic Restenosis

Angiographic Restenosis
• EMORY—A >50% diameter stenosis at follow-up. • NHLBI I—An increase in diameter stenosis > 30% at follow-up from the diameter stenosis immediately after PTCA. • NHLBI II—A residual stenosis <50% after PTCA increasing to a stenosis >70% at follow-up. • NHLBI III—An increase in stenosis severity at follow-up to within 10% or less of the stenosis severity before PTCA. • NHLBI IV—A >50% loss of the initial gain achieved. • Thoraxcenter II—A > 0.72 mm lumen loss at follow-up
Clinical Restenosis
• Target site revascularization • Target vessel revascularization

BALLOON ANGIOPLASTY AND STENTING

The word "stent" was introduced in 1916 by Johannes Esser, a Dutch plastic surgeon, to describe oral splints developed to scaffold the mouth by Charles Stent, a British dentist.[1,2] Other theories regarding the origin of the world stent trace it as back as the late 14th century to the Anglo-French word **extente**, ("valuation of land, stretch of land") and derived from the old French extendre "extend" and from Latin "extendere."[3,4] As of today, the definitions according to the Oxford English Living Dictionaries include (1) "A splint placed temporarily inside a duct, canal, or blood vessel to aid healing or relieve an obstruction" and "An impression or cast of a part or body cavity, used to maintain pressure so as to promote healing, especially of a skin graft" originating from the name of Charles Stent. (2) An assessment of property made for purposes of taxation. (From Old French estente "valuation," related to Anglo-Norman French extente.)[5]

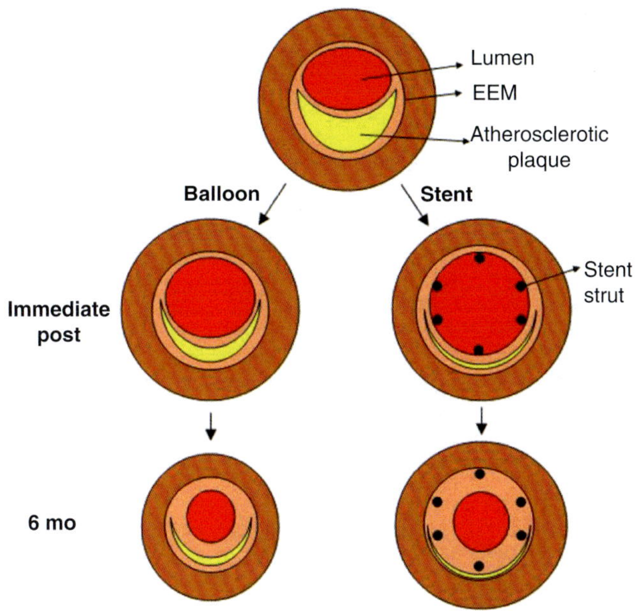

FIGURE 20.2 Illustration of differences in mechanisms of restenosis between plain balloon angioplasty and stenting. In balloon angioplastied vessels, restenosis is caused by a combination of neointimal growth and negative remodeling. Stented arteries have lower rates of restenosis despite incurring greater neointimal growth owing to their ability to achieve a larger initial lumen size and the elimination of negative remodeling. From Kern MJ. *SCAI Interventional Cardiology Board Review*. 2nd ed. Philadelphia, PA: Wolters Kluwer; 2013.

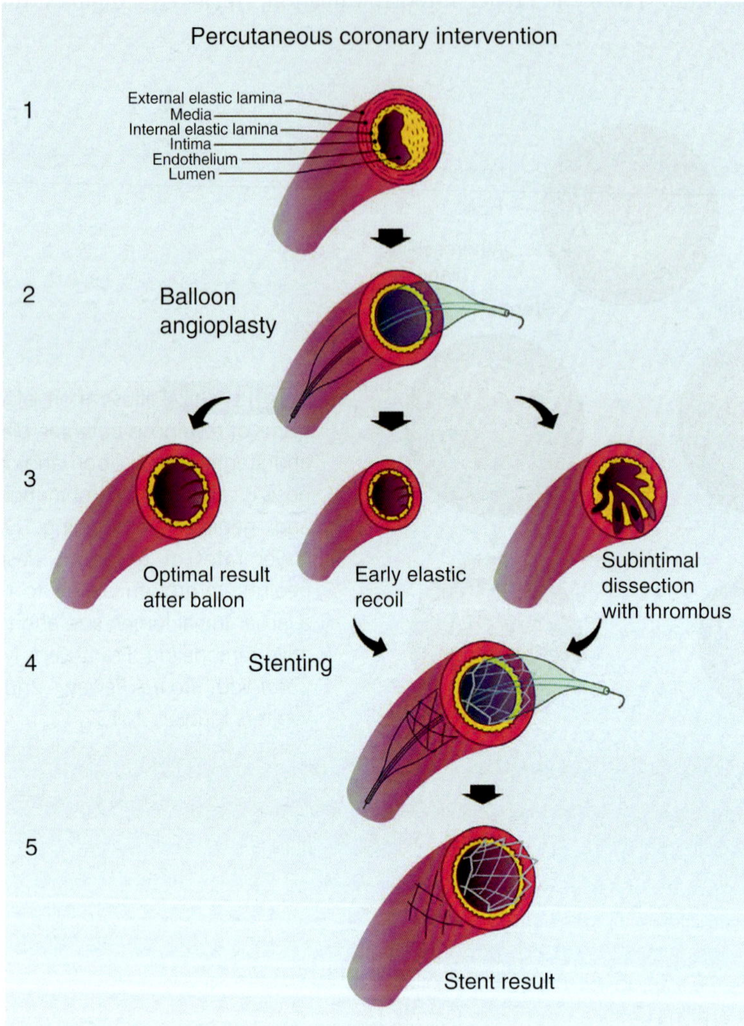

FIGURE 20.3 Benefits of stenting when compared with percutaneous transluminal balloon angioplasty. By providing a scaffolding system at the treated site, coronary stents prevent elastic recoil, prevent negative remodeling, and reduce significantly the risk of abrupt closure and emergency coronary artery bypass graft (CABG). Reproduced with permission from Windecker S, Meier B. Intervention in coronary artery disease. *Heart*. 2000;83(4):481-90.

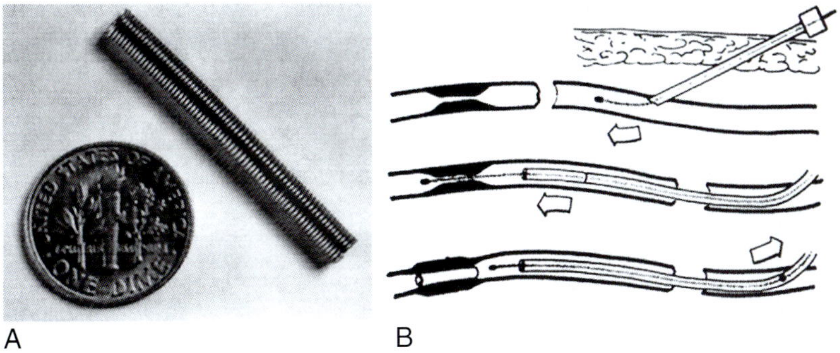

FIGURE 20.4 **A and B**, Coil spring tubular prosthesis and percutaneous placement described by Charles Dotter in 1969. In an attempt to overcome the frequent reocclusion of the femoral artery following angioplasty, Dotter begun experimenting with the insertion of different type of tubing. He found that while various plastic tubes would clot, an open coil-spring configuration promoted long-term patency.[6] Reproduced with permission from Dotter CT. Transluminally-placed coilspring endarterial tube grafts. Long-term patency in canine popliteal artery. *Invest Radiol*. 1969;4:329-332.

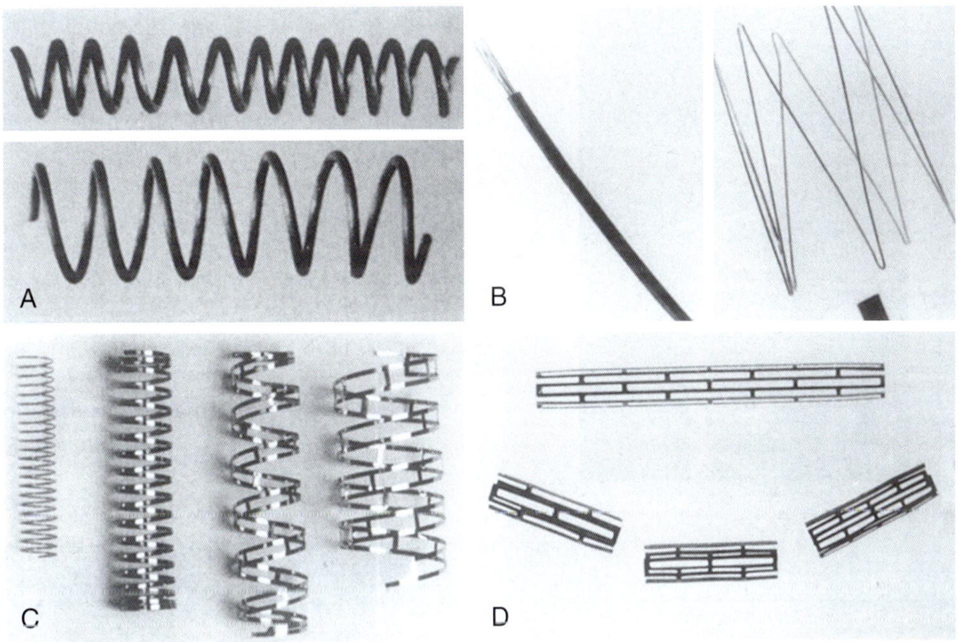

FIGURE 20.5 Four early endovascular stents. **A**, The upper left panel show Dotter's early nitinol coil wire stent compacted for placement and after heat-induced expansion to its predetermined dimensions[7]. **B**, The zigzag expanding stainless steel stent described by Wright et al.[8] shown in the upper right panel in both its sheathed and unsheathed forms. **C**, The lower left panel shows the stents developed by Maass et al.[9] **D**, The lower right panel shows the balloon expandable stainless steel Palmaz stent.[10] Reproduced with permission from Ruygrok PN, Serruys PW. Intracoronary stenting. *Circulation*. 1996;94:882-890.

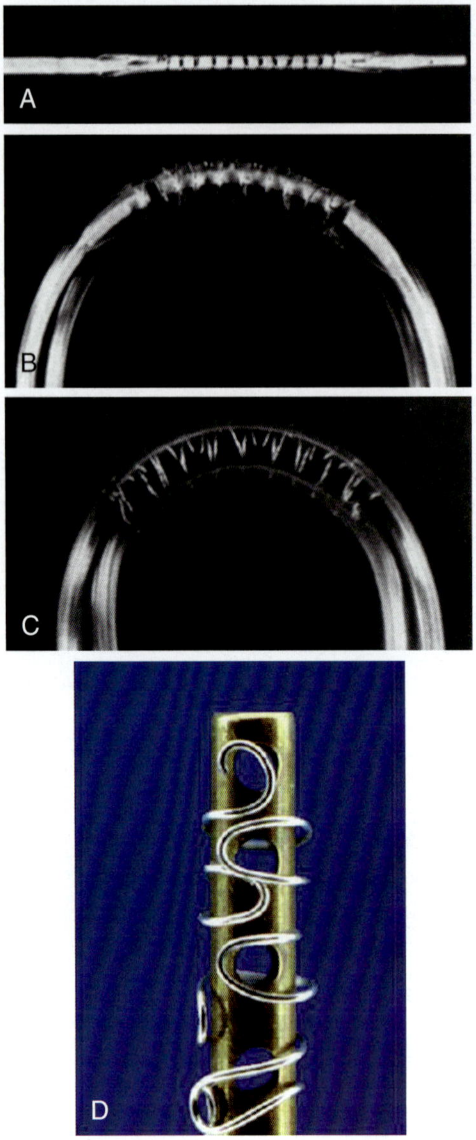

FIGURE 20.6 The Gianturco-Roubin Stent was the first stent approved in the United States for the management of abrupt closure.[11-13] At that time it was estimated that 2% to 11% of the ~300,000 patients receiving coronary angioplasties annually would develop vessel closure or threatened closure, making the device potentially useful in 6000-33,000 patients per year. **A**, Stent coil wrapped firmly on standard PTCA balloon catheter prepared for use. **B**, Stent fully expanded by maximally inflated balloon catheter demonstrated in transparent flexible tubing. **C**, Stent fully expanded after removal of deflated balloon catheter.[14] **D**, Stainless steel sutures were coiled around a cylindrical rod to shape the wire, resulting in a clamshell design. **A-C**, Reproduced with permission from Roubin GS, Robinson KA, King SB III, et al. Early and late results of intracoronary arterial stenting after coronary angioplasty in dogs. *Circulation*. 1987;76(4):891-897; **D**, Reproduced with permission from Moscucci M, ed. *Grossman & Baim's Cardiac Catheterization Angiography and Intervention*. Philadelphia: Lippincott Williams and Wilkins; 2014.

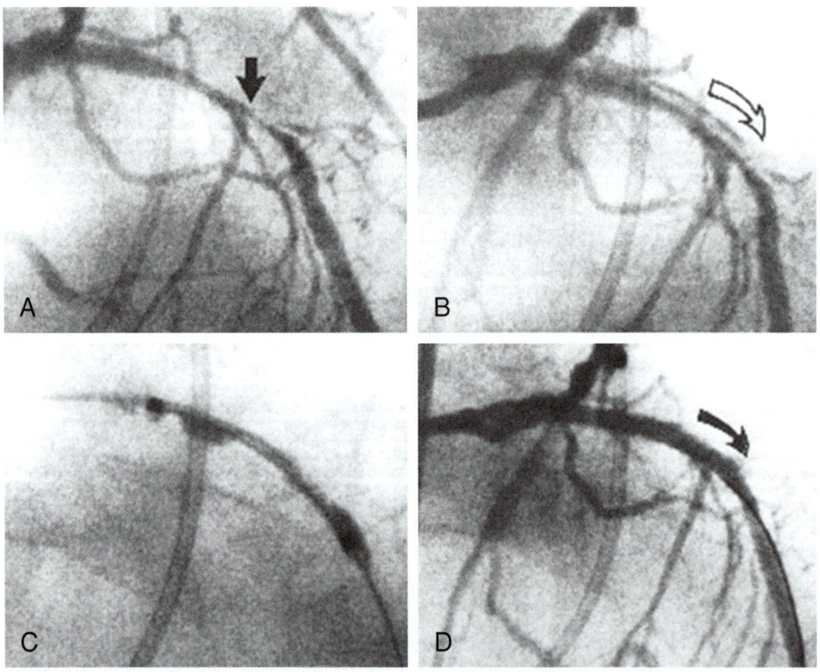

FIGURE 20.7 Early example of placement of a Gianturco-Roubin coil stent for threatened abrupt closure. **A**, A long lesion is present in the left anterior descending (top left, arrow), with a long dissection after angioplasty **(B)** (open arrow, upper right); placement of a coil stent **(C)** (bottom left) results in effacement of the dissection and elimination of the need for emergency bypass graft surgery **(D)** (bottom right, arrow). Reproduced with permission from Baim DS. *Grossman's Cardiac Catheterization, Angiography, and Intervention*. 7th ed. Philadelphia: Lippincott Williams & Wilkins; 2006.

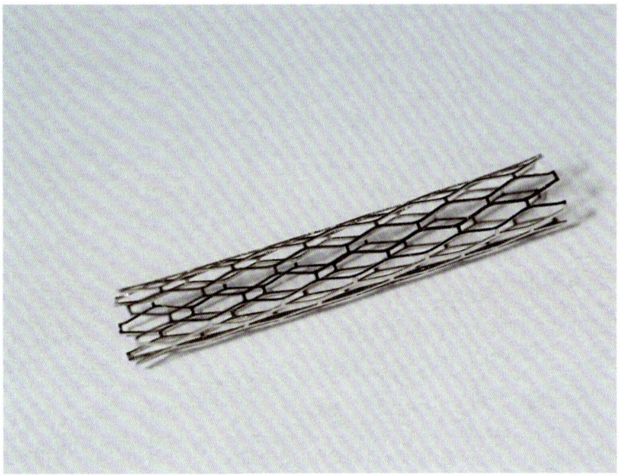

FIGURE 20.8 Palmaz stent. The original Palmaz stent was developed for stenting of the biliary tract. It was a relatively rigid, laser-cut slotted tube made of stainless steel L 316. It had a high radial strength, but owing to its rigidity, it was less suitable for tortuous anatomy.

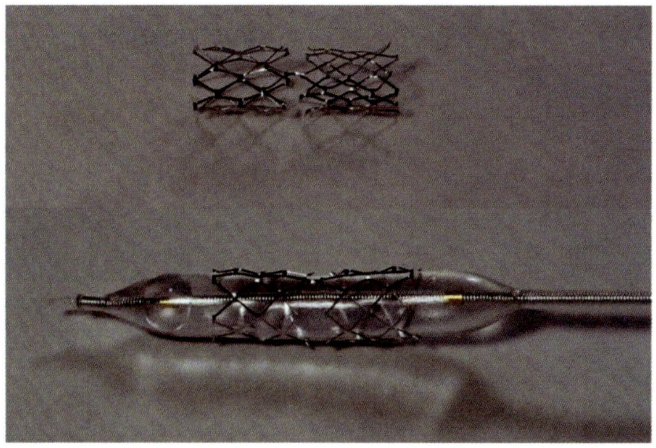

FIGURE 20.9 Palmaz-Schatz stent. The Palmaz-Schatz was an evolution of the original Palmaz stent, and it was developed for the management of coronary artery disease. It was made by 2 7-mm segments joined by a 1-mm articulation site, which made the stent more flexible and able to navigate more tortuous anatomy. Following the results of the STRESS (STent REStenosis Study)[15] and BENESTENT (Belgian Netherlands Stent)[16] clinical trials comparing stent implantation with PTCA in the prevention of restenosis, the Palmaz-Schatz stent was approved for the treatment of de novo coronary artery stenosis.

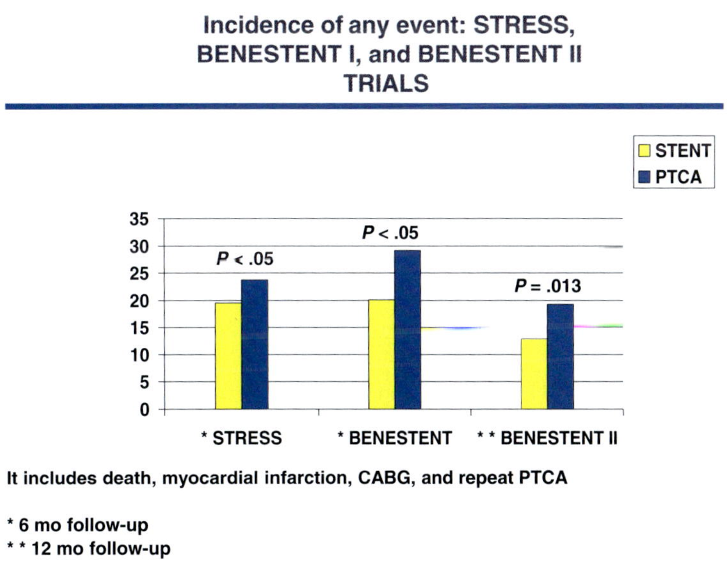

FIGURE 20.10 Incidence of any event in the STRESS, BENESTENT I, and BENESTENT II TRIALS. In the "Randomized comparison of coronary-stent placement and balloon angioplasty in the treatment of coronary artery disease. Stent Restenosis Study Investigators" 410 patients with symptomatic coronary disease were randomized to elective placement of a Palmaz-Schatz stent or to standard balloon angioplasty.[15] The BENESTENT 1 trial randomized a total of 520 patients with stable angina and a single coronary artery lesion to either stent implantation (262 patients) or standard balloon angioplasty (258 patients),[16] while in the BENESTENT II trial 827 patients were randomized to heparin-coated stents or balloon angioplasty.[17] Each trial showed a clear benefit of stent implantation when compared with balloon angioplasty in the reduction of "hard" events including death, myocardial infarction, CABG, and repeat PTCA.

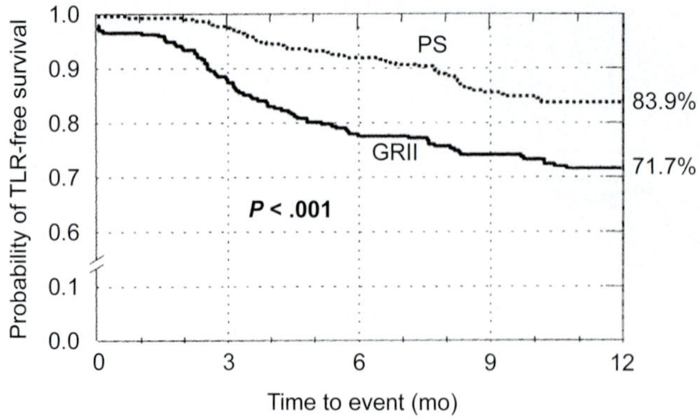

FIGURE 20.11 Restenosis rates and stent design. Randomized comparison of GR-II Stent and Palmaz-Schatz stent for elective treatment of coronary stenoses, target-lesion revascularization (TLR)–free survival: Kaplan-Meier estimate of overall survival free of TLR. Freedom from TLR at 12 months was 71.7% for GR-II stent versus 83.9% for PS stent ($P < .001$). Reproduced with permission from Lansky AJ, Roubin GS, O'Shaughnessy CD, et al. Randomized comparison of GR-II stent and Palmaz-Schatz stent for elective treatment of coronary stenoses. *Circulation*. 2000;102(12):1364-1368. doi:10.1161/circ.102.12.1364. The data supported the hypothesis that stent design can affect restenosis.

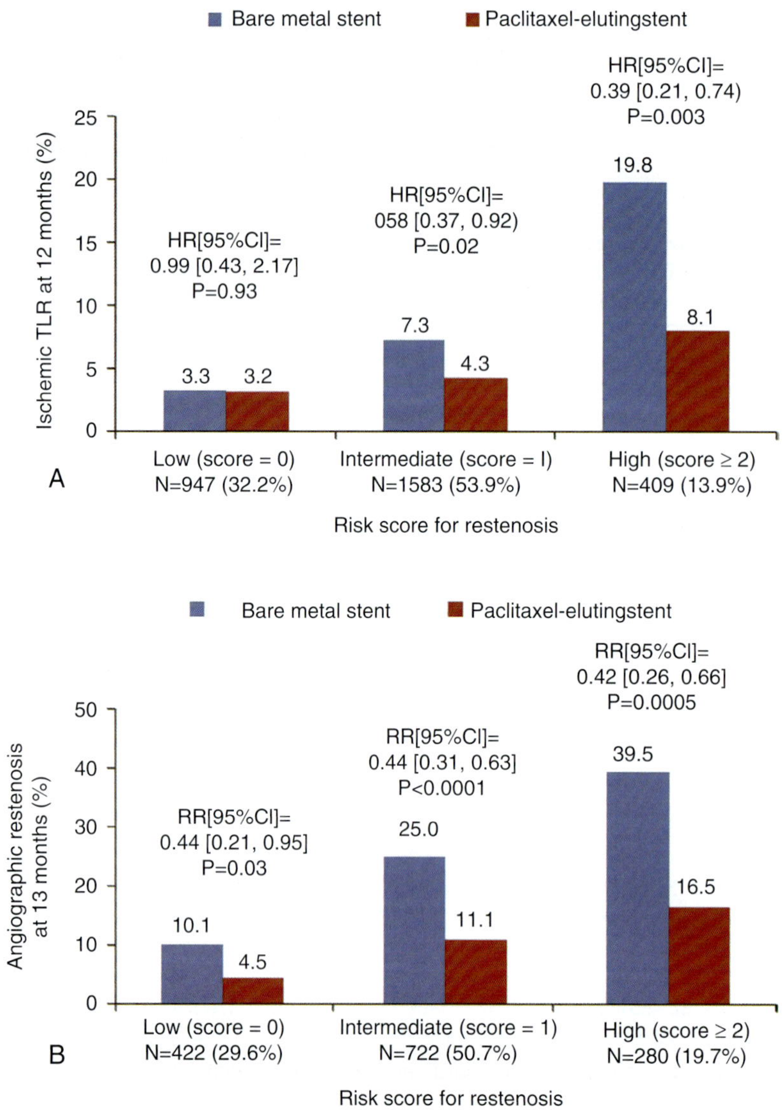

FIGURE 20.12 Risk for restenosis comparing DESs and BMSs in the HORIZONS-AMI study. Rates of 12-mo TLR (target lesion revascularization) and 13-month angiographic restenosis. **A**, Rates of 12-mo ischemic TLR and **(B)** 13-mo angiographic restenosis in patients randomly allocated to paclitaxel-eluting stents (red bars) or to bare-metal stents (blue bars), according to the risk strata for restenosis. BMSs, bare-metal stents; CI, confidence interval; DESs, drug-eluting stents; HR, hazard ratio; RR, relative risk; RVD, reference vessel diameter. Low-, intermediate-, and high-risk groups for restenosis were created using 3 variables (1 point each): **(A)** RVD <3.0 mm, **(B)** lesion length >30 mm, and **(C)** insulin-treated diabetes. Patients with 0, 1, and >2 of these 3 risk factors were defined as being at low, intermediate, or high risk for TLR and restenosis, respectively. Reprinted with permission from Stone GW, Parise H, Witzenbichler B, et al. Selection criteria for drug-eluting vs bare-metal stents and the impact of routine angiographic follow-up: 2-year insights from the HORIZONS-AMI (Harmonizing Outcomes With Revascularization and Stents in Acute Myocardial Infarction) trial. *J Am Coll Cardiol*. 2010;56:1597-1604.

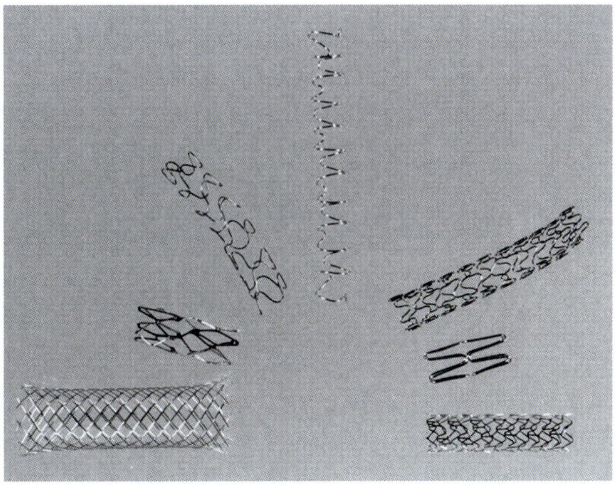

FIGURE 20.13 Stent geometry and evolution of coronary stents. Early to late 90s. Seven coronary stents, clockwise from bottom left: Wallstent, Palmaz-Schatz stent, Wiktor stent, Gianturco-Roubin stent, Cordis stent, AVE stent, and multilink stent. Early stent designs were classified as slotted tube (Palmaz stent) or coils (Gianturco-Roubin stent). Additional geometries include the helical spiral, the woven geometry (Wallstent), individual rings, and sequential rings. Helical spiral geometries have minimal internal connection points and are very flexible. Sequential rings have either connections at every inflection point around the circumference (closed-cell design) or periodic connections where connected inflections points alternate with unconnected inflection points (open-cell design). Reproduced with permission from Ruygrok PN, Serruys PW. Intracoronary stenting. *Circulation*. 1996;94:882-890.

TABLE 20.3

Risk Factors for In-Stent Restenosis

- Diabetes
- Small vessels
- Multiple stents
- Total occlusion
- Ostial location
- ±Prior restenosis
- LAD location
- Stent design

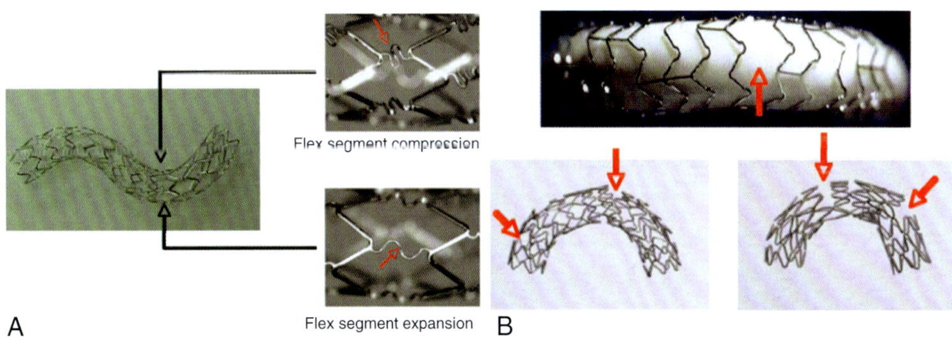

FIGURE 20.14 Stent design. Closed-cell design indicates a sequential ring construction where all the internal inflection points of the structural members are connected by bridging elements. The early Palmaz stent is a typical example of closed-cell design. The major advantage of a closed cell design is optimal scaffolding and a uniform surface, at the expense of reduced flexibility when compared with a similar open-cell design. With an open cell construction, some of the internal inflection points of the structural members are not connected by bridging elements. This provides enhanced flexibility at the expense of scaffolding characteristics and dishomogeneous coverage particularly around bends. **A**, Closed-cell design with a detailed view of the bridge demonstrating the flexibility and conformability after expansion. **B**, Larger open-cell–designed stents may not provide adequate scaffolding in a complex bend (red arrows) but do provide conformability. Open-cell design at the concave surface of the stent. Modified with permission from Wholey MH, Finol EA. Designing the ideal stent. Stent cell geometry and its clinical significance in carotid stenting. *Endovasc Today*. 2007.

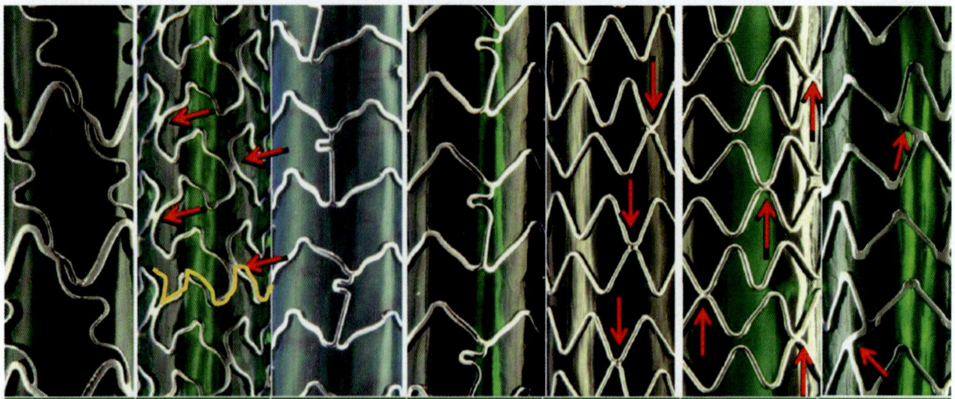

Cypher Select	Liberte	Vision Xience V	MultiLink 8 Xience Prime	Driver Endeavor	Integrity Resolute	Omega Promus Elem
Stainless steel	Stainless steel	Cobalt Chromium	Cobalt Chromium	Cobalt Chromium	Cobalt Chromium	Platinum Chromium
140 µ	**100 µ**	**81 µ**	**81 µ**	**91 µ**	**91 µ**	**81 µ**
6	3	3	3	2	2	2

FIGURE 20.15 Stent design and longitudinal integrity. Longitudinal integrity is an important characteristic of stent design. Shown are photographs of the stent designs, their names, the metal they are constructed from, strut thickness in microns, and the number of connectors between hoops for each design. The Cypher Select, cut from a stainless steel tube, has a strut thickness of 140 µm. Its design is out-of-phase sinusoidal hoops linked by 6 sinusoidal bridges that are orientated about 30° from the stent long axis. The Liberte, cut from a stainless steel tube, has struts100 µm thick. Its apparently complex design is fundamentally out-of-phase hoops (yellow line) that are joined directly by 3 links (red arrows). The Vision and MultiLink 8 and their drug-eluting counterparts, Xience V and Xience Prime, are cut from a cobalt chromium tube and have struts 81 µm thick. The design is in-phase sinusoidal hoops linked by 3 bridges that are aligned with the stent long axis. Each connector has a U-shaped loop to improve flexibility. The 3-mm driver (and the drug-eluting version, Endeavor or Resolute) has sinusoidal, largely out-of-phase hoops linked by 2 welds (red arrows). The Integrity and its Resolute drug-eluting counterpart has a single sinusoidal cobalt chromium component that winds helically from 1 end of the stent to the other with 2 welds between adjacent "hoops" (red arrows). The Omega (bare-metal version) and Promus Element (everolimus-eluting version) and the paclitaxel-eluting version (Taxus Element, called "ION" in the United States) have sinusoidal hoops made from platinum chromium. These are linked by 2 straight bridges per hoop that are aligned at an angle of about 45° from the stent long axis (red arrows). Reproduced with permission from Ormiston JA, Webber B, Webster MW. Stent longitudinal integrity bench insights into a clinical problem. *JACC Cardiovasc Interv*. 2011;4:1310-1317.

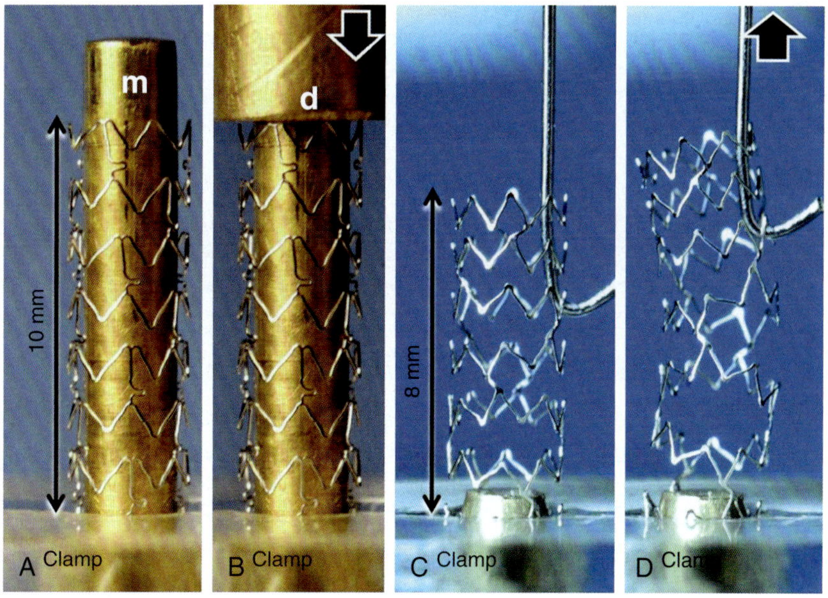

FIGURE 20.16 Compression and elongation tests In **(A)**, for the compression test, the expanded stent was placed over a 2.60-mm diameter mandrel (m) and clamped so that 10 mm of stent was exposed. In **(B)**, a donut-shaped component (d) attached to an Instron universal testing machine was lowered over the mandrel to make contact with the stent. The force required to compress the stent 5 mm was plotted against compression distance. In **(C)**, for the elongation test, a stent was clamped so that 8 mm was exposed. In **(D)**, a hook attached to the Instron was passed through the side of a stent below the third hoop. The force to elongate the stent 4 mm was plotted against elongation distance. Reproduced with permission from Ormiston JA, Webber B, Webster MW. Stent longitudinal integrity bench insights into a clinical problem. *JACC Cardiovasc Interv*. 2011;4:1310-1317.

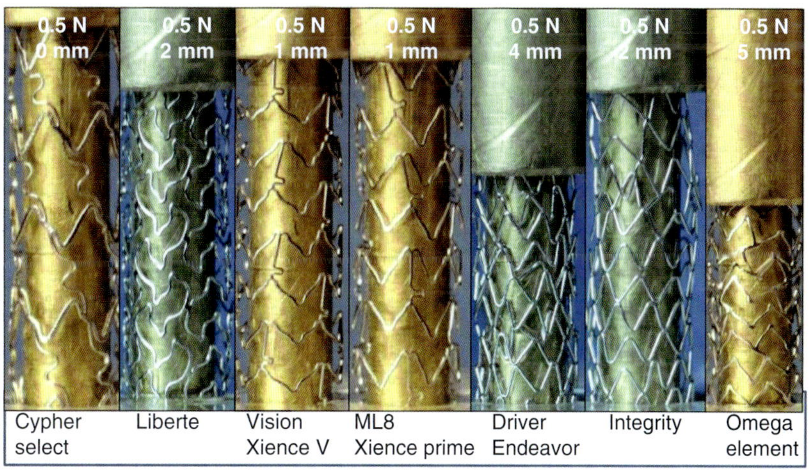

FIGURE 20.17 Comparative stent longitudinal shortening and distortion with 0.5 N compressing force. The 0.5 N force did not compress the Cypher Select stent, and the Liberte was compressed 2 mm. The Vision/Xience and MultiLink 8/Xience Prime were compressed 1 mm with minimal distortion. The Integrity shortened by 2 mm, with a small amount of strut overlap. The most shortening was with the Driver/Endeavor (4 mm) and Omega/Element (5 mm), and these stents experienced the most longitudinal distortion, with strut overlap. Reproduced with permission from Ormiston JA, Webber B, Webster MW. Stent longitudinal integrity bench insights into a clinical problem. *JACC Cardiovasc Interv*. 2011;4:1310-1317.

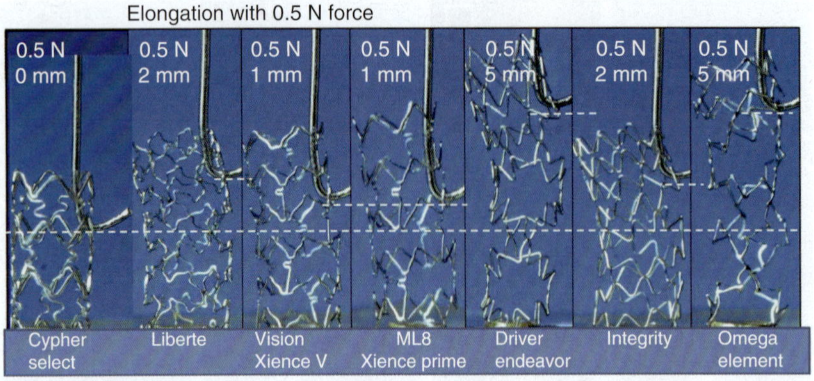

FIGURE 20.18 Comparative stent elongation and distortion with 0.5 N elongating force demonstrated by microcomputed tomography. The magnitude of elongation in millimeters for each stent design subjected to a 0.5-N elongating force is shown at the top of the image of that stent. The stent was secured by clamping the portion of stent below the broken line onto the mandrel, so this portion was not exposed to disruptive forces. The Cypher Select had the greatest longitudinal stability with no elongation in response to 0.5-N force, and the Driver/Endeavor and Omega/Element had the least longitudinal stability, with 5-mm elongation in response to 0.5-N force. Reproduced with permission from Ormiston JA, Webber B, Webster MW. Stent longitudinal integrity bench insights into a clinical problem. *JACC Cardiovasc Interv*. 2011;4:1310-1317.

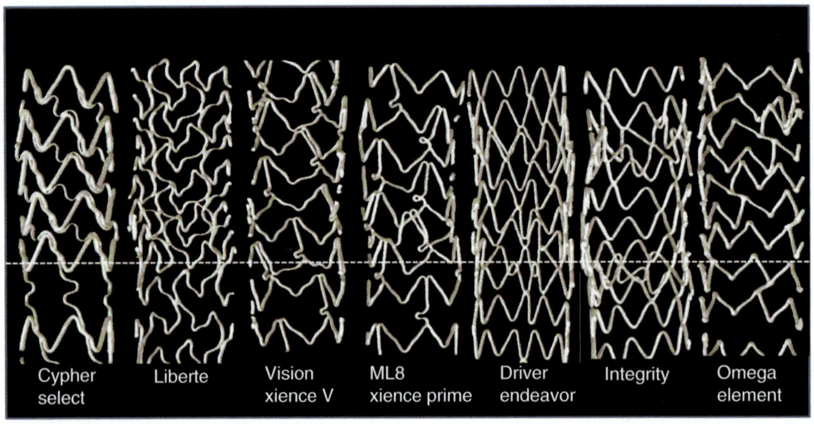

FIGURE 20.19 Stent appearances after 5-mm shortening. Shown are microcomputed tomographic images cut electronically longitudinally after the stents had been compressed by 5 mm. Of course, different magnitudes of force were required to compress different designs by 5 mm. The lower portions of the stents below the broken line were clamped, hence were not subjected to compressive forces and serve as normal stent comparators for insights into mechanisms of shortening. For the Cypher Select the hoops were able to bunch as the wavelength of the sinusoidal connectors shortened and the connectors angulated and became less aligned with the long axis. For the Vision and MultiLink 8 designs, the hoops were pushed together where there are no connectors. In addition, the connectors became angulated and less aligned with the long axis of the stent. Furthermore, especially with the MultiLink 8, the U-shaped loop in the connector closed up. The Liberte, Driver, and Integrity designs have only 2 connectors between hoops, and these are direct connections, so there was little to prevent struts bunching and overlapping in response to compressive forces. With only 2 connectors between hoops, there is again little to prevent Omega/Element struts being pushed together. Additionally, connector orientation changed, becoming more aligned with the stent long axis. Reproduced with permission from Ormiston JA, Webber B, Webster MW. Stent longitudinal integrity bench insights into a clinical problem. *JACC Cardiovasc Interv*. 2011;4:1310-1317.

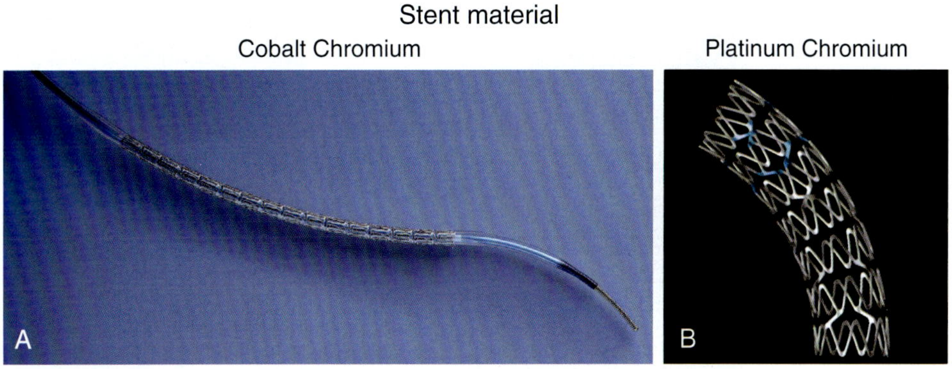

FIGURE 20.20 Experimental evidence has shown that thinner struts cause less arterial wall injury. In addition, a lower struts thickness can increase the flexibility of the stent. The past decade has been characterized by the development of newer metal alloys such as cobalt chromium and platinum chromium, aimed at reducing struts thickness without affecting radial strength and improving visibility. This new alloys are currently used both for bare-metal and drug-eluting stents platforms. **A**, The MULTI-LINK MINI VISION Coronary Stent System is Abbott Vascular's cobalt chromium stent for small vessels. Cobalt chromium allows MULTI-LINK MINI VISION to have thin struts and a low stent metal volume while maintaining radial strength, and radiopacity. **B**, REBEL Stent System. The REBEL stent is made with a platinum chromium alloy. It has been designed to provide visibility, radial strength, and deliverability. **A**, MULTI-LINK MINI VISION and St. Jude Medical are trademarks of St. Jude Medical, LLC or its related companies. Reproduced with permission of St. Jude Medical, © 2018. All rights reserved. **B**, Image provided courtesy of Boston Scientific. ©2018 Boston Scientific Corporation or its affiliates. All rights reserved.

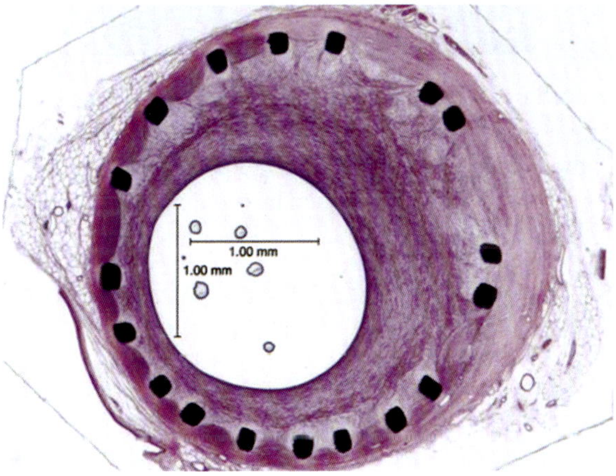

FIGURE 20.21 Stent-induced neointimal hyperplasia. Cross-section of uncoated arterial stent (H and E stain). The lumen is narrowed by neointimal ingrowth. As the stent remains fully expanded, elastic recoil or constrictive remodeling are not components of in-stent restenosis. Reprinted with permission from Geschwind J, Dake M. *Abrams' Angiography*. 3rd ed. Philadelphia, PA: Wolters Kluwer; 2013.

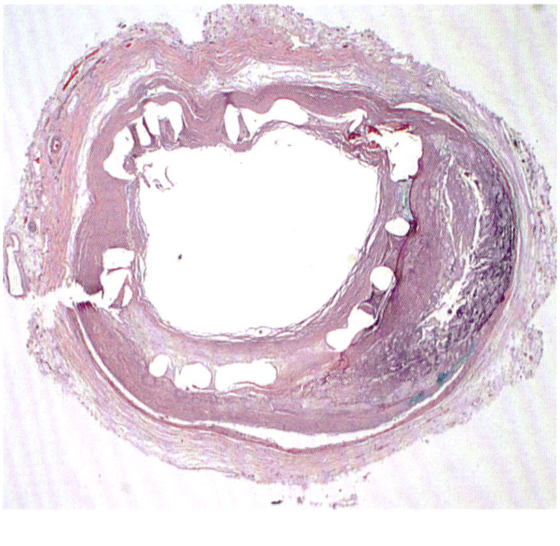

FIGURE 20.22 Overlapping stents. In this example, there are multiple stent struts seen circumferentially around the lumen, with minimal restenosis. The increased number of struts reflects the fact that the section was taken at an overlapping segment. Reprinted with permission from Burke AP, Tavora F. *Practical Cardiovascular Pathology*. Philadelphia, PA: Wolters Kluwer; 2010.

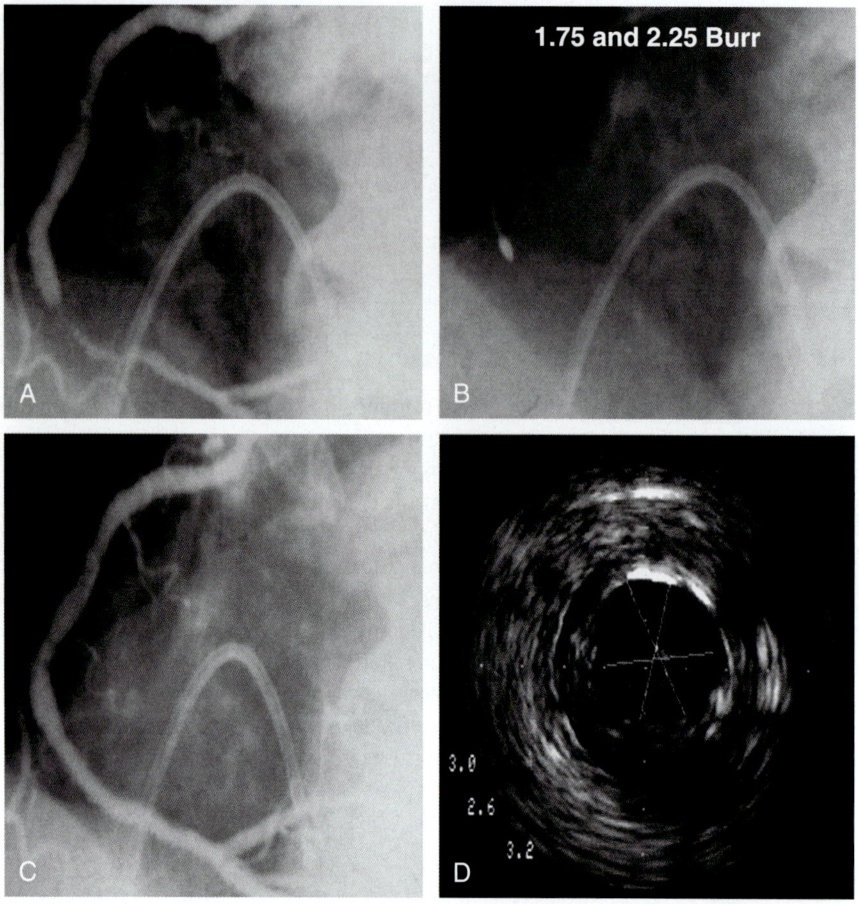

FIGURE 20.23 **A-D**, Rotational atherectomy for in-stent restenosis. Given the high restenosis rate following conventional balloon angioplasty for in-stent restenosis, several debulking approaches including rotational atherectomy, directional atherectomy, and laser atherectomy were proposed in the late 1990s. The images illustrate a case of in-stent restenosis managed by rotational atherectomy and adjunctive balloon angioplasty.

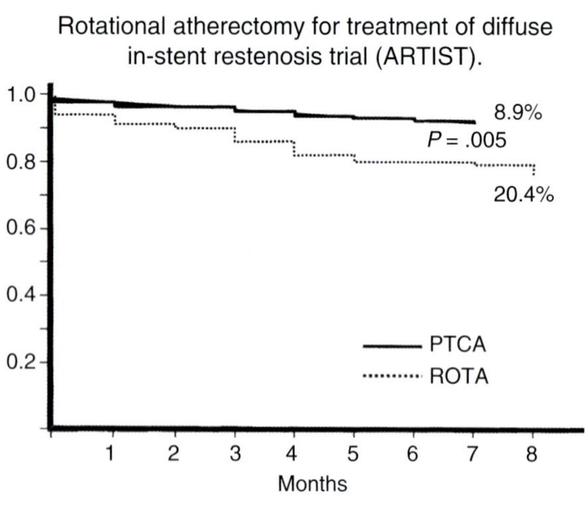

FIGURE 20.24 The ARTIST trial randomized patients with in stent restenosis to rotational atherectomy (recommended burr to artery [stent] ratio >0.7) plus adjunctive balloon angioplasty or to PTCA. At 6 mo follow-up, the event free survival was significantly higher after PTCA (91.3%) compared with rotational atherectomy (79.6%, P = .0052). Reproduced with permission from vom Dahl J, Dietz U, Haager PK, et al. Results of the angioplasty vs rotational atherectomy for treatment of diffuse in-stent restenosis trial (ARTIST). *Circulation*. 2002;105:583-588.

"Candy wrapper" in-stent restenosis

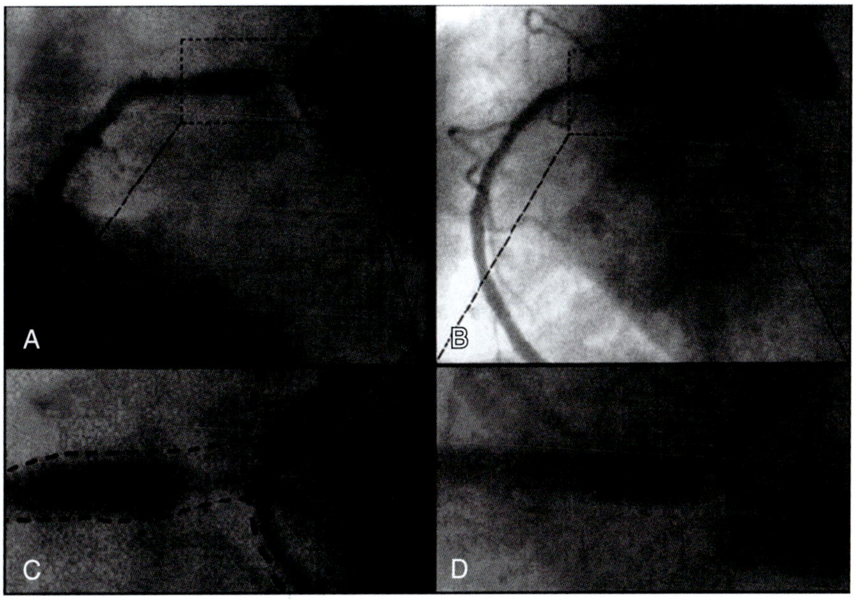

FIGURE 20.25 The battle against restenosis included the development of radioactive β-emitting stents. They were shown to reduce the degree of intrastent intimal hyperplasia, but they were associated with edge restenosis mostly due to negative remodeling and introduced the new term of "candy wrapper" stent restenosis possibly due to an interaction between low activity level of radiation at the edges of the stent and an aggressive approach to stenting.[19,20] Pattern of restenosis in 2 patients at 6-mo follow-up who had intrastent restenosis after implantation of a radioactive stent with an initial activity level of 18.16 mCi **(A)** and 12.36 mCi **(B)**. Magnified views of areas shown in dotted lines are shown in **C and D**, Restenosis occurred in both patients at the ostium of the right coronary artery. Note that in the first patient, the proximal edge of the stent was placed in the aorta (**C**; outlined with dotted lines). Modified with permission from Albiero R, Nishida T, Adamian M, et al. Edge restenosis after implantation of high activity 32P radioactive b-emitting stents. *Circulation*. 2000;101:2454-2457; Albiero R, Adamian M, Kobayashi N, et al. Short- and intermediate-term results of (32)P radioactive beta-emitting stent implantation in patients with coronary artery disease: the Milan Dose-Response Study. *Circulation*. 2000;101(1):18-26.

START trial

476 patients

	Beta	Placebo
N	244	232
DM	32 %	31%
Prior MI	47%	48 %
Debulk	49 %	47 %
Add stent	22 %	21 %
LAD	43%	41%
Lesion length(mm)	16.3	16.0
Device success	98%	97%

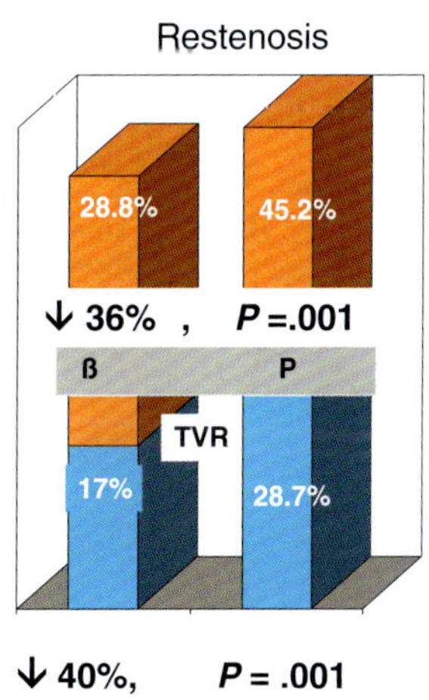

FIGURE 20.26 β-radiation for in-stent restenosis. In the Stents and Radiation Therapy (START) investigators trial, patients with in-stent restenosis were randomized to Beta-Cath System with $^{90}Sr/^{90}Y$ or placebo. Debulking and restenting permitted at operator discretion. Dual antiplatelet therapy was continued for 1 to 3 mos. The primary end point was 8 months TVR. As shown in the figure, β-radiation was associated with a significant reduction in TVR (17% vs 28.7%) and restenosis (28.8% vs 45.1%).[20]

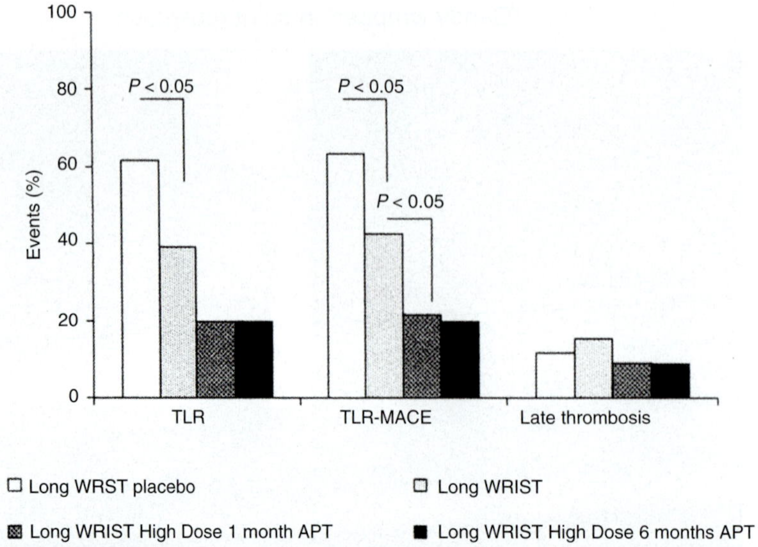

FIGURE 20.27 Intracoronary γ-radiation for long lesions—Long WRIST trial.[21] A total of 120 patients with diffuse in-stent restenosis in native coronary arteries (lesion length, 36-80 mm) were randomized for either radiation with ^{192}Ir with 15 Gy at 2 mm from the source axis or placebo. After enrollment, 120 additional patients with the same inclusion criteria were treated with ^{192}Ir with 18 Gy and included in the Long WRIST High Dose registry. Antiplatelet therapy was initially prescribed for 1 month and was extended to 6 months in the last 60 patients of the Long WRIST High Dose registry. Primary clinical end points at 12 months. TLR indicates target lesion revascularization. APT indicates antiplatelet therapy. Reproduced with permission from Waksman R. Intracoronary radiation therapy improves the clinical and angiographic outcomes of diffuse in-stent restenotic lesions: results of the Washington Radiation for In-Stent Restenosis Trial for Long Lesions (Long WRIST) Studies. *Circulation*. 2003;107(13):1744-1749.

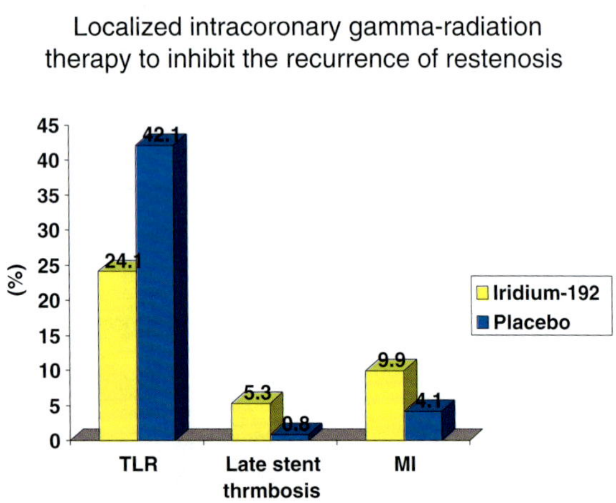

FIGURE 20.28 Localized intracoronary γ-radiation therapy to inhibit The recurrence of restenosis. The benefit of intracoronary radiation in reducing recurrent restenosis was documented in several clinical trials and registry analysis. Unfortunately, in the "Localized intracoronary gamma-radiation therapy to inhibit the recurrence of restenosis" trial, the new issue of late stent thrombosis emerged. It was an important complication of the initial experience with radiation therapy. Avoidance of implantation of a second stent and prolonged antiplatelet therapy were steps taken to reduce the risk. Data from Leon MB, Teirstein PS, Moses JW, et al. Localized intracoronary gamma-radiation therapy to inhibit the recurrence of restenosis after stenting. *N Engl J Med*. 2001;344(4):250-256.

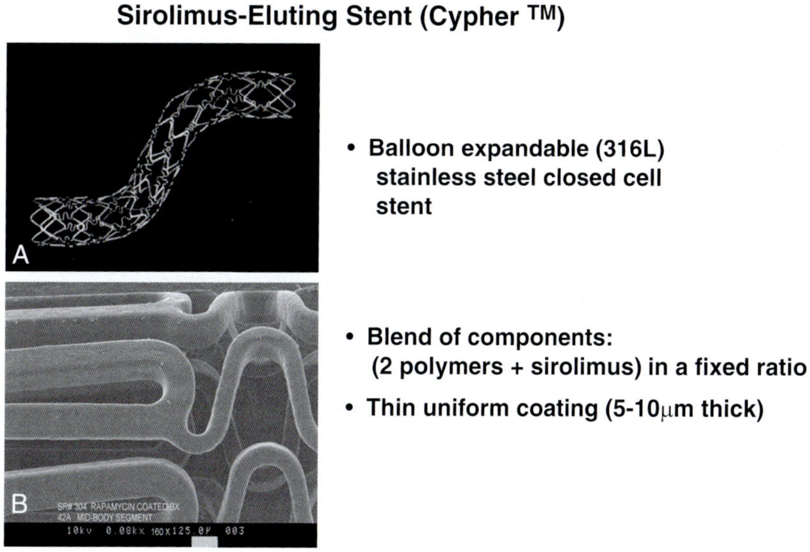

FIGURE 20.29 **A and B**, Drug-eluting stents. The sirolimus eluting Cypher stent was the first drug-eluting stent approved for the prevention of restenosis. It was a balloon-expandable 316 L steel closed-cell stent, with a coating including the blend of 2 polymers and sirolimus. The stent was loaded with 140 µg of sirolimus per square centimeter of metal surface area. A layer of drug-free polymer was applied on top of the drug-polymer matrix to prolong the release of the drug.[23] Courtesy of Cordis.

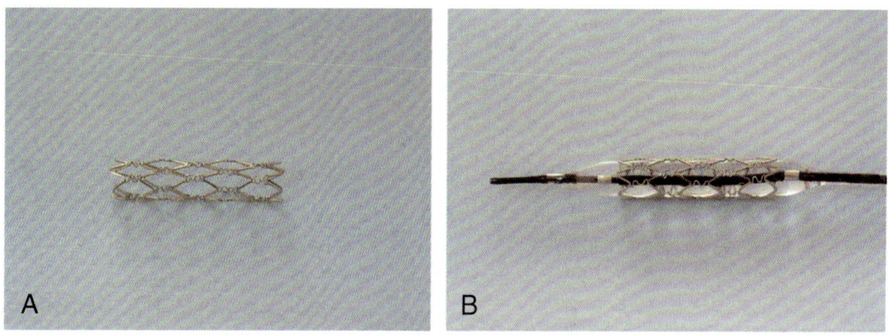

FIGURE 20.30 **A and B**, Cypher stent.

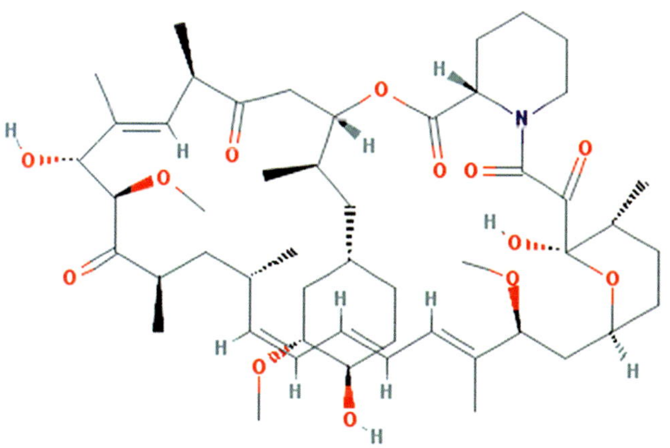

FIGURE 20.31 Rapamycin. Rapamycin (sirolimus) is a naturally occurring antibiotic, which was developed for prevention of renal transplant rejection (Rapamune). It is a selective inhibitor of cell proliferation, and it prevents vascular hyperplasia in transplant and angioplasty models. The mechanism is based on inhibition of the early phase of the cell cycle. Reproduced from National Center for Biotechnology Information. PubChem Compound Database; CID=5284616, https://pubchem.ncbi.nlm.nih.gov/compound/5284616. Accessed September 14, 2018).

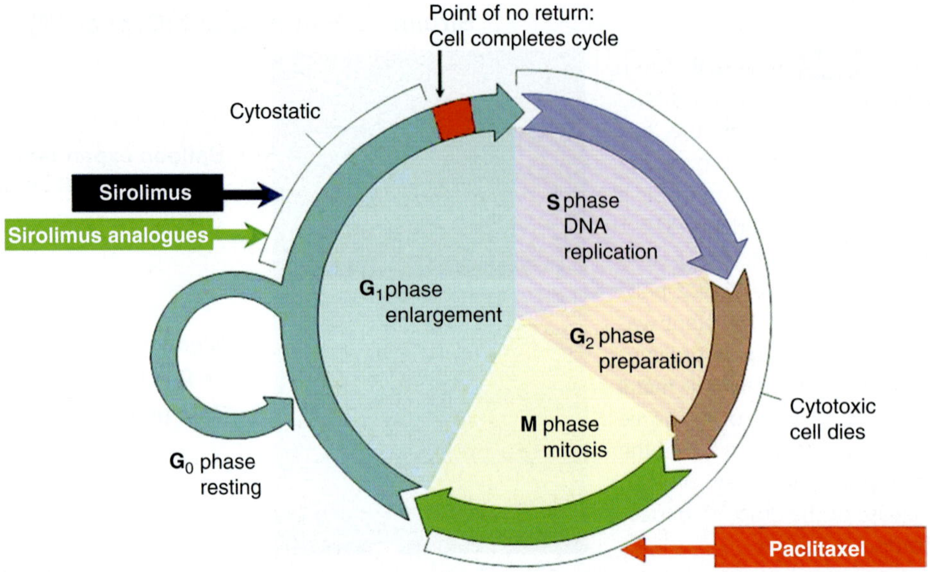

FIGURE 20.32 Diagram of the cell cycle, showing the different phases where sirolimus or its analogues (phase G1) and paclitaxel (phase M) exert their mechanisms of action. Reproduced with permission from Seabra-Gomes R. Percutaneous coronary interventions with drug eluting stents for diabetic patients. *Heart*. 2006;92:410-419.

FIGURE 20.33 Event-free survival at 1 y for target lesion revascularization, MACE, and target vessel failure in the sirolimus-eluting stents versus standard stents in patients with stenosis in a native coronary artery (Sirius) trial. In the Sirius trial, a total of 1101 patients with de novo coronary lesions were randomized to the BX-Velocity bare-metal stent (556 patients) or to the Cipher drug-eluting stent (545 patients).[24] The study included an angiographic substudy with the first 850 patients, follow-up at 8 months, and an IVUS substudy with 250 patients at selected sites. Courtesy of Cordis.

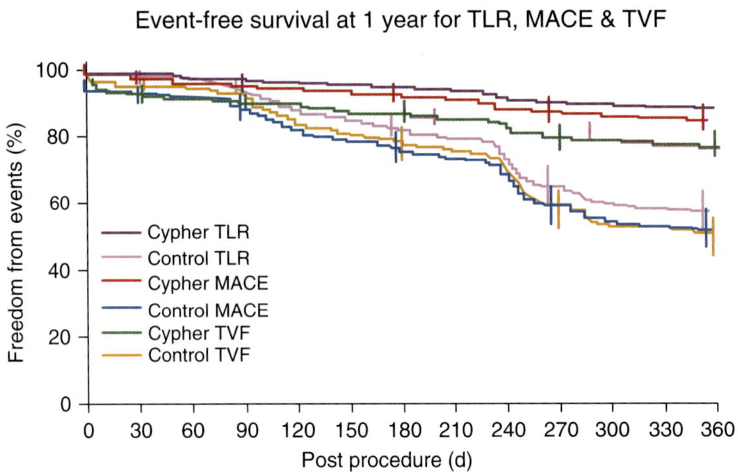

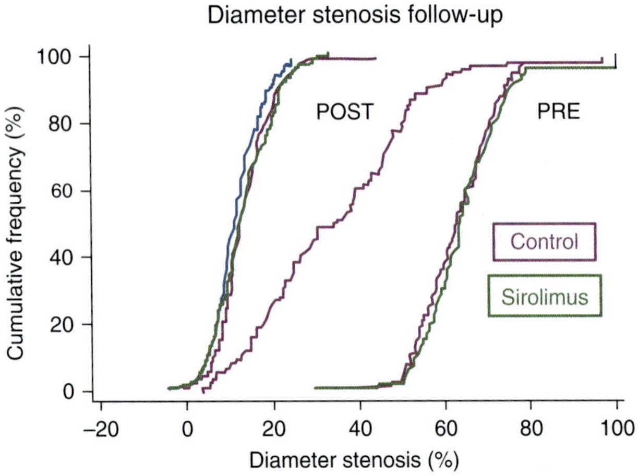

FIGURE 20.34 RAVEL study (randomized study with the sirolimus-coated Bx velocity balloon-expandable stent in the treatment of patients with de novo native coronary artery lesions). Diameter stenosis before stenting, after stenting and at follow-up.

FIGURE 20.35 Comparison of the diameter stenosis at follow-up in the BENESTENT 1 balloon arm, BENESTENT 1 stent arm, BENESTENT II stent arm, and in the RAVEL sirolimus arm. In the RAVEL study, 238 patients with single, primary lesions in native coronary arteries were randomized to sirolimus drug-eluting stent or to bare-metal stent implantation.[23] The primary end point was in-stent late luminal loss (the difference between the minimal luminal diameter immediately after the procedure and the diameter at 6 months). As the cumulative distribution curves show, the diameter stenosis at follow-up was lower in the RAVEL Sirolimus group when compared with the other historical controls.

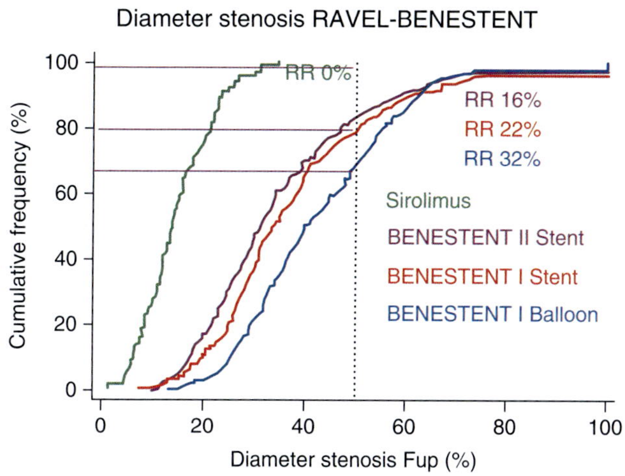

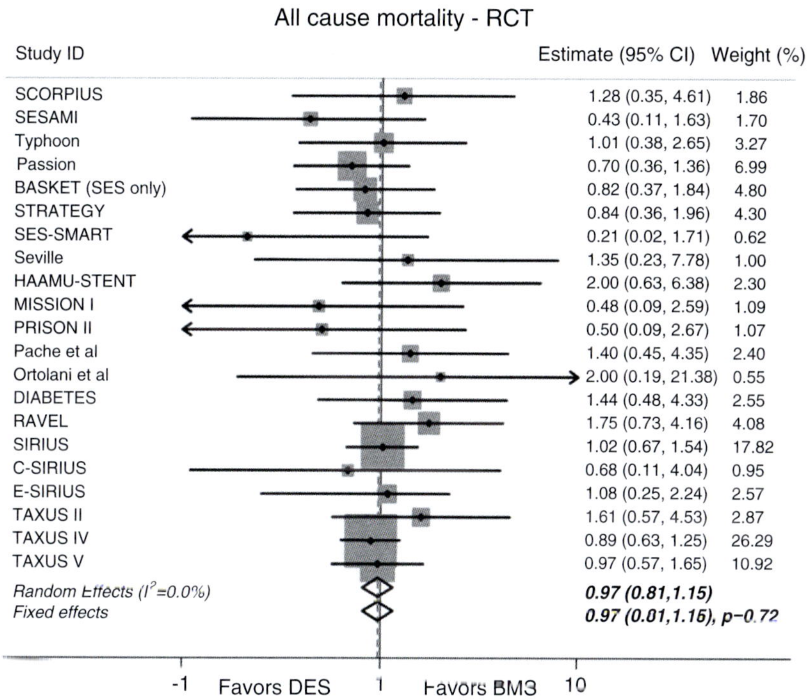

FIGURE 20.36 Safety of drug-eluting stents. All-cause mortality in randomized clinical trials. In 2006, concerns about late subacute stent thrombosis and an increase risk of death and myocardial infarction with drug-eluting stents were raised. The concerns prompted a series of large analysis, which showed no evidence of an increased risk of mortality or myocardial infarction with drug-eluting stents when compared with bare-metal stents. Reproduced with permission from Kirtane A, Gupta A, Iyengar S, et al. Safety and efficacy of drug-eluting and bare metal stents: comprehensive meta-analysis of randomized trials and observational studies. *Circulation*. 2009;119(25):3198-3206.

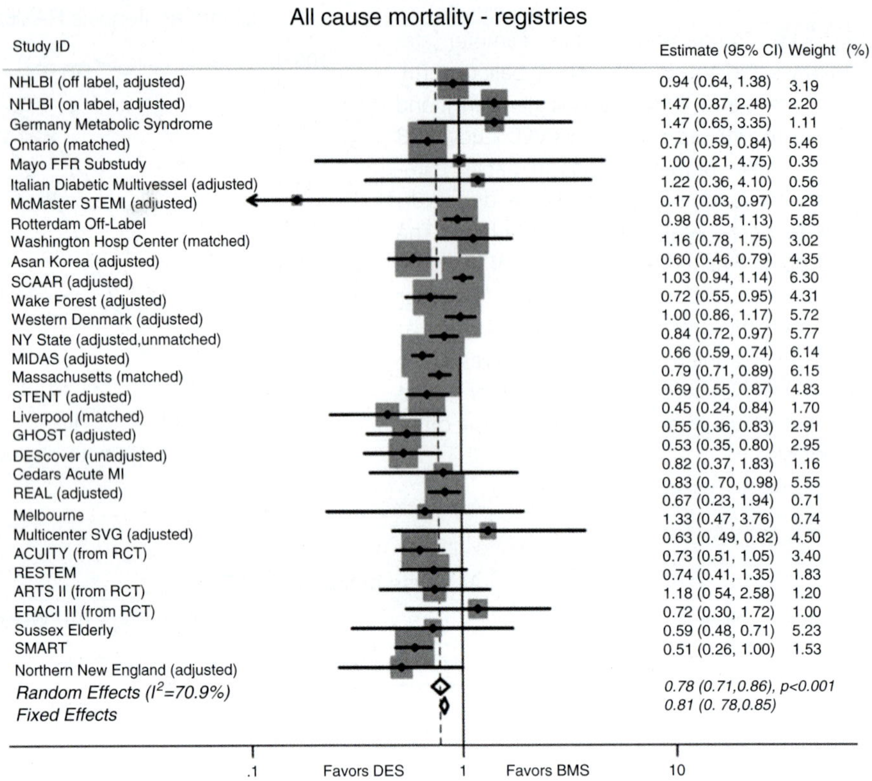

FIGURE 20.37 Safety of drug-eluting stents. All-cause mortality in registries. Reproduced with permission from Kirtane A, Gupta A, Iyengar S, et al. Safety and efficacy of drug-eluting and bare metal stents: comprehensive meta-analysis of randomized trials and observational studies. *Circulation*. 2009;119(25):3198-3206.

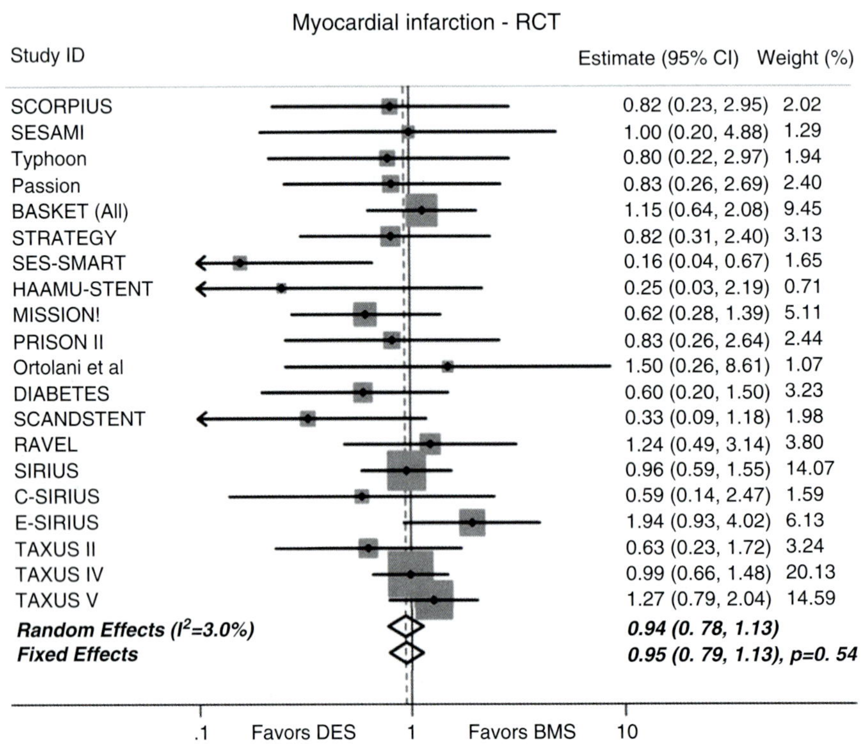

FIGURE 20.38 Safety of drug-eluting stents. All-cause mortality in myocardial infarction in randomized clinical trials. Reproduced with permission from Kirtane A, Gupta A, Iyengar S, et al. Safety and efficacy of drug-eluting and bare metal stents: comprehensive meta-analysis of randomized trials and observational studies. *Circulation*. 2009;119(25):3198-3206.

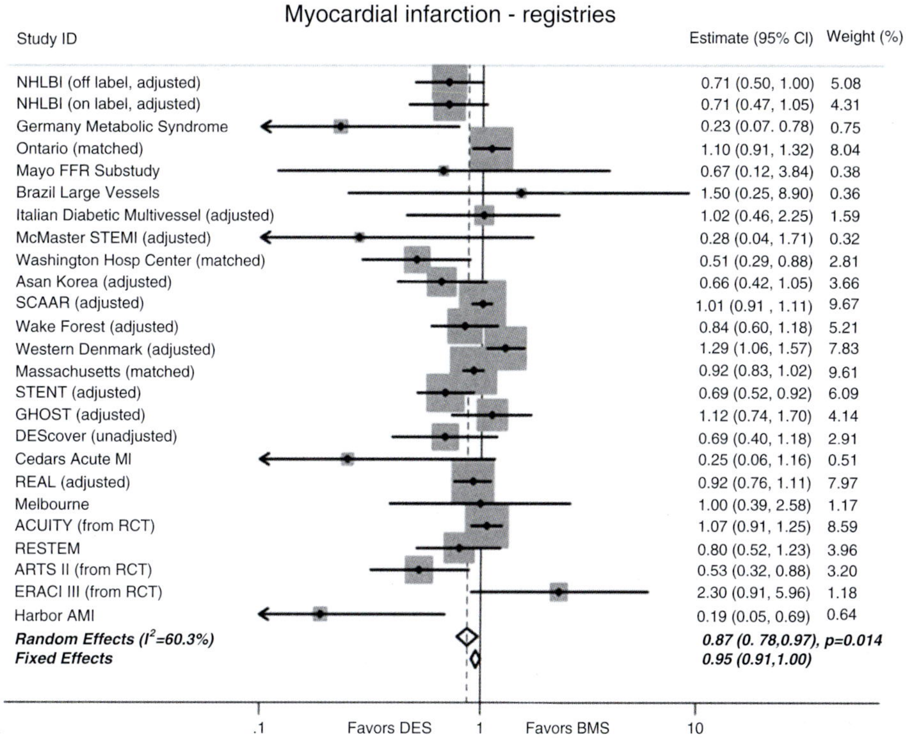

FIGURE 20.39 Safety of drug-eluting Stents. All-cause mortality in myocardial infarction registries. Reproduced with permission from Kirtane A, Gupta A, Iyengar S, et al. Safety and efficacy of drug-eluting and bare metal stents: comprehensive meta-analysis of randomized trials and observational studies. *Circulation*. 2009;119(25):3198-3206.

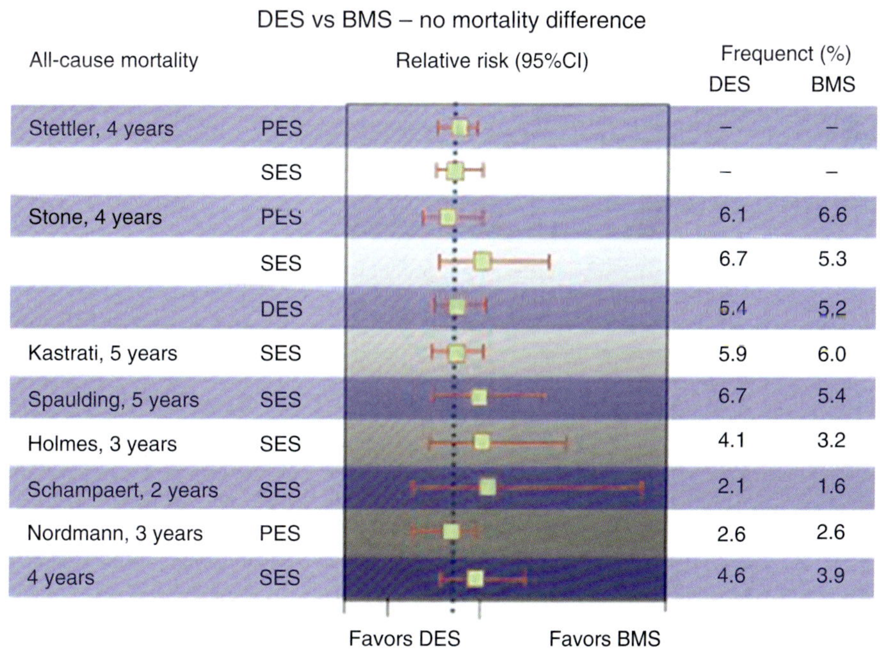

FIGURE 20.40 Drug-eluting versus bare-metal stents. Mortality risk. Adapted from Bavry AA, Bhatt DL. Appropriate use of drug-eluting stents: balancing the reduction in restenosis with the concern of late thrombosis. *Lancet*. 2008;371:2134-2143.

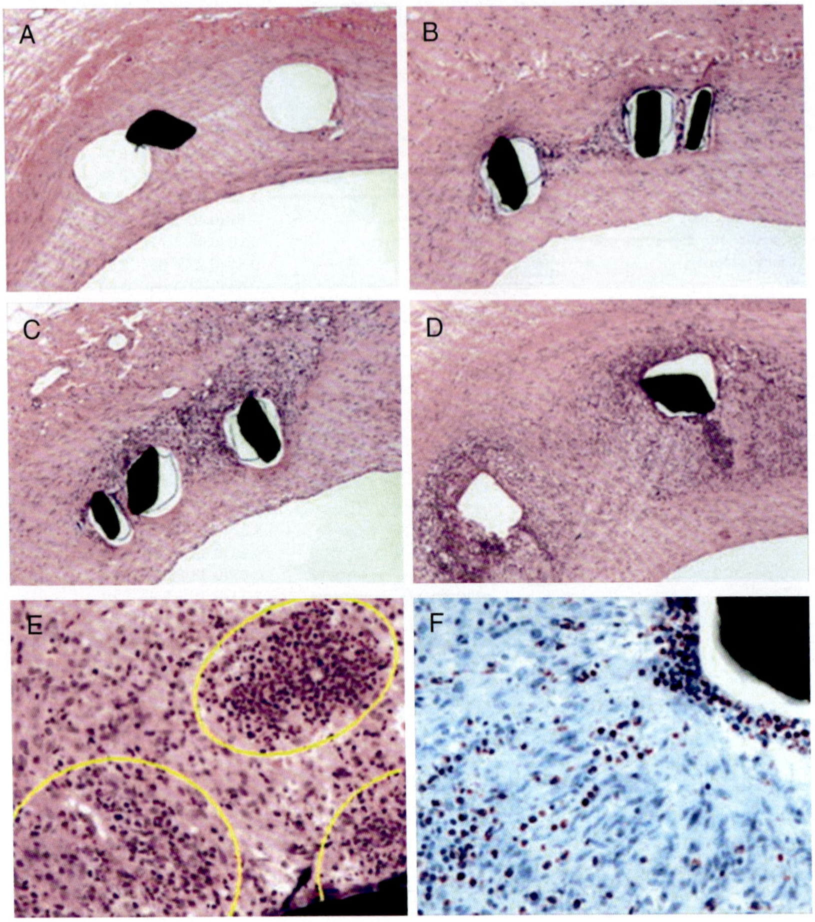

FIGURE 20.41 Inflammatory response after implantation of sirolimus- and paclitaxel-eluting stents. There has been recently strong interest in the possibility that the polymer and metallic stents that remain in the vessel can lead to a local inflammatory response leading to vasomotor dysfunction, in-stent neoatherosclerosis and potentially late thrombosis. Showing in this slide is a grading scale for inflammation, which was developed in a porcine model. Grading scale for inflammation. Minimal **(A)**, mild **(B)**, moderate **(C)**, and severe (which includes granuloma formation; **D** through **F**), with many eosinophils (**E**; large aggregates of eosinophils circled) stained with Luna eosinophil stain **(F)** showing granules as red. Reproduced with permission from Wilson GJ, Nakazawa G, Schwartz RS, et al. Comparison of inflammatory response after implantation of sirolimus- and paclitaxel-eluting stents in porcine coronary arteries. *Circulation*. 2009;120(2):141-149.

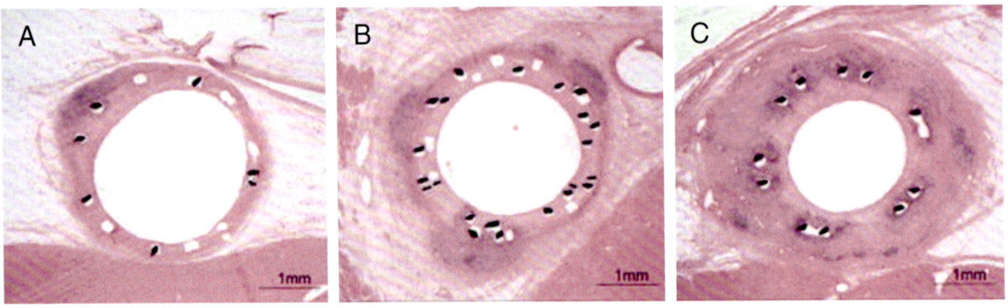

FIGURE 20.42 Regional patterns of granulomatous inflammation (GI). One focus of GI involving no more than 1 quadrant (90°) of the circumference was designated unifocal GI **(A)**. Two or more foci of GI involving no more than 3 quadrants (270° maximum) of the circumference were designated multifocal GI **(B)**. Several foci of GI involving all 4 quadrants for circumference were designated circumferential granulomatous inflammation (CGI) **(C)**. In CGI, usually every strut was involved. Reproduced with permission from Wilson GJ, Nakazawa G, Schwartz RS, et al. Comparison of inflammatory response after implantation of sirolimus- and paclitaxel-eluting stents in porcine coronary arteries. *Circulation*. 2009;120(2):141-149.

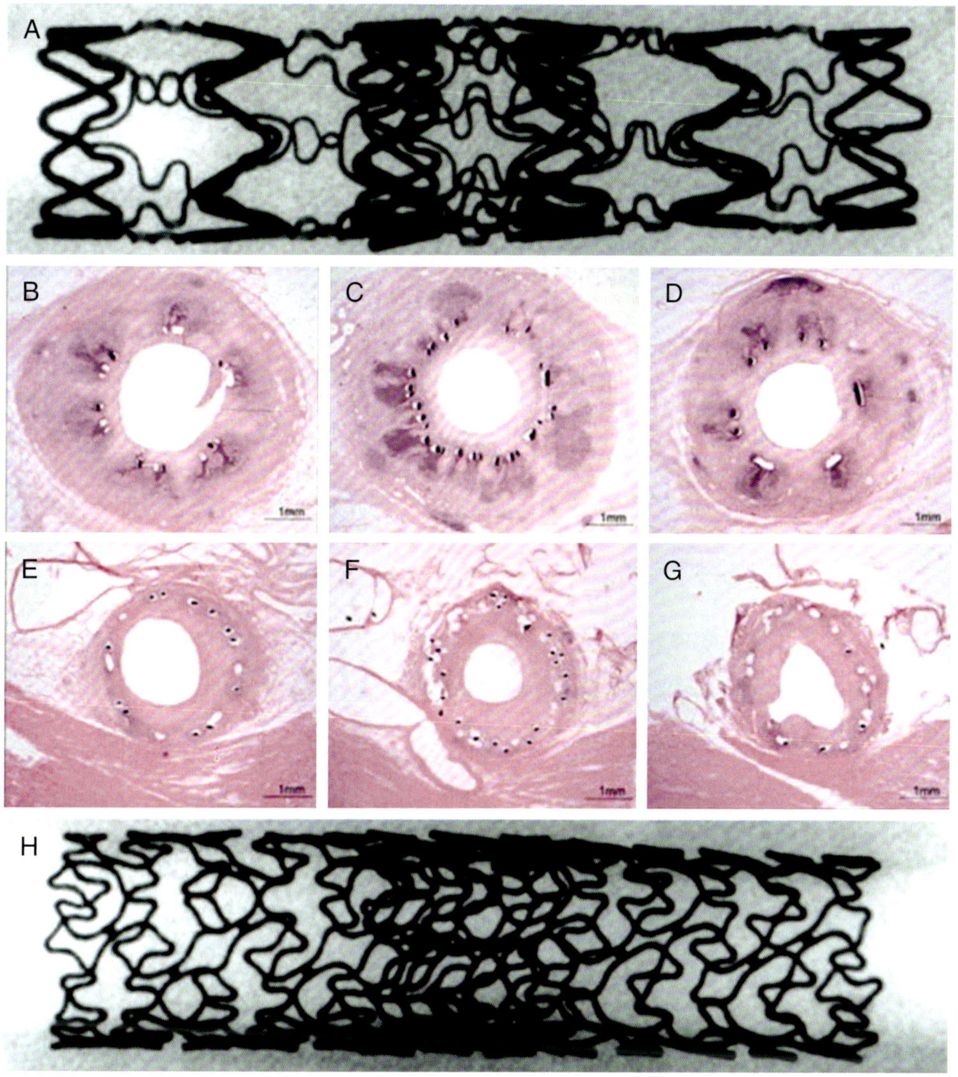

FIGURE 20.43 CYPHER versus TAXUS comparison of CGI in all 3 stented vessel segments: proximal, overlap, and distal. Radiographs of CYPHER- **(A)** and TAXUS- (H) stented segments. Histological sections through a CYPHER stent are shown in **B** (proximal), **C** (overlap), and **D** (distal). In all 3, the CGI extends into the adventitia, where there is severe adventitial fibrosis and a greatly expanded vessel cross-sectional area (positive remodeling). Histological sections through the 1 TAXUS-stented vessel segment that showed CGI in the proximal **(E)**, overlap **(F)**, and distal **(G)** sections show less extensive inflammatory activity and less positive remodeling than seen with CYPHER. **H**, All hematoxylin and eosin-stained sections are shown at the same magnification. Reproduced with permission from Wilson GJ, Nakazawa G, Schwartz RS, et al. Comparison of inflammatory response after implantation of sirolimus- and paclitaxel-eluting stents in porcine coronary arteries. *Circulation*. 2009;120(2):141-149.

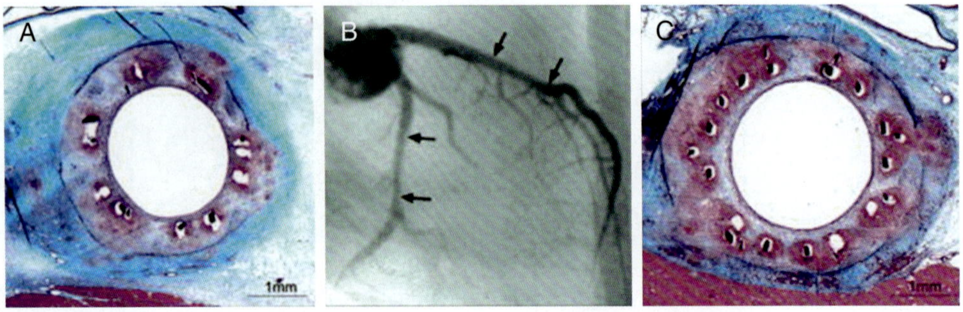

FIGURE 20.44 Angiography compared with histology of CGI. The 90-day angiogram **(B)** shows the locations (arrows) of 2 stented porcine coronary arteries from this study with modest narrowing. Angiography provides no insight into the existing CGI with extension into the adventitia, breakdown of the black elastica (EEL), and fibrosis (blue areas) in the elastic trichrome-stained sections **(A and C)**. Reproduced with permission from Wilson GJ, Nakazawa G, Schwartz RS, et al. Comparison of inflammatory response after implantation of sirolimus- and paclitaxel-eluting stents in porcine coronary arteries. *Circulation*. 2009;120(2):141-149.

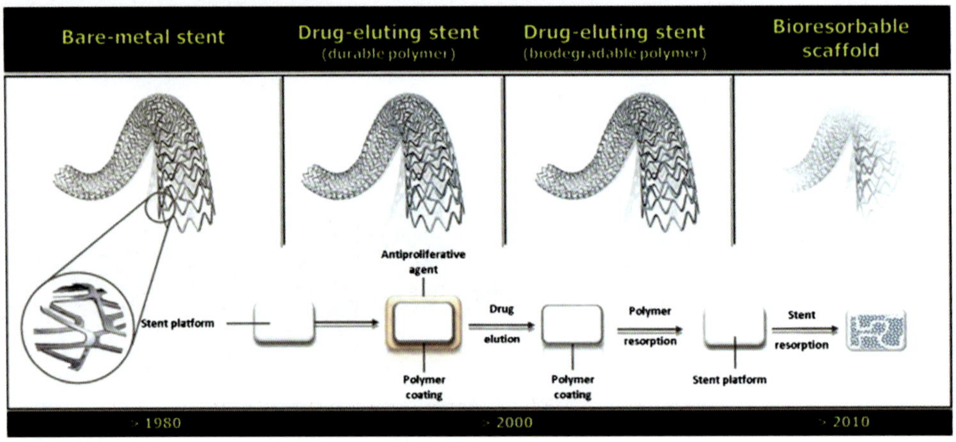

FIGURE 20.45 Stent platform components and evolving innovations. The continuous evolution in stent technology has enhanced the efficacy and safety of drug-eluting stents. That said, the concerns regarding local inflammatory responses to the polymer and metal struts have led to the development of bioreabsorbable platforms with biodegradable polymers. Reproduced with permission from Gogas BD, McDaniel M, Samady H, King SB III. Novel drug-eluting stents for coronary revascularization. *Trends Cardiovasc Med*. 2014;24(7):305-313.

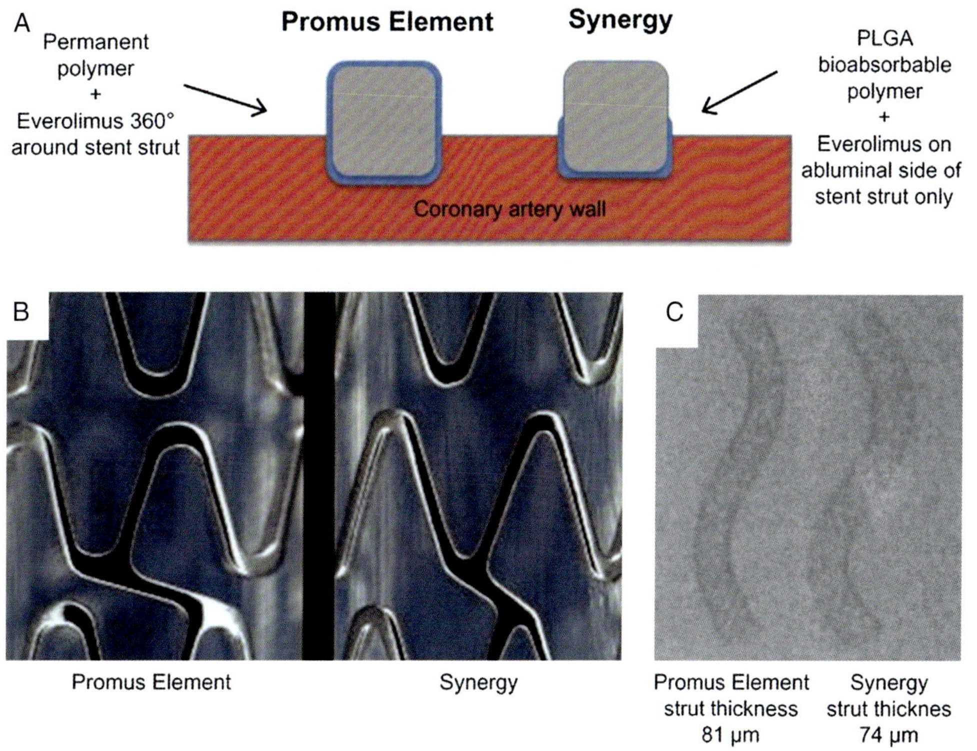

FIGURE 20.46 Contemporary stent platforms. Key differences between the Promus Element and Synergy stent. In the thinner-strut Synergy stent, the drug and bioabsorbable poly-DL-lactide-co-glycolide (PLGA) polymer are applied to the abluminal stent surface only **(A)**. The Synergy stent has different strut thickness, connector angle, and peak radius diameters, resulting in an enhanced stent platform **(B)**. Panel **(C)** shows similar radiopacity between the stents despite reduced strut thickness in the Synergy stent. Reproduced with permission from Bennett J, Dubois C. A novel platinum chromium everolimus-eluting stent for the treatment of coronary artery disease. *Biologics*. 2013:7:149-159. Dove Press.

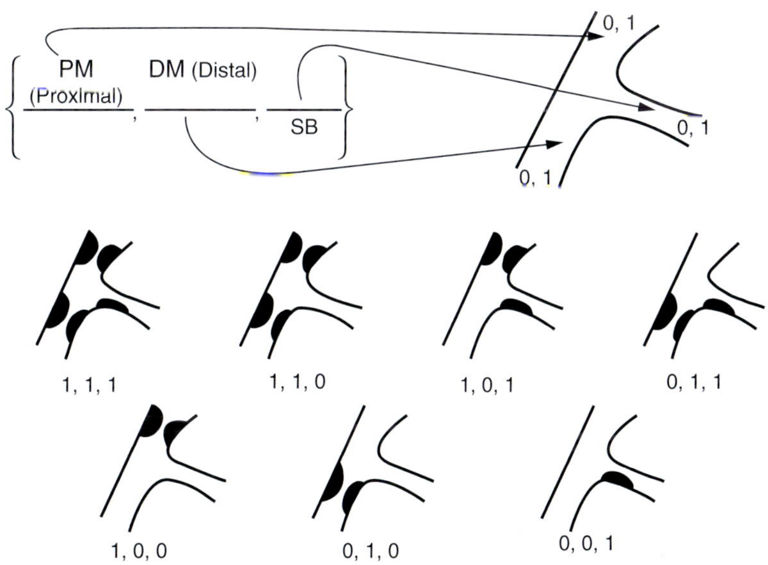

FIGURE 20.47 Bifurcation stenting. Medina classification of bifurcation stenosis. The approach to bifurcation lesions continues to be a major challenge of contemporary stenting. Depending on the type and location of the lesion, different techniques have been proposed. Reprinted from EuroIntervention Vol 6 (Supplement J), Louvard Y et al. Definition and classification of bifurcation lesions and Treatments. Pages No. J31-J35, Copyright (2010), with permission from Europa Digital & Publishing.

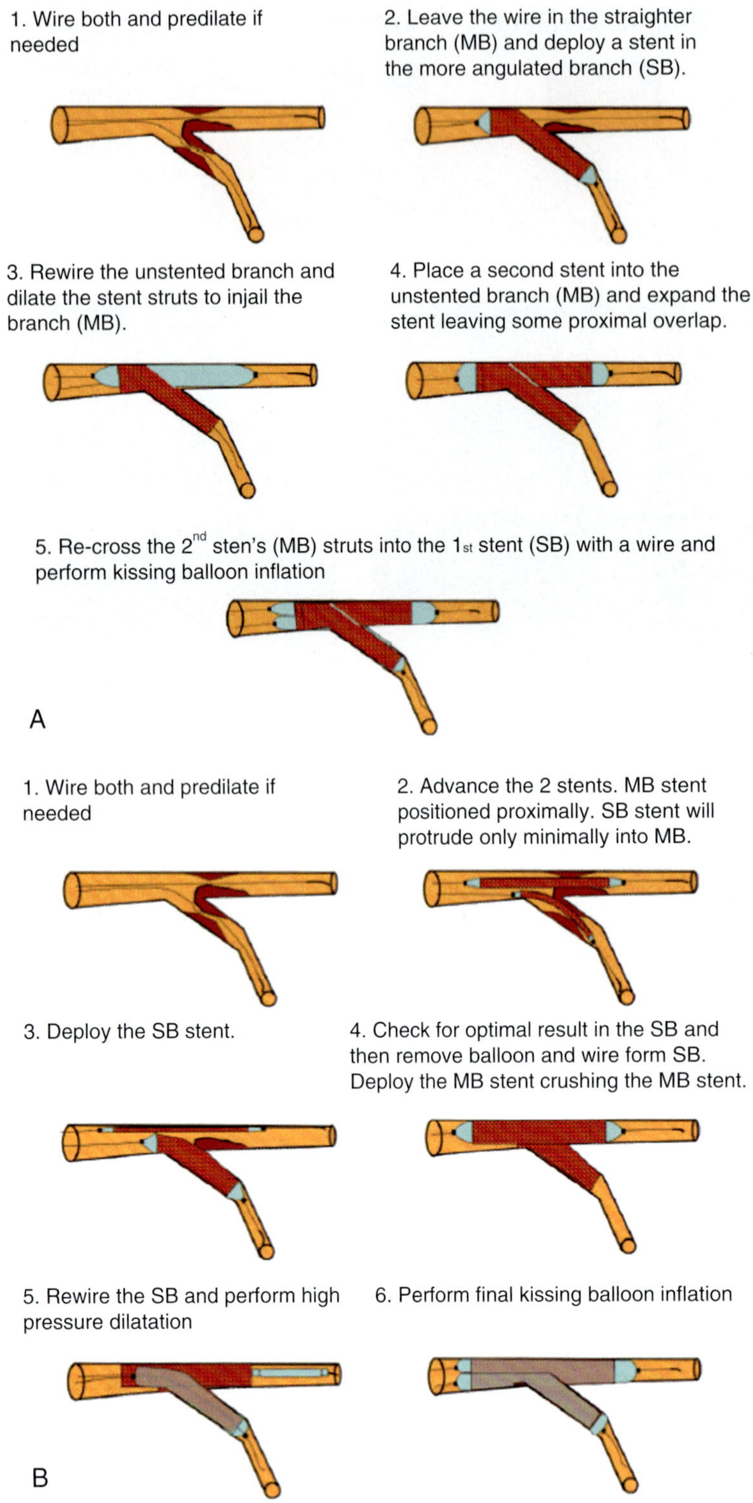

FIGURE 20.48 Schematic representation of the **(A)** Culotte technique and **(B)** Mini-Crush technique. Reprinted from EuroIntervention Vol 6 (Supplement J), Latib A et al. When are two stents needed? Which technique is the best?. Pages No. J81-J87, Copyright (2010), with permission from Europa Digital & Publishing.

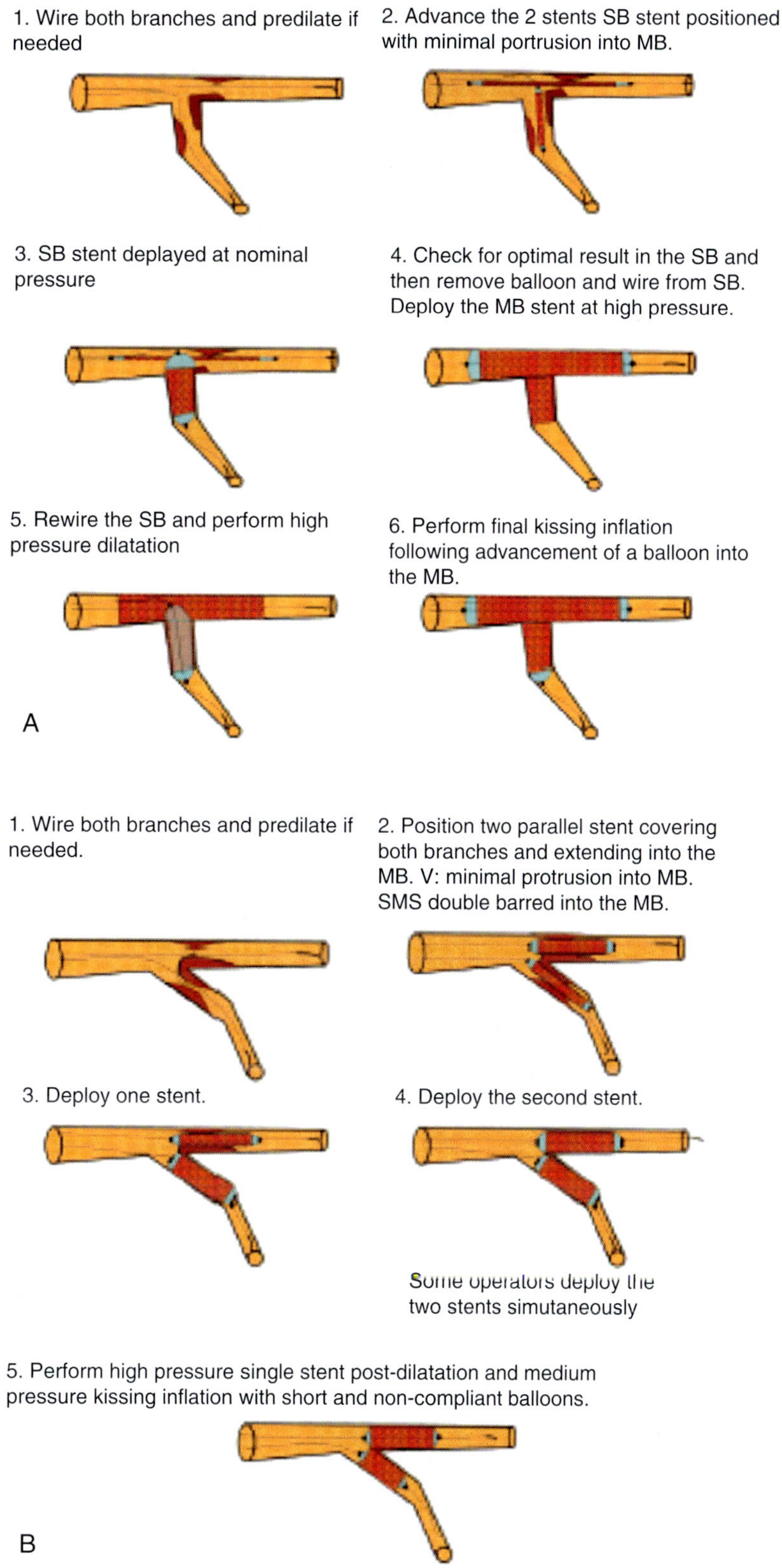

FIGURE 20.49 Schematic representation of the **(A)** modified T-stenting technique and **(B)** V-stenting technique. Reprinted from EuroIntervention Vol 6 (Supplement J), Latib A et al. When are two stents needed? Which technique is the best?. Pages No. J81-J87, Copyright (2010), with permission from Europa Digital & Publishing.

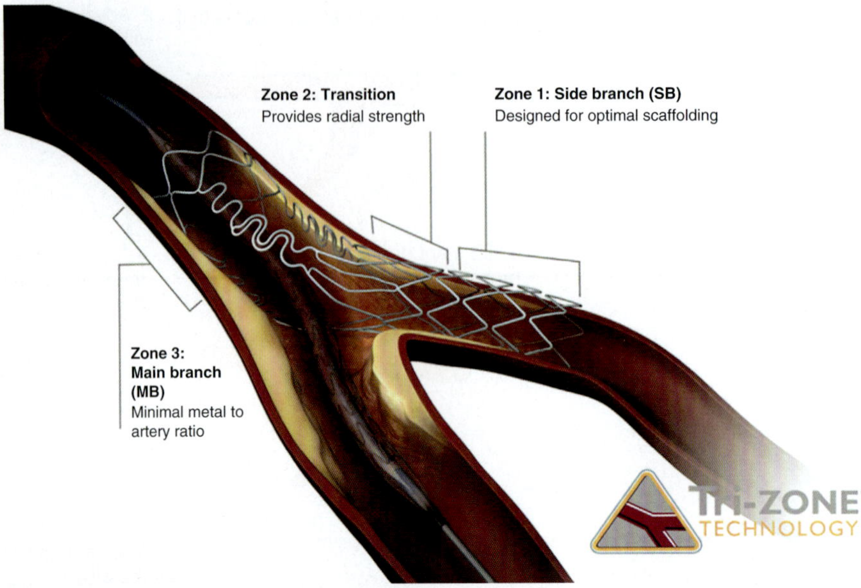

FIGURE 20.50 Tryton stent. The Tryton stent is the first stent approved for the treatment of bifurcation lesions. It is a chromium cobalt, bare-metal stent, and its concept is based on the "reverse culotte" technique. The side branch is secured with the placement of this dedicated stent in the proximal main vessel, across to the side branch, and the stent facilitates the positioning of a conventional stent in the proximal to distal main vessel. Reproduced with permission form Tryton Medical, Inc.

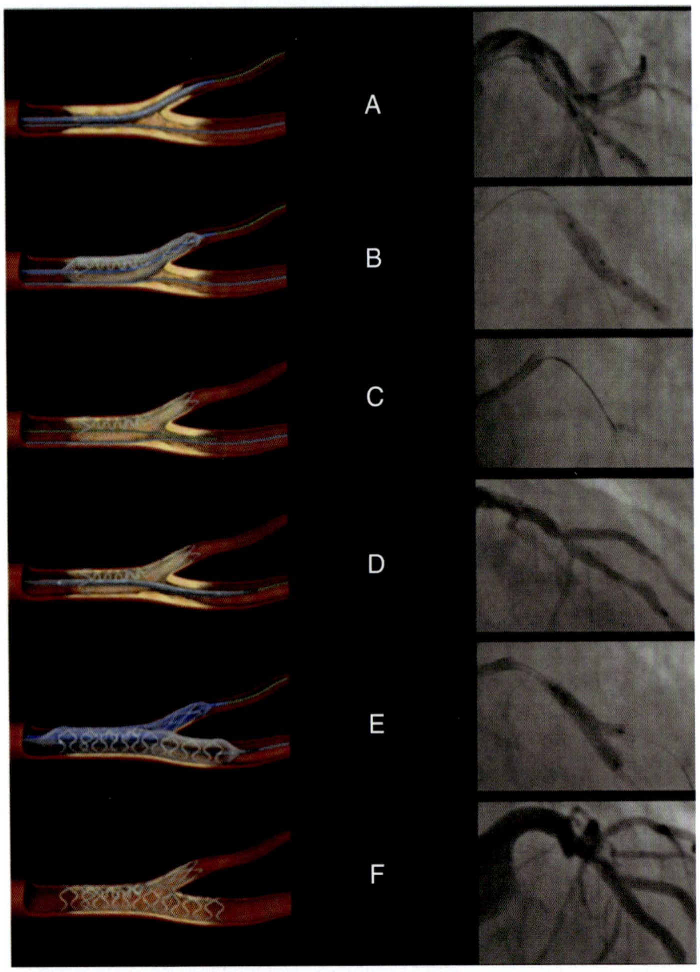

FIGURE 20.51 Schematic illustration of the reverse culotte stenting technique with the Tryton Side Branch Stent and a corresponding angiographic appearance from a patient treated for a left anterior descending/diagonal bifurcation lesion. **A**, Positioning of the Tryton stent is optimized by placing the middle markers equidistant from the carina; **(B)** inflation of the stepped balloon deploys the stent; **(C)** retraction of the side branch wire and recross into the distal main vessel; **(D)** positioning of the main vessel stent is followed by deployment of the stent; **(E)** wire recross into the side branch allows final kissing balloon inflation; **(F)** final result. Reprinted from EuroIntervention Vol 6 (Supplement J), Magro M et al. The Tryton Side Branch Stent EuroIntervention Supplement. Pages No. J147-J150, Copyright (2010), with permission from Europa Digital & Publishing.

REFERENCES

1. Esser JF. Studies in plastic surgery of the face: I. Use of skin from the neck to replace face defects. II. Plastic operations about the mouth. III. The epidermic inlay. *Ann Surg*. 1917;65(3):297-315.
2. Roguin A. Stent: the man and word behind the coronary metal prosthesis. *Circ Cardiovasc Interv*. 2011;4(2):206-209.
3. Ambekar S, Nanda A. Charles Stent and the mystery behind the word "stent". *J Neurosurg*. 2013;119(3):774-777.
4. Hedin M. The origin of the word stent. *Acta Radiol*. 1997;38(6):937-939.
5. https://en.oxforddictionaries.com/definition/stent.
6. Dotter CT. Transluminally-placed coilspring endarterial tube grafts. Long-term patency in canine popliteal artery. *Invest Radiol*. 1969;4(5):329-332.
7. Dotter CT, Buschmann RW, McKinney MK, Rosch J. Transluminal expandable nitinol coil stent grafting: preliminary report. *Radiology*. 1983;147(1):259-260.
8. Wright KC, Wallace S, Charnsangavej C, Carrasco CH, Gianturco C. Percutaneous endovascular stents: an experimental evaluation. *Radiology*. 1985;156(1):69-72.
9. Maass D, Zollikofer CL, Largiader F, Senning A. Radiological follow-up of transluminally inserted vascular endoprostheses: an experimental study using expanding spirals. *Radiology*. 1984;152(3):659-663.
10. Palmaz JC, Sibbitt RR, Reuter SR, Tio FO, Rice WJ. Expandable intraluminal graft: a preliminary study. Work in progress. *Radiology*. 1985;156(1):73-77.
11. George BS, Voorhees WD III, Roubin GS, et al. Multicenter investigation of coronary stenting to treat acute or threatened closure after percutaneous transluminal coronary angioplasty: clinical and angiographic outcomes. *J Am Coll Cardiol*. 1993;22(1):135-143.
12. Lincoff AM, Topol EJ, Chapekis AT, et al. Intracoronary stenting compared with conventional therapy for abrupt vessel closure complicating coronary angioplasty: a matched case-control study. *J Am Coll Cardiol*. 1993;21(4):866-875.
13. Roubin GS, Cannon AD, Agrawal SK, et al. Intracoronary stenting for acute and threatened closure complicating percutaneous transluminal coronary angioplasty. *Circulation*. 1992;85(3):916-927.
14. Roubin GS, Robinson KA, King SB III, et al. Early and late results of intracoronary arterial stenting after coronary angioplasty in dogs. *Circulation*. 1987;76(4):891-897.
15. Fischman DL, Leon MB, Baim DS, et al. A randomized comparison of coronary-stent placement and balloon angioplasty in the treatment of coronary artery disease. Stent Restenosis Study Investigators. *N Engl J Med*. 1994;331(8):496-501.
16. Serruys PW, de Jaegere P, Kiemeneij F, et al. A comparison of balloon-expandable-stent implantation with balloon angioplasty in patients with coronary artery disease. Benestent Study Group. *N Engl J Med*. 1994;331(8):489-495.
17. Serruys PW, van Hout B, Bonnier H, et al. Randomised comparison of implantation of heparin-coated stents with balloon angioplasty in selected patients with coronary artery disease (Benestent II). *Lancet*. 1998;352(9129):673-681.
18. Albiero R, Nishida T, Adamian M, et al. Edge restenosis after implantation of high activity (32)P radioactive beta-emitting stents. *Circulation*. 2000;101(21):2454-2457.
19. Albiero R, Adamian M, Kobayashi N, et al. Short- and intermediate-term results of (32)P radioactive beta-emitting stent implantation in patients with coronary artery disease: the Milan Dose-Response Study. *Circulation*. 2000;101(1):18-26.
20. Popma JJ, Suntharalingam M, Lansky AJ, et al. Randomized trial of 90Sr/90Y beta-radiation versus placebo control for treatment of in-stent restenosis. *Circulation*. 2002;106(9):1090-1096.
21. Waksman R, Cheneau E, Ajani AE, et al. Intracoronary radiation therapy improves the clinical and angiographic outcomes of diffuse in-stent restenotic lesions: results of the Washington Radiation for In-Stent Restenosis Trial for Long Lesions (Long WRIST) Studies. *Circulation*. 2003;107(13):1744-1749.
22. Leon MB, Teirstein PS, Moses JW, et al. Localized intracoronary gamma-radiation therapy to inhibit the recurrence of restenosis after stenting. *N Engl J Med*. 2001;344(4):250-256.
23. Morice MC, Serruys PW, Sousa JE, et al. A randomized comparison of a sirolimus-eluting stent with a standard stent for coronary revascularization. *N Engl J Med*. 2002;346(23):1773-1780.
24. Moses JW, Leon MB, Popma JJ, et al. Sirolimus-eluting stents versus standard stents in patients with stenosis in a native coronary artery. *N Engl J Med*. 2003;349(14):1315-1323.

chapter 21

Percutaneous Interventions for Valvular Heart Disease

HONG JUN (FRANCISCO) YUN, MD and STANLEY J. CHETCUTI, MD

TRANSCATHETER AORTIC VALVE INTERVENTIONS

Aortic stenosis is the most common valvular heart disease in developed countries, with increasing prevalence as the population ages. Left untreated, severe, symptomatic aortic stenosis has a poor prognosis with mortality rates approaching 50% at 2 years.[1] Traditionally, surgical aortic valve replacement (SAVR) represented the only treatment available to relieve the left ventricular outflow obstruction, alleviate symptoms, and improve survival.[2] Despite the class I indication from the American College of Cardiology/American Heart Association (ACC/AHA) guidelines for aortic valve replacement in patients with severe, symptomatic aortic stenosis, nearly one-third of patients are not referred for or declined treatment, often due to multiple comorbidities as well as anatomic factors that make patients poor candidates for SAVR.[3] The emergence of transcatheter aortic valve replacement (TAVR) over the past decade has provided a feasible and lower-risk option for the frail and elderly who are deemed poor candidates for surgery.

Currently, 2 TAVR platforms have been approved by the U.S. Food and Drug Administration: the CoreValve Revalving System (Medtronic, Minneapolis, MN) and the Edwards Sapien System (Edwards Lifesciences, Irvine, CA). The landmark Placement of AoRTic TraNscathetER Valve Trial (PARTNER) demonstrated the superiority of TAVR using the balloon-expandable Edwards Sapien valve compared with medical therapy in extreme surgical risk patients (all-cause mortality, 71.8% vs 93.6% for TAVR vs medical therapy [Hazard Ratio 0.50, 95% CI 0.39-0.65, *P* < .0001]), as well as noninferiority of TAVR to SAVR in high-risk patients (all-cause mortality, 67.8% vs 62.4% for TAVR vs SAVR [HR 1.04, 95% CI 0.86-1.24; *P* = .76]) at 5 years.[4,5] Subsequently the US Pivotal CoreValve trials using the self-expanding valve prosthesis not only showed favorability for TAVR in the extreme surgical risk patients but also demonstrated superiority of TAVR to SAVR in the high-risk patient population (all-cause mortality, 14.2% vs 19.1% absolute risk reduction 4.9%, *P* = .04 for superiority).[6,7] Given the promising results of these landmark trials using the first generation platforms, further studies have been carried out to define the role of TAVR in lower-risk patients. The PARTNER-2 trial showed noninferiority of the Edwards Sapien XT valve in intermediate surgical risk patients with severe aortic stenosis randomized to SAVR versus TAVR (primary endpoint of all-cause death or stroke, 19.3% vs 21.1% [HR 0.89, 95% CI 0.73-1.09, *P* = .25]).[8] TAVR also compared favorably with surgery in terms of lower rates of bleeding, kidney injury, and new-onset atrial fibrillation. Although TAVR was associated with higher rates of paravalvular regurgitation (PVR), the Sapien XT valves resulted in better hemodynamics with lower gradients and larger valve areas compared with surgical valves. Similarly, the Safety and Efficacy Study of the Medtronic CoreValve® System in the Treatment of Severe, Symptomatic Aortic Stenosis in Intermediate Risk Subjects Who Need Aortic Valve Replacement (SURTAVI) trial, an intermediate risk study using the second generation Medtronic CoreValve, demonstrated noninferiority of TAVR versus SAVR with respect to the primary endpoint of all-cause death or disabling stroke (12.6% vs 14.0%; 95% credible interval [Bayesian analysis] for difference, −5.2%-2.3%; posterior probability of noninferiority, >0.999).[9]

Based on the results of these trials, advances to newer generation devices, and refinements in the procedural approach, TAVR provides an effective, minimally invasive therapeutic option for patients with severe aortic stenosis, who previously were left untreated. This paradigm shift has been reflected in the most recent 2017 valvular heart disease guidelines endorsed by the ACC/AHA that recommend either surgical AVR or TAVR for high-risk patients (class I) and make TAVR a reasonable alternative to SAVR in intermediate-risk patients (class IIa) after assessment by a heart valve team.[10]

TRANSCATHETER AORTIC VALVE REPLACEMENT: EDWARDS SAPIEN VALVE

Edwards Sapien Valve and Commander Delivery System (Figure 21.1)

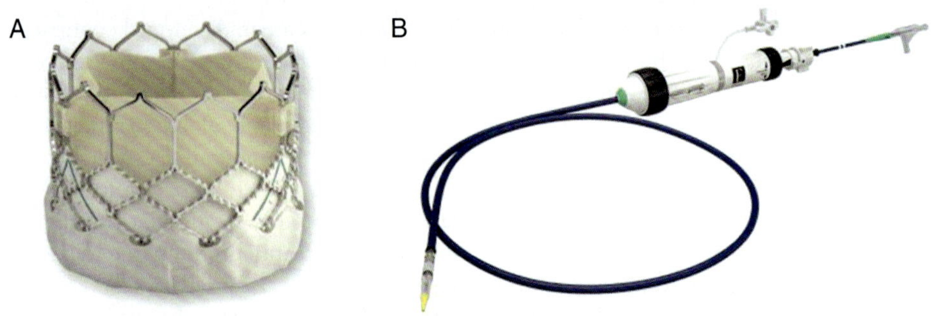

FIGURE 21.1 **A**, The Edwards Sapien valve is a trileaflet bovine pericardial valve mounted on a balloon-expandable, radio-opaque cobalt chromium stent. The low frame height and open cell geometry promote access to the coronary arteries for future interventions. The newest generation Edwards Sapien 3 valve includes a polyethylene terephthalate outer skirt to reduce PVR, and it is available in 4 sizes (20, 23, 26, and 29 mm). **B**, The Commander delivery system incorporates a nose-cone-tipped inner balloon catheter on which the prosthesis is crimped and an outer deflectable flex catheter. An attached handle incorporates a rotating wheel used to deflect the flex catheter tip, a fine adjustment wheel for fine alignment of the prosthesis during valve alignment, a balloon lock knob to secure the balloon catheter to the flex catheter, and a flush port. The balloon catheter contains radio-opaque valve alignment markers, defining the valve alignment position and working length of the balloon. A central radio-opaque marker in the balloon assists in valve positioning. The delivery system allows for advancing or retracting the valve several millimeters up or down within the annulus by rotating the fine alignment wheel.

Preprocedural Planning Using MDCT (Figure 21.2)

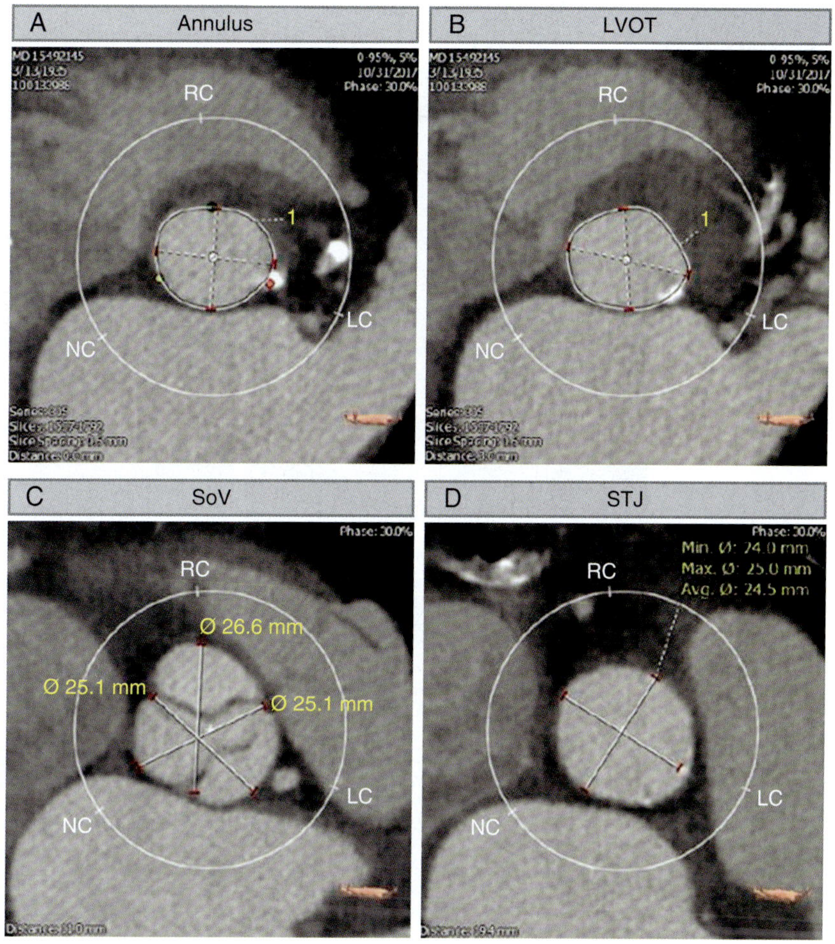

FIGURE 21.2 Key measurements to determine appropriate sizing of the TAVR are shown at the levels of the **(A)** annulus (perimeter: 64 mm, area: 3.2 cm2), **(B)** left ventricular outflow tract (LVOT), **(C)** sinus of Valsalva, **(D)** sinotubular junction (STJ).

Successful Deployment

Preprocedural planning using MDCT is integral to successful device deployment (**FIGURE 21.3**.)

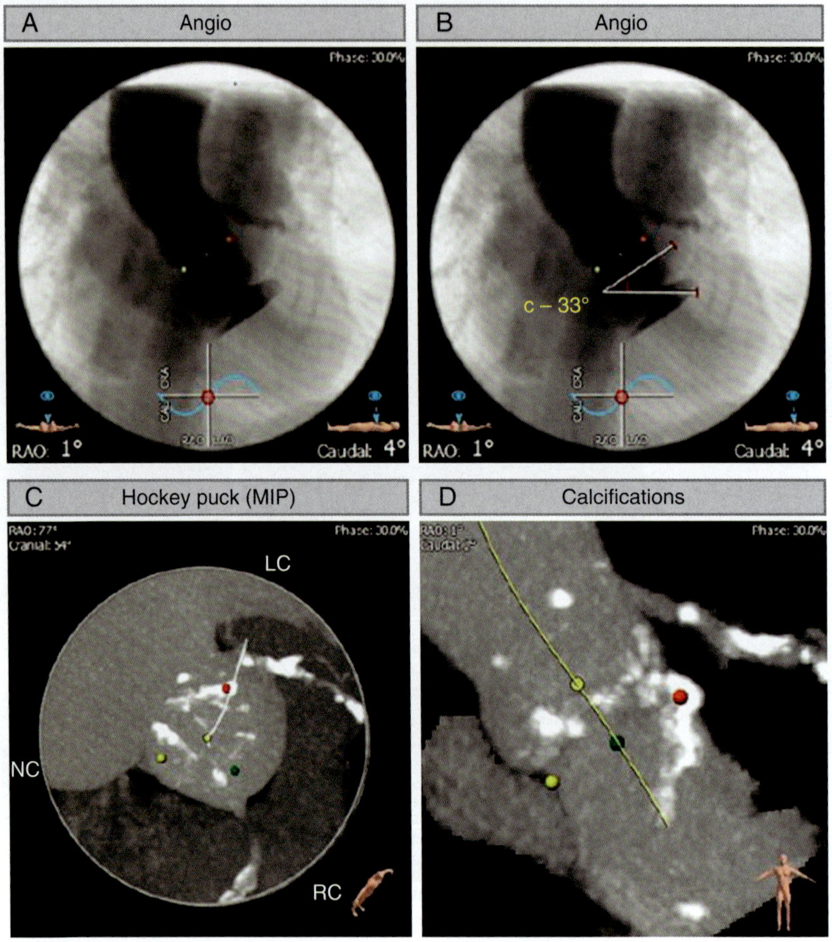

FIGURE 21.3 **A and B**, Multidetector computed tomography (MDCT) reconstruction of the optimal fluoroscopic implant view or "coplanar" view, where all 3 cusps are seen in a line, and the aortic root orientation. **B**, The aortoventricular angle is best determined from the coronal view by determining the angle of the horizontal plane at the level of the ventricle and aortic annulus angulation. **C and D**, MDCT demonstrating the burden of calcification of the native aortic valve leaflets, annulus, and LVOT. Excessive leaflet calcification is a potential risk for coronary obstruction while increased LVOT or annular calcification is a risk factor for PVR (especially asymmetric calcification) and annular rupture.[11] The burden of calcium at the aortic annulus has been directly correlated to rates of complete heart block, degree of PVR, risk of annular rupture, and, in certain circumstances, residual post-implant gradients.[12-14]

Peripheral Vascular Access

Imaging of the peripheral vascular system using MDCT is crucial to access vessels for implantation and minimize the risk of vascular complications. Multiple measurements are taken along the common iliac, external iliac, common femoral, innominate, subclavian, and proximal axillary arteries bilaterally. **FIGURE 21.4** displays a 3D computed tomography (CT) reconstruction of the peripheral vasculature with sequential axial cuts, illustrating lumen size, tortuosity, and calcification. The vessel anatomy is suitable for a 23 mm Edwards Sapien 3 valve through a 14 FR delivery system.

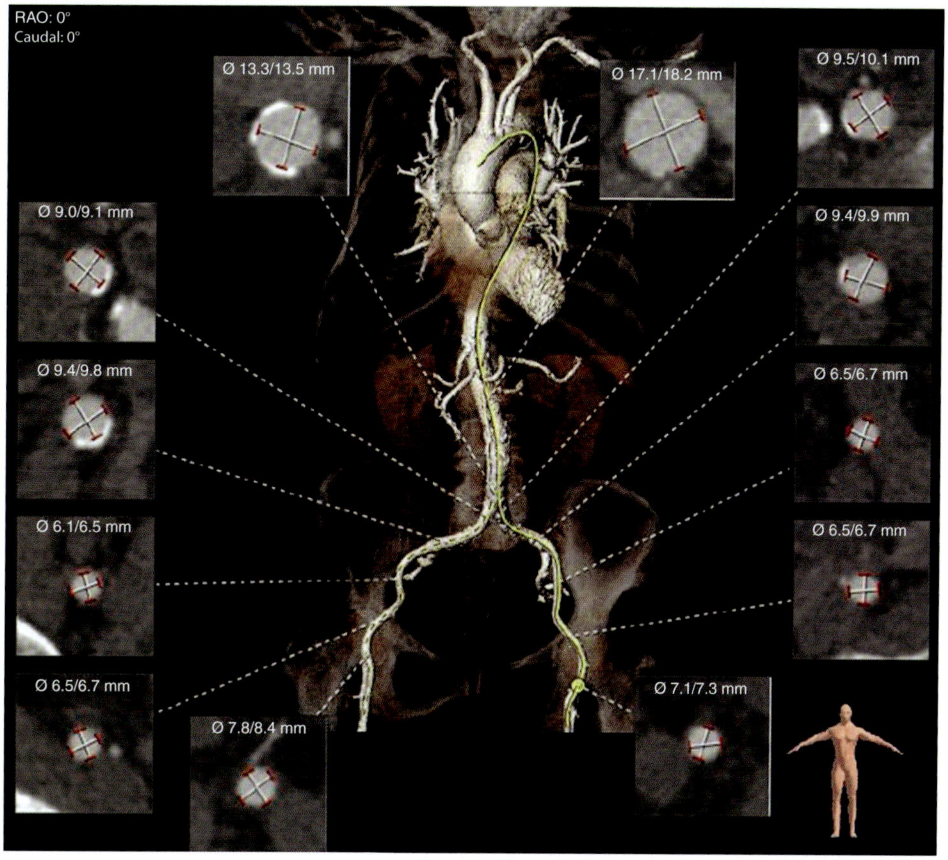

FIGURE 21.4 MDCT of peripheral vasculature access vessels.

CASE 1 *Patient With Severe Aortic Stenosis*

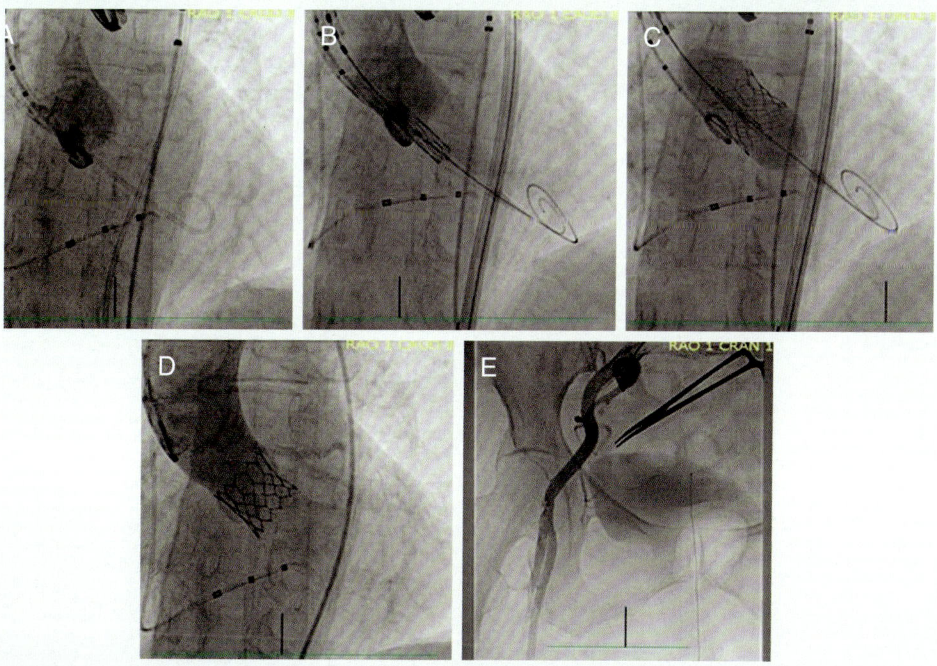

FIGURE 21.5 Transfemoral transcatheter aortic valve replacement in a patient with severe aortic stenosis using 23 mm Edwards Sapien 3 valve.

As shown in **FIGURE 21.5A**, a pigtail catheter placed in the noncoronary cusp, an aortogram is performed in the optimal deployment projection or coplanar (Video 21.1). In **FIGURE 21.5B**, the aortic valve prosthesis and delivery system are advanced over a preshaped Safari guide wire (Boston Scientific, Marlborough, MA, USA). The retroflex catheter is activated to allow the passage of the valve through the aortic arch. Correct positioning is confirmed with fluoroscopy and transesophageal echocardiography (TEE) (Video 21.2). The valve is deployed during rapid ventricular pacing at 180 beats per minute (bpm) (**FIGURE 21.5C**, Video 21.3). A final aortogram is performed and confirms optimal valve position, mild aortic insufficiency, and unrestricted coronary flow (**FIGURE 21.5D**, Video 21.4). **E**, Iliofemoral angiography shows no vascular complications, and percutaneous closure is performed using Perclose ProGlide sutures (Abbott Vascular, Santa Clara, California, USA).

Hemodynamic Tracings

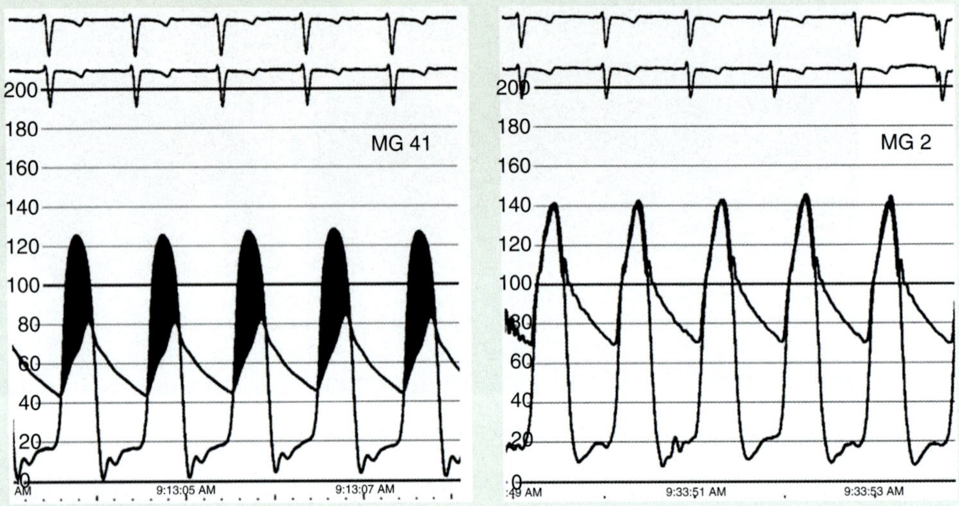

FIGURE 21.6 Hemodynamic tracings before and after successful transcatheter aortic valve replacement with an Edwards Sapien 3 valve in a patient severe aortic stenosis.

In **FIGURE 21.6**, simultaneous aortic and left ventricular pressures are measured before (left panel) and after (right panel) device implantation. Before TAVR, a large LV-AO gradient, slow aortic pressure upstroke, and absence of a dicrotic notch are evident. After successful device deployment, the hemodynamic tracing reveals a minimal pressure gradient across the valve, recovery of brisk aortic upstroke, and a crisp dicrotic notch. The mean gradient across the aortic valve has decreased from 41 to 2 mm Hg.

Assessment of Transcatheter Heart Valves (THV)

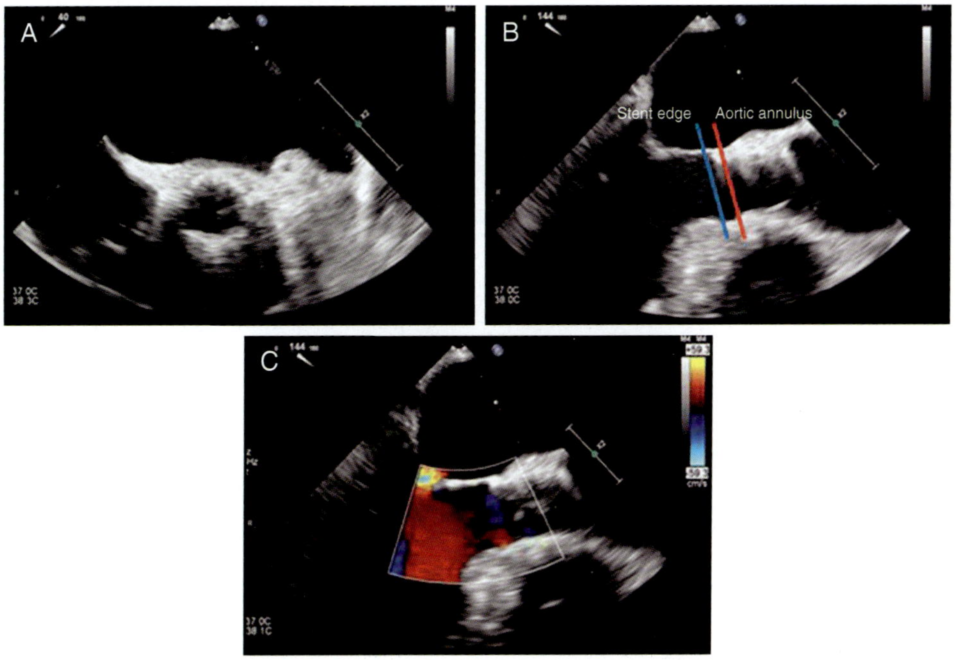

FIGURE 21.7 Echocardiography in the assessment of THV.

Post-TAVR echocardiographic assessment guidelines were reviewed in a joint statement of the American and European Societies of Echocardiography and further endorsed by the Valve Academic Research Consortium (VARC).[15,16] Follow-up echocardiography should be performed predischarge (or within 30 days after transapical TAVR), at 6 and 12 months, and then yearly. A systematic approach to imaging at follow-up includes visual inspection, hemodynamic assessment of the transcatheter heart valves (THV), assessment of adjacent cardiac structures, and assessment of ventricular function. This approach allows accurate diagnosis of common THV-related complications.[17]. In FIGURES 21.7AB, 2D TEE images of an Edwards Sapien 3 valve immediately after deployment in short- and long-axis views illustrating the circular appearance of the new valve prosthesis deployed below the native aortic valve annulus. There is no evidence of paravalvular aortic regurgitation on color Doppler (FIGURE 21.7C).

TRANSCATHETER AORTIC VALVE REPLACEMENT: MEDTRONIC COREVALVE EVOLUT

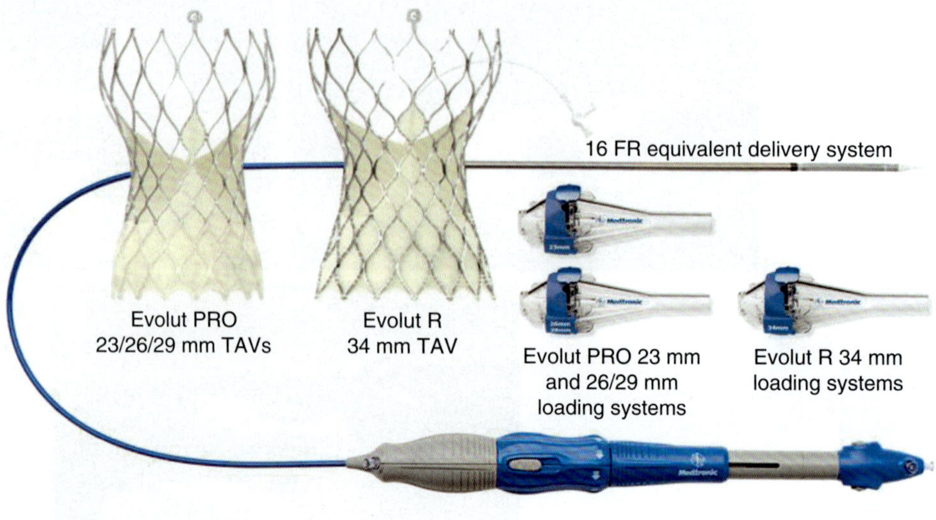

FIGURE 21.8 The Medtronic Evolut CoreValve and EnVeo Delivery Catheter System.

The Medtronic CoreValve Evolut System is made of a trileaflet, supra-annular porcine tissue valve on a self-expanding nitinol frame (**FIGURE 21.8**). The nitinol frame conforms and seals to the noncircular annulus while preserving circularity at the height of the functioning valve. The nitinol frame geometry provides consistent radial force across the treated annulus. The newest generation Evolut Pro bioprosthesis has an added external porcine pericardial wrap to increase surface area contact and minimize paravalvular leak. The open frame geometry can accommodate a 10 FR catheter for future coronary access. The Evolut valve is mounted on 14 and 16 FR EnVeo Delivery Catheter System (DCS) with an integrated inline sheath that allows for access without a separate introducer sheath. The EnVeo DCS provides uniform and controlled valve expansion in the annulus and the option to recapture and reposition up to 3 times. The device is able to treat annuli up to 30 mm and is available in 4 sizes (23, 26, and 29 mm Evolut Pro and 34 mm Evolut R).

Measurements and Assessments

Aortic Valve, sinuses of valsalva and coronary arteries

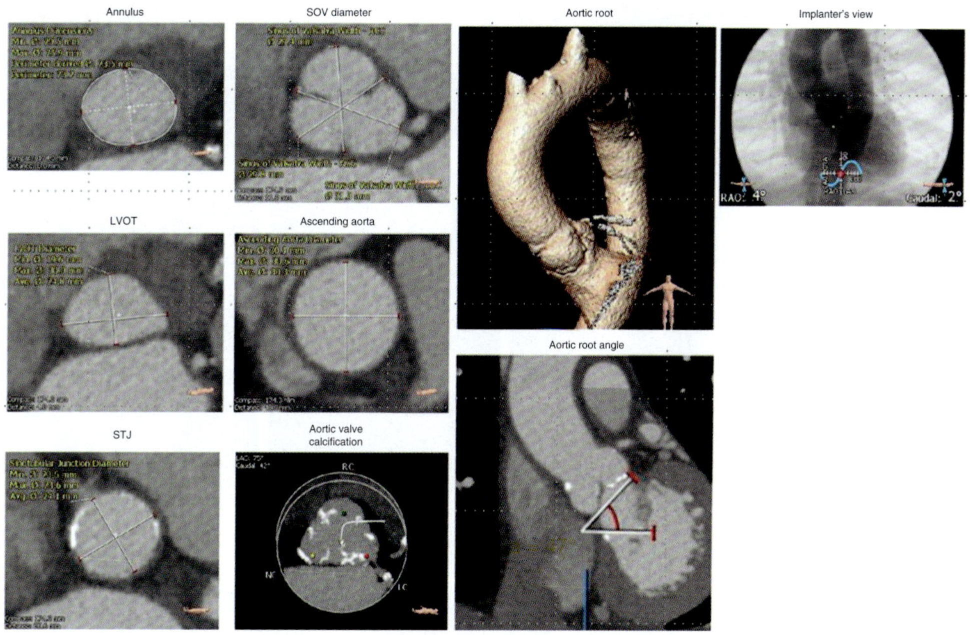

FIGURE 21.9 MDCT measurements and assessment of the aortic valve complex.

Accurate aortic annular measurements are key to determining the size of device and also in reducing the impact of paravalvular regurgitation (FIGURE 21.9). Adequate sinus of Valsalva width and height is required to avoid coronary occlusion. Other anatomic considerations include burden of calcification in the aortic valve apparatus, adequate aortoventricular angle less than 70° for iliofemoral and left subclavian access routes, and less than 30° for the right subclavian approach. MDCT reconstruction of the optimal fluoroscopic implant view or "coplanar" view is shown here. Key measurements to determine appropriate sizing of the TAVR are shown at the levels of the aortic valve annulus (min: 20.5 mm, max: 25.9 mm, perimeter: 73.7 mm), LVOT, sinus of Valsalva, and STJ. The perimeter is the preferred sizing measurement for the CoreValve Evolut platform. A 29 mm CoreValve Evolut Pro THV was chosen based on the above characteristics.

Peripheral Vascular Assessment

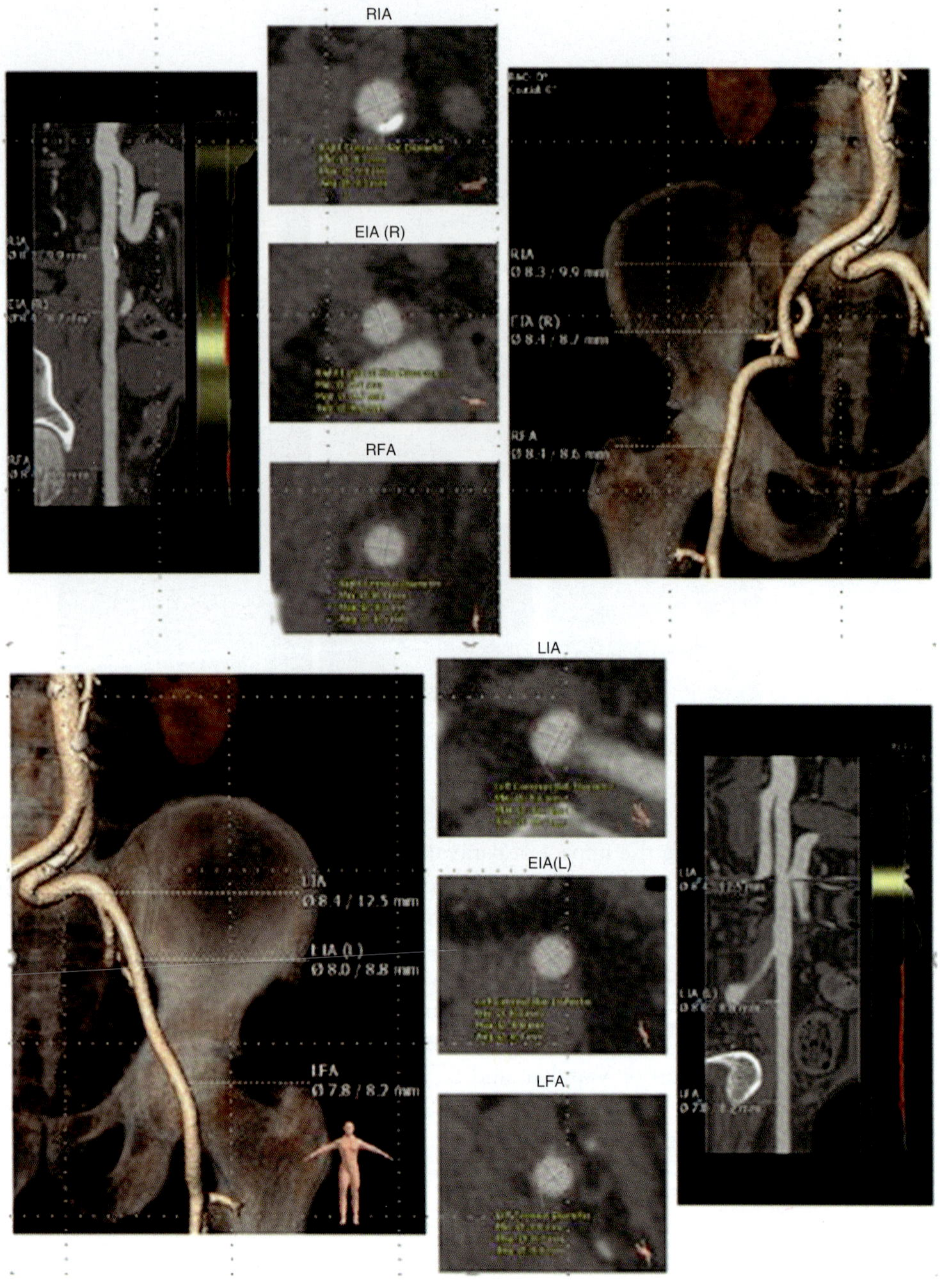

FIGURE 21.10 Peripheral vascular assessment using MDCT.

Important procedural considerations for vascular access include vessel size, degree and location of calcification, and tortuosity of the target vessels. CT with 3D reconstruction of the peripheral vasculature and sequential axial cuts, illustrating lumen size, tortuosity, and calcification of vessels, is shown here. Careful evaluation will determine the preferred side for access to deliver the THV in addition to the optimal location for common femoral artery puncture (ie, at sites absent of calcification) to allow for preclosure using Perclose ProGlide percutaneous sutures (**FIGURE 21.10**).

CASE 2 *Patient with Severe Aortic Atenosis*

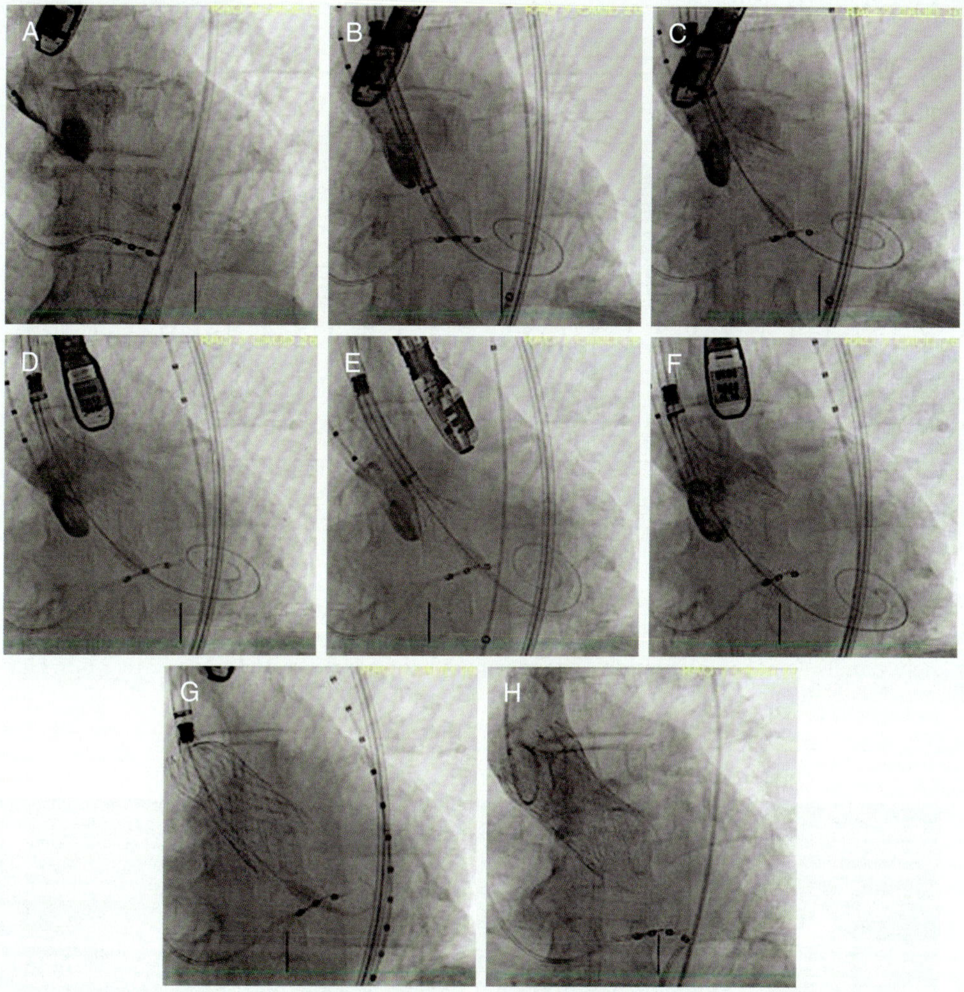

FIGURE 21.11 Transfemoral transcatheter aortic valve replacement in an 80-year-old patient with severe aortic stenosis and moderate risk for an open procedure using a 29 mm CoreValve Evolut Pro.

A pigtail catheter is placed at the bottom of the noncoronary cusp, and a diagnostic aortogram is performed in the coplanar view (**FIGURE 21.11A**, Video 21.5). A 29 mm CoreValve Evolut Pro prosthesis and delivery system are advanced over a preshaped Safari guide wire to the level of implantation under fluoroscopy. The projection is adjusted to view the radiopaque marker band as a straight line before deployment (**FIGURE 21.11B**, Video 21.6). Using the linear markings on the valve, the valve is positioned 3 to 5 mm below the patient's native valve and slowly released with pacing at 110 bpm using a Tempo (Biotrace, Menlo Park, CA) active fixation temporary pacemaker to maintain stability during valve deployment (**FIGURE 21.11C**, Video 21.7). At the 80% position and before the point of no recapture, an aortogram is performed revealing that the bioprosthesis has migrated above the native valve annulus and the decision is made to recapture the valve (**FIGURE 21.11D**, Video 21.8). A second deployment is initiated with the bioprosthesis again positioned 3 to 5 mm below native annulus (**FIGURE 21.11E**, Video 21.9). An aortogram is performed at the point of no recapture and shows the bioprosthesis at the optimal implant depth (**FIGURE 21.11F**, Video 21.10). The position of the valve is further confirmed by TEE before release. The remaining portion of the valve is fully deployed and confirmation of complete release of the valve from the loading system is confirmed on fluoroscopy (**FIGURE 21.11G**, Video 21.11). A final aortogram verifies that the CoreValve is deployed at the 5 mm mark with minimal aortic regurgitation (**FIGURE 21.11H**, Video 21.12).

Hemodynamic Tracings

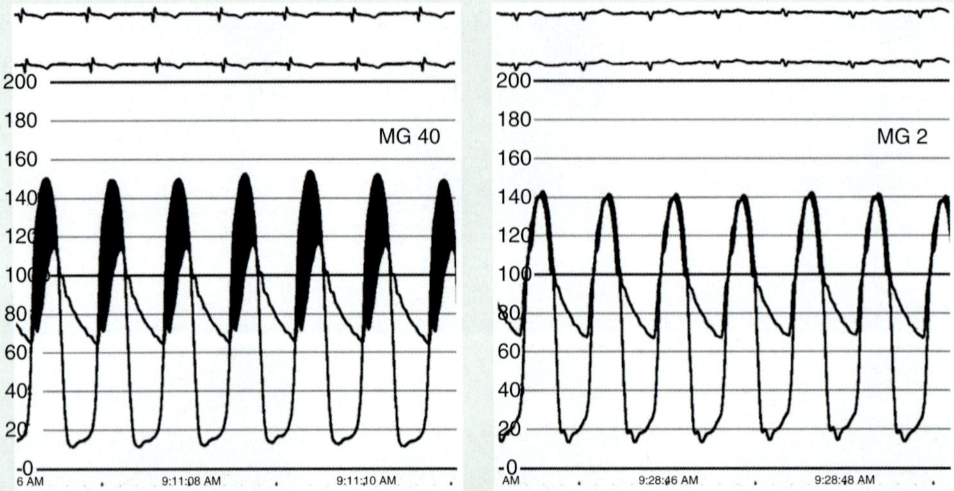

FIGURE 21.12 Hemodynamic changes after successful transcatheter aortic valve replacement using a 29 mm CoreValve Evolut Pro valve.

In **FIGURE 21.12**, simultaneous aortic and left ventricular pressures measurements are shown before (left panel) and after (right panel) device implantation. The mean gradient has decreased from 40 to 2 mm Hg.

TEE

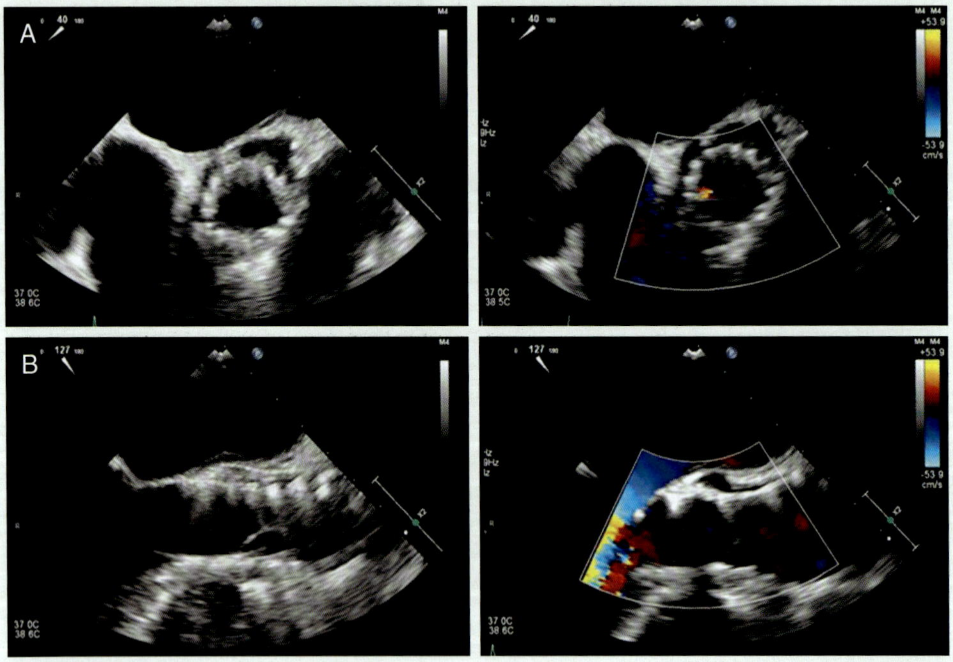

FIGURE 21.13 Real-time assessment of THV deployment using TEE.

In addition to fluoroscopy, echocardiography provides real-time assessment of the valve position, leaflet motion, paravalvular regurgitation, and mitral valve function. In the setting of hemodynamic collapse, echocardiography is crucial to identify potential etiologies such as aortic root catastrophes, left and right ventricular dysfunction, or cardiac tamponade. Intraprocedural TEE immediately after deployment of a 29 mm CoreValve Evolut

Pro valve is shown in short (**FIGURE 21.13A**) and long (**FIGURE 21.13B**) axis views with color Doppler. TEE is used to confirm adequate implant depth, paravalvular aortic regurgitation, and function of the new prosthesis. Note the circular appearance of the new valve prosthesis with minimal protrusion into the LVOT and no impingement on the mitral valve leaflets. To assess for paravalvular regurgitation, color Doppler should always be performed in both the long and short axis projections, with visualization of all jets entering the left ventricle. The short axis views are particularly useful to identify jets around the perimeter of the valve. Multiple guidelines endorse use of a multiwindow, multiparametric approach taking into account the total circumferential extent of jets, width, number, and path of the jets along with presence of proximal flow convergence.[16] Note that small paravalvular jets following TAVR may spontaneously regress over 10 to 15 minutes and require no further intervention as seen for this patient.[18]

TRANSCATHETER VALVE-IN-VALVE INTERVENTIONS

Improvements in durability and the desire to avoid anticoagulation have made the bioprosthetic tissue valves the most commonly implanted surgical heart valves (SHV). However, within 10 to 20 years these valves will degenerate resulting in stenosis or regurgitation or both. Conventional therapy for bioprosthetic failure has been reoperation and surgical aortic valve replacement, but patients requiring redo valvular surgery are at increased risk for adverse events related to technical challenges, chest wall adhesions, advanced age, and high burden of comorbid conditions. Operative mortality for redo valve surgery may exceed 20% in high-risk patients.[19] With favorable clinical outcomes associated with TAVR in treatment of native aortic valve disease, transcatheter valve-in-valve (VIV) implantation has recently emerged as a practical and safe option for treatment of failing surgical bioprostheses. The PARTNER-2 VIV registry showed a low, overall 30-day and 1-year mortality of 2.7% and 12.4%, respectively, in high-risk patients, with an observed-to-expected mortality ratio of 0.3 when using the Society of Thoracic Surgeons (STS) predicted risk model. The results also compared favorably to the earlier native valve PARTNER experiences using first generation devices in the treatment of native aortic valve disease. There was a steep learning curve associated with this procedure, reflected by the decrease in 1-year mortality from the initial registry to the subsequent continued access registry (19.7% vs 9.8%, respectively; $P = .006$).[20]

Transcatheter VIV interventions have been described using both the Edwards Sapien and Medtronic CoreValve THVs. The Melody transcatheter valve is a bovine jugular venous valve attached to a platinum-iridium stent scaffold designed for use in the pulmonary circulation. Unlike the self-expanding valves, the Edwards Sapien valve is suitable for both retrograde and anterograde approaches. Device malposition, coronary occlusion, and elevated postprocedural gradients have been observed more commonly in aortic VIV procedures compared with native aortic valve replacement.[21] Familiarity of the surgical bioprosthesis previously implanted including type and exact internal dimensions are essential for successful implantation and to minimize adverse events. In this regard, obtaining a detailed surgical operative note is crucial before the procedure.

AORTIC BIOPROSTHETIC VALVE-IN-VALVE: EDWARDS SAPIEN VALVE

CASE 3 *Patient with Rheumatic Heart Disease*

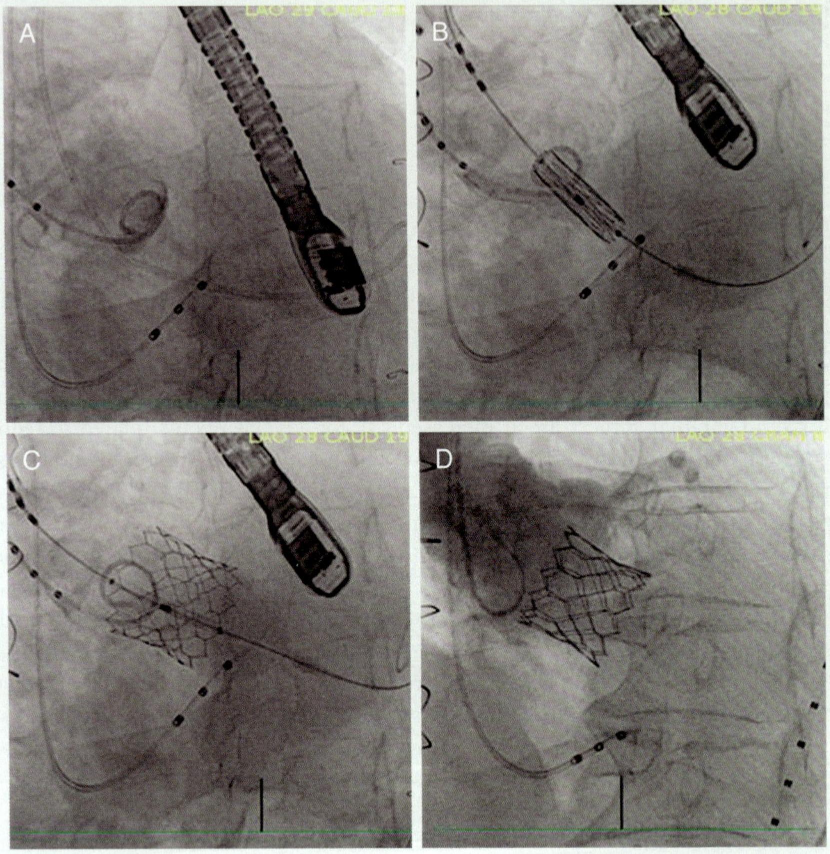

FIGURE 21.14 Transcatheter aortic VIV implantation using an Edwards Sapien valve.

A 63-year-old male with rheumatic heart disease and 2 prior surgical aortic valve replacements (most recently, a 29 mm Freestyle inclusion root and ascending aorta replacement) developed severe bioprosthetic aortic insufficiency (AI) and was planned for a transfemoral TAVR using a 29 mm Edwards Sapien 3 valve. The optimal placement of a transcatheter valve inside of a surgical heart valve is at the level of the sewing ring, which is the narrowest portion of all surgical valves. The use of this reference plane or "neo-annulus" and the fluoroscopic relationship between the surgical heart valve and the level of the sewing ring must be fully elucidated to achieve overlap with the THV.[22] The stentless Freestyle root, as depicted in this figure, poses several technical challenges including lack of radiopaque markers, difficulty measuring coronary ostial clearance and often lack of calcium or a frame to anchor the new TAVR. A pigtail catheter is placed in the noncoronary sinus and aortography shows severe, bioprosthetic AI (FIGURE 21.14A, Video 21.13). The aortic valve prosthesis is positioned across the previous bioprosthetic aortic valve and overlap with the prosthetic sewing ring (FIGURE 21.14B, Video 21.14). The valve is deployed during rapid ventricular pacing (FIGURE 21.14C, Video 21.15). Control aortography shows no aortic insufficiency, and the mean transvalvular gradient is measured at 4 mm Hg (FIGURE 21.14D, Video 21.16).

AORTIC AND MITRAL VALVE-IN-VALVE: EDWARDS SAPIEN VALVE

CASE 4 *Patient with Severe Bioprosethic Aortic and Mitral Stenosis*

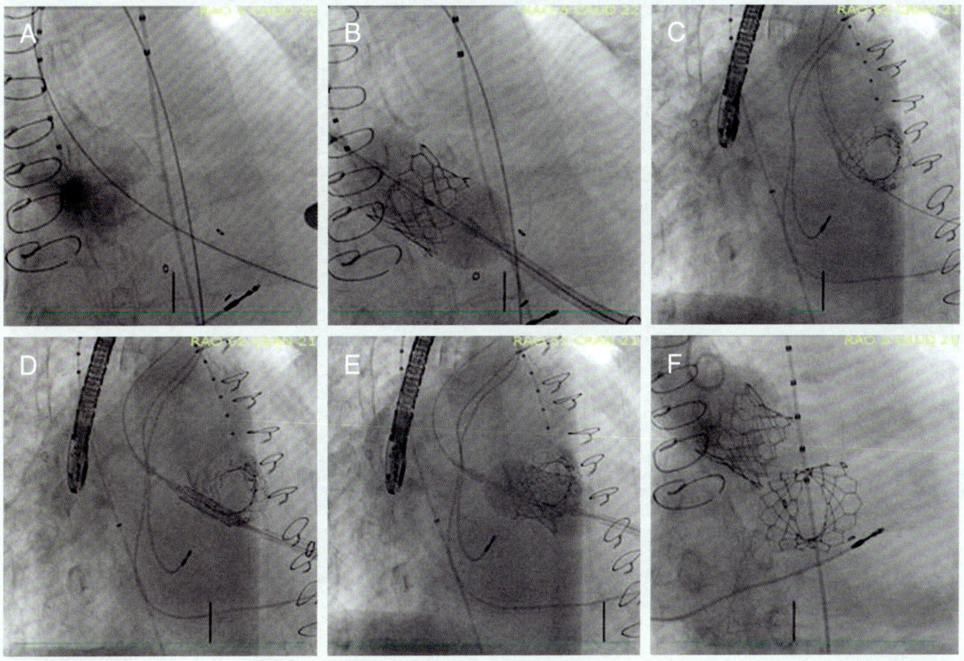

FIGURE 21.15 Transcatheter aortic and mitral VIV implantation using an Edwards Sapien valve via transapical access.

A 54-year-old male with severe bioprosthetic aortic (#25 Homograft) and mitral (#29 Medtronic Mosaic) stenosis who was deemed high risk for an open procedure underwent transcatheter aortic and mitral valve replacement with an Edwards Sapien 3 via transapical access. Through a left minithoracotomy, the left ventricular apex is exposed, and a Certitude sheath is placed over an Amplatz Extra Stiff wire. A transfemoral diagnostic aortogram is performed in preparation for placement of the transthoracic aortic valve prosthesis (**FIGURE 21.15A**, **Video 21.17**). A 29 mm Edwards Sapien 3 valve is positioned so that the midline of the Sapien valve is at the annular level, and the valve is deployed during rapid ventricular pacing (**FIGURE 21.15B**, **Video 21.18**). A J-tipped wire is then directed across the mitral valve, into the left superior pulmonary vein, and subsequently exchanged for an Amplatz Extra Stiff wire (**FIGURE 21.15C**). A 29 mm Edwards Sapien 3 valve is positioned across the old bioprosthetic mitral valve using fluoroscopic and TEE guidance (**FIGURE 21.15D**, **Video 21.19**). The Edwards Sapien 3 valve is deployed across the old mitral bioprosthesis during rapid ventricular pacing (**FIGURE 21.15E**, **Video 21.20**). Control aortography shows appropriate valve position and no AI (**FIGURE 21.15F**, **Video 21.21**). TEE also reveals minimal mitral regurgitation (MR) and a gradient of 2 and 3 mm Hg across the aortic and mitral valves, respectively.

TEE

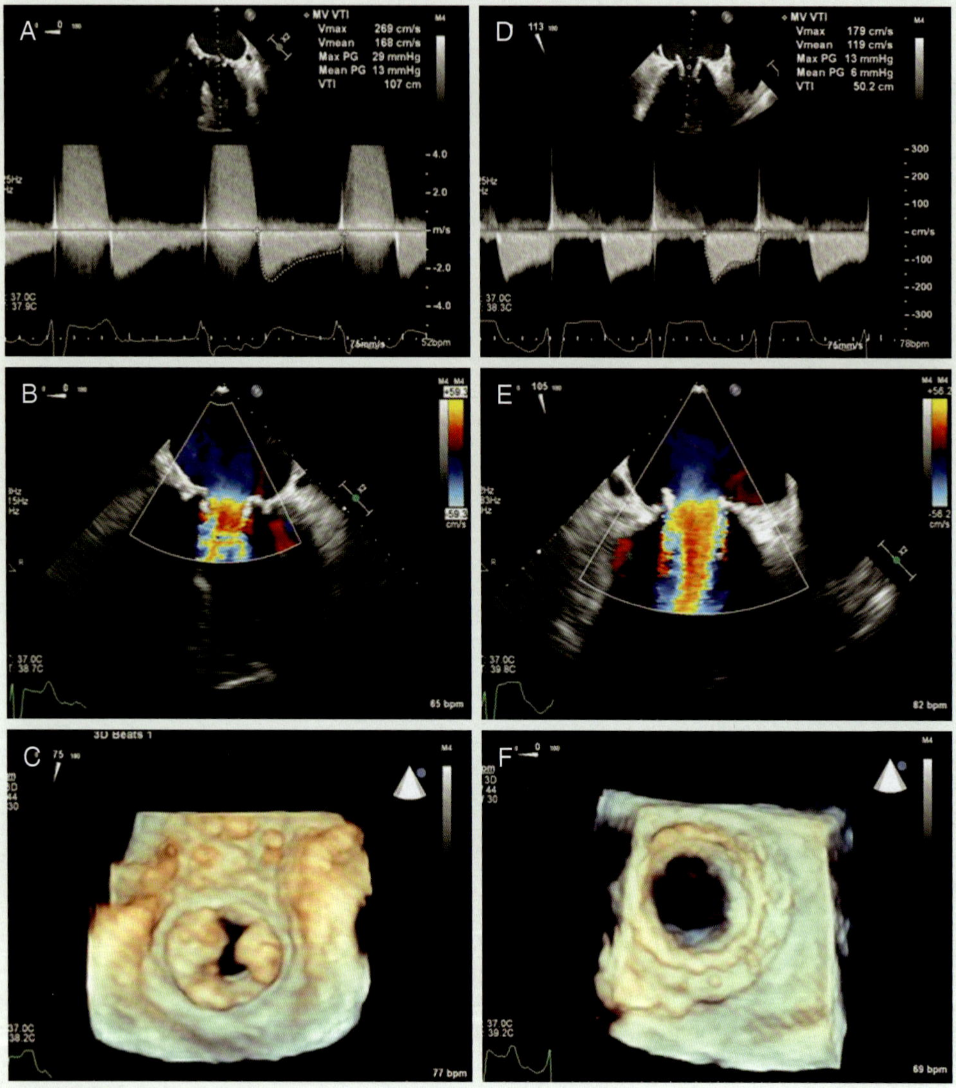

FIGURE 21.16 **A**, The mitral gradient as assessed by continuous wave Doppler shows severe mitral stenosis with a mean gradient of 13 mm Hg. **B**, Color flow Doppler displays a high-velocity jet across a stenotic mitral valve. **C**, 3D TEE showing a severe, bioprosthetic mitral stenosis. **D**, Continuous wave Doppler immediately after transcatheter mitral valve replacement shows a mitral gradient of 6 mm Hg. **E**, Color flow Doppler after valve implantation shows no MR. **F**, 3D TEE after valve implantation shows a well-functioning valve-in-valve prosthesis.

In **FIGURE 21.16**, TEE images of severe, bioprosthetic mitral valve stenosis before and after implantation of an Edwards Sapien 3 valve are shown.

TRICUSPID BIOPROSTHETIC VALVE-IN-VALVE: EDWARDS SAPIEN VALVE

Echocardiography

For an example of severe tricuspid stenosis see FIGURE 21.17.

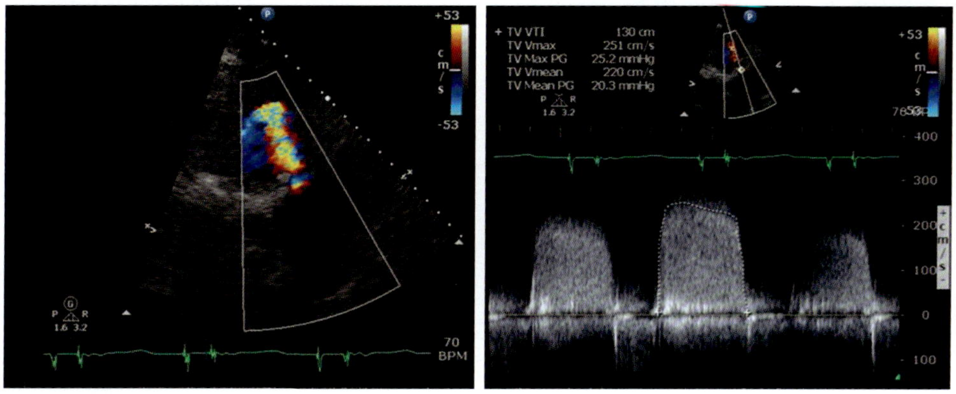

FIGURE 21.17 Transthoracic echocardiography shows a bioprosthetic tricuspid valve with an inflow VTI of 130 cm and a diastolic mean gradient of 20 mm Hg consistent with severe stenosis.

In FIGURE 21.18, an example of transesophageal echocardiography of a degenerated 31 mm Carpentier-Edwards bioprosthetic tricuspid valve is shown.

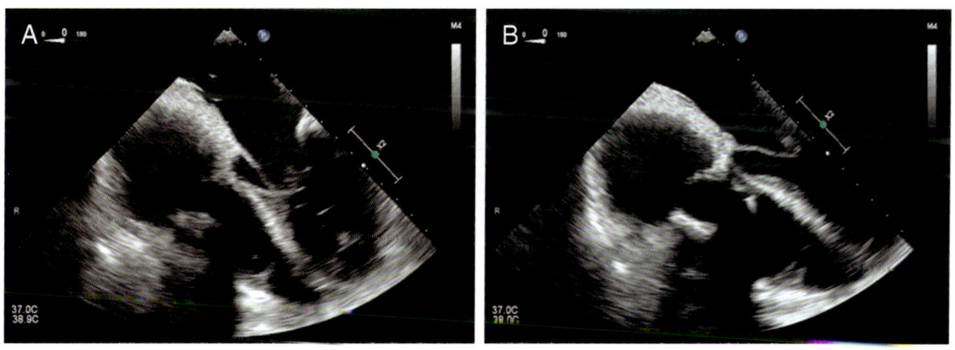

FIGURE 21.18 **A**, Before and **B**, after transcatheter VIV implantation using a 29 mm Edwards Sapien 3 valve.

CASE 5 *Patient with Severe Tricuspid Stenosis*

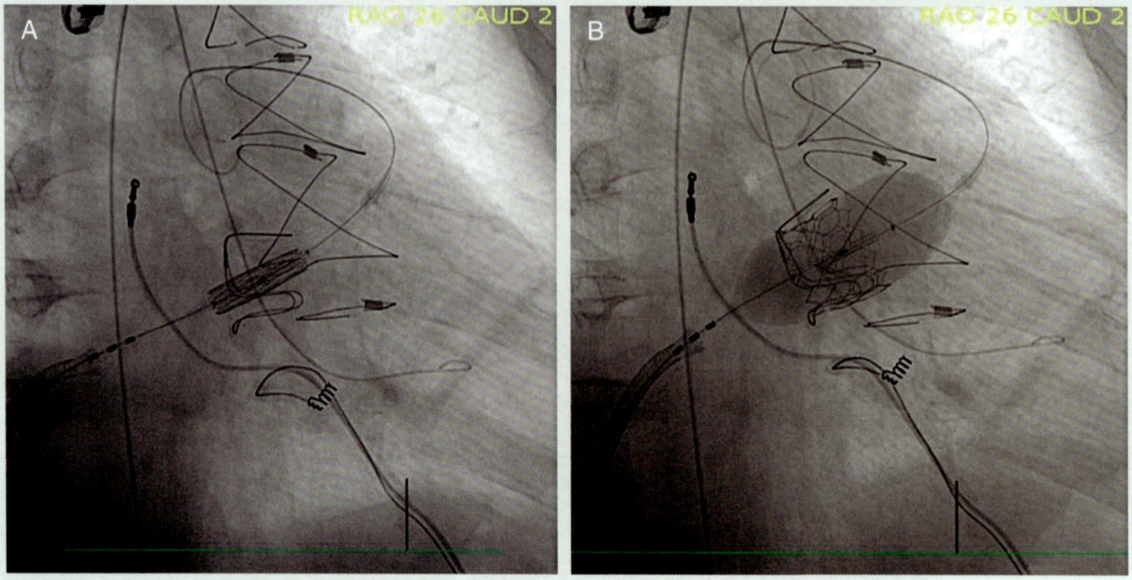

FIGURE 21.19 Transcatheter tricuspid VIV implantation using a 29 mm Edwards Sapien valve.

A 58-year-old male with 31 mm Carpentier-Edwards bioprosthetic tricuspid valve for endocarditis developed severe tricuspid stenosis and underwent a percutaneous transcatheter VIV procedure. As shown in **FIGURE 21.19A**, Because conventional right ventricular temporary pacing cannot be performed, arterial access is obtained and rapid pacing is provided via a 0.035″ J-tip starter wire in the left ventricular apex insulated by a multipurpose catheter. Alternatively, the percutaneous tricuspid valve replacement can be performed without rapid ventricular pacing or with temporary pacing leads placed in the right atrium, coronary sinus, or pericardium. This stented bioprosthesis is shown in the coaxial plane with the radiopaque components shown in a straight line. Over a preshaped Confida wire in the right pulmonary artery, a 29 mm Edwards Sapien 3 valve is positioned into the bioprosthetic tricuspid valve (**Video 21.22**). The Edwards Sapien 3 valve is inflated during rapid pacing at 180 bpm (**FIGURE 21.19B**, **Video 21.23**). No tricuspid regurgitation is noted on transesophageal echocardiography and simultaneous pressure measurements across the THV showed a transtricuspid valve mean gradient of 5 mm Hg.

AORTIC BIOPROSTHETIC VALVE-IN-VALVE: MEDTRONIC COREVALVE EVOLUT

CASE 6 *Patient with Coronary Artery Disease*

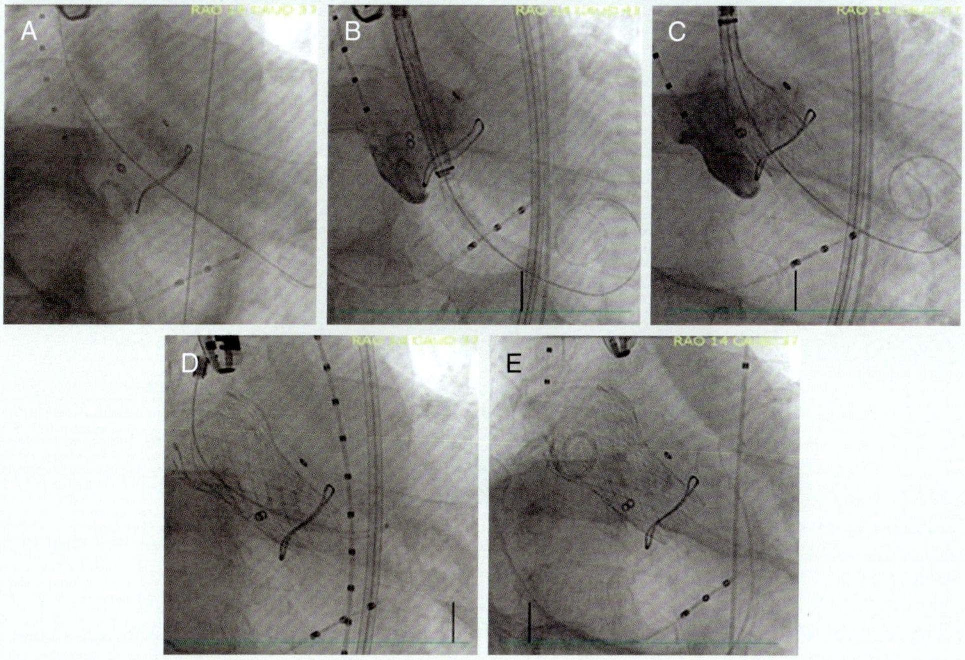

FIGURE 21.20 Transcatheter aortic VIV implantation using a CoreValve Evolut valve.

A 72-year-old male with coronary artery disease and previous stented aortic valve bioprosthesis (27 mm Hancock II) developed severe, symptomatic bioprosthetic aortic valve stenosis and was referred for a transfemoral TAVR using a 29 mm CoreValve Evolut Pro THV. Similar to conventional TAVR, the optimal fluoroscopic view perpendicular to the bioprosthetic annular plane is obtained by lining up the bioprosthetic fluoroscopic ring (**FIGURE 21.20A**, **Video 21.24**). Note that the sewing ring is not radiopaque. A marker pigtail is placed into the noncoronary cusp, and a preshaped Confida guide wire is placed in the left ventricle. An aortogram is performed as the valve is slowly released from the loading device after initially positioned 4 mm below the bioprosthetic annular plane (**FIGURE 21.20B**, **Video 21.25**). Controlled pacing is performed at 110 bpm. Deployment is continued to the point of no recapture, hemodynamics are assessed, and the position of the valve is confirmed by angiography and TEE (**FIGURE 21.20C**). **D**, Once position and stable hemodynamics are confirmed, the pigtail catheter in the noncoronary sinus is pulled back into the distal ascending aorta and the remaining portion of the valve is deployed (**FIGURE 21.20D**, **Video 21.26**). Complete release of the valve loading system from the valve is confirmed on fluoroscopy (**FIGURE 21.20E**, **Video 21.27**).

TEE

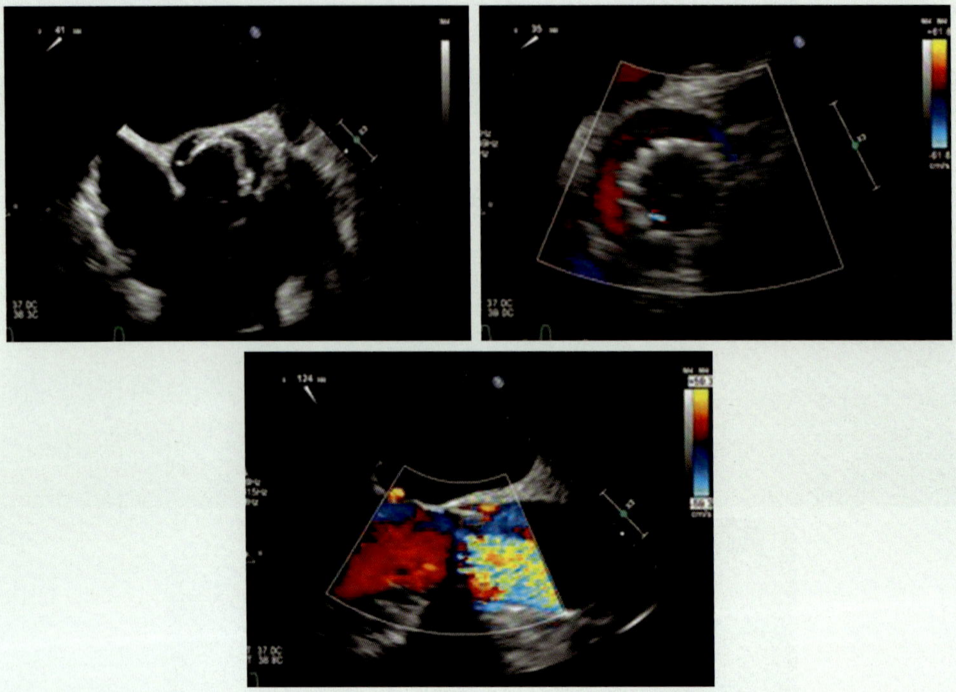

FIGURE 21.21 2D TEE images immediately after deployment of a 29 mm CoreValve Evolut Pro valve in short- and long-axis views.

TEE is used to confirm adequate implant depth, paravalvular aortic insufficiency, and function of the new prosthesis (**FIGURE 21.21**). Color Doppler shows no paravalvular aortic regurgitation.

TRANSCATHETER AORTIC VALVE REPLACEMENT FOR SEVERE AORTIC INSUFFICIENCY AFTER LEFT VENTRICULAR ASSIST DEVICE PLACEMENT: MEDTRONIC COREVALVE EVOLUT

CASE 7 *Patient with End-Stage Nonischemic Cardiomyopathy*

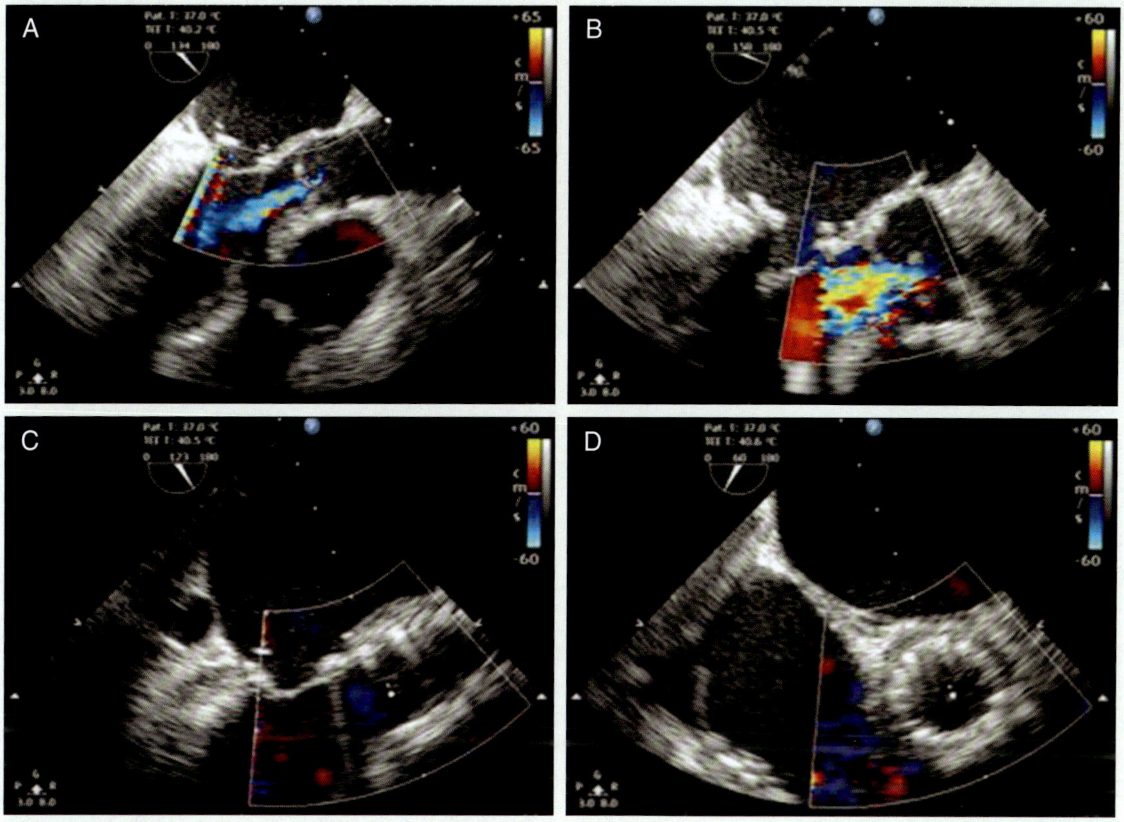

FIGURE 21.22 Early, severe AI after LVAD placement. **A**, Midesophageal long-axis image revealing continuous, moderate AI. **B**, With the LVAD system turned down, there is opening of the native aortic valve with severe AI. Long **(C)** and short **(D)** axis images after TAVR reveal a well seated 26 mm CoreValve Evolut R with no residual AI.

In **FIGURE 21.22**, 2D images of a 73-year old female with end-stage nonischemic cardiomyopathy and destination therapy with a HeartWare left ventricular assist device (LVAD) who developed early, severe AI after LVAD implantation is shown. She was considered prohibitive risk by the heart valve team and was referred for a TAVR using a CoreValve Evolut THV. AI tends to progress with the duration of LVAD support, and 49% of subjects are free of moderate or worse AI at 18 months.[23] Significant AI can create futile cycles and lead to ineffective LVAD function owing to the recycling of regurgitant blood and secondary upregulation of pump flow volume to maintain adequate systemic flow.

TEE

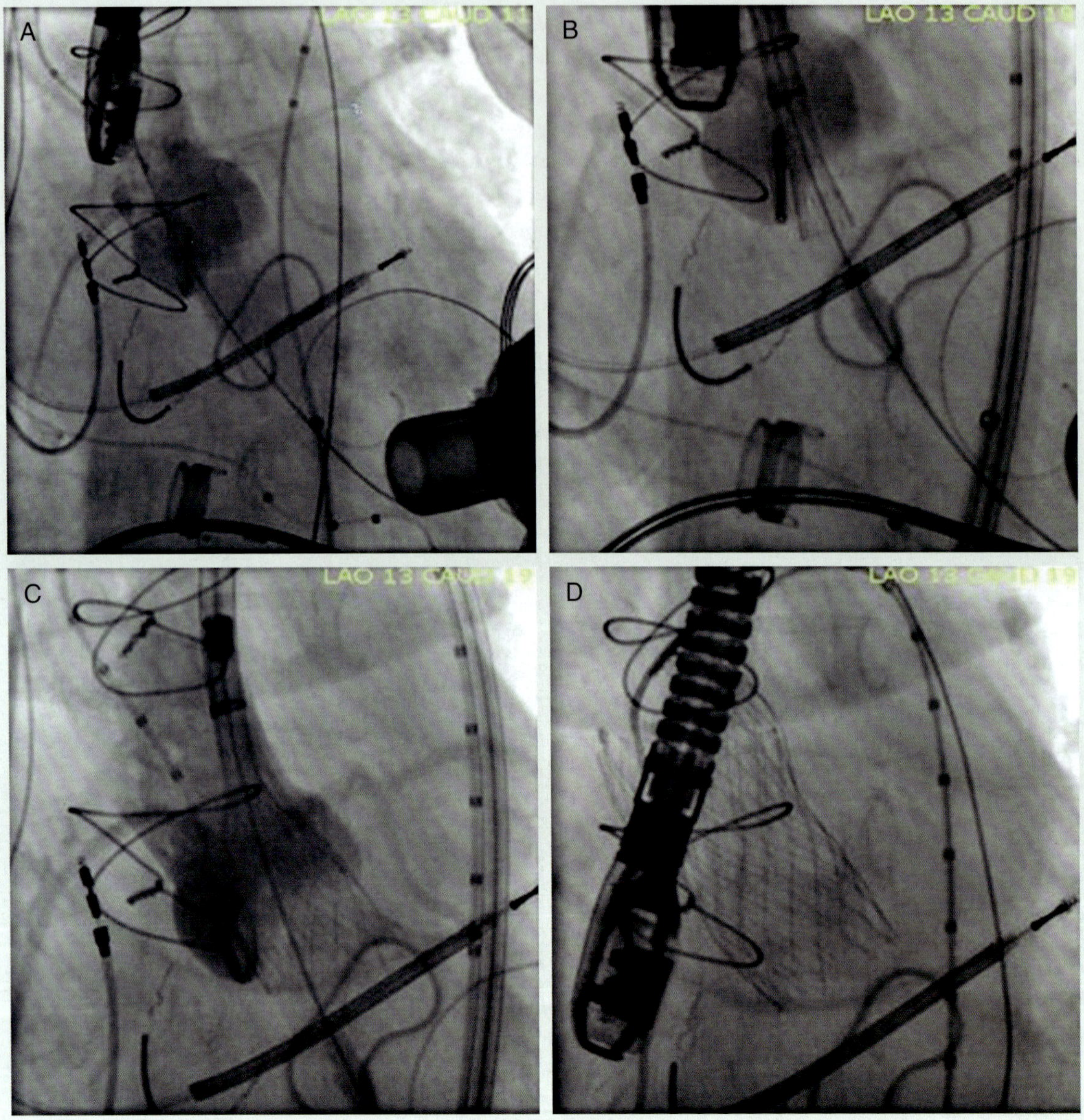

FIGURE 21.23 Transcatheter aortic valve replacement for severe AI after HeartMate LVAD placement.

A pigtail catheter is placed at the bottom of the noncoronary cusp A diagnostic aortogram is performed in the coplanar view with the LVAD turned down, showing severe AI (**FIGURE 21.23A**, Video 21.28). A 26 mm CoreValve Evolut Pro prosthesis and delivery system are advanced over a preshaped Confida guide wire to the level of implantation and slowly released (**FIGURE 21.23B**, Video 21.29). An aortogram is performed to confirm the valve is positioned 3 to 5 mm below the patient's native valve (Video 21.30). At the 80% position and before the point of no recapture, another aortogram is performed and confirms that the bioprosthesis is at the optimal implant depth (**FIGURE 21.23C**, Video 21.31). The valve position is also confirmed by TEE. The LVAD flows are turned back up, and the valve position on fluoroscopy is reassessed to ensure stability of the THV (**FIGURE 21.23D**, Video 21.32). TEE showed no aortic regurgitation.

PERCUTANEOUS MITRAL BALLOON VALVULOPLASTY FOR MITRAL STENOSIS

Despite a decreasing prevalence in industrialized nations, rheumatic valvular heart disease remains a major cause of cardiovascular morbidity in developing countries. While cardiac surgery and percutaneous options are both available for the treatment of severe, symptomatic mitral stenosis, percutaneous mitral balloon valvuloplasty (PMV) is the preferred treatment of choice in those with suitable anatomy, particularly in developing countries and in select patients such as pregnant women and acutely ill patients in cardiogenic shock. PMV or more appropriately percutaneous mitral commissurotomy (balloon dilation works to increase valve orifice by separating the fused mitral commissures) provides immediate hemodynamic improvements and has been associated with low complication rates. The immediate and long-term results have been promising, with 62% of patients remaining free of reintervention after successful PMV at a median follow-up of 12 years. Moreover, of those requiring percutaneous reintervention, cardiovascular survival without surgery was 60% ± 7% at 10 years, thus supporting the notion that PMV is an effective treatment for mitral stenosis and that reintervention is a safe procedure that allows further postponement of surgery.[24]

CASE 8 *Patient with Atrial Fibrillation and Severe, Symptomatic Rheumatic Mitral Stenosis*

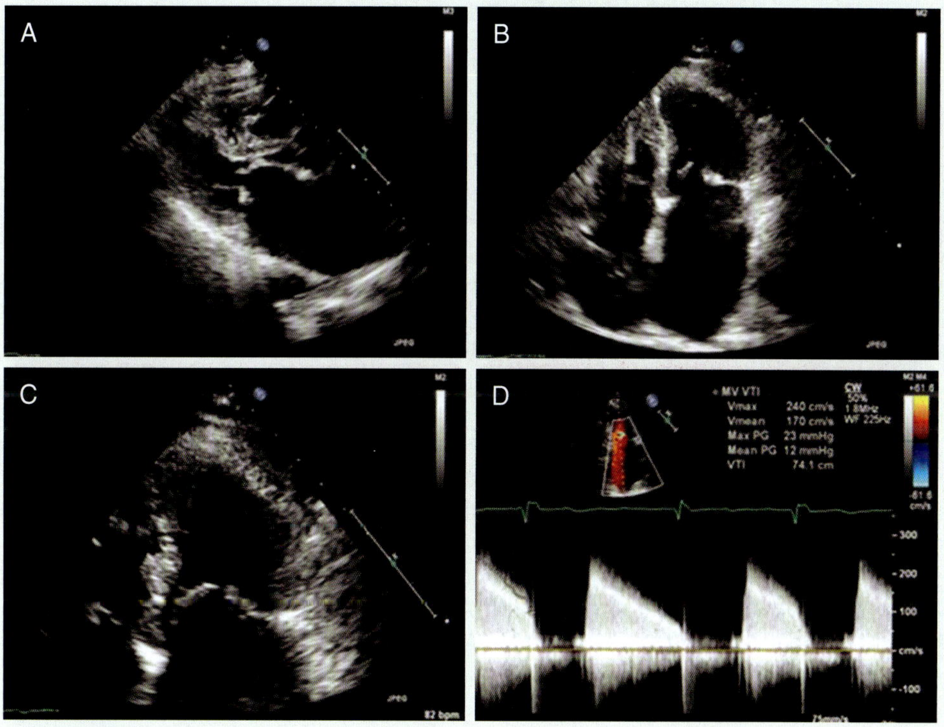

FIGURE 21.24 **A**, Parasternal long images show thickened mitral valve leaflets with diastolic doming of the anterior mitral leaflet consistent with rheumatic mitral disease. **B and C**, Apical 4 chamber view demonstrates dense calcification of the posterior mitral leaflet and chordal thickening without calcification. There is also massive left atrial enlargement. **D**, Determination of the mean mitral gradient using Doppler diastolic mitral flow in a patient with severe mitral stenosis and atrial fibrillation. The mean gradient varies according to the length of diastole and should be calculated as the average of 5 cycles in patients with atrial fibrillation (12 mm Hg in this patient). Echocardiographic scores can be calculated to identify abnormalities of the mitral valve apparatus and predict immediate and long-term outcomes with PMV. The most used score developed by Wilkins et al, incorporates leaflet rigidity, leaflet thickening, valvular calcification, and subvalvular disease, each one graded from 0 to 4. The best outcomes occur in patients with echocardiographic sores ≤8.[25,26]

In **FIGURE 21.24**, transthoracic echocardiography images of an 81-year-old female with atrial fibrillation and severe, symptomatic rheumatic mitral stenosis is shown.

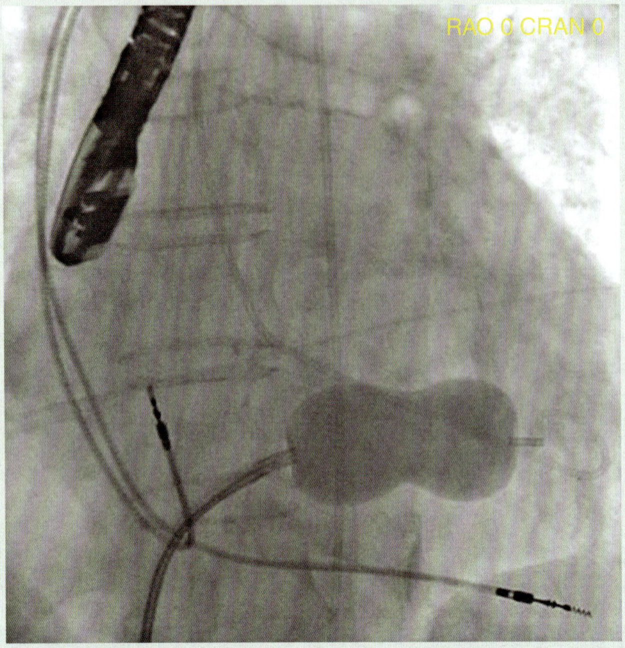

FIGURE 21.25 Percutaneous mitral balloon valvuloplasty using the Inoue technique.

As shown in **FIGURE 21.25**, a diagnostic right and transseptal left heart catheterization is performed per usual technique. A pigtail catheter is placed in the left ventricle, and direct left atrial-left ventricular gradients are measured confirming severe mitral stenosis (12 mm Hg). Systemic anticoagulation is achieved by administration of weight-based unfractionated heparin bolus, and an Inoue wire is placed in the left atrium. The atrial septum is dilated using a 12 FR dilator in preparation for balloon insertion. The Inoue-Balloon Catheter (Toray, Tokyo, Japan) has a 12 FR shaft with a balloon made up of 2 latex layers and interposed polyester micromesh. Two proximally positioned stopcocks accomplish balloon inflation and catheter venting. A balloon catheter is chosen on the basis of the patient's weight, height, and estimated mitral valve area. The balloon catheter is advanced over the guide wire into the left atrium. The distal portion of the balloon is then partially inflated and advanced across the mitral valve and into the left ventricle with the aid of a stylet. The distal balloon is fully inflated and pulled, seating the balloon on the mitral valve. Rapid inflation is performed with full balloon expansion at 22 mm and quickly deflated. During initial inflation, the balloon resembles an hourglass shape, which centers the balloon on the valve and prevents migration (**Videos 21.33-21.35**). TEE confirms no significant MR, and repeat balloon inflations are performed at 23 and 24 mm. Final mitral valve gradient has decreased to 2.5 mm Hg. Postprocedure TEE reveals increased mobility of the anterior mitral leaflet without evidence of significant MR.

PERCUTANEOUS TREATMENT FOR MITRAL REGURGITATION: THE MITRAL CLIP

Nonrheumatic MR is a heterogeneous disorder resulting from degenerative valve disease, such as prolapse, chordal rupture, myxomatous degeneration, or functional etiologies from underlying left ventricular dysfunction and annular dilation. It has a 2% prevalence in the general population, with increasing frequency in the elderly.[27] Surgical repair or replacement is the standard of care for patients with symptomatic, severe MR. Unfortunately, a significant proportion of eligible patients are denied surgery owing to high operative risk.[28] While there is growing demand for minimally invasive, catheter-based therapies in this population, device development for percutaneous treatment has been challenging owing to the complex and dynamic interplay between the structures of the mitral valve apparatus (mitral annulus, chordae tendineae, papillary muscles, left ventricle, and left atrium).

The MitraClip System (Abbott Vascular Structural Heart, Menlo Park, CA) is based on the surgical Alfieri edge-to-edge repair, which involves suturing together the middle segments of the anterior and posterior mitral valve leaflets, thereby creating a "double orifice" MR area.[29] The MitraClip system uses a cobalt chromium clip covered with a polypropylene fabric that grasps both the anterior and posterior mitral valve leaflets, thereby reducing MR by increasing the coaptation between the regurgitant valve leaflets. The safety and efficacy was shown in the EVEREST I nonrandomized trial (Endovascular Valve Edge-to-Edge Repair Study). In the randomized, controlled, EVEREST II trial, the 5-year composite endpoint of freedom from death, surgery, or 3+ or 4+ MR was 44.2% versus 64.3% in the percutaneous repair and surgical groups, respectively ($P = .01$). The difference was driven by increased rates of 3+ to 4+ MR (12.3% vs 1.8%; $P = .02$) and surgery (27.9% vs 8.9%; $P = .003$) in patients undergoing percutaneous repair within the first year. At 1- and 5-year follow-up, the rates of surgery, moderate-to-severe MR, and mortality were similar between the 2 repair techniques.[30]

CASE 9 *Patient with History of Remote CABG and Severe MR*

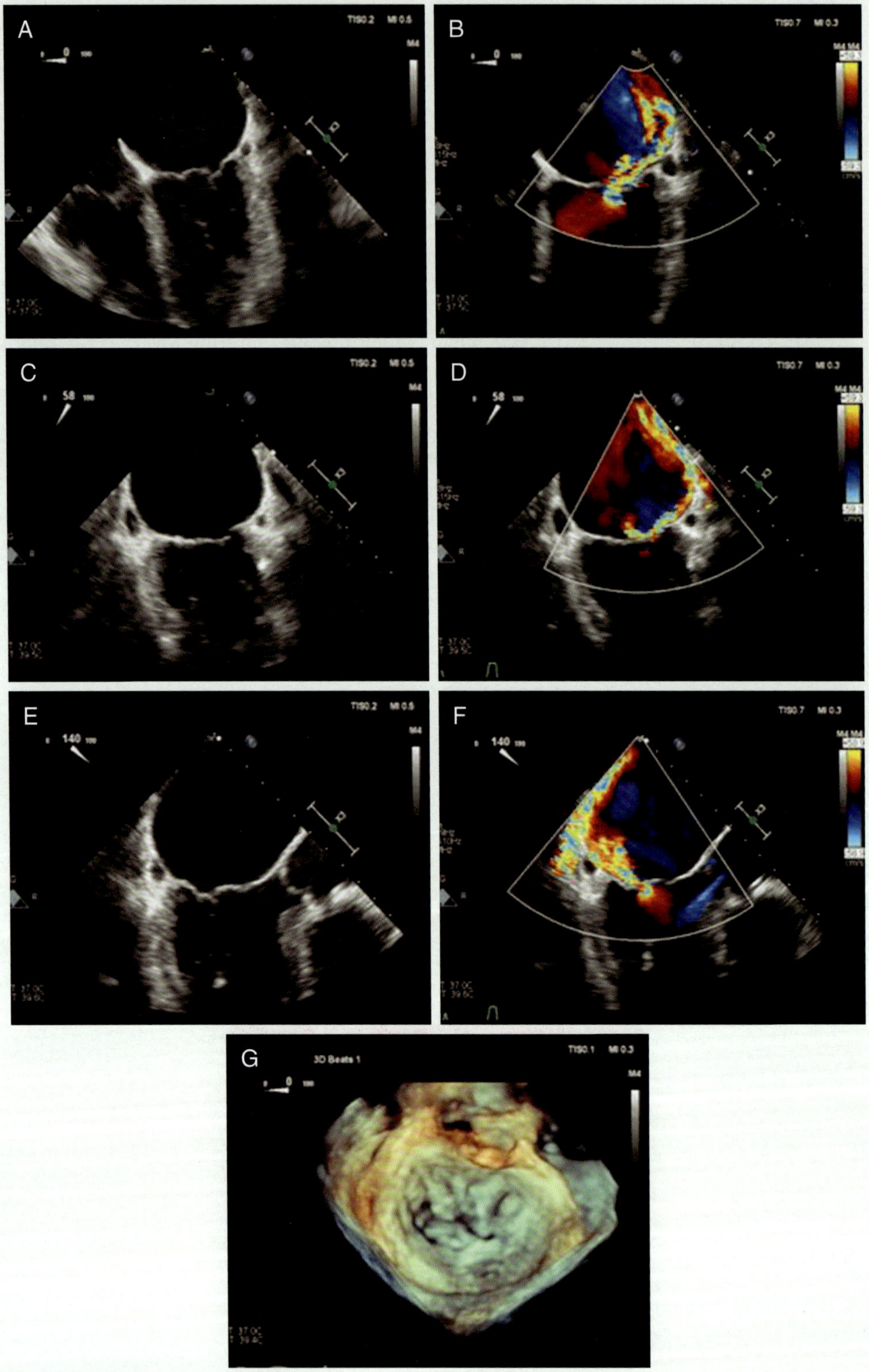

FIGURE 21.26 Procedural planning with TEE is crucial for MitraClip interventions. **A and B**, Midesophageal 4 chamber view with accompanying color Doppler. **C and D**, Midesophageal intercommissural (IC) view with accompanying color Doppler. **E and F**, Midesophageal long-axis view with accompanying color Doppler. **G**, 3D TEE with anterior leaflet prolapse.

In **FIGURE 21.26**, TEE of a 74-year old patient with a previous history of remote CABG with severe MR who was deemed high risk for surgical mitral valve and was referred for percutaneous MitraClip. Baseline TEE images show a restricted posterior leaflet and prolapse of the anterior leaflet with severe, eccentric MR. An effective regurgitant orifice area of 0.42 cm^2 and regurgitant volume of 60 mL is consistent with severe MR.

TEE

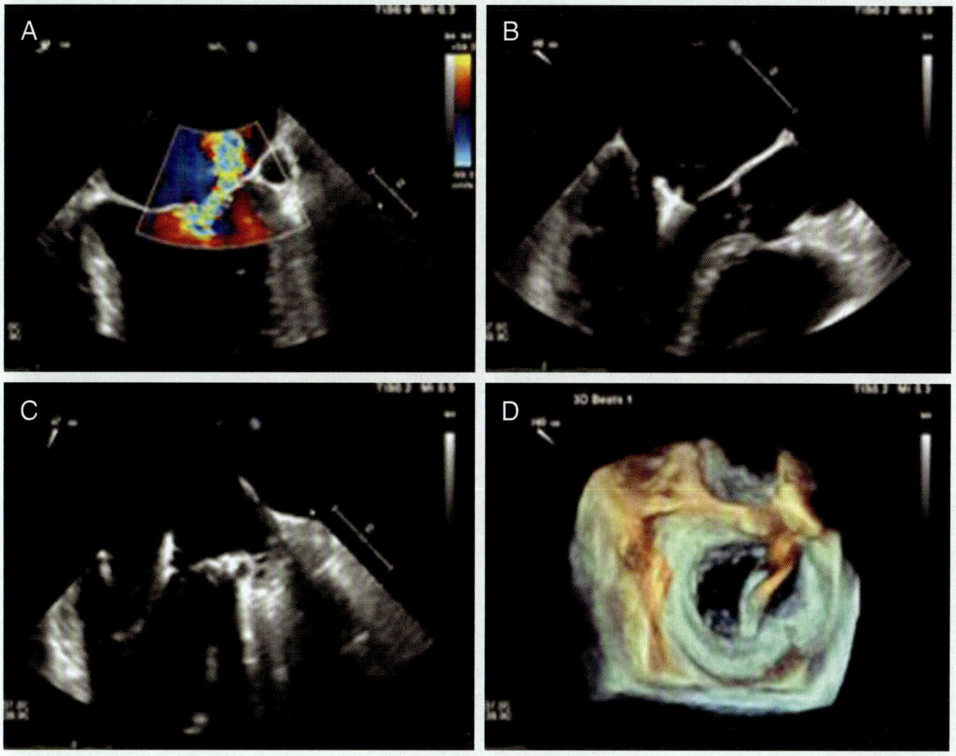

FIGURE 21.27 TEE guidance during MitraClip implantation. **A**, 2D TEE shows severe, posteriorly directed MR secondary to anterior leaflet prolapse and restricted posterior leaflet before intervention. **B and C**, The open MitraClip is advanced into the left ventricle using fluoroscopy and TEE IC and LVOT views while observing the anterioposterior and medial-lateral positions. In the IC view, no part of the Clip arm should appear whereas in the LVOT view, both Clip arms are seen of equal length. Proper axial alignment of the MitraClip splitting the MR jet and perpendicular alignment to the line of coaptation are essential for a successful grasp.[30] **D**, A 3D TEE en-face view displays direct views of the MitraClip in relation to the mitral valve and the line of coaptation. **E**, Both leaflets are identified above the Clip before closure. **F**, After optimal alignment is verified in all views, the leaflets are captured in between the Clip arms and the grippers. Color Doppler shows satisfactory coaptation and insertion of both leaflets along with reduction of MR. **G**, The transvalvular diastolic gradient assessed by continuous wave Doppler shows a mean gradient of 3 mm Hg. **H**, Color Doppler shows residual moderate MR after deployment of a single MitraClip. **I**, A second Clip is implanted lateral to the previously deployed clip with further reduction of MR to mild. **J**, Final 3D TEE shows a double valve orifice with 2 adjacent MitraClips and a reduction in regurgitation from severe to mild.

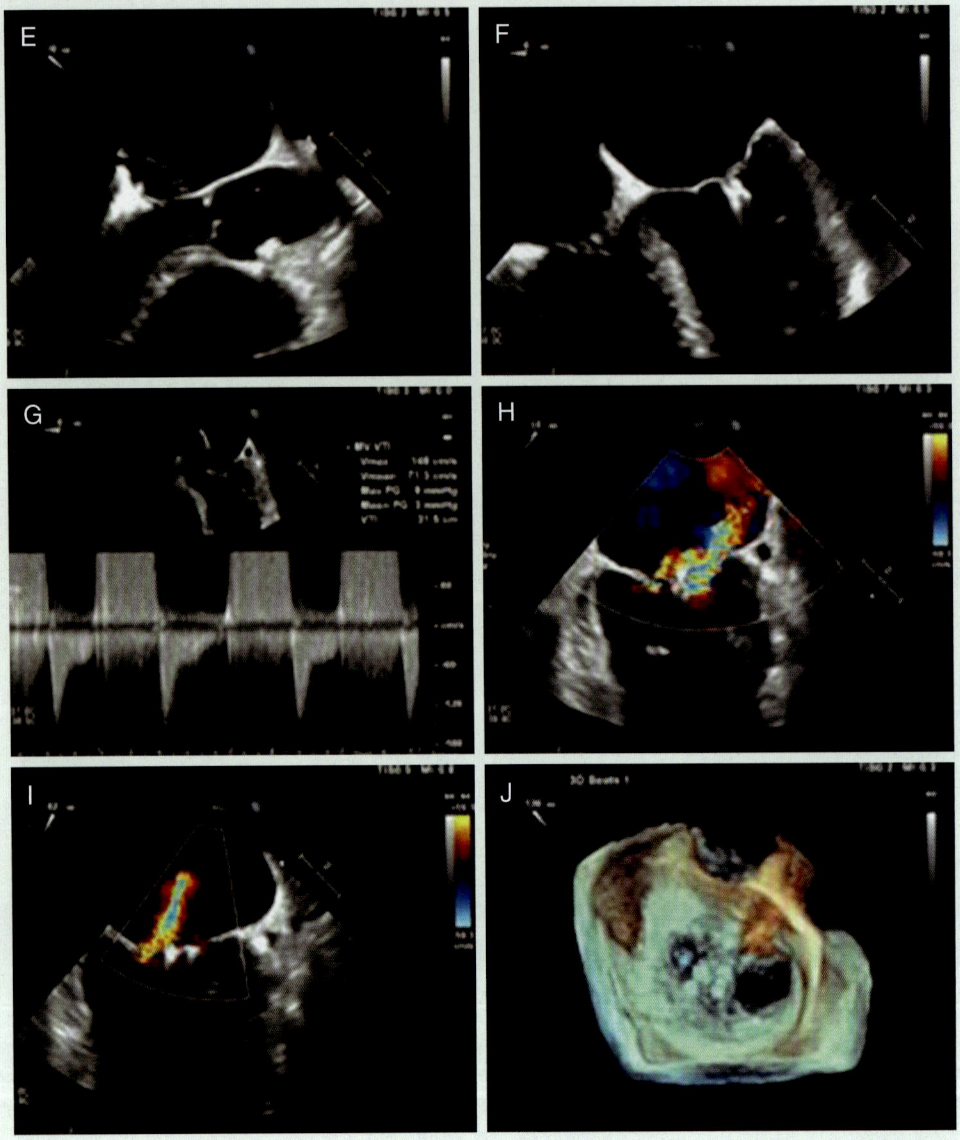

FIGURE 21.27 (Continued)

As shown in **FIGURE 21.27**, use of echocardiography is is essential for procedural success, as the mitral leaflets cannot be assessed by fluoroscopy.

Fluoroscopic Views

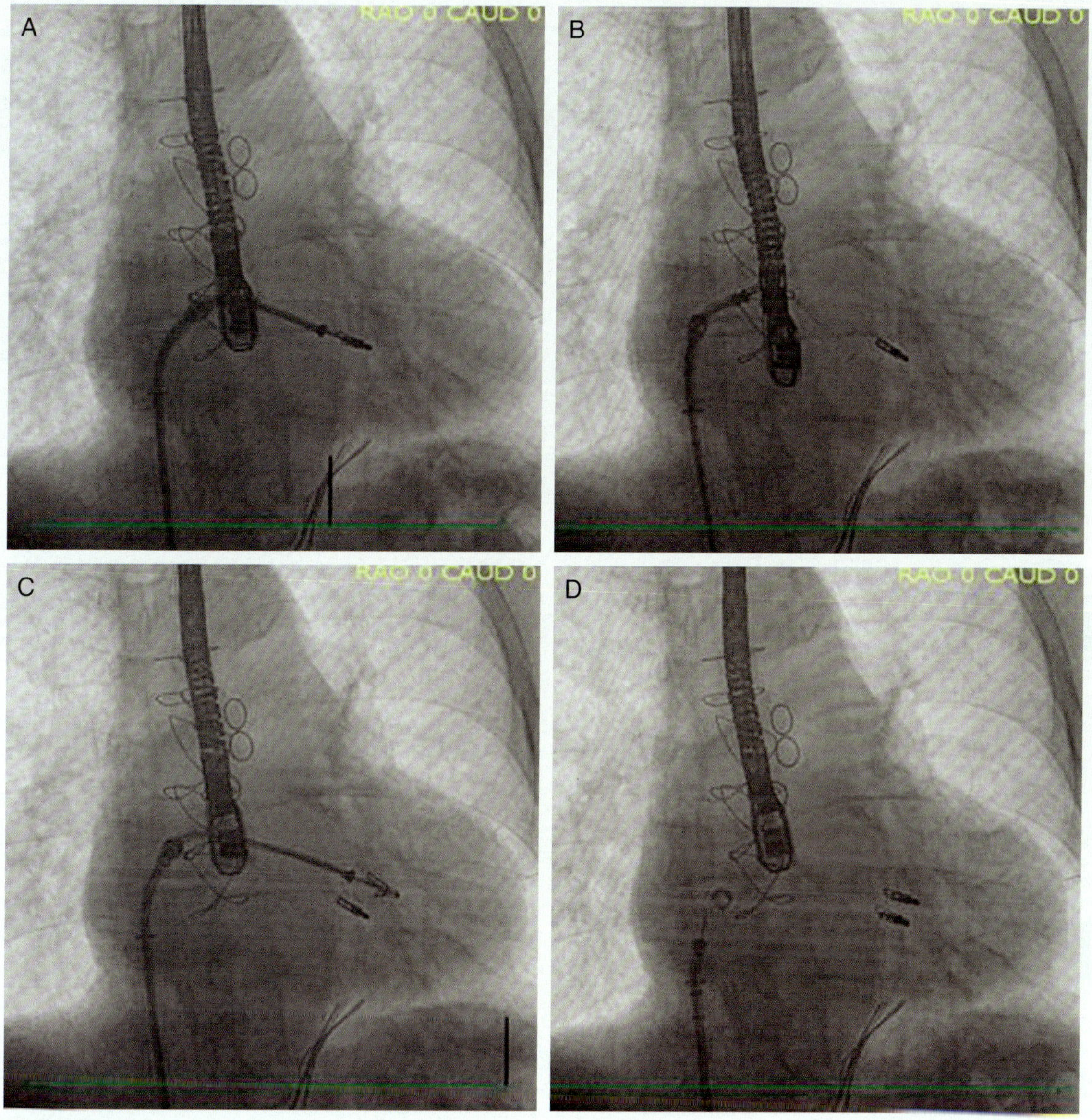

FIGURE 21.28 Fluoroscopic views of the MitraClip procedure. **A**, The MitraClip is advanced into the left ventricle under fluoroscopic and TEE guidance. After successful grasp and leaflet insertion, the MitraClip is closed. **B**, The delivery catheter shaft is fully detached from the Clip and removed from the body. **C**, A second Clip is inserted into the left ventricle with partially open Clip arms. **D**, Final fluoroscopic image after deployment of 2 clips.

Fluoroscopic views of the MitraClip procedure are shown in **FIGURE 21.28**.

REFERENCES

1. Ross J, Braunwald E. Aortic stenosis. *Circulation*. 1968;38(suppl 1):61-67.
2. Schwarz F, Baumann P, Manthey J, et al. The effect of aortic valve replacement on survival. *Circulation*. 1982;66(5):1105-1110.
3. Iung B, Cachier A, Baron G, et al. Decision-making in elderly patients with severe aortic stenosis: why are so many denied surgery? *Eur Heart J*. 2005;26(24):2714-2720.
4. Mack MJ, Leon MB, Smith CR, et al. 5-year outcomes of transcatheter aortic valve replacement or surgical aortic valve replacement for high surgical risk patients with aortic stenosis (PARTNER 1): a randomised controlled trial. *Lancet*. 2015;385(9986):2477-2484.
5. Kapadia SR, Leon MB, Makkar RR, et al. 5-year outcomes of transcatheter aortic valve replacement compared with standard treatment for patients with inoperable aortic stenosis (PARTNER 1): a randomised controlled trial. *Lancet*. 2015;385(9986):2485-2491.
6. Popma JJ, Adams DH, Reardon MJ, et al. Transcatheter aortic valve replacement using a self-expanding bioprosthesis in patients with severe aortic stenosis at extreme risk for surgery. *J Am Coll Cardiol*. 2014;63(19):1972-1981.
7. Adams DH, Popma JJ, Reardon MJ, et al. Transcatheter aortic-valve replacement with a self-expanding prosthesis. *N Engl J Med*. 2014;370(19):1790-1798.
8. Leon MB, Smith CR, Mack MJ, et al. Transcatheter or surgical aortic-valve replacement in intermediate-risk patients. *N Engl J Med*. 2016;374(17):1609-1620.
9. Reardon MJ, Van Mieghem NM, Popma JJ, et al. Surgical or transcatheter aortic-valve replacement in intermediate-risk patients. *N Engl J Med*. 2017;376(14):1321-1331.
10. Nishimura RA, Otto CM, Bonow RO, et al. 2017 AHA/ACC focused update of the 2014 AHA/ACC guideline for the management of patients with valvular heart disease. *J Am Coll Cardiol*. 2017;70(2):252-289.
11. Al-Najafi S, Sanchez F, Lerakis S. The crucial role of cardiac imaging in transcatheter aortic valve replacement (TAVR): pre- and post-procedural assessment. *Curr Treat Options Cardiovasc Med*. 2016;18(12):70.
12. Mauri V, Reimann A, Stern D, et al. Predictors of permanent pacemaker implantation after transcatheter aortic valve replacement with the SAPIEN 3. *JACC Cardiovasc Interv*. 2016;9(21):2200-2209.
13. Athappan G, Patvardhan E, Tuzcu EM, et al. Incidence, predictors, and outcomes of aortic regurgitation after transcatheter aortic valve replacement: meta-analysis and systematic review of literature. *J Am Coll Cardiol*. 2013;61(15):1585-1595.
14. Gunning PS, Saikrishnan N, McNamara LM, Yoganathan AP. An in vitro evaluation of the impact of eccentric deployment on transcatheter aortic valve hemodynamics. *Ann Biomed Eng*. 2014;42(6):1195-1206.
15. Zamorano JL, Badano LP, Bruce C, et al. EAE/ASE recommendations for the use of echocardiography in new transcatheter interventions for valvular heart disease. *Eur Heart J*. 2011;32(17):2189-2214.
16. Kappetein AP, Head SJ, Généreux P, et al. Updated standardized endpoint definitions for transcatheter aortic valve implantation: the Valve Academic Research Consortium-2 consensus document. *J Am Coll Cardiol*. 2012;60(15):1438-1454.
17. Pislaru SV, Nkomo VT, Sandhu GS. Assessment of prosthetic valve function after TAVR. *JACC Cardiovasc Imaging*. 2016;9(2):193-206.
18. Daneault B, Koss E, Hahn RT, et al. Efficacy and safety of postdilatation to reduce paravalvular regurgitation during balloon-expandable transcatheter aortic valve replacement. *Circ Cardiovasc Interv*. 2013;6(1):85-91.
19. Kirsch M, Nakashima K, Kubota S, Houël R, Hillion ML, Loisance D. The risk of reoperative heart valve procedures in Octogenarian patients. *J Heart Valve Dis*. 2004;13(6):991-996; discussion 996.
20. Webb JG, Mack MJ, White JM, et al. Transcatheter aortic valve implantation within degenerated aortic surgical bioprostheses: PARTNER 2 valve-in-valve registry. *J Am Coll Cardiol*. 2017;69(18):2253-2262.
21. Dvir D, Barbanti M, Tan J, Webb JG. Transcatheter aortic valve-in-valve implantation for patients with degenerative surgical bioprosthetic valves. *Curr Probl Cardiol*. 2014;39(1):7-27.
22. Bapat VN, Attia RQ, Condemi F, et al. Fluoroscopic guide to an ideal implant position for Sapien XT and CoreValve during a valve-in-valve procedure. *JACC Cardiovasc Interv*. 2013;6(11):1186-1194.
23. Cowger J, Pagani FD, Haft JW, et al. The development of aortic insufficiency in LVAD supported patients. *Circ Heart Fail*. 2010;3(6):668-674.
24. Bouleti C, Iung B, Himbert D, et al. Reinterventions after percutaneous mitral commissurotomy during long-term follow-up, up to 20 years: the role of repeat percutaneous mitral commissurotomy. *Eur Heart J*. 2013;34(25):1923-1930.
25. Abascal VM, Wilkins GT, O'Shea JP, et al. Prediction of successful outcome in 130 patients undergoing percutaneous balloon mitral valvotomy. *Circulation*. 1990;82(2):448-456.
26. Wilkins GT, Weyman AE, Abascal VM, Block PC, Palacios IF. Percutaneous balloon dilatation of the mitral valve: an analysis of echocardiographic variables related to outcome and the mechanism of dilatation. *Br Heart J*. 1988;60(4):299-308.
27. Nkomo VT, Gardin JM, Skelton TN, Gottdiener JS, Scott CG, Enriquez-Sarano M. Burden of valvular heart diseases: a population-based study. *Lancet*. 2006;368(9540):1005-1011.
28. Mirabel M, Iung B, Baron G, et al. What are the characteristics of patients with severe, symptomatic, mitral regurgitation who are denied surgery? *Eur Heart J*. 2007;28(11):1358-1365.
29. Maisano F, La Canna G, Colombo A, Alfieri O. The evolution from surgery to percutaneous mitral valve interventions: the role of the edge-to-edge technique. *J Am Coll Cardiol*. 2011;58(21):2174-2182.
30. Feldman T, Kar S, Elmariah S, et al. Randomized comparison of percutaneous repair and surgery for mitral regurgitation: 5-year results of EVEREST II. *J Am Coll Cardiol*. 2015;66(25):2844-2854.

chapter 22

Interventions for Adult Structural Heart Disease

HONG JUN (FRANCISCO) YUN, MD and STANLEY J. CHETCUTI, MD

PERCUTANEOUS REPAIR OF PARAVALVULAR LEAKS

Because of an aging population, the burden of valvular heart disease is increasing. With the advent of transcatheter therapies, more patients are being referred for transcatheter aortic valve replacement (TAVR) and valve-in-valve (VIV) procedures besides the >100,000 surgical valve procedures performed annually in the United States.[1] Paravalvular leak (PVL) is not an uncommon complication of mechanical or bioprosthetic surgical valves, occurring in 2% to 17% of all cases.[2] At least moderate PVL has been reported in 22% of cases in patients undergoing TAVR with the Edwards Sapien or the Medtronic CoreValve.[3] PVL is related to an abnormal gap between the outer edge of the prosthetic valve and the native valve annulus leading to turbulent flow. Although many patients with mild PVL remain asymptomatic, signs of more severe PVL include heart failure, LV enlargement, and hemolytic anemia. The occurrence of PVL is an important factor for TAVR devices, as the development of at least moderate PVL has been associated with impaired survival.[4] Traditional therapy for the management of PVL has been open surgery, but the growth of safe, minimally invasive percutaneous techniques with experienced operators has obviated the need for surgery in many cases (**FIGURES 22.1-22.3**).

PERCUTANEOUS CLOSURE OF VENTRICULAR SEPTAL DEFECTS

Ventricular septal defects (VSDs) are one of the most common congenital heart lesions and occur in ~50% of all patients with congenital heart disease.[4] Although most small defects close spontaneously within the first 2 years, undiagnosed and untreated defects may persist into adulthood. The natural history of untreated VSDs is related to the size of the defect. Patients may present with a murmur, endocarditis, heart failure, or pulmonary hypertension. Acquired VSDs, iatrogenic, traumatic, or postmyocardial infarction (MI), are much less common. VSDs complicating an acute myocardial infarction are a rare event, occurring in 0.17% of patients in the era of percutaneous coronary intervention (PCI) reperfusion therapy.[5] Although the presentation may be insidious, patients with post-MI VSD can become acutely ill and develop cardiogenic shock. Thus, early identification is crucial because mechanical repair is the only effective treatment and mortality rates can approach 100% in patients who are treated medically.[6] Although surgery has been the mainstay for VSD closure, transcatheter approaches have been demonstrated as viable alternatives since the first percutaneous VSD closure was performed in 1987 using the Rashkind double-umbrella device.[7] Currently, the Amplatzer Muscular VSD Occluder is the most commonly used percutaneous device and has been associated with low mortality and high success rates, ranging from 93% to 100% (**FIGURES 22.4-22.7**).[8]

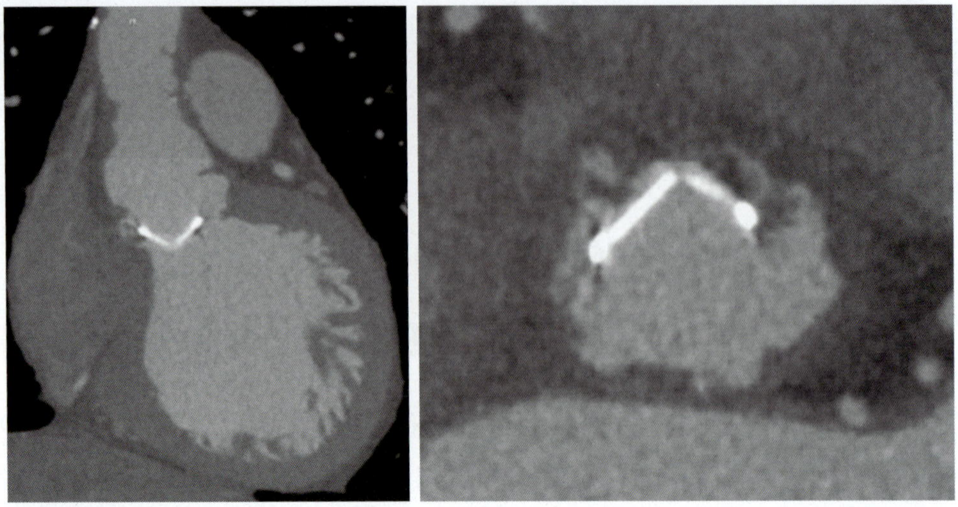

FIGURE 22.1 Cardiac CT angiography shows a #23 St Jude mechanical aortic valve with a severe PVL. There is irregular pooling of contrast and a path of contrast continuity around the mechanical aortic valve prosthesis concerning for a PVL.

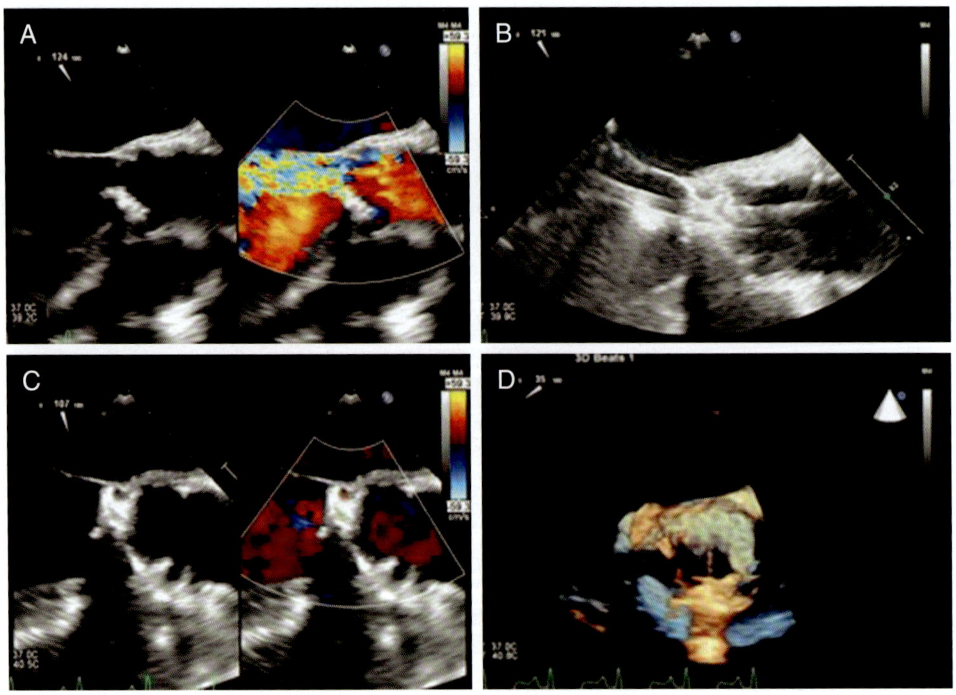

FIGURE 22.2 Percutaneous repair of an aortic PVL using Amplatzer VSD Occluder Devices (St Jude Medical, St Paul, MN) under TEE and fluoroscopic guidance. **A**, TEE shows a bileaflet tilting-disc mechanical aortic valve with dehiscence and severe paravalvular aortic regurgitation. **B**, Three guide wires are advanced through the paravalvular space and into the left ventricle. **C**, One 4 mm and three 6 mm Amplatzer VSD Occluder devices are deployed with no residual paravalvular regurgitation. TEE and fluoroscopy show stability of the devices and a normally functioning mechanical valve with no impingement of leaflet excursion. **D**, 3D TEE shows the 4 VSD Occluder devices in the paravalvular space.

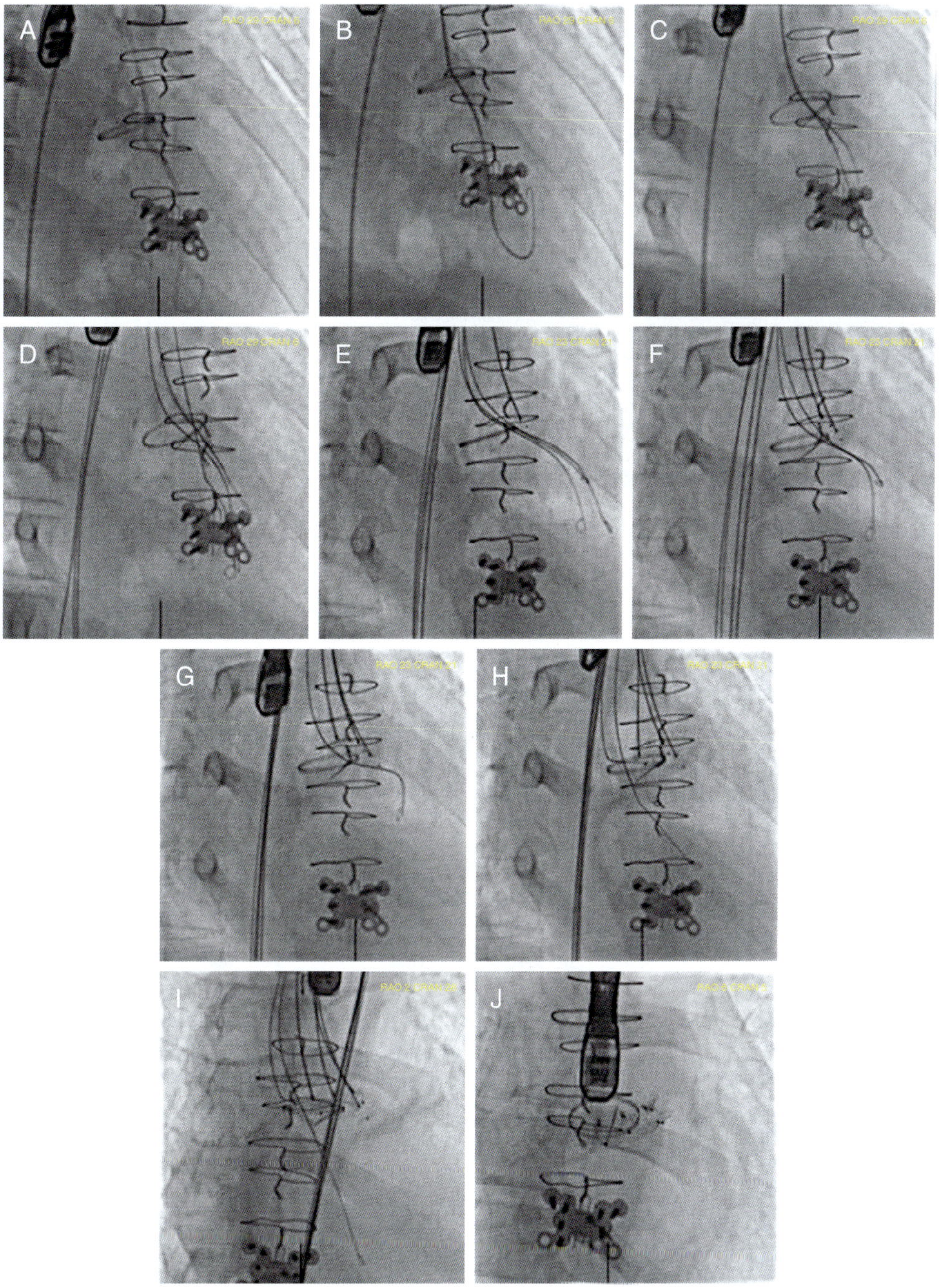

FIGURE 22.3 Step-by-step approach to transfemoral PVL closure using Amplatzer VSD Occluder devices. Severe aortic PVL closure via a retrograde transfemoral approach in a 32-year-old man with bicuspid aortic valve and prior valve sparing ascending aorta replacement and aortic valve repair followed by 2 subsequent AVRs (last with a 23 mm St Jude mechanical valve). **A**, A 6 FR AL1 catheter is used to cross the PVL using a J tipped guide wire and a 6 FR pigtail catheter is advanced into the left ventricle (Video 22.1). **B**, Through the pigtail catheter, a J tipped Rosen wire is advanced into the left ventricle (Video 22.2). **C and D**, 6 FR 90 cm Shuttle Sheath is then advanced into the LV to allow direct passage of 3 additional J tipped Rosen wires through the paravalvular space into the ventricle (Video 22.3). **E**, Using a 5 FR Amplatzer TorqVue 180 Delivery System, a 4 mm VSD Occluder is positioned within the PVL and confirmed by TEE (Videos 22.4 and 22.5). **F-I**, Three additional 6 mm VSD Occluder devices are positioned in the paravalvular space using the corresponding guide wires (Video 22.6). A fifth J tipped Rosen wire is advanced into the left ventricle to maintain access of the paravalvular space. **J**, Once appropriate position of the occluding devices and reduction of the PVL is verified by fluoroscopy and TEE, the Rosen wire is removed and the VSD Occluder devices are deployed (Video 22.7).

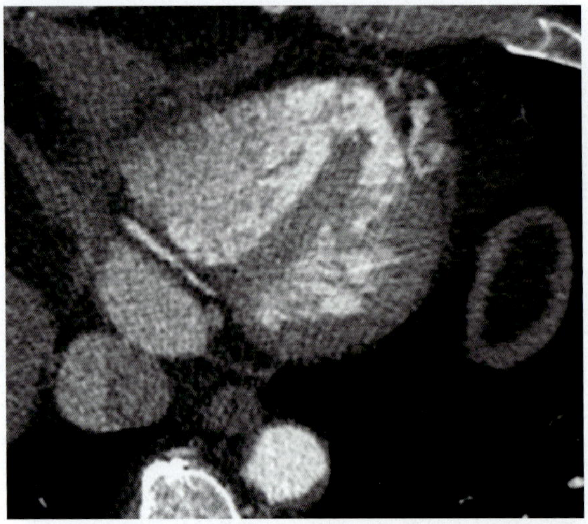

FIGURE 22.4 Post-MI VSD with residual defect after surgical repair. Computed tomography image showing postsurgical changes at the cardiac apex with at least 1 cm residual ventricular septal defect along the inferoapical septum.

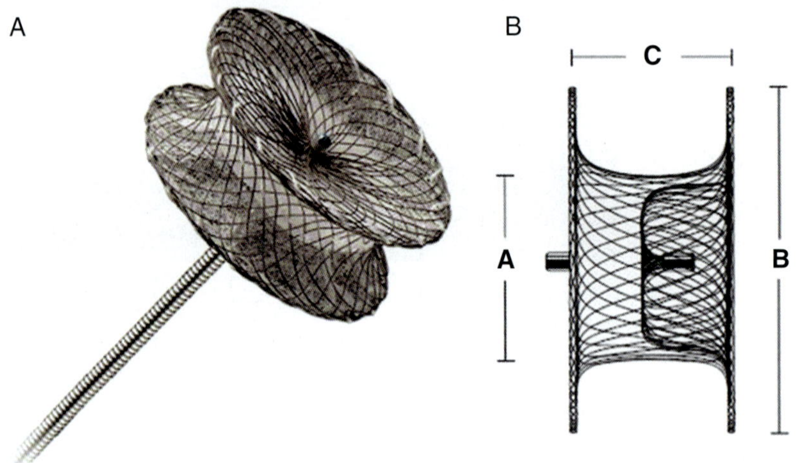

FIGURE 22.5 **A**, Amplatzer Muscular VSD Occluder. It is a self-expanding, double-disc device made of nitinol and interwoven polyester to promote occlusion and tissue ingrowth. It has a 7 mm waist length to accommodate the muscular ventricular septal wall. **B**, The device comes in a variety of sizes (4-18 mm at the waist, corresponding to disc diameters of 9-26 mm). A, device size at the waist. B, length of the proximal disc. C, length of the waist. The Amplatzer Muscular VSD Occluder is implanted with either a 45° or a 180° Amplatzer TorqVue Delivery System accommodating 5-9 F access vessels.

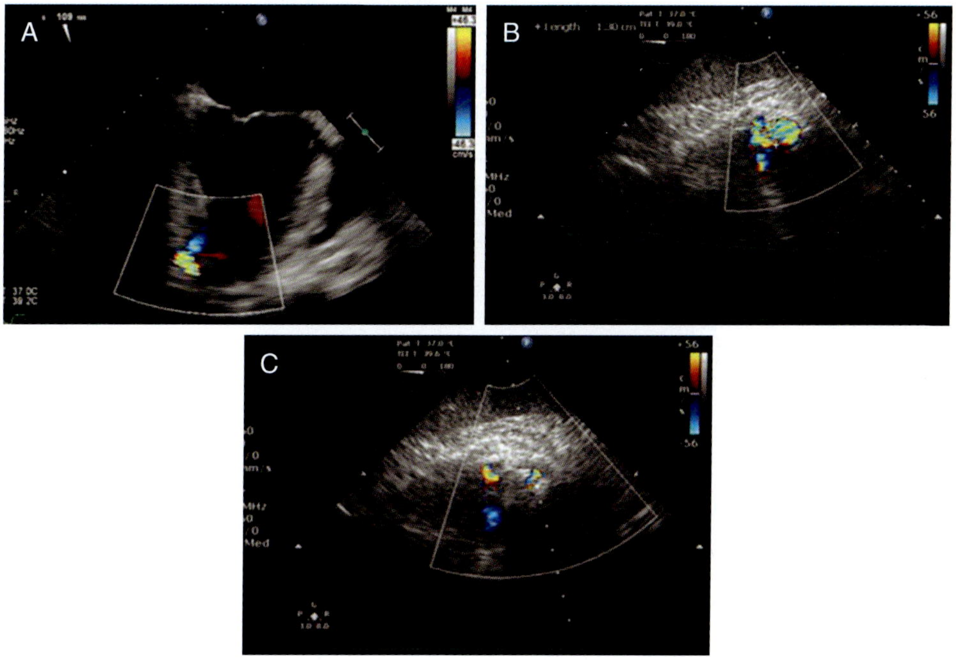

FIGURE 22.6 Transesophageal echocardiography images of an inferoapical VSD, measuring 1.0 to 1.3 mm. **A and B**, Left-to-right shunting is seen on color Doppler before intervention. **C**, TEE images after VSD closure reveal no evidence of shunt on color Doppler.

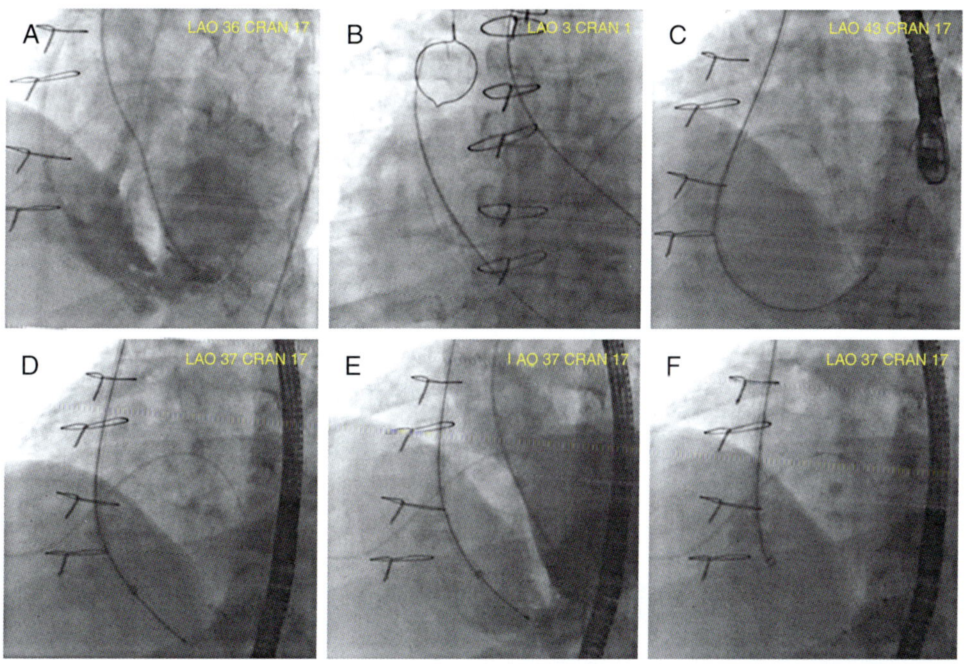

FIGURE 22.7 Fluoroscopic views of an apical VSD closure in a 59-year-old patient who underwent VSD repair after a STEMI and had a residual VSD with left-to-right shunting (Qp:Qs was measured at 1.8:1). **A**, Left ventricular angiography shows a large apical VSD (**Video 22.8**). **B**, A JR4 catheter is used to direct a J tipped wire through the VSD and the wire is then snared through the right internal jugular vein sheath, thus creating an arteriovenous loop formed by externalizing the J tipped wire through the VSD (**Video 22.9**). **C**, Using a venous approach, the Amplatzer VSD Occluder device is advanced through the VSD and the left ventricular disc is deployed. **D**, The right ventricular disc is semi-deployed. **E**, Left ventricular angiography shows appropriate position of the left disc and trivial residual shunt (**Video 22.10**). **F**, The right disc is then fully deployed and the device is released (**Video 22.11**).

PERCUTANEOUS CLOSURE OF PATENT FORAMEN OVALE

The foramen ovale is an important structure during fetal development and facilitates flow of oxygenated blood from the right atrium to the left atrium. At birth, most people have functional closure of the foramen ovale by apposition of the septum primum on the left against the septum secundum on the right. The prevalence of a patent foramen ovale (PFO) is very common and has been estimated to be 25% in autopsy and community-based transesophageal echocardiography (TEE) studies.[9,10] Most of them are asymptomatic, but PFOs have been associated with cryptogenic strokes, platypnea-orthodeoxia syndrome, decompression sickness, and migraines. The main indication for percutaneous PFO closure is to prevent recurrent cryptogenic strokes, particularly in young patients if there is no other cause of stroke after extensive evaluation. In 2014, the American Heart Association guidelines concluded that the evidence did not support routine PFO closure for secondary stroke prevention and this was reiterated by the American Academy of Neurology in 2016.[11,12] Recently, extended follow-up from the RESPECT trial along with 2, new randomized clinical trials, REDUCE and CLOSE, strongly suggest that PFO closure reduces the risk of recurrent stroke in young, carefully selected patients with cryptogenic stroke, when no alternative etiology of stroke is present. Although the annual risk of stroke recurrence is low and the absolute benefit of closure is modest, cumulative lifetime risk reduction is likely meaningful in young patients.[13-15] At this time, the 2 most commonly used percutaneous devices are the Amplatzer PFO Occluder (St Jude Medical, St Paul, MN) and the Gore Helex or Cardioform Septal Occluders (WL Gore & Associates, Flagstaff, AZ) (**FIGURES 22.8-22.11**).

PERCUTANEOUS CLOSURE OF PATENT DUCTUS ARTERIOSUS

The ductus arteriosus is a persistent, vascular connection between the left pulmonary artery near its origin and the aorta, just distal to the left subclavian artery. It is a fetal structure that spontaneously closes after delivery in more than 95% of full-term infants during the first 72 hours of life, completing the conversion of the fetal circulation to the normal postnatal circulation. It can be isolated or may be present in association with other forms of congenital heart disease. Clinical manifestations of persistent patent ductus arteriosus (PDA) are related to the degree of left-to-right shunting. Significant and prolonged aortopulmonary shunting may result in LV dilation and ultimately left-sided heart failure. Left untreated, large left-to-right shunts may additionally lead to irreversible pulmonary hypertension and progress to Eisenmenger physiology with right-to-left shunting at the level of the PDA.[16] The ACC/AHA Task Force on Practice Guidelines recommend routine follow-up for patients with a small PDA without evidence of left-sided heart volume overload. Closure of the PDA, through either a transcatheter or surgical approach, is recommended in patients with left atrial and/or left ventricular enlargement, or in the presence of a net left-to-right shunt, or a history of endarteritis.[16] Since the first surgical closure of a PDA by Gross and Hubbard in 1939, and

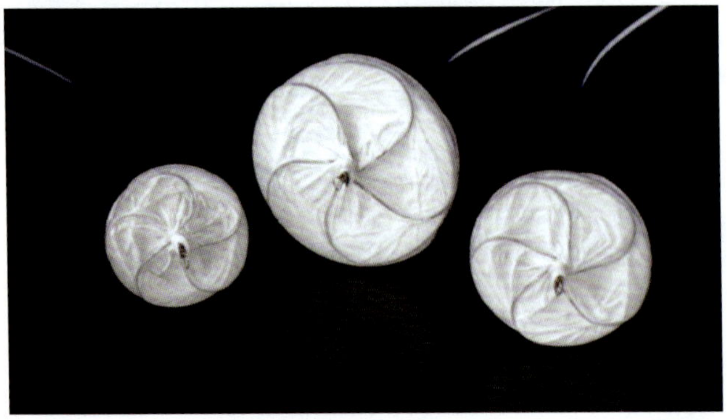

FIGURE 22.8 Gore Cardioform Septal Occluder. These devices comprise a nitinol wire frame covered with expanded polytetrafluorethylene (ePTFE). A locking loop connects the right and left discs and stabilizes the device within the septum. The handle also allows repositioning and retrieval of the Occluder via the retrieval cord, if necessary.

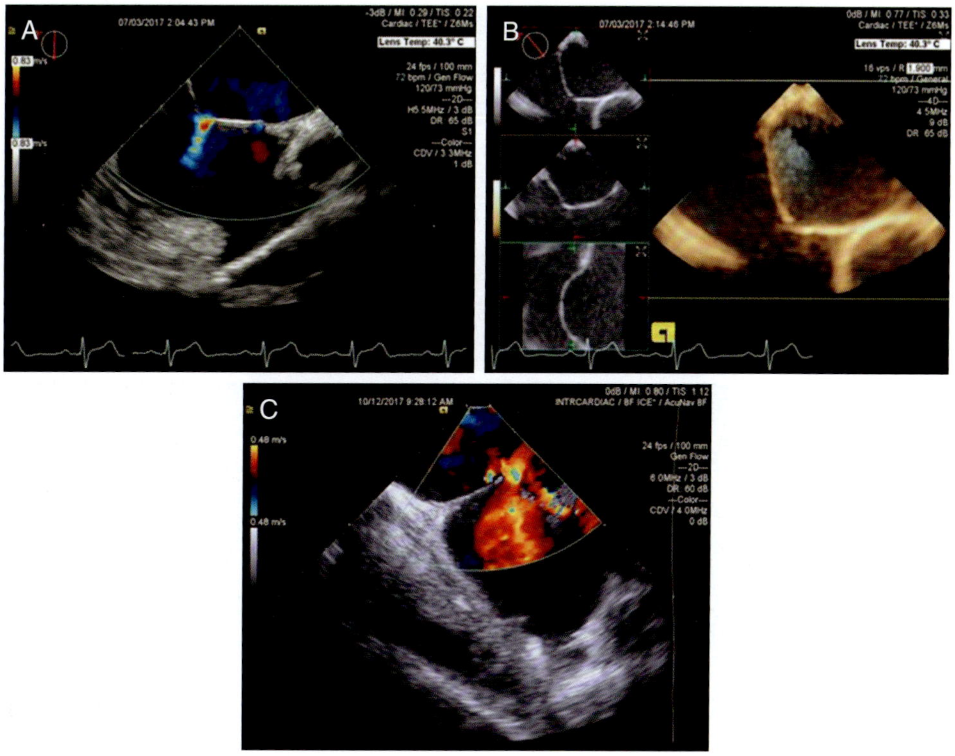

FIGURE 22.9 **A**, TEE with color doppler showing 2 atrial septal defects (ASDs) with left-to-right shunting and a PFO. **B**, 3D echocardiography shows an aneurysmal, mobile interatrial septum with an ASD superior to the PFO. **C**, Intracardiac echocardiography (ICE) performed during the procedure verifies the presence of 2 ASDs and concomitant PFO.

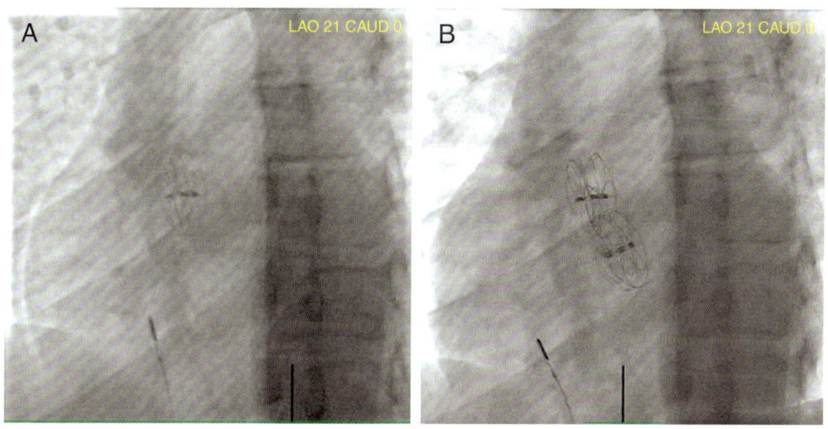

FIGURE 22.10 PFO and ASD closure in an 18-year-old man with a cryptogenic, posterior circulation stroke. Percutaneous PFO and ASD closure is performed using ICE guidance to visualize the location and anatomy of the PFO and to determine the presence or absence of ASDs. A multipurpose catheter is introduced through a venous sheath to access the left atrium via the defect and secured in the left upper pulmonary vein (LUPV). The use of a sizing balloon is common, although not required during percutaneous PFO closure. Over the 11 FR sheath and a J tipped Rosen wire, a 25 mm Cardioform Septal Occluder device is advanced across the PFO under fluoroscopic and ICE guidance. The left disc is first deployed with simultaneous retraction of the delivery system while minimizing advancement of the Occluder and risk of perforation. Gentle pull of the handle brings the left atrial disc onto the surface of the left atrial septum and the right atrial disc is subsequently deployed. Once fluoroscopy and ICE confirms planar appearance of both discs and apposition to the septum, the Occluder is fully released from the delivery system. Next, the ASD is crossed using a JR4 catheter and a Rosen wire is advanced into the LUPV. A second 25 mm Cardioform Septal Occluder device is then advanced across the ASD and successfully deployed under fluoroscopic and ICE guidance. Fluoroscopy image in the left anterior oblique projection showing **(A)** a Gore Cardioform Septal Occluder across the PFO and **(B)** a second Gore Cardioform Septal Occluder to close the ASDs.

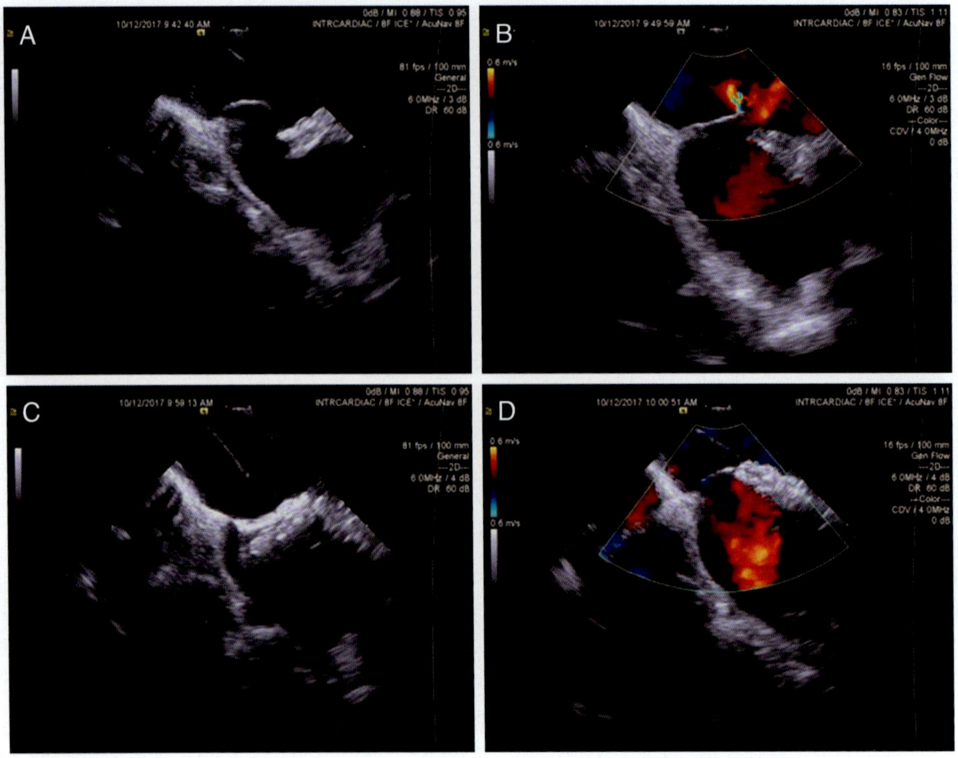

FIGURE 22.11 ICE of 2 Gore Cardioform Septal Occluders. **A and B**, ICE demonstrates an ASD and a 25 mm Gore Cardioform Septal Occluder device across the PFO. **C and D**, A second, 25 mm Gore Cardioform Septal Occluder device is deployed to cover the ASDs. ICE reveals 2, well-seated devices and no residual shunt on color doppler.

later transcatheter closure by Portsmann in 1967, there have been significant advances in device development, making transcatheter closure the preferred approach in contemporary practice. The Amplatzer Occluders are the most commonly used device to treat moderate to large PDAs. Coil embolization has also been successfully used to close PDAs of 2 mm or smaller at the narrowest portion (**FIGURES 22.12-22.14**).

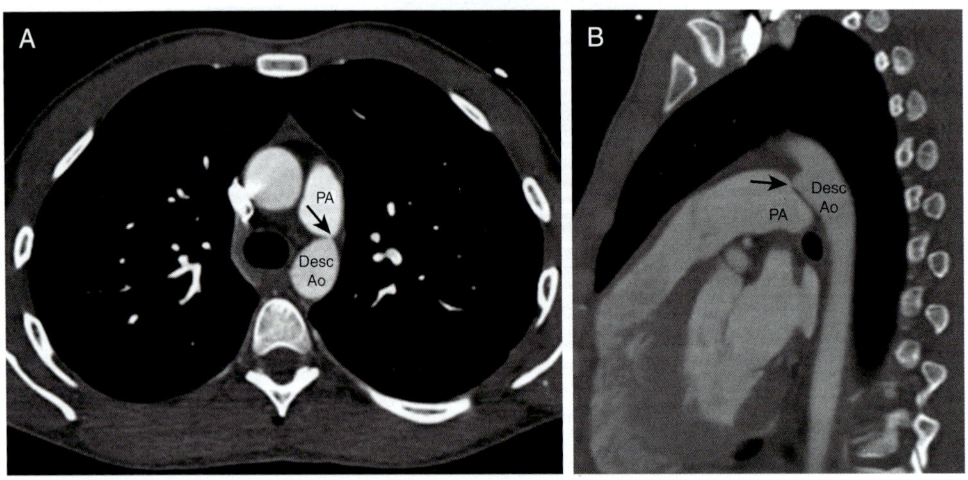

FIGURE 22.12 The Krichenko classification.[16] Type A: conical ductus, prominent aortic ampulla with narrowing at pulmonary artery end; Type B: window, short and wide ductus with blending of pulmonary artery; Type C: long tubular ductus with no constrictions; Type D: multiple constrictions with complex ductus; Type E: elongated ductus with remote constriction. **A**, Computed tomography showing a PDA (Krichenko Type A) with a 2 mm communication between the descending aorta and the main pulmonary artery. **B**, Sagittal images of the PDA connection to the descending aorta.

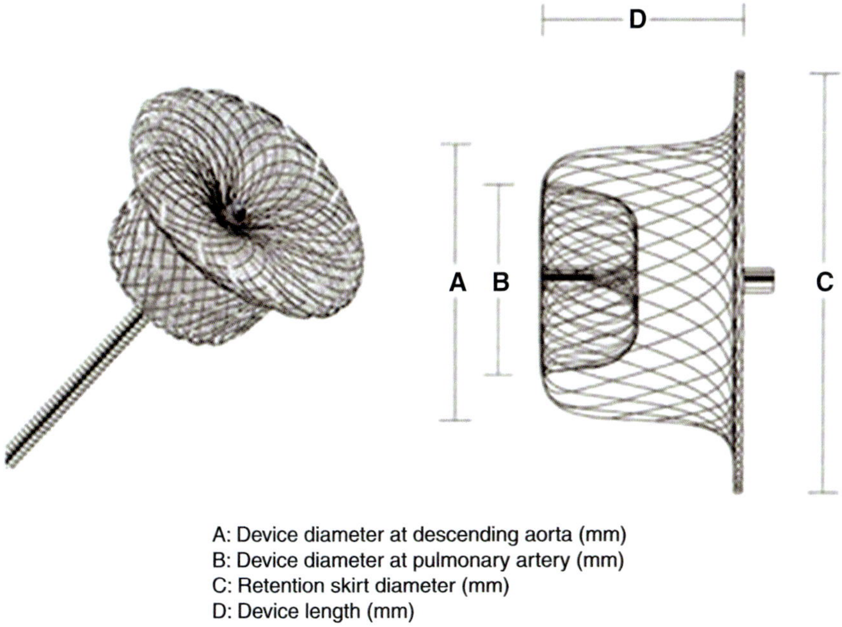

FIGURE 22.13 Amplatzer Duct Occluder.

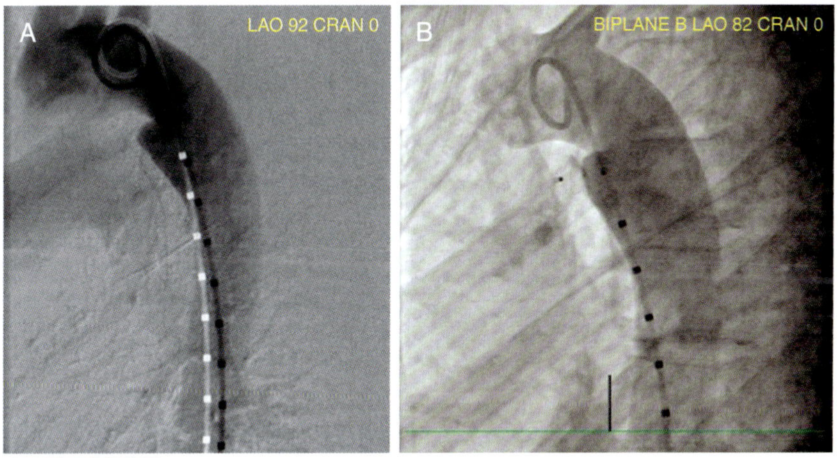

FIGURE 22.14 Transcatheter closure in a 28 year old man with a PDA and biventricular enlargement. A pigtail catheter is advanced into the aortic arch and a lateral angiogram is performed to visualize the PDA (Video 22.12). **A**, Attempts to cross the PDA from the venous side are unsuccessful. Therefore, the PDA is crossed from the aortic side using a J tipped guide wire and a JR4 catheter. The wire is then snared and externalized through the femoral vein. Through the venous sheath, an AMPLATZER TorqVue LP Delivery System with 10 mm retention disc is advanced through the PDA and successfully deployed across the PDA (Video 22.13). **B**, A final aortogram confirms device placement and stability across the PDA with minimal flow (Video 22.14).

PERCUTANEOUS PULMONARY VEIN STENOSIS INTERVENTION

Atrial fibrillation remains the most common cardiac arrhythmia presenting with a wide spectrum of symptoms and severity. The use of catheter-based ablative therapy to the left atrial wall and pulmonary veins has been largely successful in reducing the burden of atrial fibrillation and restoring sinus rhythm. Despite advances in technology and modification of ablative techniques, pulmonary vein stenosis (PVS) has been described as a rare, but severe complication of ablation. In the early studies of ablative therapy, PVS was reported in up to 30% to 40% of patients, but using contemporary techniques, the incidence has decreased to approximately 1%.[17-19] Clinical symptomatology is variable, ranging from dyspnea, cough, and chest pain to hemoptysis and recurrent lung infections, and as such requires a high index of suspicion. CT or MRI has been used as gold standard to assess for PV stenosis because they provide accurate delineation of the pulmonary vein anatomy. Other imaging modalities include echocardiography, ventilation/perfusion (V/Q) scan, and rarely pulmonary vein angiography. Although there is no standard definition of PVS on echocardiography, an increased maximum PV doppler flow velocity (>1.1 m/s) combined with color doppler turbulence may be a reliable index.[20] A V/Q scan is useful for detecting hemodynamically significant PVS, as perfusion of a pulmonary lobe draining to a PV with a significant stenosis (ie, >50%) may be decreased and detected.

Transcatheter therapy with or without stent placement is the most common approach for treatment of symptomatic patients with severe PVS. Treatment of asymptomatic patients remains controversial, but reasons for early intervention include eventual progression to thrombotic occlusion and inadequate pulmonary arterial flow leading to ischemia and edema of the surrounding alveoli and subsequent pulmonary hypertension (**FIGURES 22.15-22.18**).[21]

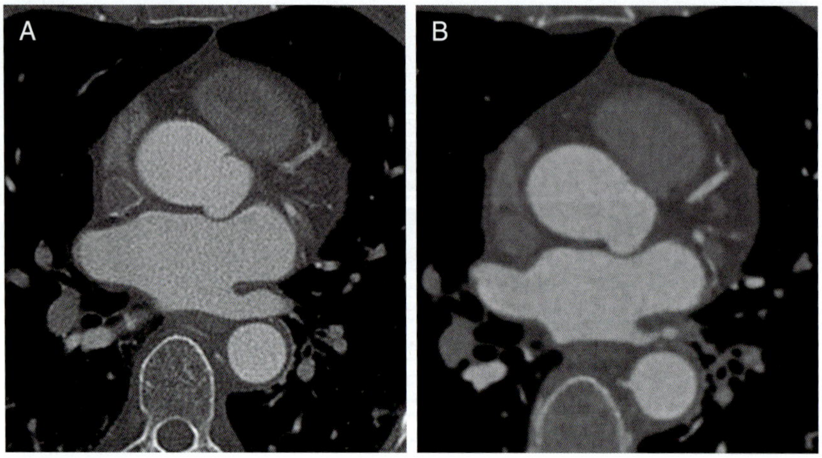

FIGURE 22.15 Computed tomography showing severe stenosis in the left inferior pulmonary vein (LIPV) after catheter-based ablation. The LIPV is shown before **(A)** and after **(B)** AF ablation.

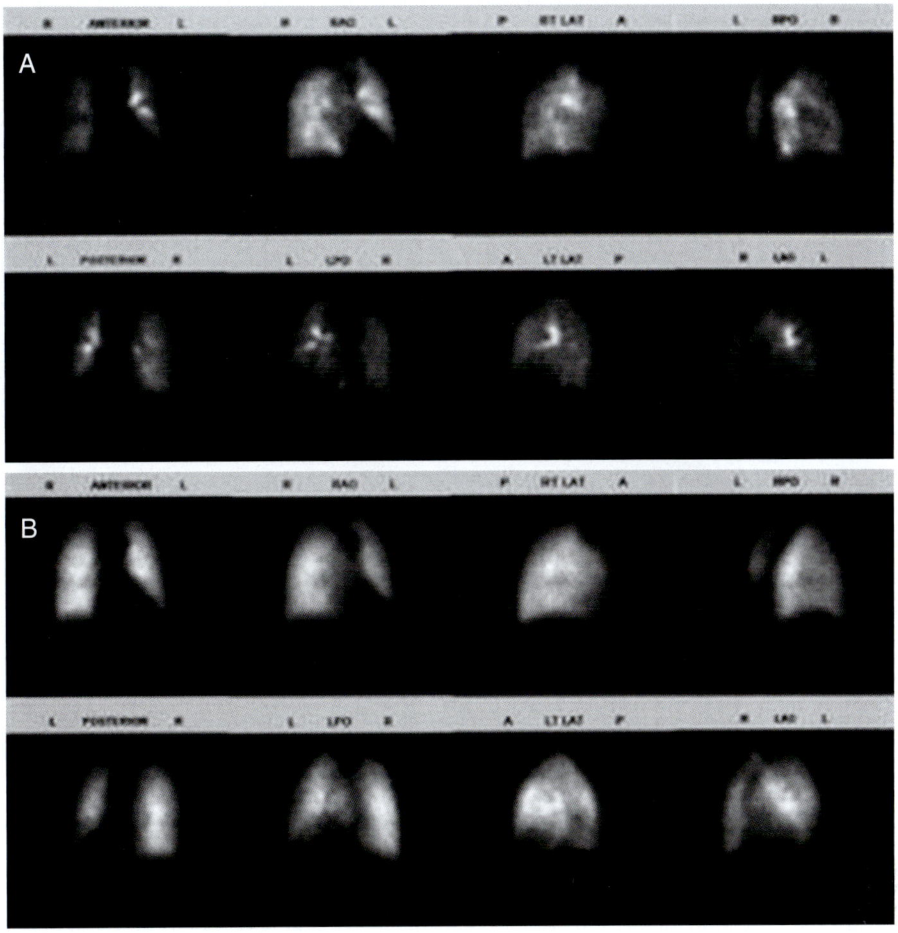

FIGURE 22.16 Ventilation/perfusion scan showing a large mismatched defect with severe reduction in perfusion in the left lower lobe secondary to the known left inferior pulmonary stenosis. **A**, Normal ventilation. **B**, Hypoperfusion of the left lower lobe involving the superior, posterior basal, and lateral basal segments.

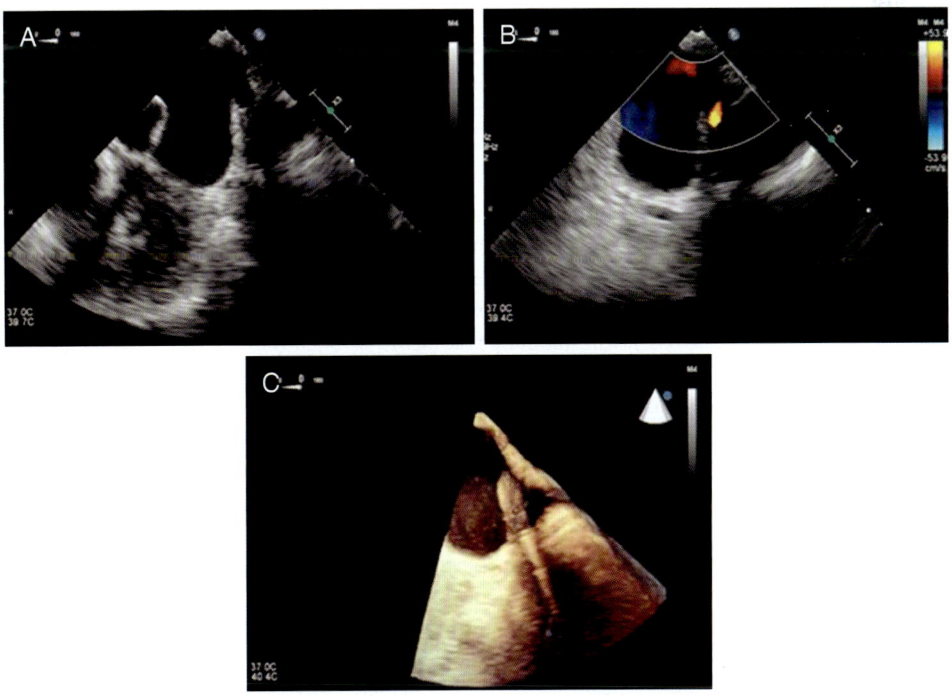

FIGURE 22.17 2D TEE in a patient with severe PVS. **A**, 2D images show severe stenosis in the proximal, LIPV. **B**, Color doppler shows turbulent flow across the proximal PVS. **C**, Echocardiography is helpful to help guide transseptal puncture and verify the pulmonary vein (PV) of interest, as seen in this 3D TEE image showing a wire across the PV lesion.

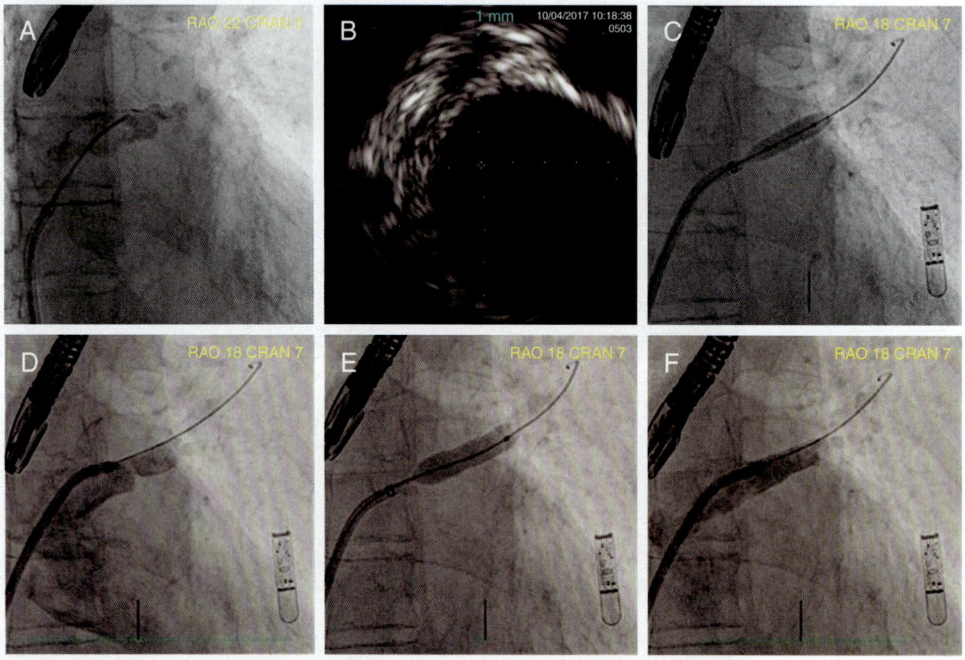

FIGURE 22.18 Transseptal puncture is performed using standard techniques and TEE guidance (**Video 22.15**). Over an 8.5 F SL-1 sheath secured in the left atrium and through a multipurpose catheter, a guide wire is advanced into the LIPV. **A**, Selective pulmonary venography is performed using hand injections over the multipurpose catheter and a glide catheter is used to measure a pressure gradient of 10 mm Hg across the lesion (**Videos 22.16 and 22.17**). **B**, Intravascular ultrasound is performed for sizing of the vessel (10 mm) as well as assessing lesion length and severity. **C**, A standard J tipped guide wire is reintroduced into the LIPV and the lesion is angioplastied using an 8.0 × 20 mm balloon (**Video 22.18**). **D**, Repeat selective angiography is performed using the SL-1 sheath (**Video 22.19**). **E**, The lesion is stented using a 10 × 25 mm bare metal stent (**Video 22.20**). **F**, Final angiography reveals excellent stent expansion and no evidence of complications (**Video 22.21**).

TRANSCATHETER LEFT ATRIAL APPENDAGE OCCLUSION: WATCHMAN DEVICE

Atrial fibrillation is the most common cardiac arrhythmia, affecting 1% to 2% of the general population. Patients with atrial fibrillation have a 5-fold higher risk of stroke, and >90% of the thromboembolic source appears to originate from the left atrial appendage (LAA).[22,23] Several scoring systems have been developed to assess the risk of stroke in atrial fibrillation. The $CHADS_2$-VASc score, a modified version of the original $CHADS_2$ score, has been used to categorize patients as low risk (score of 0), intermediate risk (score of 1), and high risk (score of 2 or greater) based on the 1 year per patient, thromboembolic event rate of 0, 0.46, and 1.71, respectively ($P < .0001$).[24] Oral anticoagulation is the standard of care for embolic prevention in patients with atrial fibrillation (class I, level of evidence A). Yet, warfarin has a narrow therapeutic range and requires frequent monitoring and dose adjustments. In addition, warfarin has significant interactions with other medications and some foods that may affect its effectiveness. Newer direct thrombin and Factor Xa inhibitors are available and do not require monitoring, but like warfarin, are associated with major bleeding. To mitigate the risks of bleeding, particularly in those patients who are at high risk, alternative therapies such as surgical ligation, LAA clips, and more recently endovascular closure of the LAA have become available. The WATCHMAN device (Boston Scientific, St Paul, MN) is a percutaneously inserted device that reduces the risk of stroke by closing off the LAA. Pooled meta-analysis of PROTECT-AF and PREVAIL studies, evaluating the safety and efficacy of the WATCHMAN device compared with warfarin at 5 years, demonstrate that LAA closure with WATCHMAN provides comparable outcomes to warfarin in stroke prevention for nonvalvular atrial fibrillation (cardiovascular death, stroke, or systemic embolism occurred in 2.8% of the device group vs 3.4% of the warfarin group [$P = .27$]) (**FIGURES 22.19-22.22**).[25]

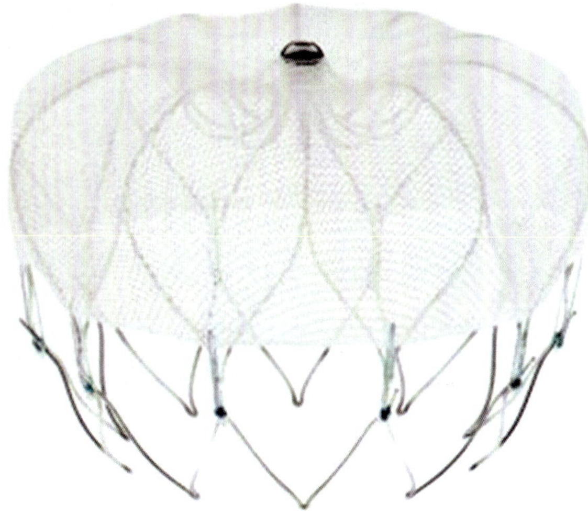

FIGURE 22.19 The WATCHMAN Device. The WATCHMAN Device is made of a nitinol frame that radially expands to maintain position in the LAA and has 10 active fixation anchors to engage the LAA tissue. A 160-micron polyethylene terephthalate cap is designed to block emboli from exiting the LAA and promote healing.

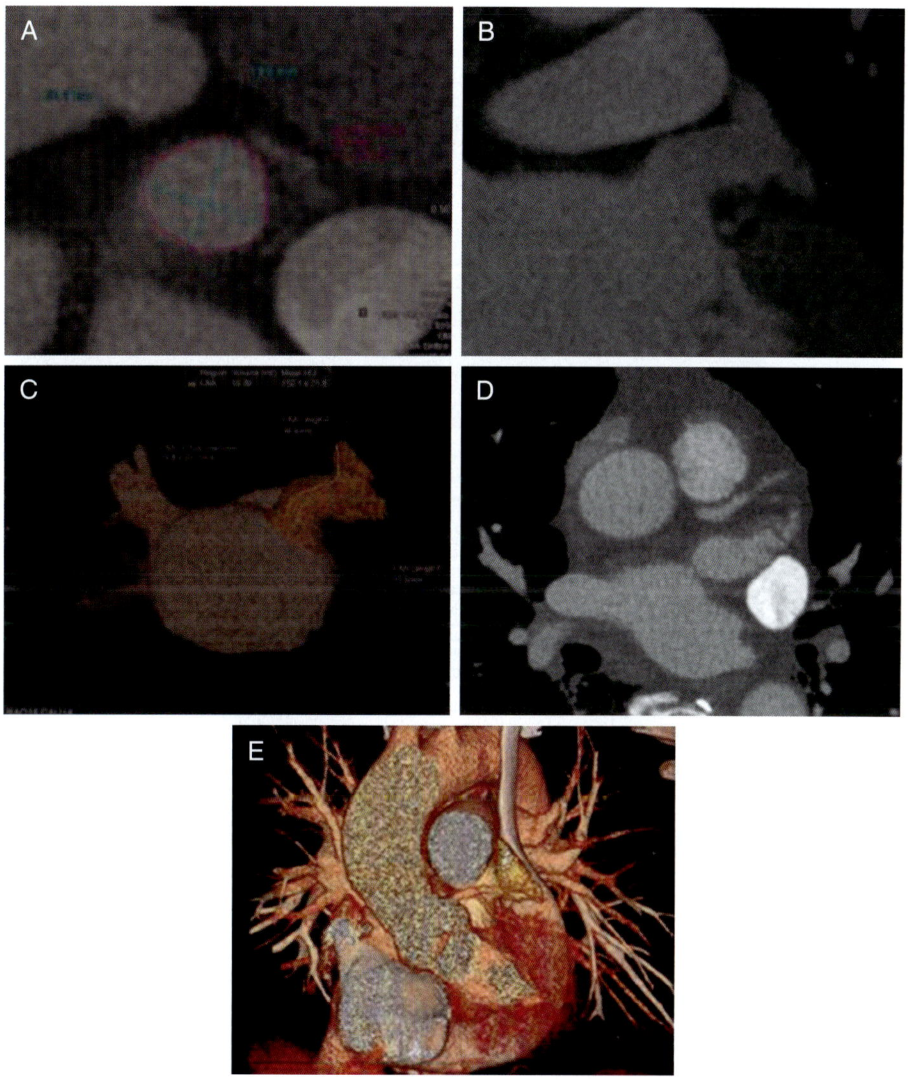

FIGURE 22.20 Cardiac CT can provide important information to assess the suitability of patients for percutaneous LAA closure. Contrast enhanced CT images of the LAA before closure with a WATCHMAN occlusion device. **A**, Measurement of the LAA os or landing zone dimensions for the WATCHMAN device. The orifice has a minimum diameter of 19.9 mm and maximum of 23.1 mm with an area of 342 mm^2. **B**, Oblique images illustrating the LAA. **C**, 3D volume-rendered images of the LAA. Note the angulated, chicken wing appearance of this appendage. **D**, Axial images displaying the location and anatomy of the LAA. In this patient, the LAA runs posterior to the main pulmonary trunk and the left anterior descending artery. **E**, Volume-rendered images depicting the LAA and surrounding structures. The LAA courses behind the main PA trunk and the left anterior descending artery.

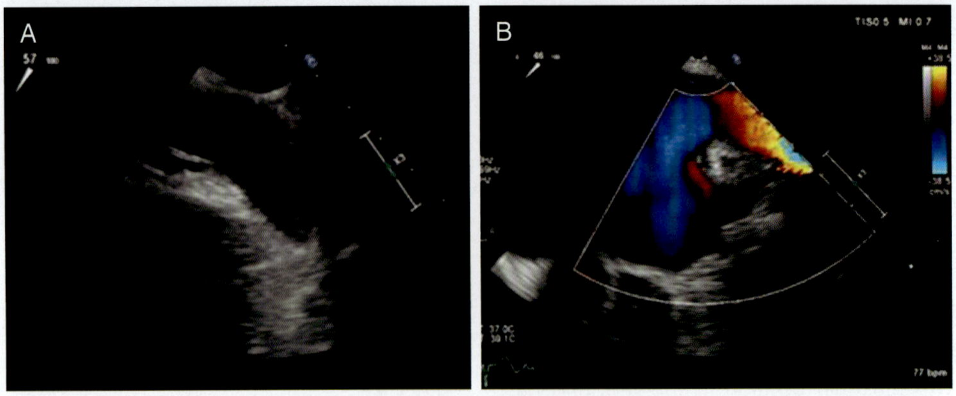

FIGURE 22.21 TEE images are required to confirm the LAA size and to select the appropriate WATCHMAN device. TEE guidance is used to measure the LAA ostium width and depth in 4 views (0°, 45°, 90°, 135°). **A**, The LAA ostium was measured at 23 mm in multiple views. **B**, The 3-month postprocedure TEE shows a well-seated WATCHMAN device with complete seal and no residual leak on color doppler. There is no evidence of any intracardiac thrombus. Warfarin is stopped and the patient is continued on aspirin and clopidogrel and at 6 months, he is continued on aspirin only.

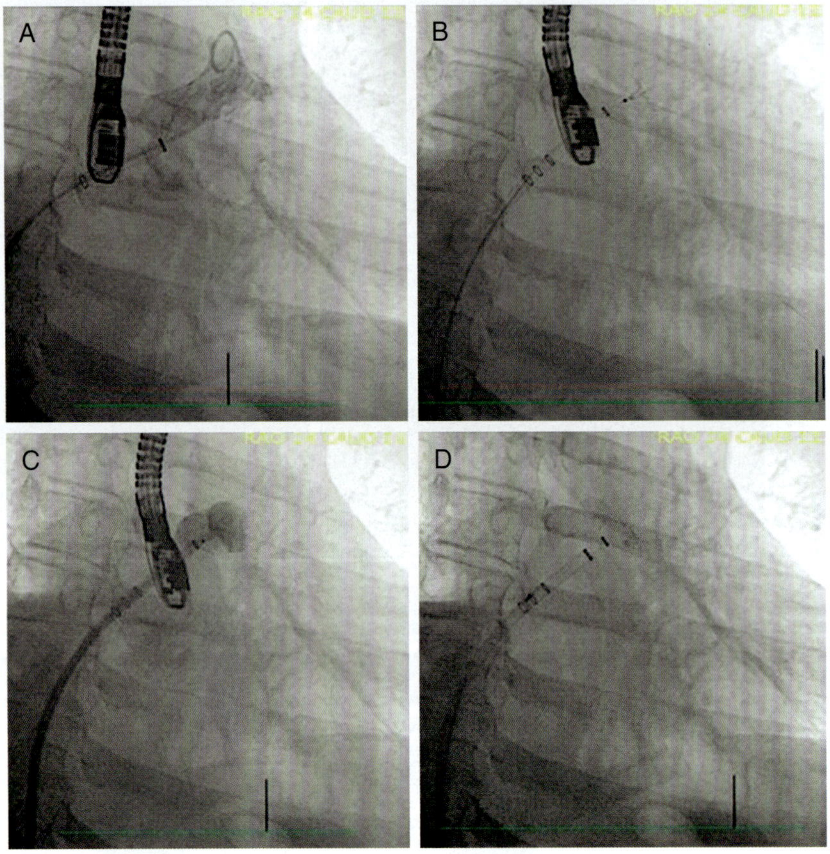

FIGURE 22.22 Endovascular closure of the LAA using a WATCHMAN device in a 63-year-old patient with nonvalvular atrial fibrillation, previous stroke, and recurrent gastrointestinal bleeding. A transseptal puncture is performed using standard techniques under TEE and fluoroscopic guidance. An Amplatz Extra Stiff wire is then inserted into the LUPV. Over the Amplatz Extra Stiff wire, the 14 FR Watchman Access Sheath (AS) is inserted into the left atrium. **A**, Through the Watchman AS a pigtail catheter is advanced into the LAA and LAA angiography is performed (Video 22.22). Accounting for the 8% to 20% device compression and CT/TEE measurements, a size 27 mm WATCHMAN device is selected. The AS is then advanced over the pigtail catheter into the LAA until the correct sizing marker band is situated at the ostium (ie, middle marker band corresponds to the 27 mm device). Under fluoroscopic guidance, the Delivery System (DS) is advanced through the AS until the most distal marker band on the DS and the most distal marker on the AS are aligned (Video 22.23). The AS is slowly retracted and subsequently snapped onto the DS. **B**, The WATCHMAN device is deployed by holding the deployment knob stationary while slowly retracting the AS/DS assembly. **C**, An angiogram is performed through the assembly to verify seal with the device (Video 22.24). **D**, After confirmation of position, stability, compression, and seal of the device on fluoroscopy and TEE, the WATCHMAN device is fully released in the LAA by rotating the deployment knob counterclockwise 3 to 5 turns (Video 22.25).

ENDOVASCULAR TREATMENT OF SAPHENOUS VEIN GRAFTS ANEURYSMS

Coronary artery pseudoaneurysms are rare and usually caused by prior iatrogenic manipulation (either prior bypass surgery or PCIs), blunt trauma, or infection. Rapidly enlarging pseudoaneurysms carry the risk of rupture and tamponade, along with thrombosis and subsequent distal embolization. Patients may have variable presentations, ranging from asymptomatic to a chest pain syndrome and myocardial infarction.[26] Although there are no well-established guideline recommendations for surgical or percutaneous treatment of large aneurysms, management is largely driven by patency of the feeder vessel and the size of the myocardium at risk. If the vessel supplies significant myocardial tissue, the pseudoaneurysm may be excluded using a covered stent. Alternatively, in a large number of patients, the affected graft is occluded when the patent aneurysmal vessel supplies a small territory. In this subset, preservation of myocardial blood supply is not a concern, and embolization of the feeder vessels can be achieved with coils or a vascular plug. In the presence of mechanical complications such as fistula, rupture, compression of other structures, or concomitant valve surgery, cardiac surgery may be the preferred or only option. Thus, patients should always be assessed by a heart team comprising a cardiac surgeon and an interventional cardiologist experienced in structural heart disease (**FIGURES 22.23-22.25**).

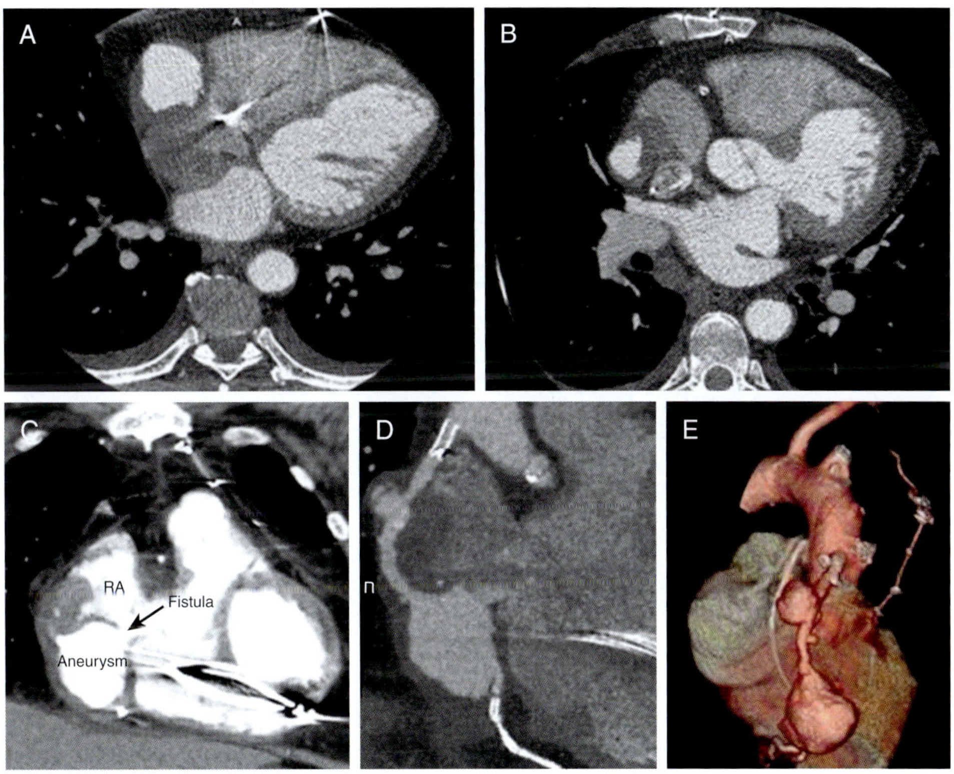

FIGURE 22.23 Pre-intervention cardiac CT with multiplanar reconstruction demonstrating 2 large, saphenous vein graft (SVG) aneurysms with mass effect and fistulous connection to the right atrium (RA). **A**, Axial images show a partially thrombosed distal aneurysm measuring 5.3 × 4.3 × 5 cm with significant mass effect on the RA. **B**, Axial images show a smaller, partially thrombosed, proximal aneurysm measuring 3.0 × 2.4 and 3.9 cm. **C**, Coronal images show a fistulous communication with the inferolateral wall of the RA. The mouth of the fistulous communication measures approximately 14 mm. **D**, Multiplanar reconstruction displays the 2 large saphenous vein aneurysms with the fistulous connection between the distal aneurysm and the RA. There is a patent stent in the proximal body of the SVG and multiple stents in the right posterior descending artery (RPDA) distal to the graft anastomosis that appear to be occluded. **E**, 3D volume-rendered images displaying the 2 large SVG to RPDA aneurysms

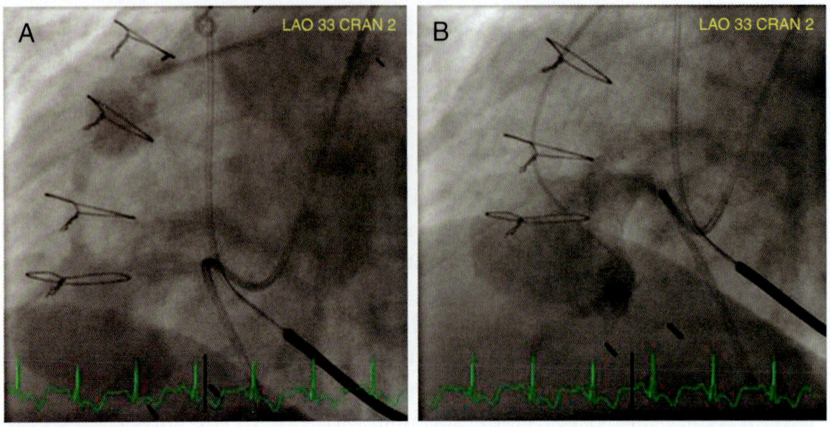

FIGURE 22.24 Diagnostic angiogram of a 56-year-old man with a remote history of CABG who presented with a NSTEMI. **A**, Selective graft injections are performed using a multipurpose catheter (Video 22.26). **B**, Over a coronary guide wire the multipurpose catheter is carefully advanced into the distal aneurysm. Hand injections demonstrate minimal flow into the native right coronary artery. A right heart catheterization is performed and shows a Qp to Qs ratio of 1.2 to 1.

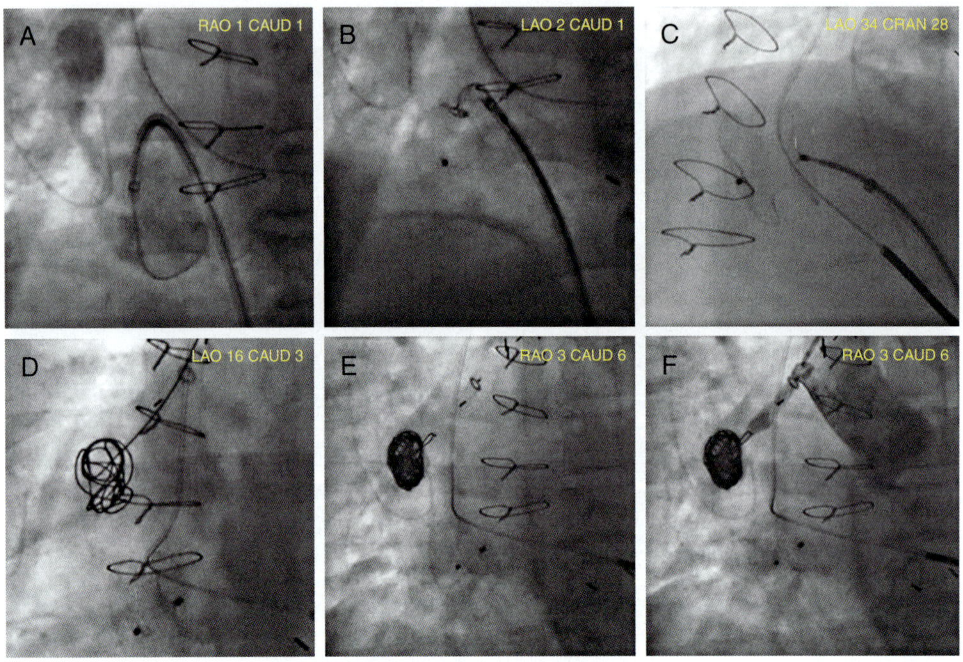

FIGURE 22.25 Endovascular closure of large, SVG aneurysms with a fistula to the RA. Femoral arterial and venous access is obtained. **A**, Through the venous sheath and over a 5 F IMA catheter, a J tipped wire is directed from the RA and into the distal aneurysm, allowing for advancement of a 9 F Amplatzer TorqVue deliver catheter (Video 22.27). **B and C**, A 24 mm Amplatzer Septal Occluder is deployed across the SVG to RA fistula. The delivery system is slowly retracted and the distal disc is first deployed. The entire assembly (delivery cable and sheath) is pulled into the fistula and the delivery catheter is slowly withdrawn while maintaining the position of the distal disc, gradually unsheathing the proximal disc (Videos 22.28 and 22.29). **D**, A 6 F multipurpose guide catheter is used to engage the aorto-ostium of the vein graft and two 20 mm framing coils are deployed in the superior fistula (Video 22.30). **E**, A 5 mm Amplatzer Ductal Occluder is deployed in the proximal graft to ensure complete closure of the vessel (Video 22.31). **F**, Final angiography shows adequate positioning of all deployed devices and minimal flow into the distal vein graft.

REFERENCES

1. Nishimura RA, Otto CM, Bonow RO, et al. 2014 AHA/ACC guideline for the management of patients with valvular heart disease: a report of the American College of Cardiology/American Heart Association Task Force on Practice Guidelines. *J Am Coll Cardiol.* 2014;63:e57-e185.
2. Hammermeister K, Sethi GK, Henderson WG, Grover FL, Oprian C, Rahimtoola SH. Outcomes 15 years after valve replacement with a mechanical versus a bioprosthetic valve: final report of the Veterans Affairs randomized trial. *J Am Coll Cardiol.* 2000;36:1152-1158.
3. Hayashida K, Lefèvre T, Chevalier B, et al. Impact of post-procedural aortic regurgitation on mortality after transcatheter aortic valve implantation. *JACC Cardiovasc Interv.* 2012;5:1247-1256.
4. Kodali SK, Williams MR, Smith CR, et al. Two-year outcomes after transcatheter or surgical aortic-valve replacement. *N Engl J Med.* 2012;366:1686-1695.
5. French JK, Hellkamp AS, Armstrong PW, et al. Mechanical complications after percutaneous coronary intervention in ST-elevation myocardial infarction (from APEX-AMI). *Am J Cardiol.* 2010;105:59-63.
6. Crenshaw BS, Granger CB, Birnbaum Y, et al. Risk factors, angiographic patterns, and outcomes in patients with ventricular septal defect complicating acute myocardial infarction. GUSTO-I (Global Utilization of Streptokinase and TPA for Occluded Coronary Arteries) Trial Investigators. *Circulation.* 2000;101:27-32.
7. Lock JE, Block PC, McKay RG, Baim DS, Keane JF. Transcatheter closure of ventricular septal defects. *Circulation.* 1988;78:361-368.
8. Minette MS, Sahn DJ. Ventricular septal defects. *Circulation.* 2006;114:2190-2197.
9. Hagen PT, Scholz DG, Edwards WD. Incidence and size of patent foramen ovale during the first 10 decades of life: an autopsy study of 965 normal hearts. *Mayo Clin Proc.* 1984;59:17-20.
10. Meissner I, Whisnant JP, Khandheria BK, et al. Prevalence of potential risk factors for stroke assessed by transesophageal echocardiography and carotid ultrasonography: the SPARC study. Stroke Prevention Prevalence of potential risk factors for stroke assessed by transesophageal echocardiography and carotid ultrasonography: Prevalence of potential risk factors for stroke assessed by transesophageal echocardiography and carotid ultrasonography:Assessment of Risk in a Community. *Mayo Clin Proc.* 1999;74:862-869.
11. Kernan WN, Ovbiagele B, Black HR, et al. Guidelines for the prevention of stroke in patients with stroke and transient ischemic attack: a guideline for healthcare professionals from the American Heart Association/American Stroke Association. *Stroke.* 2014;45:2160-2236.
12. Messé SR, Gronseth G, Kent DM, et al. Practice advisory: recurrent stroke with patent foramen ovale (update of practice parameter): report of the guideline development, dissemination, and implementation subcommittee of the American Academy of Neurology. *Neurology.* 2016;87:815-821.
13. Mas J-L, Derumeaux G, Guillon B, et al. Patent foramen ovale closure or anticoagulation vs. antiplatelets after stroke. *N Engl J Med.* 2017;377:1011-1021.
14. Saver JL, Carroll JD, Thaler DE, et al. Long-term outcomes of patent foramen ovale closure or medical therapy after stroke. *N Engl J Med.* 2017;377:1022-1032.
15. Søndergaard L, Kasner SE, Rhodes JF, et al. Patent foramen ovale closure or antiplatelet therapy for cryptogenic stroke. *N Engl J Med.* 2017;377:1033-1042.
16. Warnes CA, Williams RG, Bashore TM, et al. ACC/AHA 2008 guidelines for the management of adults with congenital heart disease. *J Am Coll Cardiol.* 2008;52:e143-e263.
17. Arentz T, Jander N, von Rosenthal J, et al. Incidence of pulmonary vein stenosis 2 years after radiofrequency catheter ablation of refractory atrial fibrillation. *Eur Heart J.* 2003;24:963-969.
18. Cappato R, Calkins H, Chen S-A, et al. Updated worldwide survey on the methods, efficacy, and safety of catheter ablation for human atrial fibrillation. *Circ Arrhythm Electrophysiol.* 2010;3:32-38.
19. Chen SA, Hsieh MH, Tai CT, et al. Initiation of atrial fibrillation by ectopic beats originating from the pulmonary veins: electrophysiological characteristics, pharmacological responses, and effects of radiofrequency ablation. *Circulation.* 1999;100:1879-1886.
20. Obeid AI, Carlson RJ. Evaluation of pulmonary vein stenosis by transesophageal echocardiography. *J Am Soc Echocardiogr.* 1995;8:888-896.
21. Saad EB, Rossillo A, Saad CP, et al. Pulmonary vein stenosis after radiofrequency ablation of atrial fibrillation: functional characterization, evolution, and influence of the ablation strategy. *Circulation.* 2003;108:3102-3107.
22. Thambidorai SK, Murray RD, Parakh K, et al. Utility of transesophageal echocardiography in identification of thrombogenic milieu in patients with atrial fibrillation (an ACUTE ancillary study). *Am J Cardiol.* 2005;96:935-941.
23. Wolf PA, Abbott RD, Kannel WB. Atrial fibrillation as an independent risk factor for stroke: the Framingham Study. *Stroke.* 1991;22:983-988.
24. Lip GYH, Frison L, Halperin JL, Lane DA. Identifying patients at high risk for stroke despite anticoagulation: a comparison of contemporary stroke risk stratification schemes in an anticoagulated atrial fibrillation cohort. *Stroke.* 2010;41:2731-2738.
25. Reddy VY, Doshi SK, Kar S, et al. 5-year outcomes after left atrial appendage closure: from the PREVAIL and PROTECT AF trials. *J Am Coll Cardiol.* 2017;70:2964-2975.
26. Ramirez FD, Hibbert B, Simard T, et al. Natural history and management of aortocoronary saphenous vein graft aneurysms: a systematic review of published cases. *Circulation.* 2012;126(18):2248-2256.

chapter 23

Peripheral Interventions

JAYENDRAKUMAR S. PATEL, MD, SAMIR R. KAPADIA, MD, and MEHDI H. SHISHEHBOR, DO, MPH, PHD

INTRODUCTION

Peripheral artery and venous disorders are becoming more prevalent and clinically apparent in developed countries owing to the growth of the aging population. Advanced age and comorbid conditions prohibit many patients with peripheral vascular disorders from conventional surgical therapies. For such cases, percutaneous options have become first-line. Over the past decade, the field of peripheral intervention has realized significant advances in technique, devices, and pharmacotherapy making it possible to treat complex disease. In this chapter, we present a technical review of the most common arterial and venous peripheral interventions.

ARTERIAL INTERVENTIONS

Carotid Arteries

Carotid artery stenting (CAS) has been shown to offer similar or possibly better long-term outcomes in carefully selected patients with symptomatic or asymptomatic carotid stenosis when performed by experienced centers with low periprocedural morbidity and mortality rates (<6%).[1,2] Age ≥70 to 80 years, presence of chronic kidney disease, complex plaque morphology (including long lesion length), and calcified complex arch anatomy have been associated with higher rates of stroke or death at 1 month.[1,3-5] Current American Heart Association/American Stroke Association guidelines recommend CAS for symptomatic patients who have internal carotid artery stenosis of 70% to 99% by noninvasive imaging or 50% to 99% by angiography.[6] Asymptomatic patients who undergo CAS should have 70% to 99% stenosis by Doppler or 60% to 99% stenosis by angiography.[6]

Noninvasive Imaging

See **FIGURES 23.1** and **23.2**.

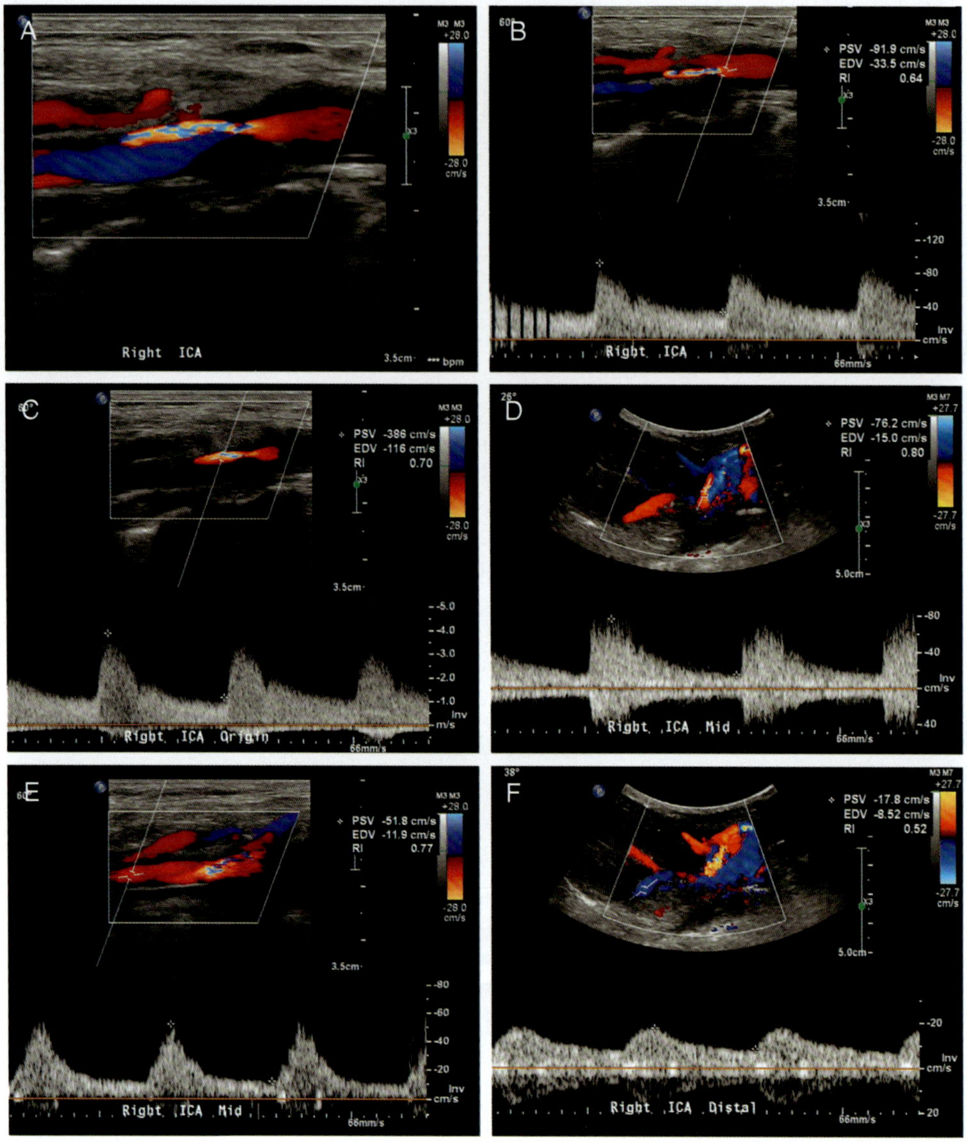

FIGURE 23.1 Abnormal carotid artery duplex ultrasound. An arterial duplex is often the first test that is obtained for patients with suspected carotid artery stenosis and is highly sensitive and specific (>85%-90%).[7] Areas of severe stenosis will typically exhibit aliasing on color flow Doppler owing to flow acceleration. In this study, mosaic color is observed in the right internal carotid artery and is due to high-velocity blood flow **(A)**. Spectral Doppler waveform of the distal common carotid artery reveals a normal peak-systolic velocity of 92 cm/s with brisk upstroke **(B)**. However, the peak-systolic and diastolic velocities at the origin of the internal carotid artery are markedly elevated **(C)**. There is also evidence of turbulent flow on spectral waveform (flow below the baseline during systole and filing of the spectral window **(D)**. In the distal segment of the internal carotid artery, spectral waveform demonstrates a parvus-tardus pattern **(E and F)**. Importantly, duplex ultrasound may not be able to differential subtotal from complete occlusions.[7]

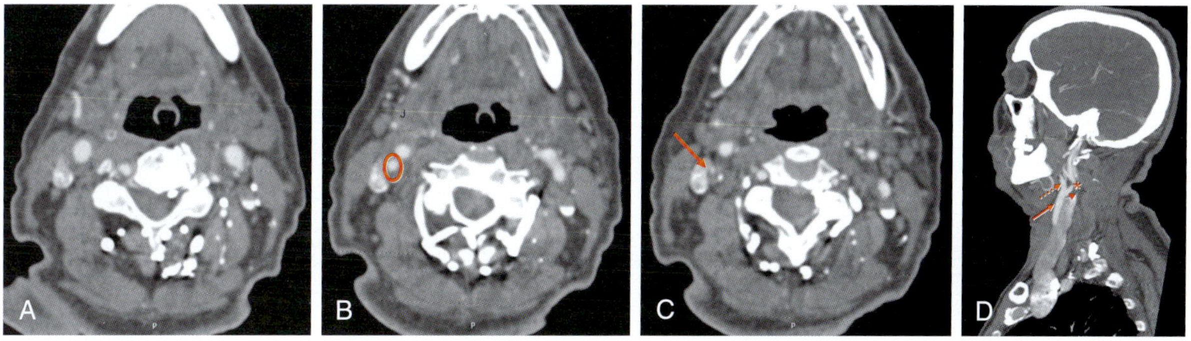

FIGURE 23.2 Computed tomography angiography (CTA), axial slices. In cases where duplex ultrasound is equivocal or nondiagnostic, CTA can be quite helpful but requires intravenous contrast and ionizing radiation.[7] The test has a high sensitivity and negative predictive value[7]. **A**, demonstrates both common carotid arteries without significant stenosis. **B**, shows the right internal carotid artery (red circle). A focal area of severe stenosis (red arrow) is seen just distal to the origin of the right internal carotid artery **(C)**. **D**, CTA, sagittal slice. The right common carotid (solid arrow), internal carotid (arrowhead), and external carotid arteries (broken arrow) are labeled. A 99% stenosis (asterisk) demonstrating the string sign is seen just distal to the origin of the right internal carotid artery.

Angiographic Evaluation and Treatment

See FIGURES 23.3-23.8.

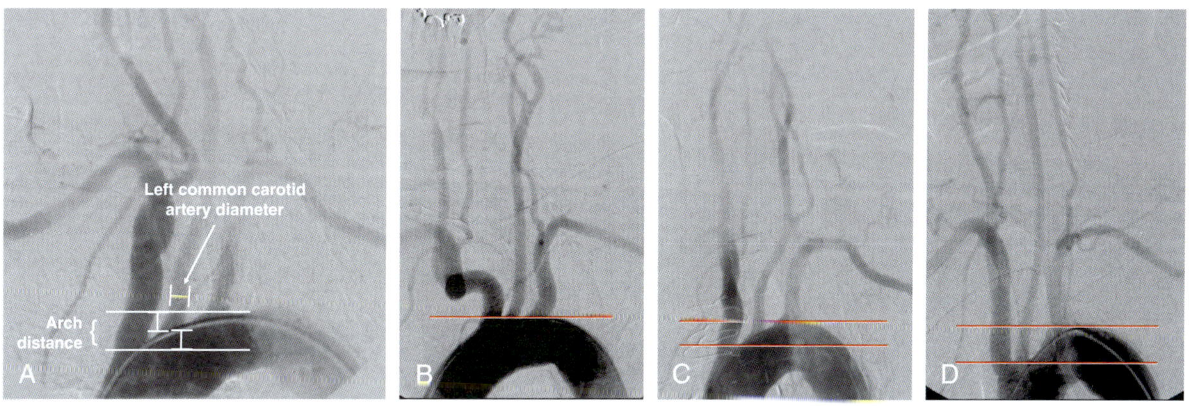

FIGURE 23.3 Arch aortography. At the start of the procedure, arch aortography is performed and carefully studied to understand the extent and location of aortic atheroma and assess the complexity of arch anatomy. The aortic arch is classified based on the vertical distance from the origin of the innominate artery to the outer curvature, with the reference diameter being the width of the left common carotid artery **(A)**. The type I arch is most common, with arch vessels arising from the outer curvature in the same plane **(B)**. In a type II arch, the vertical distance from the outer curvature of the arch to the origin of the innominate artery is 1-2 diameters of the left common carotid artery **(C)**. In a type III arch, the vertical distance from the origin of the innominate artery to the outer curvature is >2 diameters of the left common carotid artery **(D)**. A type III aortic arch and proximal common carotid tortuosity portends a difficult procedure and is associated with higher rates of periprocedural stroke, death, and other complications.[3,8,9]

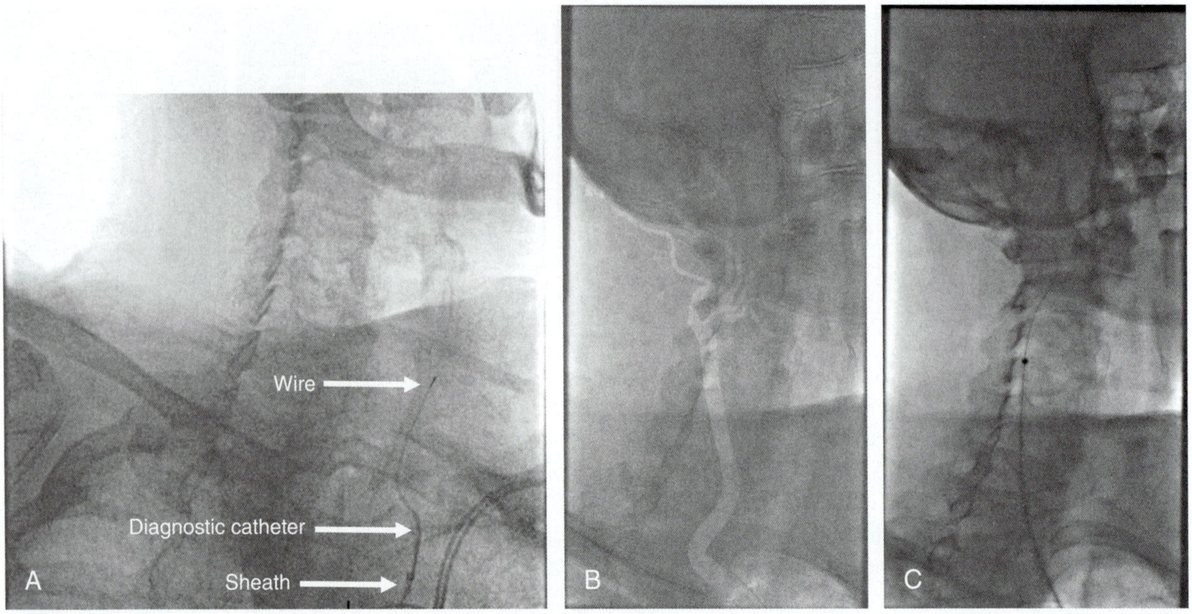

FIGURE 23.4 **A**, Engaging the carotid artery. After administering heparin to a therapeutic activated clotting time of 250-300 s, the carotid artery can be engaged. A diagnostic preshaped catheter (JR, Simons, V Tek) is used to engage the carotid or innominate artery. Selective carotid angiography is performed to create a roadmap reference image **(B)**. A Wholey or glidewire is advanced into the external carotid artery to ensure that the sheath will not touch the internal carotid artery lesion. The diagnostic catheter is advanced into the external carotid artery, and the sheath is subsequently advanced over the diagnostic catheter up to the proximal innominate or common carotid artery **(C)**. After reaching the desired location, the diagnostic catheter and wire are slowly removed, the system is de-aired, and selective carotid and cerebral angiography are performed. Courtesy of Samir Kapadia and Jay S. Patel, Cleveland Clinic Non Invasive Vascular Laboratory.

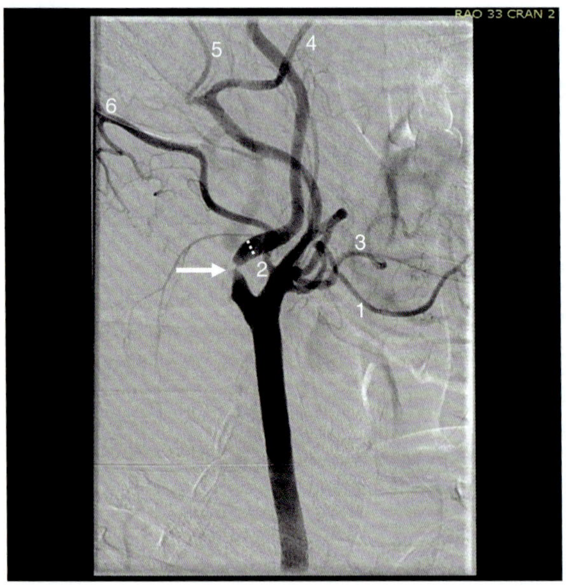

FIGURE 23.5 Selective angiography of the common carotid artery. Note the presence of a string sign in the internal carotid artery (arrow). Percent stenosis of the target lesion is most commonly calculated by using the North American Symptomatic Carotid Endarterectomy Trial (NASCET) method, where the reference diameter is the region distal to the stenosis (dashed line).[7] Branches of the external carotid artery are outlined. Lingual artery (1). Ascending pharyngeal artery (2). Facial artery (3). Maxillary artery (4). Superficial temporal artery (5). Occipital artery (6).

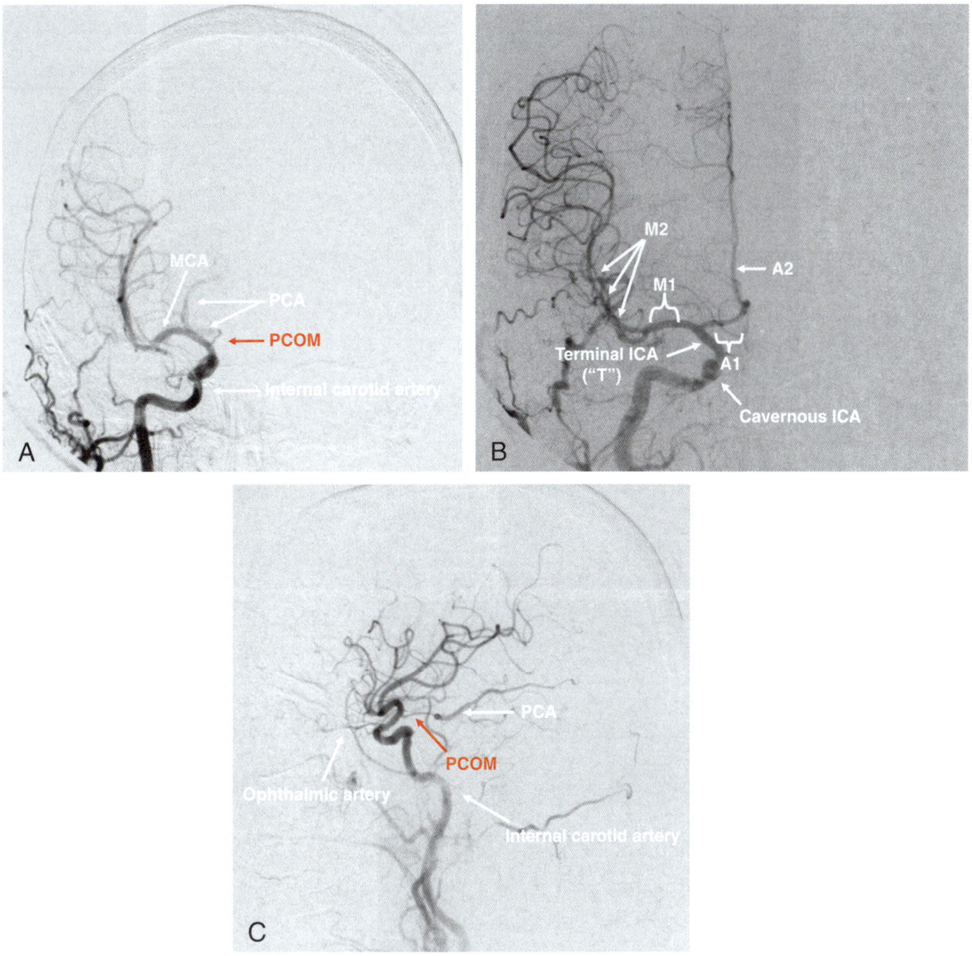

FIGURE 23.6 **A-C**, Selective angiography of the internal carotid artery is routinely performed both before and after CAS. Terminal branches of the internal carotid artery are labeled. ICA, internal carotid artery; MCA, middle cerebral artery; PCA, posterior cerebral artery; PCOM, posterior communicating artery.

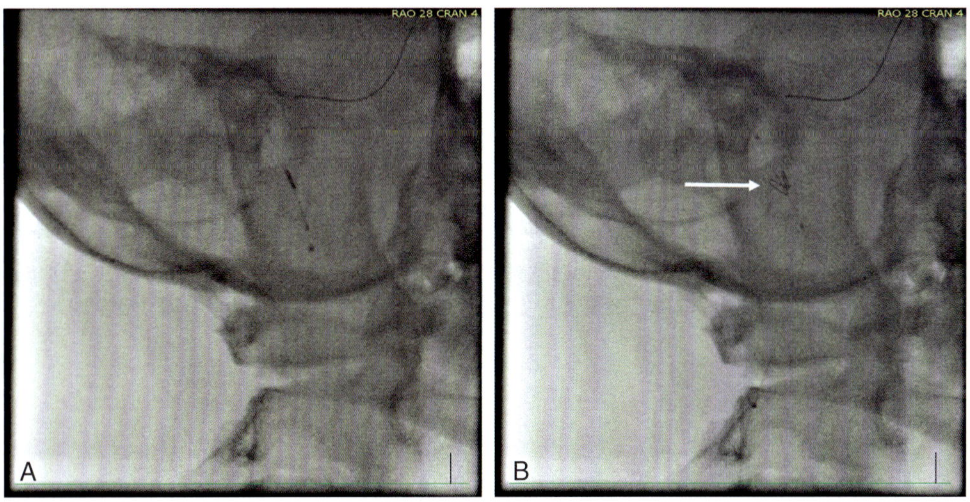

FIGURE 23.7 Positioning and deployment of distal embolic protection device. A distal embolic protection device is carefully advanced in the collapsed configuration into the distal segment of the internal carotid artery **(A)** and is subsequently deployed (**B**, arrow). An attempt should be made to deploy the filter in a segment of the internal carotid artery that is free of disease and vertical. Courtesy of Samir Kapadia and Jay S. Patel, Cleveland Clinic Non Invasive Vascular Laboratory.

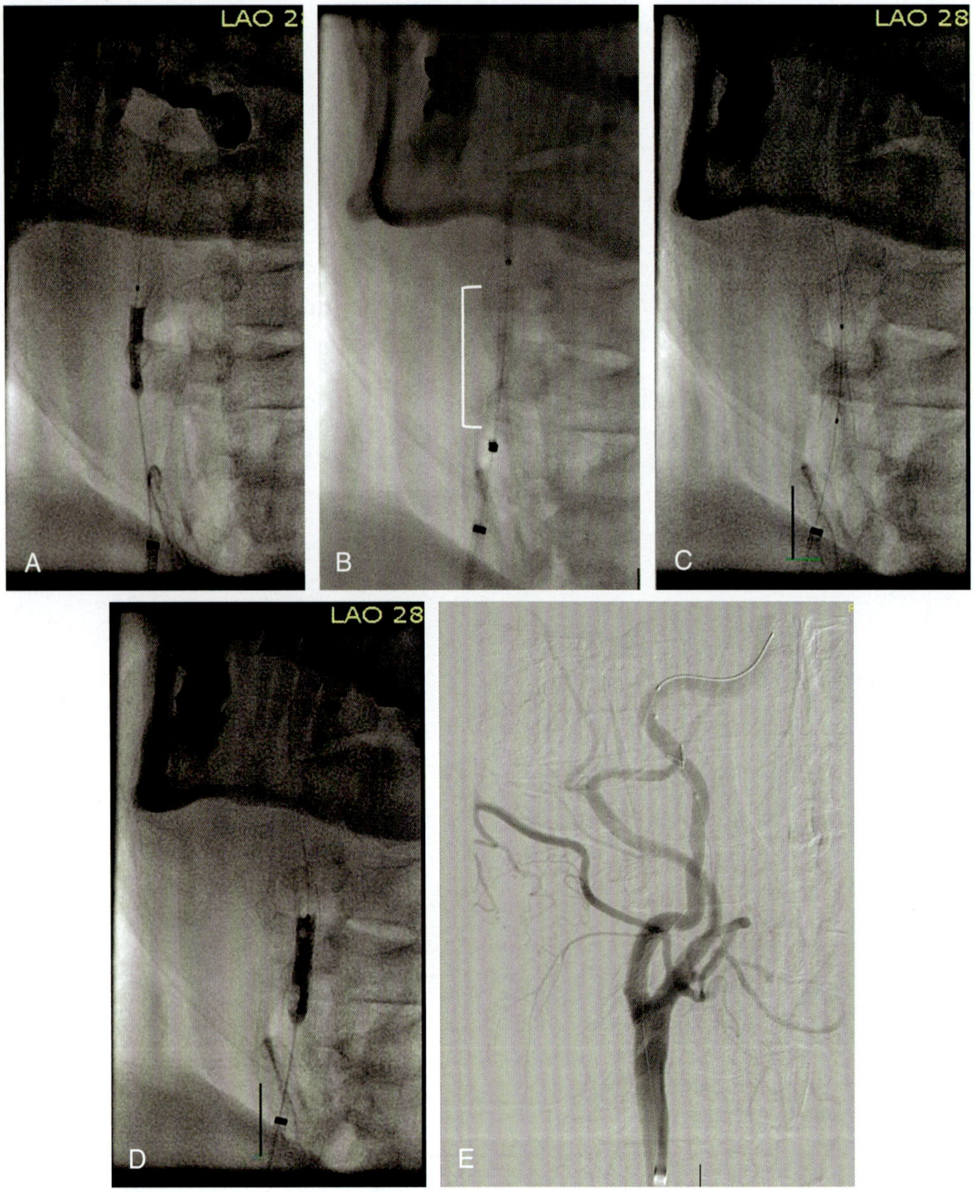

FIGURE 23.8 Carotid stenting. After deployment of the embolic protection device, the severe internal carotid artery lesion is predilated at low pressure **(A)** to facilitate passage of the stent and ensure deformation of the lesion. A self-expanding stent is then positioned using a roadmap image and slowly deployed (**B**, bracket), taking care to avoid placing the distal edge of the stent at areas of extreme tortuosity. The stent is subsequently postdilated at the lesion site at nominal pressures, taking care to avoid the stent edge **(C and D)**. Bradycardia may occur during stent deployment or balloon dilation owing to baroreceptor activation. The embolic protection device is retrieved. It is acceptable to have a residual 10%-20% stenosis, and further postdilation is not advisable **(E)**.

Subclavian Arteries

Patients with severe subclavian artery stenosis due to atherosclerosis are usually asymptomatic and often incidentally diagnosed with the finding of differential arm blood pressures on routine physical examination. Those with symptoms may experience arm claudication or ischemia, syncope/neurologic symptoms (subclavian steal syndrome), or chest pain (coronary-subclavian steal) during arm exertion. Current American College of Cardiology/American Heart Association (ACC/AHA) guidelines give a class IIa recommendation for revascularization in patients with symptomatic severe subclavian artery stenosis.[7] Revascularization should also be considered for patients before coronary bypass surgery to improve flow into the mammary arteries or to preserve axillary graft or dialysis conduits. Revascularization for asymptomatic patients carries a class III level of evidence C recommendation.[7] The choice between surgical and percutaneous revascularization depends on anatomical and lesion characteristics, surgical risk, and patient preference. However, percutaneous revascularization is associated with a high success rate and low complication rate and is typically pursued for focal or short proximal stenoses that avoid the vertebral artery.

Noninvasive Imaging

See FIGURE 23.9.

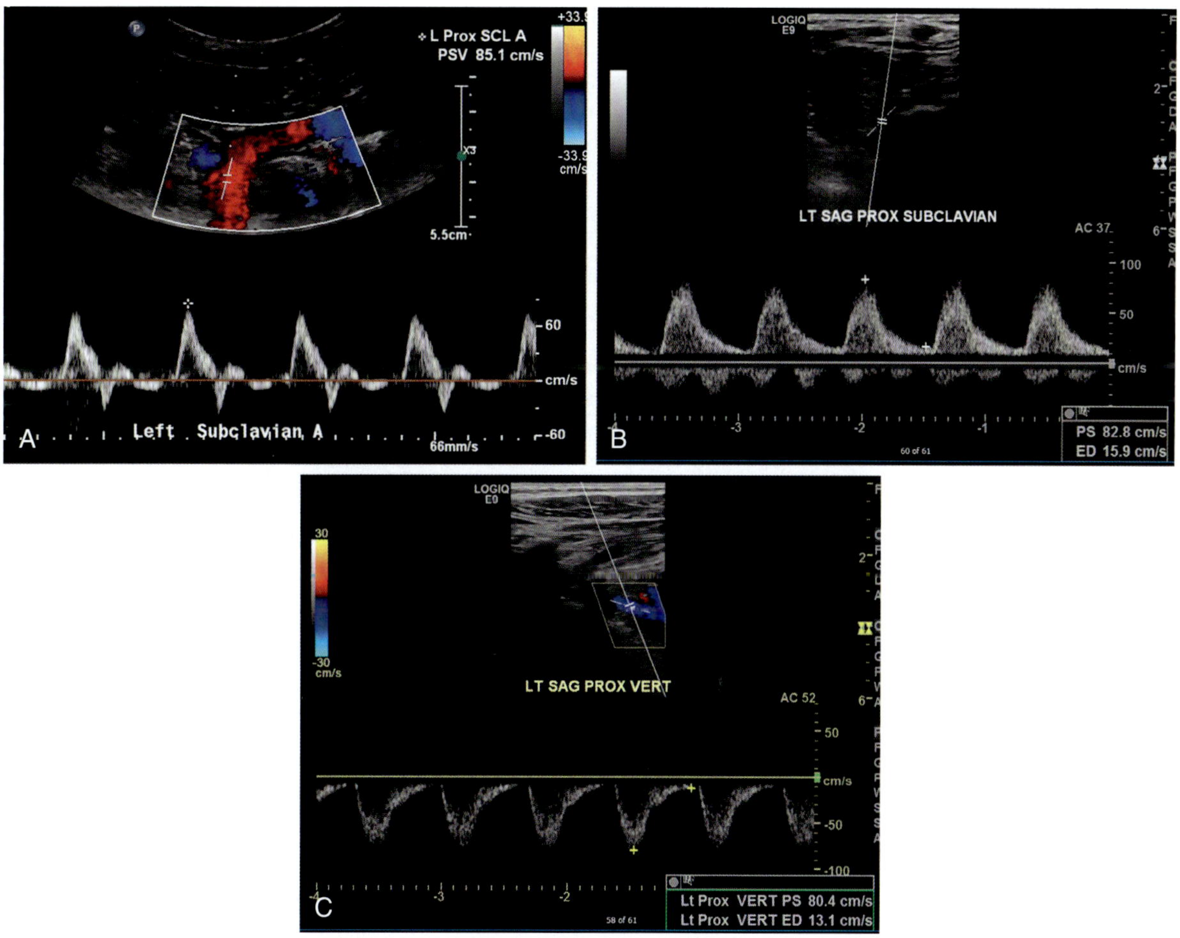

FIGURE 23.9 Abnormal subclavian arterial duplex ultrasound. **A**, Demonstrates normal triphasic waveform with brisk upstroke. Note the absence of aliasing and spectral broadening (both characteristics of turbulent flow). **B**, shows a typical poststenotic waveform with delayed upstroke (tardus-parvus) and spectral broadening. Interrogation of the ipsilateral vertebral artery **(C)** demonstrates retrograde flow, consistent with subclavian steel.

Angiographic Evaluation and Treatment

See FIGURES 23.10-23.13.

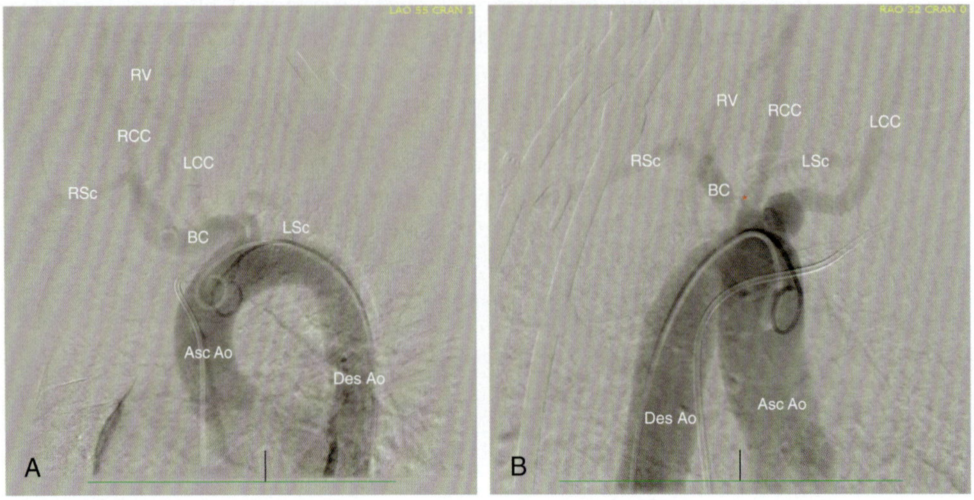

FIGURE 23.10 Arch aortography. An arch aortogram is performed in standard fashion in the LAO **(A)** and RAO **(B)** projections to create a roadmap for selective engagement of the subclavian artery and for treatment planning. Ascending aorta (Asc Ao), descending aorta (Des Ao), brachiocephalic (BC), right subclavian (RSc), right vertebral (RV), right common carotid (RCC), left common carotid (LCC), left subclavian (LSc) vessels are labeled. Note the severe stenosis at the origin of the left subclavian artery (red asterisk).

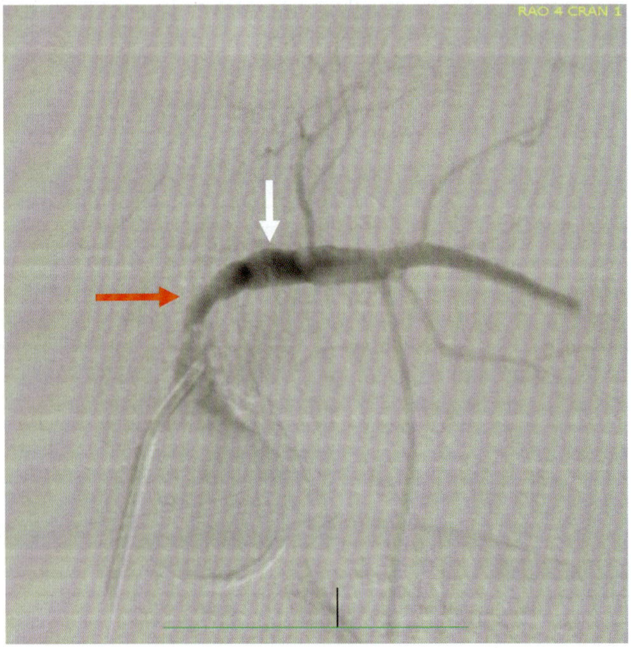

FIGURE 23.11 Selective left subclavian angiography. For nonocclusive lesions, a diagnostic catheter (typically JL4) is used to engage the ostium of the subclavian artery. Angiography is then performed, taking note of lesion severity and location with respect to the ostium of the subclavian artery and proximity to vertebral and internal mammary artery. Note the presence of a severe proximal stenosis denoted by the red arrow and the absence of the vertebral artery likely due to retrograde flow (white arrow).

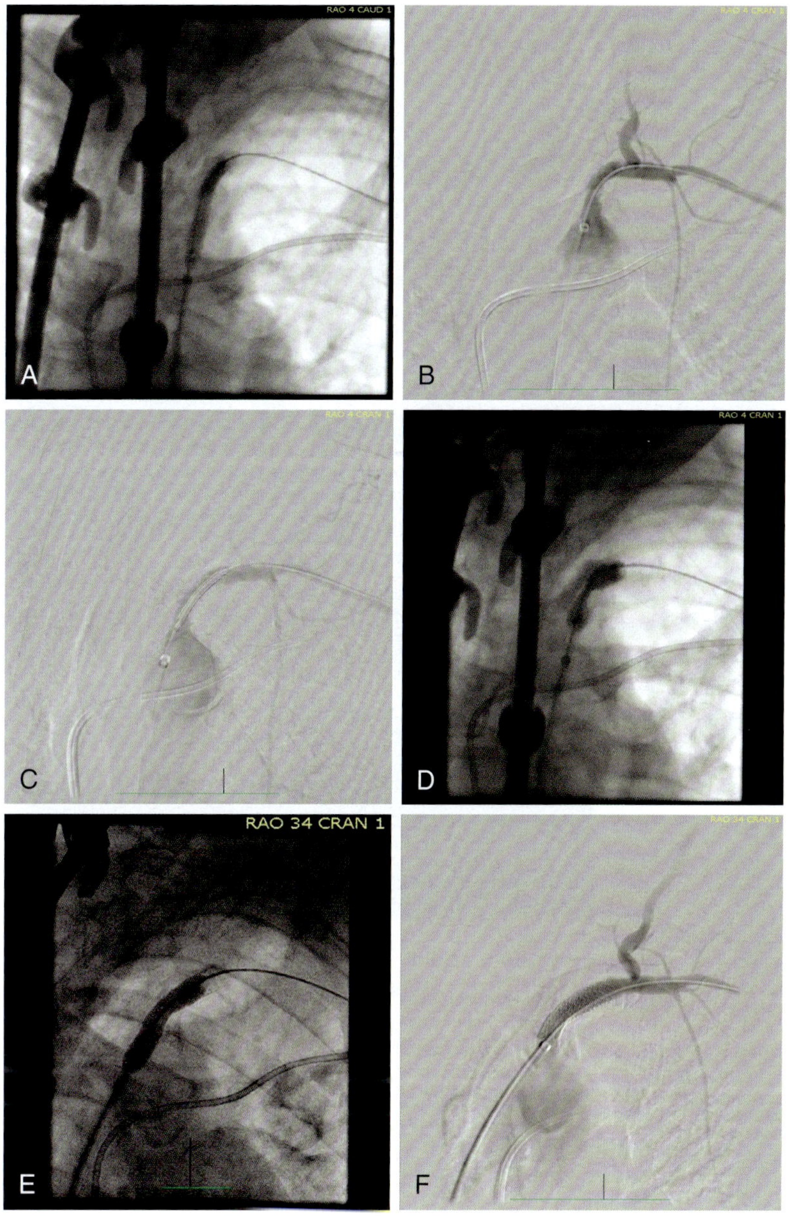

FIGURE 23.12 Left subclavian angioplasty and stenting. Intervention can be performed via the femoral approach using a 5- to 8 Fr guide. For total occlusions, a retrograde brachial artery approach may be warranted. A smaller caliber diagnostic catheter is telescoped through the guide (eg, H-1 or JR4) and the subclavian artery is subsequently engaged with the diagnostic catheter. After selective subclavian angiography, the lesion is crossed using a heavy-support coronary or 0.035-inch stiff angle glidewire or, if possible, a Wholey wire advanced into the axillary artery. The diagnostic catheter and sheath are gently advanced over the wire and positioned just proximal to the lesion. The glidewire can then be exchanged for a 0.035-inch Wholey wire if the lesion was not initially crossed with the Wholey. An undersized (typically 4-6 mm) balloon is then advanced into position, and predilation is performed to assist with sizing and ensure that the stent will expand **(A)**. Angiography is then performed to assess for dissection or perforation **(B)**, and a balloon-expandable stent is then advanced into position **(C and D)**, taking care to avoid jailing of the vertebral or internal mammary arteries. Although randomized controlled trials are lacking, stent placement appears to be associated with lower rates of restenosis.[10-13] The choice between balloon-expandable and self-expanding stents depends, in part, on lesion location, degree of calcification, and vessel anatomy. For ostial or proximal segment disease, balloon-expandable stents are preferred due to more precise positioning. Distal segment disease (past the internal mammary artery) or tortuous anatomy may be best treated with self-expanding stents. The stent is then deployed **(E)** and carefully postdilated **(F)** to match the size of the subclavian artery (usually between 5 and 8 mm). Further dilation should be avoided if the patient experiences pain.

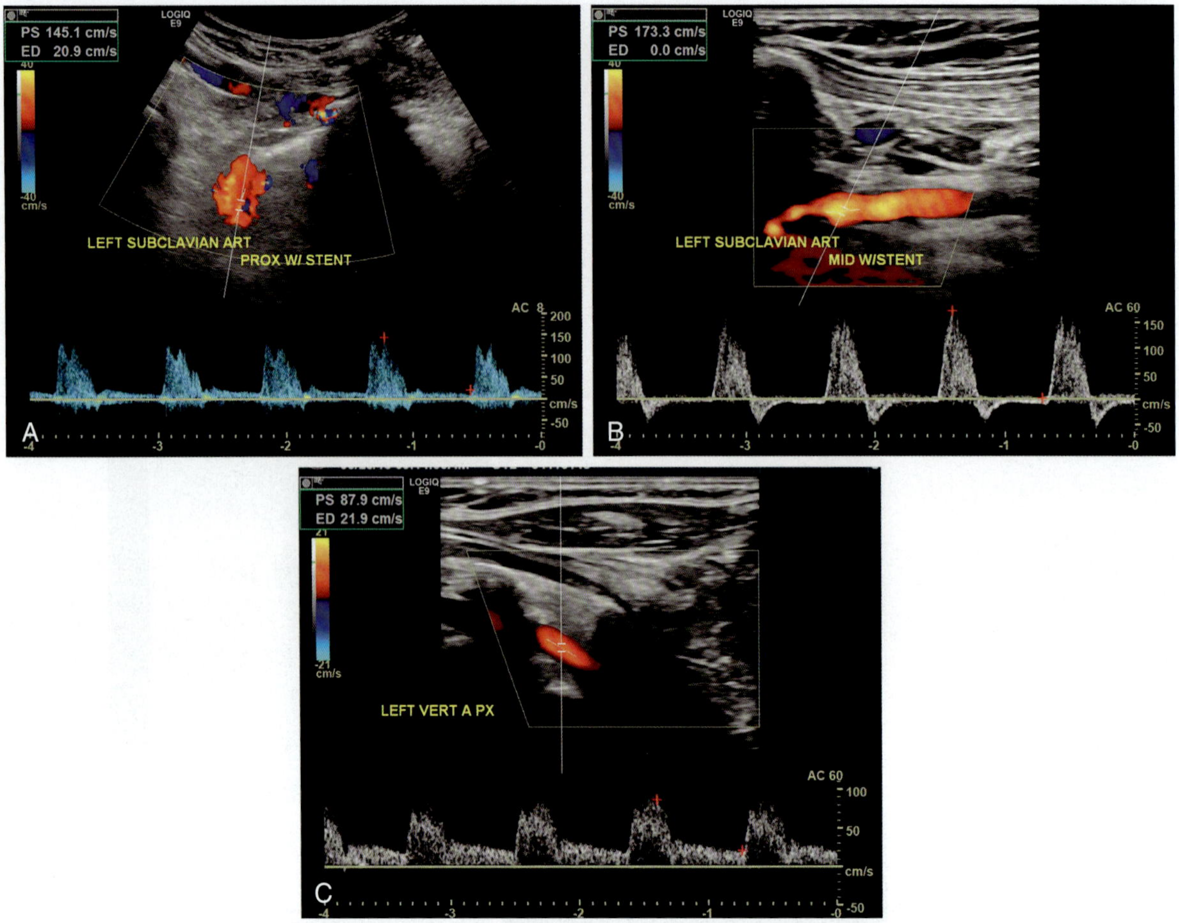

FIGURE 23.13 Postprocedure subclavian arterial duplex ultrasound. **A and B**, Demonstrate normalization of the waveform with no evidence of color aliasing. Flow in the vertebral artery is now normal and antegrade **(C)**.

Renal Arteries

Renal artery stenosis is most commonly due to atherosclerosis or fibromuscular dysplasia (FMD) and can result in treatment-resistant or malignant hypertension, recurrent flash pulmonary edema, or ischemic nephropathy. Invasive management of atherosclerotic renal artery stenosis remains somewhat controversial owing to lack of strong evidence of benefit from randomized trials. Indeed, the only class I indication for revascularization is in patients with hemodynamically significant stenosis and recurrent unexplained heart failure or pulmonary edema.[14] However, it may also be beneficial in cases of failed medical therapy with fairly recent onset hypertension or progressive renal failure secondary to suspected ischemic nephropathy. There are no randomized trials available to guide revascularization for patients with FMD; however, hypertension is markedly and durably improved with angioplasty in the majority of patients. As such, revascularization is usually recommended for FMD if anatomically feasible. A percutaneous approach is preferred, with surgery reserved only for those patients with complex anatomy (eg, concomitant periaortic disease requiring surgery, aneurysmal disease, dissection).

Noninvasive Imaging

See FIGURES 23.14 and 23.15

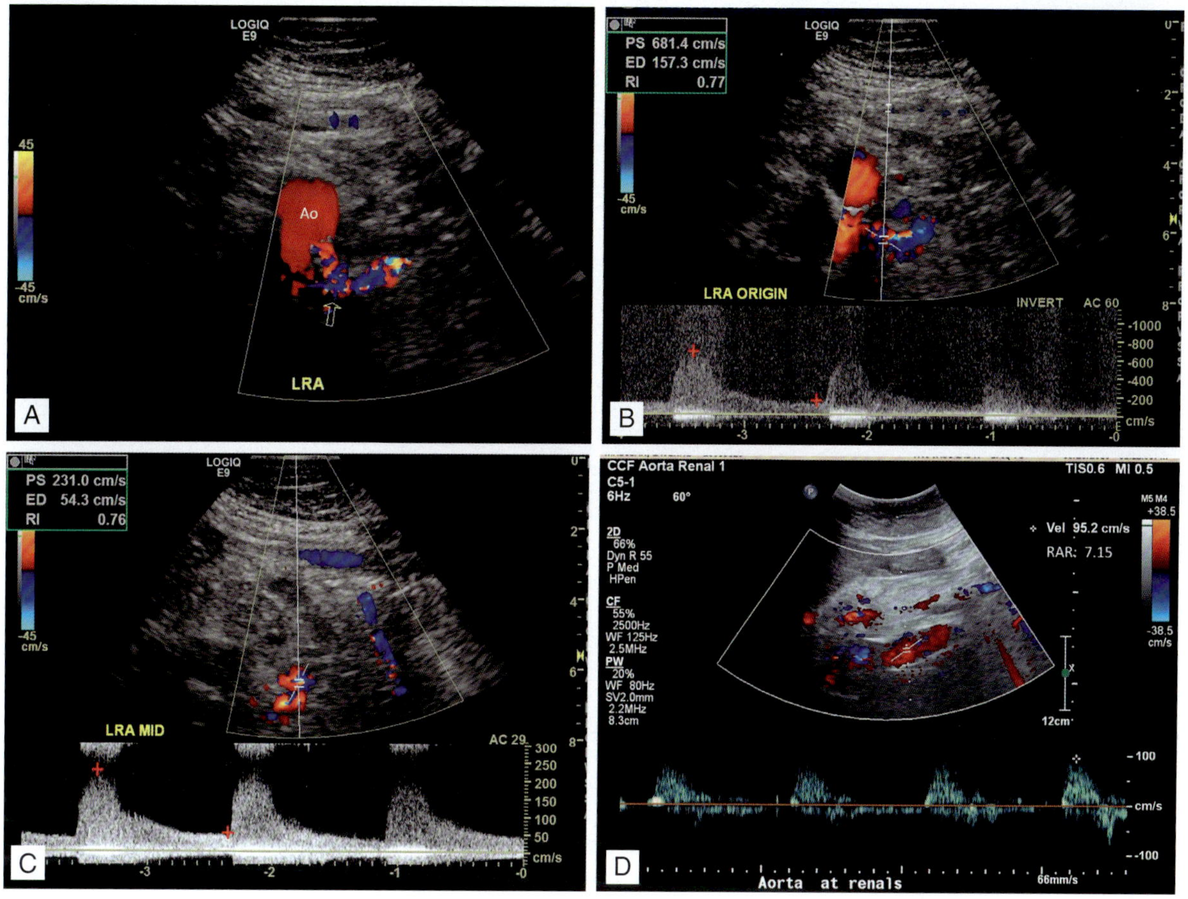

FIGURE 23.14 Abnormal renal artery duplex ultrasound in a patient with atherosclerotic renal artery stenosis. Renal artery duplex ultrasound is relatively inexpensive and provides both anatomical and functional information.[15] **A,** Demonstrates laminar flow within the Ao at the level of the left renal artery (LRA). Color aliasing is noted at the proximal segment of the LRA and is suggestive of nonlaminar blood flow. Peak-systolic and end-diastolic flow velocities at the origin of the LRA are markedly elevated and consistent with a severe stenosis **(B)**. Note the parvus-tardus waveform along with spectral broadening and turbulence in **(C)**. The renal aortic ratio **(D)** can be calculated by comparing the peak systolic velocity of the renal artery to the Ao. Values >3.5 are considered to be consistent with severe stenosis. The resistive index **(B and C)** can also be calculated and may be a useful prognostic tool.[16,17]

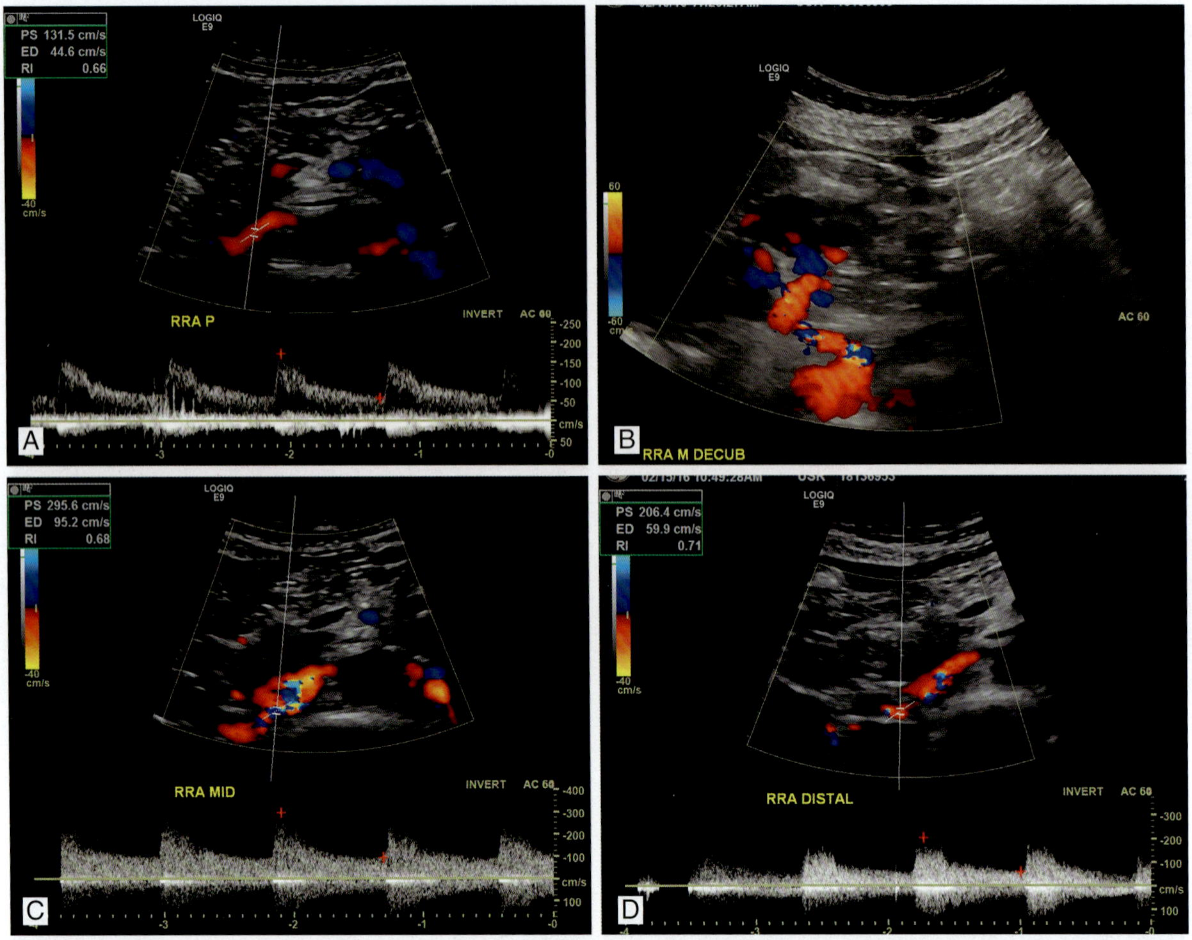

FIGURE 23.15 Abnormal renal artery duplex ultrasound in a patient with renal artery stenosis due to FMD. Unlike atherosclerotic disease, FMD typically involves the mid to distal segments of the renal arteries. **A**, Demonstrates normal peak-systolic velocity and waveform at the proximal segment of the right renal artery (RRA), and inspection of color Doppler reveals laminar flow without evidence of color aliasing. However, color Doppler assessment at the mid segment **(B)** reveals multiple areas of aliasing suggestive of turbulent flow and possible stenosis. This is corroborated by markedly elevated peak-systolic velocities recorded at the mid and distal segments **(C and D)** along with spectral broadening of the Doppler waveform.

Angiographic Evaluation and Treatment

See **FIGURES 23.16-23.18.**

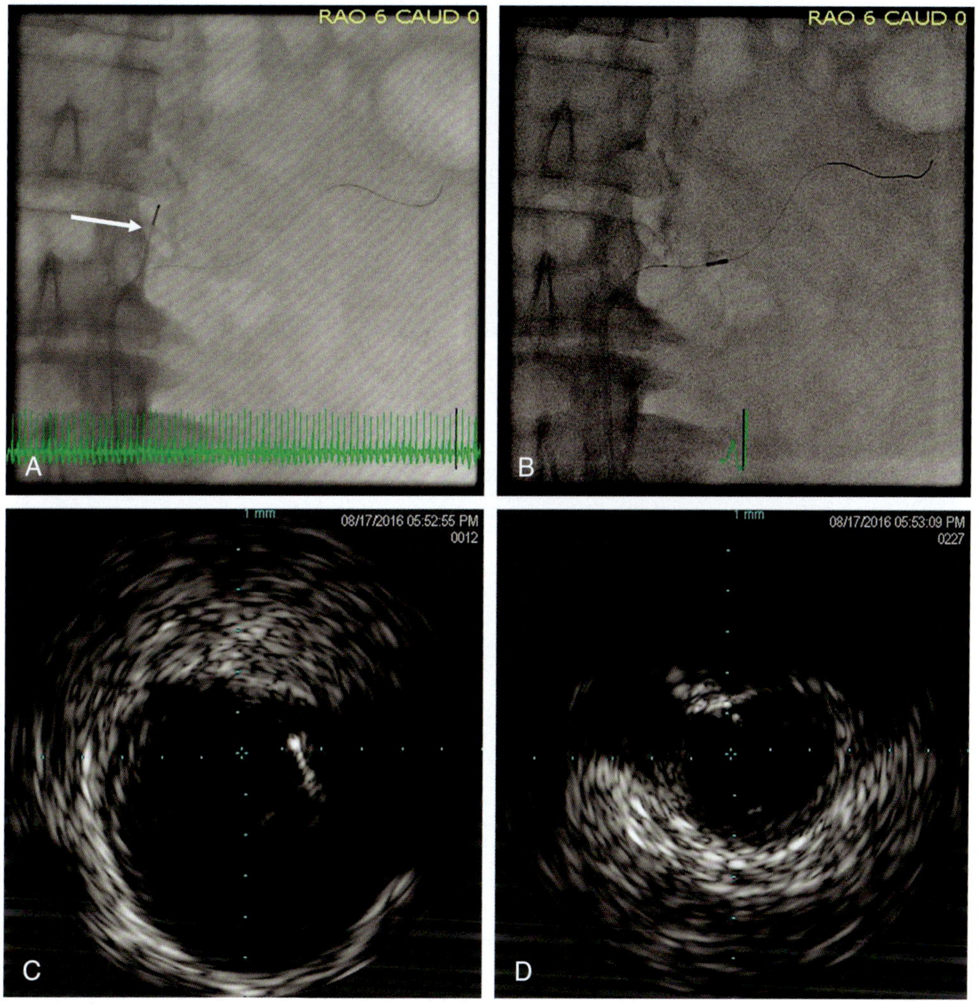

FIGURE 23.16 Invasive renal artery assessment. We routinely perform renal angiography and intervention using the "no-touch" technique to minimize contrast use and reduce aortic wall trauma.[18] A 0.035-inch wire (**A**, white arrow) is first placed well above the renal arteries in the Ao and the guide catheter is then advanced over the wire to the L1-2 vertebral body level. While the 0.035-inch wire is still in place, the renal artery is wired using a 0.014-inch guide wire or fractional flow reserve (FFR) wire. The artery is subsequently engaged by retracting the 0.035-inch wire into the guide and advancing the guide over the 0.014-inch guide wire. Selective renal angiography can then be performed with 3 mL of contrast mixed with 3-4 mL of heparinized saline flush under digital subtraction angiography. Intravascular ultrasound (IVUS) **(B)** is then used to assess reference vessel size **(C)**, plaque characteristics, and lesion severity and identify the true ostium. Once the true ostium is identified on IVUS **(D)**, a fluoroscopic image is obtained to mark the ostium and guide stent placement. FFR assessment using a 0.014-inch pressure wire should be performed if there is a question of hemodynamic significance for stenoses between 50%-70% severity. A resting mean pressure gradient >10 mm Hg, systolic hyperemic pressure gradient >20 mm Hg, or Pd/Pa ≤0.80 is considered to be flow limiting.[19,20] Intrarenal dopamine (*not* adenosine) or papaverine can be used to induce maximal hyperemia.

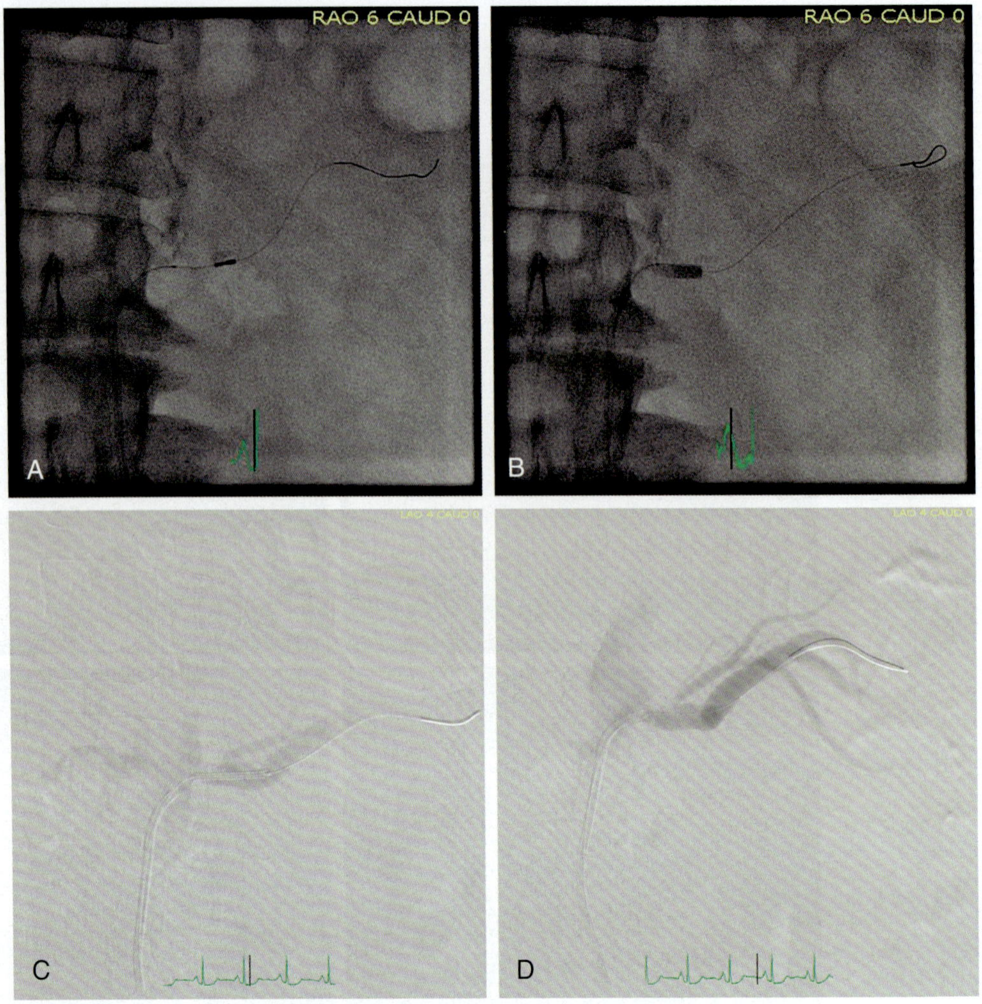

FIGURE 23.17 Renal artery stent positioning and deployment. Several studies have shown lower restenosis rates associated with stenting compared with angioplasty alone, and current ACC/AHA guidelines recommend stent placement if revascularization is performed for atherosclerotic renal artery stenosis.[21-25] We routinely use IVUS to assess plaque characteristics and vessel size and identify the true ostium **(A)** as under-sizing or over-sizing leads to suboptimal results.[26] A reference fluoroscopic image marking the true ostium is created and used to optimally position the stent. Careful predilation is performed using an undersized balloon if there is concern that the lesion will not expand during stent placement **(B)**. An appropriately sized stent is then advanced into position (with about 1-2 mm extension into the Ao) using the reference image and deployed **(C)**. We then perform angiography and IVUS to assess for edge dissection and malapposition. **D**, Shows final angiographic result after stent deployment.

Mesenteric Arteries

The most common cause of mesenteric artery stenosis is atherosclerosis, but other causes should be considered including median arcuate ligament compression, FMD, vasculitis, or dissection. Owing to the extensive collateral network of the mesenteric arterial system, severe stenosis in 1 artery rarely results in symptoms. Occasionally, patients can present with postprandial abdominal pain (intestinal angina), especially after a fatty meal, that tends to resolve over several hours. If left untreated, the patient may experience significant weight loss or develop intestinal infarction. Percutaneous angioplasty with stent placement is the preferred method of revascularization in severely symptomatic patients, and the superior mesenteric artery (SMA) is often targeted for treatment.[27]

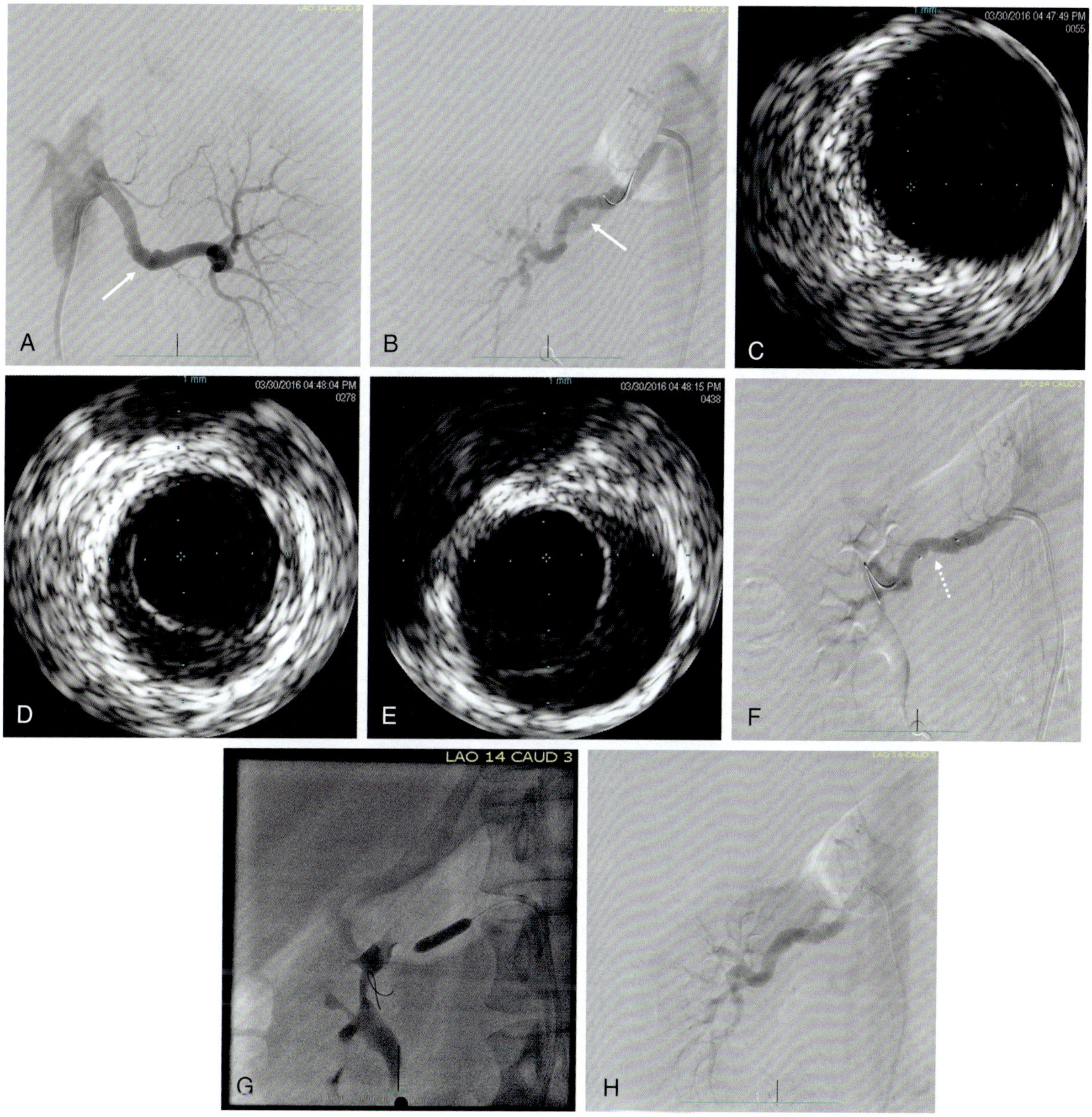

FIGURE 23.18 FMD. Typical "string of beads" finding on renal angiography (**A and B,** white arrowhead). Note that the ostial and proximal segments of the artery are spared, which is characteristic in FMD. We routinely use IVUS preintervention to assess reference vessel size **(C)**, visualize coexisting plaque burden, and identify the segment(s) with most severe stenosis. **D and E**, Demonstrate significant fibrous bands that are seen in FMD. In cases where it is unclear which renal artery requires intervention, we perform FFR assessment with the caveat that a false-negative result may be obtained if the webs are easily compressible by the FFR wire. In this case, mean resting pressure gradient in the LRA was 2 mm Hg, while gradient in the RRA was 20 mm Hg. Balloon angioplasty was subsequently performed on the RRA at the segment with the most severe narrowing identified by IVUS (**F and G**; arrowhead). We often perform FFR and IVUS assessment after angioplasty to document adequate treatment in cases where angiography is ambiguous or residual stenosis >30% suspected **(H)**. Postangioplasty FFR assessment, in this case, demonstrated a residual gradient of >15 mm Hg. After repeat angioplasty, the residual gradient was <6 mm Hg. Note that stenting is reserved for failure or complications resulting from balloon angioplasty.

Noninvasive Imaging

See **FIGURES 23.19** and **23.20**.

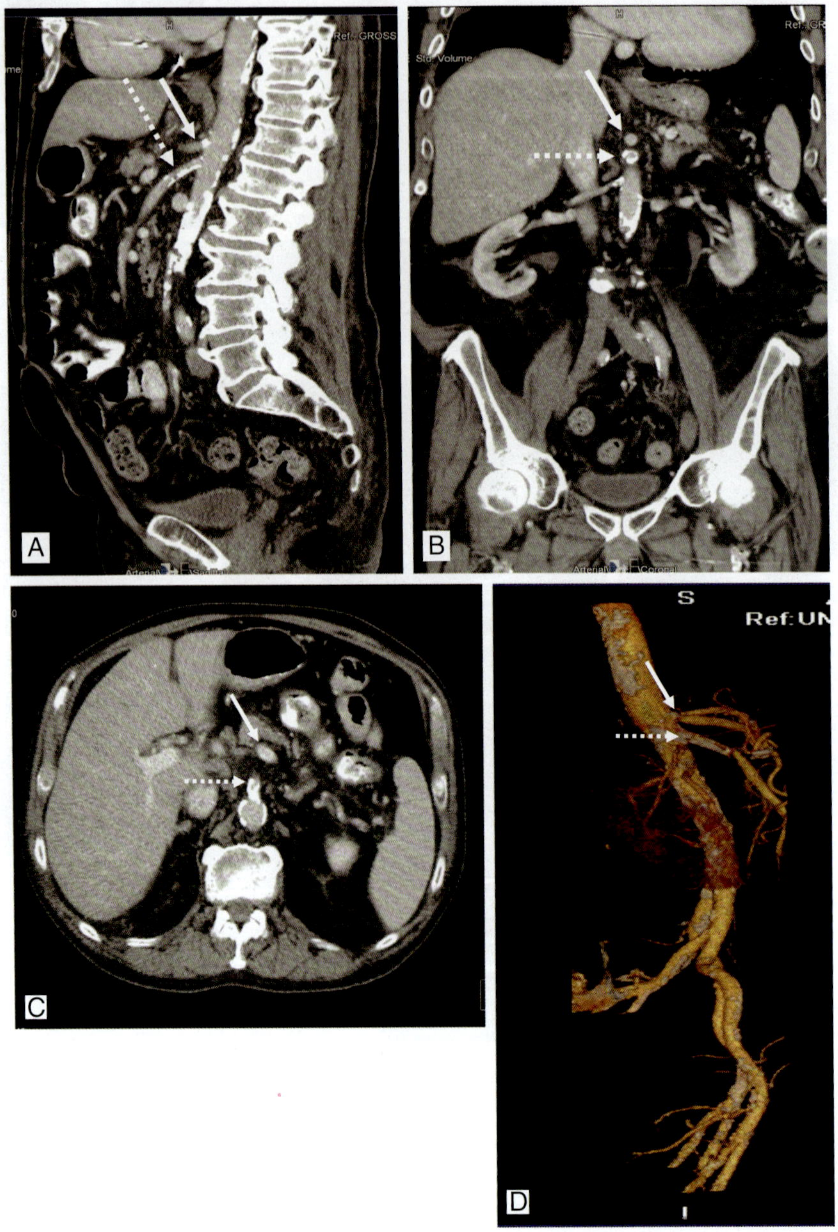

FIGURE 23.19 CT of the abdominal Ao. CT is often the initial diagnostic test performed in patients with suspected mesenteric ischemia, as it can simultaneously assess disease in multiple branch vessels and the degree of collateralization and highlight additional abdominal pathology that could be related to symptomatology (eg, malignancy). Sagittal slice of the abdominal Ao at the level of the celiac artery (CA, solid arrow) and SMA (dashed arrow) are presented in **(A)**. There is extensive calcification and severe narrowing of the Ao and ostium of both the CA and SMA. Coronal and axial slices **(B and C)** demonstrate severe calcification and narrowing extending into the proximal segment of the SMA. Reconstruction of the abdominal aorta showing the CA (solid arrow) and SMA (dashed arrow) **(D)**.

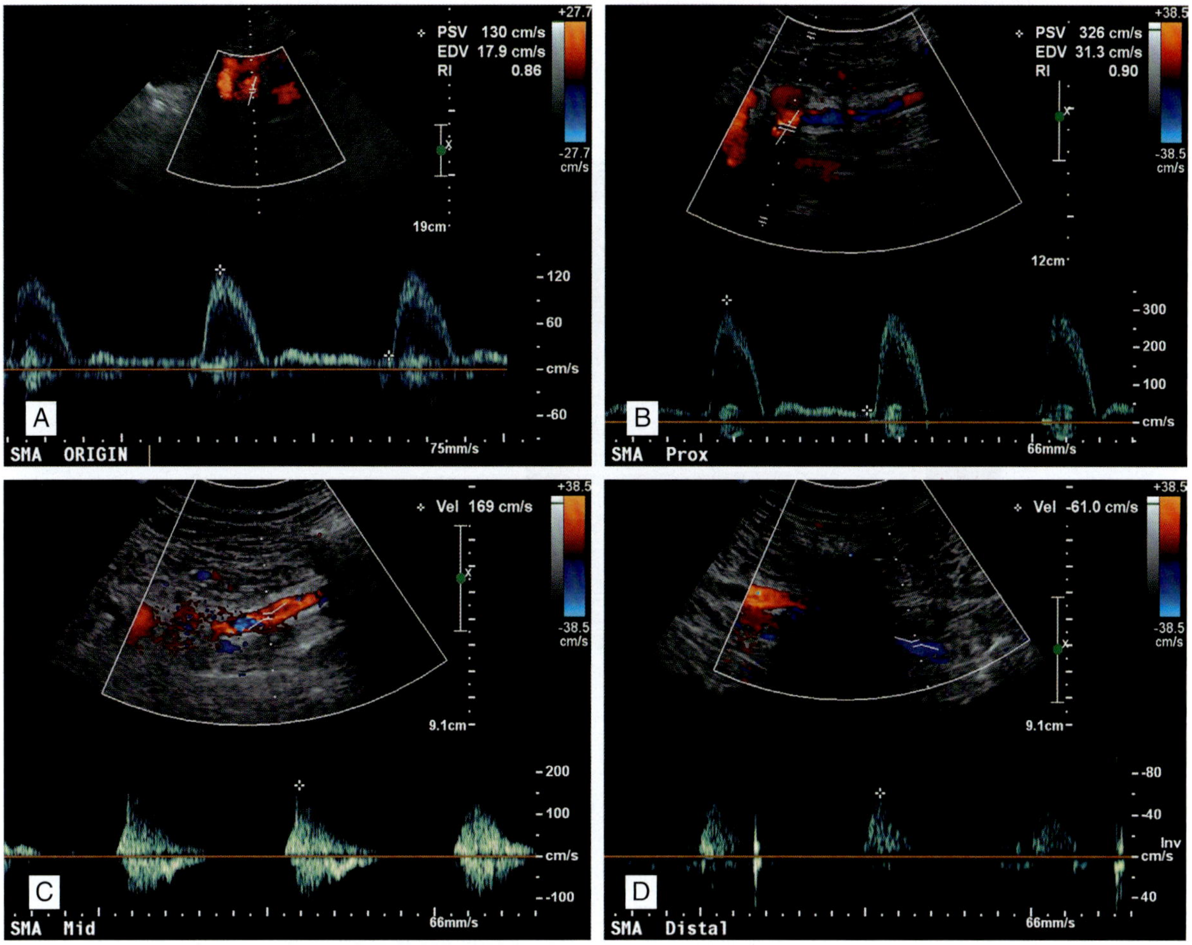

FIGURE 23.20 Abnormal mesenteric arterial duplex ultrasound. Arterial duplex ultrasound is relatively inexpensive, avoids intravenous contrast, can identify collateralization, and has high sensitivity (>90%) and negative predictive value (>99%). In **(A)**, Doppler interrogation at the origin of the SMA reveals laminar flow with normal peak-systolic velocity. Interrogation at the proximal segment, however, reveals a significant step-up in peak-systolic velocity to >275 cm/s and is suggestive of high-grade (≥70%) stenosis **(B)**. The Doppler waveforms at the mid and distal segments **(C and D)** have a typical poststenotic parvus-tardus pattern with evidence of turbulent flow (spectral broadening and color aliasing).

Angiographic Evaluation and Treatment

See **FIGURES 23.21** and **23.22**.

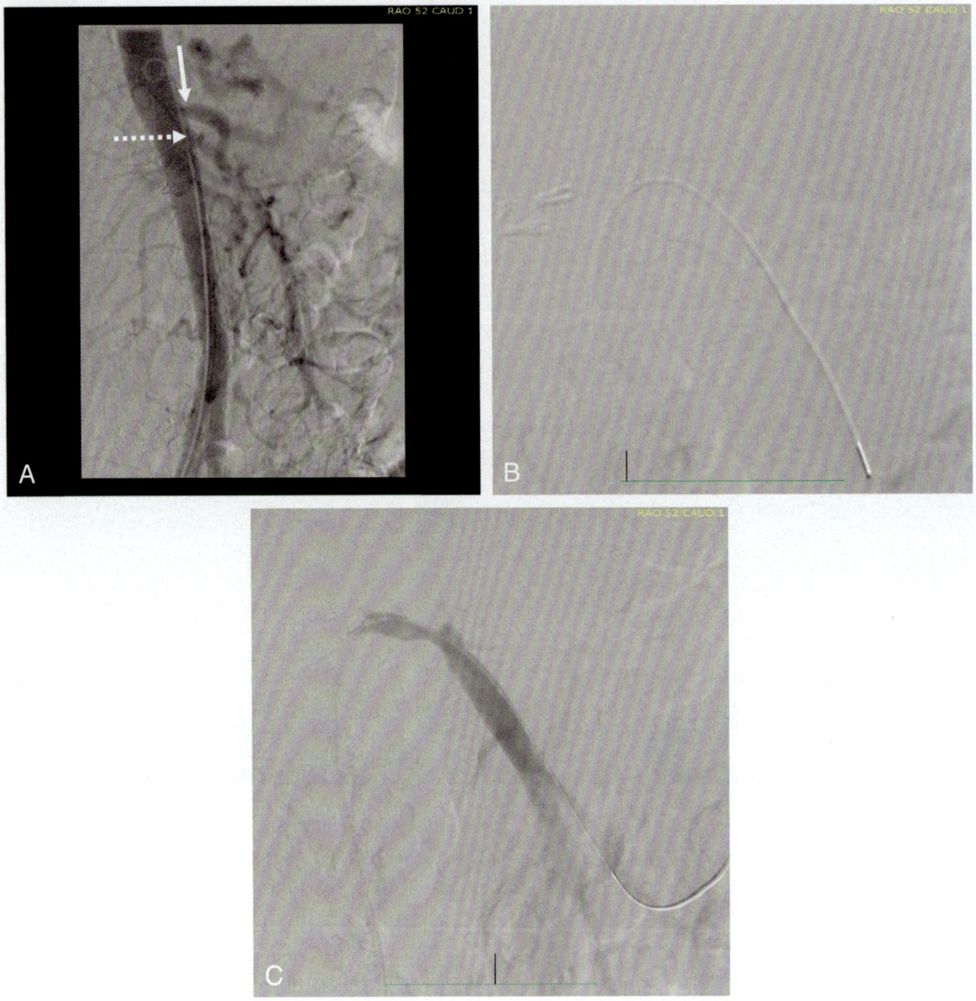

FIGURE 23.21 Selective SMA angiography. Mesenteric artery angiography and intervention should ideally be performed from the radial or brachial arteries owing to their anterior and inferior takeoff. With the arms positioned above the patient's head, a pig-tail catheter is placed just proximal to the L1 vertebral body, and abdominal aortography is performed in a steep oblique or lateral projection **(A)**. This image can serve as a reference for selective intubation of the mesenteric vessel of interest. The CA (solid arrows) has a moderate ostial narrowing, and the SMA (dashed arrow) has disease that is difficult to determine on this nonselective injection. The SMA can then be carefully wired with an atraumatic 0.035-inch Wholey wire using the roadmap image created earlier **(B)**. A JR4 guide catheter is then slowly advanced over the wire into the ostium of the SMA, and selective angiography can be performed **(C)**. The Wholey wire can be exchanged for a 0.014-inch coronary guide wire to facilitate further assessment with IVUS or intervention.

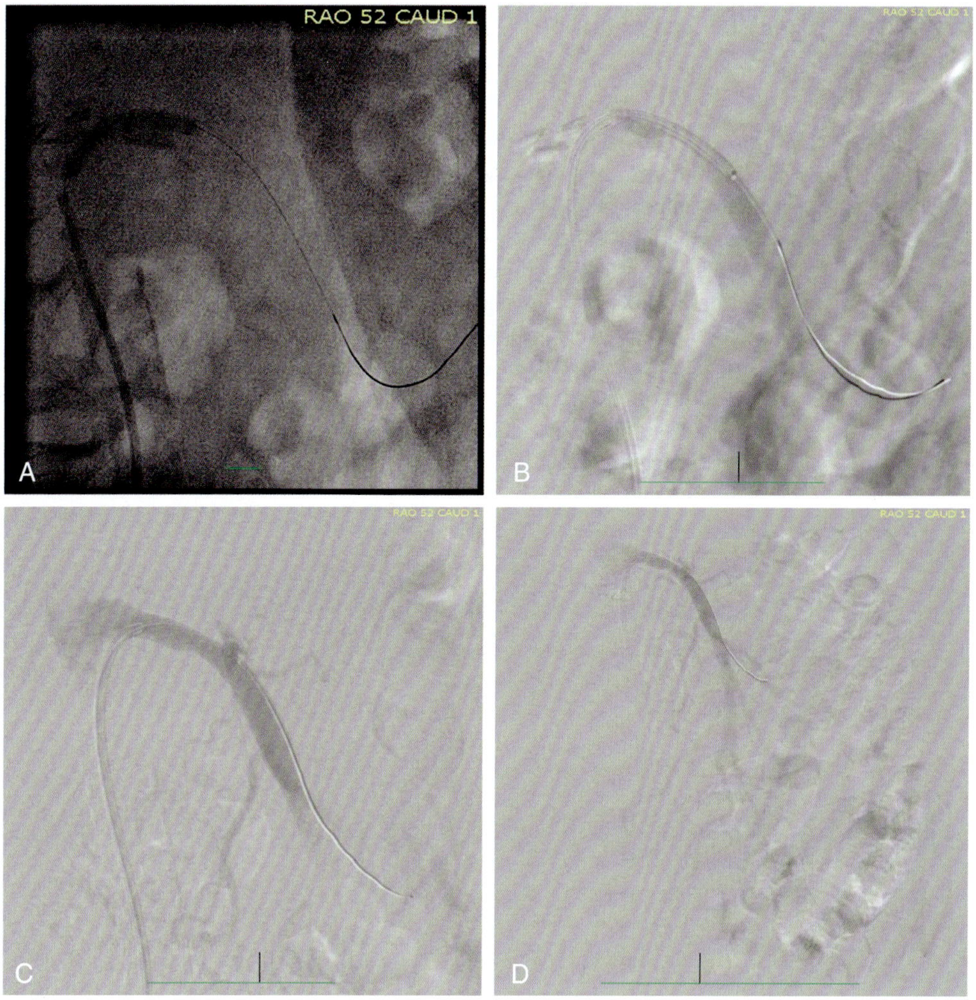

FIGURE 23.22 Antegrade SMA intervention. Owing to a lower observed restenosis rate, stenting is preferred over angioplasty alone when feasible.[28-31] After administering heparin to a therapeutic ACT of 250-300 s, the SMA is wired using a 0.014-inch coronary guide wire. We routinely perform predilation to assess the adequacy of lesion expansion before stent placement **(A)**. A balloon-expandable stent is then advanced into the appropriate position using fluoroscopic guidance with or without IVUS **(B)**. While a balloon-expandable stent placement is preferable at the aorto-ostial location owing to superior radial strength, a self-expanding stent may be more appropriate at the mid to distal segments owing to the curvature of the artery. Mesenteric artery stenoses commonly involve the aorto-ostium, and IVUS can be very helpful in the identifying the true ostium and with precise stent positioning. After deploying the stent, angiography with or without IVUS is performed to assess for residual stenosis, edge dissection, thrombosis, and other complications **(C and D)**.

NORMAL LOWER EXTREMITY ARTERIAL ANATOMY (FIGURE 23.23)

Aortoiliac Occlusive Disease

Patients with aortoiliac occlusive disease often present with limb claudication in the distribution of the hip, buttock, or thigh muscles, rest pain, or even critical limb ischemia with development of ischemic ulcers or gangrene. Men can experience erectile dysfunction. Although medical management plus a supervised exercise program should be prescribed for all patients, revascularization is warranted for those with lifestyle-limiting symptoms, rest pain, distal embolization, nonhealing wounds, or those that require access to more proximal vascular beds for other procedures.[14,32-34] Given lower risk and good patency rates, endovascular therapy is generally preferred over surgical revascularization in most cases as long as there is a reasonable landing zone for a stent without compromise of the renal arteries.[35-40] In most cases, endovascular therapy does not preclude later surgical revascularization. Surgical revascularization is preferred when the renal arteries or suprarenal aorta (Ao) is involved.

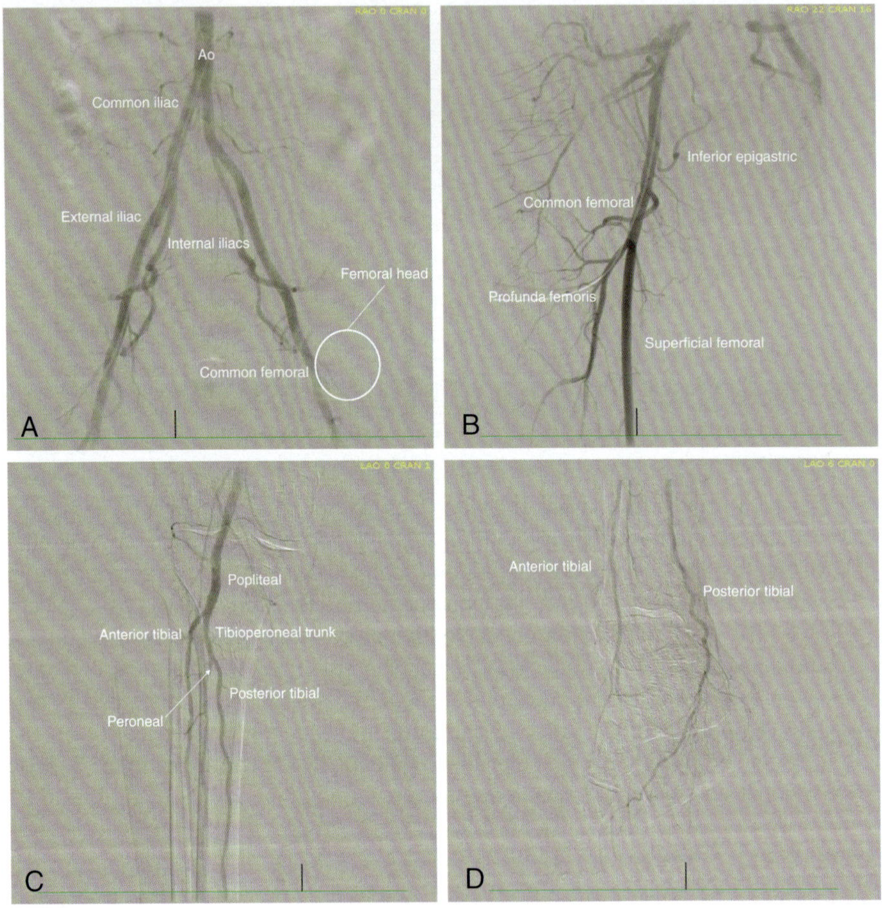

FIGURE 23.23 Normal lower extremity arterial angiogram with runoff. **A**, Demonstrates distal Ao and common iliac, external iliac, and internal iliac arteries. Important branches off the external iliac artery are the inferior epigastric, superficial, and deep circumflex iliac arteries. Below the inguinal ligament, the external iliac becomes the common femoral artery **(B)**, which bifurcates into the superficial and profunda femoris arteries. The superficial femoral artery continues on to become the popliteal artery at the level of the knee **(C)** and typically trifurcates into the anterior tibialis, posterior tibialis, and peroneal arteries. The anterior tibial artery supplies the anterior compartment of the leg and continues on to form the dorsal pedis artery **(D)**. The posterior tibial artery supplies the posterior compartment of the leg and continues on to supply lateral and plantar aspect of the foot.

Noninvasive Imaging

See **FIGURES 23.24** and **23.25**.

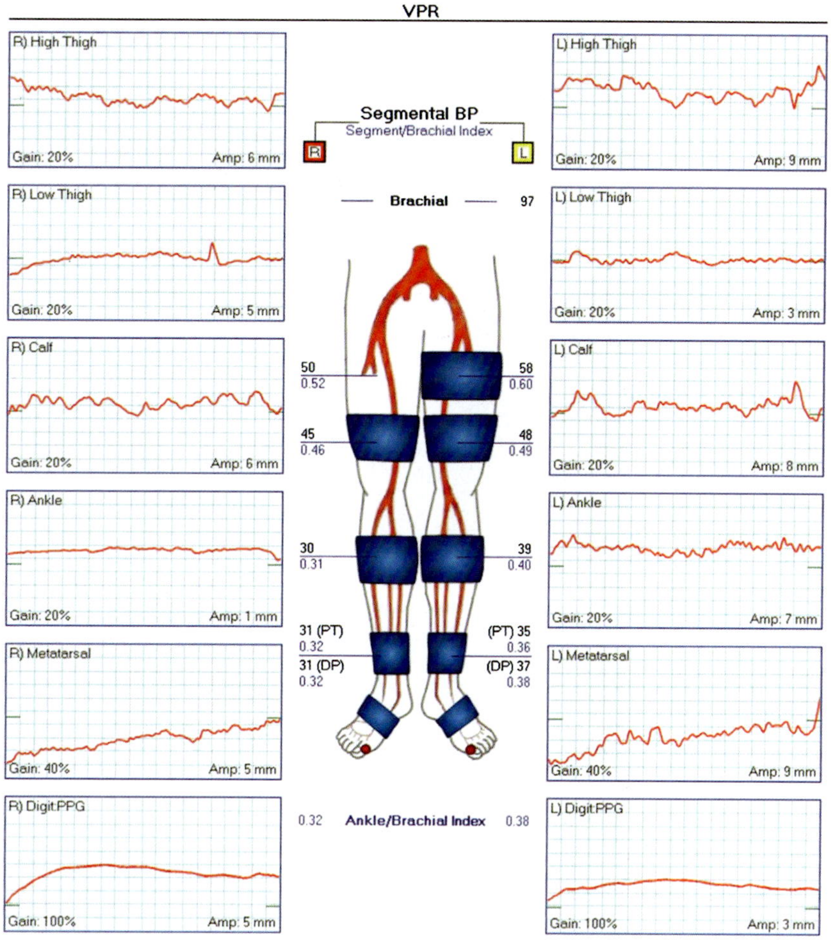

Segmental BP

Right		Index	Left		Index
Brachial:			**Brachial:**	97	
High Thigh:	50	0.52	**High Thigh:**	58	0.60
Low Thigh:	45	0.46	**Low Thigh:**	48	0.49
Calf:	30	0.31	**Calf:**	39	0.40
Ankle (PT):	31	0.32	**Ankle (PT):**	35	0.36
Ankle (DP):	31	0.32	**Ankle (DP):**	37	0.38

FIGURE 23.24 Ankle-brachial index, segmental limb pressures, and pulse volume recording waveforms. Ankle-brachial index with or without exercise is highly accurate, relatively inexpensive, noninvasive, and generally considered the initial test of choice in patients with suspected peripheral arterial disease.[32] Angiography or further imaging is typically not required until revascularization is contemplated. The level of disease can be ascertained by inspecting segmental limb pressure measurements and pulse volume recording waveforms. The center column demonstrates severe bilateral peripheral arterial disease as evident by the markedly abnormal ABI in both limbs (<0.4). In general, high thigh pressures should exceed brachial artery pressure by at least 20 mm Hg. In this case, the high thigh-brachial index is <1.0 and consistent with significant aortoiliac or bilateral iliofemoral disease. Pulse volume recording waveforms complement segmental pressure data and are consistent with aortoiliac or bilateral iliofemoral disease. There is no significant (ie, >20 mm Hg) pressure gradient between adjacent segments within the same leg. Adapted from the Cleveland Clinic Non Invasive Vascular Laboratory.

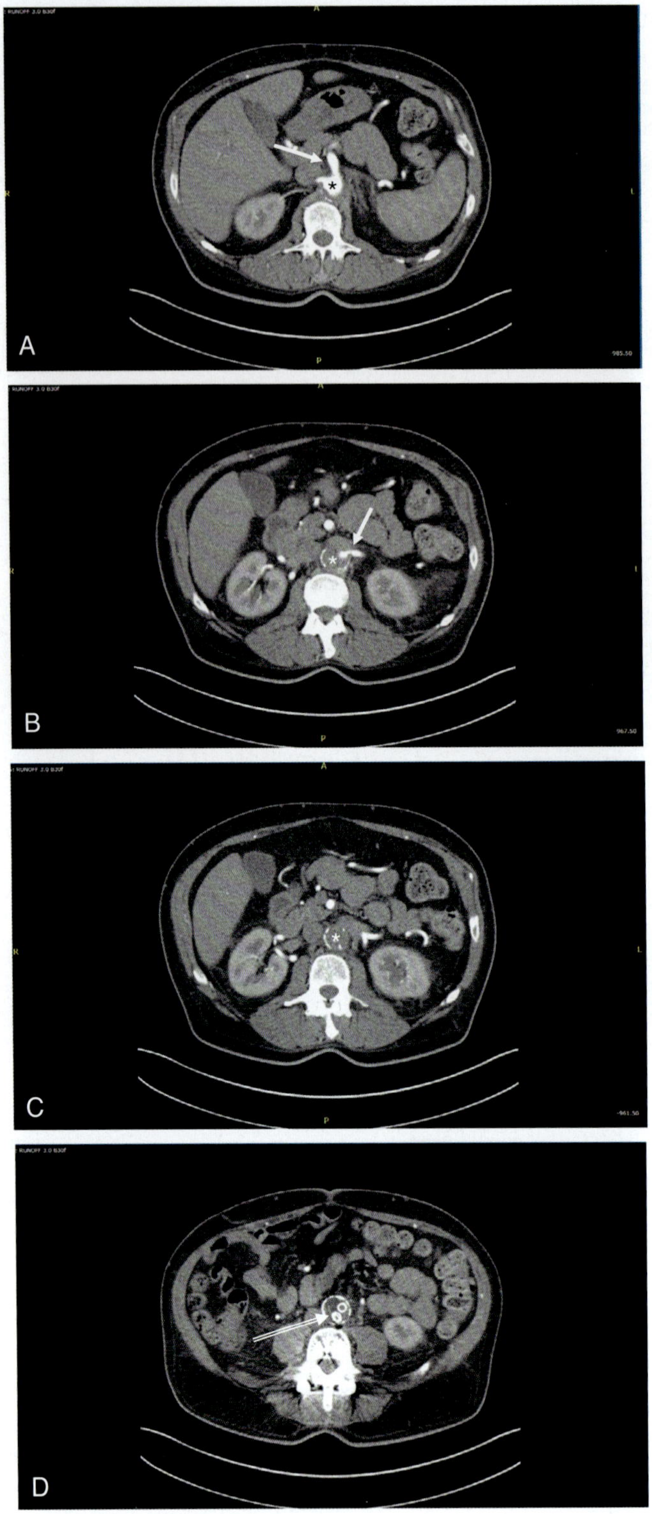

FIGURE 23.25 CTA of the abdominal Ao with bilateral iliofemoral runoff. CT can noninvasively provide a detailed anatomic roadmap that may be used for planning treatment. The abdominal Ao (asterisk) is patent but severely diseased with plaque and calcium at the takeoff of the mesenteric (solid arrow) and RRAs **(A)**. The Ao (asterisk) is completely occluded at the takeoff of the LRA (arrow; **B and C**). The patient has a history of aorto-bi-iliac stent placement which are also occluded (double line arrow, **D**) and plans were for bilateral axillary-femoral artery bypass; however, the patient was deemed to be a poor surgical candidate due to severe heart failure and endovascular therapy was pursued.

Angiographic Evaluation and Treatment

See FIGURE 23.26.

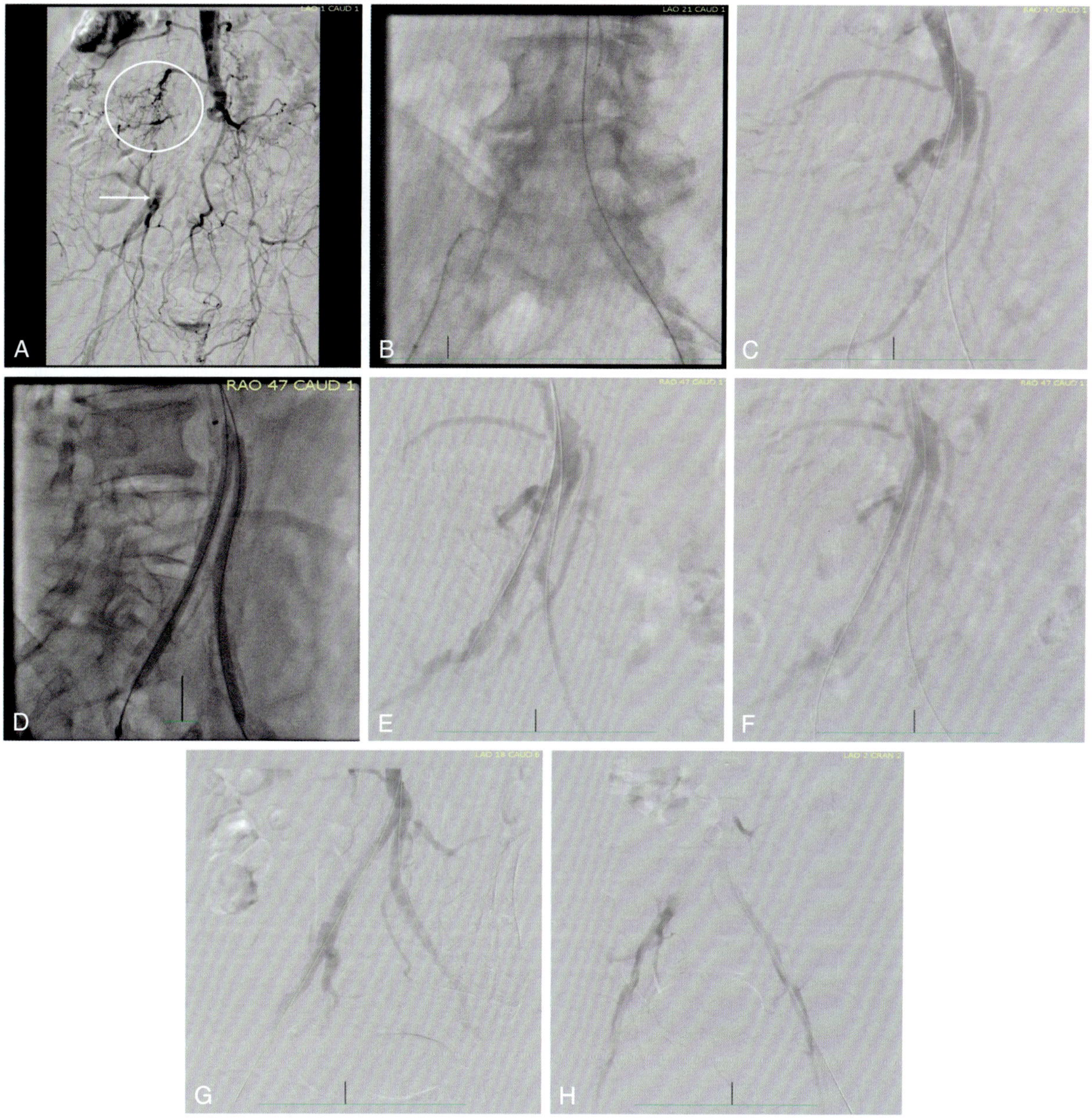

FIGURE 23.26 Reconstruction of distal Ao and bilateral iliac system. For occlusive disease, we access the ipsilateral common femoral and the left brachial arteries. In the case presented, both common femoral arteries were accessed to facilitate bilateral intervention. A 0.035-inch Wholey guide wire is advanced from the left brachial artery to the distal descending Ao, and a pig-tail catheter is then advanced over the wire to the level of the renal arteries. Aortography is performed and shows complete occlusion of the distal Ao and both common iliac arteries **(A)**. There is extensive collateral formation (circle) with reconstitution of the distal right common iliac (arrow) and left common femoral arteries. Retrograde recanalization via the left and right common femoral arteries is then carefully performed with a 0.035-inch stiff angle glidewire with a support catheter **(B)**. We attempt to stay intraluminal while traversing the lesion; however, the glidewire may enter the subintimal space. If this occurs, a subintimal approach is appropriate but the true lumen must be entered as soon as the lesion is completely traversed. Re-entry should be above the common femoral artery to prevent jailing of the profunda femoral artery. Luminal entry should be confirmed by aspiration of blood and angiography. The glidewire is then exchanged for a 0.035-inch Wholey wire, and the aortoiliac bifurcation and iliac arteries are predilated **(C and D)**. Stents are positioned and deployed simultaneously (**E and F**). Compared with angioplasty, stenting is associated with higher success and patency rates and lower complication rates.[41,42] Balloon-expanding stents are typically used for the common iliac artery while self-expanding stents are preferred for the external iliac artery.[43] For Trans-Atlantic Inter-Society Consensus (TASC) C and D lesions, there is evidence of superiority of covered stents over self-expanding stents.[44] Postdilation is performed to optimize stent apposition, and final angiography is performed (**G and H**).

Superficial Femoral and Popliteal Arteries

Superficial femoral and popliteal segment disease is notoriously challenging to treat with endovascular techniques owing to the mechanical stress and deformations created by knee flexion and ambulation. Such forces, in addition to lesion characteristics, are felt to be the cause of higher rates of stent fracture and restenosis compared with other arterial segments.[45] Revascularization is thus best reserved for patients with disabling claudication or ischemic wounds.[32,34] Percutaneous revascularization is often the preferred initial approach in the current era, even for long chronic total occlusions, as success rates are high and surgical bypass is still possible if restenosis occurs. Options include primary angioplasty with drug-coated balloon (with or without atherectomy) or primary stenting with nitinol self-expanding stents (with or without drug elution), wire-interwoven nitinol stents, or covered stents. A clear advantage of one treatment modality over another has not been demonstrated, and choice of therapy should depend on lesion location, length, degree of calcification, postangioplasty angiogram, size of the vessel, and clinical presentation.[46-48] In general, short to moderate length lesions, especially at the distal segment, can probably be treated with angioplasty alone using a drug-coated balloon (with provisional stenting), whereas long (>20 cm) severely calcified lesions or chronic total occlusions are likely best treated with self-expanding or interwoven nitinol stents.[48,49] The proximal segment can also be treated with drug-coated balloons with provisional drug-eluting or self-expanding stent placement unless there are complex plaque characteristics.

Noninvasive Imaging

See FIGURES 23.27 and 23.28.

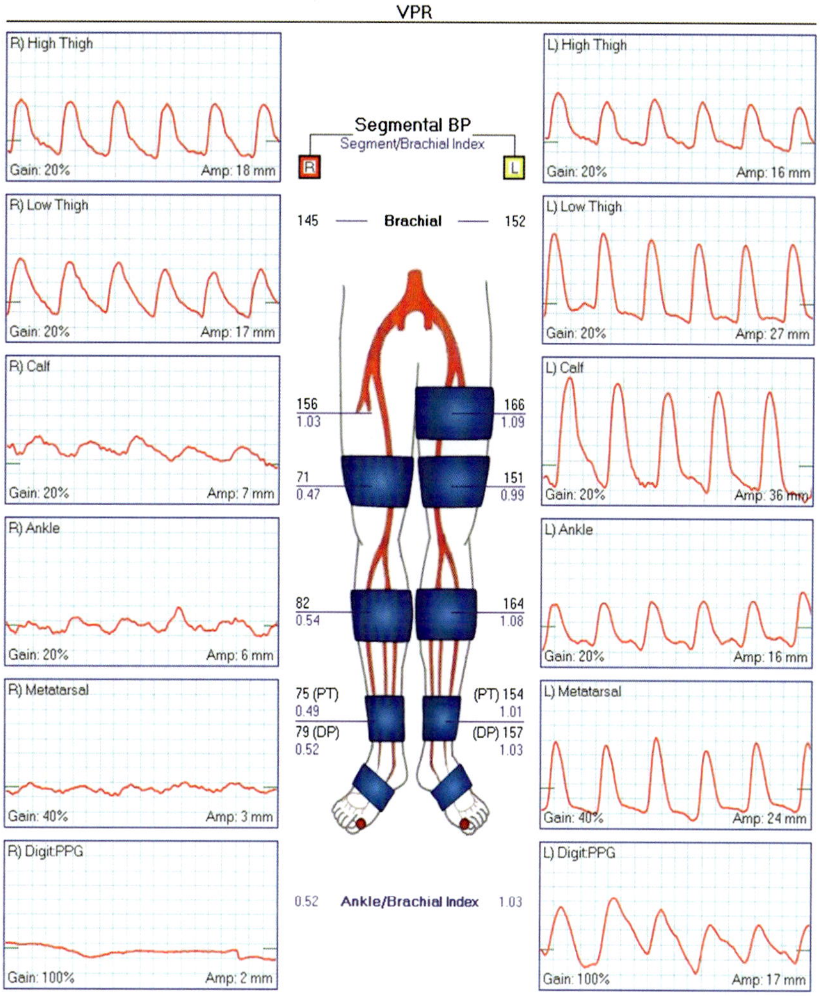

Segmental BP

Right			Left		
		Index			Index
Brachial:	145		Brachial:	152	
High Thigh:	156	1.03	High Thigh:	166	1.09
Low Thigh:	71	0.47	Low Thigh:	151	0.99
Calf:	82	0.54	Calf:	164	1.08
Ankle (PT):	75	0.49	Ankle (PT):	154	1.01
Ankle (DP):	79	0.52	Ankle (DP):	157	1.03

A

FIGURE 23.27 Abnormal ankle-brachial index and pulse volume recording in a patient with SFA-popliteal segment disease. **A**, The ankle-brachial index of the right leg is 0.52 and consistent with peripheral arterial disease of at least moderate severity. There is significant pressure gradient (>20 mm Hg) between the high and the low thigh segments in the right leg, indicating disease at the SFA level. Additionally, the pulse volume waveform of the right leg is normal at the high thigh but is moderately damped at the low thigh and calf segments when compared with the same level at the left side. **B**, After revascularization of the right distal SFA, the ankle-brachial index is improved but considered to be borderline abnormal. There is marked improvement in pulse volume waveforms on the right side. There is residual disease at the level of the SFA and popliteal arteries as indicated by a significant pressure gradient between the high and low thigh segments and low thigh and calf segments. SFA, superficial femoral artery. Adapted from the Cleveland Clinic Non Invasive Vascular Laboratory.

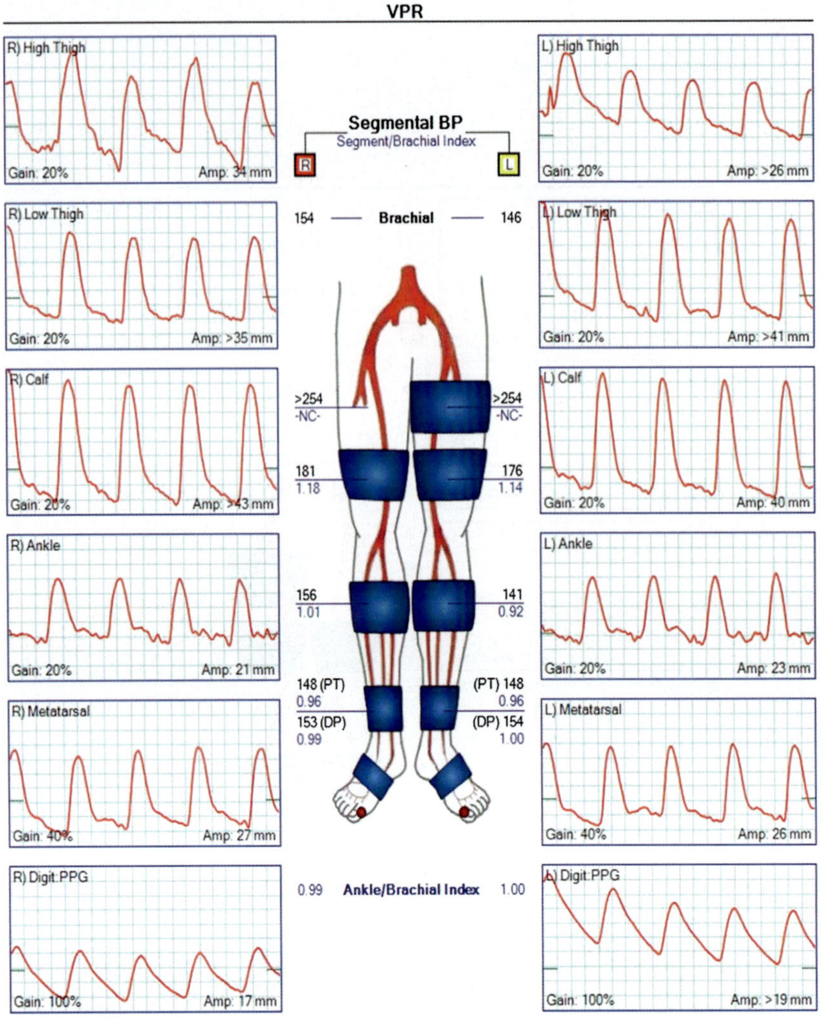

Segmental BP

Right			Left		
		Index			Index
Brachial:	154		**Brachial:**	146	
High Thigh:	>254	-NC-	**High Thigh:**	>254	-NC-
Low Thigh:	181	1.18	**Low Thigh:**	176	1.14
Calf:	156	1.01	**Calf:**	141	0.92
Ankle (PT):	148	0.96	**Ankle (PT):**	148	0.96
Ankle (DP):	153	0.99	**Ankle (DP):**	154	1.00

B

FIGURE 23.27 (Continued)

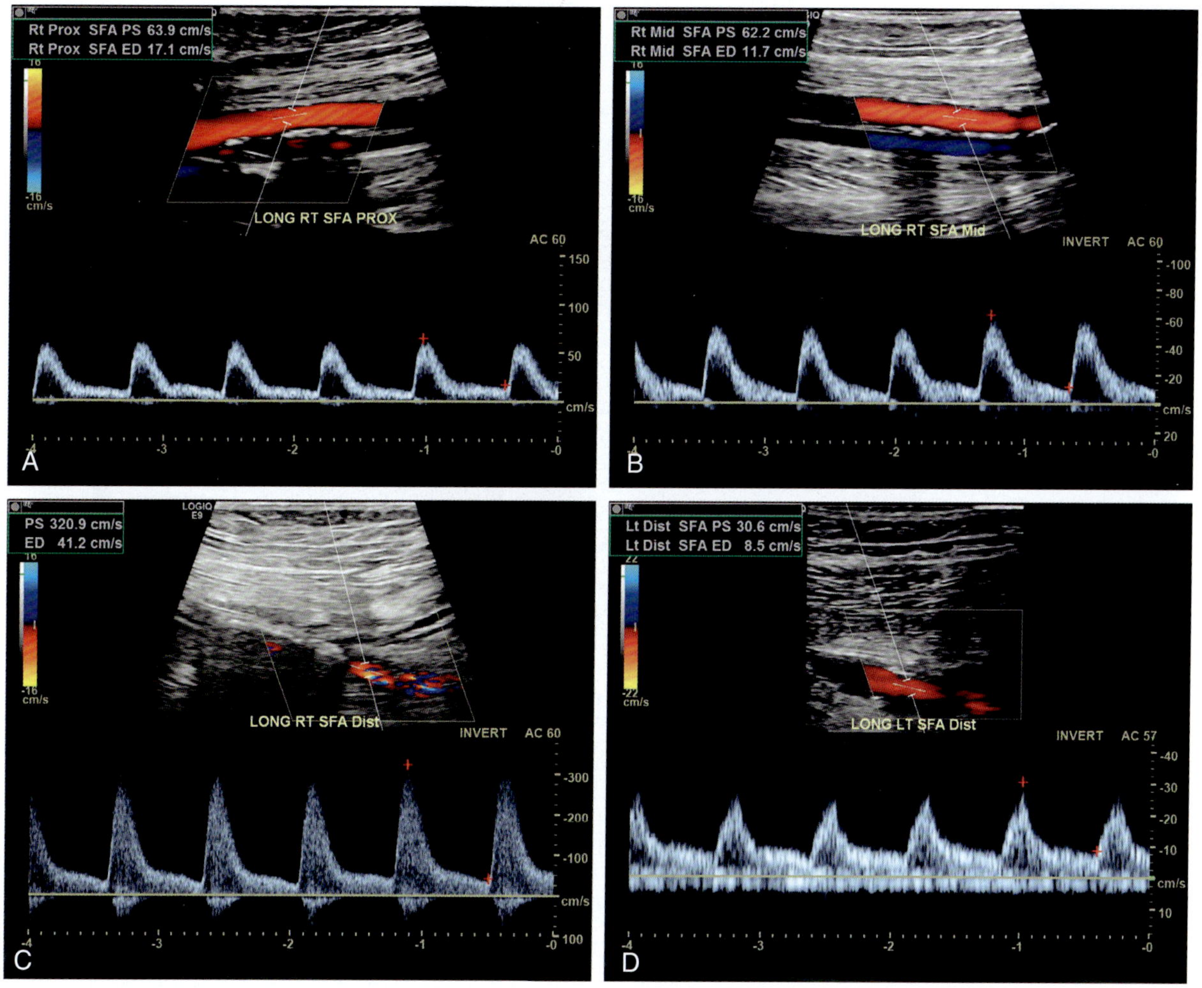

FIGURE 23.28 Abnormal superficial femoral arterial duplex ultrasound. Arterial duplex ultrasound is time intensive and operator dependent but can be quite useful in identifying the location, severity, and extent of disease in proximal segments. Hence, this modality is usually performed before intervention or as follow-up after intervention. **A and B**, Show monophasic waveforms with normal peak-systolic velocities at the proximal and mid SFA segments, and color Doppler shows laminar flow. Compared with the mid segment, there is greater than 4-fold increase in peak-systolic velocity, spectral broadening, and evidence of turbulent flow on color Doppler at the distal SFA **(C)**. These findings suggest significant stenosis of >75% severity at the distal SFA. Often, the segment distal to a severe obstruction will exhibit delayed upstroke (parvus-tardus) with blunted peak **(D)**.

Angiographic Evaluation and Treatment

See **FIGURES 23.29-29.32.**

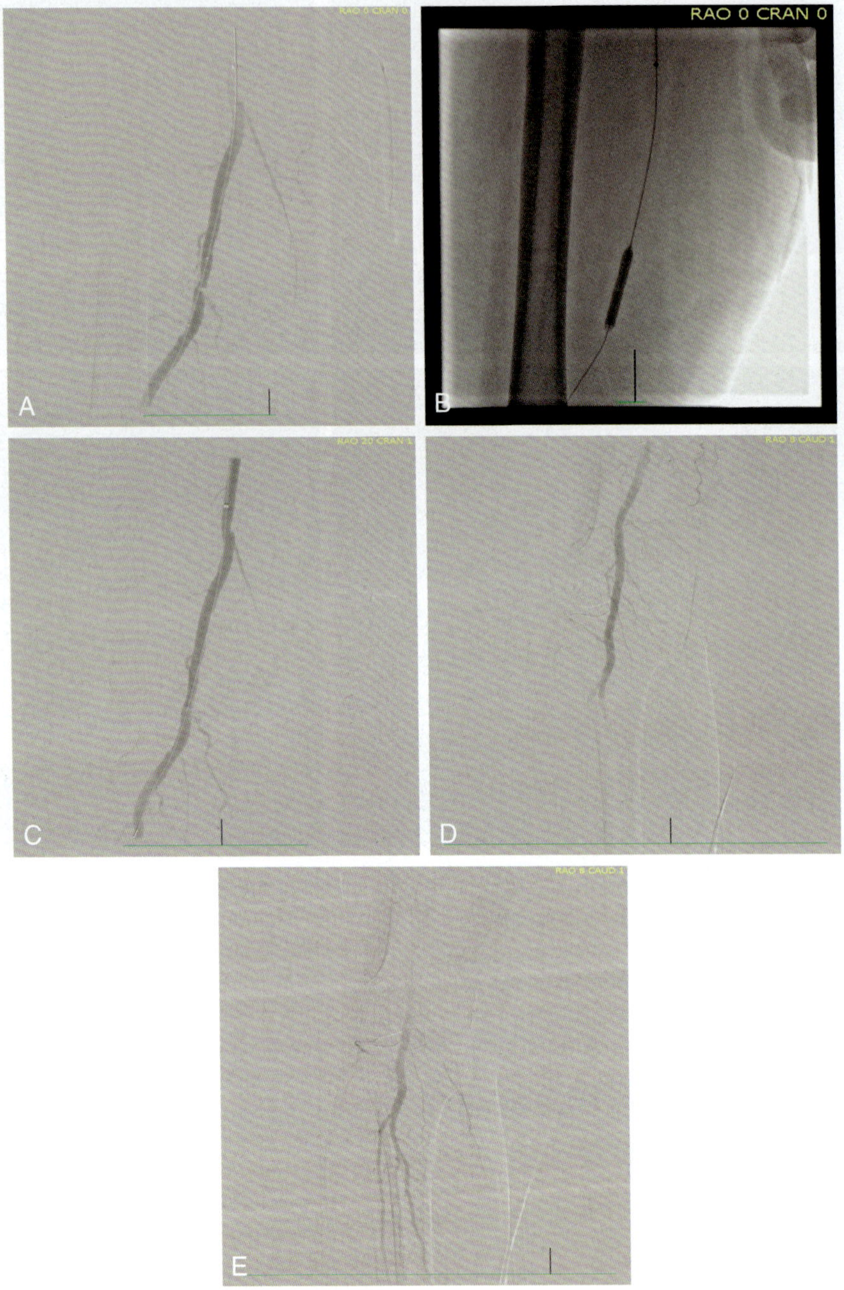

FIGURE 23.29 Selective right superficial femoral angiography with intervention of a TASC type A lesion using the contralateral crossover technique. Access is most commonly obtained via the contralateral common femoral artery with placement of a 6 Fr sheath. A 0.035-inch Wholey wire is advanced to the level of the aortic bifurcation, and a diagnostic catheter such as a JR4 or IMA is used to direct the Wholey wire down the contralateral common iliac artery. The diagnostic catheter is then advanced into the contralateral common iliac artery and the Wholey wire is exchanged for a stiff angled glidewire. The diagnostic catheter can then be positioned at the level of the common femoral artery and angiography can be performed. Before intervention, a kink-resistant sheath is exchanged for the diagnostic catheter. **A**, Demonstrates an eccentric severe focal stenosis at the distal segment of the SFA. Given the short segment of stenosis and lack of severe calcification, primary angioplasty using a drug-coated balloon is undertaken **(B)**. Postangioplasty angiography with runoff shows <10% residual stenosis without dissection or perforation **(C)** and no downstream complications at the popliteal artery **(D)** or infrapopliteal segments **(E)**.

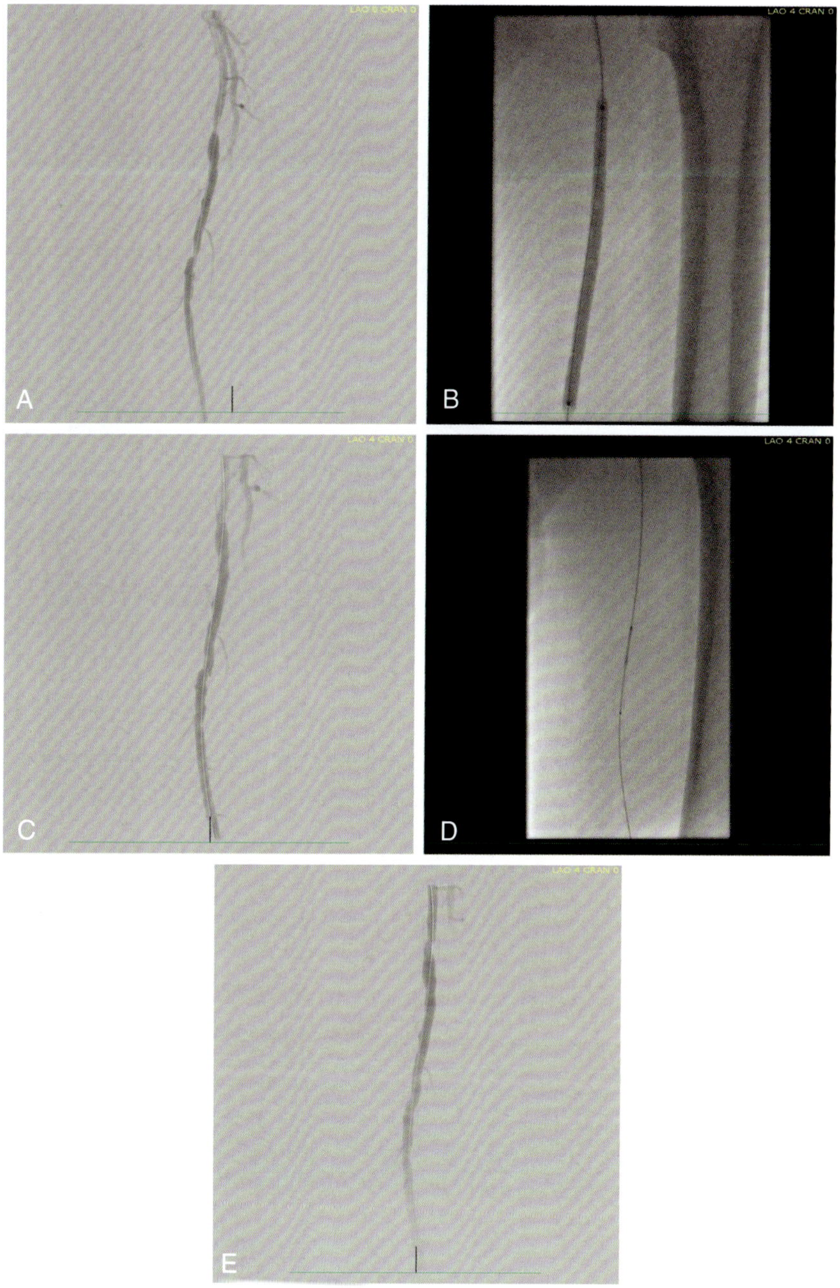

FIGURE 23.30 Revascularization of a left superficial femoral artery TASC type B lesion using ipsilateral antegrade access. **A**, Demonstrates a 70% stenosis followed by a 90% stenosis in the proximal and mid SFA. Given the moderate length of disease and degree of calcification, primary angioplasty using a drug-coated balloon is undertaken **(B)**. Postangioplasty angiography reveals focal dissection at the mid SFA **(C)**. A bare-metal nitinol self-expanding stent is deployed at the site of dissection **(D)**, and final angiography shows no perforation or additional dissections **(E)**.

Infrapopliteal Arteries

Many patients with chronic critical limb ischemia will have severe infrapopliteal disease alone or, more commonly, coexistent with more proximal disease. Revascularization of 2- or 3-vessel infrapopliteal disease is appropriate for Rutherford category 4 to 6 disease and can ideally be directed by the involved angiosome when possible.[34,50-53] Revascularization of 1-vessel infrapopliteal disease may be appropriate for Rutherford category 4 and 5. Importantly, in patients with rest pain all significant proximal disease should be addressed first. In the current era, many individuals can undergo an endovascular-first approach with angioplasty with or without drug-coated balloon and provisional drug-eluting stent placement.

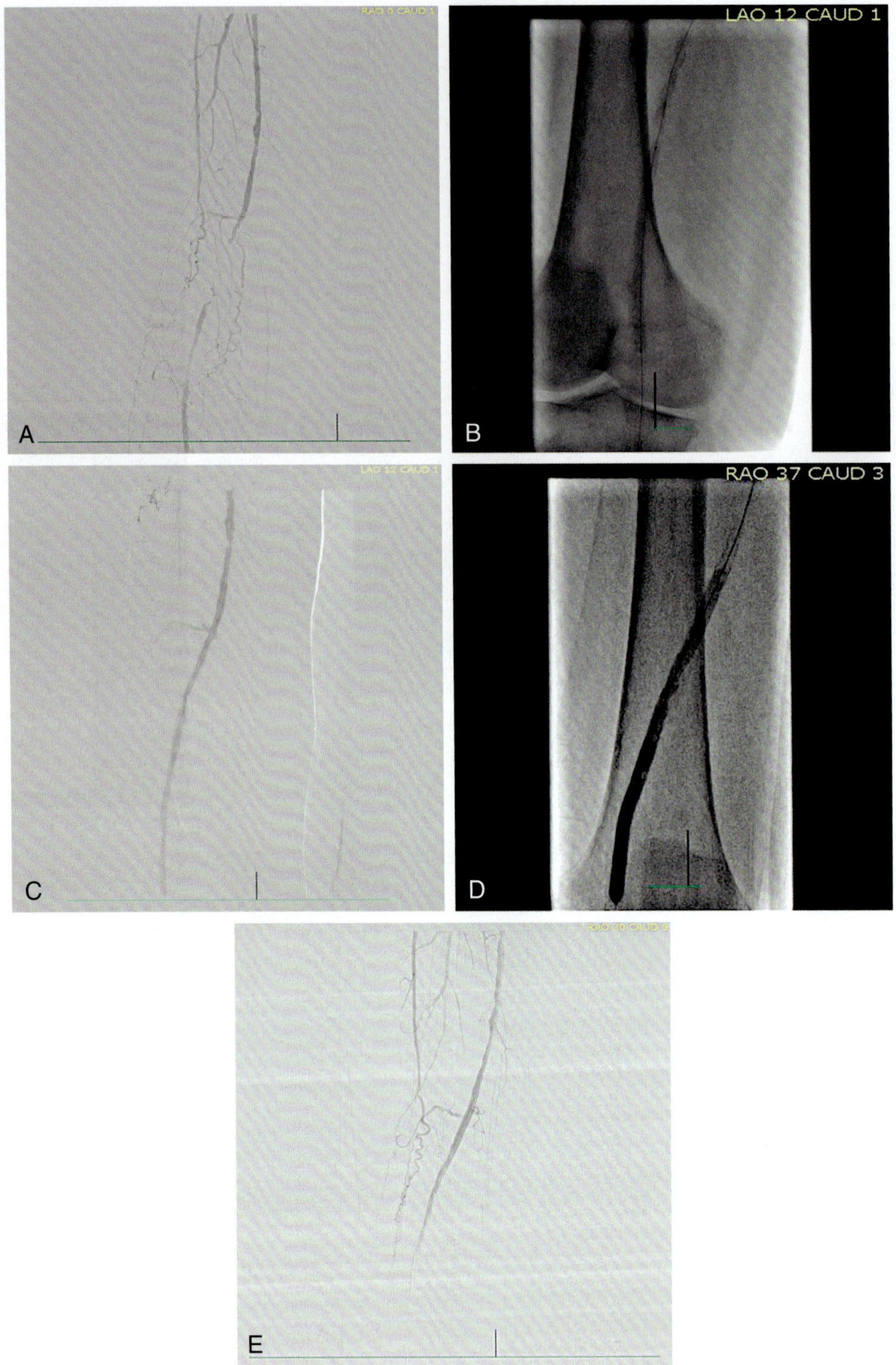

FIGURE 23.31 Revascularization of a right superficial femoral and popliteal artery chronic total occlusion (TASC type D lesion) using contralateral crossover technique. Selective SFA angiography demonstrates a moderately long total occlusion at the distal segment that extends into the P1 segment of the popliteal artery **(A)**. The proximal popliteal artery reconstitutes via collaterals. A hydrophilic coated 0.035-inch guide wire is used to carefully cross the occlusive lesions with the support of a microcatheter **(B)**. We take care to enter the true lumen as soon as the occlusion has been crossed. Angioplasty using an undersized non–drug-coated balloon is then performed to facilitate the passage of devices. Angioplasty using an appropriately sized drug-coated balloon is then performed and a picture is obtained **(C)**. A nitinol interwoven stent is then deployed from the distal SFA into the proximal popliteal artery and post-dilated **(D)**. Final angiography reveals no dissection or perforation with good runoff **(E)**.

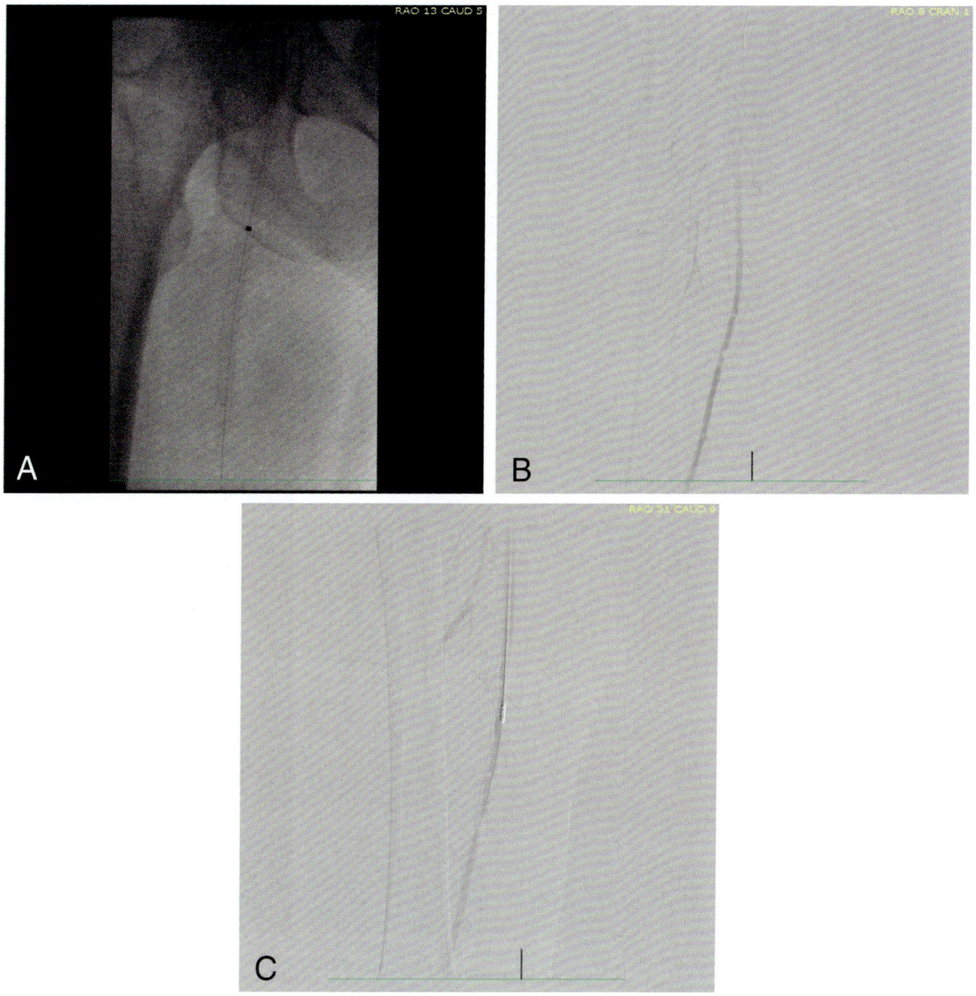

FIGURE 23.32 Atherectomy devices used in lower extremity arterial interventions. Several different atherectomy devices are currently available for use in the lower extremity arterial system. Atherectomy modifies an atherosclerotic plaque and, in theory, may prevent significant plaque shift, dissection, lesion recoil, or incomplete stent expansion. Such devices may be used with or without distal embolization protection devices. At present, little high-quality data exist to suggest improvement in outcomes with use of atherectomy devices. However, there is great interest in combining atherectomy with drug-coated balloon angioplasty and several studies are ongoing. In **(A)**, laser atherectomy is used to assist with crossing and debulking a totally occluded SFA stent. The application of laser atherectomy is particularly useful for in-stent restenosis and chronic total occlusions. **B**, Demonstrates severe tandem stenoses at the mid segment of the SFA. Rotational atherectomy is used in this situation, as it can debulk lesions without predilation because the cutting blades are at the tip of the catheter **(C)**. In addition, the Jetstream device offers continuous aspiration and may also be beneficial in thrombotic lesions.

Angiographic Evaluation and Treatment

See **FIGURE 23.33**.

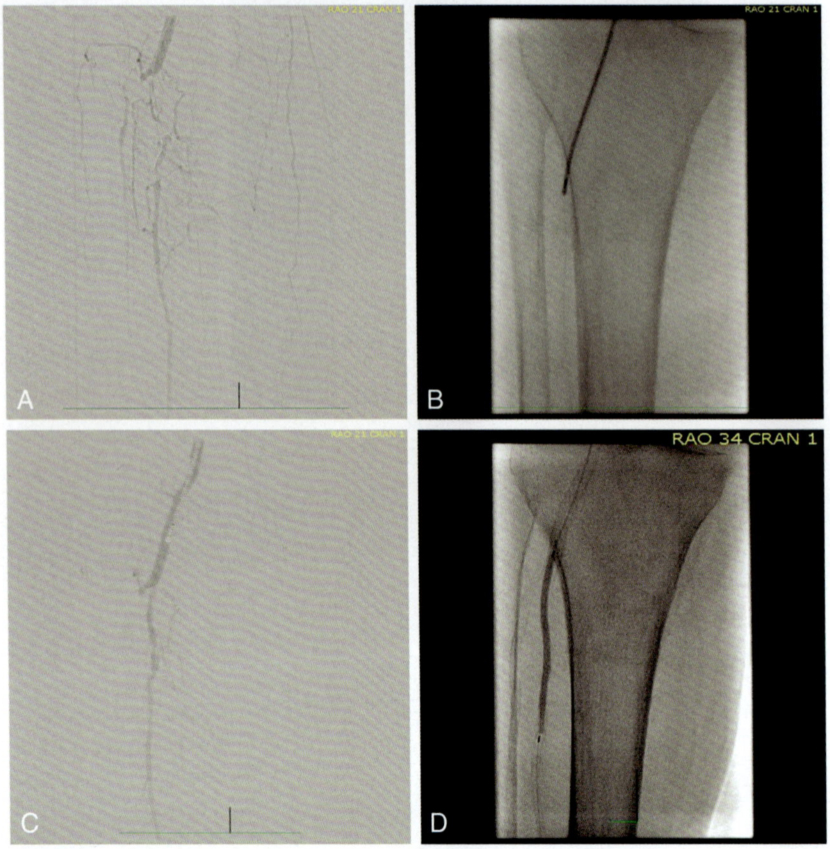

FIGURE 23.33 Reconstruction of peroneal and anterior tibial chronic total occlusions in a patient with Rutherford category 5 disease. We routinely perform interventions with ipsilateral antegrade common femoral arterial access for better guide wire control and device deliverability. However, infrapopliteal interventions can be done with contralateral crossover technique. Ipsilateral antegrade popliteal or retrograde tibio-pedal access may be required in some cases. A kink-resistant sheath is inserted over a Wholey wire, and a catheter is subsequently advanced to the level of the popliteal artery. Selective angiography of the infrapopliteal segment is then performed. **A**, Shows 3-vessel (anterior tibial, peroneal, and posterior tibial) occlusion. When possible, we attempt to target revascularization based on the diseased angiosome. A 0.014- or 0.018-inch guide wire with a support microcatheter is used to carefully cross the occluded peroneal artery. Coronary chronic total occlusion (CTO) guide wires may be required for difficult to cross lesions. In this case, we used a Pilot 200 coronary guide wire. Once intraluminal position is confirmed with aspiration and gentle contrast injection, atherectomy can performed **(B)** if there is severe calcification. Notably, there is a lack of high-quality evidence for the use of atherectomy devices in infrapopliteal disease. A postatherectomy angiogram is performed **(C)** to assess for dissection or perforation. If no complications are present, then balloon angioplasty can be performed **(D)**. A postangioplasty angiogram is performed **(E)** to assess for complications, and a stent can be deployed if needed. Attention is then turned to the anterior tibial artery occlusion, which is carefully crossed using a support microcatheter. Once intraluminal position is confirmed, devices or adjunct therapies can be delivered. In this case, balloon angioplasty is performed **(F)**. Final angiography reveals successful reconstruction of 2 tibial arteries with in-line flow to the foot **(G)**.

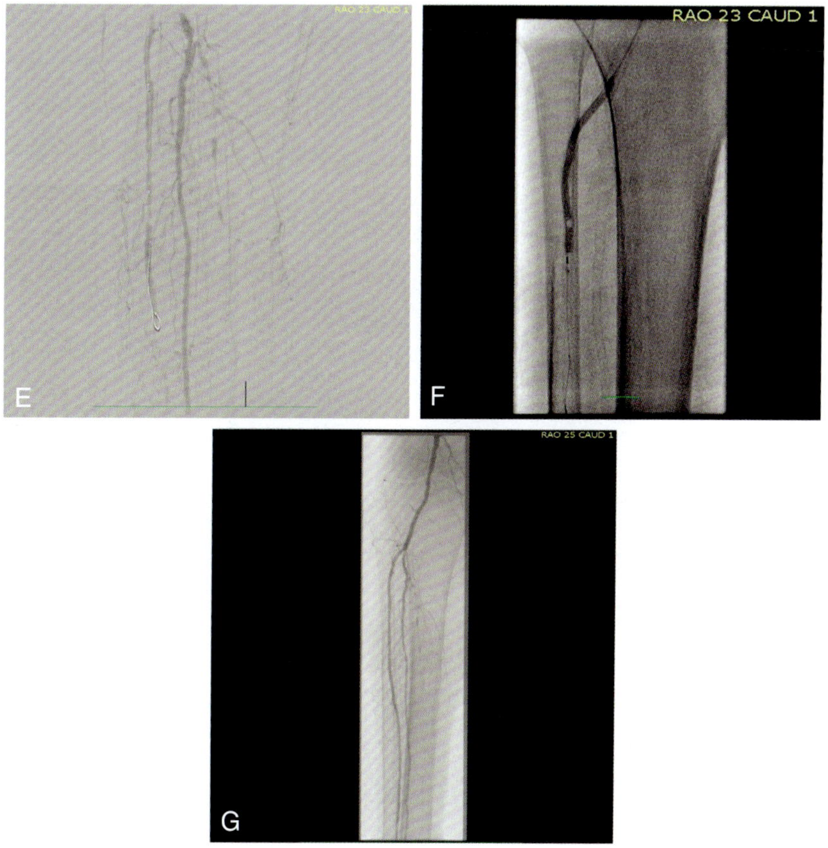

FIGURE 23.33 (Continued)

VENOUS INTERVENTIONS

Inferior Vena Cava Filter

Therapeutic anticoagulation is the treatment of choice for venous thromboembolic disease. However, inferior vena cava filter placement should be considered for patients who absolutely cannot tolerate therapeutic anticoagulation or if there is failure of anticoagulation.[54,55] The primary purpose of filter insertion is to prevent recurrent pulmonary embolism. Although high-quality evidence is lacking, small retrospective studies and prospective trials suggest that use of IVC filters in patients with contraindications to anticoagulation may reduce recurrent pulmonary embolism but has no effect on mortality.[56-58] Unfortunately, filters can serve as a nidus for development of deep venous thrombus, and so we prefer inserting retrievable filters when possible, especially because no studies have demonstrated superiority of one type of filter over another.[56,59]

Angiographic Evaluation and Treatment

See **FIGURES 23.34** and **23.35**.

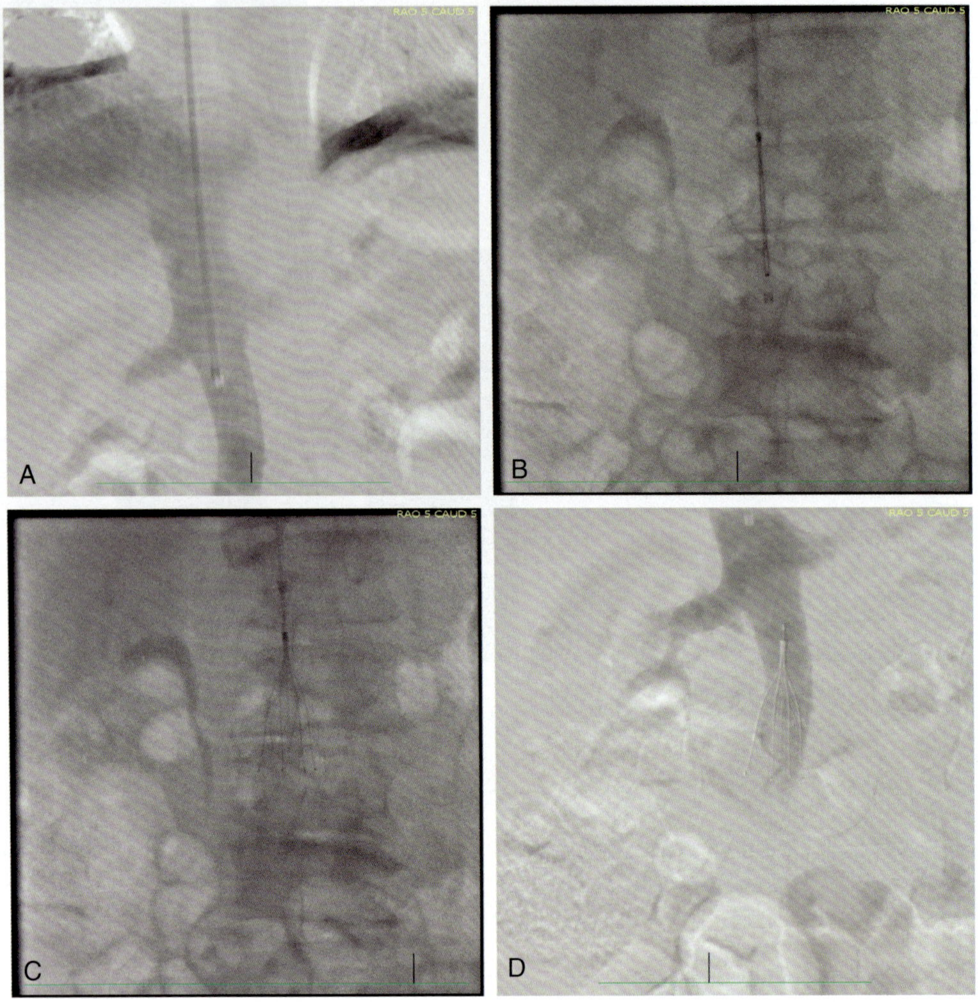

FIGURE 23.34 Vena cavogram and filter placement. Access is obtained in the right internal jugular vein under ultrasound guidance, and a 5 Fr sheath is inserted. A 0.035-inch Wholey wire is advanced into the inferior vena cava, and a straight flush diagnostic catheter is advanced over the guide wire below the level of L2-3 vertebral bodies (ideally in the left common iliac vein). Digital subtraction vena cavogram is then performed using 3-5 mL of contrast with 5 mL of saline **(A)** or with carbon dioxide. The cavogram is studied for the presence, extent, and location of thrombus, diameter of IVC, position of the renal veins, caval duplication, and other anomalies. The diameter of the IVC should be confirmed in the lateral projection if the anteroposterior diameter seems too large for the selected filter. The diagnostic catheter is exchanged for the device catheter over the guide wire. The guide wire is removed, and the device is then placed at the target location **(B)** using bony landmarks. We routinely position the tip of the filter at or just below the inflow of the renal veins. If double left renal veins are present, then we position the tip of the filter below the lower limb. If significant thrombus is near or within the renal veins, then suprarenal placement may be indicated. The device is then slowly unsheathed, taking care to watch for migration or suboptimal positioning, and deployed **(C)**. Final vena cavogram is performed to document position and identify complications **(D)**. After filter placement, physicians should assess the need for the device on a frequent basis and be referred for retrieval as soon as the contraindication to anticoagulation resolves.

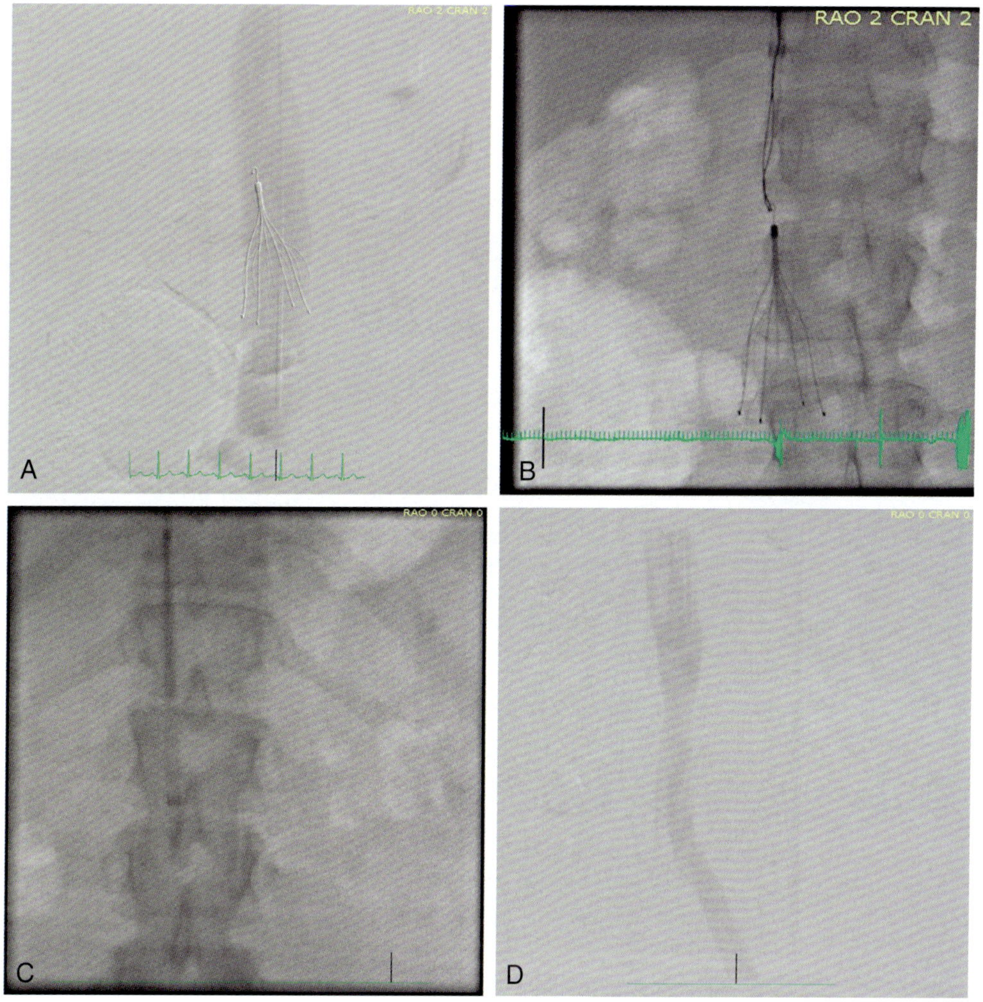

FIGURE 23.35 Filter retrieval. We highly recommend filter retrieval if feasible as soon as possible once contraindication to anticoagulation has resolved, as longer dwell times may result in dense adherence of the filter to the IVC wall. The procedure is performed with local analgesia and light sedation, so it may be possible to monitor the patient for abdominal pain during retrieval. The right internal jugular vein is accessed under ultrasound guidance, and a Wholey wire is carefully advanced to the inferior vena cava. A catheter (eg, straight flush, pig tail, etc) is subsequently advanced below the filter to the level of the iliocaval confluence and a vena cavogram is performed **(A)**. Images are carefully reviewed for the presence and amount of clot, degree of filter tilt, and anatomical issues that may portend difficult retrieval. If the filter is not full of significant amount of clot (<25%), then the catheter is exchanged for the retrieval sheath and placed just proximal to the filter. A snare or retrieval cone is used to grasp the hook **(B)** and gentle traction is applied, as the retrieval sheath is simultaneously advanced over the filter **(C)**. If significant abdominal pain is experienced, retrieval should be halted and a cavogram performed. Final vena cavogram is performed via the sheath to assess for vascular injury **(D)**.

Chronic Inferior Vena Cava Occlusion

Chronic inferior vena cava occlusion can occur as a consequence of deep vein thrombosis or extrinsic compression and is difficult to treat. Patients who present with disabling postthrombotic syndrome (Clinical, Etiology, Anatomy, Pathophysiology [CEAP] classification >3) and have failed conservative medical therapy may warrant consideration for intervention.[60,61] Diagnostic studies often include venous duplex ultrasound, computed tomography (CT) venography, magnetic resonance venography, or transfemoral venography. Most partial or complete occlusions are located at the infrarenal segment, and there is often iliac vein involvement.[62] Percutaneous therapy is preferred over surgical techniques, and primary stenting with predilation is typically performed. Although high-quality evidence for vena cava stenting is lacking, several series have reported reasonable intermediate-term patency rates.[60,63-67]

Angiographic Evaluation and Treatment

See **FIGURE 23.36**.

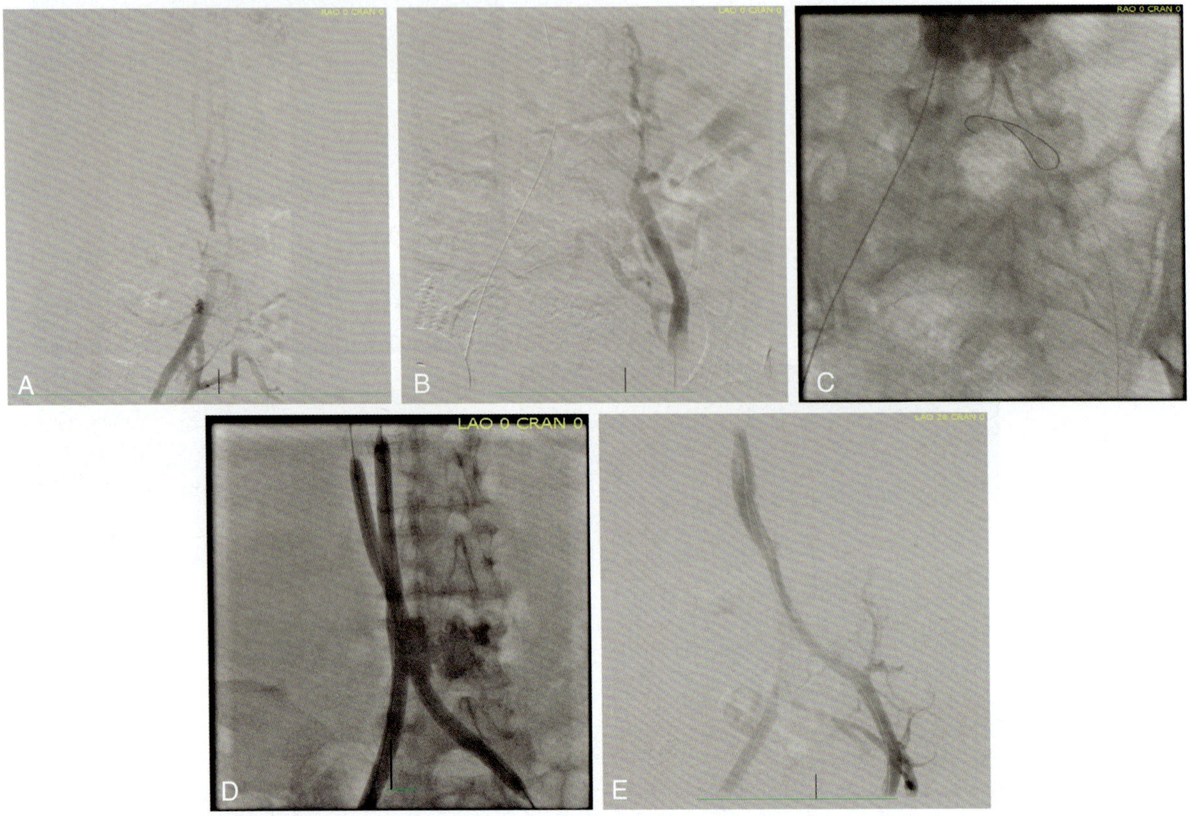

FIGURE 23.36 Percutaneous angioplasty and stenting of an extrinsically compressed ilio-vena cava system. Venous access is typically obtained at the superficial femoral vein in cases of occlusion owing to thrombotic disease to allow for adequate evaluation and treatment of more proximal segments. In this case, there was extrinsic compression of the ilio-vena cava from metastatic adenopathy and so bilateral common femoral veins were accessed. Transfemoral venography with or without IVUS is performed to evaluate the extent of disease. **A and B**, Demonstrate complete occlusion of the distal IVC, severe stenoses of bilateral common iliac veins, and extensive paravertebral collateral formation. The occlusion is carefully crossed using a stiff glidewire with supporting microcatheter **(C)**. True luminal position is confirmed with aspiration and injection of dilute contrast. The glidewires are then exchanged for Wholey wires, and serial balloon dilations are performed with or without kissing technique. Two Wallstents are then deployed **(D)** from the distal vena cava into both iliac veins, and postdilation is performed. Final venography demonstrates <20% residual stenosis without vascular injury **(E)**. Anticoagulation duration for the procedure is generally 1-3 mo. Otherwise, duration of further anticoagulation should be directed by the underlying disease process.

Acute and Subacute Inferior Vena Cava Occlusion

Acute (<14 days) and subacute (<28 days) inferior vena cava occlusion most often results from proximal extension of deep venous thrombus. Usually, patients present with symptoms secondary to thromboembolism and massive burden of clot is subsequently discovered by noninvasive lower extremity imaging. Occasionally, patients may present with acute profound bilateral lower extremity edema or rarely phlegmasia alba or cerulea dolens. In such patients, catheter-directed thrombolysis (CDT) with or without adjunct therapies may result in rapid and more complete dissolution of clot with lower rates of postthrombotic syndrome.[68-70] Although the risk of bleeding is not trivial, there has been a significant reduction in major bleeding events owing to greater experience.[55]

Noninvasive Imaging

See FIGURE 23.37.

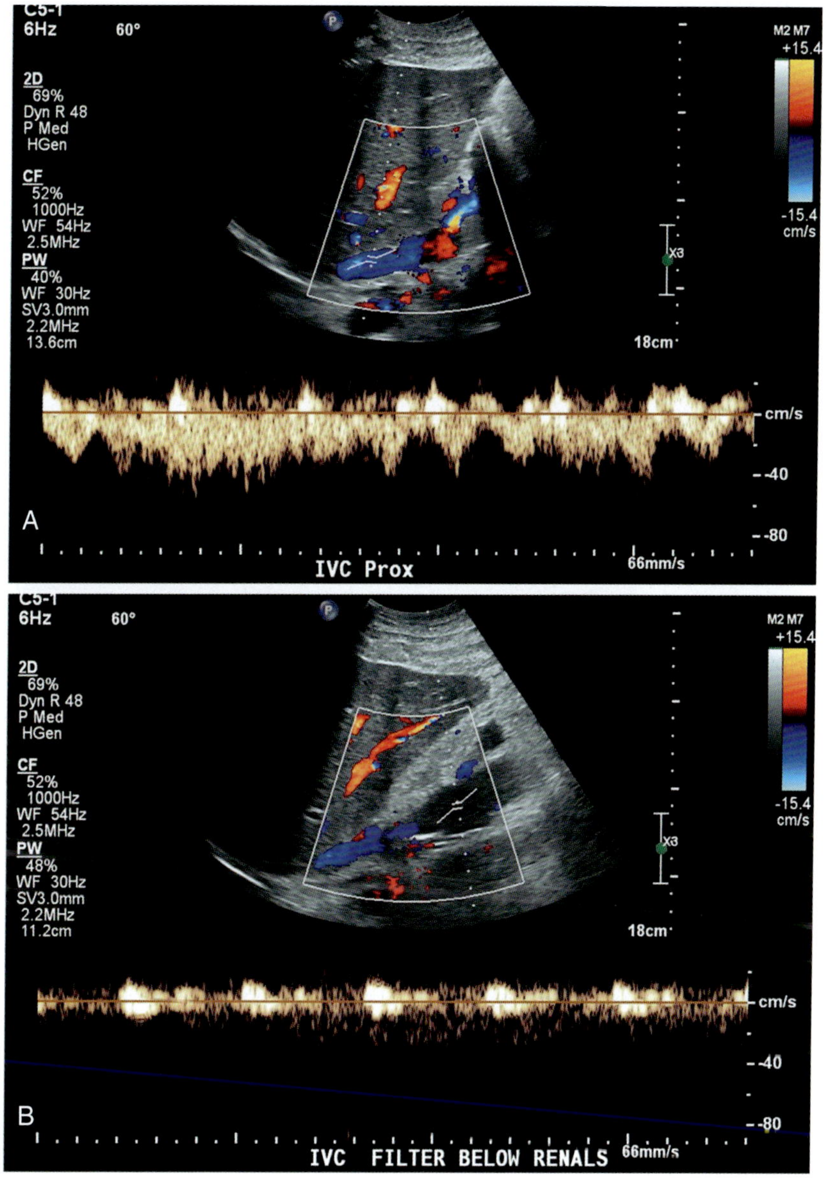

FIGURE 23.37 Abnormal venous duplex ultrasound. **A**, Demonstrates patent inferior vena cava at the proximal segment with normal color Doppler and waveform. **B**, At the mid and distal segments, there is near absence of flow on color Doppler and waveform, suggestive of thrombus.

Angiographic Evaluation and Treatment

See FIGURE 23.38.

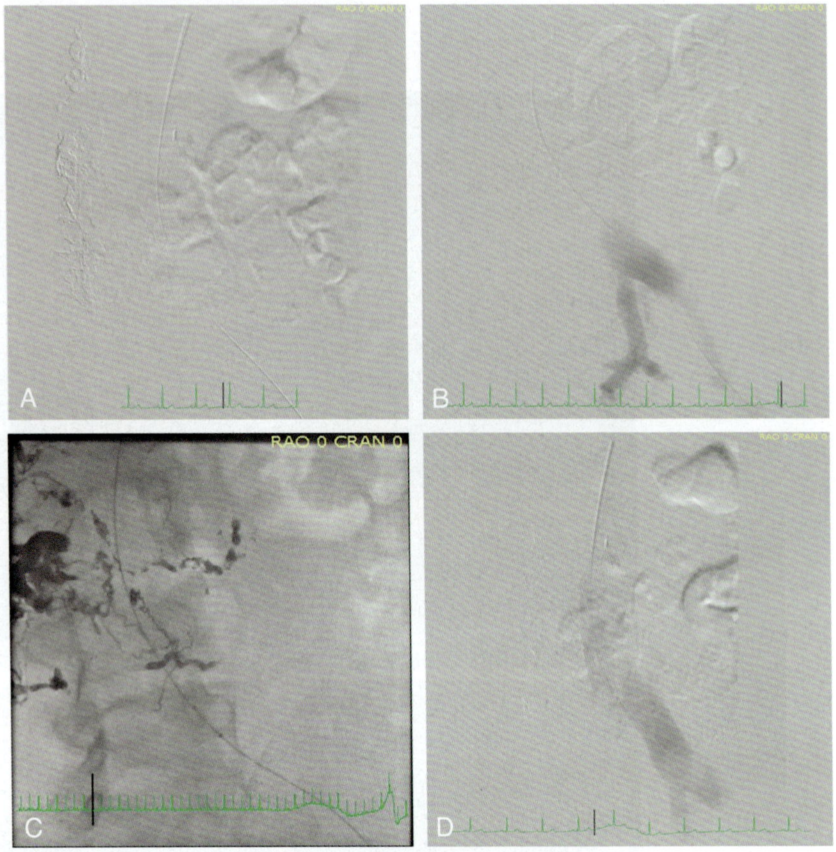

FIGURE 23.38 Percutaneous treatment of acute massive iliofemoral and IVC thrombus using pharmacomechanical CDT. Pharmacomechanical CDT appears to be quite effective and uses a lower dose of thrombolytic agent.[71-73]. Noninvasive imaging (see FIGURE 23.37) shows occlusion of the distal IVC with clot in bilateral common iliac veins. Hence, the right internal jugular vein is accessed and a 0.035-inch Wholey wire is advanced across the IVC into the left common iliac vein with use of a supporting catheter **(A)**. The catheter is advanced into the left external iliac vein and venography is performed, demonstrating slow flow and complete occlusion of the distal IVC **(B)**. Several passes are then made with a rheolytic thrombectomy device and balloon angioplasty is performed **(C)**, resulting in partial recanalization of the distal IVC **(D)**. Thrombus is observed as a filling defect in the left common and external iliac vein. The Wholey wire is subsequently redirected into the right iliac vein and venography is performed. This shows extensive thrombus in the right common iliac vein and at the IVC filter **(E)**. Balloon angioplasty is performed at the IVC filter **(F)** to treat any organized material, but extensive clot is present **(G)**. As a result, an ultrasound-enhanced CDT catheter is inserted across the distal IVC into the right common iliac vein **(H)**. Continuous thrombolytic is infused through the catheter and a thrombolytic check can be performed at 24 h.

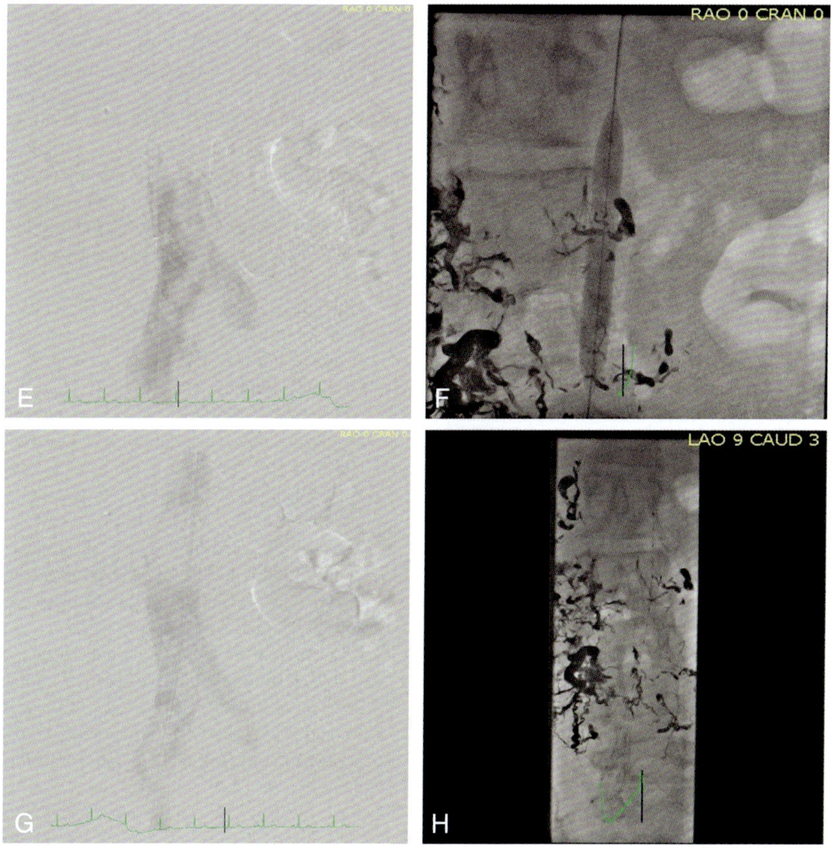

FIGURE 23.38 (Continued)

REFERENCES

1. Bonati LH, Lyrer P, Ederle J, Featherstone R, Brown MM. Percutaneous transluminal balloon angioplasty and stenting for carotid artery stenosis. *Cochrane Database Syst Rev.* 2012:CD000515.
2. Brott TG, Howard G, Roubin GS, et al. Long-term results of stenting versus endarterectomy for carotid-artery stenosis. *N Engl J Med.* 2016;374:1021-1031.
3. Bijuklic K, Wandler A, Varnakov Y, Tuebler T, Schofer J. Risk factors for cerebral embolization after carotid artery stenting with embolic protection: a diffusion-weighted magnetic resonance imaging study in 837 consecutive patients. *Circ Cardiovasc Interv.* 2013;6:311-316.
4. Hofmann R, Niessner A, Kypta A, et al. Risk score for peri-interventional complications of carotid artery stenting. *Stroke.* 2006;37:2557-2561.
5. Hawkins BM, Kennedy KF, Giri J, et al. Pre-procedural risk quantification for carotid stenting using the CAS score: a report from the NCDR CARE Registry. *J Am Coll Cardiol.* 2012;60:1617-1622.
6. Kernan WN, Ovbiagele B, Black HR, et al. Guidelines for the prevention of stroke in patients with stroke and transient ischemic attack: a guideline for healthcare professionals from the American Heart Association/American Stroke Association. *Stroke.* 2014;45:2160-2236.
7. Brott TG, Halperin JL, Abbara S, et al. 2011 ASA/ACCF/AHA/AANN/AANS/ACR/ASNR/CNS/SAIP/SCAI/SIR/SNIS/SVM/SVS guideline on the management of patients with extracranial carotid and vertebral artery disease: executive summary: a report of the American College of Cardiology Foundation/American Heart Association Task Force on Practice Guidelines, and the American Stroke Association, American Association of Neuroscience Nurses, American Association of Neurological Surgeons, American College of Radiology, American Society of Neuroradiology, Congress of Neurological Surgeons, Society of Atherosclerosis Imaging and Prevention, Society for Cardiovascular Angiography and Interventions, Society of Interventional Radiology, Society of NeuroInterventional Surgery, Society for Vascular Medicine, and Society for Vascular Surgery. Developed in collaboration with the American Academy of Neurology and Society of Cardiovascular Computed Tomography. *Catheter Cardiovasc Interv.* 2013;81:E76-E123.
8. Macdonald S, Lee R, Williams R, Stansby G, Delphi Carotid Stenting Consensus Panel. Towards safer carotid artery stenting: a scoring system for anatomic suitability. *Stroke.* 2009;40:1698-1703.
9. Madhwal S, Rajagopal V, Bhatt DL, Bajzer CT, Whitlow P, Kapadia SR. Predictors of difficult carotid stenting as determined by aortic arch angiography. *J Invasive Cardiol.* 2008;20:200-204.
10. Chatterjee S, Nerella N, Chakravarty S, Shani J. Angioplasty alone versus angioplasty and stenting for subclavian artery stenosis–a systematic review and meta-analysis. *Am J Ther.* 2013;20:520-523.
11. De Vries JP, Jager LC, Van den Berg JC, et al. Durability of percutaneous transluminal angioplasty for obstructive lesions of proximal subclavian artery: long-term results. *J Vasc Surg.* 2005;41:19-23.
12. Sixt S, Rastan A, Schwarzwalder U, et al. Results after balloon angioplasty or stenting of atherosclerotic subclavian artery obstruction. *Catheter Cardiovasc Interv.* 2009;73:395-403.
13. Patel SN, White CJ, Collins TJ, et al. Catheter-based treatment of the subclavian and innominate arteries. *Catheter Cardiovasc Interv.* 2008;71:963-968.

14. Rooke TW, Hirsch AT, Misra S, et al. Management of patients with peripheral artery disease (compilation of 2005 and 2011 ACCF/AHA guideline recommendations): a report of the American College of Cardiology Foundation/American Heart Association Task Force on Practice Guidelines. *J Am Coll Cardiol*. 2013;61:1555-1570.
15. Olin JW, Piedmonte MR, Young JR, DeAnna S, Grubb M, Childs MB. The utility of duplex ultrasound scanning of the renal arteries for diagnosing significant renal artery stenosis. *Ann Intern Med*. 1995;122:833-838.
16. Radermacher J, Chavan A, Bleck J, et al. Use of Doppler ultrasonography to predict the outcome of therapy for renal-artery stenosis. *N Engl J Med*. 2001;344:410-417.
17. Mukherjee D, Bhatt DL, Robbins M, et al. Renal artery end-diastolic velocity and renal artery resistance index as predictors of outcome after renal stenting. *Am J Cardiol*. 2001;88:1064-1066.
18. Feldman RL, Wargovich TJ, Bittl JA. No-touch technique for reducing aortic wall trauma during renal artery stenting. *Catheter Cardiovasc Interv*. 1999;46:245-248.
19. Gross CM, Kramer J, Weingartner O, et al. Determination of renal arterial stenosis severity: comparison of pressure gradient and vessel diameter. *Radiology*. 2001;220:751-756.
20. Parikh SA, Shishehbor MH, Gray BH, White CJ, Jaff MR. SCAI expert consensus statement for renal artery stenting appropriate use. *Catheter Cardiovasc Interv*. 2014;84:1163-1171.
21. American College of Cardiology and Foundation, American Heart Association Task Force on Practice Guidelines, Society for Cardiovascular Angiography and Interventions, et al. 2011 ACCF/AHA focused update of the guideline for the management of patients with peripheral artery disease (updating the 2005 guideline). *Vasc Med*. 2011;16:452-476.
22. Tuttle KR, Chouinard RF, Webber JT, et al. Treatment of atherosclerotic ostial renal artery stenosis with the intravascular stent. *Am J Kidney Dis*. 1998;32:611-622.
23. van de Ven PJ, Kaatee R, Beutler JJ, et al. Arterial stenting and balloon angioplasty in ostial atherosclerotic renovascular disease: a randomised trial. *Lancet*. 1999;353:282-286.
24. Blum U, Krumme B, Flugel P, et al. Treatment of ostial renal-artery stenoses with vascular endoprostheses after unsuccessful balloon angioplasty. *N Engl J Med*. 1997;336:459-465.
25. Rocha-Singh K, Jaff MR, Rosenfield K, Investigators A-T. Evaluation of the safety and effectiveness of renal artery stenting after unsuccessful balloon angioplasty: the ASPIRE-2 study. *J Am Coll Cardiol*. 2005;46:776-783.
26. Lederman RJ, Mendelsohn FO, Santos R, Phillips HR, Stack RS, Crowley JJ. Primary renal artery stenting: characteristics and outcomes after 363 procedures. *Am Heart J*. 2001;142:314-323.
27. Steinmetz E, Tatou E, Favier-Blavoux C, et al. Endovascular treatment as first choice in chronic intestinal ischemia. *Ann Vasc Surg*. 2002;16:693-699.
28. Tallarita T, Oderich GS, Macedo TA, et al. Reinterventions for stent restenosis in patients treated for atherosclerotic mesenteric artery disease. *J Vasc Surg*. 2011;54:1422-1429.e1.
29. Aburahma AF, Campbell JE, Stone PA, et al. Perioperative and late clinical outcomes of percutaneous transluminal stentings of the celiac and superior mesenteric arteries over the past decade. *J Vasc Surg*. 2013;57:1052-1061.
30. Matsumoto AH, Angle JF, Spinosa DJ, et al. Percutaneous transluminal angioplasty and stenting in the treatment of chronic mesenteric ischemia: results and longterm followup. *J Am Coll Surg*. 2002;194:S22-S31.
31. Sarac TP, Altinel O, Kashyap V, et al. Endovascular treatment of stenotic and occluded visceral arteries for chronic mesenteric ischemia. *J Vasc Surg*. 2008;47:485-491.
32. Hirsch AT, Haskal ZJ, Hertzer NR, et al. ACC/AHA 2005 Practice guidelines for the management of patients with peripheral arterial disease (lower extremity, renal, mesenteric, and abdominal aortic): a collaborative report from the American Association for Vascular Surgery/Society for Vascular Surgery, Society for Cardiovascular Angiography and Interventions, Society for Vascular Medicine and Biology, Society of Interventional Radiology, and the ACC/AHA Task Force on Practice Guidelines (Writing Committee to develop guidelines for the management of patients with peripheral arterial disease): endorsed by the American Association of Cardiovascular and Pulmonary Rehabilitation; National Heart, Lung, and Blood Institute; Society for Vascular Nursing; TransAtlantic Inter-Society Consensus; and Vascular Disease Foundation. *Circulation*. 2006;113:e463-e654.
33. Murphy TP, Hirsch AT, Cutlip DE, et al. Claudication: exercise vs endoluminal revascularization (CLEVER) study update. *J Vasc Surg*. 2009;50:942-945.e2.
34. Gerhard-Herman MD, Gornik HL, Barrett C, et al. 2016 AHA/ACC guideline on the management of patients with lower extremity peripheral artery disease: executive summary: a report of the American College of Cardiology/American Heart Association Task Force on Clinical Practice Guidelines. *J Am Coll Cardiol*. 2017;69(11):1465-1508.
35. Klonaris C, Katsargyris A, Tsekouras N, Alexandrou A, Giannopoulos A, Bastounis E. Primary stenting for aortic lesions: from single stenoses to total aortoiliac occlusions. *J Vasc Surg*. 2008;47:310-317.
36. Kashyap VS, Pavkov ML, Bena JF, et al. The management of severe aortoiliac occlusive disease: endovascular therapy rivals open reconstruction. *J Vasc Surg*. 2008;48:1451-1457, 1457.e1-3.
37. Burke CR, Henke PK, Hernandez R, et al. A contemporary comparison of aortofemoral bypass and aortoiliac stenting in the treatment of aortoiliac occlusive disease. *Ann Vasc Surg*. 2010;24:4-13.
38. Wilson SE, Wolf GL, Cross AP. Percutaneous transluminal angioplasty versus operation for peripheral arteriosclerosis. Report of a prospective randomized trial in a selected group of patients. *J Vasc Surg*. 1989;9:1-9.
39. Holm J, Arfvidsson B, Jivegard L, et al. Chronic lower limb ischaemia. A prospective randomised controlled study comparing the 1-year results of vascular surgery and percutaneous transluminal angioplasty (PTA). *Eur J Vasc Surg*. 1991;5:517-522.
40. Ye W, Liu CW, Ricco JB, Mani K, Zeng R, Jiang J. Early and late outcomes of percutaneous treatment of TransAtlantic Inter-Society Consensus class C and D aorto-iliac lesions. *J Vasc Surg*. 2011;53:1728-1737.
41. Goode SD, Cleveland TJ, Gaines PA, Collaborators St. Randomized clinical trial of stents versus angioplasty for the treatment of iliac artery occlusions (STAG trial). *Br J Surg*. 2013;100:1148-1153.
42. Bosch JL, Hunink MG. Meta-analysis of the results of percutaneous transluminal angioplasty and stent placement for aortoiliac occlusive disease. *Radiology*. 1997;204:87-96.
43. Leung DA, Spinosa DJ, Hagspiel KD, Angle JF, Matsumoto AH. Selection of stents for treating iliac arterial occlusive disease. *J Vasc Interv Radiol*. 2003;14:137-152.
44. Mwipatayi BP, Thomas S, Wong J, et al. A comparison of covered vs bare expandable stents for the treatment of aortoiliac occlusive disease. *J Vasc Surg* 2011;54:1561-1570.
45. Scheinert D, Scheinert S, Sax J, et al. Prevalence and clinical impact of stent fractures after femoropopliteal stenting. *J Am Coll Cardiol*. 2005;45:312-315.
46. Shishehbor MH, Jaff MR. Percutaneous therapies for peripheral artery disease. *Circulation* 2016;134:2008-2027.
47. Shishehbor MH, White CJ, Gray BH, et al. Critical limb ischemia: an expert statement. *J Am Coll Cardiol*. 2016;68:2002-2015.
48. Shishehbor MH. Endovascular treatment of femoropopliteal lesions: so many options, little consensus. *J Am Coll Cardiol*. 2015;66:2339-2342.
49. Acin F, de Haro J, Bleda S, Varela C, Esparza L. Primary nitinol stenting in femoropopliteal occlusive disease: a meta-analysis of randomized controlled trials. *J Endovasc Ther* 2012;19:585-595.

50. Shishehbor MH, Reed GW. Personalized approach to revascularization of critical limb ischemia. *Circ Cardiovasc Interv*. 2014;7:642-644.
51. Stegman BM, Shishehbor MH. Commentary: optimal revascularization for critical limb ischemia: one approach doesn't always fit all. *J Endovasc Ther*. 2015;22:482-484.
52. Bunte MC, Shishehbor MH. Treatment of infrapopliteal critical limb ischemia in 2013: the wound perfusion approach. *Curr Cardiol Rep*. 2013;15:363.
53. Shishehbor MH. Acute and critical limb ischemia: when time is limb. *Cleve Clin J Med*. 2014;81:209-216.
54. Jaff MR, McMurtry MS, Archer SL, et al. Management of massive and submassive pulmonary embolism, iliofemoral deep vein thrombosis, and chronic thromboembolic pulmonary hypertension: a scientific statement from the American Heart Association. *Circulation*. 2011;123:1788-1830.
55. Kearon C, Akl EA, Comerota AJ, et al. Antithrombotic therapy for VTE disease: antithrombotic therapy and prevention of thrombosis, 9th ed: American College of Chest Physicians Evidence-Based Clinical Practice Guidelines. *Chest*. 2012;141:e419S-e494S.
56. White RH, Brunson A, Romano PS, Li Z, Wun T. Outcomes after vena cava filter use in noncancer patients with acute venous thromboembolism: a population-based study. *Circulation*. 2016;133:2018-2029.
57. Muriel A, Jimenez D, Aujesky D, et al. Survival effects of inferior vena cava filter in patients with acute symptomatic venous thromboembolism and a significant bleeding risk. *J Am Coll Cardiol*. 2014;63:1675-1683.
58. Girard P, Stern JB, Parent F. Medical literature and vena cava filters: so far so weak. *Chest*. 2002;122:963-967.
59. Mismetti P, Laporte S, Pellerin O, et al. Effect of a retrievable inferior vena cava filter plus anticoagulation vs anticoagulation alone on risk of recurrent pulmonary embolism: a randomized clinical trial. *J Am Med Assoc*. 2015;313:1627-1635.
60. Neglen P, Hollis KC, Olivier J, Raju S. Stenting of the venous outflow in chronic venous disease: long-term stent-related outcome, clinical, and hemodynamic result. *J Vasc Surg*. 2007;46:979-990.
61. Delis KT, Bjarnason H, Wennberg PW, Rooke TW, Gloviczki P. Successful iliac vein and inferior vena cava stenting ameliorates venous claudication and improves venous outflow, calf muscle pump function, and clinical status in post-thrombotic syndrome. *Ann Surg*. 2007;245:130-139.
62. Meissner AJ, Huszcza S. Surgical strategy for management of deep venous thrombosis of the lower extremities. *World J Surg*. 1996;20:1149-1155.
63. Wahlgren CM, Wahlberg E, Olofsson P. Endovascular treatment in postthrombotic syndrome. *Vasc Endovascular Surg*. 2010;44:356-360.
64. AbuRahma AF, Perkins SE, Wulu JT, Ng HK. Iliofemoral deep vein thrombosis: conventional therapy versus lysis and percutaneous transluminal angioplasty and stenting. *Ann Surg*. 2001;233:752-760.
65. Knipp BS, Ferguson E, Williams DM, et al. Factors associated with outcome after interventional treatment of symptomatic iliac vein compression syndrome. *J Vasc Surg*. 2007;46:743-749.
66. Hartung O, Otero A, Boufi M, et al. Mid-term results of endovascular treatment for symptomatic chronic nonmalignant iliocaval venous occlusive disease. *J Vasc Surg*. 2005;42:1138-1144; discussion 44.
67. Hartung O, Loundou AD, Barthelemy P, Arnoux D, Boufi M, Alimi YS. Endovascular management of chronic disabling ilio-caval obstructive lesions: long-term results. *Eur J Vasc Endovasc Surg*. 2009;38:118-124.
68. Rao AS, Konig G, Leers SA, et al. Pharmacomechanical thrombectomy for iliofemoral deep vein thrombosis: an alternative in patients with contraindications to thrombolysis. *J Vasc Surg*. 2009;50:1092-1098.
69. Baekgaard N, Broholm R, Just S, Jorgensen M, Jensen LP. Long-term results using catheter-directed thrombolysis in 103 lower limbs with acute iliofemoral venous thrombosis. *Eur J Vasc Endovasc Surg*. 2010;39:112-117.
70. Enden T, Haig Y, Klow NE, et al. Long-term outcome after additional catheter-directed thrombolysis versus standard treatment for acute iliofemoral deep vein thrombosis (the CaVenT study): a randomised controlled trial. *Lancet*. 2012;379:31-38.
71. Martinez Trabal JL, Comerota AJ, LaPorte FB, Kazanjian S, DiSalle R, Sepanski DM. The quantitative benefit of isolated, segmental, pharmacomechanical thrombolysis (ISPMT) for iliofemoral venous thrombosis. *J Vasc Surg*. 2008;48:1532-1537.
72. Parikh S, Motarjeme A, McNamara T, et al. Ultrasound-accelerated thrombolysis for the treatment of deep vein thrombosis: initial clinical experience. *J Vasc Interv Radiol*. 2008;19:521-528.
73. O'Sullivan GJ, Lohan DG, Gough N, Cronin CG, Kee ST. Pharmacomechanical thrombectomy of acute deep vein thrombosis with the Trellis-8 isolated thrombolysis catheter. *J Vasc Interv Radiol*. 2007;18:715-724.

chapter **24**

Thoracic Aortic Endovascular Repair

ARNOUD KAMMAN, MD, KAREN M. KIM, MD, DAVID M. WILLIAMS, MD, and HIMANSHU J. PATEL, MD

INTRODUCTION

Thoracic endovascular aortic repair (TEVAR), introduced by Dake et al in 1994,[1] has emerged as the preferred management strategy for multiple pathologic entities in the descending thoracic aorta such as complicated type B aortic dissection, fusiform and saccular aortic aneurysm, penetrating aortic ulcer, and blunt traumatic rupture.[2,3] TEVAR is less invasive than conventional open aortic repair and has also been successfully applied in more frail patients who are not candidates for conventional open repair. Unlike open repair, which requires significant physiologic reserve, TEVAR has anatomical constraints, such as adequate landing zones and access vessels needed for device delivery. Although open surgical repair is commonly used when TEVAR is not possible, several advances such as branched/fenestrated devices[4] and controlled rupture of iliofemoral vessels[5] have made endovascular procedures possible in these more complicated clinical scenarios. Complications unique to TEVAR include endoleak, stent graft–induced new entry tears, and less commonly, stent migration.[6-9] Neurologic complications such as spinal cord ischemia can occur after extensive coverage of the descending thoracic aorta.[10] In this chapter we will illustrate the use of TEVAR in several case scenarios and in stepwise complexity from treatment of an isolated descending aortic aneurysm to one encompassing use of branched endografts. For each case, we will present images in sequence from preoperative diagnosis to intraoperative angiograms and postoperative results. The accompanying legends will provide explanation about the specific phase of the procedure.

CASE 1 *TEVAR in an isolated saccular thoracic aortic aneurysm (FIGURES 24.1-24.11)*

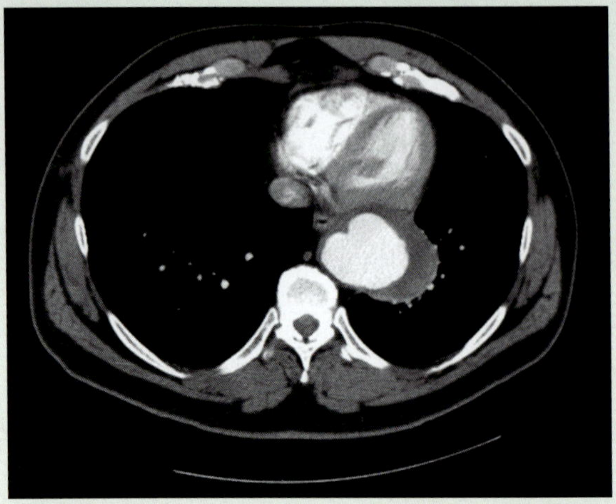

FIGURE 24.1 A 55-year old man presented with a saccular aneurysm measuring 7.8 × 5.7 × 5.6 cm in maximum diameter in the mid-descending thoracic aorta. He was evaluated for an elective standard TEVAR procedure.

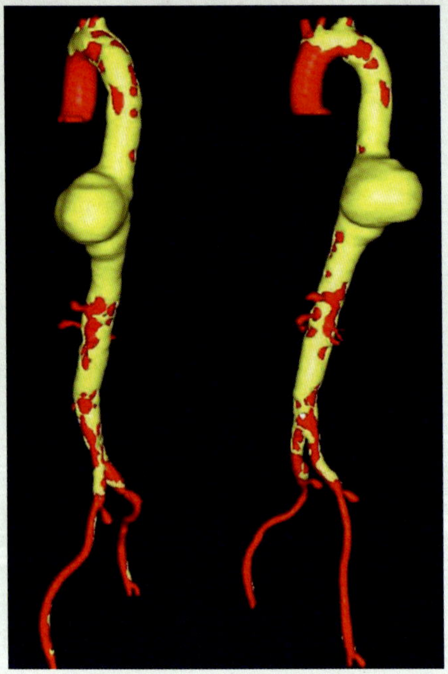

FIGURE 24.2 The iliofemoral vessels were straight and of adequate size for vascular access. The proximal landing zone was at least 2 cm, noncalcified, uniform in diameter, without mural thrombus and without aneurysmal involvement. The distal landing zone was straight and of sufficient length.

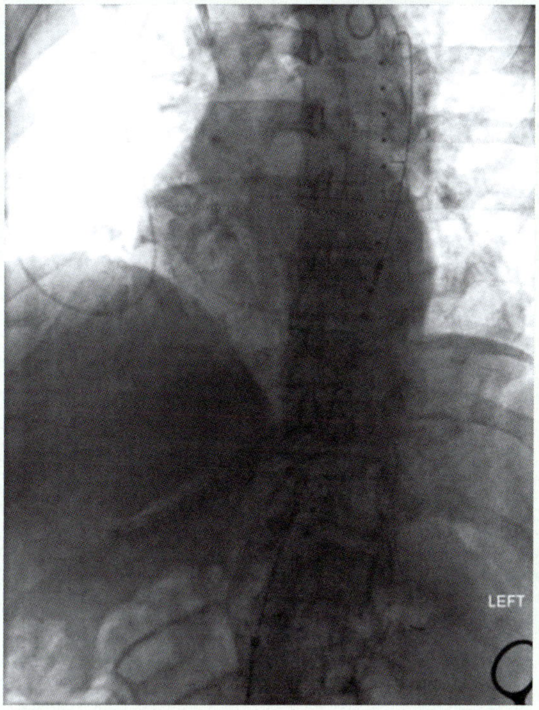

FIGURE 24.3 The left femoral artery was exposed for access and the right femoral artery was accessed percutaneously under ultrasound guidance.

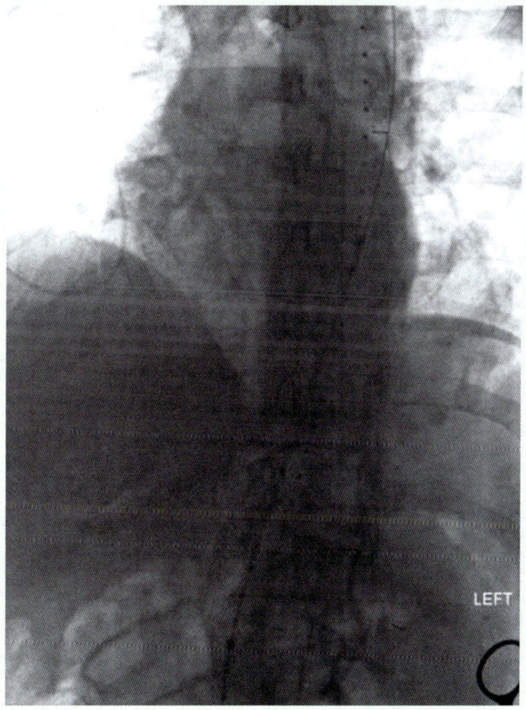

FIGURE 24.4 A guide wire was placed into the distal arch aorta via the right femoral artery.

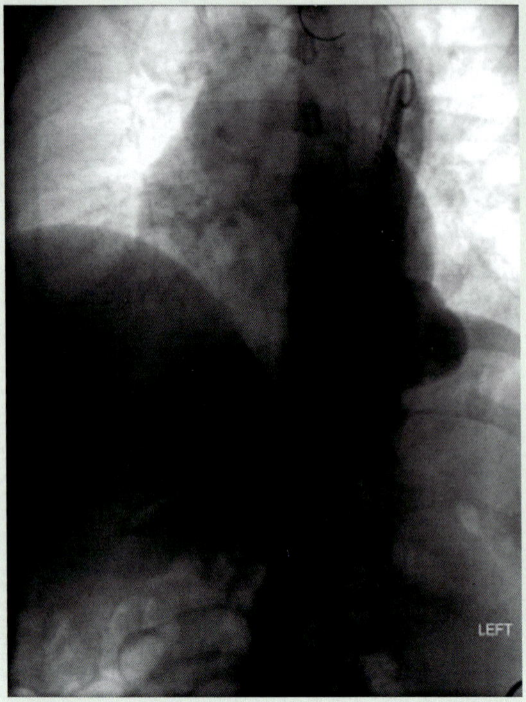

FIGURE 24.5 Intravascular ultrasound examination (not shown) confirmed the location of the large saccular aneurysm with no evidence of intramural hematoma or acute dissection. Thoracic aortography shows undeployed endograft centered on bilobed aneurysm in the distal descending aorta.

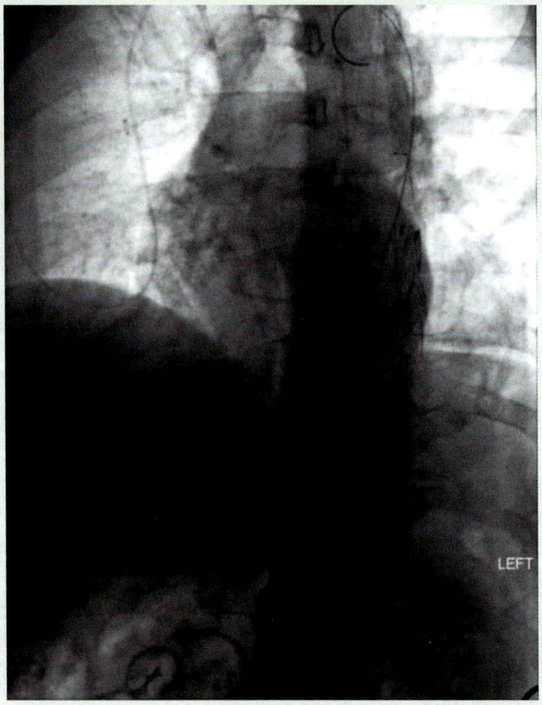

FIGURE 24.6 A 32 × 28 mm tapered Medtronic Valiant distal main stent graft, 150 mm in length, was selected for repair. The stent graft was placed approximately 1 cm above the location of the celiac artery to provide a 3 cm distal landing zone. The proximal edge of the stent graft was within 1 cm of the proximal landing zone.

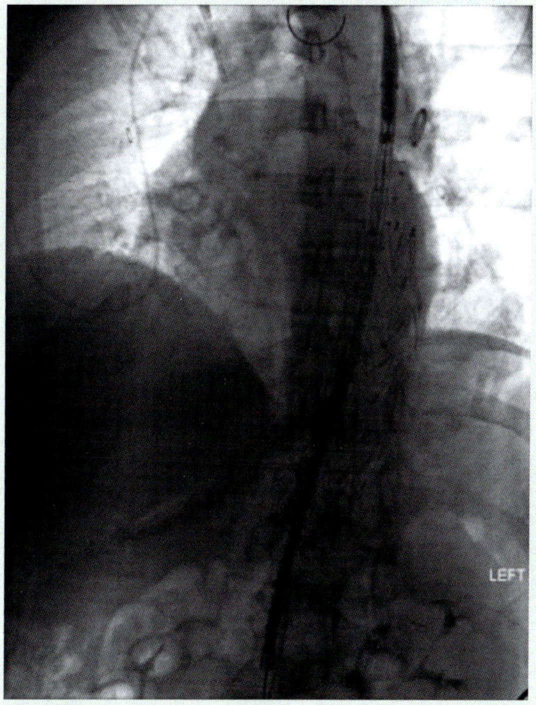

FIGURE 24.7 A second Medtronic Valiant proximal non-tapered main stent graft (32 mm diameter, 117 mm length) was then used with approximately a 6 to 7 cm overlap.

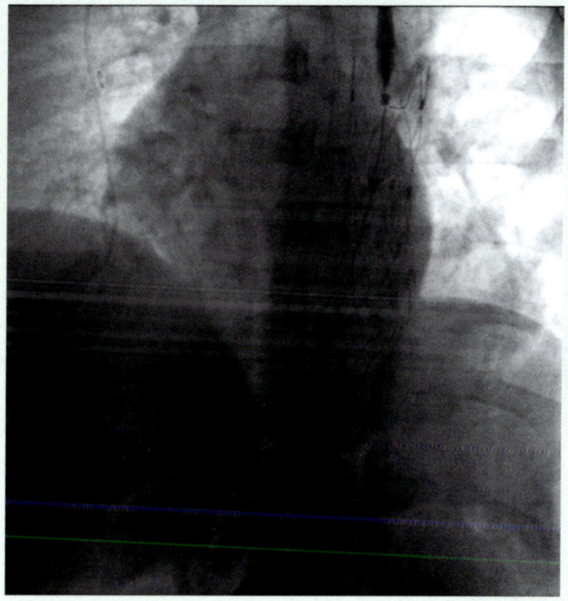

FIGURE 24.8 This device was then deployed.

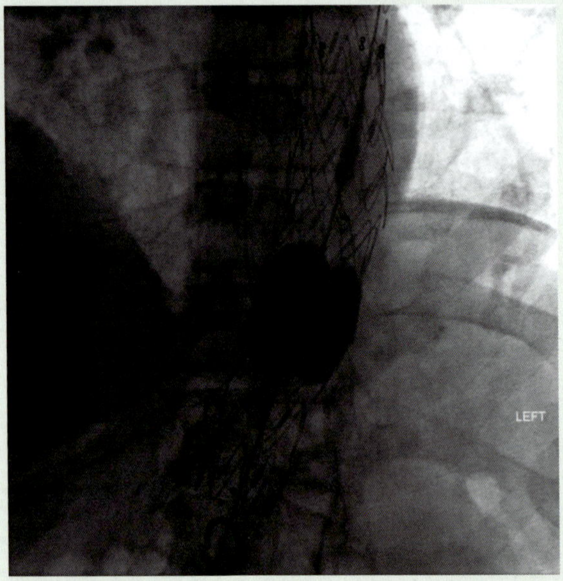

FIGURE 24.9 The overlap zones were balloon dilated to profile.

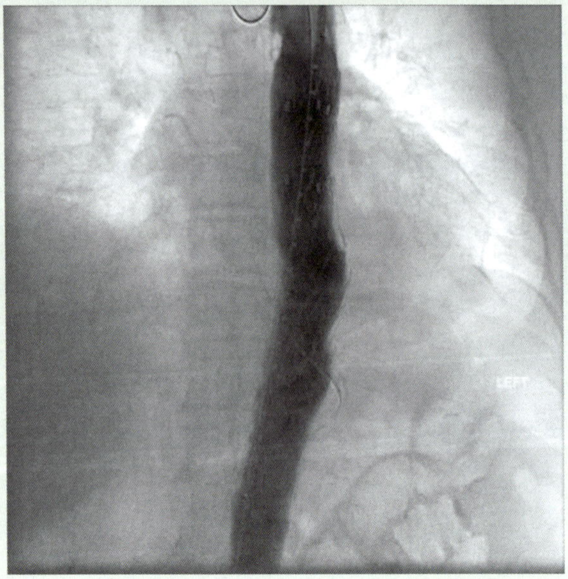

FIGURE 24.10 Completion of thoracic aortography revealed a sluggish type 4 endoleak and the opinion was that it was due to graft porosity and would resolve after heparin reversal.

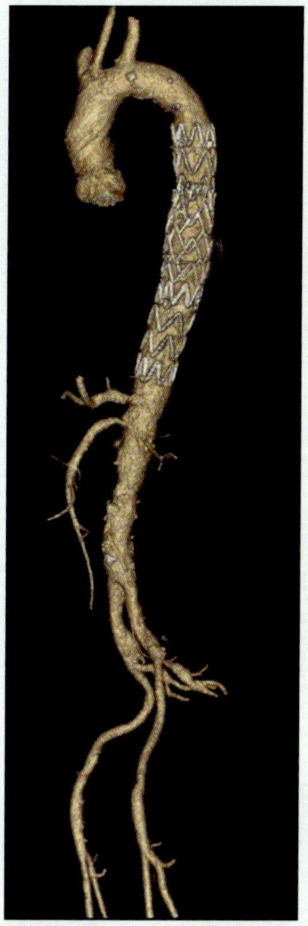

FIGURE 24.11 3D rendering of the postoperative result showed a patent stent graft with good apposition and exclusion of the aneurysm.

CASE 2 *TEVAR in an isolated thoracic aortic aneurysm with intramural thrombus (FIGURES 24.12-24.22)*

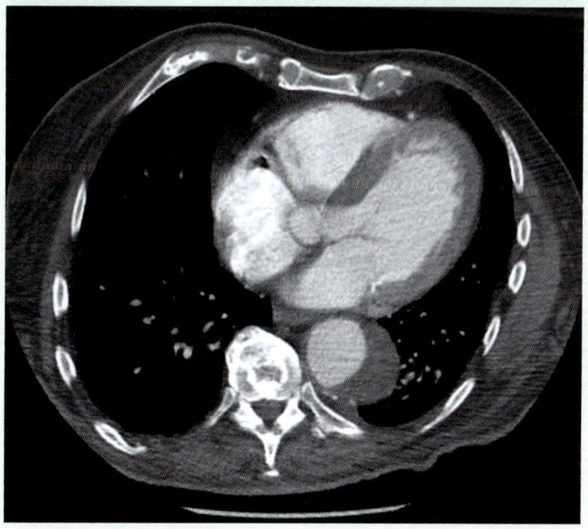

FIGURE 24.12 A 73-year old man presented to the ER with symptoms resembling an aortic dissection. CT-imaging revealed a descending aortic aneurysm, measuring 62 mm in diameter. He was evaluated for an elective TEVAR procedure.

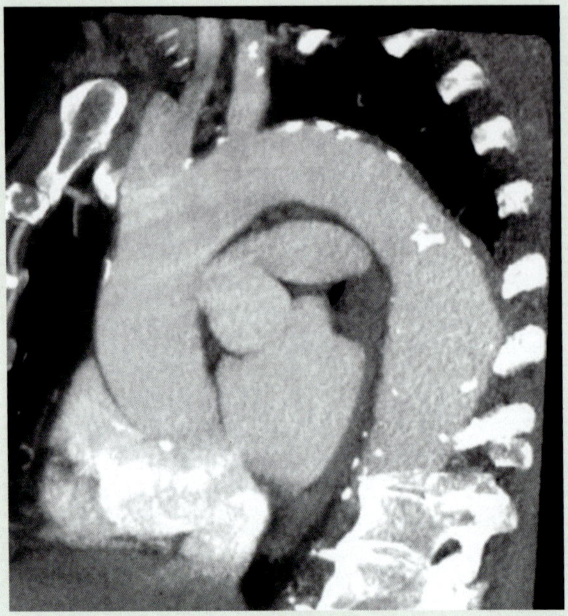

FIGURE 24.13 A proximal landing zone was identified of sufficient length (at least 2 cm noncalcified, uniform diameter, no mural thrombus) and without aneurysmal involvement, making this case suitable for a standard TEVAR procedure.

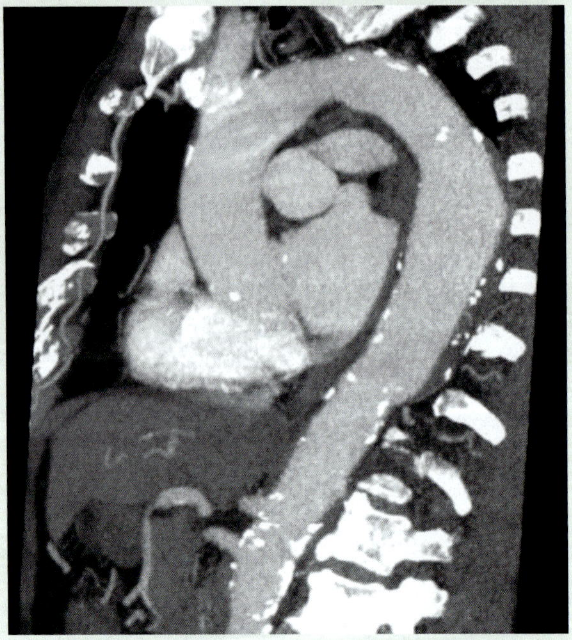

FIGURE 24.14 The distal landing zone was also of sufficient length, and the visceral vessels were not involved in the aortic aneurysm.

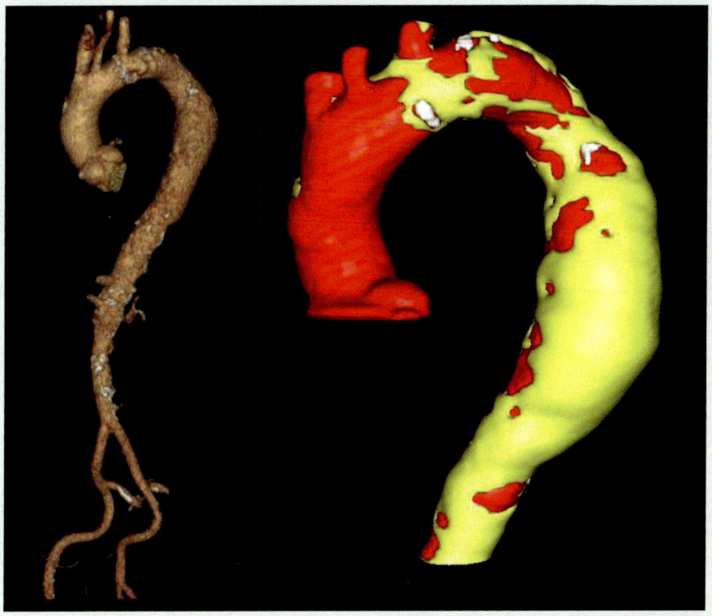

FIGURE 24.15 3D rendering and reconstruction with thrombus (yellow) of the aorta, demonstrating the descending aortic aneurysm. Both left and right iliofemoral vessels showed appropriate size, and lack of tortuosity and calcium for vascular access.

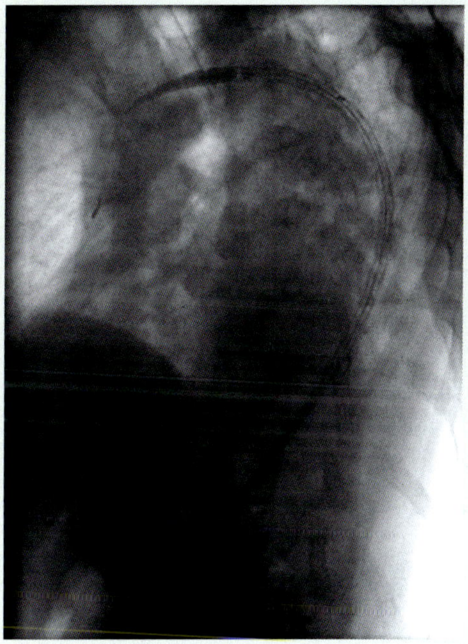

FIGURE 24.16 Both left and right femoral vessels were accessed and a pigtail and Lunderquist guide wire advanced. The endograft (Medtronic Valiant 36 × 36 × 200) was advanced over the stiff Lunderquist wire from the right femoral artery into the descending aorta. A thoracic aortogram was performed delineating the origin of the celiac artery.

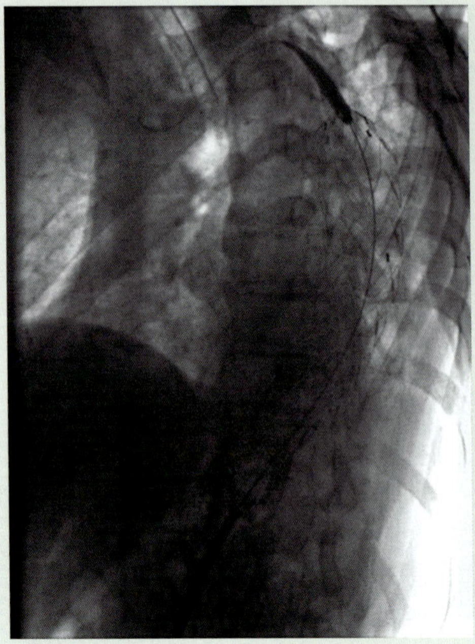

FIGURE 24.17 This device was then deployed approximately 3 cm above the celiac artery.

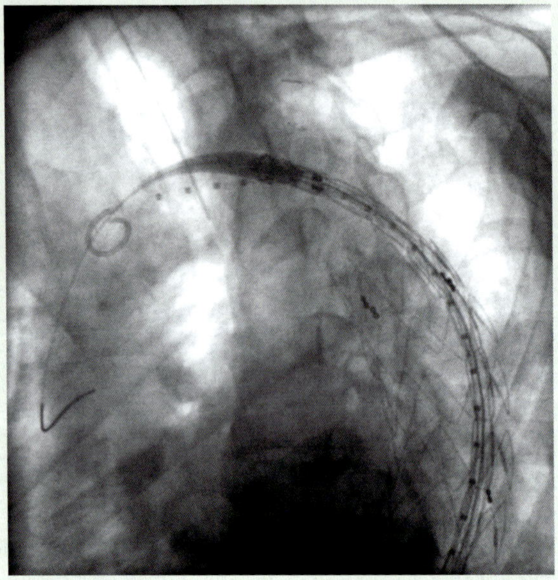

FIGURE 24.18 Proximal extension was deemed necessary and a second Medtronic thoracic stent graft was advanced (36 × 36 × 150 proximal main device).

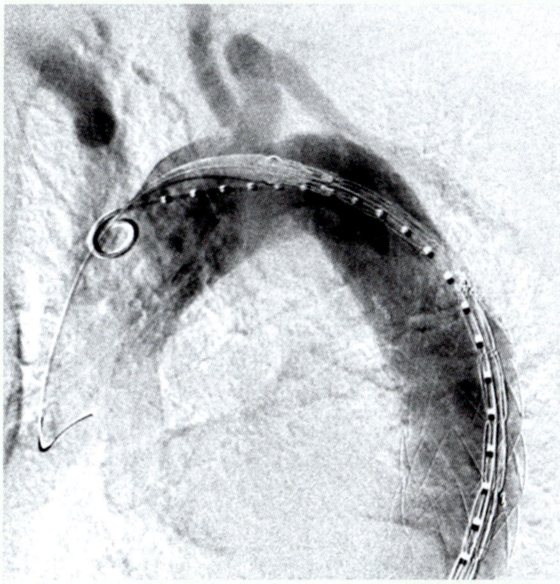

FIGURE 24.19 An intravascular ultrasound was performed and the location of the intraluminal thrombus as well as the left subclavian artery was noted.

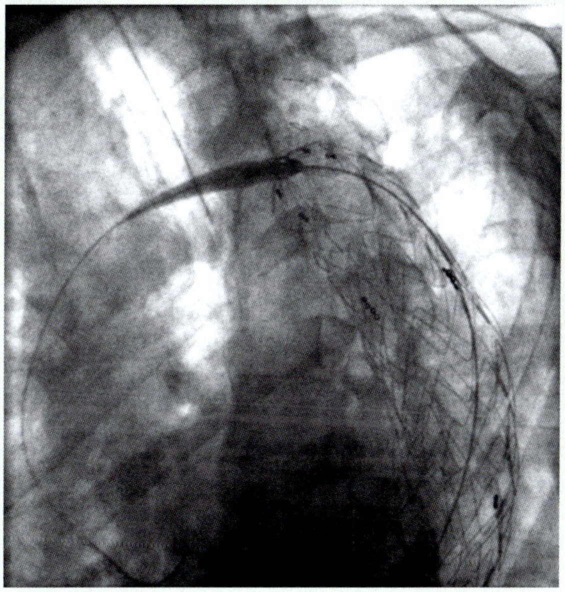

FIGURE 24.20 The second device was then deployed such that the proximal bare-metal flares were placed just distal to the origin of the mid–arch thrombus.

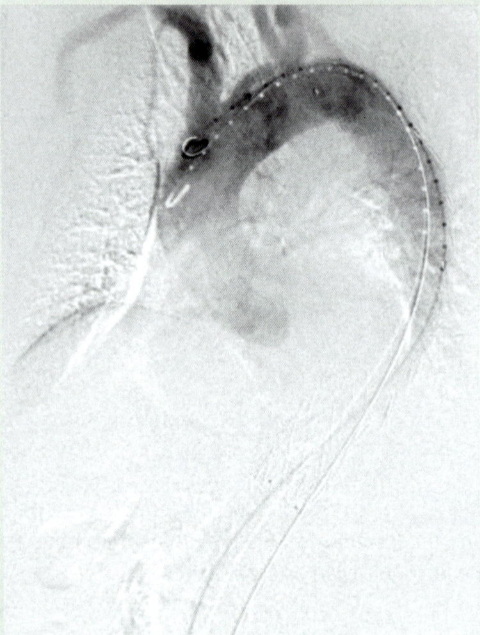

FIGURE 24.21 Completion thoracic aortography revealed brisk filling of the arch vessels and the celiac artery, and satisfactory exclusion of the thoracic aneurysm.

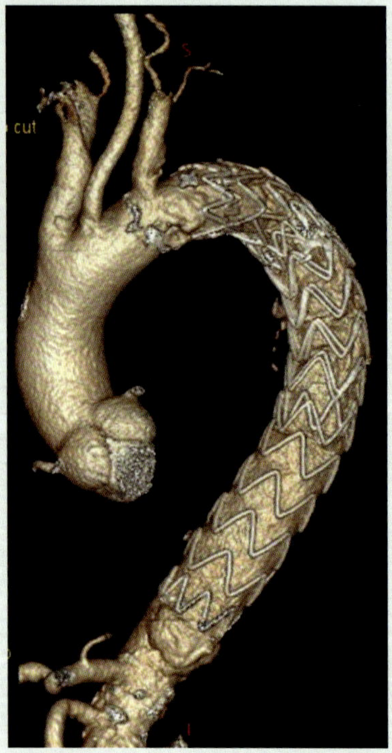

FIGURE 24.22 3D rendering showed good proximal position of the patent endograft as well as patent arch vessels.

CASE 3 *TEVAR for aortic aneurysm encroaching on the left subclavian artery necessitating revascularization (FIGURES 24.23-24.34)*

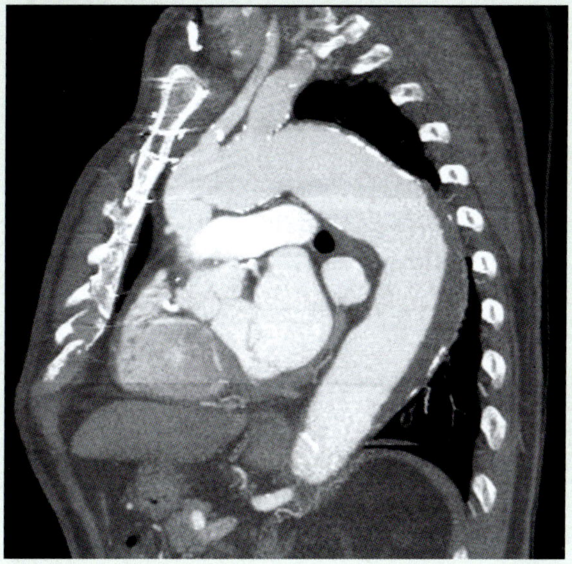

FIGURE 24.23 A 74-year old man with previous proximal aortic repair presented with degeneration of his descending aorta, measuring 5.5 cm. TEVAR was deemed appropriate and preoperative imaging was performed.

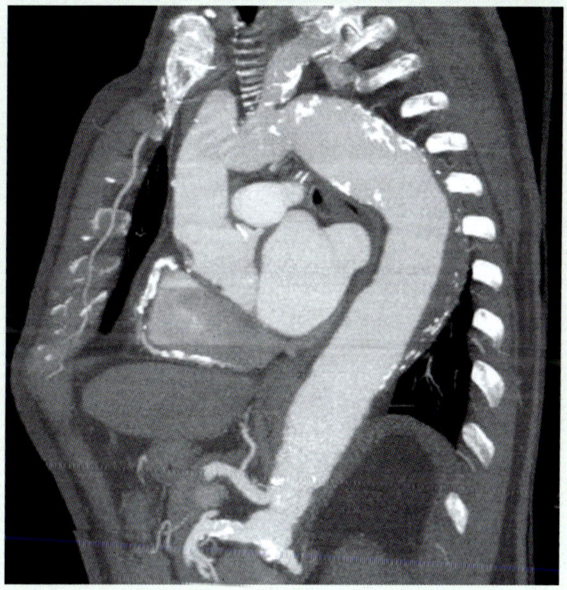

FIGURE 24.24 Preoperative CT imaging showed involvement of the distal arch/proximal descending aorta, requiring coverage of the left subclavian artery to achieve adequate proximal landing zone. Because of a patent LIMA to LAD bypass, a left carotid to left subclavian artery bypass was performed before TEVAR.

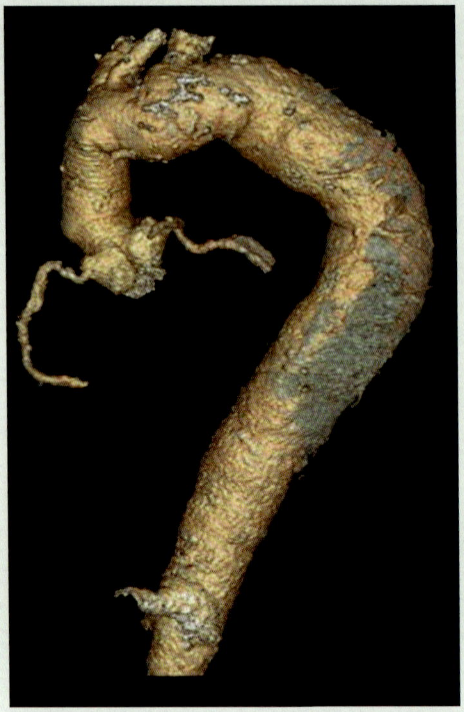

FIGURE 24.25 3D rendering showing involvement of the distal arch/proximal descending aorta and calcification along the entire descending aorta.

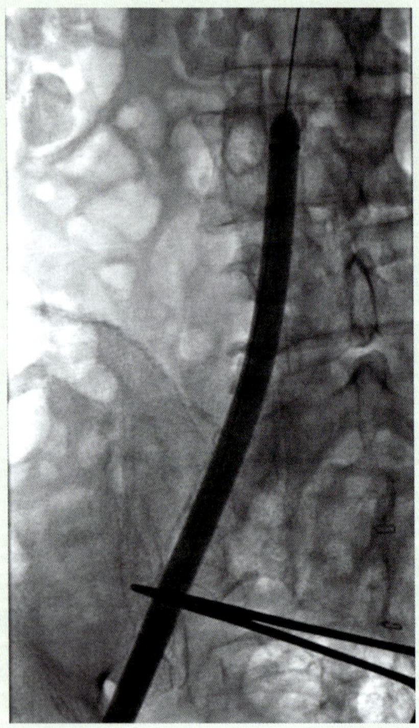

FIGURE 24.26 The femoral vessels were investigated and were of appropriate size and were not tortuous, allowing for femoral access. The right femoral artery was used as access vessel and the distal component (45 × 20 mm Gore C-TAG device) was advanced over a Lunderquist wire into the aortic arch.

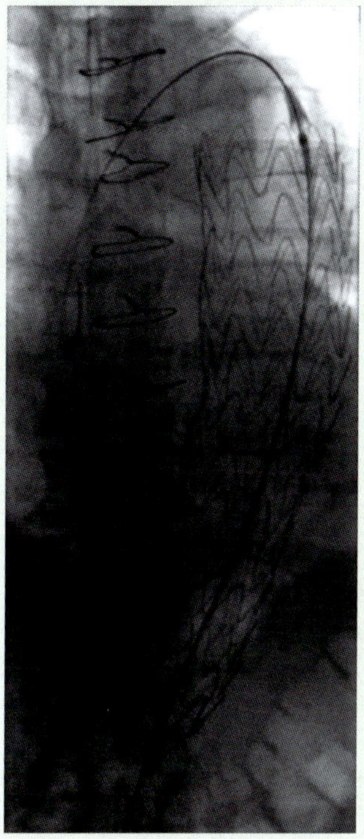

FIGURE 24.27 The distal component was then deployed approximately 3 cm above the celiac artery. Intravascular ultrasound was then used to find the orifice of the left carotid artery.

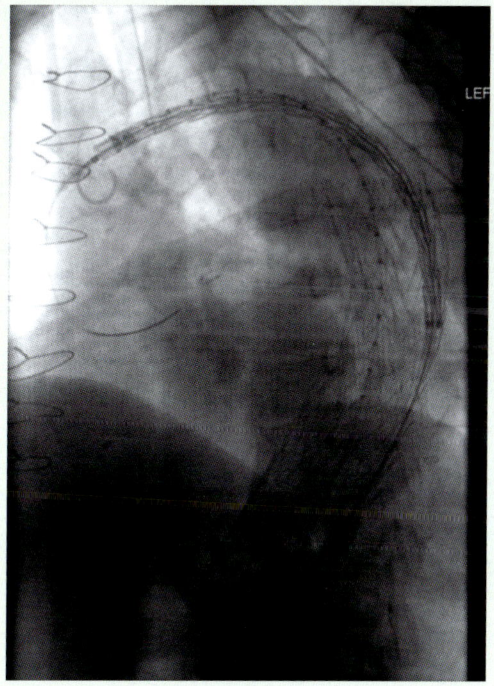

FIGURE 24.28 Another 45 × 20 Gore C-TAG device was advanced to rest within the aortic arch.

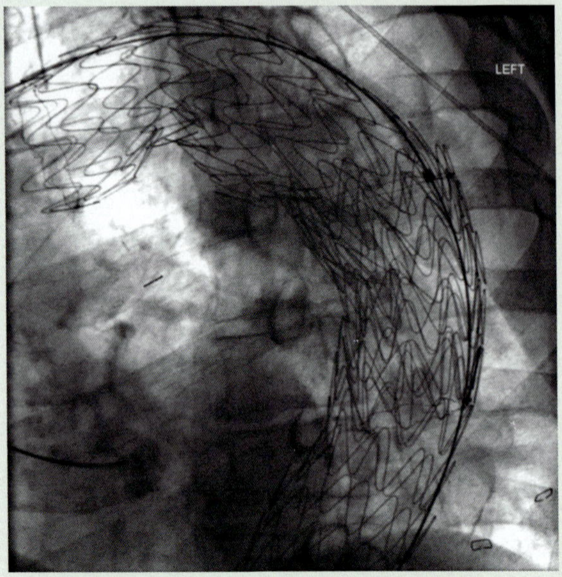

FIGURE 24.29 The proximal thoracic endograft was deployed to lie just distal to the origin of the left carotid artery.

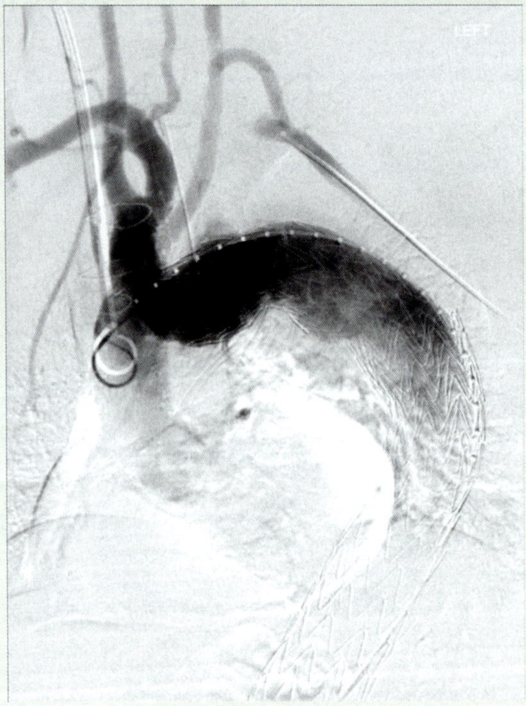

FIGURE 24.30 Completion angiogram showed brisk filling of the left carotid and innominate artery, as well as filling of the left subclavian artery via the bypass.

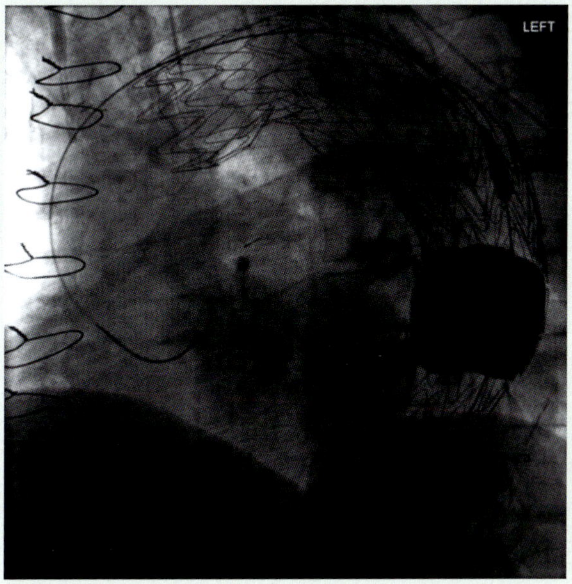

FIGURE 24.31 The overlap between the proximal and distal components was ballooned for adequate sealing.

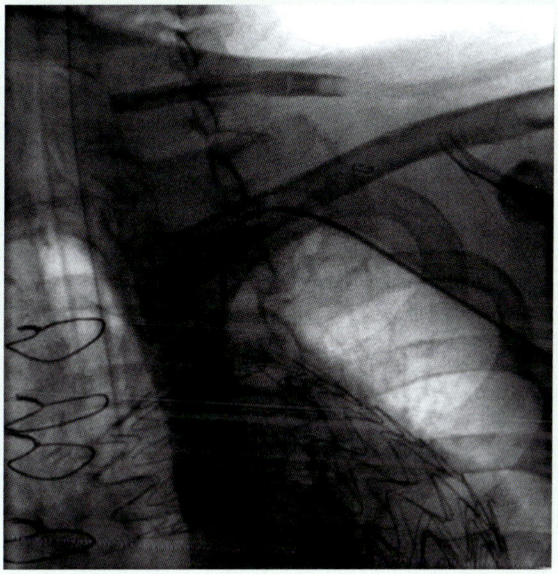

FIGURE 24.32 Because the aneurysm in the proximal landing zone encompassed the left subclavian artery origin, coil embolization was indicated. A catheter was advanced via the left brachial access toward the ostium of the left subclavian artery. An alternative approach could have been plug occlusion of the left subclavian artery orifice before TEVAR placement.

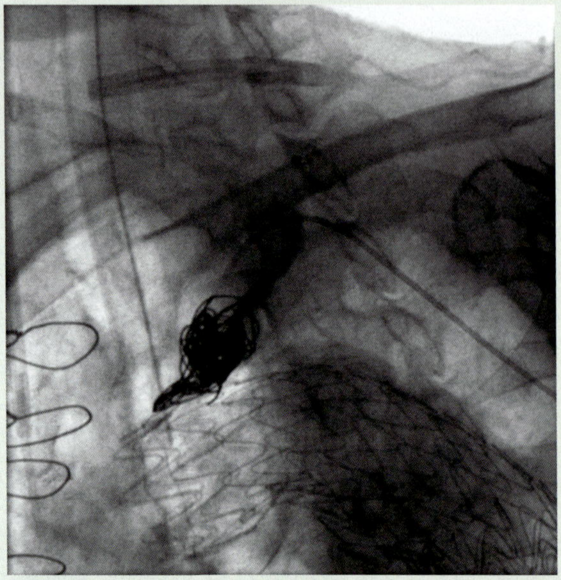

FIGURE 24.33 Several Nester coils (Cook, Incorporated, Bloomington IN) were deployed to ensure no retrograde type 2 endoleaks would occur after the procedure. Patency of the left vertebral artery was confirmed after coiling.

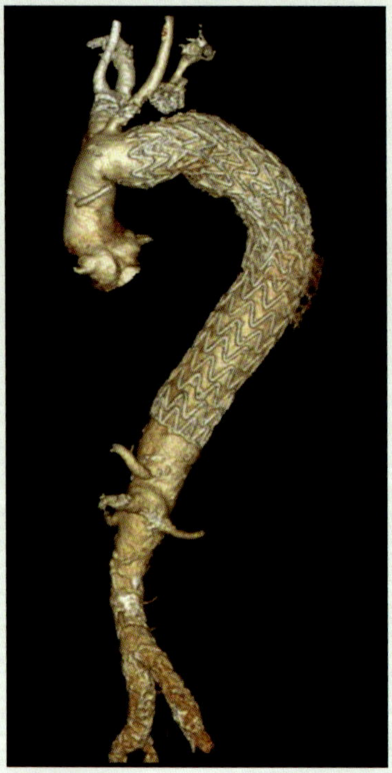

FIGURE 24.34 3D rendering of postoperative result with visible coils in the orifice of the left subclavian artery.

CASE 4 *TEVAR for ulcerlike lesion in proximity of left subclavian artery and with poor femoral access (FIGURES 24.35-24.49)*

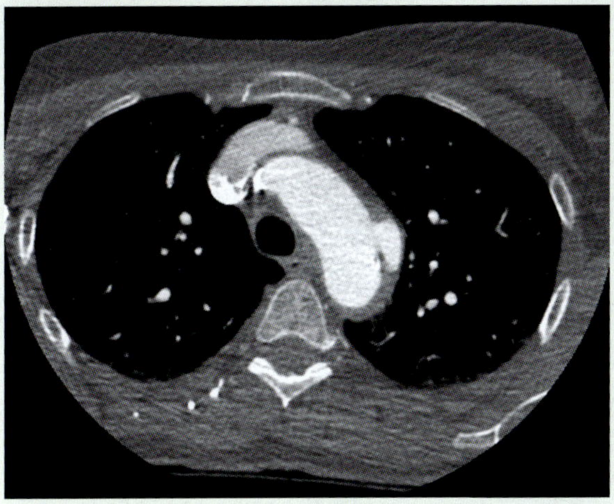

FIGURE 24.35 A 51-year-old woman presented with sudden onset of pain. Aortic imaging revealed a penetrating aortic ulcer in the arch with saccular aneurysm formation, in close proximity of the left subclavian artery.

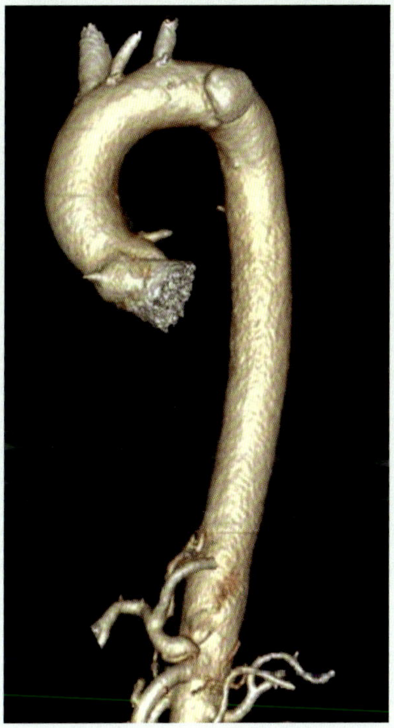

FIGURE 24.36 3D rendering of the aorta, showing the penetrating aortic ulcer with an appropriate straight distal landing zone. The proximal landing zone was not long enough to spare the left subclavian artery. Therefore the decision was made to perform a left subclavian to left carotid artery transposition prior to TEVAR.

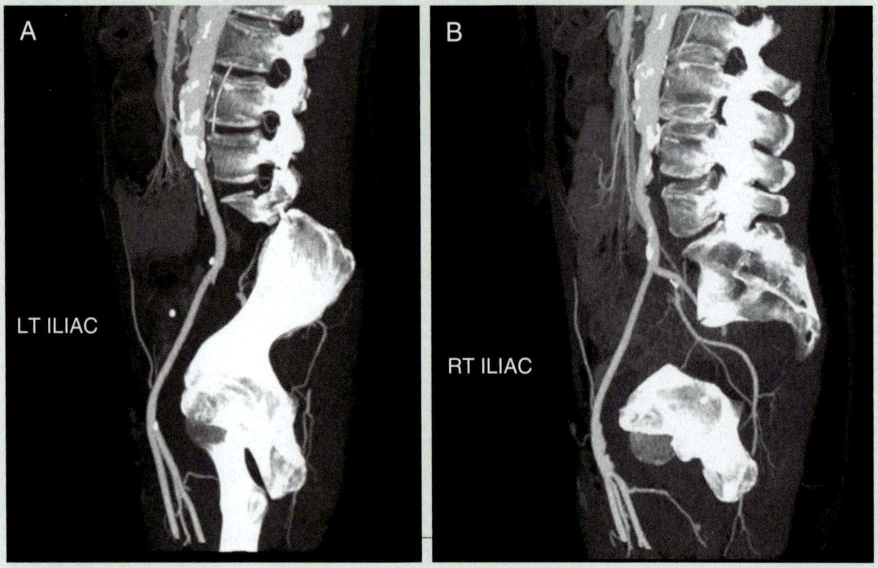

FIGURE 24.37 **A** and **B**, On the CT scan of the access vessels, both femoral arteries and external iliac arteries were 5 to 6 mm. Therefore, planned controlled pre-rupture of the right iliac artery was discussed. This has been shown to be a useful adjunct in selected cases of difficult iliofemoral access and can be done to avoid the morbidity of construction of a retroperitoneal iliac artery conduit.[5]

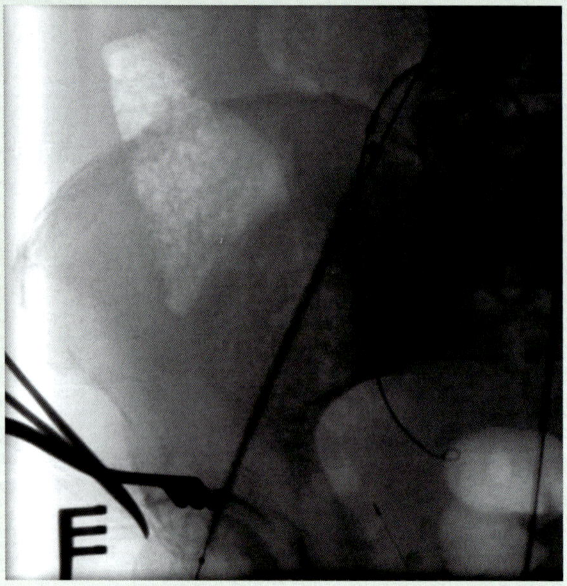

FIGURE 24.38 The right femoral artery was exposed and surrounded with vessel loops distally and proximally. The size of the external iliac artery was about 5 mm.

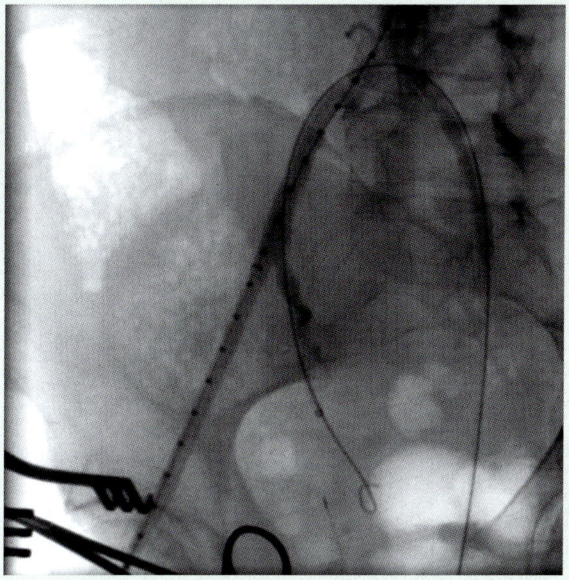

FIGURE 24.39 The left femoral artery was accessed. A 5 FR sheath was placed. An occlusion balloon was inserted from the left femoral artery into the right common and internal iliac arteries.

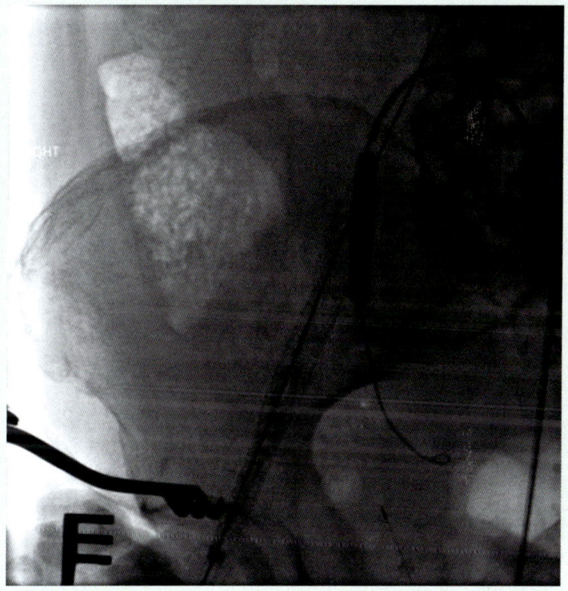

FIGURE 24.40 The balloon was inflated to occlude flow from the right common and internal iliac arteries. A 10 mm Viabahn stent graft was placed from the bifurcation of the right common iliac artery to the distal right internal iliac artery and femoral artery junction. The external iliac artery was then ruptured in controlled fashion with a noncompliant balloon.

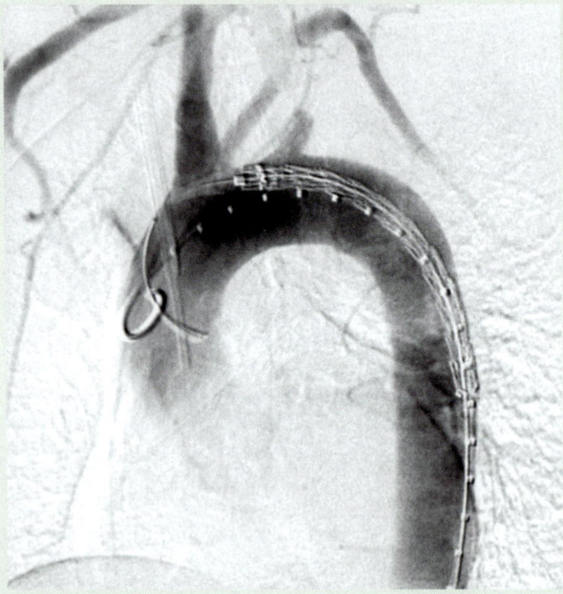

FIGURE 24.41 After obtaining controlled rupture access, the endograft was advanced over a Lunderquist wire and position checked. Filling of the innominate and left carotid artery can be seen, as well as filling of the left subclavian artery via the transposition.

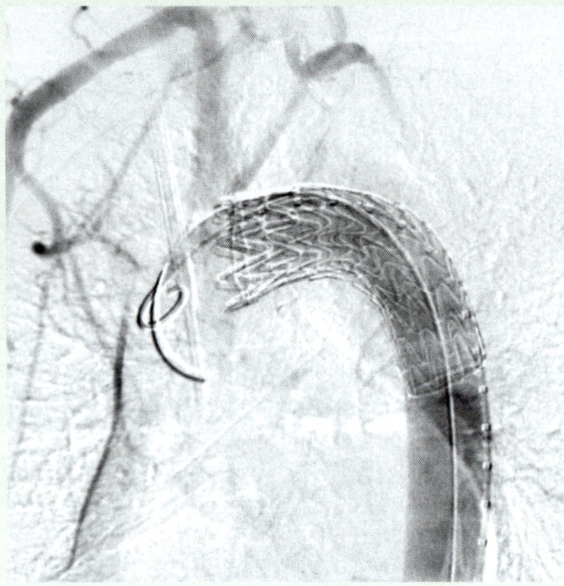

FIGURE 24.42 The endograft was then deployed, and it was noted to have jumped proximally to partially cover the orifice of the left carotid artery.

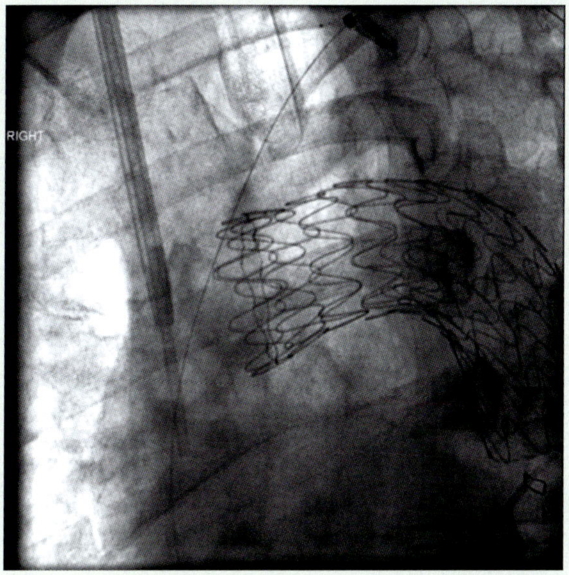

FIGURE 24.43 Left brachial access was used to advance a bare stent into the left carotid artery via the left carotid to left subclavian artery transposition and this was then deployed to ensure patency of the branch.

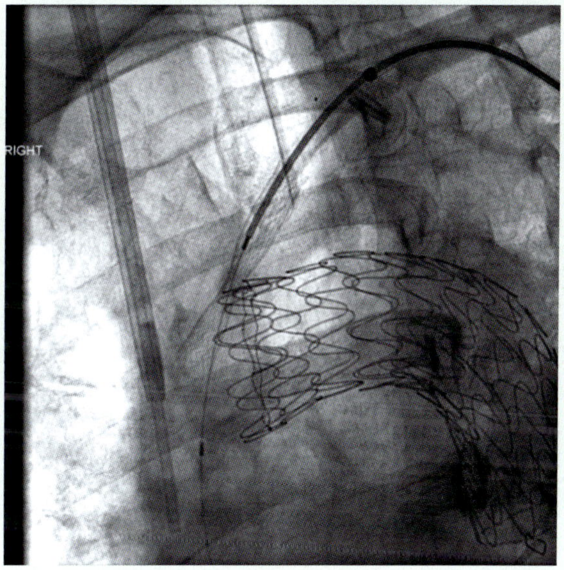

FIGURE 24.44 A second bare stent was needed to prevent collapse of the left carotid artery stent and also to ensure adequate caliber of the origin of the left carotid artery.

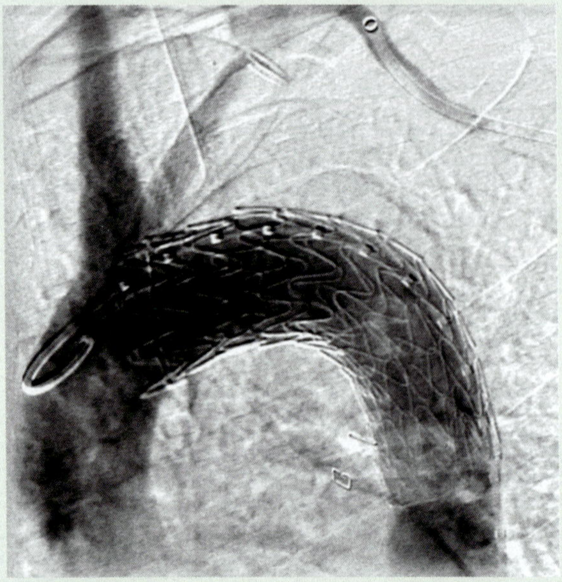

FIGURE 24.45 Filling of the left subclavian artery can be seen through the transposition performed before the TEVAR procedure.

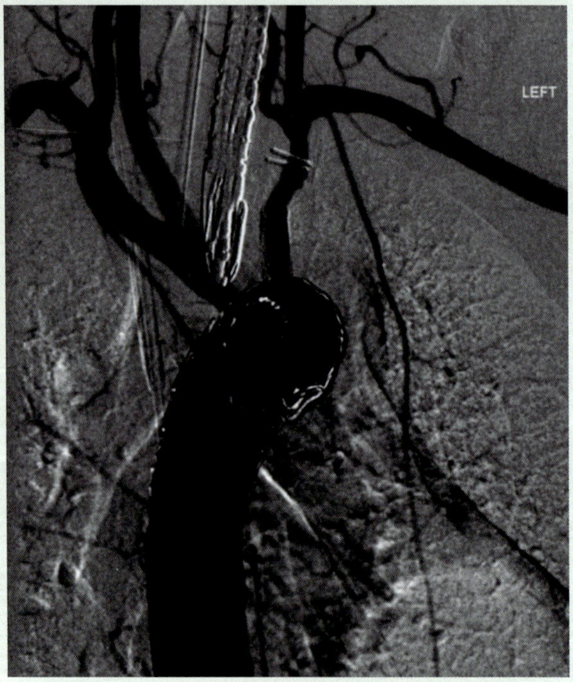

FIGURE 24.46 Completion angiogram shows brisk filling of all the arch vessels.

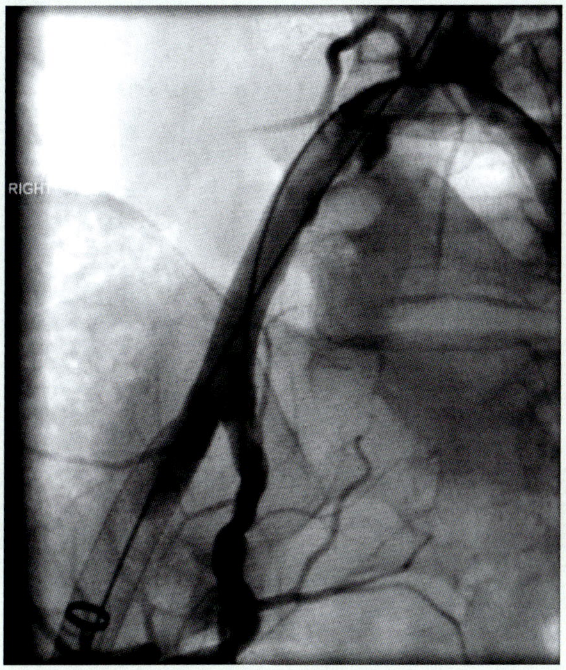

FIGURE 24.47 A bovine pericardial patch was used to repair the right external iliac and femoral arteries with 5-0 Prolene in running suture fashion. This angiogram shows a patent Viabahn graft in the right iliofemoral region. The sheath prevents outflow of contrast into the right leg but does show an intact iliac artery bifurcation.

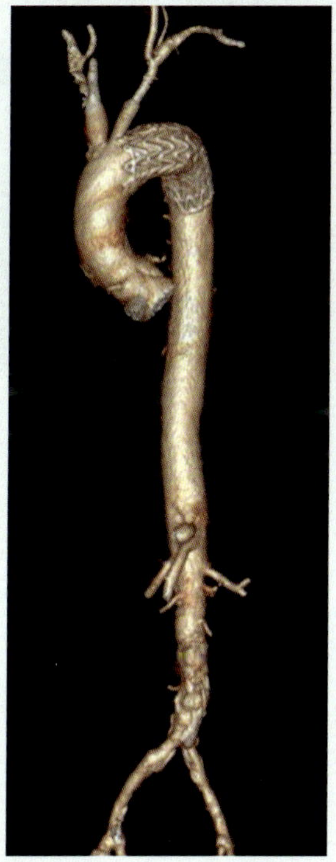

FIGURE 24.48 3D rendering showing a patent left carotid artery and correct positioning of the endograft in the descending aorta.

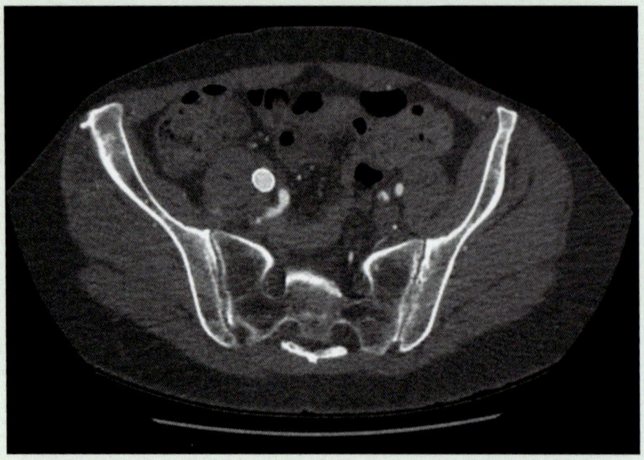

FIGURE 24.49 The Viabahn stent in the right iliofemoral section was widely patent.

CASE 5 *TEVAR with necessity of distal extension requiring celiac stenting (snorkel stent graft) (FIGURES 24.50-24.59)*

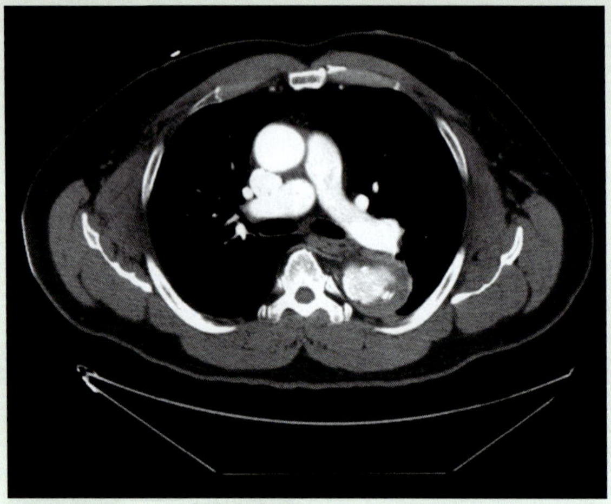

FIGURE 24.50 A 65-year-old was treated previously with TEVAR in an outside hospital for a descending thoracic aneurysm.

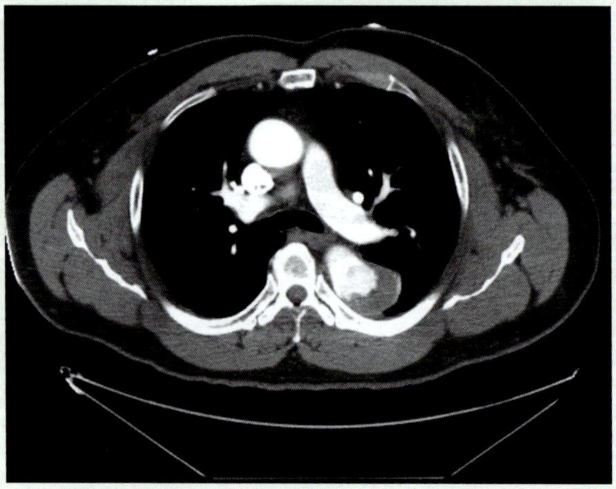

FIGURE 24.51 He underwent TEVAR with implantation of 2 devices. At that time he did not have any endoleaks or other procedure-related problems.

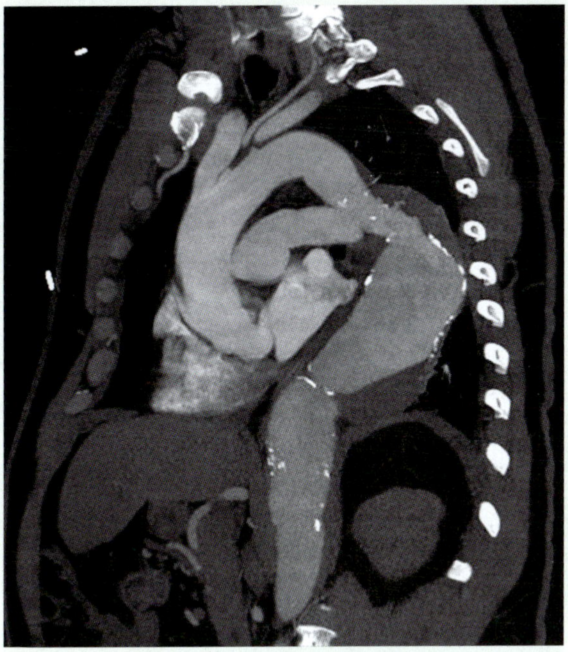

FIGURE 24.52 Sagittal view of the original un treated thoracic aneurysm. In 2015 he presented with a type 1B endoleak, and a secondary TEVAR procedure was planned. Snorkeling of the celiac artery was deemed necessary to preserve this vessel.

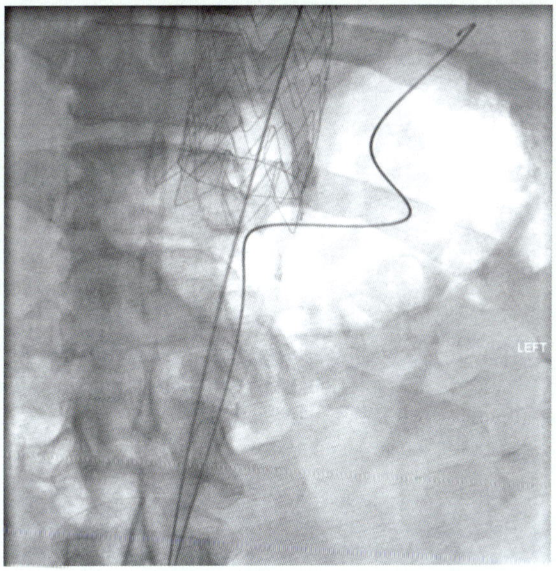

FIGURE 24.53 Intraoperative angiogram showing the previously deployed endograft in the descending aorta. A Rosen wire was advanced into the celiac artery and a Lunderquist into the aorta.

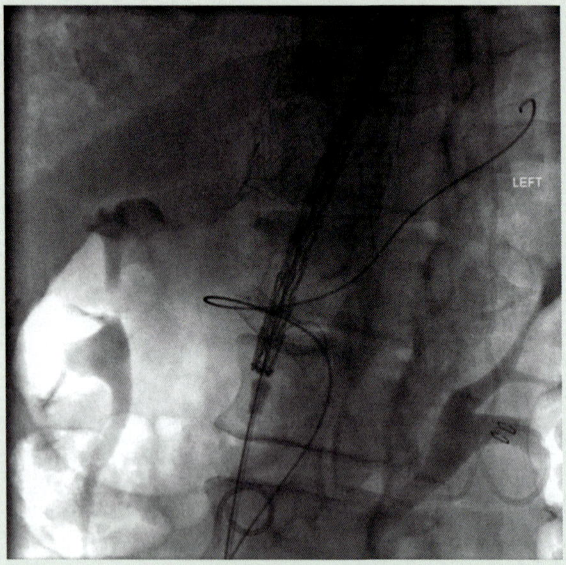

FIGURE 24.54 The distal extension endograft (37 × 15 Gore C-TAG) was positioned in the distal descending aorta, while the guide wire in the celiac artery is kept in place.

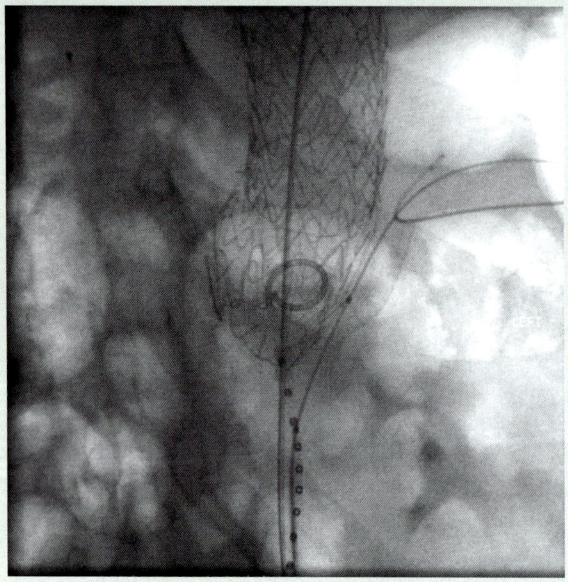

FIGURE 24.55 The celiac artery stent graft (11 × 5 Viabahn) was then deployed and a balloon placed in the orifice. The distal extension (37 × 15 Gore C-TAG) was subsequently deployed over the native celiac artery orifice.

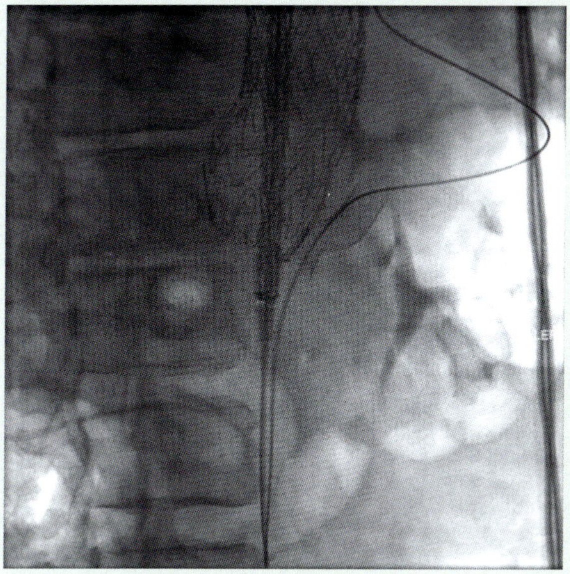

FIGURE 24.56 Another extension of both the aortic segment and the celiac stent graft was needed because of a persistent type 1B endoleak.

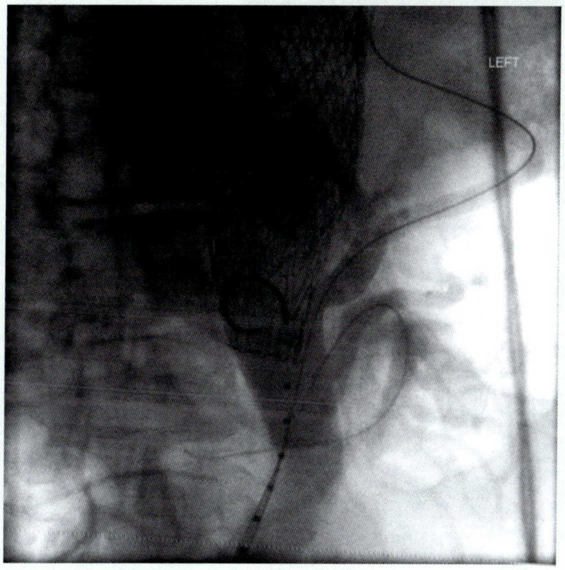

FIGURE 24.57 After this extension, the intraoperative angiogram showed a patent celiac artery and no endoleaks.

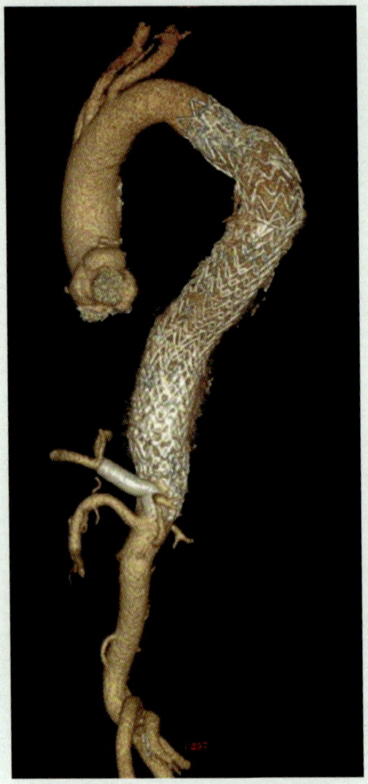

FIGURE 24.58 3D rendering of the completed procedure; the stent in the celiac artery can be clearly observed.

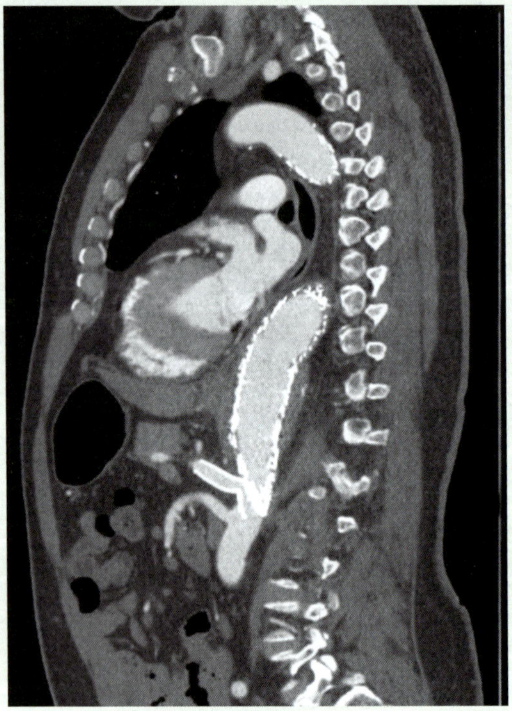

FIGURE 24.59 Clear patency of the celiac trunk can be observed on postoperative CT scans.

CASE 6 *Branched TEVAR procedure for arch lesion (FIGURES 24.60-24.73)*

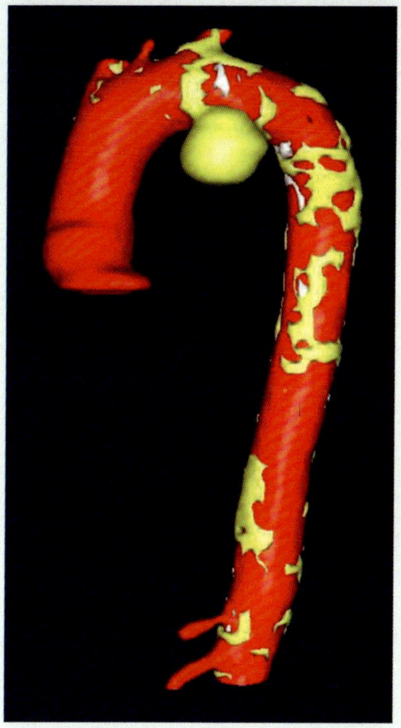

FIGURE 24.60 A 77-year-old man presented with an incidental finding of a saccular aortic aneurysm in the aortic arch measuring 3.6 × 3.7 cm and encroaching on the arch vessels. Because of the location of the disease, the inferior aortic arch, and a saccular aneurysm, an intervention was deemed appropriate. The patient consented for a clinical trial for placement of a Thoracic Branched Endoprosthesis (W.L. Gore). Thrombus can be seen within the saccular aneurysm of the aortic arch (yellow).

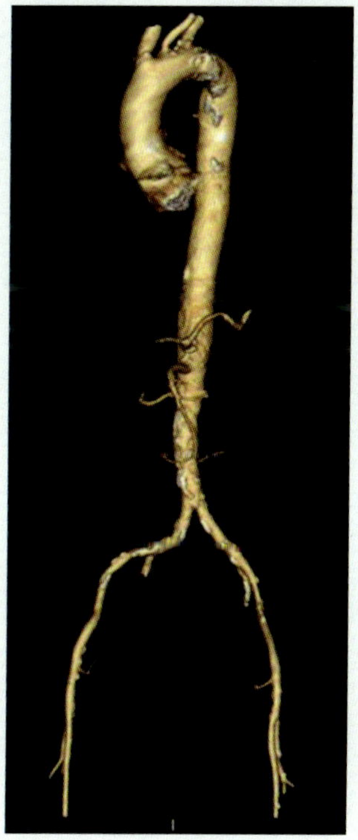

FIGURE 24.61 Both iliac vessels showed iliac anatomy suitable for vascular access.

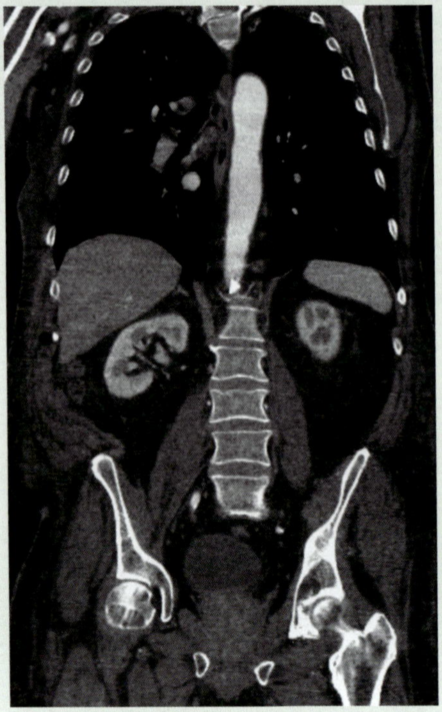

FIGURE 24.62 The distal landing zone is straight and of sufficient length.

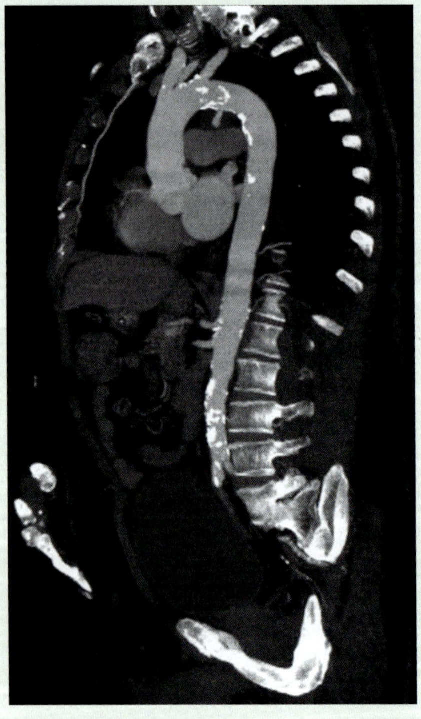

FIGURE 24.63 The arch contains some calcifications, but is of sufficient length to allow stent graft apposition in zone 2.

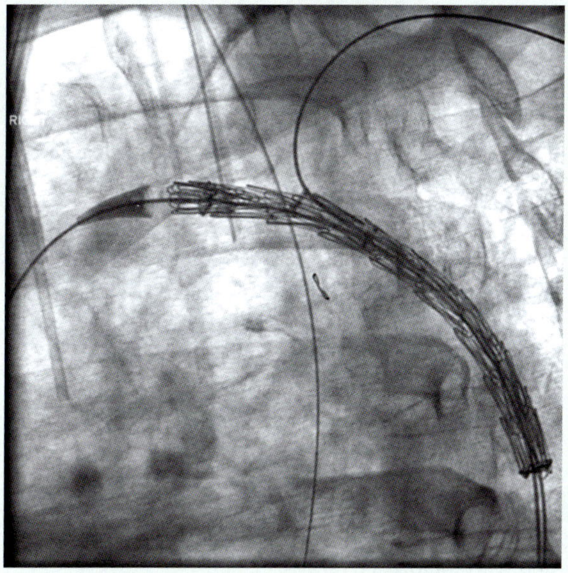

FIGURE 24.64 Both femoral and the left brachial arteries were used for vascular access. Through and through access for the side branch component was obtained via a snare in the ascending aorta. This wire was then exchanged for an Amplatz Super Stiff wire.

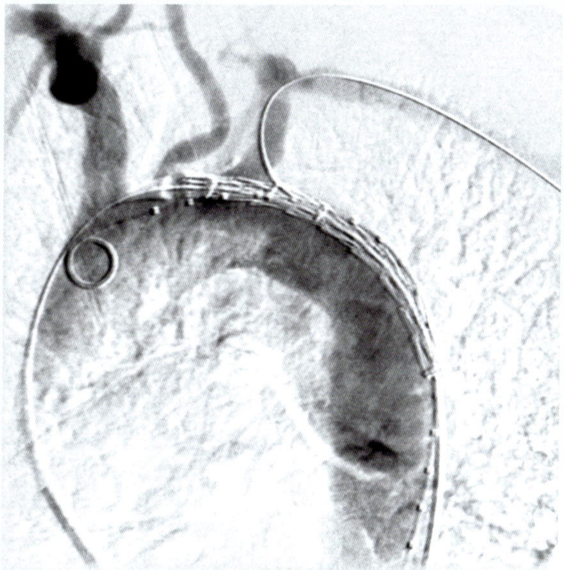

FIGURE 24.65 The branched endograft was precannulated and advanced over both wires into the aortic arch, with the branch guide wire in the left subclavian artery. The position of the stent graft was checked via angiogram.

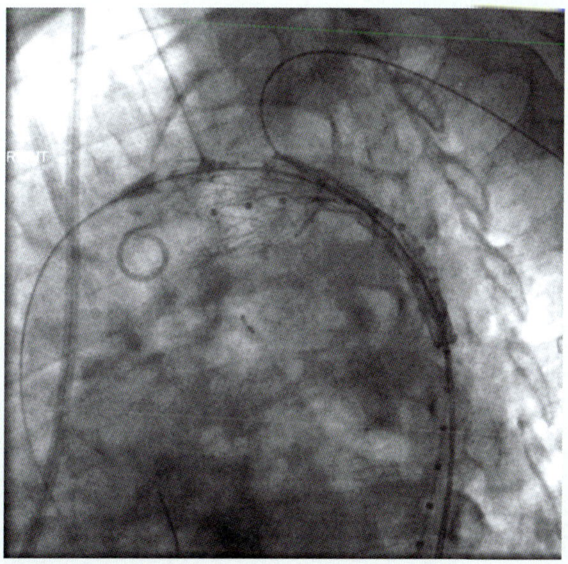

FIGURE 24.66 The main body (37 × 10 Gore TBE, 8 mm portal) was then deployed in the appropriate position, paying special attention to the branch.

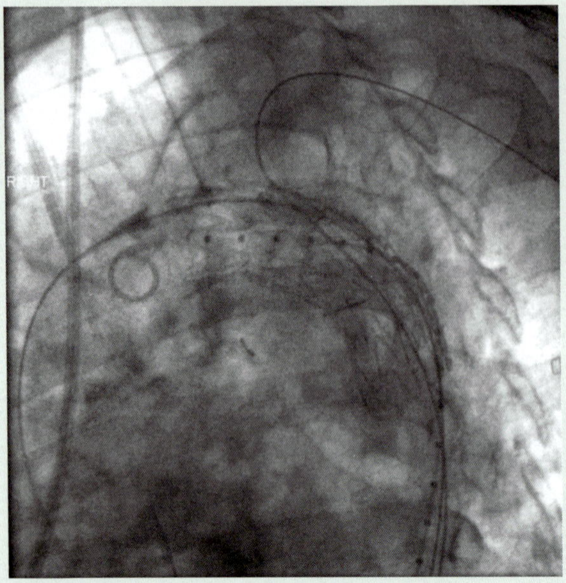

FIGURE 24.67 The through and through wire was exchanged for a Rosen wire and the side branch cannulated with the branch device.

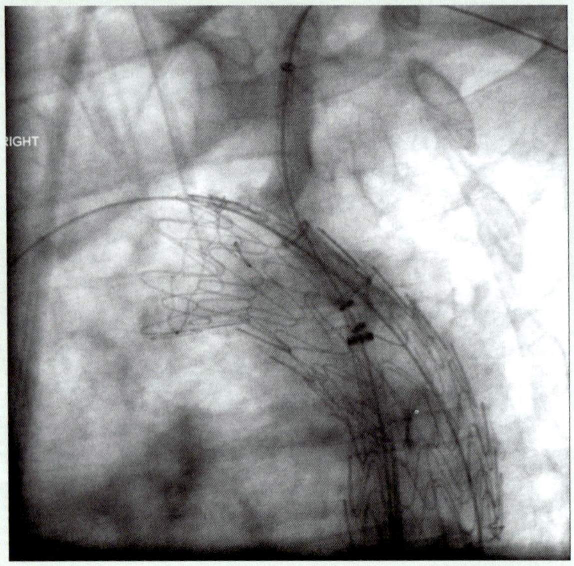

FIGURE 24.68 This side branch endograft (8 mm portal, 12 mm diameter, 6 cm length) was then deployed in the left subclavian artery.

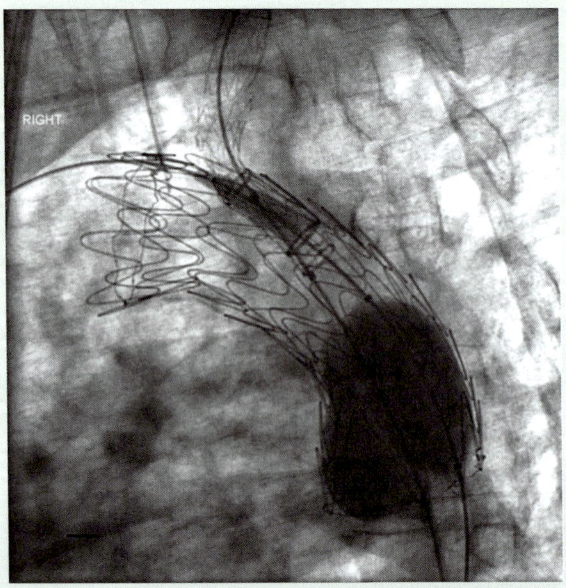

FIGURE 24.69 The distal and proximal landing zones were then balloon dilated.

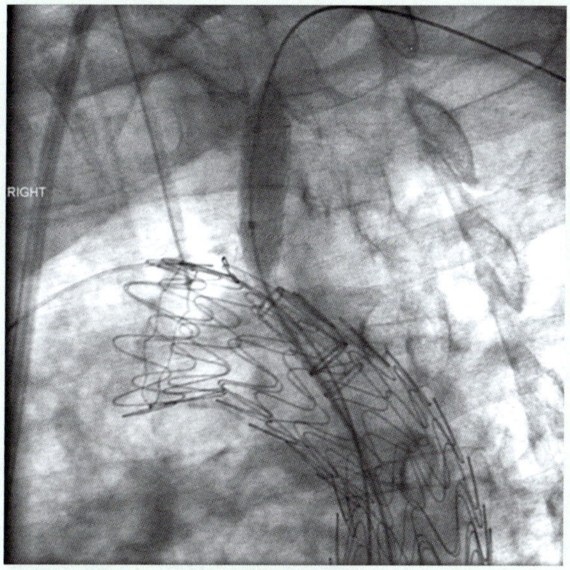

FIGURE 24.70 The branch vessel was then ballooned at the proximal and distal landing zones, as well as in the portal.

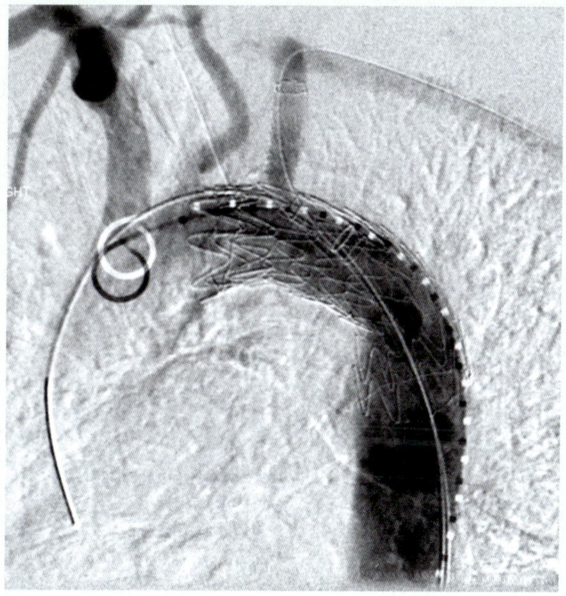

FIGURE 24.71 Completion of thoracic aortography revealed no evidence of endoleak and brisk filling of all arch vessels.

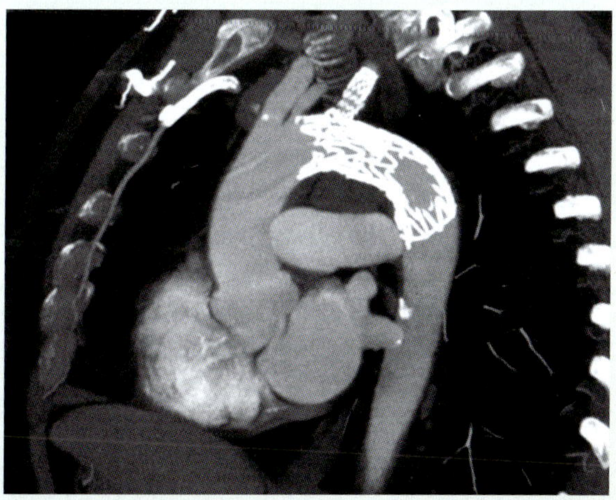

FIGURE 24.72 Postoperative results showing good positioning of the left subclavian artery branch and patency of the graft.

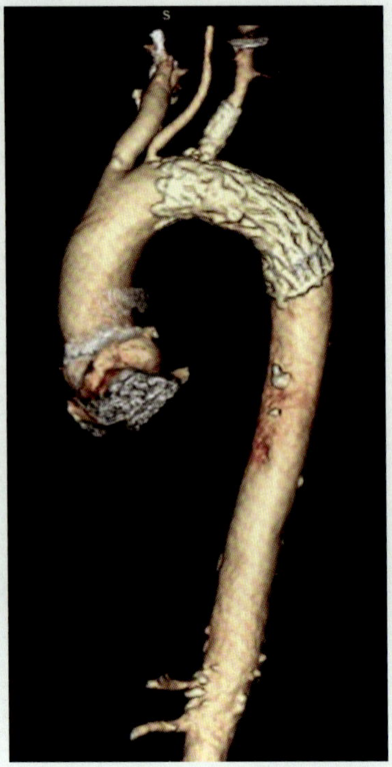

FIGURE 24.73 3D rendering of the postoperative result.

POSSIBLE CONFLICT OF INTEREST

Dr Patel has consulting relationship with W.L. Gore, Medtronic, and Terumo. Dr Williams discloses financial relationships with W.L. Gore and Boston Scientific.

ACKNOWLEDGMENTS

Dr Patel was generously supported by the David Hamilton Fund and the Phil Jenkins Breakthrough Fund in Cardiac Surgery at the University of Michigan Frankel Cardiovascular Center.

REFERENCES

1. Dake MD, Miller DC, Semba CP, Mitchell RS, Walker PJ, Liddell RP. Transluminal placement of endovascular stent-grafts for the treatment of descending thoracic aortic aneurysms. *N Engl J Med*. 1994;331(26):1729-1734.
2. Erbel R, Aboyans V, Boileau C, et al. 2014 ESC Guidelines on the diagnosis and treatment of aortic diseases: document covering acute and chronic aortic diseases of the thoracic and abdominal aorta of the adult. The Task Force for the Diagnosis and Treatment of Aortic Diseases of the European Society of Cardiology (ESC). *Eur Heart J*. 2014;35(41):2873-2926.
3. Hiratzka LF, Bakris GL, Beckman JA, et al. 2010 ACCF/AHA/AATS/ACR/ASA/SCA/SCAI/SIR/STS/SVM guidelines for the diagnosis and management of patients with thoracic aortic disease: a report of the American College of Cardiology Foundation/American Heart Association Task Force on Practice Guidelines, American Association for Thoracic Surgery, American College of Radiology, American Stroke Association, Society of Cardiovascular Anesthesiologists, Society for Cardiovascular Angiography and Interventions, Society of Interventional Radiology, Society of Thoracic Surgeons, and Society for Vascular Medicine. *Circulation*. 2010;121(13):e266-e369.
4. Verhoeven EL, Paraskevas KI, Oikonomou K, et al. Fenestrated and branched stent-grafts to treat post-dissection chronic aortic aneurysms after initial treatment in the acute setting. *J Endovasc Ther*. 2012;19(3):343-349.
5. van Bogerijen GH, Williams DM, Eliason JL, Dasika NL, Deeb GM, Patel HJ. Alternative access techniques with thoracic endovascular aortic repair, open iliac conduit versus endoconduit technique. *J Vasc Surg*. 2014;60(5):1168-1176.
6. Dong Z, Fu W, Wang Y, et al. Stent graft-induced new entry after endovascular repair for Stanford type B aortic dissection. *J Vasc Surg*. 2010;52(6):1450-1457.
7. Eggebrecht H, Thompson M, Rousseau H, et al. Retrograde ascending aortic dissection during or after thoracic aortic stent graft placement: insight from the European registry on endovascular aortic repair complications. *Circulation*. 2009;120(suppl 11):S276-S281.
8. Yunoki J, Kuratani T, Shirakawa Y, et al. Mid-term results of endovascular treatment with the Gore TAG device for degenerative descending thoracic aortic aneurysms. *Gen Thorac Cardiovasc Surg*. 2015;63(1):38-42.
9. Foley PJ, Criado FJ, Farber MA, et al. Results with the talent thoracic stent graft in the VALOR trial. *J Vasc Surg*. 2012;56(5):1214-1221.e1.
10. Czerny M, Eggebrecht H, Sodeck G, et al. Mechanisms of symptomatic spinal cord ischemia after TEVAR: insights from the European registry of endovascular aortic repair complications (EuREC). *J Endovasc Ther*. 2012;19(1):37-43.

chapter **25**

Percutaneous Epicardial Techniques

JUAN F. VILES-GONZALEZ, MD, FACC, FAHA, FHRS and ANDRÉ D'AVILA, MD

Percutaneous access to the pericardial cavity (pericardiocentesis) is typically performed for drainage of pericardial effusions. In the absence of effusion, epicardial access can also be obtained during epicardial ablation of arrhythmias, certain structural heart disease procedures such as percutaneous closure of the left atrial appendage, and, more rarely, balloon pericardiotomy.[1-7] A systematic approach to the patient evaluated for such procedures is paramount (**FIGURE 25.1**). The presence of adhesions (more frequent in patients with prior cardiac surgery or history of pericarditis) can complicate percutaneous access to the pericardial space.[7] In this situation, surgical consultation for possible pericardial window and lysis of adhesions should be considered.

The pericardial cavity is a virtual space between the parietal and visceral layers of the serous pericardium. It is continuous with the epicardium and reflects around the roots of the great vessels and onto the visceral surface of the fibrous pericardium. The visceral surface of the pericardium is continuous with the adventitia of the great vessels superiorly, and it is related posteriorly to the bronchi, esophagus, descending thoracic aorta, and mediastinal surface of each lung. The phrenic nerves descend between the visceral pericardium and the mediastinal pleural layers that adhere to its lateral sides (**FIGURE 25.2**).[6]

The oblique sinus, a recess located behind the left atrium, is formed as the pericardium envelopes the pulmonary veins and vena cava. Within it lies the vein of Marshall, connected by the fetal remnant of the duct of Cuvier to the highest left intercostal vein and draining into the coronary sinus. The transverse sinus is located superior to the heart between the arterial mesocardium, which envelopes the ascending aorta and pulmonary trunk anteriorly, and the venous mesocardium, which covers the superior vena cava (SVC), left atrium, and pulmonary veins posteriorly and inferiorly (**FIGURE 25.2**).[6]

Although most of the pericardial cavity can be easily accessed using standard catheters, reaching the posterior wall of the left atrium (LA) can be challenging given the complex pericardial reflections that form the pulmonary vein (PV) recesses and the 2 major sinuses. On the other hand, the epicardial surfaces of both ventricles are free of reflections. In the absence of prior severe pericarditis or cardiac surgery, this allows for simple manipulation of the catheters during epicardial procedures. The inferior and anterior approach taken during percutaneous epicardial access allows for easier access to the respective surfaces of the heart (**FIGURE 25.2**).[1-5]

The technique for safely accessing the normal pericardial space for the purposes of epicardial interventions was first described by Sosa and colleagues using a modification of the traditional method.[1,2] This approach allows free access to the entire ventricular surfaces, the right atrium, and the majority of the right and left atrium (**FIGURES 25.3-25.10**).

Conceptually, entering the pericardial space is simple when draining pericardial effusions. However, in the absence of an effusion, epicardial access can be challenging, as there is little room for error. The normal pericardial cavity contains only 20 to 25 cc of physiologic fluid with only virtual space. Thus, there is an increased risk of perforating the right ventricle (RV) wall and/or of damaging epicardial vessels when attempts are made to access the space percutaneously with a regular pericardiocentesis needle. In a series of 200 patients, Sosa et al reported a bleeding rate of 10% and "dry" RV puncture rate of 4.5% that decreases with experience.[1-4]

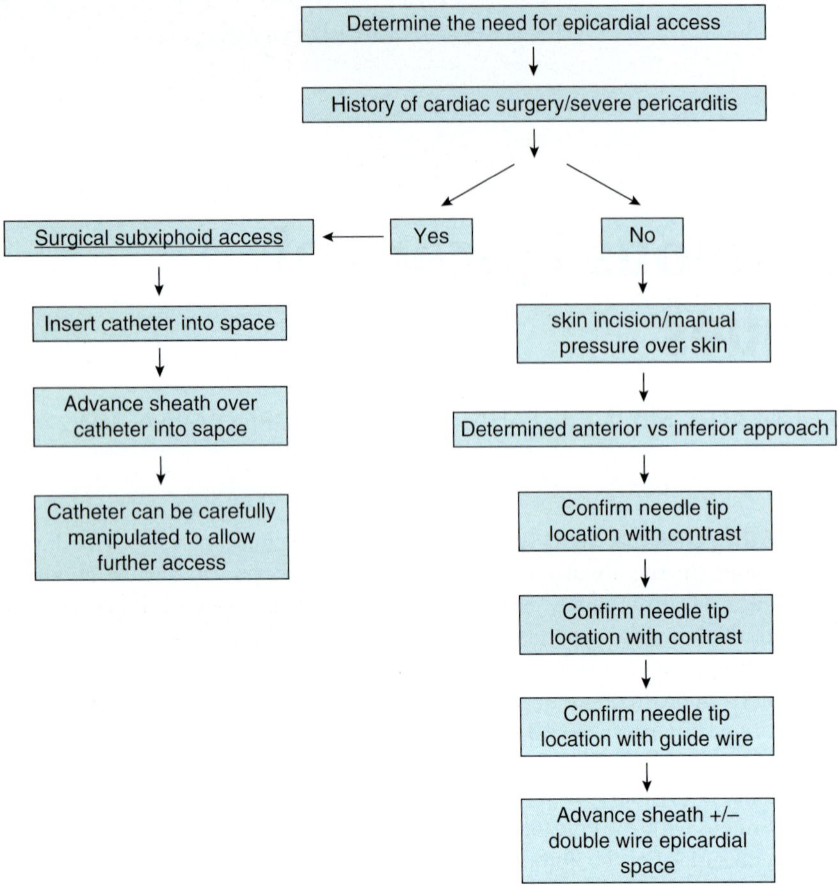

FIGURE 25.1 Percutaneous epicardial access: step-by-step approach.

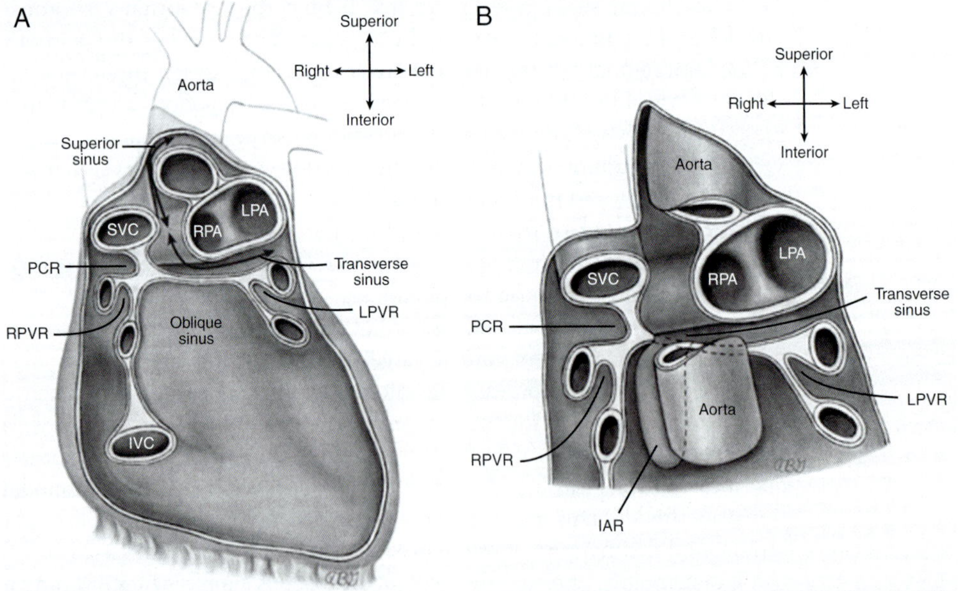

FIGURE 25.2 **A and B**, The anatomy of the pericardium and its reflections along the great vessels, sinuses, and recesses are shown in an anterior view after removal of the heart. The transverse sinus is limited by a pericardial reflection between the superior pulmonary veins. The oblique sinus is confined by the pericardial reflections around the pulmonary veins and the inferior vena cava. IVC, inferior vena cava; LPA, left pulmonary artery; PCR, postcaval recess; RPA, right pulmonary artery; RPVR and LPVR, right and left pulmonary vein recesses; SVC, superior vena cava.

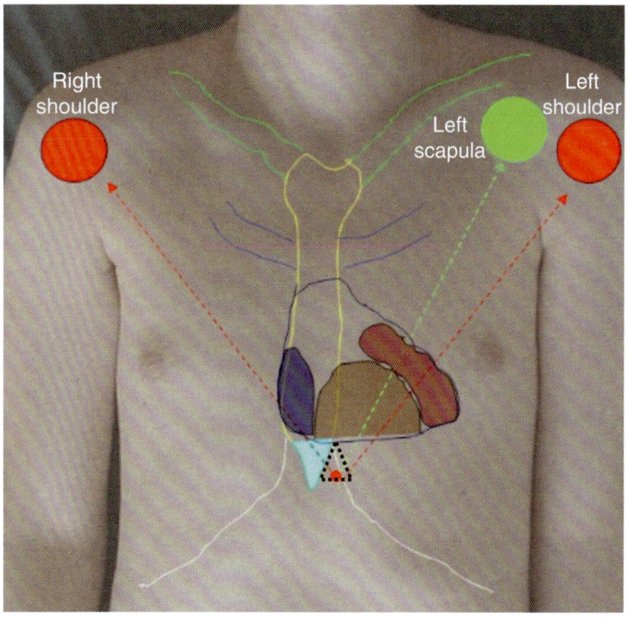

FIGURE 25.3 Anterior chest wall depicting the normal cardiac location within the chest. The angulation of the needle for percutaneous epicardial access should be aimed in the direction of the left scapula and/or the left shoulder. The light blue triangle represents the xiphoid process, the white lines mark the caudal border of the rib cage, and the triangle in black dotted lines marks a soft tissue area lateral to the xiphoid process typically used for initial needle puncture.

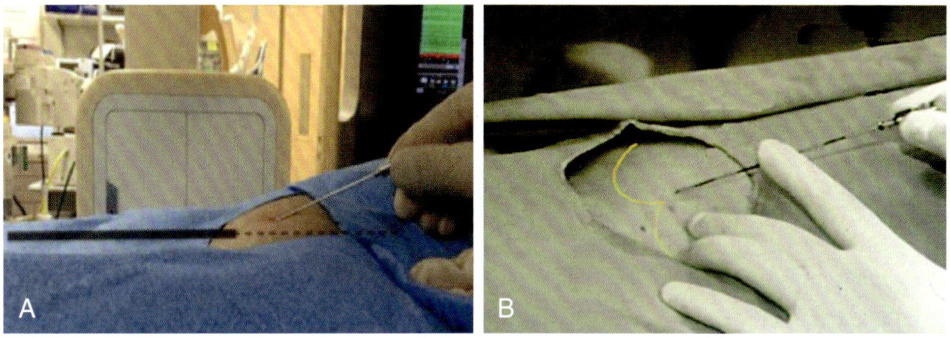

FIGURE 25.4 Anterior chest wall depicting the angle and initial puncture site for the anterior and inferior percutaneous pericardiocentesis approach. The angulation of the needle for percutaneous epicardial access should be aimed in the direction of the left scapula and/or the left shoulder as shown in **FIGURE 25.3**. **A**, The anterior approach appears to have a slightly higher rate of RV puncture and vascular structures in the anterior mediastinum including the left internal mammary artery. **B**, The inferior approach on the other hand is associated with inadvertent puncture of subdiaphragmatic structures including the liver and abdominal vessels. LIMA, Left internal mammary artery.

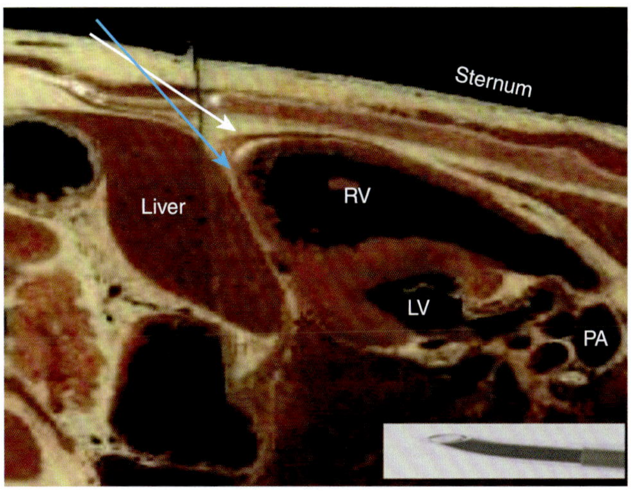

FIGURE 25.5 Sagittal cross section of the chest illustrating the relationship of the sternum with the RV, the liver, the dome of the diaphragm over the liver, and more posterior the LV and the PA. The white arrow depicts the ideal angle for an anterior percutaneous approach (landing on the anterior aspect of the apex); the light blue arrow shows the angle required for an inferior approach.

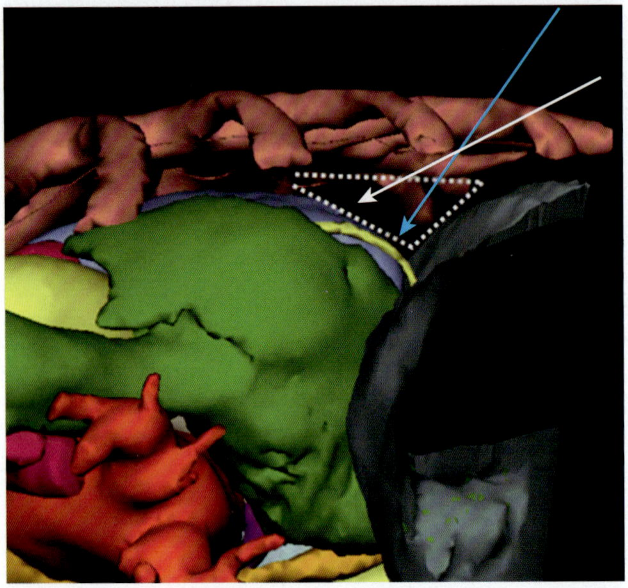

FIGURE 25.6 Sagittal cross section of a 3D reconstruction of a chest computed tomography (CT) (from a right lateral view) illustrating the relationship of the sternum and rib cage (in light brown) with the right ventricle (in blue), the right atrium (in green), the dome of the diaphragm over the liver (in gray), and more posterior the left atrium (in red) and the PA. The white arrow depicts the ideal angle for an anterior percutaneous approach (landing on the anterior aspect of the apex); the light blue arrow shows the angle required for an inferior approach. The triangular space is known as Larrey space (white dotted line).

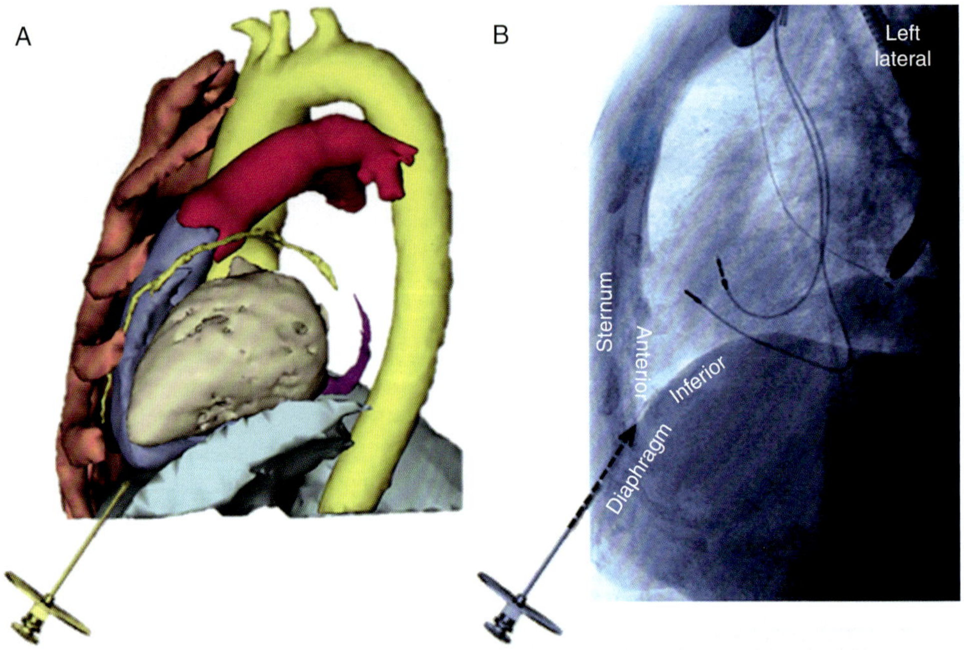

FIGURE 25.7 **A**, shows a sagittal cross section of a 3D reconstruction of a chest CT (from a left lateral view) illustrating the relationship of the sternum and rib cage (in red) with the RV (in blue), the LV (in light brown), the dome of the diaphragm over the liver (in gray), and the pericardiocentesis needle entering Larrey space. **B**, shows a fluoroscopic left lateral projection illustrating the relationship of the RV with the diaphragm and the sternum. The epicardial puncture may be performed in various fluoroscopic projections, per the discretion of the operator. Some operators prefer the use of a left lateral projection, as this can assist with guiding an anterior versus an inferior puncture approach and can help circumvent unintentional diaphragmatic puncture by the pericardiocentesis needle.

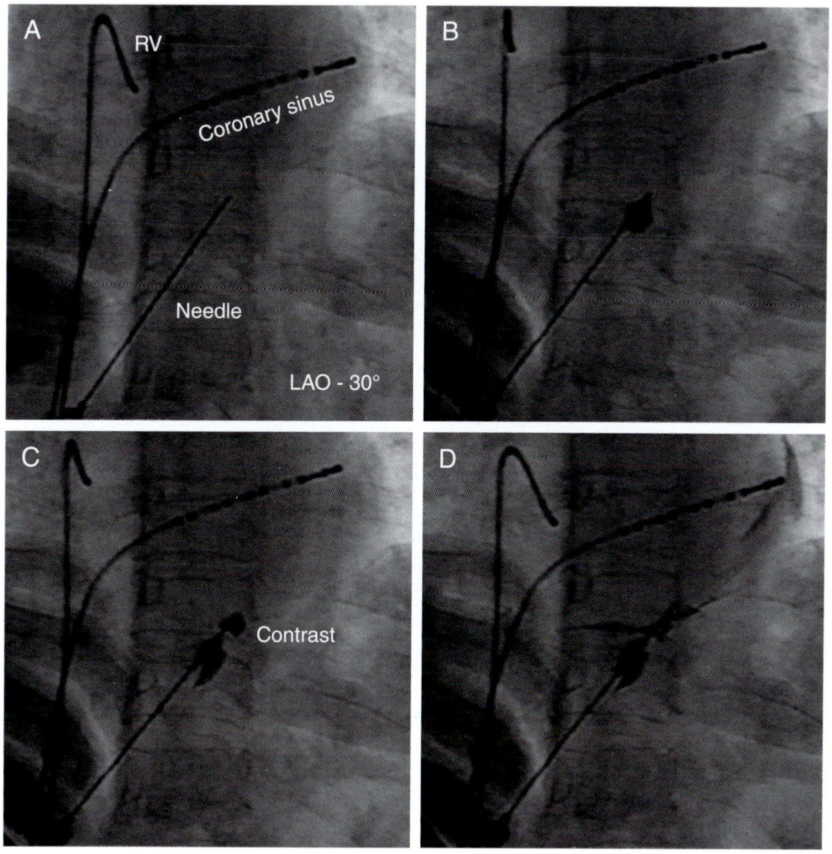

FIGURE 25.8 LAO fluoroscopic projection illustrating the approach of the tip of the needle to the inferior aspect of the cardiac silhouette **(A)**. In **B,** a small amount of contrast has been injected to visualize the amount of tenting against the cardiac border. The needle is further advanced until a pop is felt or the cardiac motion is perceived by the operator, and at this point, additional contrast is injected, which now layers on the dependent aspect of the epicardial space **(C and D)**. At this point, it is safe to advance a guide wire.

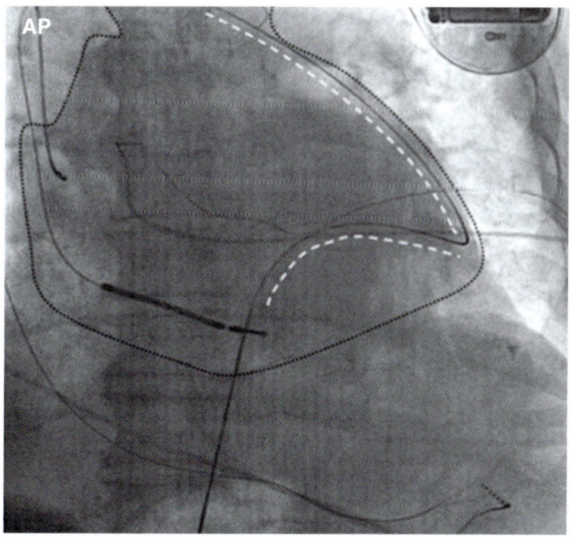

FIGURE 25.9 AP fluoroscopic projection illustrating the cardiac silhouette (black dotted line) and a guide wire through the epicardial needle during an anterior approach forming a large loop (white dashed line) that lies along the cardiac silhouette suggesting pericardial location.

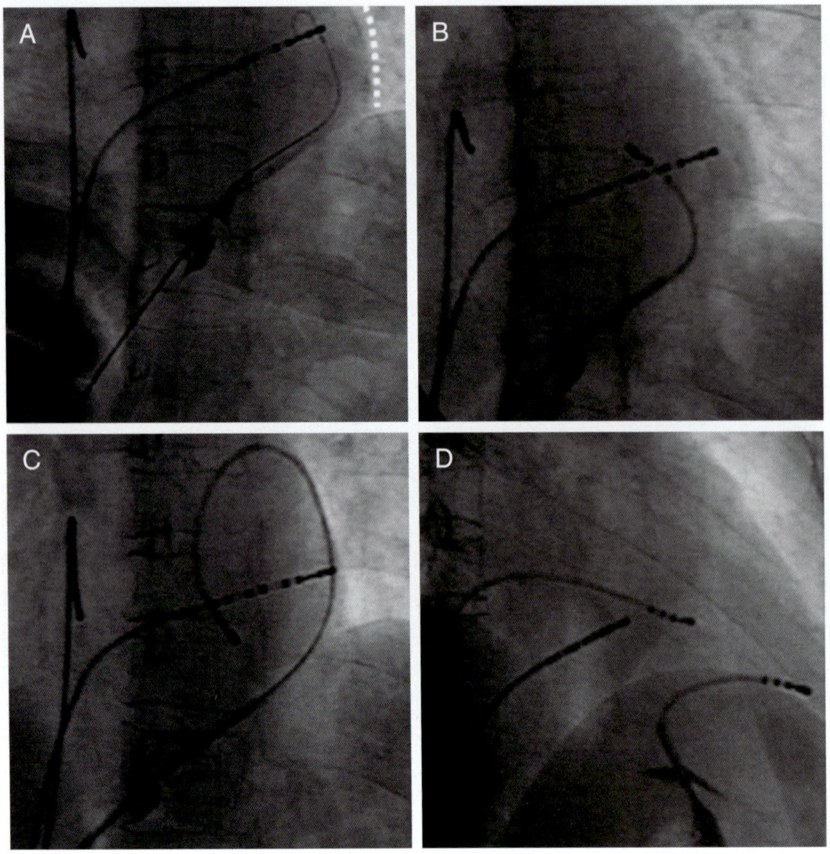

FIGURE 25.10 Irrespective of the projection chosen to guide the puncture, it is essential to always validate the guide wire position in the LAO projection **(A)** before advancement of the introducer sheath inside the pericardium. Confirmation of guide wire passage along the left cardiac border in the LAO projection (white dotted line) virtually excludes the possibility of advancement inside the RV, as in the case of an inadvertent RV puncture. **B and C** show the advancement of an ablation catheter via an introducer sheath in the LAO projection. Note the ablation following the left lateral border of the pericardial space in LAO projection in **C**. In **D**, the RAO projection shows the inferior site of access into the pericardial space.

After a small incision is made on the skin of the subxiphoid area using an 11 blade, a blunt-tipped epidural needle (Tuohy) designed to enter virtual spaces is routinely used. The skin incision is often made to allow easy entry of the needle into the deeper tissues, and it also helps in transmitting the tactile sensation of various structures encountered on the way, especially the contracting walls of the heart (**FIGURES 25.3** and **25.4**). The needle is then advanced gently at an angle (depending on whether an anterior or inferior approach is required) aiming for the left scapula with the patient in the supine position. The preferred entry point is 2 to 3 cm below a line that joins the xiphoid process and the costal margin, left of the midline (**FIGURES 25.4-25.8**). Under fluoroscopic guidance, the needle is continually advanced until the operator can feel cardiac motion. X-ray can be deceiving especially in one view. Often, as one reaches the border of the heart, small injections of contrast are made to delineate proximity to the pericardium (**FIGURE 25.8**).[1]

It is preferable to perform percutaneous access after induction of general anesthesia, which can allow a more controlled puncture during apnea. A small amount of contrast may be then injected to demonstrate entry of the needle into the pericardial space (**FIGURE 25.10**). Occasionally, the parietal pericardium can be stained and tenting of the pericardium can be seen before the needle suddenly enters the space. The appearance of layering of the contrast medium within the pericardial space indicates that the needle is correctly positioned within the pericardial cavity. This transition into virtual space is usually accompanied by a sensation of "give," which is noted with experience (**FIGURES 25.8-25.10**).[1]

Once within the pericardial space, a guide wire is passed through the needle. This step again allows confirmation of entry within pericardial space (**FIGURE 25.9**). Occasionally, in some patients, cardiac motion and/or the sensation of "give" is difficult to perceive and direct entry into the RV cavity may occur inadvertently. In such cases, aspiration of blood or passage of the guide wire into the RV/right ventricular outflow tract (RVOT) accompanied by salvoes of premature ventricular contractions indicates entry into the RV cavity. If this occurs, the needle should be slowly withdrawn a few millimeters, and the guide wire should be pulled back into the needle tip and readvanced. This can be repeated until one gains entry into the pericardial space as opposed to withdrawing the needle entirely.[1]

As a general rule, as the guide wire is advanced, it should slide unrestricted over the epicardial surface until it outlines the fluoroscopic left-sided heart border (**FIGURES 25.9** and **25.10**). This is usually achieved and confirmed in the left anterior oblique (LAO) view by advancing the guide wire, forcing it into a loop and observing the loop glide across the various chambers until it outlines the cardiac silhouette. Once the wire position within the pericardial space is confirmed beyond any doubt, the introducer and sheath are advanced over the wire under fluoroscopy maintaining adequate length of guide wire distal to the sheath tip (**FIGURE 25.10**). The introducer/guide wire is then removed, and a standard ablation/pigtail catheter is advanced through the sheath and manipulated into the pericardial space. Double wiring of the epicardial space to avoid inadvertent loss of pericardial access during sheath manipulation is often helpful. The pigtail catheter is particularly useful to accurately assess the presence of hemopericardium, which has implications for subsequent anticoagulation with heparin.[1]

The guide wire is always advanced under fluoroscopy typically in the anteroposterior (AP)/LAO projection. When the AP projection is chosen, it is difficult to discriminate whether the guide wire is actually in the pericardium along the lateral surface of the LV or it is instead advanced into a dilated RV and pulmonary artery (PA) (**FIGURE 25.9**). The operator can be sure that the guide wire is wrapping around the heart only in the LAO projection (**FIGURE 25.10**). When it occurs, inadvertent RV puncture with the epidural needle or the guide wire does not cause severe complications. However, if the sheath is inadvertently advanced into the RV, surgical repair may be required to control the resulting hemopericardium. Thus, until the location of the guide wire is confirmed by fluoroscopic visualization in the LAO projection, the sheath should not be placed.[1]

Special care should be taken when contrast is injected, as an excessive amount of contrast can obscure relevant fluoroscopic details. In this situation, the operator should consider waiting until the contrast dissipates, thus allowing clear visualization of the cardiac silhouette before attempting another puncture. Some operators try not to use contrast. However, it can be difficult to confirm the correct access without contrast using current tools.[1] Once the sheath has been inserted, it is important to ensure that the lumen of the sheath is always occupied by either an ablation catheter or a pigtail catheter to prevent the distal edge of the sheath from causing local trauma.

ANTERIOR AND INFERIOR APPROACH

Depending on the indication and/or the location of the potential ablation target, either an inferior or an anterior approach to pericardial puncture may be chosen (**FIGURES 25.11-25.13**). Typically, an inferior puncture (**FIGURE 25.11**) allows for better mapping and ablation of the inferolateral wall of the ventricles and the posterior wall of the LA or for epicardial LV lead

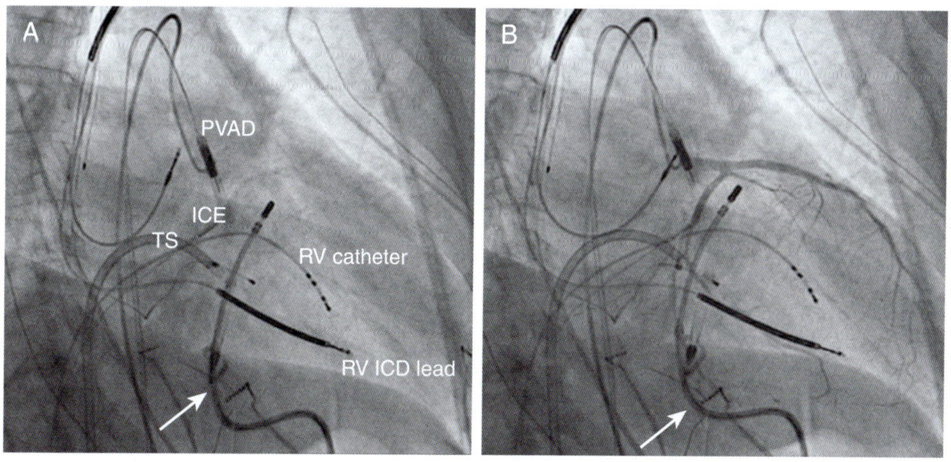

FIGURE 25.11 This picture shows an inferior approach in the RAO projection. A transseptal sheath (TS), intracardiac echocardiography probe (ICE), percutaneous ventricular assist device (PVAD), RV quadripolar diagnostic catheter, and ICD lead can be identified in **A**. **B** shows the relationship of these elements with the epicardial puncture and the left coronary artery. White arrows show epicardial sheath with ablation catheter inside. ICD, Implantable cardiac defibrillator.

placement. Conversely, an anterior puncture (**FIGURE 25.12**) may be preferable when the anterior walls of the heart, such as the anterior RV or the left and right atrial appendages are the target regions. When needle access is attempted with prior cardiac surgery, inferior access maybe attempted. To enter at the inferior surface of the pericardium, the puncture can be performed in LAO projection because it gives the operator a better view of the inferior wall of the heart. When an anterior puncture is chosen (**FIGURE 25.12**), the entering point should be 3 to 4 cm below the junction of the xiphoid appendage and the costal bone and the needle should be advanced in a slightly shallow approach angle, often with gentle downward pressure to keep the left lobe of the liver away from the needle path. In this situation, the AP projection may facilitate visualization of the free wall of the RV.[1]

When performing an epicardial left atrial appendage (LAA) closure procedure, the anterior approach is mandatory and a more lateral angulation is preferred to approach the LAA with the catheters from a more favorable and stable position.[5] The anterior approach is associated with a higher incidence of RV free puncture, which, however, is less likely to occur when a pericardial effusion is present (**FIGURES 25.13** and **25.14**). The inferior approach is associated with a higher incidence of diaphragmatic puncture and subdiaphragmatic injury/intra-abdominal complications (such as hepatic or phrenic vascular injury) (**FIGURES 25.13** and **25.15**).

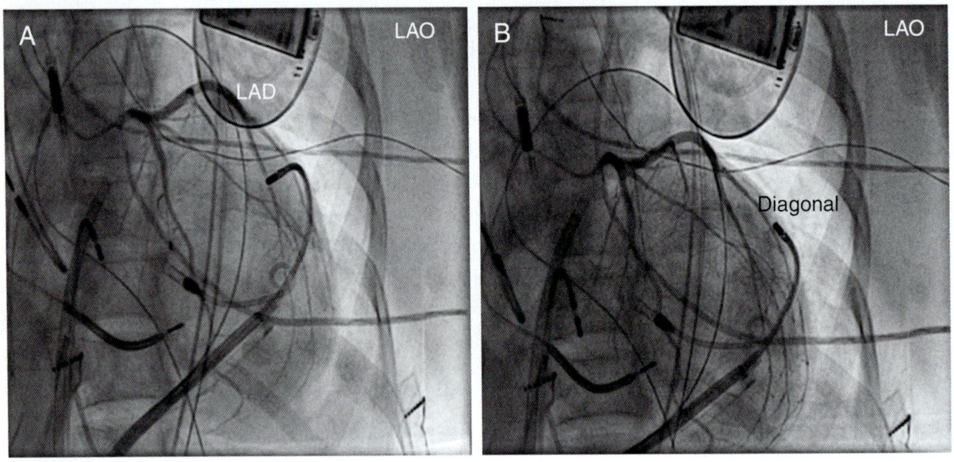

FIGURE 25.12 This picture shows an anterior approach in the RAO projection. A TS, ICE, PVAD, RV quadripolar diagnostic catheter, and ICD lead can be identified in **Panel A**. **Panel B** shows the relationship of these elements with the epicardial puncture and the left anterior descending coronary artery **(A)** and diagonal branch **(B)**. LAD, Left anterior descending.

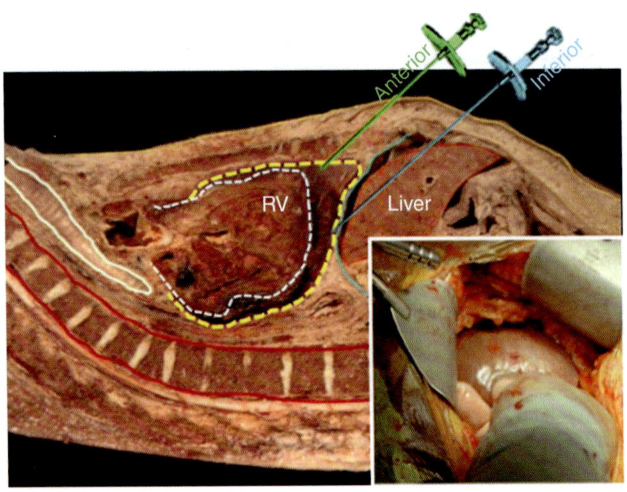

FIGURE 25.13 Sagittal cross section of the chest illustrating the relationship of the sternum with the RV, the liver, the dome of the diaphragm over the liver, and more posterior the LV and the PA. The green needle depicts the ideal angle for an anterior percutaneous approach (landing on the anterior aspect of the apex); the light blue needle shows the angle required for an inferior approach. It should be noted that if this angle is too steep, it can result in advertent liver puncture (as illustrated on the frame in the right lower corner). The anterior approach is associated with a higher incidence of RV free puncture. The inferior approach is associated with a higher incidence of diaphragmatic puncture and subdiaphragmatic injury/intra-abdominal complications (such as hepatic or phrenic vascular injury).

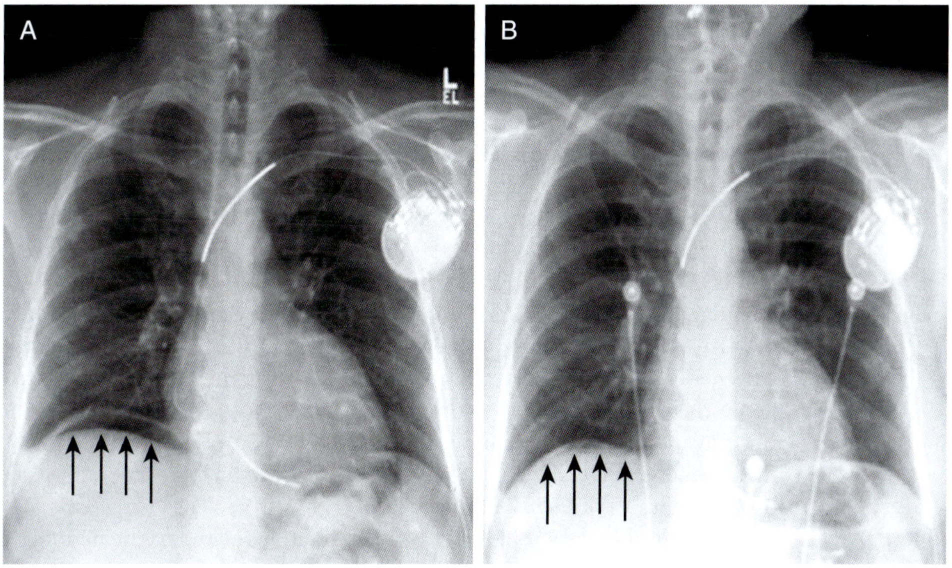

FIGURE 25.14 **A and B**, This AP chest X-ray shows the presence of air (black arrows) under the right hemidiaphragm, consistent with pneumoperitoneum in a patient who underwent percutaneous pericardiocentesis.

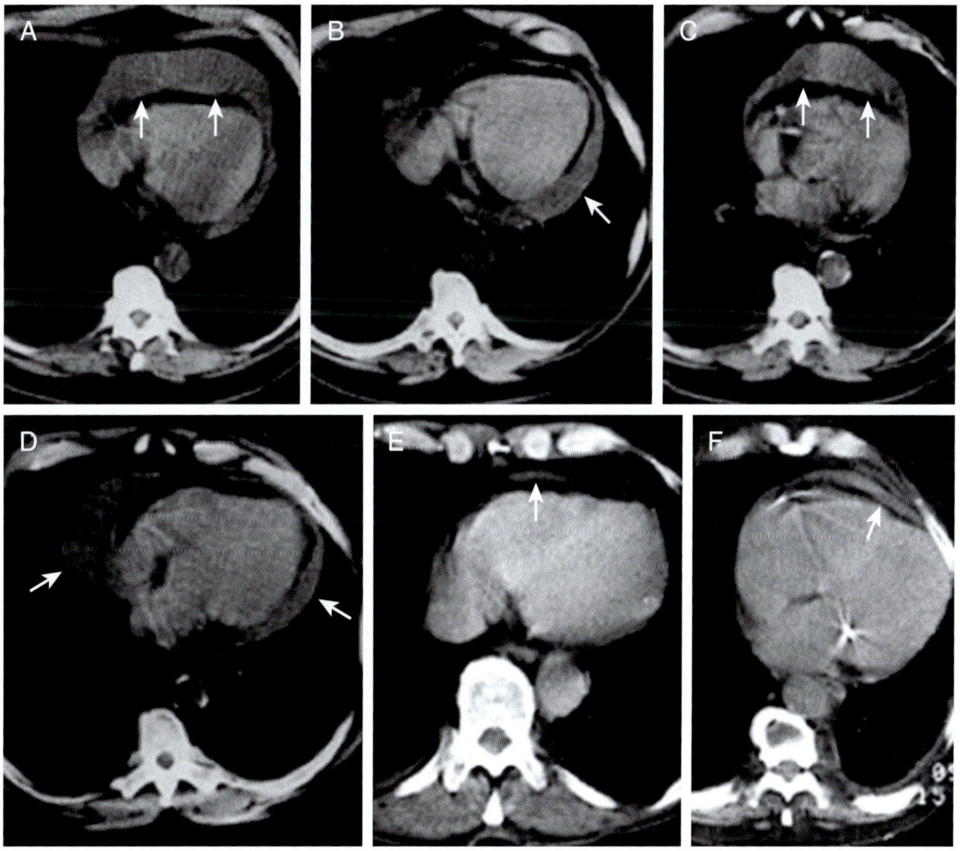

FIGURE 25.15 Archimedes principle states that the upward buoyant force that is exerted on a body immersed in a fluid, whether fully or partially submerged, is equal to the weight of the fluid that the body displaces and acts in the upward direction at the center of mass of the displaced fluid. Therefore, the distribution of the pericardial fluid in the pericardial space is a function of the fluid volume and the heart mass (assuming there are no adhesions). These images from a cardiac CT in a patient with pericardial effusion show that with the patient in supine position the fluid is located solely or predominantly anterior to the right ventricle. Hence, percutaneous pericardiocentesis in a patient with a large pericardial effusion without adhesions is less likely to result in inadvertent RV puncture.

FLUOROSCOPIC NAVIGATION OF THE EPICARDIAL SPACE

The right anterior oblique (RAO) and LAO positions project the heart in its anatomic sagittal and coronal planes such that in RAO, the left and right sides are superimposed, but there is good atrioventricular differentiation, whereas in LAO there is left-right differentiation, but the atria and ventricles are superimposed (**FIGURES 25.8-25.12**). A catheter placed in the coronary sinus marks the mitral valve annulus from the interatrial septum medially (**FIGURE 25.10**). These landmarks can be used to determine the position of the epicardial catheter as it is navigated within the pericardial space. Once the catheter is inserted into the pericardial space, it can be moved freely laterally, anteriorly, and inferiorly over various parts of the ventricle ranging from the RVOT to the posterior crux. Damage to the coronary arteries during ablation is a major concern, particularly when it becomes necessary to ablate at the base of the heart or septum, for example, in the case of accessory pathways that could not otherwise be ablated with an endocardial or intravenous approach. Fluoroscopic identification of anatomic landmarks, supplemented by intracardiac catheters, including retrograde placement of a catheter in the aortic root, will help in avoiding this (**FIGURES 25.11** and **25.12**).[3]

The mitral and tricuspid annuli are intimately related to the major arteries and veins of the heart. The mitral annulus is outlined by the coronary sinus catheter, and the tricuspid annulus is identified by the endoluminal diagnostic quadripolar RV catheter, while the septum is defined fluoroscopically by the diagnostic catheter placed in the His bundle area. Any remaining doubt regarding proximity to a coronary artery should prompt performing coronary angiography. It is important to also appreciate the close relation of the RVOT to the proximal coronary arteries and distal coronary veins. The LAA is easily reached and is the first atrial structure to be encountered when a catheter is advanced laterally and cranially, being identifiable by the characteristic change in intracardiac electrograms. Understanding its fluoroscopic anatomy is important because of its close proximity to the RVOT and the proximal coronary arterial system. It should be noted that the left ventricular outflow tract (LVOT) cannot be reached using this approach because it is covered by the RVOT anteriorly and the mitral valve or the left atrium posteriorly.[3]

The blind-ending oblique sinus can be reached by passing the catheter superiorly behind the heart, its opening being bounded by the 2 inferior pulmonary veins. Its importance in contemporary ablation practice of atrial arrhythmias is related to its unique anatomic location behind the pulmonary venous atrium and the posterior left atrial wall. Within it rests the vein of Marshall, which can itself be a source of arrhythmia amenable to ablation. The esophagus is directly behind the left atrium and subject to thermal injury.[3]

The transverse sinus lies superior to the oblique sinus and can be reached by passing the catheter around the lateral wall of the left ventricle and left atrium, and then under the pulmonary arteries. It is of functional importance because a catheter placed at this site may ablate the roof of the left atrium or Bachmann bundle and important sites for certain atrial arrhythmias. It is intimately related to the aorta, which arches around it, the pulmonary arteries, and left atrium. The floor of the transverse sinus is formed by the pericardial reflection between the right and left superior pulmonary veins, which separates it from the oblique sinus and the roof of the left atrium, where the Bachmann bundle is located. It allows access to the anterior LVOT, as it communicates with the epicardial aspect of the noncoronary and right coronary aortic cusps via the inferior aortic recess. It also communicates with the vena cava by way of the aortocaval sinus, a small virtual space between the SVC and the ascending aorta that in some individuals is large enough to bypass with a catheter and reach the right-sided heart border.[3]

The percutaneous epicardial puncture technique is now well established and has been embraced by electrophysiologists owing to the importance of the epicardial substrate for arrhythmias and other interventional procedures such as percutaneous LAA occlusion. In experienced hands, it has an acceptable complication rate. It is important to note that this safety profile reflect practices at centers that specialize in arrhythmia management and may not be applicable to less experienced operators or centers. With up to a 20% risk for ventricular perforation, careful patient selection is important, and the procedure should be solely performed by experienced operators with surgical backup.[3]

REFERENCES

1. Sosa E, Scanavacca M, d'Avila A, Oliveira F, Ramires JA. Nonsurgical transthoracic epicardial catheter ablation to treat recurrent ventricular tachycardia occurring late after myocardial infarction. *J Am Coll Cardiol*. 2000;35:1442-1449.
2. Sosa E, Scanavacca M, D'Avila A, et al. Endocardial and epicardial ablation guided by nonsurgical transthoracic epicardial mapping to treat recurrent ventricular tachycardia. *J Cardiovasc Electrophysiol*. 1998;9:229-239.
3. d'Avila A, Koruth JS, Dukkipati SD, Reddy VY. Epicardial access for the treatment of cardiac arrhythmias. *Europace*. 2012;(suppl 2):ii13-ii18.
4. Sacher F, Roberts-Thomson K, Maury P, et al. Epicardial ventricular tachycardia ablation a multicenter safety study. *J Am Coll Cardiol*. 2010;55:2366-2372.
5. Syed F, Lachman N, Christensen K, et al. The pericardial space: obtaining access and an approach to fluoroscopic anatomy. *Card Electrophysiol Clin*. 2010;2:9-23.
6. Asirvatham SJ. Correlative anatomy for the invasive electrophysiologist: outflow tract and supravalvar arrhythmia. *J Cardiovasc Electrophysiol*. 2009;20:955-968.
7. Soejima K, Couper G, Cooper JM, et al. Subxiphoid surgical approach for epicardial catheter-based mapping and ablation in patients with prior cardiac surgery or difficult pericardial access. *Circulation*. 2004;110:1197-1201.

Index

Note: Page numbers followed by "f" indicate figures, "t" indicate tables and "b" indicate boxes.

B

D

K

L

M

R

S

T

CCS1118